Critical Limb Ischemia

Robert S. Dieter • Raymond A. Dieter, Jr
Raymond A. Dieter, III • Aravinda Nanjundappa
Editors

Critical Limb Ischemia

Acute and Chronic

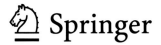 Springer

Editors
Robert S. Dieter, MD, RVT
Loyola University Medical Center
Maywood, IL, USA

Edward Hines, Jr. VA Hospital
Hines, IL, USA

Raymond A. Dieter, III, MD
The University of Tennessee Medical Center
Knoxville, TN, USA

Raymond A. Dieter, Jr., MD, MS
Northwestern Medicine
Central DuPage Hospital
Glen Ellyn, IL, USA

Aravinda Nanjundappa, MD, RVT
West Virginia University
Charleston, WV, USA

Videos can also be accessed at http://link.springer.com/book/10.1007/978-3-319-31991-9

ISBN 978-3-319-31989-6   ISBN 978-3-319-31991-9   (eBook)
DOI 10.1007/978-3-319-31991-9

Library of Congress Control Number: 2016941740

Printed on acid-free paper

This Springer imprint is published by Springer Nature
The registered company is Springer International Publishing AG Switzerland

To my wonderful wife who has been patient and supportive through all my training and pursuits,
my children who bring a smile to my face every day,
my parents and family who taught me to always strive to do my best,
and to God who makes it all possible.

The Dieters

I dedicate this endeavor to my parents Lakshmidevamma and Nanjundappa who have been wonderfully supportive of my pursuits, without whom, none of this would be possible.

Aravinda Nanjundappa

Foreword

As a long-term colleague and friend of Raymond A. Dieter, Jr., I applaud the superb contributions that he and his sons, Raymond A. Dieter, III and Robert S. Dieter, have made to the art, science, and literature of vascular care. Their careers span the entire gamut of this specialty. Raymond A. Dieter, Jr., is a pioneer of angiography, endovascular procedures, and hybrid surgical/endovascular procedures. Raymond A. Dieter, III is a cardiothoracic and vascular surgeon, and Robert S. Dieter is an interventional cardiologist with an emphasis on vascular disease. Over the past 7 years, the three of them have produced a series of textbooks designed to cover all aspects of this subject: *Peripheral Arterial Disease* (2009), *Venous and Lymphatic Diseases* (2011), and *Endovascular Interventions* (2013). I have had the privilege of writing the foreword to each of these volumes.

This textbook, *Critical Limb Ischemia: Acute and Chronic*, complements the previous volumes by addressing the most severe stage of peripheral arterial disease. Unfortunately, critical limb ischemia (CLI) is one of the most underdiagnosed and undertreated cardiovascular maladies. Patients with CLI have high rates of mortality and morbidity, including limb loss. These patients often are elderly and have serious comorbid conditions, such as diabetes mellitus, heart disease, and cerebrovascular disease. Delays in the diagnosis and treatment of CLI are associated with poor results, including a high incidence of heart attack and stroke. In addition to taking a heavy human toll, CLI is responsible for increased utilization of medical resources. As the average age of the Western population continues to rise, the ravages of this disease can be expected to increase.

In editing this volume, the Dieters were joined by cardiologist Aravinda Nanjundappa. The result is an outstanding textbook that builds on its predecessors and conforms to their high standard. As a guide to the diagnosis and successful management of CLI, this work will be an important resource not only for vascular and endovascular surgeons but also for nonvascular clinicians, who play a crucial role in the early recognition of CLI and prompt referral for specialized care.

Houston, TX, USA
Denton A. Cooley, MD
Founder and President Emeritus
Texas Heart Institute

Preface

This textbook, our fourth on vascular disease and fifth medical textbook overall, is focused on critical limb ischemia. We have purposefully included both acute and chronic conditions in critical limb ischemia. These two disease processes share many common features, yet are unique enough in their presentation and treatment that they deserve separation in their diagnosis and treatment discussions. It is our intent that one volume that covers both entities will be a valuable resource to clinicians.

Although once the sole purview of vascular surgeons, the therapeutics of critical limb ischemia has been significantly advanced through the multidisciplinary approach to the patient and disease. Overall, limb and patient care are enhanced by the current group of specialists who provide care for these patients.

Our book systematically addresses the afflicted patient and the disease process leading to the very real concern—critical limb ischemia—that may torment the patient, the family, and the consulting physician. Loss of an extremity, or a portion thereof, is not necessarily a life-ending process, but it certainly is a debilitating experience whether involvement is of the upper or the lower extremity.

Depending on the etiology, the list of specialties requiring involvement is long, and the required multiple specialty disease/patient physician programs become apparent as the disease progresses. Diabetic, renal, and even oncological consultations are administered concomitantly with the vascular physician, with all working to salvage an extremity, to avoid a prosthesis and lifetime without an arm or leg.

We have included the most frequent as well as the more unusual etiological processes that may lead to the most dreaded concern of a patient and family—amputation. Atherosclerotic diseases of the smoker and the diabetic patient, malignancy-induced occlusive disease, and vasculitic as well as the iatrogenic disorders, while unexpected, are all part of the much larger etiological group endangering the patient and the extremity.

Physicians face these concerns with recognition of the life and lifestyle changes presenting to the family and the patient with extremity ischemia. Diagnosis, diagnostic approaches, and therapeutic options become a major and timely focus for all involved. The multiple disciplines and specialty recognition of the authors and chapter contributors define the majority of the disease complex and the goal for salvage whenever possible.

Maywood, IL, USA   Robert S. Dieter, MD, RVT
Glen Ellyn, IL, USA   Raymond A. Dieter, Jr., MD, MS
Knoxville, TN, USA   Raymond A. Dieter, III, MD
Charleston, WV, USA   Aravinda Nanjundappa, MD, RVT

Contents

1   **Epidemiology of Acute Critical Limb Ischemia**.. 1
Martyn Knowles and Carlos H. Timaran

2   **Epidemiology of Chronic Critical Limb Ischemia**.. 9
Akhil Gulati, Lawrence Garcia, and Subasit Acharji

3   **Classification Systems for Acute and Chronic Limb Ischemia**........................... 15
Taishi Hirai, Amit S. Dayal, Rie Hirai, Timothy E. Tanke, and Robert S. Dieter

4   **Pathologic Aspects of Ischemic Limb Disease**....................................... 23
Arno A. Roscher, Raymond A. Dieter, Jr., and Beth L. Johnson

5   **History and Physical Exam of Acute Limb Ischemia**.. 29
Nancy Panko and Matthew Blecha

6   **History and Physical Exam of Chronic Critical Limb Ischemia**....................... 37
Rajmony Pannu and Steven M. Dean

7   **Vascular Anatomy of the Upper Limbs**.. 45
Rand S. Swenson, Norman J. Snow, and Brian Catlin

8   **Vascular Anatomy of the Lower Limbs**... 57
Rand S. Swenson, Norman J. Snow, and Brian Catlin

9   **Overlap of Atherosclerotic Disease**... 71
Natalie Gwilliam and Ross Milner

10   **Differential Diagnosis of Upper Extremity Ischemia**.................................... 79
Laura Drudi and Kent MacKenzie

11   **Differential Diagnosis for Lower Extremity Ischemia and Ulcerations:
Focus on Non-atherosclerotic Etiologies**.. 95
Sara E. Clark and Faisal Aziz

12   **Cardiac Causes of Acute and Chronic Limb Ischemia**.................................. 109
Raymond A. Dieter, III, Tjuan L. Overly, Madhur A. Roberts,
and Juan J. Gallegos Jr.

13   **Progression of Peripheral Artery Disease to Critical Limb Ischemia**................ 121
Michael J. McArdle, Jay Giri, and Emile R. Mohler, III

14   **Basic Science of Wound Healing**.. 131
Stephanie R. Goldberg and Robert F. Diegelmann

15   **Diagnostic Approach to Chronic Critical Limb Ischemia**.............................. 133
Tadaki M. Tomita and Melina R. Kibbe

16 **Diagnostic Approach to Acute Limb Ischemia**...................................... 159
Carlo Setacci, Gianmarco de Donato, Giuseppe Galzerano, Maria Pia Borrelli,
Giulia Mazzitelli, and Francesco Setacci

17 **CT Evaluation of Critical Limb Ischemia** 171
Suraj Rao, Shankho Ganguli, and Mark G. Rabbat

18 **Magnetic Resonance Imaging in Acute and Chronic Limb Ischemia**............... 183
Rajeev R. Fernando, Lara Bakhos, and Mushabbar A. Syed

19 **Noninvasive Imaging in Critical Limb Ischemia**................................... 199
John H. Fish, III and Teresa L. Carman

20 **Invasive Imaging in Critical Limb Ischemia** 211
Sohail Ikram and Prafull Raheja

21 **Vascular Trauma to the Extremity: Diagnosis and Management** 217
Julia M. Boll, Andrew J. Dennis, and Elizabeth Gwinn

22 **Iatrogenic Extremity Ischemia with the Potential for Amputation**.................... 241
Raymond A. Dieter, Jr., George B. Kuzycz, Raymond A. Dieter, III,
and Dwight W. Morrow

23 **Thromboangiitis Obliterans**.. 249
Federico Bucci, Francesco Sangrigoli, and Leslie Fiengo

24 **Critical Ischemia in Patients with Raynaud's Phenomenon**............................ 257
Michael Hughes, Ariane Herrick, and Lindsay Muir

25 **Hypercoagulable Conditions Leading to Limb Ischemia**................................ 267
Arjun Jayaraj, Waldemar E. Wysokinski, and Robert D. McBane

26 **Vasculitis** 279
Michael Czihal and Ulrich Hoffmann

27 **Cholesterol Emboli**.. 293
Muhamed Saric and Rose Tompkins

28 **Venous Etiologies of Acute Limb Ischemia**.. 305
John R. Hoch

29 **Malignant and Benign Tumor-Induced Critical Limb Ischemia**........................ 323
Raymond A. Dieter, Jr., George B. Kuzycz, Marcelo C. DaSilva,
Raymond A. Dieter, III, Anthony M. Joudi, and Morgan M. Meyer

30 **Frostbite**.. 333
Stephen M. Milner, Julie A. Caffrey, and Syed F. Saquib

31 **Vascular Issues in Thermal Injury**... 337
Michael J. Feldman and Michael Fiore Amendola

32 **Diabetic Foot**.. 349
Joseph C. Babrowicz Jr., Richard F. Neville, and Anton N. Sidawy

33 **Critical Limb Ischemia and the Angiosome Model** 367
Alexander Turin and Robert S. Dieter

34 **Principles of Endovascular Treatment of Critical Limb Ischemia**...................... 373
Robert S. Dieter

35 **Endovascular Technologies for Chronic Critical Limb Ischemia** 387
Ambrose F. Panico, Asif Jafferani, Paul A. Johnson, John J. Lopez,
John R. Laird, and Robert S. Dieter

36 Surgical Revascularization of Chronic Limb Ischemia.................................... 413
Sarah P. Pradka, Vahram Ornekian, and Cameron M. Akbari

37 Importance of Pedal Arch in Treatment of Critical Limb Ischaemia................ 427
Hani Slim, Elias Khalil, Hiren Mistry, Raghvinder Singh Gambhir,
Domenico Valenti, and Hisham Rashid

**38 Endovascular and Thrombolytic Therapy for Upper
and Lower Extremity Acute Limb Ischemia**... 441
Sarah S. Elsayed and Leonardo C. Clavijo

39 Surgical Treatment for Acute Limb Ischemia.. 451
Pegge M. Halandras

**40 Sympathectomy Revisited: Current Status in the Management
of Critical Limb Ischemia**.. 459
Pawan Agarwal and Dhananjaya Sharma

41 Spinal Cord Stimulation.. 465
Pawan Agarwal and Dhananjaya Sharma

**42 Omental Transplant for Revascularization in Critical Ischemic
Limbs and Tissues**.. 469
V. K. Agarwal, Jyoti Bindal, and Swati Bhargava

43 Hyperbaric Oxygen Therapy for Critical Limb Ischemia................................. 483
Raymond C. Shields

44 Gene and Cell Therapy for Critical Limb Ischemia.. 491
Surovi Hazarika and Brian H. Annex

45 Lower Extremity Ulceration: Evaluation and Care... 503
Rodney M. Stuck, Coleen Napolitano, Daniel Miller, and Francis J. Rottier

46 Diagnosis and Management of Wound Infections... 517
Alfredo J. Mena Lora, Jesica A. Herrick, Bradley Recht,
and Ivette Murphy-Aguilu

47 Wound Care: Maggot Debridement Therapy... 531
Taku Maeda and Chu Kimura

48 Medical Therapy for Critical Limb Ischemia.. 537
Gianluca Rigatelli, Sara R. Shah, Amsa Arshad, Nisa Arshad,
and Thach Nguyen

49 Endocrine Considerations in Critical Limb Ischemia...................................... 543
Ioanna Eleftheriadou, Nicholas Tentolouris, and Edward B. Jude

50 Renal Considerations in Critical Limb Ischemia.. 561
Pranav Sandilya Garimella, Amit M. Kakkar, and Prakash Muthusami

51 Upper Extremity Amputation.. 571
Nikola Babovic and Brian T. Carlsen

52 Amputations in the Foot and Ankle.. 587
Rodney M. Stuck, Coleen Napolitano, and Francis J. Rottier

53 Major Amputation of the Lower Extremity for Critical Limb Ischemia........... 603
Ryan P. Ter Louw, Benjamin J. Brown, and Christopher E. Attinger

54 Extremity Replantation or Transplantation 619
Raymond A. Dieter, Jr., George B. Kuzycz, and Raymond A. Dieter, III

55 The Importance of a Multidisciplinary Approach to Leg Ulcers 625
Albeir Mousa, Mehiar El Hamdani, Raymond A. Dieter, Jr.,
Aravinda Nanjundappa, Mohamed A. Rahman, David J. Leehey,
Raymond A. Dieter, III, James S. Walter, Scott T. Sayers, Sanjay Singh,
Morgan M. Meyer, Amit S. Dayal, Amir Darki, and Robert S. Dieter

56 Appropriate Endpoints for Chronic Limb Ischemia 629
Dustin Y. Yoon, Alejandro Garza, and Heron E. Rodriguez

57 Economic Burden of Chronic Critical Limb Ischemia 637
Taishi Hirai, Benjamin Ross Weber, John P. Pacanowski Jr.,
Miguel F. Montero Baker, and Raymond A. Dieter, IV

58 The Long-Term Care of Patients with Critical Limb Ischemia (CLI) 641
Larry J. Diaz-Sandoval

Index 651

Contributors

Subasit Acharji, MD Section of Interventional Cardiology and Vascular Intervention, Vascular Medicine, Department of Cardiovascular Medicine, St. Elizabeth's Medical Center, Boston, MA, USA

Pawan Agarwal, MS, MCh, DNB, MNAMS, PhD Department of Surgery, NSCB Government Medical College, Jabalpur, MP, India

V.K. Agarwal, MBBS, MS Surgery, M.G.M. Medical College, Sanjivini Nursing Home, Indore, MP, India

Cameron M. Akbari, MD Vascular Surgery, Georgetown University Hospital, Washington, DC, USA

Michael Fiore Amendola, MA, MD Division of Vascular Surgery, Department of Surgery, VCU Medical Center, McGuire VA Medical Center, Richmond, VA, USA

Brian H. Annex, MD Division of Cardiovascular Medicine, University of Virginia, Charlottesville, VA, USA

Amsa Arshad, MD Cardiology, St. Mary's Medical Center, Hobart, IN, USA

Nisa Arshad, MD Cardiology, St. Mary's Medical Center, Hobart, IN, USA

Christopher E. Attinger, MD Department of Plastic Surgery, Medstar Georgetown University Hospital, Washington, DC, USA

Faisal Aziz, MD, RVT, RPVI Heart and Vascular Institute, Penn State Hershey Medical Center, Hershey, PA, USA

Nikola Babovic, MD Orthopaedic Surgery, Allegheny Health Network, Pittsburgh, PA, USA

Joseph C. Babrowicz Jr., MD Division of Vascular Surgery, Medical Faculty Associates/ GWU, Washington, DC, USA

Lara Bakhos, MD Division of Cardiology, Department of Medicine, Loyola University Medical Center, Maywood, IL, USA

Swati Bhargava, MBBS, MS (OBGY) Obstetrics and Gynaecology, M.G.M. Medical College, Indore, MP, India

Jyoti Bindal, MBBS, MS, LLB. PGDHM Obstetrics and Gynecology, G.R. Medical College, Gwalior, MP, India

Matthew Blecha, MD Section of Vascular Surgery and Endovascular Therapy, University of Chicago Medical Center, Chicago, IL, USA

Julia M. Boll, MD Department of General Surgery, John H. Stroger Hospital of Cook County, Rush University Medical Center, Chicago, IL, USA

Maria Pia Borrelli, MD Department of Medicine, Surgery and Neuroscience, Unit of Vascular Surgery, University of Siena, Siena, Italy

Benjamin J. Brown, MD Plastic Surgery, Gulf Coast Plastic Surgery, Pensacola, FL, USA

Federico Bucci, MD Vascular Surgery Department, Polyclinique Bordeaux Rive Droite, Bordeaux, France

Julie A. Caffrey, DO, MS Department of Plastic and Reconstructive Surgery, Johns Hopkins University School of Medicine, Baltimore, MD, USA

Brian T. Carlsen, MD Orthopedic and Plastic Surgery, Mayo Clinic, Rochester, MN, USA

Teresa L. Carman, MD Vascular Medicine, University Hospitals Case Medical Center, Cleveland, OH, USA

Brian Catlin, MD Anatomy, Geisel School of Medicine at Dartmouth, Hanover, NH, USA

Sara E. Clark, MD Heart and Vascular Institute, Penn State Hershey Medical Center, Hershey, PA, USA

Leonardo C. Clavijo, MD, PhD Interventional Cardiology, Cardiovascular Medicine, University of Southern California, Los Angeles, CA, USA

Denton A. Cooley, MD, PhD Health Science Center, University of Tennessee, College of Medicine, Memphis, TN, USA

Michael Czihal, MD Division of Vascular Medicine, Medical Clinic and Policlinic IV, Hospital of the Ludwig Maximilians-University Hospital, Munich, Germany

Amir Darki, MD, MSc Medicine Cardiology, Loyola University Medical Center, Maywood, IL, USA

Marcelo C. DaSilva, MD Thoracic Surgery, Harvard Medical School, Brigham and Women's Hospital, Boston, MA, USA

Amit S. Dayal, MD Medicine, Stritch School of Medicine, Loyola University Chicago, Maywood, IL, USA
Medicine, Edward Hines Jr. VA Hospital, Hines, IL, USA

Steven M. Dean, DO, RPVI Division of Cardiovascular Medicine, Department of Internal Medicine, The Ohio State University Wexner Medical Center, Columbus, OH, USA

Gianmarco de Donato, MD Department of Medicine, Surgery and Neuroscience, Unit of Vascular Surgery, University of Siena, Siena, Italy

Andrew J. Dennis, DO Surgery, Division of Pre-Hospital and Emergency Trauma Services, Department of Trauma and Burn, JSH Cook County Hospital, Rush Medical College, Chicago, IL, USA

Larry J. Diaz-Sandoval, MD Department of Medicine, Michigan State University, Wyoming, MI, USA

Robert F. Diegelmann, PhD Biochemistry and Molecular Biology, Virginia Commonwealth University Medical Center, Richmond, VA, USA

Raymond A. Dieter, Jr., MD, MS Northwestern Medicine, Central DuPage Hospital, Glen Ellyn, IL, USA
International College of Surgeons, Cardiothoracic and Vascular Surgery, Glen Ellyn, IL, USA

Raymond A. Dieter, III, MD Division of Cardiothoracic Surgery, The University of Tennessee Medical Center, Knoxville, TN, USA

Raymond A. Dieter, IV, BA Health Science Center, University of Tennessee, College of Medicine, Memphis, TN, USA

Robert S. Dieter, MD, RVT Medicine, Cardiology, Vascular and Endovascular Medicine, Loyola University Medical Center, Maywood, IL, USA

Laura Drudi, MD, CM Division of Vascular Surgery, McGill University, Montreal, QC, Canada

Mehiar El Hamdani, MD Medicine, Marshall University School of Medicine, Huntington, WV, USA

Ioanna Eleftheriadou, MD, PhD Internal Medicine, 1st Department of Propaedeutic and Internal Medicine, Laiko General Hospital, Medical School, University of Athens, Athens, Greece

Sarah S. Elsayed, MD Interventional Cardiology, Cardiovascular Medicine, University of Southern California, Los Angeles, CA, USA

Michael J. Feldman, MD Division of Plastic and Reconstructive Surgery, Critical Care Hospital, Virginia Commonwealth University, Richmond, VA, USA

Rajeev R. Fernando, MD Division of Cardiology, Department of Medicine, Loyola University Medical Center, Maywood, IL, USA

Leslie Fiengo, MD, PhD Department of Surgery, La Sapienza University of Rome, Rome, Italy

John H. Fish III, MD Anticoagulation Services, Aurora Cardiovascular, Vascular Medicine, Aurora St. Luke's Medical Center, Milwaukee, WI, USA

Juan J. Gallegos, Jr., MD General Surgery, University of Tennessee Medical Center, Knoxville, TN, USA

Giuseppe Galzerano, MD Department of Medicine, Surgery and Neuroscience, Unit of Vascular Surgery, University of Siena, Siena, Italy

Raghvinder Singh Gambhir, MD Department of Vascular Surgery, King's College Hospital, London, UK

Shankho Ganguli, MD Cardiology, Aurora St. Luke's Medical Center, Milwaukee, WI, USA Cardiology, Aurora Sinai Medical Center, Milwaukee, WI, USA

Lawrence Garcia, MD Section of Interventional Cardiology and Vascular Intervention, Vascular Medicine, Department of Cardiovascular Medicine, St. Elizabeth's Medical Center, Boston, MA, USA

Pranav Sandilya Garimella, MD, MPH Division of Nephrology, Tufts Medical Center, Boston, MA, USA

Alejandro Garza, MD Division of Plastic Surgery, Northwestern University Feinberg School of Medicine, Chicago, IL, USA

Jay Giri, MD, MPH Cardiovascular Division, Department of Medicine, Hospital of the University of Pennsylvania, Perelman School of Medicine, University of Pennsylvania, Philadelphia, PA, USA

Stephanie R. Goldberg, MD Surgery Department, Virginia Commonwealth University Medical Center, Richmond, VA, USA

Akhil Gulati, MD Section of Interventional Cardiology and Vascular Intervention, Vascular Medicine, Department of Cardiovascular Medicine, St. Elizabeth's Medical Center, Boston, MA, USA

Natalie Gwilliam, MD General Surgery, University of Chicago, Chicago, IL, USA

Elizabeth Gwinn, MD Department of Trauma and Burn, JSH Cook County Hospital, Chicago, IL, USA

Pegge M. Halandras, MD Division of Vascular Surgery and Endovascular Therapy, Department of Surgery, Loyola University Chicago, Maywood, IL, USA

Surovi Hazarika, MBBS, PhD Division of Cardiovascular Medicine, University of Virginia, Charlottesville, VA, USA

Ariane Herrick, MD Centre for Musculoskeletal Research, The University of Manchester and Salford Royal NHS Foundation Trust, Manchester, UK

Jesica A. Herrick, MD, MS Department of Medicine, Section of Infectious Diseases, Immunology, and International Medicine, University of Illinois at Chicago, Chicago, IL, USA

Rie Hirai, MD Internal Medicine, Loyola University Medical Center, Maywood, IL, USA

Taishi Hirai, MD Division of Cardiology, Department of Medicine, Stritch School of Medicine, Loyola University Medical Center/Loyola University Chicago, Maywood, IL, USA

John R. Hoch, MD University of Wisconsin School of Medicine and Public Health, Madison, WI, USA

Ulrich Hoffmann, MD Division of Vascular Medicine, Medical Clinic and Policlinic IV, Hospital of the Ludwig Maximilians-University Hospital, Munich, Germany

Michael Hughes, MSc(Hons), MSc, MBBS Centre for Musculoskeletal Research, The University of Manchester and Salford Royal NHS Foundation Trust, Manchester, UK

Sohail Ikram, MBBS Invasive and Interventional Cardiology and Peripheral Vascular Interventions, School of Medicine, University of Louisville, Louisville, KY, USA

Asif Jafferani, MBBS Cardiology, University of Wisconsin, Madison, WI, USA

Arjun Jayaraj, MBBS, MPH, RPVI Division of Vascular and Endovascular Surgery, Mayo Clinic, Rochester, MN, USA

Beth L. Johnson, MD Northwestern Medicine, At Central DuPage Hospital, Winfield, IL, USA

Paul A. Johnson, BS Loyola University Chicago, Stritch School of Medicine, Loyola University, Maywood, IL, USA

Anthony M. Joudi, MD Loyola University Medical Center, Stritch School of Medicine, Maywood, IL, USA

Edward B. Jude, MBBS, MD Diabetes and Endocrinology, Tameside Hospital NHS Foundation Trust, Lancashire, UK

Amit M. Kakkar, MD Department of Medicine, Albert Einstein College of Medicine, Bronx, NY, USA

Department of Medicine, Jacobi Medical Center, Bronx, NY, USA

Elias Khalil, MD, MSc Department of Vascular Surgery, King's College Hospital, London, UK

Melina R. Kibbe, MD Department of Surgery, University of North Carolina, Chapel Hill, NC, USA

Chu Kimura, Doctor Plastic and Reconstructive Surgery, Hakodate General Central Hospital, Hakodate City, Hokkaido, Japan

Martyn Knowles, MD Division of Vascular Surgery, University of North Carolina, Chapel Hill, NC, USA

George B. Kuzycz, MD Thoracic and Cardiovascular Surgery, Cadence Hospital of Northwestern System, Winfield, IL, USA

John R. Laird, MD Internal Medicine, Cardiovascular Medicine UC Davis Vascular Center, Sacramento, CA, USA

David J. Leehey, MD Medicine, Loyola University Medical Center and Hines VA, Mayhood, IL, USA

John J. Lopez, MD Medicine, Cardiology, Loyola University Medical Center, Maywood, IL, USA

Ryan P. Ter Louw, MD Department of Plastic Surgery, Medstar Georgetown University Hospital, Washington, DC, USA

Kent MacKenzie, MD Program Director, Vascular Surgery Residency and Fellowship, McGill University Health Center – Royal Victoria Hospital-Glen Site, Montreal, QC, Canada

Taku Maeda, Doctor Plastic and Reconstructive Surgery, Hakodate General Central Hospital, Hakodate City, Hokkaido, Japan

Giulia Mazzitelli, MD Department of Medicine, Surgery and Neuroscience, Unit of Vascular Surgery, University of Siena, Siena, Italy

Michael J. McArdle, MD Department of Internal Medicine, University of Pennsylvania, Philadelphia, PA, USA

Robert D. McBane, MD Department of Cardiovascular Diseases, Gonda Vascular Center, Mayo Clinic, Rochester, MN, USA

Alfredo J. Mena Lora, MD Department of Medicine, Section of Infectious Diseases, University of Illinois at Chicago, Chicago, IL, USA

Morgan M. Meyer, MD Internal Medicine, Illinois State Medical Society, Lombard, IL, USA

Anar Mikailov, MD Harvard Combined Medicine – Dermatology Residency Program, Boston, MA, USA

Daniel Miller, DPM Podiatry, St. Joseph Medical Center, Kansas City, MO, USA

Ross Milner, MD Vascular Surgery, Center for Aortic Diseases, University of Chicago, Chicago, IL, USA

Stephen M. Milner, MBBS, BDS Department of Plastic and Reconstructive Surgery, Johns Hopkins University School of Medicine, Baltimore, MD, USA

Hiren Mistry, MBBS Department of Vascular Surgery, King's College Hospital, London, UK

Emile R. Mohler, III, MD Cardiovascular Division, Department of Medicine, Hospital of the University of Pennsylvania, Perelman School of Medicine, University of Pennsylvania, Philadelphia, PA, USA

Miguel F. Montero Baker, MD Vascular Surgery, Pima Vascular, Tucson, AZ, USA

Dwight W. Morrow, MD Pathology, Edward Hospital, Naperville, IL, USA

Albeir Mousa, MD, MPH, MBA Surgery, Charleston Area Medical Center, WVU Physicians of Charleston, Charleston, WV, USA

Lindsay Muir, MB, MChOrth Hand Surgery, Salford Royal NHS Foundation Trust, Lancashire, UK

Ivette Murphy-Aguilu, DO Infectious Disease, Alexian Brothers Medical Center, Chicago, IL, USA

Prakash Muthusami, MD Division of Diagnostic Imaging, The Hospital for Sick Children, Toronto, ON, Canada

Aravinda Nanjundappa, MD, RVT Medicine and Surgery, West Virginia University, Charleston, WV, USA

Coleen Napolitano, DPM Podiatry Division, Department of Orthopaedic Surgery and Rehabilitation, Loyola University Stritch School of Medicine, Maywood, IL, USA

Richard F. Neville, MD Department of Surgery, Vascular Surgery, George Washington University Hospital, MFA, Washington, DC, USA

Thach Nguyen, MD Cardiology, Cardiovascular Clinics, Merrillville, IN, USA

Vahram Ornekian, MD, MS Vascular Surgery, Washington Hospital Center, Washington, DC, USA

Tjuan L. Overly, MD Cardiovascular Disease, University Cardiology, The University of Tennessee Medical Center, Knoxville, TN, USA

John P. Pacanowski, Jr., MD Vascular Surgery, Pima Vascular, Tucson, AZ, USA

Ambrose F. Panico, DO Internal Medicine, Loyola University Medical Center, Maywood, IL, USA

Nancy Panko, MD General Surgery, St. Joseph Hospital, Chicago, IL, USA

Rajmony Pannu, MD Vascular & Endovascular Medicine, Columbus Vascular Vein & Wound Center, Columbus, OH, USA

Sarah P. Pradka, MD Vascular Surgery, Washington Hospital Center, Washington, DC, USA

Mark G. Rabbat, MD Department of Cardiology, Loyola University Chicago, Maywood, IL, USA

Prafull Raheja, MBBS Interventional Cardiology, Department of Medicine, School of Medicine, University of Louisville, Louisville, KY, USA

Mohamed A. Rahman, MD Medicine, Nephrology, Hines VA Hospital, Loyola University, Hines, IL, USA

Suraj Rao, MD Department of Cardiology, Scripps, San Diego, CA, USA

Hisham Rashid, MSc Department of Vascular Surgery, King's College Hospital, London, UK

Bradley Recht, MD Department of Internal Medicine, Jesse Brown VA, Chicago, IL, USA

Gianluca Rigatelli, MD, PhD Cardiovascular Diagnosis and Endoluminal Interventions Unit, Rovigo General Hospital, Rovigo, Italy

Madhur A. Roberts, MD Cardiovascular Disease, University Cardiology, The University of Tennessee Medical Center, Knoxville, TN, USA

Heron E. Rodriguez, MD Division of Vascular Surgery, Northwestern University Feinberg School of Medicine, Chicago, IL, USA

Arno A. Roscher, MD Surgical Pathology and Laboratory Medicine, Keck School of Medicine (Ret), University of Southern California (USC), Chatsworth, CA, USA

Francis J. Rottier, DPM Podiatry Division, Department of Orthopaedic Surgery and Rehabilitation, Loyola University Stritch School of Medicine, Maywood, IL, USA

Francesco Sangrigoli, MD Vascular Department, King's College Hospital, London, UK

Syed F. Saquib, MD Department of Plastic and Reconstructive Surgery, Johns Hopkins University School of Medicine, Baltimore, MD, USA

Muhamed Saric, MD, PhD Echocardiography Lab, Leon H. Charney Division of Cardiology, Department of Medicine, New York University Langone Medical Center, New York, NY, USA

Scott T. Sayers, PhD Department of Thoracic and Cardiovascular Surgery, Loyola University Medical Center, Maywood, IL, USA

Carlo Setacci, MD Department of Medicine, Surgery and Neuroscience, Unit of Vascular Surgery, University of Siena, Siena, Italy

Francesco Setacci, MD Department of Surgery "P. Valdoni", Sapienza University of Rome, Rome, Italy

Sara R. Shah Department of Cardiology, Community Hospital, Munster,, IN, USA

Dhananjaya Sharma, MS, PhD, DSc Department of Surgery, Government NSCB Medical College, Jabalpur, MP, India

Raymond C. Shields, MD Department of Medicine, College of Medicine, Mayo Clinic, Rochester, MN, USA
Division of Cardiovascular Diseases, Mayo Clinic, Rochester, MN, USA

Anton N. Sidawy, MD, MPH Department of Surgery, George Washington University, Washington, DC, USA

Sanjay Singh, MS, PhD Research Service, Edward Hines Jr., VA Hospital, Hines, IL, USA

Hani Slim, MD Department of Vascular Surgery, King's College Hospital, London, UK

Norman J. Snow, MD Anatomy, Geisel School of Medicine at Dartmouth, Hanover, NH, USA

Rodney M. Stuck, DPM Podiatry Section, Department of Orthopaedic Surgery and Rehabilitation, Loyola University University Stritch School of Medicine, Maywood, IL, USA
Hines Veterans Administration Hospital, Hines, IL, USA

Rand S. Swenson, MD, PhD Anatomy and Neurology, Geisel School of Medicine at Dartmouth, Hanover, NH, USA

Mushabbar A. Syed, MD Departments of Medicine (Cardiology), Radiology and Cell and Molecular Physiology, Loyola University Medical Center, Maywood, IL, USA

Timothy E. Tanke, MD Cardiology Department, Bellin Hospital, Green Bay, WI, USA

Nicholas Tentolouris, MD Internal Medicine and Diabetes, 1st Department of Propaedeutic and Internal Medicine, Laiko General Hospital, Medical School, University of Athens, Athens, Greece

Carlos H. Timaran, MD Division of Vascular and Endovascular Surgery, University of Texas Southwestern Medical Center, Dallas, TX, USA

Tadaki M. Tomita, MD Department of Surgery, Northwestern University Feinberg School of Medicine, Chicago, IL, USA

Rose Tompkins, MD Department of Cardiology, New York University Langone Medical Center, New York, NY, USA

Alexander Turin, MD Internal Medicine, Loyola University Medical Center, Maywood, IL, USA

Domenico Valenti, DM, PhD Department of Vascular Surgery, King's College Hospital, London, UK

James S. Walter, PhD Research Service, Hines VA Hospital, Hines, IL, USA

Benjamin Ross Weber, MD Internal Medicine, University of Chicago, Chicago, IL, USA

Waldemar E. Wysokinski, MD, PhD Department of Cardiovascular Diseases, Gonda Vascular Center, Mayo Clinic, Rochester, MN, USA

Dustin Y. Yoon, MD Division of Vascular Surgery, Northwestern University Feinberg School of Medicine, Chicago, IL, USA

Epidemiology of Acute Critical Limb Ischemia

Martyn Knowles and Carlos H. Timaran

Introduction

Acute limb ischemia (ALI) is defined as any sudden decrease in limb perfusion causing a potential threat to limb viability [1]. The incidence of ALI is 9–16 cases per 100,000 persons per year for the lower extremity [2–4] and around 1–3 cases per 100,000 persons per year for the upper extremity [5]. Etiology includes embolism, in situ thrombosis with coexisting peripheral arterial disease (PAD), graft/stent thrombosis, trauma, or peripheral aneurysm with embolism or thrombosis. ALI management makes up 10–16% of the vascular workload for the average vascular specialist. Amputation and mortality rates are historically high in these patients, however, with advances in anticoagulation and surgical therapy that have decreased over time.

Background

Population-based studies have traditionally shown that 3–12% of the worldwide population suffers from PAD [1, 6–8]. It is estimated that approximately 8 million Americans have impeded lower extremity blood flow, and around half are symptomatic [9, 10]. Smokers, diabetics over the age of 50, renal failure patients, and those over age 70 are particularly at risk [11–14]. Patients with PAD have a significant risk of myocardial infarction, cerebrovascular accident, or death [15, 16]. Symptoms can vary from no symptoms to pain with walking (intermittent claudication), rest pain, and subsequently tissue loss. The majority of patients with claudication will remain stable at 5 years (70–80%), with 10–20% developing worsening claudication and only 1–2% progressing to critical limb ischemia [17].

Critical limb ischemia (CLI) is a more advanced state of arterial occlusive disease, which places the extremity at risk for loss of function, gangrene, or limb loss. In 2003, more than 2.5 million Americans had CLI, which resulted in more than 240,000 amputations in the United States and Europe [18, 19]. Critical limb ischemia can be split into acute or chronic and has different etiologies and natural histories.

Acute limb ischemia (ALI) refers to an abrupt cutoff in the circulation to an extremity—in the absence of trauma or iatrogenic injury—caused by either embolism or thrombosis Cases of CLI with onset <14 days are deemed acute. The significance of ALI is seen in the high limb loss and mortality rates, thus early recognition and treatment is essential to salvage the ischemic extremity [20].

Incidence and Prevalence of Acute Limb Ischemia

The true incidence of ALI is difficult to ascertain. Much of the literature is historical data with no recent updates and has been summarized in multiple texts [21, 22]. Scandinavia has been pivotal in population data regarding ALI. In 1984, Dryjski and Swedenborg [3] investigated the incidence of lower extremity ALI in Stockholm, with a population around 1.5 million. They found an overall annual incidence of nine per 100,000 people. This incidence was related to age; 0.4 per 100,000 for those 20–30 years old, with a peak incidence of 180 per 100,000 in patients over 90. More recently, the Swedish Vascular Registry identified the national incidence of ALI to be 13 per 100,000 people in 1998 [3]. Ljungman et al. focused on temporal trends in ALI over a 19-year period from 1965 to 1983 in Uppsala. They showed an annual increase in ALI from 2.7 to 3.9%, which remained after age adjustments were made with a 2.7% annual increase in men [23]. This increase over time was felt to be likely due to an aging population.

M. Knowles, MD
Division of Vascular Surgery, University of North Carolina, Chapel Hill, NC, USA

C.H. Timaran, MD (✉)
Division of Vascular and Endovascular Surgery, University of Texas Southwestern Medical Center, 5909 Harry Hines Blvd., Dallas, TX 75390-9157, USA

© Springer International Publishing Switzerland 2017
R.S. Dieter et al. (eds.), *Critical Limb Ischemia*, DOI 10.1007/978-3-319-31991-9_1

The other major epidemiological data for ALI have originated from British studies. Clason et al. showed in 1989 the incidence for lower extremity ALI in an area of Scotland to be 3.7 per 100,000 [24]. Later, the incidence was assessed from the entire county of Gloucestershire, England, from a single year in 1994. All data was prospectively gathered including hospital and general practice records, for a total population of 540,000. They found that the incidence during that period was one per 7000 and rose to one per 6000 when bypass grafts were included (14.3 per 100,000 and 16.7 per 100,000, respectively) [4].

Acute upper limb ischemia accounts for 16.6 %, approximately one-fifth of all ALI [5]. Upper extremity ALI occurs with an incidence of 1.2–3.5 cases per 100,000 people per year; however, this estimate is an underestimation as it only includes those that underwent intervention [5]. Dryjski and Swedenborg identified a risk of 1.13 per 100,000 people that included all admissions to the hospital. The patients who develop upper extremity ischemia tended to be slightly older than those with lower extremity ALI, with mean ages of 74 compared to 70 [25], and have a higher ratio of female to male at 2:1. The female to male preponderance was noted in a Danish study over a 13-year period that showed the incidence of upper extremity thromboembolectomy was 3.3 per 100,000 person-years among men and 5.2 per 100,000 person-years among women; however, they did not look at any patients that underwent conservative management [26].

Presentation

Campbell et al. showed that 75 % of patients with ALI presented from home, with 10 % coming from another ward or 8 % from another hospital [27]. Only 3 % presented from a nursing home. They additionally noted that 14 % of ALI patients presented with bilateral lower extremity ischemia and that a similar number of left and right legs were affected. Furthermore, Campbell et al. showed that 40 % of patients had a delay in presentation with equal numbers due to patient, primary care physician, and transport delays [27]. Thirty-five percent had a delay in referral to a vascular specialist. There does not appear to be a significant seasonal variation with ALI; however, there is a trend toward a higher presentation in the winter [28].

Patients with ALI present in different stages of severity. Three stages were developed for ALI standardization (Table 1.1) [29]. Stage I is termed "viable." The limb is not immediately threatened, without continuing ischemic pain, without neurologic deficit, and clear audible arterial signal in the pedal arteries. Stage II is termed "threatened." Within this stage there are two levels, split for managing therapies. Stage IIa is marginally threatened and IIb is immediately threatened. Neither have clear audible signals in the pedal arteries. Those patients in IIa will have transient or minimal sensory loss which is usually limited to the toes. Those in IIb have persistent ischemic rest pain, sensory loss above the toes, and any motor disturbance. Stage III is termed "irreversible." These patients have permanent neuromuscular damage with profound sensory loss and muscle paralysis, absent venous, and capillary flow distally. Typically there are skin changes such as skin marbling and muscle. The distribution of the stages of ALI at presentation is shown in Fig. 1.1 [1].

Etiology

The etiology of lower extremity ALI is traditionally either embolism, in situ thrombosis with preexisting peripheral arterial disease (PAD), graft/stent thrombosis, trauma, or peripheral aneurysm with embolism or thrombosis. The frequency of these etiologies is shown in Fig. 1.2 [1, 27]. The timing of presentation depends on the severity of ischemia, which is linked to the etiology. Patients with embolism, trauma, and popliteal aneurysms present early (hours), compared to those with in situ thrombosis presenting later (days) [1]. Reconstructions—either bypass grafts, stents, or angioplasty

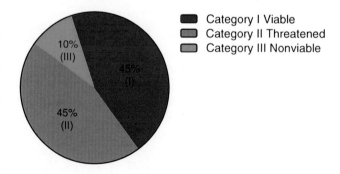

Fig. 1.1 Categories of ALI on presentation. Data from Norgren et al. [1]

Table 1.1 Classification of acute limb ischemia

Ischemic stage	Sensory deficit	Motor deficit	Arterial signal	Venous signal	Treatment
Stage 1	Absent	Absent	Audible	Present	Urgent workup
Stage 2a	None—minimal	Absent	Absent (often)	Present	Urgent surgery
Stage 2b	Moderate	Mild—moderate	Absent (usually)	Present	Emergent surgery
Stage 3	Profound	Profound	Absent	Absent	Amputation

Data from Rutherford et al. [29]

Fig. 1.2 Etiology of acute limb ischemia. Data from Norgren et al. [1] and Campbell et al. [27]

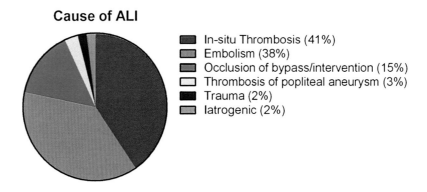

Cause of ALI

- In-situ Thrombosis (41%)
- Embolism (38%)
- Occlusion of bypass/intervention (15%)
- Thrombosis of popliteal aneurysm (3%)
- Trauma (2%)
- Iatrogenic (2%)

Table 1.2 Differential diagnosis of the mechanism of ALI

Embolism	Thrombosis
Atherosclerotic heart disease	Atherosclerosis
Coronary heart disease	Low-flow states
Acute myocardial infarction	Congestive heart failure
Arrhythmia	Hypovolemia
Valvular heart disease	Hypotension
Rheumatic	Hypercoagulable states
Degenerative	Vascular grafts
Congenital	Progression of disease
Bacterial	Intimal hyperplasia
Prosthetic	Mechanical
Artery to artery	Arterial plaque rupture
Aneurysm	Trauma
Atherosclerotic plaque	Aortic/arterial dissection
Idiopathic	HIV arteriopathy
Iatrogenic	Arteritis with thrombosis
Paradoxical embolus	Popliteal adventitial cyst with thrombosis
Trauma	Popliteal entrapment with thrombosis
Other	Vasospasm with thrombosis (e.g., ergotism, cocaine)
Air	External compression
Amniotic fluid	Iatrogenic
Fat	
Tumor	
Chemicals	
Drugs	

Data from Norgren et al. [1] and O'Connell et al. [30]

Table 1.3 Mechanism of acute limb ischemia according to anatomic location

Sites of limb ischemia	Embolism (%)	Thrombosis (%)
Axillary artery	3	0
Brachial artery	14	3
Aortic bifurcation	3	9
Iliac bifurcation	9	16
Femoral bifurcation	57	53
Popliteal artery	14	19

Data from Hallett et al. [21] and Dryjski et al. [32]

the upper extremities. The heart is the usual source of the embolism, ranging from 58 to 93 %, and atrial fibrillation is the usual etiology [5]. Although the source of the atrial fibrillation has changed from valve disease to ischemic heart disease or myocardial infarction, the incidence has remained relatively unchanged. Other rare causes include atrial myxoma, ventricular aneurysm, cardiac failure, and paradoxical embolus.

Changing Patterns

Over the last 30 years, there has been a change in the pattern of etiology for ALI. Dryjski et al. identified that 81 % of the cases they saw in their patient population were embolic, and 19 % were thrombotic [3]. In the most contemporary data, embolism now only accounts for 14 % of all cases of ALI [33, 34].

The reasons that arterial embolism has decreased in incidence are multifactorial. There has been a relative decrease of rheumatic fever and subsequently rheumatic heart disease (RHD) in the developed world, though it is still a significant cause of cardiovascular morbidity and mortality in the young in the less developed world. Additionally, aggressive surgical management of rheumatic heart lesions has increased the lifespan and decreased cardiovascular sequelae from RHD. Furthermore, advances in the management of cardiac valve disease and anticoagulation for atrial fibrillation have vastly decreased the number of cardiac embolisms.

Because of the higher prevalence of PAD and an increasingly aging population, arterial thrombosis has increased over time.

sites—can present early or late given whether it is an acute thrombosis or in situ thrombosis with neointimal hyperplasia or atherosclerosis. This timing of presentation is generally related to the presence of or lack of collateral flow, something chronic PAD that typically affords individuals over time. The other differential diagnosis for ALI is shown in Table 1.2 [1, 31]. The typical sites for ALI involvement are shown in Table 1.3 [21, 32].

Upper extremity ALI, in contrast to acute lower extremity ALI, is almost all from embolism, between 72 and 90 % [5]. This is likely due to the relative absence of atherosclerosis in

Current studies show as little as 9% of ALI cases being caused by embolism [35]. This has, however, not been an acute change with evidence in the decline of embolism since the 1980s. SWEDVASC, the Swedish Vascular Registry, showed a decline of embolism over time from 65 to 43% (Fig. 1.3) [36]. A British study evaluated the management of ALI in 1998 and found that 41% were from thrombosis in situ, 38% from embolism, and 15% from graft or angioplasty occlusion [27]. Luther and Albäck evaluated the population of Helsinki between 1980 and 1991, reporting increases in the frequency of thrombosis by 91% and graft occlusions by 130%, with no change in the incidence of embolism [37].

Current data supports this shift in etiology over time. Ouriel et al. compared the use of urokinase versus surgical intervention for ALI, with thrombosis being the main indication for treatment in 85.6% and embolism in 14.4% [33].

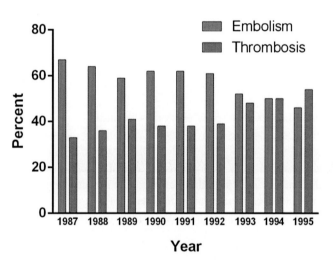

Fig. 1.3 Change in the pattern of embolic and thrombotic disease over time. Data from Bergqvist et al. [36]

Byrne et al. showed the indication for intervention for ALI: thrombosed bypass (36.4%), thrombosed stent (26.6%), native artery thrombosis (24%), embolization (14.3%), and thrombosed popliteal aneurysm (3.2%) [34]. These more current studies show a modern incidence of around 14% for embolism, a stark contrast from 81% in the 1980s (Fig. 1.4).

Natural History

Mortality for lower extremity ALI ranges from 15 to 20% [1]. Major morbidity includes bleeding in 10–15%, major amputation up to 25%, fasciotomy in 5–25%, and renal insufficiency in up to 20%. Campbell et al. evaluated the results from a Vascular Surgical Society of Great Britain and Ireland survey looking at ALI results after 30 days. Thirty-five percent (35%) had died in the follow-up period of 2 years [38]. The cause of death was thromboembolic in 28% including myocardial infarction (15.5%), limb ischemia (5.6%), stroke (4.2%), and mesenteric infarct (2.8%). Further causes of death included cardiac failure (7%), malignant disease (14.1%), and ruptured abdominal aortic aneurysms (2.8%). Twenty-seven percent (27%), however, had an unknown cause of death. Further ALI was noted in 11% of patients; vascular intervention was required in 11% of patients including open surgery, angioplasties, and thrombolytic therapy. Amputation was noted in a further 11% of patients. Of the patients who represented with ALI, 62% required amputations. Survival rates after ALI depend on the etiology. The 5-year survival rate after embolism was 17% and after thrombosis was 44%. This was likely related to an older patient age and higher cardiac risk in the embolism group [30]. Age also appears to affect survival, with older patients doing significantly worse than younger patients. In patients over the age of 80 years, there was an operative

Fig. 1.4 Changes in the pattern of ALI etiology

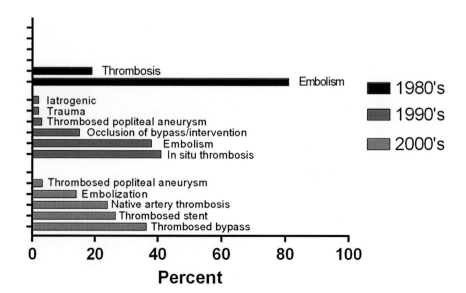

mortality of 50 %; this is in contrast to 5 % in those under the age of 60 [3].

Acute limb ischemia appears to be a slightly more benign event than lower extremity ALI. Conservative management was undertaken prior to the ability to perform an embolectomy. All patients that had upper extremity ALI maintained their arm without the need for amputation, and in hospital mortality was 17 % [39, 40]. Operative mortality has improved with the use of thromboembolectomy; however, there has been little contemporary data evaluating conservative management.

Results with Intervention

With surgical intervention, morbidity and mortality have traditionally been high. In 1948, a series from Massachusetts General Hospital showed an amputation rate of 71 %, with mostly conservative management [39]. In those that received heparin, 38 % underwent amputation. These poor results early on and the introduction of anticoagulants ushered in nonsurgical management with similar results between anticoagulation and surgery [41]. A later review from the same investigators at Massachusetts General Hospital showed an earlier referral for treatment, subsequent higher surgical treatment, and limb survival of 86 % [42]. Over later years in the 1960s and 1970s, there were increasing numbers of arterial embolectomies after the introduction of a balloon-tipped catheter. In the early experience with embolectomies, only 23 % survived without amputation [43]. In a later experience over 20 years in Sweden, ending in 1999, 1-month survival without amputation was 55 % with arterial embolectomy [44]. Kendrick et al. identified similar mortality and amputation rates and were related to the timing of embolectomy [45]. If the patient was operated on within 6 h of the onset of symptoms, mortality was 15 % and the amputation rate was 4 %. In those that were operated on after 12 h, the mortality rate was 48 % and the amputation rate was 52 %.

With increasing advances in anticoagulation, long-term use of anticoagulation, and operative techniques, operative mortality has improved. In 1998, operative mortality for embolism was 17 % and was 14 % for thrombosis [30]. More recent results show a survival rate of 84 % at 1 year after intervention with a major amputation rate of 15 % [34]. The periprocedural amputation rate was lower at 6.4 %. Time to presentation was noted to be associated with worse outcomes. The risk of amputation was four times higher if presentation was more than 25 h after the onset of symptoms [36].

Thromboembolectomy is the treatment of choice for ALI from embolism. Amputation rates have been 0–8 % since the introduction of the embolectomy balloon with a mortality rate up to 20 %. Recent data suggests a 0–3 % risk of amputation and 0–4.8 % risk of death [26, 46–48]. There is a risk of stroke with upper limb embolectomies of up to 19 % [26]. Greater than 95 % of patients are symptom free after embolectomy, but over time up to 50 % can develop claudication [49]. Recurrent embolization can occur in around 10 % of people who are anticoagulated and 1/3 of those who are off anticoagulation, most likely due to continued atrial fibrillation [50]. Recurrent episodes are associated with higher mortality.

Summary

Acute limb ischemia is a harbinger of significant morbidity and mortality. Despite advances in the medical and surgical treatment over the last century, limb amputation and mortality remain high. Furthermore, long-term follow-up of patients after ALI show a significant risk of cardiovascular morbidity and loss of life. The etiology for lower extremity ALI has changed over the last 30 years, with a decrease in the rate of embolic events, likely related to aggressive anticoagulation for valvular and cardiac complaints. Embolism remains the predominant cause of upper extremity ALI. Vascular intervention for ALI is a significant part of any vascular practice and is likely to increase in an aging population. Expeditious presentation and operative management, whether with open or endovascular techniques, yield the best results.

References

1. Norgren L, Hiatt WR, Dormandy JA, et al. Inter-society consensus for the management of peripheral arterial disease (TASC II). J Vasc Surg. 2007;45(Suppl S):S5–67.
2. Creager MA, Kaufman JA, Conte MS. Clinical practice. Acute limb ischemia. N Engl J Med. 2012;366:2198–206.
3. Dryjski M, Swedenborg J. Acute ischemia of the extremities in a metropolitan area during one year. J Cardiovasc Surg. 1984; 25:518–22.
4. Davies B, Braithwaite BD, Birch PA, Poskitt KR, Heather BP, Earnshaw JJ. Acute leg ischaemia in Gloucestershire. Br J Surg. 1997;84:504–8.
5. Eyers P, Earnshaw JJ. Acute non-traumatic arm ischaemia. Br J Surg. 1998;85:1340–6.
6. Olin JW, Sealove BA. Peripheral artery disease: current insight into the disease and its diagnosis and management. Mayo Clin Proc. 2010;85:678–92.
7. Hirsch AT, Haskal ZJ, Hertzer NR, et al. ACC/AHA 2005 guidelines for the management of patients with peripheral arterial disease (lower extremity, renal, mesenteric, and abdominal aortic): executive summary a collaborative report from the American Association for Vascular Surgery/Society for Vascular Surgery, Society for Cardiovascular Angiography and Interventions, Society for Vascular Medicine and Biology, Society of Interventional Radiology, and the ACC/AHA Task Force on Practice Guidelines (Writing Committee to Develop Guidelines for the Management of Patients With Peripheral Arterial Disease) endorsed by the American Association of Cardiovascular and Pulmonary Rehabilitation; National Heart, Lung, and Blood Institute; Society for Vascular Nursing; TransAtlantic Inter-Society Consensus; and Vascular Disease Foundation. J Am Coll Cardiol. 2006;47:1239–312.

8. Novo S. Classification, epidemiology, risk factors, and natural history of peripheral arterial disease. Diabetes Obes Metab. 2002;4 Suppl 2:S1–6.

9. Allison MA, Ho E, Denenberg JO, et al. Ethnic-specific prevalence of peripheral arterial disease in the United States. Am J Prev Med. 2007;32:328–33.

10. Rosamond W, Flegal K, Furie K, et al. Heart disease and stroke statistics—2008 update: a report from the American Heart Association Statistics Committee and Stroke Statistics Subcommittee. Circulation. 2008;117:e25–146.

11. O'Hare AM, Glidden DV, Fox CS, Hsu CY. High prevalence of peripheral arterial disease in persons with renal insufficiency: results from the National Health and Nutrition Examination Survey 1999–2000. Circulation. 2004;109:320–3.

12. Ostchega Y, Paulose-Ram R, Dillon CF, Gu Q, Hughes JP. Prevalence of peripheral arterial disease and risk factors in persons aged 60 and older: data from the National Health and Nutrition Examination Survey 1999–2004. J Am Geriatr Soc. 2007;55: 583–9.

13. Hirsch AT, Criqui MH, Treat-Jacobson D, et al. Peripheral arterial disease detection, awareness, and treatment in primary care. JAMA. 2001;286:1317–24.

14. Criqui MH, Fronek A, Klauber MR, Barrett-Connor E, Gabriel S. The sensitivity, specificity, and predictive value of traditional clinical evaluation of peripheral arterial disease: results from noninvasive testing in a defined population. Circulation. 1985;71:516–22.

15. Muluk SC, Muluk VS, Kelley ME, et al. Outcome events in patients with claudication: a 15-year study in 2777 patients. J Vasc Surg. 2001;33:251–7. discussion 7–8.

16. Weatherley BD, Nelson JJ, Heiss G, et al. The association of the ankle-brachial index with incident coronary heart disease: the Atherosclerosis Risk in Communities (ARIC) study, 1987–2001. BMC Cardiovasc Disord. 2007;7:3.

17. Hirsch AT, Haskal ZJ, Hertzer NR, et al. ACC/AHA 2005 practice guidelines for the management of patients with peripheral arterial disease (lower extremity, renal, mesenteric, and abdominal aortic): a collaborative report from the American Association for Vascular Surgery/Society for Vascular Surgery, Society for Cardiovascular Angiography and Interventions, Society for Vascular Medicine and Biology, Society of Interventional Radiology, and the ACC/AHA Task Force on Practice Guidelines (Writing Committee to Develop Guidelines for the Management of Patients With Peripheral Arterial Disease): endorsed by the American Association of Cardiovascular and Pulmonary Rehabilitation; National Heart, Lung, and Blood Institute; Society for Vascular Nursing; TransAtlantic Inter-Society Consensus; and Vascular Disease Foundation. Circulation 2006;113:e463–654.

18. Allie DE, Hebert CJ, Lirtzman MD, et al. Critical limb ischemia: a global epidemic. A critical analysis of current treatment unmasks the clinical and economic costs of CLI. EuroIntervention. 2005;1:75–84.

19. Dormandy J, Heeck L, Vig S. Major amputations: clinical patterns and predictors. Semin Vasc Surg. 1999;12:154–61.

20. Baril DT, Patel VI, Judelson DR, et al. Outcomes of lower extremity bypass performed for acute limb ischemia. J Vasc Surg. 2013;58:949–56.

21. Hallett JW, Mills JL, Earnshaw J, Reekers JA, Rooke T. Comprehensive vascular and endovascular surgery: expert consult—online and print. UK: Elsevier Health Sciences; 2009.

22. Cronenwett JL, Johnston KW. Rutherford's vascular surgery, 2-volume set: expert consult—print and online. UK: Elsevier—Health Sciences Division; 2014.

23. Ljungman C, Adami HO, Bergqvist D, Sparen P, Bergstrom R. Risk factors for early lower limb loss after embolectomy for acute arterial occlusion: a population-based case–control study. Br J Surg. 1991;78:1482–5.

24. Clason AE, Stonebridge PA, Duncan AJ, Nolan B, Jenkins AM, Ruckley CV. Acute ischaemia of the lower limb: the effect of centralizing vascular surgical services on morbidity and mortality. Br J Surg. 1989;76:592–3.

25. Stonebridge PA, Clason AE, Duncan AJ, Nolan B, Jenkins AM, Ruckley CV. Acute ischaemia of the upper limb compared with acute lower limb ischaemia: a 5-year review. Br J Surg. 1989;76:515–6.

26. Andersen LV, Mortensen LS, Lindholt JS, Faergeman O, Henneberg EW, Frost L. Upper-limb thrombo-embolectomy: national cohort study in Denmark. Eur J Vasc Endovasc Surg. 2010;40:628–34.

27. Campbell WB, Ridler BM, Szymanska TH. Current management of acute leg ischaemia: results of an audit by the Vascular Surgical Society of Great Britain and Ireland. Br J Surg. 1998;85:1498–503.

28. Kuukasjarvi P, Salenius JP, Lepantalo M, Luther M, Ylonen K, Finnvasc Study Group. Weekly and seasonal variation of hospital admissions and outcome in patients with acute lower limb ischaemia treated by surgical and endovascular means. Int Angiol. 2000;19:354–7.

29. Rutherford RB, Baker JD, Ernst C, et al. Recommended standards for reports dealing with lower extremity ischemia: revised version. J Vasc Surg. 1997;26:517–38.

30. Aune S, Trippestad A. Operative mortality and long-term survival of patients operated on for acute lower limb ischaemia. Eur J Vasc Endovasc Surg. 1998;15:143–6.

31. O'Connell JB, Quinones-Baldrich WJ. Proper evaluation and management of acute embolic versus thrombotic limb ischemia. Semin Vasc Surg. 2009;22:10–6.

32. Dryjski M, Swedenborg J. Acute nontraumatic extremity ischaemia in Sweden. A one-year survey. Acta Chir Scand. 1985;151:333–9.

33. Ouriel K, Veith FJ, Sasahara AA, Thrombolysis or Peripheral Arterial Surgery (TOPAS) Investigators. A comparison of recombinant urokinase with vascular surgery as initial treatment for acute arterial occlusion of the legs. N Engl J Med. 1998;338:1105–11.

34. Byrne RM, Taha AG, Avgerinos E, Marone LK, Makaroun MS, Chaer RA. Contemporary outcomes of endovascular interventions for acute limb ischemia. J Vasc Surg. 2014;59:988–95.

35. Bergqvist D, Troeng T, Elfstrom J, et al. The Steering Committee of Swedvasc. Auditing surgical outcome: ten years with the Swedish Vascular Registry—Swedvasc. Eur J Surg Suppl. 1998;581:3–8.

36. Bergqvist D, Troeng T, Elfstrom J, et al., The Steering Committee of Swedvasc. Auditing surgical outcome: ten years with the Swedish Vascular Registry—Swedvasc. Eur J Surg Suppl. 1998;(581):3–8.

37. Luther M, Alback A. Acute leg ischaemia—a case for the junior surgeon? Ann Chir Gynaecol. 1995;84:373–8.

38. Campbell WB, Ridler BM, Szymanska TH. Two-year follow-up after acute thromboembolic limb ischaemia: the importance of anticoagulation. Eur J Vasc Endovasc Surg. 2000;19:169–73.

39. Warren R, Linton RR. The treatment of arterial embolism. N Engl J Med. 1948;238:421–9.

40. Abbott WM, Maloney RD, McCabe CC, Lee CE, Wirthlin LS. Arterial embolism: a 44 year perspective. Am J Surg. 1982;143:460–4.

41. Haimovici H. Peripheral arterial embolism; a study of 330 unselected cases of embolism of the extremities. Angiology. 1950;1:20–45.

42. Warren R, Linton RR, Scannell JG. Arterial embolism: recent progress. Ann Surg. 1954;140:311–7.

43. Key E. Embolectomy on the vessels of the extremities. Br J Surg. 1936;24:350–61.

44. Jivegard L, Wingren U. Management of acute limb ischaemia over two decades: the Swedish experience. Eur J Vasc Endovasc Surg. 1999;18:93–5.

45. Kendrick J, Thompson BW, Read RC, Campbell GS, Walls RC, Casali RE. Arterial embolectomy in the leg. Results in a referral hospital. Am J Surg. 1981;142:739–43.
46. Karapolat S, Dag O, Abanoz M, Aslan M. Arterial embolectomy: a retrospective evaluation of 730 cases over 20 years. Surg Today. 2006;36:416–9.
47. Ueberrueck T, Marusch F, Schmidt H, Gastinger I. Risk factors and management of arterial emboli of the upper and lower extremities. J Cardiovasc Surg (Torino). 2007;48:181–6.
48. Gossage JA, Ali T, Chambers J, Burnand KG. Peripheral arterial embolism: prevalence, outcome, and the role of echocardiography in management. Vasc Endovascular Surg. 2006;40:280–6.
49. Galbraith K, Collin J, Morris PJ, Wood RF. Recent experience with arterial embolism of the limbs in a vascular unit. Ann R Coll Surg Engl. 1985;67:30–3.
50. Clason AE, Stonebridge PA, Duncan AJ, Nolan B, Jenkins AM, Ruckley CV. Morbidity and mortality in acute lower limb ischaemia: a 5-year review. Eur J Vasc Surg. 1989;3:339–43.

Epidemiology of Chronic Critical Limb Ischemia

Akhil Gulati, Lawrence Garcia, and Subasit Acharji

Introduction

Peripheral artery disease (PAD) is often referred to as a continuum of disease of occlusive arterial syndromes that can range from asymptomatic obstructive disease through occlusive disease requiring amputation. This entire spectrum of PAD has prevalence as high as 20% of the general population [1]. This spectrum becomes more progressive and symptomatic as the disease causes an imbalance of distal perfusion pressure to the tissue and metabolic demands within that tissue. On the latter end of this continuum, chronic critical limb ischemia (CLI) has a prevalence that is more difficult to define and is quite variable in the published literature. Unlike asymptomatic PAD or exertional claudication, CLI occurs with inadequate perfusion at rest [2].

Like most of the terminology of peripheral vascular disease, the definitions of CLI have evolved over the years, with first an increasing need to classify the entire continuum of PAD, the need to further classify those undergoing surgical procedures, and then to include more objective measures as well as the clinical presentation. In this chapter, we will discuss the epidemiology of CLI. We will present the historical background of CLI and the risk factors along with its clinical presentations and then after the epidemiology and prevalence of CLI along with its risk stratification and prognostic data before discussing the socioeconomic impact of this disease.

A. Gulati, MD • L. Garcia, MD (✉) • S. Acharji, MD
Section of Interventional Cardiology and Vascular Intervention, Vascular Medicine, Department of Cardiovascular Medicine, St. Elizabeth's Medical Center, 736 Cambridge St., Boston, MA 02135, USA

Definition of Chronic Critical Limb Ischemia

The definition of CLI has evolved over time. It has been classically defined as greater than 2 weeks of extremity rest pain, ulcers, or extremity gangrene, secondary to objectively proven peripheral artery disease. In its most extreme case, CLI can lead to limb loss [1, 2].

Several criteria are often used for objective evidence of CLI, but most commonly involve: (a) ankle-brachial index (ABI) of 0.4 or less, (b) ankle systolic pressure of 50 mmHg or less, (c) toe systolic pressure of 30 mmHg or less, (d) toe-brachial index (TBI) of 0.25 or less, and (e) reduced supine forefoot transcutaneous oxygen pressure (TcPO2) less than 30 mmHg [3, 4]. Although not an exact definition, CLI would be seen as corresponding with stages III and IV of Fontaine Classification and categories 4 through 6 of the Rutherford classification system [5, 6] (see Table 2.1).

While the Fontaine and Rutherford classification systems originally were implemented to categorize peripheral arterial disease by symptoms several decades ago, objective criteria were adapted as technology has developed and several consensus documents have then evolved the definition of CLI [7].

The first consensus document was the Second European Meeting Consensus Document on CLI (1991) that used two definitions for CLI based on clinical use and on research use [4] as written below:

1. CLI, in both diabetic and nondiabetic patients, is defined by either of the following two criteria:
   a. Persistently recurring ischemic rest pain requiring regular adequate analgesia for more than 2 weeks with an ankle systolic pressure ≤50 mmHg and/or toe systolic pressure ≤30 mmHg
   b. Ulceration or gangrene of the foot or toes, with an ankle systolic pressure ≤50 mmHg or toe systolic pressure ≤30 mmHg
2. A more precise description of the type and severity of CLI is also necessary for the design and reporting of

Table 2.1 Fontaine's stages and Rutherford categories for lower limb symptom classification

Fontaine's stages		Rutherford categories		
Stage	Clinical presentation	Grade	Category	Clinical presentation
I	Asymptomatic	0	0	Asymptomatic
IIa	Mild claudication	I	1	Mild claudication
IIb	Moderate to severe		2	Moderate claudication
	Claudication		3	Severe claudication
III	Ischemic rest pain	II	4	Ischemic rest pain
IV	Ulceration or gangrene	III	5	Minor tissue loss
			6	Major tissue loss

clinical trials. In addition to the above definition, the following information is also desirable:

a. Arteriography to delineate the anatomy of the large vessel disease throughout the leg and foot
b. Toe arterial pressure in all patients, including those who are not diabetic
c. A technique for quantifying the local microcirculation in the ischemia area (e.g., capillary microscopy, transcutaneous oxygen pressure [TcPO2], or laser Doppler)

There has been some debate on the value of ankle pressures. However these definitions have been generally agreed upon as the threshold to be used.

The next large summary consensus was the Trans-Atlantic Inter-Society Consensus (TASC) Document on Management of Peripheral Arterial Disease (2000) that did continue the method of having a clinical definition, as well as a research definition. It also changed the thresholds for some of the objective criteria [8]:

1. Clinical definition of critical limb ischemia (CLI): The term critical limb ischemia should be used for all patients with chronic ischemic rest pain, ulcers, or gangrene attributable to objectively proven arterial occlusive disease. The CLI implies chronicity and is to be distinguished from acute limb ischemia.
2. Trials and reporting standards definition of CLI: A relatively inclusive entry criterion is favored, the aim being to ensure that the ulceration, gangrene, or rest pain is indeed caused by peripheral arterial disease and that most would be expected to require a major amputation within the next 6 months to a year in the absence of a significant hemodynamic improvement. To achieve this, it is suggested to use absolute pressures of either ankle pressure <50–70 mmHg or toe pressure <30–50 mmHg or reduced supine forefoot TcPO2 <30–50 mmHg.

Here, there is an emphasis on CLI being defined by symptoms and showing objective-proven arterial occlusive

disease. The thresholds for ankle pressure were raised, possibly to answer some of the critics of the 1991 European Consensus Document. However, the toe pressure and TcPO2 pressure thresholds were also raised.

The ACC/AHA created practice guidelines in 2005 for management of patients with peripheral artery disease and also addressed the definition of CLI using some of the other consensus statements [9]. It uses the TASC clinical definition as above and points out that most vascular clinicians would define CLI as those patients in whom the untreated natural history would lead to a major limb loss within 6 months [9].

The most recent consensus statement is the TASC Document that was updated (TASC II 2007) that simplified the definition: "The term critical limb ischemia should be used for all patients with chronic ischemic rest pain, ulcers or gangrene attributable to objectively proven arterial occlusive disease. The term CLI implies chronicity and is to be distinguished from acute limb ischemia" [3]. It also stresses that ischemic rest pain will most often occur with ankle pressures <50 mmHg and toe pressures <30 mmHg but that in situations where healing is needed (if a venous or traumatic ulcer is not healing well due to poor arterial flow), often ankle pressures less than 70 mmHg and toe pressures less than 50 mmHg are insufficient [3]. There is not complete consensus as to the objective vascular parameters to be used for CLI, but the thresholds we have mentioned are the most commonly used in various clinical practices, as well as for various research articles and publications.

CLI is most often caused by, and associated with, obstructive atherosclerotic arterial disease. While most risk factor modification, research, and focus are on this disease process, it is important to note that since CLI results from the imbalance between supply of nutrients and metabolic demand in distal tissues, there are other causes that can result in CLI. Other causes can include atheroembolic/thromboembolic disease, thrombosis resulting from hypercoagulable states, vasculitides, thromboangiitis obliterans, cystic adventitial disease, Buerger's disease, thoracic outlet syndrome, popliteal entrapment syndrome, trauma, and more [9, 10]. There are also multiple risk factors to CLI as well as contributing factors to the acceleration of the disease process that will be addressed elsewhere.

Epidemiology of Chronic Critical Limb Ischemia

Peripheral arterial occlusive disease has been well studied over the last several decades with most research dealing with symptomatic disease, including intermittent claudication through the extreme of limb loss. It has been noted that there is a prevalence of 8–10 million Americans who suffer from arterial occlusive disease [3]. While the reported prevalence of peripheral arterial disease (PAD) may depend on the particular population studied, and the modality used to diagnose it (subjective and objective criteria), if one uses PAD to be defined by an ankle-brachial index of <0.90, then it may likely be present in up to 4–10 % of patients in the USA and Europe [11–13] and involving a prevalence of an estimated 27 million people in those same areas [14].

There is widespread data about the incidence and prevalence of PAD as an entity; however, there is limited data regarding chronic critical limb ischemia. It is difficult to obtain specific epidemiologic data for CLI for several reasons [7]. First, the identification of CLI is more difficult than identifying some other conditions (like PAD as defined by ABI <0.90). As stated above, a general definition that most clinicians use is by attributing rest pain, ulcers, or extremity gangrene to a peripheral arterial occlusive disease, and that lasts longer than 2 weeks. This requires a level of proficiency and diagnostic assessments that are not often readily available in large epidemiological studies [7].

Secondly, as noted, the definition of CLI has evolved over time. There is a heterogeneity of many studies using different definitions and often without the objective parameters to define that CLI has been published. There are often major differences between the various studies that can make the data inconsistent. Lastly, the actual numerical epidemiological data that is usually used and cited is often inferred from other markers, such as the incidence of amputations (which assumes that a quarter of CLI patients undergo this procedure). Data is often presented from assumptions of the natural history of PAD (i.e., perhaps the estimate that 5–10 % of patients with either asymptomatic PAD or claudication will go on to become CLI at 5 years time) [3, 7].

An Italian study by Catalano et al. tried to confront the difficult problem of getting accurate epidemiological data for CLI [15]. The study used three different methods to obtain data. They first created a prospective study on the incidence of CLI in 200 patients who had been suffering from claudication and in 190 controls that showed an incidence of 450 per million people per year for CLI and 112 per million people per year for amputations in those above the age of 45. They also did a 3-month prospective study on CLI hospitalizations in a sample of hospitals in Lombardy, Italy (Northern Italy region), that showed an incidence of 642 per million people per year for CLI and 160 per million people per year in those over the age of 45. Lastly, they also looked at the number of amputations performed in hospitals of two regions (6 years in Lombardy and 2 years in Emilia Romagna) that showed an incidence of 577 per million people per year for CLI and 172 per million people per year for amputations in Lombardy and 530 per million people per year for CLI and 154 per million people per year for amputations in Emilia Romagna. Interestingly, the results revealed an incidence of both CLI and amputation rates that were lower

than expected, with authors suggesting this to be explained by the area of Italy studied being one with a known high rate of "cardiovascular protection" [15].

While epidemiological data may be difficult to obtain, compare, and contrast, much of the data that is available is still fairly useful and reveals the scope of the disease, the natural history of PAD, and the serious effects of CLI and the socioeconomic impact of this disease.

The TASC II guidelines have estimated that the incidence of CLI, as inferred from the natural history of PAD and amputation rates, is approximately 500–1000 per million per year in a European or North American population (150,000 cases per year in the USA) [3]. As noted, some of the large prospective population studies have shown an incidence of 220 new cases per million per year in the general population [15, 16]. The prevalence of CLI is often estimated between 0.5 and 1.2 % in various studies and registries. One particular European cross-sectional study done in Sweden used an age-standardized randomly selected population sample of men and women aged 60–90 years with 5080 subjects included (64 % participation rate) to answer questionnaires on medical history, medication, and symptoms as their ABI was also measured [17]. The study also gave special attention to critical limb ischemia and gender differences. The prevalence of CLI was found to be approximately 1.2 %, with women having a slightly higher prevalence than men (1.5 % vs 0.8 %, $p < 0.008$), although other studies may show the opposite. This study also showed that prevalence of CLI increased as age increased, as one would expect.

In attempting to determine the prevalence of CLI and the risk factors associated with developing CLI, the largest published population study was done in Norway (HUNT 2 Study) between 1995 and 1997 with a questionnaire for the 20,291 participants between the age of 40 and 69 that was specifically aimed at identifying CLI [18]. Questionnaires were sent to all patients over age 20, but the focus was on those 40–69 years of age, and thus the study population consisted of 9640 men and 10,651 women. For the purpose of the study, CLI was defined as having ulcers on toes, feet, or ankles that have failed to heal or persistent pain in the forefoot while in the supine position but with relief of the pain when standing up. The study revealed a prevalence of CLI in this population of 0.24 % (0.26 % for men and 0.24 % for women), with the age-adjusted prevalence of CLI increasing with age as expected. Tobacco use conferred a 2.3 times increased risk of CLI compared to those participants who never smoked, and diabetes mellitus conferred a 4.4 times increased risk of developing CLI compared to the general population. Other risk factors that were independently associated with increased risk of CLI included older age, elevated total cholesterol, elevated serum triglyceride, higher body mass index (BMI), and angina. The prevalence of CLI was found to be 2500 per million inhabitants, similar between both genders and increasing with age. The study did note, however, that it may be easier and necessary to identify CLI by symptoms and clinical signs (rather than with objective measurements). This does cause drawbacks where one may include patients with non-PAD ulcers or pain in the CLI category. The study may also include some patients with acute limb ischemia (ALI) in the CLI category by the questions that were used in the questionnaire.

Another study was a population-based, prospective cohort study of the comparative value of modern risk stratification techniques for cardiac events and studied 4814 subjects aged 45–75 [19]. As part of this study, PAD was assessed by obtaining ABI and peak ankle artery pressures for all patients, and this data was used (along with patient acknowledging a history of specific PAD or CLI) to determine prevalence. In this study, CLI was considered present if the highest ankle artery pressure measured <70 mmHg. The prevalence of CLI in this population was 0.11% with a trend toward increased association with age. The study did have some limitations that may have lowered the prevalence by not including some of the more severely ill subjects, not including the subjects that could not get an ABI performed (patients with ulcers or wounds that would already qualify them as CLI subjects) and the overall low response rate that may have been a selection bias against CLI, as well.

The TASC II study noted that 5–10% of patients with asymptomatic PAD or claudication will progress to CLI within 5 years. Up to 1–3% of patients with PAD present initially with CLI [3]. This group is often characterized as patients who are older or sedentary and thus have not exerted themselves to get claudication symptoms. Also, these are often patients with sensory neuropathy or patients with other medical issues such as heart failure. Some studies have shown that possibly half of CLI patients in the general population may not have any PAD symptoms even 6 months prior to the onset of clinical CLI [7, 20].

CLI is the initial clinical presentation in only 1–3% of PAD cases, although arteriographic progression has been documented in up to 60% of PAD patients after 5 years of follow-up. Other studies have shown that 40–50% of those affected present with atypical leg pains, 10–35% with intermittent claudication, and 20–50% with no symptoms at all [9, 21].

One of the studies that attempted to show the natural history of those with intermittent claudication was the Edinburgh Artery Study in 1988, where 1592 participants between ages 55 and 74 were randomly selected and the presence of PAD was determined by questionnaire on claudication, ABI and a reactive hyperemia test. This cohort was then followed over 5 years for subsequent vascular events. In this cohort, 116 new cases of claudication were identified, and of those 4.1% underwent vascular surgery/arterial reconstruction, 4.1%

underwent amputation, and 1.4% developed leg ulceration at 5 years time [22]. Limitations in this study were the small incidence noted of intermittent claudication in the population and the variable regional practices regarding when to perform amputation.

A much larger and longer study was done over a 15 year period by Aquino et al. who collected data on 1244 men with intermittent claudication with a mean follow-up of 45 months (with some statistically valid data followed for as long as 12 years) [23]. The group collected data on demographics, clinical risk factors, ABI and serially followed ABI, self-reported walking distance, and monitored patients for ischemic rest pain and ischemic ulceration. Results revealed that ABI declined an average of 0.014 per year. The cumulative 10-year risk of development of ischemic ulcers was 23%, and the 10-year risk of ischemic rest pain was 30%. Lower ABI and diabetes mellitus were identified as significant predictors of ischemic ulcers, with smoking added as a predictor as well for ischemic rest pain. The study was limited by only following a male population (study done at a Veterans Administration Center), and there was possibly a selection bias (in that it may be likely that sicker patients were the ones referred to the vascular lab). Of note, the study also identified a particularly higher risk of limb event subset of patients who were diabetic with ABI<0.3 [24, 25].

Risk Factors, Stratification, and Prognosis of Chronic Critical Limb Ischemia

Chronic critical limb ischemia (CLI) is the result of atherosclerotic peripheral arterial occlusive disease and thus shares many of the same risk factors of atherosclerotic disease in other vascular territories. The risk factors include hypertension, hypercholesterolemia, cigarette smoking, and diabetes mellitus. The latter two are more strongly associated with progressive CLI than others [3]. Diabetic patients develop early onset and more rapidly progressive disease with the involvement of distal vessels. The aorta and iliac arteries are relatively spared when compared to profunda femoris and popliteal and tibial arteries, which may be less amenable to revascularization, thus along with presence of diabetic neuropathy leads to higher rates of amputation compared to nondiabetic. Similarly among smokers, the risk of developing CLI increases directly proportionally to the amount of cigarettes smoked [26].

Transcutaneous oxygen tension (TcPO2), determined by blood flow and arterial oxygen tension (PaO2), can be a marker of total distal runoff (arterial and arteriolar runoff) or perfusion reserve in forefoot and may predict changes in blood flow to an extremity when flow is severely restricted [27]. Recently a risk stratification tool based on TcPO2 has been suggested [7]:

- Degree 1: 10 mmHg < forefoot TcPO2 ≤ 35 mmHg in supine position
- Degree 2: forefoot TcPO2 ≤ 10 mmHg in supine position but clear improvement (≤40 mmHg) in sitting position or under oxygen inhalation
- Degree 3: forefoot TcPO2 ≤ 10 mmHg in supine position and inadequate or no improvement (<30–40 mmHg) in sitting position or under oxygen inhalation
- Degree 4: forefoot TcPO2 ≤ 10 mmHg in supine and in sitting position and/or under oxygen inhalation (very poor prognosis)

While a quarter of),patients presenting with CLI are alive without clinical CLI and major amputation at one year, 20–25 % of patients will have died, 25–30 % will have had major amputation, and 20 % will still be in CLI state [3].

Socioeconomic Impact of Chronic Critical Limb Ischemia

Patients with CLI experience a rapid functional decline and 6 min walk performance [28]. The functional impairment affects quality of life and may lead to depressed mood [29].

The financial burden of caring for patients with CLI is sobering. While the yearly cost of clinical care of a patient with CLI was $43,000 per patient in 1990 [30], the cost of surgical revascularization for CLI was £23,322 sterling in BASIL trial [31]. Although there is an initial cost saving with endovascular revascularization of CLI when compared to surgical option, higher rates of subsequent revascularization offsets the cost advantage later [31, 32]. Ultimately, the yearly cost of managing a patient with CLI undergoing amputation is actually double that of undergoing a limb salvage procedure [30].

Conclusion

Chronic critical limb ischemia is a vastly important disease process and part of the peripheral arterial occlusive disease spectrum. Much of our data regarding vascular disease covers the entire continuity of PAD as a whole, but there is more limited data regarding the distinct process of CLI. This may often be due to the difficulty and evolution of the CLI definition over the years, including subjective and objective descriptions of the disease. However, there is data that can be used in either population studies as well as inferred data from natural history of PAD and data from both surgical and endovascular studies that extrapolate CLI. Understanding the scope of CLI allows us to not only improve our diagnostic abilities but also our treatment including prevention. Understanding the devastating

effects of the end-stage vascular disease as a social effect, as well as economic effect, will also allow us to further determine cost-effective treatment (medical, endovascular, and surgical) and rehabilitation.

References

1. Bitar FG, Garcia LA. Critical limb ischemia: an overview of the epidemiologic and clinical implications. Vasc Dis Manag. 2010;7:E182–4.
2. Alonso A, McManus DD, Fisher DF. Peripheral vascular disease. Sudbury, MA: Jones and Bartlett Publishers; 2011.
3. Norgren L, Hiatt WR, Dormandy JA, et al. Inter-society consensus for the management of peripheral arterial disease (TASC II). Eur J Vasc Endovasc Surg. 2007;45(Suppl):S5–67.
4. Second European consensus document on chronic critical leg ischemia. Circulation. 1991;84 4 Suppl:1–26.
5. Fontaine R, Kim M, Kieny R. Surgical treatment of peripheral circulation disorders. Helv Chir Acta. 1954;21:499–533. German.
6. Rutherford RB, Baker JD, Ernst C, et al. Recommended standards for reports dealing with lower extremity ischemia: revised version. J Vasc Surg. 1997;26:517–38.
7. Becker F, Robert-Ebadi H, Ricco JB, et al. Chapter I: definitions, epidemiology, clinical presentation and prognosis. Eur J Vasc Endovasc Surg. 2011;45 Suppl 2:S4–12.
8. Dormandy JA, Rutherford RB. Management of peripheral arterial disease (PAD). TASC Working Group. TransAtlantic Inter-Society Consensus (TASC). J Vasc Surg. 2000;31:S1–296.
9. Hirsch AT, Haskal ZJ, Hertzer NR, Bakal CW, Creager MA, Halperin JL, Hiratzka LF, Murphy WR, Olin JW, Puschett JB, Rosenfield KA, Sacks D, Stanley JC, Taylor LM Jr, White CJ, White J, White RA, Antman EM, Smith SC Jr, Adams CD, Anderson JL, Faxon DP, Fuster V, Gibbons RJ, Hunt SA, Jacobs AK, Nishimura R, Ornato JP, Page RL, Riegel B. ACC/AHA 2005 Practice Guidelines for the management of patients with peripheral arterial disease (lower extremity, renal, mesenteric, and abdominal aortic): a collaborative report from the American Association for Vascular Surgery/Society for Vascular Surgery, Society for Cardiovascular Angiography and Interventions, Society for Vascular Medicine and Biology, Society of Interventional Radiology, and the ACC/AHA Task Force on Practice Guidelines (Writing Committee to Develop Guidelines for the Management of Patients With Peripheral Arterial Disease): endorsed by the American Association of Cardiovascular and Pulmonary Rehabilitation; National Heart, Lung, and Blood Institute; Society for Vascular Nursing; TransAtlantic Inter-Society Consensus; and Vascular Disease Foundation. Circulation. 2006;113(11):e463–654.
10. DeBakey ME, Crawford ES, Garrett E, et al. Occlusive disease of the lower extremities in patients 16 to 37 years of age. Ann Surg. 1964;159:873–90.
11. Criqui MH, Fronek A, Barrett-Conner E, et al. The prevalence of peripheral arterial disease in a defined population. Circulation. 1985;71(3):510–5.
12. Selvin E, Erlinger TP. Prevalence of and risk factors for peripheral arterial disease in the United States: results from the national Health and Nutrition Examination Survey, 1999–2000. Circulation. 2004;110:738–43.
13. Hirsch AT, Criqui MH, Treat-Jacobson D, et al. Peripheral arterial disease detection, awareness, and treatment in primary care. JAMA. 2001;286:1317–24.
14. Hankey GJ, Norman PE, Eikelboom JW. Medical treatment of peripheral arterial disease. JAMA. 2006;295:547–53.

15. Catalano M. Epidemiology of critical limb ischaemia: north Italian data. Eur J Med. 1993;2:11–4.

16. C S. Critical limb ischemia. New developments and perspectives. Turin: Edizioni Minerva Medica; 2010.

17. Sigvant B, Wiberg-Hedman K, Bergqvist D, et al. A population-based study of peripheral arterial disease prevalence with special focus on critical limb ischemia and sex differences. J Vasc Surg. 2007;45:1185–91.

18. Jensen SA, Vatten LJ, Myhre HO. The prevalence of chronic critical lower limb ischemia in a population of 20,000 subjects 40–69 years of age. Eur J Vasc Endovasc Surg. 2006;32:60–5.

19. Kroger K, Stang A, Kondratieva J, et al., Heinz Nixdorf RECALL Study Group. Prevalence of peripheral arterial disease—results of the Heinz Nixdorf Recall Study. Eur J Epidemiol. 2006; 21:279–85.

20. Varu VN, Hogg ME, Kibbe MR. Critical limb ischemia. J Vasc Surg. 2010;51:230–41.

21. Ouriel K. Peripheral arterial disease. Lancet. 2001;358:1257–64.

22. Leng GC, Lee AJ, Fowkes FG, et al. Incidence, natural history and cardiovascular events in symptomatic and asymptomatic peripheral arterial disease in the general population. Int J Epidemiol. 1996;25:1172–81.

23. Aquino R, Johnnides C, Makaroun M, Whittle JC, et al. Natural history of claudication: long-term serial follow-up study of 1244 claudicants. J Vasc Surg. 2001;34:962–70.

24. Jelnes R, Gaardsting O, Hougaard Jensen K, et al. Fate in intermittent claudication: outcome and risk factors. Br Med J. 1986;293: 1137–40.

25. Naschitz JE, Ambrosio DA, Chang JB. Intermittent claudication: predictors and outcomes. Angiology. 1988;39:16–22.

26. Rajagopalan S, Grossman PM. Management of chronic critical limb ischemia. Cardiol Clin. 2002;20:535–45.

27. Moosa HH, Makaroun MS, Peitzman AB, et al. TcPO2 values in limb ischemia: effects of blood flow and arterial oxygen tension. J Surg Res. 1986;40(5):482–7.

28. McDermott MM, Liu K, Greenland P, et al. Functional decline in peripheral arterial disease: associations with the ankle brachial index and leg symptoms. JAMA. 2004;292(4):453–61.

29. Arseven A, Guralnik JM, O'Brien E, et al. Peripheral arterial disease and depressed mood in older men and women. Vasc Med. 2001;6(4):229–34.

30. Singh S, Evans L, Datta D, et al. The costs of managing lower limb-threatening ischaemia. Eur J Vasc Endovasc Surg. 1996; 12(3):359–62.

31. Adam DJ, Beard JD, Cleveland T, et al. Bypass versus angioplasty in severe ischaemia of the leg (BASIL): multicentre, randomised controlled trial. Lancet. 2005;366(9501):1925–34.

32. Stoner MC, Defreitas DJ, Manwaring MM, et al. Cost per day of patency: understanding the impact of patency and reintervention in a sustainable model of healthcare. J Vasc Surg. 2008;48(6):1489–96.

Taishi Hirai, Amit S. Dayal, Rie Hirai, Timothy E. Tanke,
and Robert S. Dieter

Anatomic Classifications

Joint Endovascular and Noninvasive Assessment of Limb Perfusion (JENALI) Classification

JENALI scoring system divides each tibial vessel (anterior tibial artery, posterior tibial artery, and peroneal artery) into proximal, mid-, and distal segments [1]. The segment is considered patent and assigned a score of 1 if contrast is visualized within the vessel. If the segment is occluded, it is assigned a score of 0. The segment will be considered patent, so long as there is constant contrast line regardless if it fills through direct antegrade flow or indirect retrograde flow. A maximum score of 9 signifies that all the tibial vessels are patent, and a minimum score of 0 signifies that none of the segment is angiographically patent. The strength of the scoring system lies in its simplicity [1].

T. Hirai, MD (✉)
Division of Cardiology, Department of Medicine, Stritch School of Medicine, Loyola University Medical Center/Loyola University Chicago, 2160 1st Ave., Maywood, IL 60153, USA

A.S. Dayal, MD
Medicine, Stritch School of Medicine, Loyola University Chicago, Maywood, IL, USA

Medicine, Edward Hines Jr. VA Hospital, Hines, IL, USA

R. Hirai, MD
Internal Medicine, Loyola University Medical Center, Maywood, IL, USA

T.E. Tanke, MD
Cardiology Department, Bellin Hospital, Green Bay, WI, USA

R.S. Dieter, MD, RVT
Medicine, Cardiology, Vascular and Endovascular Medicine, Loyola University Medical Center, Maywood, IL, USA

Angiosomes

In 1987, Dr. Taylor, the anatomist and plastic surgeon, introduced the angiosome concept, separating the body into distinct three-dimensional blocks of tissue fed by source arteries [2]. Angiosomes of the foot are defined by different branches of the three main arteries (Fig. 3.1) [3, 4]. The *anterior tibial artery* supplies the anterior ankle which turns into the dorsalis pedis and subsequently supplies the dorsum of the foot. The *posterior tibial artery* supplies the heel through the calcaneal artery, instep through the medial plantar artery, while the lateral plantar artery supplies the lateral midfoot and forefoot. The *peroneal artery* breaks off into two segments which are the anterior perforating branch which supplies lateral anterior portion of the ankle and calcaneal branch which supplies the plantar portion of the heel.

TransAtlantic Inter-Society Consensus (TASC) Document II Classification

The foundations for TASC were laid in 2000 in an attempt to discuss how to treat arterial disease [5]. In an attempt to discuss key aspects of diagnosis and management, update the research, and provide more emphasis on management for the population with diabetes, the TASC group reconvened and updated the guideline in 2007 (TASC II system) [6]. TASC II system has graphically presented and thus is more easily and uniformly applied. Classifications of aortoiliac lesions and femoral-popliteal lesions are summarized in Figs. 3.2 and 3.3, respectively.

Endovascular therapy is the treatment of choice for type A lesions, and surgery is the treatment of choice for type D lesions. Endovascular treatment is the preferred treatment for type B lesions, and surgery is the preferred treatment for good-risk type C lesions. The patient's comorbidities, the fully informed patient preference, and the local operators' long-term success rates must be considered when making treatment recommendations for TASC B and C lesions.

© Springer International Publishing Switzerland 2017
R.S. Dieter et al. (eds.), *Critical Limb Ischemia*, DOI 10.1007/978-3-319-31991-9_3

Angiosomes of the lower extremity

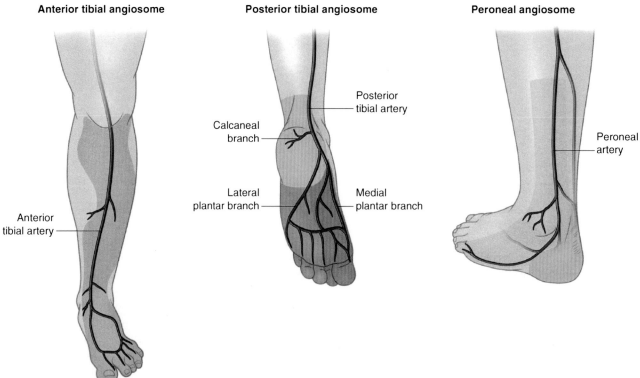

Fig. 3.1 Angiosome defined by arterial supply

Symptom Classifications

Critical limb ischemia (CLI) is a manifestation of peripheral artery disease that describes patients with typical chronic ischemic pain [6]. The Rutherford and Fontaine symptom classification systems are the most widely used [7, 8]. The walking distance that defines mild, moderate, and severe claudication is not specified in the Rutherford classification but is part of the Fontaine classification.

Rutherford Classification

Grade 0	Category 0: Asymptomatic
	Category 1: Mild claudication
Grade I	Category 2: Moderate Claudication
	Category 3: Severe Claudication
Grade II	Category 4: Rest pain
Grade III	Category 5: Ischemic ulceration not exceeding ulcer of the digits of the foot
	Category 6: Severe ischemic ulcers or frank gangrene

Fontaine Classification

| Stage 1: No symptoms |
| Stage 2: Intermittent claudication subdivided into: |
| Stage 2a: Claudication at a distance greater than 200 m |
| Stage 3b: Claudication at a distance less than 200 m |
| Stage 3: Nocturnal and/or rest pain |
| Stage 4: Tissue necrosis and/or gangrene in the limb |

Wound, Ischemia, and Foot Infection (WIfI) Classification

Rutherford and Fontaine classifications are based on symptom severity from perfusion. However, perfusion is only one determinant of outcome. Wound extent and the presence and severity of infection also greatly impact the threat to a limb. Therefore, a new classification was implemented by the Society for Vascular Surgery Lower Extremity Guidelines Committee [9]. The estimated risk of amputation of each stage is summarized in Fig. 3.4.

Type A lesions

- Unilateral or bilateral stenoses of CIA
- Unilateral or bilateral single short (≤3 cm) stenosis of EIA

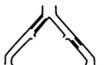

Type B lesions:

- Short (≤3cm) stenosis of infrarenal aorta
- Unilateral CIA occlusion
- Single or multiple stenosis totaling 3–10 cm involving the EIA not extending into the CFA
- Unilateral EIA occlusion not involving the origins of internal iliac or CFA

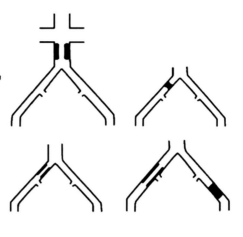

Type C lesions

- Bilateral CIA occlusions
- Bilateral EIA stenoses 3–10 cm long not extending into the CFA
- Unilateral EIA stenosis extending into the CFA
- Unilateral EIA occlusion that involves the origins of internal iliac and/or CFA
- Heavily calcified unilateral EIA occlusion with or without involvement of origins of internal iliac and/or CFA

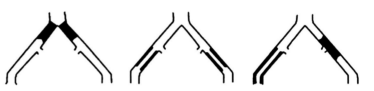

Type D lesions

- Infra-renal aortoiliac occlusion
- Diffuse disease involving the aorta and both iliac arteries requiring treatment
- Diffuse multiple stenoses involving the unilateral CIA, EIA, and CFA
- Unilateral occlusions of both CIA and EIA
- Bilateral occlusions of EIA
- Iliac stenoses in patients with AAA requiring treatment and not amenable to endograft placement or other lesions requiring open aortic or iliac surgery

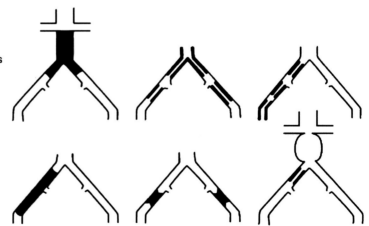

Fig. 3.2 TASC classification of aortoiliac lesions. *CIA* common iliac artery, *EIA* external iliac artery, *CFA* common femoral artery, *AAA* abdominal aortic aneurysm. From Norgren et al. Inter-Society Consensus for the Management of Peripheral Arterial Disease (TASC II). Journal of Vascular surgery 45:1 Supplement 2007. With permission from Elsevier Science and Technology Journals

Type A lesions

- Single stenosis ≤10 cm in length
- Single occlusion ≤5 cm in length

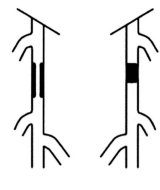

Type B lesions:

- Multiple lesions (stenoses or occlusions), each ≤5 cm
- Single stenosis or occlusion ≤15 cm not involving the infrageniculate popliteal artery
- Single or multiple lesions in the absence of continuous tibial vessels to improve inflow for a distal bypass
- Heavily calcified occlusion ≤5 cm in length
- Single popliteal stenosis

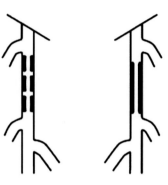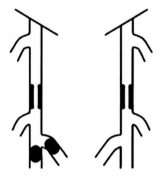

Type C lesions

- Multiple stenoses or occlusions totaling >15 cm with or without heavy calcification
- Recurrent stenoses or occlusions that need treatment after two endovascular interventions

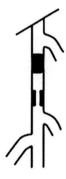

Type D lesions

- Chronic total occlusions of CFA or SFA (>20 cm, involving the popliteal artery)
- Chronic total occlusion of popliteal artery and proximal trifurcation vessels

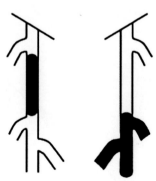

Fig. 3.3 TASC classification of femoral-popliteal lesions. *CFA* common femoral artery, *SFA* superficial femoral artery. From Norgren et al. Inter-Society Consensus for the Management of Peripheral Arterial Disease (TASC II). Journal of Vascular surgery 45:1 Supplement 2007. With permission from Elsevier Science and Technology Journals. For the tibial lesions, the unshaded region is the target stenosis/occlusion. The artery within the shaded rectangle is the associated, "background," disease. Permission granted from Wiley

TASC A lesions

Single focal stenosis, ≤5 cm in length, in the target tibial artery with occlusion or stenosis of similar or worse severity in the other tibial arteries.

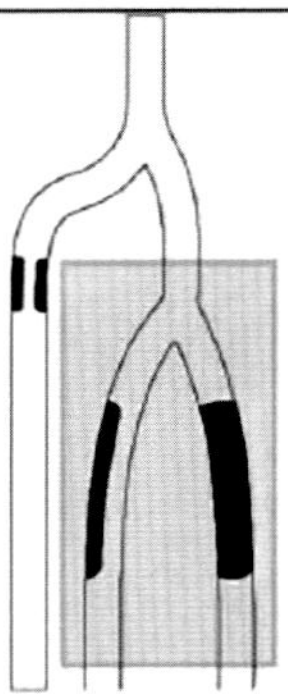

TASC B lesions

Multiple stenoses, each ≤5 cm in length, or total length ≤10 cm or single occlusion ≤3 cm in length, in the target tibial artery with occlusion or stenosis of similar or worse severity in the other tibial arteries.

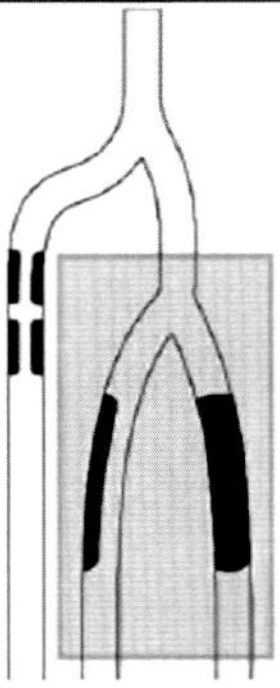

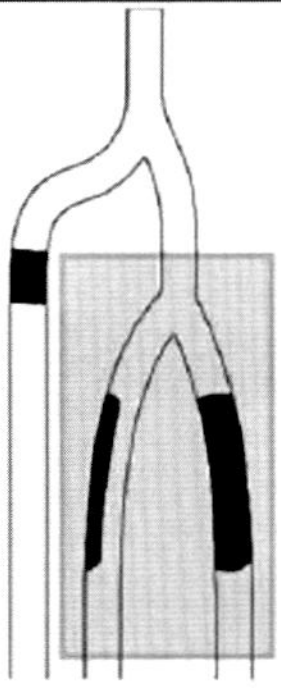

TASC C lesions

Multiple stenoses in the target tibial artery and/or single occlusion with total lesion length >10 cm with occlusion or stenosis of similar or worse severity in the other tibial arteries.

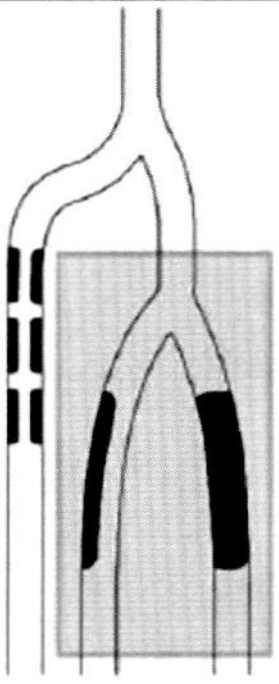

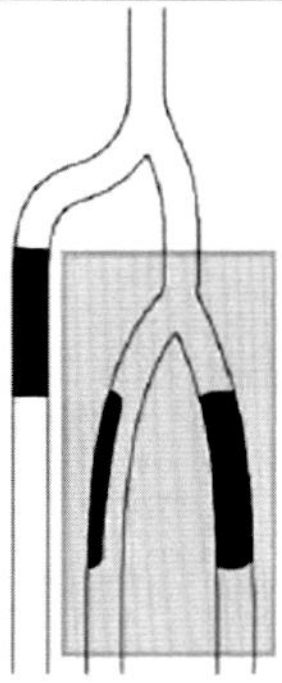

TASC D lesions

Multiple occlusions involving the target tibial artery with total lesion length >10 cm or dense lesion calcification or non-visualization of collaterals. The other tibial arteries occluded or dense calcification.

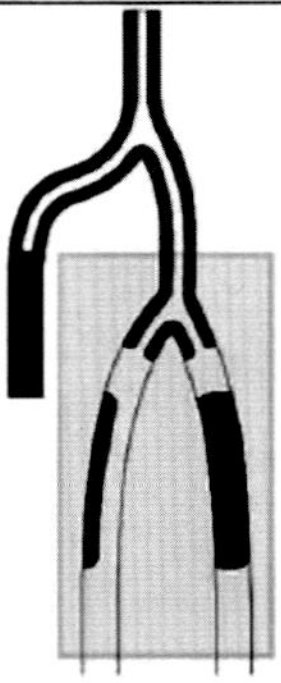

Fig. 3.3 (continued)

a, Estimate risk of amputation at 1 year for each combination

	Ischemia – 0				Ischemia – 1				Ischemia – 2				Ischemia – 3			
W-0	VL	VL	L	M	VL	L	M	H	L	L	M	H	L	M	M	H
W-1	VL	VL	L	M	VL	L	M	H	L	M	H	H	H	M	M	H
W-2	L	L	M	H	M	M	H	H	M	H	H	H	H	H	H	H
W-3	M	M	H	H	H	H	H	H	H	H	H	H	H	H	H	H
	fI-0	fI-1	fI-2	fI-3	fI-0	fI-1	fI-2	fI-3	fI-0	fI-1	fI-2	fI-3	fI-0	fI-1	fI-2	fI-3

b, Estimate likelihood of benefit of/requirement for revascularization (assuming infection can be controlled first)

	Ischemia – 0				Ischemia – 1				Ischemia – 2				Ischemia – 3			
W-0	VL	VL	VL	VL	VL	L	L	M	L	L	M	M	M	H	H	H
W-1	VL	VL	VL	VL	L	M	M	M	M	H	H	H	H	H	H	H
W-2	VL	VL	VL	VL	M	M	H	H	H	H	H	H	H	H	H	H
W-3	VL	VL	VL	VL	M	M	M	H	H	H	H	H	H	H	H	H
	f-0	fI-1	fI-2	fI-3	fI-0	fI-1	fI-2	fI-3	fI-0	fI-1	fI-2	fI-3	fI-0	fI-1	fI-2	fI-3

fI, foot Infection; I, Ischemia; W, Wound.

Premises:

1. Increase in wound class increases risk of amputation (based on PEDIS, UT, and other wound classification systems)
2. PAD and infection are synergistic (Eurodiale); infected wound + PAD increases likelihood revascularization will be needed to heal wound
3. Infection 3 category (systemic/metabolic instability): moderate to high-risk of amputation regardless of other factors (validated IDSA guidelines)

Four classes: for each box, group combination into one of these four classes

Very low = VL = clinical stage 1
Low = L = clinical stage 2
Moderate = M = clinical stage 3
High = H = clinical stage 4

Clinical stage 5 would signify an unsalvageable foot

Fig. 3.4 Risk/benefit: clinical stages by expert consensus. *IDSA* Infectious Diseases Society of America, *PAD* peripheral artery disease, *PEDIS* perfusion, extent/size, depth/tissue loss, infection, sensation, *UT* University of Texas. From Mills et al. Society for Vascular Surgery Document J. Vasc Surg 2014;59:220–34. With permission from Elsevier Science and Technology Journals

Wound

Grade 0: Rest pain; no wound, no ulcer, no gangrene
Grade 1: Small shallow ulcer(s) on the distal leg or foot, any exposed bone is only limited to distal phalanx (i.e., minor tissue loss: limb salvage possible with simple digital amputation [one or two digits] or skin coverage)
Grade 2: Deeper ulcer on distal leg or foot with exposed bone, joint, or tendon or shallow heel ulcer without involvement of the calcaneus (i.e., major tissue loss: salvageable with >3 digital amputations or standard transmetatarsal amputation plus skin coverage)
Grade 3: Extensive deep ulcer of the forefoot and/or midfoot or full-thickness heel ulcer with or without involvement of the calcaneus (i.e., extensive tissue loss: salvageable only with complex foot reconstruction or nontraditional TMA [e.g., Chopart or Lifranc amputation])

Ischemia

Grade 0: $ABI \geq 0.8$, ankle systolic pressure > 100 mmHg, toe pressure (TP)/transcutaneous oxygen ($TcPO_2$) ≥ 60
Grade 1: ABI 0.6–0.79, ankle systolic pressure 70–100 mmHg, $TP/TcPO_2$ 40–59
Grade 2: ABI 0.4–0.59, ankle systolic pressure 50–70 mmHg, $TP/TcPO_2$ 30–49
Grade 3: $ABI \leq 0.39$, ankle systolic pressure <50 mmHg, $TP/TcPO_2 < 30$

Foot Infection

Grade 0: No symptoms or signs of infection
Grade 1: Infection is present and at least two of the following are present: local swelling or induration, erythema >0.5 to ≤ 2 cm around ulcer, local tenderness or pain, local warmth, or purulent discharge. Other causes of inflammatory response of the skin have been excluded
Grade 2: Local infection is present as defined for Grade 1, but extends >2 cm around ulcer, or involves the structures deeper than the skin and subcutaneous tissues (e.g., abscess, osteomyelitis, septic arthritis, fasciitis). No clinical signs of systemic inflammatory response
Grade 3: Local infection is present as defined for Grade 2, but clinical signs of systemic inflammatory response are present as manifested by two or more of the following: temperature >38 °C or <36 °C; heart rate >90 beats per minute, respiratory rate >20 breaths per minute or $PaCO2 < 32$ mmHg; white blood cell count >12,000 or <4000 (cu/mm) or >10 % immature band forms present

Wagner Ulcer Classification System

Grade 1: Superficial diabetic ulcer
Grade 2: Ulcer extension involving the ligament, tendon, joint capsule, or fascia with no abscess or osteomyelitis
Grade 3: Deep ulcer with abscess or osteomyelitis
Grade 4: Gangrene to the portion of the forefoot
Grade 5: Extensive gangrene of the foot

Peripheral Academic Research Consortium (PARC) Classification

The goal of the PARC group was to develop standardized definitions for patients with lower extremity PAD allowing for clinical characterization and evaluation of therapies on the basis of imaging or clinical outcomes [10]. The Fontaine and Rutherford classifications were modified to use descriptive, rather than numeric, terms to classify the severity of PAD limb symptoms (Table 3.1). The limitation of current Rutherford classification system in part was felt to be due to the changing demographics of critical limb ischemia (CLI) patients with increased rates of diabetes and renal disease. PARC has also presented hemodynamic definition for CLI patients in the same article (Table 3.2).

ORC Classification

Finally, in an effort to combine anatomy, physiology, and patient comorbidities, the "ORC" scheme, initially proposed by Dr. Raymond Dieter, Jr. for oncological surgery: "O" is for operability (from a physiological stress standpoint (including renal function), which is best for patient—open surgery or endovascular therapy); "R" is for resectability, but here it would indicate the ability to revascularize either with open bypass (conduits/distal, vasculature/infection, etc.) or perform endovascular therapy; and "C" is for curability (if the patient has life-threatening gangrene or an ulceration that ultimately will never heal, then amputation rather than revascularization may be preferred). Table 3.3 summarizes ORC classification modified for CLI treatment.

Table 3.1 Proposed clinical symptom classification by PARC group

Fontaine classification					Rutherford classification		
Stage	Symptoms	<-->	Proposed PARC universal data elements	<-->	Grade	Category	Symptoms
I	Asymptomatic				0	0	Asymptomatic
II	Intermittent claudication/ other exertional limb symptoms		Mild claudication/limb symptoms (no limitation in walking)	<-->	0	1	Mild claudication
IIa		<-->	Moderate claudication/limb symptoms (able to walk without stopping >2 blocks or 200 m or 4 min)		1	2	Moderate claudication
IIb			Severe claudication/limb symptoms (only able to walk without stopping <2 blocks or 200 m or 4 min)	<-->	1	3	Severe claudication
III	Ischemic rest pain	<-->	Ischemic rest pain (pain in the distal limb at rest felt to be due to limited arterial perfusion)	<-->	II	4	Ischemic rest pain
IV	Ulceration or gangrene	<-->	Ischemic ulcers on distal leg	<-->	III	5	Ischemic ulceration
			Ischemic gangrene		III	6	Ischemic gangrene

Adapted from Patel et al. JACC 2015;65:931–41

Table 3.2 Hemodynamic definitions of critical limb ischemia

Patients with tissue loss	Patients with ischemic rest pain
Ankle pressure <80 mmHg	Ankle pressure <50 mmHg
Toe pressure <50 mmHg	Toe pressure <30 mmHg
$TcPO_2 < 40$ mmHg	$TcPO_2 < 20$ mmHg
Skin perfusion pressure <40 mmHg	Skin perfusion pressure <30 mmHg (23)

The PARC group provided hemodynamic support for the definition of CLI. Atypical leg symptoms are symptoms that are worsened by exertion but that do not meet the classic definition of intermittent claudication. These patients should have objective/confirmed evidence of PAD by noninvasive testing

CLI critical limb ischemia, *PAD* peripheral arterial disease, *PARC* Peripheral Academic Research Consortium, *TcPO2* transcutaneous oxygen pressure

Adapted from Patel et al. JACC 2015;65:931–41

Table 3.3 ORC classifications modified for CLI treatment

"O"—operability	Is the patient an acceptable candidate for either endovascular or open surgical repair
"R"—resectability	Revascularization—is there a distal target for bypass; is endovascular lesion crossing possible/trentable
"C"—curability	Will healing occur after revascularization, or are there significant comorbid conditions (e.g., infection, edema, immobility, etc.) that preclude healing

Modified from Dr. Ray Dieter's surgical oncology scheme [11]

References

1. Mustapha JA, Saab F, Diaz-Sandoval L, et al. Comparison between angiographic and arterial duplex ultrasound assessment of tibial arteries in patients with peripheral arterial disease: on behalf of the joint endovascular and non-invasive assessment of LImb perfusion (JENALI) group. J Invasive Cardiol. 2013;25:606–11.
2. Attinger CE, Evans KK, Bulan E, Blume P, Cooper P. Angiosomes of the foot and ankle and clinical implications for limb salvage: reconstruction, incisions, and revascularization. Plast Reconstr Surg. 2006;117:261S–93S.
3. Taylor GI, Pan WR. Angiosomes of the leg: anatomic study and clinical implications. Plast Reconstr Surg. 1998;102:599–616. discussion 617-8.
4. Shishehbor MH. Acute and critical limb ischemia: when time is limb. Cleve Clin J Med. 2014;81:209–16.
5. Management of peripheral arterial disease (PAD). TransAtlantic inter-society consensus (TASC). Eur J Vasc Endovasc Surg. 2000;19 Suppl A:Si–xxviii, S1–250.
6. Norgren L, Hiatt WR, Dormandy JA, et al. Inter-Society Consensus for the Management of Peripheral Arterial Disease (TASC II). J Vasc Surg. 2007;45(Suppl S):S5–67.
7. Rutherford RB, Baker JD, Ernst C, et al. Recommended standards for reports dealing with lower extremity ischemia: revised version. J Vasc Surg. 1997;26:517–38.
8. Fontaine R, Kim M, Kieny R. Surgical treatment of peripheral circulation disorders. Helv Chir Acta. 1954;21:499–533.
9. Mills JL Sr., Conte MS, Armstrong DG, et al. The society for vascular surgery lower extremity threatened limb classification system: risk stratification based on wound, ischemia, and foot infection (WIfI). J Vasc Surg. 2014;59:220-34.e1-2.
10. Patel MR, Conte MS, Cutlip DE, et al. Evaluation and treatment of patients with lower extremity peripheral artery disease: consensus definitions from peripheral academic research consortium (PARC). J Am Coll Cardiol. 2015;65:931–41.
11. Dieter Jr RA, Kuzycz GK, Dieter III RA, Dieter RS. The ORC patient/tumor classification – a new approach: a new challenge with special consideration for the lung. J Cancer Ther. 2011;2(2):172–5.

Pathologic Aspects of Ischemic Limb Disease

4

Arno A. Roscher, Raymond A. Dieter, Jr., and Beth L. Johnson

Introduction

The title ischemic limb disease affects both the upper but, in general, predominately the lower extremities. This disease entity is very multifactorial and in many of its diagnostic subsections can be very challenging. The principal diagnostic classifications include occlusive arteriosclerotic disease, with secondary thrombosis or embolism, effecting about 85 % of the cases in this category—as illustrated in Table. 4.1 [1, 2]. Miscellaneous ischemic etiologies comprise the remainder of the 15 % of clinical cases. The embolic cases, including the thrombus and tumor emboli, represent a variety of unrelated but nevertheless equally destructive clinical outcomes [3, 4]. More uncommonly, in massive trauma and extremity fractures, the rare fat and marrow embolism may be associated with extensive ischemia. Vascular dissection of major arterial channels is definitely associated with ischemic damage to distally normally perfused extremities and organs [2, 5]. Consequences of fluid, specifically amniotic fluid embolism, are significant but rarer.

Both central and peripheral ischemic vascular limb disease have been studied extensively. Figures 4.1, 4.2 and 4.3 demonstrate the underlying vascular process seen in many of these ischemic legs. An early radiologically and pathologically correlated study of the disease concepts in the study of the aortic arch and brachiocephalic vessels was presented in Tokyo in 1969 [3]. The vascular lesions were appropriately documented in a graphic design. The study was histopathologically amplified by detailed microphotographs of the classical features of occlusive atherosclerosis, gamut of cholesterol granulomas, old and recent thrombosis, as well as gitter cells (macrophages seen in brain infarcts) in the brain. Further, denoted were white versus hemorrhagic infarcts, a rare but debilitating and sometimes fatal complication of carotid endarterectomy [6]. Also of note, in relation to complications of management of atherosclerotic vessel disease is the rare but nevertheless significant occurrence of atherosclerotic embolization to distal organs, such as

A.A. Roscher, MD
Surgical Pathology and Laboratory Medicine,
Keck School of Medicine (Ret), University
of Southern California (USC), Chatsworth, CA, USA

R.A. Dieter, Jr., MD, MS (✉)
Northwestern Medicine, At Central DuPage Hospital,
Winfield, IL, USA

International College of Surgeons, Cardiothoracic
and Vascular Surgery, Glen Ellyn, IL, USA

B.L. Johnson, MD
Northwestern Medicine, At Central DuPage Hospital,
Winfield, IL, USA

Table 4.1 Pathologic considerations of critical ischemia of the extremities

Occlusive arteriosclerotic disease
Majority of patients
Embolic
Tumor
Thrombus
Fat
Marrow
Amniotic
Foreign body
Vascular dissection
Surgery
Aneurysms with clots
Raynaud's
Primary
Secondary
Other associated diseases
Buerger's/thromboangiitis obliterans (TOA)
Behcet's disease/Marco Polo disease
Coagulation defects

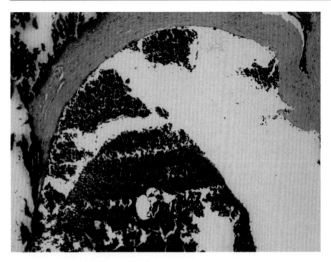

Fig. 4.1 Artery with calcified media and thrombus in patient who required a below-knee amputation for ischemia and gangrene

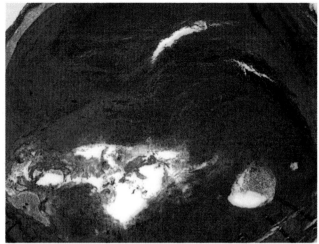

Fig. 4.3 Photomicrograph of luminal thrombus from the right femoral artery

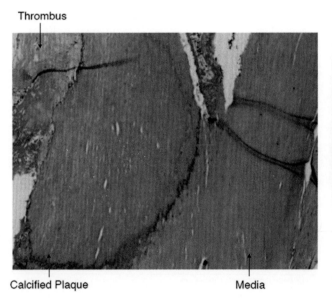

Fig. 4.2 Right femoral artery, plaque and thrombus

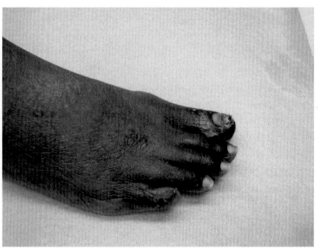

Fig. 4.4 Atherosclerotic gangrene necessitating amputation

the liver, spleen, kidneys, and extremities, especially during vascular surgery. The following paragraphs depict and mention a variety of pathological entities, which amplify the diversity of causes responsible for ischemic limb diseases, as discussed and presented in photographic form by Endlich and Roscher [4].

Many times the pathologist is the final physician to see the extremity with severe ischemic concerns. When the pathologist receives the amputated digit or extremity, the patient's options have been exhausted from the clinical and pathologic aspects in most circumstances. Despite recent advances in both diagnostic and therapeutic approaches, many patients face the consideration of amputation each year. Arteriosclerotic vascular changes with the resultant loss of the leg are illustrated in amputation specimens (Fig. 4.4). Multiple experimental and clinical programs and

products have been developed, applied, and studied with improvement but not prevention. Thus, new multicenter programs to involve multi-specialty and various conceptual programs have been initiated with multi-specialty representation to hopefully reduce and minimize the amputation rate. The etiology and variety of ischemic producing diseases are multiple, and a few of the less common such nonatherosclerotic causes of ischemic pathology are herein listed.

Raynaud's Disease

Pathological entities, such as Raynaud's disease, affecting primarily the upper extremities may lead to poor distal perfusion and remains poorly understood. The disease is clinically characterized by hypersensitivity of the skin to cold items such as cold dinnerware to the affected limb (i.e., hand or arm) and leading to vascular spasm and ischemia. Primary Raynaud's has a 75 % predilection for female patients with the 15–40 age group predominating. In this entity, there usually is no vascular pathologic damage demonstrable. Primary Raynaud's disease (white skin disease) due to the release of norepinephrine produces muscular vessel spasm and temporary limb ischemia. However, in secondary Raynaud's disease, there is an association with other diseases such as mono- and polymyositis, dermatomyositis, scleroderma, lupus, rheumatoid arthritis, and carpal tunnel syndrome. Sjogren's syndrome has also been reported to occur in patients with secondary Raynaud's disease. In the secondary form of Raynaud's, there is a 25 % incidence of a family history predilection. This implies a genetic causation for Raynaud's disease. Causative factors postulated to elicit Raynaud's symptoms include a variety of unrelated entities such as stress, cold remedies, beta blockers, and exposure to cancer chemotherapy. A very unusual example of a patient with a long history of the Raynaud's phenomenon is seen in Figs. 4.5, 4.6, 4.7, and 4.8.

Buerger's Disease

Buerger's disease (thromboangiitis obliterans, TOA) is a significant cause of distal limb disease involving primarily the fingers and toes and also involves predominately the age group of 20–40 year old patients. Although rare now in the Western industrialized world and the USA, it is still frequent in Asian countries, such as India, China, and many other Eastern Asian countries, including Indonesia, Thailand, Vietnam, Cambodia, and Taiwan as well as other developing and evolving industrialized countries of South America and Africa.

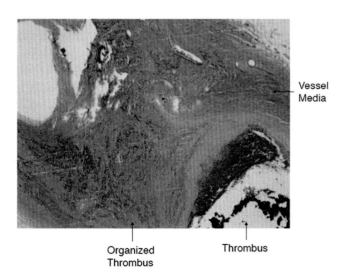

Fig. 4.5 Photomicrograph of a right ulnar artery, with thrombosis and a history of Raynaud's phenomenon

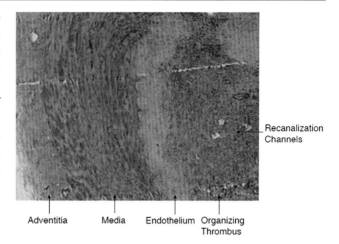

Fig. 4.6 Right ulnar artery, thrombus, and recanalization in a patient with a long history of Raynaud's phenomenon. Vessels forming in the media, the thrombus, and recanalization channels

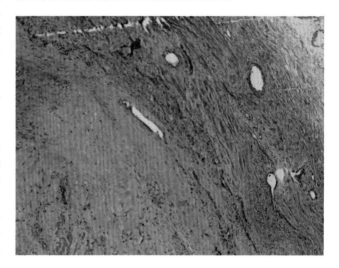

Fig. 4.7 Section of the right ulnar artery in a patient with a history of Raynaud's phenomenon showing organized thrombosis and recanalization channels. Vessels forming in both the media and the thrombus

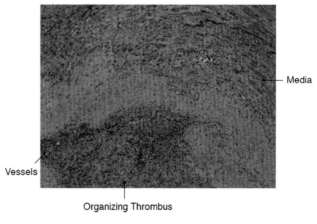

Fig. 4.8 Photomicrograph of section of right ulnar artery in a patient with a long history of Raynaud's phenomenon showing thrombosis and recanalization. Vessels showing thrombosis, organizing thrombus, and recanalization

Initially, Buerger's disease was frequently reported, as early as 1908, in the USA and Western Europe, where the disease has markedly declined over the ensuing decades and yet has shown an increased incidence in the Orient, Asia Minor, India, China, Indonesia, Korea, Japan, and the Philippines [7]. The pathogenesis of the disease remains unclassified. Acceptance as a specific disease entity has been disputed, and therefore the process has also been referred to as "Buerger's syndrome" (not to be confused with Berger disease, which is an IgA nephropathy). The clinical manifestations of overt long-standing limb ischemia, manifested by skin ulcerations to overt gangrene of the distal fingers and toes in affected patients, are readily apparent. Supporting the overt clinical damage to the affected distal hand and foot extremities is a variety of classic angiographic findings in the affected extremity vasculature, including the corkscrew appearance, the tree root pattern, and the spider leg features. In earlier stages of ischemic damage to the affected limb or extremities, plethysmography was applied to document the reduced vascular flow with the hopes to possibly forestall further ischemic tissue damage.

Thromboangiitis obliterans (TOA) is an endovasculitis causing a prothrombotic state initiated by inflammation of the lamina interna of the affected artery and/or vein vessel wall [8]. The inflammatory state is usually initiated within the lamina propria. The mechanisms leading to the endovasculitis in affected patients may be multifocal but uniformly have been associated with smoking tobacco products [7]. The patients exhibit an increased sensitivity to intradermally injected tobacco extracts and show an increased sensitivity to collagen fibers types 1 and 3. There is an elevated serum titer of anti-endothelial cell antibody, as well as impaired peripheral endothelium dependent vasorelaxation. They show an increase in HLA A9, HLA 54, and HLA B5—suggesting a genetic component to the disease [9].

In 1947, the incidence of Buerger's disease in the USA was 104 patients per 100,000 population, dropping today to a range of 12–20 per 100,000. Currently, natives of Asia and Eastern Europe, including Ashkenazi Jews, have the highest incidence of thromboangiitis obliterans (TOA). Ninety-four percent of the patients who abstain from smoking avoid amputations of any limbs. In contrast, patients who continue smoking have an 8-year amputation rate as high as 45%—implying a significant cause effect relationship. Of note, King George VI of England had advanced Buerger's disease, for which he had sympathectomy and was advised not to smoke, but he continued to smoke. In 1879, Felix von Winiwarter, an Austrian professor of surgery, was the first to implicate the risk of smoking in Buerger's disease. In 1908, Dr. Buerger was the first to describe the pathologic processes of TAO and describing the histopathologic features [6].

Bechet's Disease

Still not fully diagnosed or understood and presenting with a myriad of apparent unrelated clinical features is Behcet's disease which features uveitis, retinitis, oral stomatitis, vaginal and anal ulcerations, and peripheral ischemia. The disease is frequently seen clinically with hemorrhagic and pyo-urethritis. On account of the complex clinical manifestations, sexually transmitted disease (STD) was always strongly suspected clinically as causative, in particular if there was STD as a verified comorbidity. It is associated with an increased titer of human leukocyte antigen 51 (HLA51) suggesting the disease, but not yet proven, to belong to the autoimmune disease categories.

In addition to the clinical manifestations, there is histopathologic involvement of the micro- and macrovascular system (a vasculitis) associated with thromboembolism. A paper was presented at the 2004 World International College of Surgeons (ICS) Congress on the surgical treatment of 11 cases of abdominal aneurysms appearing in patients diagnosed with Behcet's disease [10]. Hulusi Behcet, a Turkish dermatologist who practiced in Istanbul, Turkey, first described this disorder in 1930 [10]. Behcet's disease is also referred to as Marco Polo and Silk Road disease. Today, the disease, which traveled from Turkey through the Mideast, India, China, and the far Eastern Asian continents, is readily identified in the Korean Peninsula and Japan. So, with some exaggeration, Behcet's disease can justifiably be called a historical 1000 year old disease.

Therapy

Following streptokinase, a new therapy, autologous cell therapy, in ischemic limb disease emerged as a stellar therapy to deliver progenitor cells, stem cells, in angiogenic cell therapy [11, 12]. This process works through growth factor secretion by cultured adipose tissue-derived stromal cells (ADSCs). Growth factors derived through ADSC markedly increases endothelial cell viability, with associated vascular endothelial growth factor (VEGF) secretion as well as hepatocyte growth factor (HGF) secretion. Four weeks after transplantation of ADSC-derived cells, the angiogenic score has shown significant improvement. Doppler laser image procedures (LDI) were utilized to document the increased capillary vascular flow. Using immunohistochemistry techniques, the anti CD31 antibodies were used in the study. However, ADSC injected cells did not respond to CD 31 cells, Von Willebrand factor, as well as alpha anti-smooth muscle-active-positive cells in ischemic tissue.

Coagulation

Historical and up-to-date aspects of the coagulation cascades began in the 1800s. The most pivotal discovery leading to the theory of thromboembolism from the lower extremities was embodied by Virchow's triad: (1) stasis of blood flow, (2) endothelial cell injury, and (3) hypercoagulability. This thesis was evidenced in 1850 by over 90 % of the cases of thromboembolism occurring in bedridden patients. To emphasize and amplify on this stellar discovery of Virchow's triad, a thorough and up-to-date understanding of the coagulation cascade is necessary for today's vascular surgeons.

The two major pathways, the extrinsic and the intrinsic—leading to the formation of the common pathway—will produce tissue thromboplastin with the resultant transformation of the liquid molecule of fibrinogen into fibrin with the ultimate clinical thrombus formation. The extrinsic tissue factor emanates from tissue injury converting factor 7 (proconvertin factor) to 7a (activated proconvertin factor) and platelet factor. The product of this interaction, in association with factor 10 and 10a (Stuart-Prower factor) converts prothrombin to thrombin and finally fibrinogen to fibrin and thrombus formation associated with fibrin-stabilizing factor (#13).

The intrinsic factor mechanism is dependent on the presence of factor 9 (Christmas Factor) conversion to 9a with association of factor 11 and 11a, plasma thromboplastin (an antecedent Factor) and Factor 12 (Hageman factor) resulting in prothrombin and thrombin formation with thrombus as the end product. Both pathways require Von Willebrand factor in association with platelet aggregation and factor 8 (antihemophilic factor) for clinical activation.

Heyde's Syndrome

Of great interest is the clinical Heyde's syndrome of aortic stenosis associated with hemorrhagic episodes in patients with aortic stenosis and Von Willebrand's disease. After repair of the calcific aortic stenosis, the hemorrhagic episodes disappear apparently due to the reduced mechanical degradation of the Von Willebrand factor with the eroded calcific valve surface rather than enzymatic degradation by the catabolic enzyme [Adamts #13]. Of great clinical importance for patients with Von Willebrand's disease is the large glycoprotein molecular size, which for clinical activity, it needs to be broken down by the catabolic enzyme (Adamts #13).

D-Dimer

Importance is given to the D-Dimer test to follow thromboembolism progress, which was initially described in the 1970s but not truly appreciated until the late 1990s. In general, a positive test is confirmative of thromboembolism and/or disseminated intravascular coagulation (DIC) versus a negative test ruling out the aforementioned conditions. For a more clear understanding of the mentioned clinicopathological phenomena in cardiovascular and peripheral ischemic vascular diseases, a summary of the currently used nomenclature in coagulopathies is included. Coagulation factors in today's usage include: (1) fibrinogen, (2) prothrombin, (3) thromboplastin, (4) calcium, (5) proaccelerin, (6) same as 5, (7) proconvertin, (8) antihemophilic factor, (9) Christmas factor, (10) Stuart-Prower factor, (11) plasma thromboplastin antecedent, (12) Hageman factor, and (13) fibrin-stabilizing factor.

Clotting factors and the process continue to be a challenge for physicians in the care of their patients. This is well exemplified by the efforts to predict and prevent the risks of clots in cancer patients. The Khorana risk model for detecting "at-risk" individuals has developed over the past decade as has the operable, resectable, curable (ORC) concept in the diagnosis and treatment of patients with neoplastic processes [13, 14]. Khorana, working at the Cleveland Clinic, investigated a model including two major patient factors, (1) site of malignancy (especially stomach and pancreas) and (2) body mass index (especially 35 kg/m^2 or greater), and three laboratory prechemotherapy results, ((1) leucocyte count over 11,000/mm^3, (2) hemoglobin <10g/dL, and (3) platelet count 350,000 mm^3 or greater). In studying the Khorana concept, others have added the use of D-Dimer as well as soluble p-selection in their quest to predict the risk of untoward thrombosis—especially venous thromboembolism [15].

References

1. Roscher AA, Kato NS, Quan H, Padmanabham M. Intra-atrial myxomas, clinical pathologic correlation based on two case studies, including historical review. J Cardiovasc Surg (Torino). 1996;37(6 suppl 1):131–7.
2. Stamler J. Cardiovascular diseases in the United States. Am J Cardio. 1962;10:319.
3. Endlich HL, Roscher AA. Current concepts in the study of the aortic arch and brachiocephalic vessels: a clinical and pathologic study of 300 cases, including surgical results. Twelfth Int Coll Radio. Tokyo, Japan, October 1969.
4. Endlich HL, Roscher AA. Current concepts in the study of the aortic arch and brachiocephalic bessels: a clinical and pathologic study of 300 cases, including surgical results. Int Surg. 1971;55(1): 32–41.
5. Dimmick DJ, Goho AC, Cauzze-Steinbach LS, Baumgartner I, Stausser E, Voelgelin E, Anderson SE. Imaging appearances of Buerger's disease complications in the upper and lower limbs. Clin Radiol. 2012;67(12):1207–11.
6. Millikan GH. Pathogenesis of transient focal cerebral ischemia. The Lewis A. Conner Memorial Lecture. Circulation. 1965;32: 438–50.
7. Tanaka K. Pathology and pathogenesis of Buerger's disease (TAO). Int J Cardiol. 1998;66:S237–42.

8. Dellalibera-Joiliana R, Joiliana EE, Silva JS, Evora PR. Activation of cytokines corroborates with development of inflammation and autoimmunity within thromboangiitis obliterans in patients. Clin Exp Immunol. 2012;170(1):28–35.

9. Lozarides MK, Georgiadis GS, Pappas TT, Nizolopoulos ES. Diagnostic criteria and treatment of Buerger's disease with review. Int J Low Extrem Wounds. 2006;5(2):89–95.

10. Moon IS. Abdominal aortic aneurysm repair in post kidney transplanted patients: in eleven cases of Bechet's disease. ICS World Congress. Quito, Ecuador. Oct 6–10, 2004 (page 75 of Program Booklet).

11. Goa KL, Henwood JN, Stolz KS, Langley MS, Clissold SP. Intravenous Streptokinase – a reappraisal of its therapeutic use in acute myocardial infarction. Drugs. 1990;39(5):693–719.

12. Nakagami H. Autologous cell therapy in ischemic limb disease. Dept of Gene Science Therapy, Osaka University Graduate School of Medicine. 2. 2 Yamada Osa Suite 565–0871 (Published statement) Japan.

13. Khorana AA, Kuderer NM, Culakova E, Lyman GH, Francis CW. Development and validation of a predictive model for chemotherapy – associated thrombosis. Blood. 2008; 111(10):4902–7.

14. Dieter Jr RA, Kuzycz GK, Dieter III RA, Dieter RS. The ORC patient/tumor classification – a new approach: a new challenge with special consideration for the lung. J Cancer Ther. 2011;2(2): 172–5.

15. Paxyon A. Coag quest: keying into the clot risk of cancer patients. CAP Today. 2015:(1);1–5.

History and Physical Exam of Acute Limb Ischemia

Nancy Panko and Matthew Blecha

Introduction

Acute limb ischemia occurs when there is a sudden arterial occlusion resulting in an abrupt cessation of flow to an extremity. Acute limb ischemia is a surgical emergency mandating urgent extremity revascularization to avoid the need for amputation. The potential sources of acute limb ischemia are:

1. Arterial embolus
2. In situ arterial thrombosis in the setting of advanced chronic arterial occlusive disease
3. Acute occlusion of previous vascular reconstruction
4. Peripheral artery aneurysm with distal embolization or thrombosis
5. Major arterial trauma

The clinical hallmark of acute limb ischemia is the acute onset of extremity pain in conjunction with absent pulses in the affected extremity. The severity of pain symptoms can vary dramatically depending on the etiology of the acute arterial occlusion. Patients who experience acute limb ischemia secondary to an arterial embolism versus patients who experience in situ arterial thrombosis in the setting of chronic arterial occlusive disease can have significantly different clinical presentations.

Clinical Presentation of Acute Limb Ischemia

History and Physical Exam in Acute Limb Ischemia

Occlusive arterial embolism to an otherwise normal arterial bed will nearly universally result in the abrupt onset of severe pain in the affected extremity. These patients lack collateral vessels around the flush occlusion, making the affected limb completely devoid of any arterial flow. The physical exam findings in this state are the presence of bounding "water hammer" pulses proximal to the occlusion and absent pulses distal to the occlusion. The distal extremity will be cool to touch and after 3–4 h may have neurological abnormalities (sensory loss followed by motor loss). The limb is pale with poor capillary refill. The contralateral limb in this situation will typically have normal pulses, unless the patient has underlying peripheral artery occlusive disease (PAD). Revascularization within 6 h is critical to avoid limb loss. Sources of arterial embolism are:

1. Cardiogenic (atrial fibrillation, valvular disease, cardiomyopathy)
2. Paradoxical emboli (venous emboli passing through cardiac septal defect)
3. Aortic or peripheral aneurysm with associated mural thrombus

In situ arterial thrombosis secondary to worsening chronic occlusive disease may present in a more indolent fashion. These patients experience acute primary vessel thrombosis due to either plaque rupture and secondary in situ arterial thrombosis or due to a critically low velocity flow state resulting in intra-arterial thrombosis. While the primary symptom will be limb pain, the acuity may be vaguer than patients with embolism. Physical exam findings will still be a cool, pulseless foot, often with dependent rubor instead of pallor. The contralateral pulse and Doppler exam is typically

N. Panko, MD
Department of Surgery, St. Joseph Hospital, Chicago, IL, USA

M. Blecha, MD (✉)
Section of Vascular Surgery and Endovascular Therapy, University of Chicago Medical Center, Chicago, IL 60657, USA

© Springer International Publishing Switzerland 2017
R.S. Dieter et al. (eds.), *Critical Limb Ischemia*, DOI 10.1007/978-3-319-31991-9_5

abnormal as atherosclerosis affects both limbs. The severity of pain symptoms is inversely proportional to the quality of collateral arterial flow around the occlusion.

ALI affects sensory nerves first. Therefore, loss of sensation is one of the earliest signs of ischemia. Motor nerves are affected next, and muscle weakness should be a clue to more severe disease and/or longer duration of ischemia. The skin and muscle tissue are affected last, making muscle tenderness a very late finding. In early acute ischemia, the skin distal to the affected artery will appear very pale. This can progress to a dusky blue color as capillary venodilation occurs. The skin will appear non-blanching, as the associated vessels are empty. As ischemia progresses capillary disruption occurs, leading to extravasation of blood and mottled appearance. There will be no blush with digital pressure at this point. Once ischemia has reached this stage, the skin is nonviable, and revascularization bears a significant risk of compartment syndrome and acute renal failure. Occasionally, if ALI is secondary to thrombosis, collaterals can develop over the following 6–8 h and a more normal skin color will return.

In patients with ALI secondary to peripheral arterial occlusive disease, the chief complaint may be ischemic rest pain, whereas the patient previously only had claudication. This pain may be worse when the patient is lying flat or with the affected limb elevated. Pain may be alleviated by placing the limb in a dependent position, thus allowing gravity to supplement arterial flow to the limb. Diabetic patients may not complain of pain if they have a coexisting peripheral neuropathy. This subset of patients may instead present with ischemic or gangrenous ulceration.

A complete history is essential in patients presenting with new onset ischemia, as many factors can influence the diagnosis and treatment course. Pain is most often the first symptom and chief complaint in patients with ALI. The severity of symptoms is a clue to the severity of ischemia as well as to the underlying cause; symptoms may range from claudication to severe disabling pain. Severe acute ischemia is typically an easy diagnosis, as patients present with extreme pain as well as loss of strength and sensation. Less severe ischemia can present more subtly and is often confused with musculoskeletal pain or sciatica. Duration of symptoms is a critical element of history. With severe acute ischemia, irreversible muscle necrosis can occur in 6–8 h if untreated. Onset and distribution of symptoms, prior episodes of pain, and previous functional status of the affected limb are also important components of the history. Sensory loss, followed by muscle weakness, and pain are signs of progressive severe ischemia. The history should be conducted in an attempt to determine the cause of ischemia. Therefore, it is important to ask carefully about associated factors, including cardiac disease/events (myocardial infarc-

tion, atrial fibrillation, valvular disease), hypercoagulable pathology (history of previous blood clots or malignancy), and peripheral vascular disease (rest pain, nonhealing ulcers, claudication). The history of previous vascular procedures should be ascertained. Comorbidities such as diabetes mellitus, hyperlipidemia, and hypertension are often present. Tobacco use and family history are also important contributions to the history. It is important to bear in mind that patients may have risk factors for both embolic and thrombotic disease processes; the presence of atherosclerosis cannot rule out an embolic source of ALI. Patients with acute chronic thrombus often have a history of previous intermittent claudication in either leg.

Examination of the affected limb will define the severity of ischemia. The "rule of Ps"—pain, pulse deficit, pallor, poikilothermia, paresthesias, and paralysis—is a guiding tool.

Pain is often the primary complaint and can be chronic to severe. It is important to document the severity, localization, and progression of pain symptoms. Patients with ALI often have diffuse pain throughout the affected limb. Muscle weakness and tenderness, especially in the calf, is an ominous finding. In severe cases, pain can be replaced with paresthesia as sensory nerves become ischemic.

The vascular supply can be roughly approximated by the color of the skin. Pallor is seen in the early stages of ischemia, which then progresses to cyanosis. Sluggish capillary refill is a sign that at least some degree of distal flow is present and that runoff vessels may be patent. The skin may appear mottled at this point. A severely pale limb is a late finding that indicates total ischemia. Figure 5.1 represents an acutely ischemic limb before and after revascularization.

The limb will be cool to the touch as a result of loss of distal flow. This temperature change is secondary to vasoconstriction and plays a role in the propagation of the ischemic cascade. Coolness is usually present one level below the occluded artery and should be documented at presentation to help determine progression.

Neurologic findings will also help guide classification of ischemia. Loss of sensation is a relatively early sign; be sure to test specifically for loss of fine touch and proprioception, as these small fibers is the most susceptible to ischemic changes. The first dorsal web space of the foot is often the first area to become affected.

Paralysis is an indication of limb threatening ischemia. It is important to determine the extent of paralysis; loss of dorsiflexion and plantar flexion points to a more proximal level of occlusion than paralysis of the toes only. There is a reduced chance of functional limb salvage once motor function is severely diminished, highlighting the importance of immediate revascularization in patients with an acutely painful, cold limb.

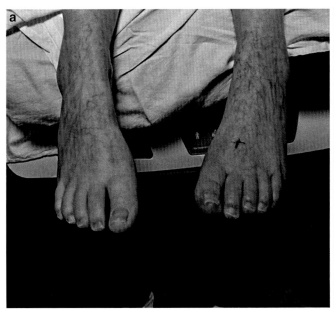 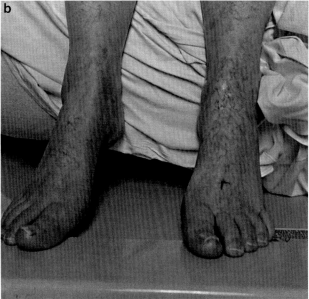

Fig. 5.1 Patient with right acute lower extremity ischemia. (**a**) Note pallor at the patient's right forefoot. Doppler tones are absent on initial exam. (**b**) Illustrating hyperemia after right leg percutaneous revascularization via percutaneous mechanical thrombectomy and thrombolytic therapy

Pulse examination can help determine the level of the occlusion. Typically pulses are present one arterial level above the occlusion; however, early clot can sometimes transduce a weak pulse. Palpable normal pulses in the contralateral limb point toward embolism as the cause of ALI. Bounding water hammer pulses may also present proximal to the level of occlusion after acute embolism, with weakened or absent pulses distally. Pedal arterial signals may be absent or reduced with bedside Doppler exam. The presence of normal triphasic Doppler signals at the pedal level largely excludes the diagnosis of ALI. Soft monophasic signals may be associated with patent distal vessels but proximal occlusion. Absent Doppler signal at the ankle is a poor prognostic sign; arteries may be patent with negligible flow or may be completely occluded. In patients with severe late ischemia, ankles will be impossible to Doppler secondary not only to lack of flow, but also to tenderness. Ankle pressures of 30–50 are expected in less severe ALI, and ABI of 0.3 is diagnostic of critical ischemia. The Doppler can also be used to measure flow in the extremity veins. Lack of venous signal in the popliteal fossa indicates popliteal venous occlusion, which is a poor prognostic sign.

Clinical Classification of ALI

The Society of Vascular Surgery and the International Society of Cardiovascular Surgery has published guidelines to help guide classification. These standards were modified in 2007 by the Trans-Atlantic Inter-Society Consensus (TASC II), which defines acute ischemia as any sudden decrease in limb perfusion causing a potential threat to limb viability [1]. Categories of ischemia are based on clinical and Doppler findings.

Class I ischemia refers to a viable limb in which there is an absence of pedal rest pain, sensory loss, or muscle weakness. Arterial and venous Doppler tones are present.

Class II ischemia refers to a threatened limb and is subdivided into class IIa and class IIb. Both of these patient groups require intervention; however, the urgency of the intervention can vary based on where ischemia falls on this spectrum. Therefore it is important to distinguish between these two groups. Class IIa is referred to as marginally threatened ischemia. Patients who fall in this category typically have a longer duration before irreversible nerve injury occurs. This category is referred to as subacute critical ischemia. Clinically, category IIa ischemia features minimal sensory loss, no muscle weakness, and faint monophasic or absent pedal Doppler tones.

Class IIb ischemia indicates a limb that is immediately threatened with sensory loss, mild or moderate muscle weakness, and absent pedal Doppler tones. These patients require urgent intervention to prevent irreversible tissue loss and are deemed to have acute critical ischemia. Class IIb is the classic acutely painful, cold limb.

Class III ischemia is severe and irreversible. Clinically it is characterized by profound sensory loss, paralysis with impending major tissue loss or permanent nerve damage. Muscle groups are rigorous, and there is pain with passive movement of the foot. Revascularization incurs a significant chance of rhabdomyolysis and acute renal failure. In these patients, amputation or palliative measures are better choices.

Confirmation of Diagnosis of Acute Limb Ischemia

Emergent arterial imaging is indicated for any patient presenting with acute onset limb pain and absent pulses. Imaging options include duplex ultrasound, CT angiography (CTA), magnetic resonance angiography (MRA), and invasive diagnostic angiogram.

Duplex ultrasound is rapid, can be performed at the bedside, and has near 100 % sensitivity for diagnosing complete arterial occlusion. Ankle-brachial index (ABI) will be near zero for patients with acute limb ischemia. Evaluating aortoiliac inflow and tibial arterial outflow vessels may be suboptimal with duplex alone.

CTA has the benefit of rapid availability, high-quality imaging which allows for precise planning of revascularization. CTA provides imaging of the entire arterial tree from the aortic inflow to the digital level. CTA typically requires 150 mL of iodinated contrast and therefore has to be used with caution in patients with baseline renal insufficiency (GFR <40). For patients with renal insufficiency, aggressive hydration before and following exam with sodium bicarbonate is recommended for CTA or invasive angiography [2].

MRA has a limited role in acute limb ischemia as the exam can be lengthy (45–60 min), is less often available outside regular work hours, and generally has poorer arterial imaging quality to 64 (or greater) slice CTA.

Invasive angiography has the advantage of allowing for simultaneous percutaneous revascularization with both mechanical thrombectomy and thrombolytic therapy.

After revascularization for embolism, patients should undergo echocardiography and aortic imaging after the limb is revascularized to investigate the proximal source of embolus.

Treatment of Acute Limb Ischemia

Before engaging in any revascularization for acute limb ischemia, the treating surgeon should perform a global patient evaluation with confirmation of ambulatory status, relative quality of life, and surgical risk. A 30-day amputation rate of 15 % [3, 4] is discussed with the patient and family.

Once quality arterial imaging has been obtained, urgent revascularization is undertaken with the goal of achieving uninterrupted in-line flow from the aorta to the affected extremity. The goal of revascularization is to achieve non-disrupted in-line flow from the aorta to the affected extremity. Lower extremity revascularization is to have at least one tibial artery patent with angiographic confirmation of outflow onto the foot. In the upper extremity, outflow to the hand via the radial or ulnar artery (ideally both) with filling of the palmar arch is the treatment goal.

If no contraindication to anticoagulation exists, the patient should be given an IV heparin bolus of 100 units per kg followed by IV heparin infusion of 15 units per kg with a goal PTT of 60–80. If a continuous thrombolytic therapy drip is initiated, then heparin dose should be reduced to prevent bleeding complications. This dosing, as well as contraindications to anticoagulation and thrombolytic therapy, is discussed below.

There are two primary treatment options for acute limb ischemia:

1. Percutaneous thrombolytic therapy with adjunctive mechanical thrombectomy
2. Surgical thrombectomy with as needed adjunctive bypass or endarterectomy

Option 1: Endovascular Percutaneous Thrombectomy and Thrombolysis for Acute Limb Ischemia

Arterial access should be achieved proximal to the arterial occlusion. Most commonly, contralateral retrograde common femoral arterial access is achieved followed by angiogram of the aortoiliac system. The primary predictor of success for percutaneous revascularization of acute limb ischemia is successful guidewire crossing through the thrombus burden. If the thrombus burden extends proximally to the aortic bifurcation, then brachial artery access may be necessary to achieve guidewire and catheter passage into the thrombus.

This is followed by catheter and sheath selection of the affected limb's iliac arterial system. Through this, sheath dedicated lower extremity angiography can then be performed. A hydrophilic guidewire with four French supporting catheter can then be used to cross into the arterial thrombus. The guidewire should be passed as distally as possible, then the angiojet catheter (Medrad/Possis) can be passed over the guidewire, activated through the thrombus burden, and the thrombus treated with both TPA bolus of 5 mg and mechanical pulse spray/suctioning with the catheter (Fig. 5.2) [5]. Figure 5.3 illustrates an acute iliac artery embolus treated with percutaneous mechanical thrombectomy. Figure 5.4 displays a patient with in situ thrombosis of the right common femoral, profunda femoral, and femoral-above knee popliteal artery bypass. Occlusion was treated with angiojet percutaneous thrombectomy of the common femoral and arterial bypass with subsequent TPA drip to resolve residual mural thrombus and tibial level thrombus.

For mechanical thrombectomy of the iliac, common femoral, superficial femoral, and popliteal arteries, .035 in. guidewires and six French thrombectomy catheters can be used. When treating tibial thrombus, smaller-caliber .018 in.

Fig. 5.2 Angiojet catheter for percutaneous mechanical thrombectomy. From Rutherford's Vascular Surgery, 7th Edition. Copyright Elsevier (2010). Reprinted with permission

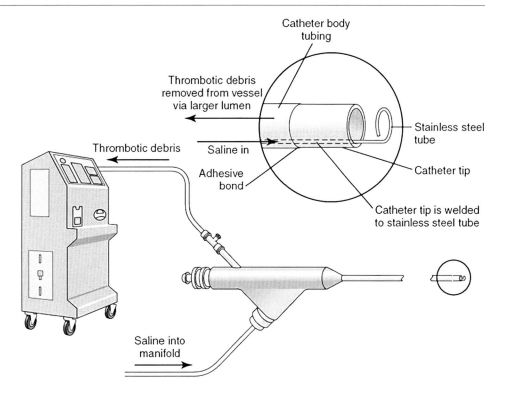

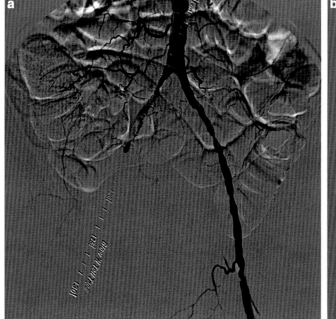

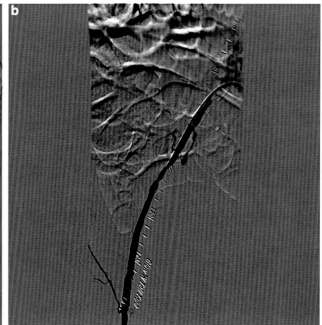

Fig. 5.3 Acute arterial embolus to the right distal common iliac artery seen on the image on the left (**a**). After 5 mg TPA bolus and percutaneous mechanical thrombectomy with angiojet device, successful resolution of the occlusion is seen on the right (**b**). The underlying external iliac stenosis would be subsequently treated with angioplasty

guidewires with three French angiojet thrombectomy catheter are utilized. The mechanical thrombectomy catheters will typically create a flow channel of adequate diameter to reperfuse the limb. Residual thrombus can then be treated as needed with continuous TPA drip of 0.05–0.1 U/kg/h.

Thrombolytic drip is performed through "side hole" infusion catheters invested into the region of thrombus. Moderate-dose IV heparin drip is also administered while patients are receiving TPA infusion. Fibrinogen level, PTT, INR, and hemoglobin should be checked every 6 h while TPA drip is

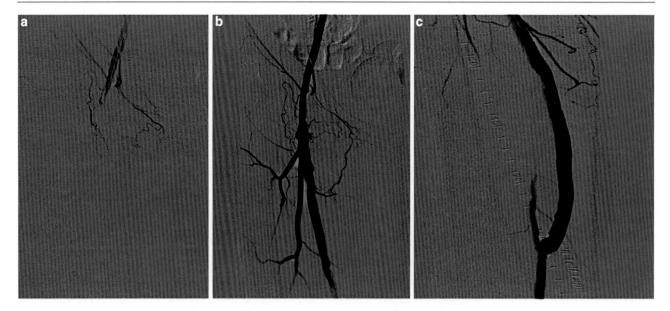

Fig. 5.4 Patient with acute thrombosis of right common femoral artery, profunda femoral artery, and fem-pop bypass. Far left image illustrating complete occlusion (**a**). Middle and right images (**b**, **c**) depicting patent common femoral, profunda femoral, and femoral-popliteal artery bypass after angiojet percutaneous thrombectomy and subsequent thrombolytic therapy (TPA) drip

ongoing. TPA should be held for fibrinogen level below 100 mg/dl and heparinized saline infused through the catheter until the next angiogram should this occur. PTT goal while the TPA drip is ongoing is 30–50 s. Higher levels are associated with increased bleeding risk.

Once follow-up angiography confirms successful lysis of the thrombus burden, any underlying arterial occlusive disease can be identified and treated percutaneously with angioplasty or if necessary surgically with bypass or endarterectomy.

Unlike anticoagulants and antiplatelet medications (heparins, warfarin, thrombin inhibitors, factor Xa inhibitors, ASA, clopidogrel) which serve to prevent thrombus formation, TPA directly induces lysis of fibrin-based clot creating significant bleeding risks for anyone with recent endothelial injury. Contraindications to thrombolytic therapy include [6–8]:

- CVA within 3 months
- Intracranial tumor or other gross pathology
- Intrathoracic, abdominal, pelvic, or thoracic surgery within 3 weeks.
- Major trauma within 3 weeks
- Severe (SBP>180 mmHG) hypertension that cannot be controlled with medication
- Cirrhosis with coagulation abnormality

Acute limb ischemia patients who are not candidates for thrombolytic therapy should undergo emergent surgical revascularization.

Option 2: Open Surgical Thrombectomy with as Needed Adjunctive Revascularization or Thrombolytic Therapy

Treatment of Acute Arterial Embolus

For patients experiencing acute embolus to an otherwise normal arterial tree, surgical embolectomy provides rapid revascularization and is an outstanding treatment option. The recommended exposure sites for acute embolus are based on anatomical location and extent of thrombus burden. Recommended dissection sites are:

- Lower extremity embolus with patent iliac, common femoral, and profunda femoral arteries: Below-knee popliteal artery cutdown with retrograde and antegrade Fogarty balloon thrombectomy. This dissection site allows for selective Fogarty balloon catheter thrombectomy of both the anterior tibial artery and the tibioperoneal trunk.
- Lower extremity embolus with occluded common femoral artery: Common femoral artery cutdown with Fogarty balloon thrombectomy of the iliac, profunda femoral, and distal arteries. Secondary cutdown at the below-knee popliteal artery to expose the origin of the tibial vessels may also be necessary after the inflow thrombectomy if remote thrombectomy does not result in at least one tibial artery being widely patent to the foot.
- Upper extremity embolus: Brachial artery cutdown at the antecubital level just above the bifurcation with control of the proximal radial and ulnar arteries

Muscular fascia should never be closed after surgical thrombectomy due to risk for compartment syndrome. Appropriate Fogarty balloon sizes are No. 5 for iliac and subclavian arteries; No. 4 for femoral, popliteal, and brachial arteries; and No. 3 for tibial, radial, and ulnar arteries. All embolectomy and thrombectomy procedures should be followed by completion angiography with confirmation of in-line flow to the affected distal limb.

If thrombectomy is unsuccessful at the tibial artery level, intraoperative direct intra-arterial distal thrombolytic therapy can be performed. A sheath or catheter can be placed in an antegrade fashion down the proximal arterial system and 5 mg of TPA injected directly into the thrombosed tibial vessel. Ten minutes later, secondary angiogram is performed to evaluate the efficacy of the TPA.

Surgical Treatment of Acute Limb Ischemia in Setting of Chronic Arterial Occlusive Disease

Surgical treatment of acute limb ischemia secondary arterial thrombosis in the setting of coexisting chronic arterial occlusive disease is a far more challenging scenario than acute embolus. It can be difficult to discern based on angiography or CTA which vessels have been occluded for several months and which arteries are acutely occluded. These patients, as mentioned above, may present with more subtle onset of pain. Essentially they are chronic arterial occlusive disease (discussed below) patients who have developed arterial thrombosis and reached a critical threshold of tissue ischemia.

Surgical treatment for these patients is "whatever it takes" to achieve in-line flow to affected extremity. The treatment armamentarium includes thrombectomy, bypass, endarterectomy, thrombolytic therapy, angioplasty, and stenting. Treatment is individualized to patient anatomy. Dissection should be carried out at the level of the most distal inflow artery which has uninterrupted proximal in-line flow. From here, attempts at distal thrombectomy can be made with the understanding that distal outflow vessel exposure, further thrombectomy, and bypass may be necessary based on post thrombectomy angiographic findings. Similarly, based on post thrombectomy imaging, subsequent sheath insertion with angioplasty can be performed if anatomically feasible. Ensuring patency of the profunda femoral artery should always be attempted to potentially prevent limb loss in the event of revascularization failure.

Percutaneous Versus Open Surgical Revascularization in Acute Limb Ischemia

Limb salvage and mortality rates were equivalent in the two largest randomized trials (STILE and TOPAS II trials) comparing surgical thrombectomy to percutaneous thrombolysis

[2, 3]. The endovascular limb in these trials, however, relied on thrombolysis alone without initial percutaneous mechanical thrombectomy. Mechanical thrombectomy achieves rapid revascularization and typically removes over 90 % of the acute thrombus burden within minutes while avoiding the morbidity of open vascular surgery [9]. The author's strong preference is to treat all acute limb ischemia patients (without contraindication to TPA) with percutaneous mechanical thrombectomy and as needed continued percutaneous thrombolytic drip.

Monitoring and Treatment for Post-revascularization Compartment Syndrome and Rhabdomyolysis

Compartment Syndrome

Patients undergoing revascularization for acute limb ischemia are at high risk for calf compartment syndrome. Reperfusion edema and the confined space of the anterior, lateral, and deep/superficial posterior compartments can result in venous compression, worsening edema, and ultimately neurologic ischemia. Risk for compartment syndrome is highest for patients with a lack of collateral vessels (embolus or trauma in a normal arterial tree) and for patients with prolonged ischemia.

The anterior and lateral compartments are the most common first symptomatic distribution, presenting with peroneal nerve distribution sensory deficit on the dorsum of the foot. The most reliable physical exam finding is pain with passive extension of the muscles of the involved compartment.

Any suspicion for compartment syndrome warrants either immediate four-compartment fasciotomy (Fig. 5.5) or measuring of compartment pressures. Any post-revascularization compartment pressure greater than 30 mmHg warrants fasciotomy. In order to avoid permanent neurologic injury, error should always be made on the side of full four-compartment fasciotomy when concerning symptoms or signs of compartment syndrome exist.

Rhabdomyolysis

Patients with prolonged (greater than 6 h) acute limb ischemia are at risk for acute renal tubular necrosis due to recirculation of the necrotic muscle breakdown product myoglobin. Oliguria and discolored (pink or red) urine should raise suspicion for rhabdomyolysis. Diagnosis can be confirmed with urine myoglobin level. Urine microscopy will be negative for RBC but urine dip will be positive for blood. Treatment is IV hydration, diuresis with mannitol, and alkalinization of urine with IV bicarbonate [10]. Urine

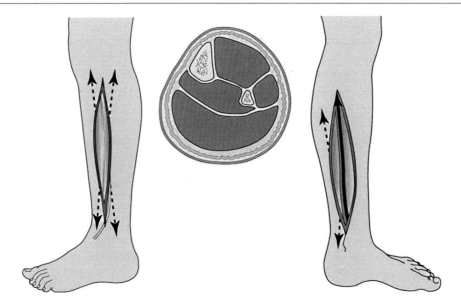

Fig. 5.5 Double-incision (anterolateral and medial) fasciotomy of the lower leg. A longitudinal incision lateral to the tibia and overlying the intermuscular septum is used to visualize the anterior and lateral compartments. Parallel fascial incisions are used to decompress these compartments. A medial incision immediately posterior to the tibia is used to access both posterior compartments. The soleus muscle must be detached from the tibia to decompress the deep posterior compartment. From Janzing H, Broos P, Rommens P. Compartment syndrome as a complication of skin traction in children with femoral fractures. J Trauma. 1996;41:156. Picture and caption from Rutherford's Vascular Surgery, 7th Edition. Page 2418, Copyright Elsevier (2010). Reprinted with permission

myoglobin levels may not be rapidly attainable in many hospitals. Similar to compartment syndrome, it is safest to empirically treat rhabdomyolysis if the diagnosis is in question.

References

1. Norgren L, Hiatt WR, Dormandy JA, Nehler MR, et al. TASC II Working Group. Inter-society consensus for the management of peripheral arterial disease (TASC II). J Vasc Surg. 2007;45:S9A
2. Merten GJ, Burgess WP, Gray LV, et al. Prevention of contrast-induced nephropathy with sodium bicarbonate: a randomized controlled trial. JAMA. 2004;291:2328.
3. The STILE Trial: results of a prospective randomized trial evaluating surgery versus thrombolysis for ischemia of the lower extremity. Ann Surg. 1994;220:251–66
4. Ouriel K, Veith FJ, Sasahara AA. A comparison of recombinant urokinase with vascular surgery as initial treatment for acute arterial occlusion of the legs for the thrombolysis or peripheral arterial surgery (TOPAS) investigators. N Engl J Med. 1998;338:1105–11.
5. Rutherford's Vascular Surgery. Chapter 85, p. 2403. Image 158-1 A. Elsevier, 2010. ISBN: 978-1-4160-5223-4.
6. Campbell WB, Rider BMF, Szymanska TH. Current management of acute leg ischemia: results of audit by the vascular surgical society of great Britain and Ireland. Br J Surg. 1998;85:1498–503.
7. Nypaver TJ, Whyte BR, Endean ED, et al. Nontraumatic lower-extremity acute arterial ischemia. Am J Surg. 1998;176:147–52.
8. Pemberton M, Varty K, Nydahl S, Bell PR. The surgical management of acute limb ischemia due to native vessel occlusion. Eur J Vasc Endovasc Surg. 1999;17:72–6.
9. Kasirajan K, Gray B, Beavers FP, et al. Rheolytic thrombectomy in the management of acute and subacute limb threatening ischemia. J Vasc Interv Radio. 2001;12:413–21.
10. Eneas JF, Schoenfield BY, Humphreys MH. The effect of infusion of mannitol-sodium bicarbonate on the clinical course of myoglobinuria. Arch Int Med. 1979;139:801.

History and Physical Exam of Chronic Critical Limb Ischemia

Rajmony Pannu and Steven M. Dean

Introduction

"Journey of thousand miles begins with a single step" Lao-tzu: 604 BC - 531 BC

History taking and physical examination are the first steps in patient evaluation. This chapter describes in detail the components of the physical exam that are essential in decision making when confronting patients with critical limb ischemia. The methods described can be applied as a stand-alone modality or in conjunction with vascular tests to diagnose and follow up vascular disease. This review will allow an astute clinician to recognize common complaints associated with critical limb ischemia and correctly associate them with the characteristic physical manifestations. Consequently, this highly morbid disease should not go unrecognized.

History

The medical history initiates the physician-patient relationship, guides the uncovering of relevant physical findings, facilitates appropriate vascular testing, and then assists treatment choices. Per one report, a skilled history can lead to the correct diagnosis 75 % of the time [1]. The most common presenting symptom for limb ischemia is pain, and knowing its severity, location, frequency, exacerbating, and/or relieving factors along with the duration assists in distinguishing vascular vs nonvascular leg discomfort.

R. Pannu, MD, RPVI
Vascular & Endovascular Medicine, Columbus Vascular Vein & Wound Center, 895 S State street, Columbus, OH 43081, USA

S.M. Dean, DO, RPVI (✉)
Division of Cardiovascular Medicine, Department of Internal Medicine, The Ohio State University Wexner Medical Center, Columbus, OH 43017, USA

Critical Limb Ischemia

A distinction must be made between chronic critical limb ischemia (cCLI) and acute critical limb ischemia (aCLI). aCLI is a medical emergency related to abrupt arterial occlusion which requires immediate treatment. The pathophysiology of cCLI is related to slowly progressive, inadequate arterial limb perfusion that is below the threshold needed to meet the metabolic demands of the limb, resulting in resting ischemia with pain, skin breakdown, and eventual tissue necrosis [2].

Acute Critical Limb Ischemia

aCLI most commonly occurs due to embolism or in situ thrombosis. Arterial dissection or trauma can also cause aCLI but at a much lower rate. Unfortunately, the presenting symptoms do not predict the cause of aCLI. Patients can present with an asymptomatic loss of pulse, acute deterioration in previously stable claudication or as sudden onset of severe rest pain in the affected limb. These symptoms may develop over several days or over few hours. Acute arterial occlusion may result in any one or all of the notorious five "Ps":

1. Pain
2. Paresthesias
3. Pallor
4. Paralysis
5. Poikilothermia

These manifestations typically occur due to lack of collateral blood flow and reestablishment of primary arterial flow in timely fashion is the key.

The pain in aCLI may be evanescent and pallor may quickly give way to cyanosis. This discomfort is very different than that of cCLI. For instance, it is not localized to the

© Springer International Publishing Switzerland 2017
R.S. Dieter et al. (eds.), *Critical Limb Ischemia*, DOI 10.1007/978-3-319-31991-9_6

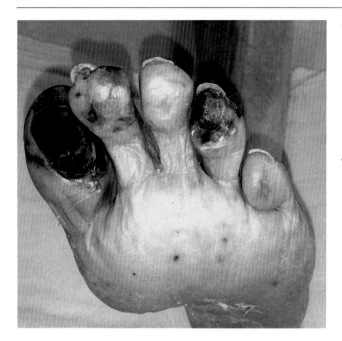

Fig. 6.1 Arterial emboli after endovascular procedure

- Paper grip test: The patient attempts to grip a standard paper sheet between two toes while the physician tries to pull it away. Patient may curl their toes to grip the paper and this action is hypothesized to activate the long extrinsic toe flexors. Therefore, the paper grip test is repeatable but has questionable validity as a measure of intrinsic weakness because is likely to be assessing both intrinsic and extrinsic muscle strength [3].

- Intrinsic positive test: The test involves the participant extending the great toe while simultaneously attempting to flex the lesser toes at the MTP joint and extend the interphalangeal joints. The strength of the intrinsic muscles is determined by the type of lesser toe flexion demonstrated which includes either (1) intrinsic positive pattern, which involves flexion at the MTP joint and extension at the interphalangeal joints, or (2) intrinsic negative pattern, where the participant is unable to actively flex the MTP joint and extend the interphalangeal joints. This test has not been extensively validated and level of strength required to perform the test is unknown [4].

More objective testing can be performed in centers that have access to a handheld dynamometer. This instrument can measure toe flexor strength [5].

The persistence of pain, particularly if followed by numbness and/or weakness suggests the threat of limb loss.

Chronic Critical Limb Ischemia

Inability of the blood flow to meet the functional demands of tissue produces pain that has two very distinct characteristics: intermittent claudication and ischemic rest pain.

Intermittent claudication is discomfort associated with exercise that is relieved by rest. Depending on the anatomical location and extent of arterial occlusive disease, the patient may present with buttock, thigh, and/or calf claudication. Calf claudication is the most common presenting symptom and is reported as cramps in the calf that are brought on by walking. This should not be confused with nocturnal cramps that some elderly people manifest. These cramps have no known vascular origin and are thought to be the result of an exaggerated neuromuscular response to stretching. Chronic exertional compartment syndrome can also produce calf tightness provoked by exercise, but the distinguishing feature is that the patient is usually a younger athlete without atherosclerotic risk factors and large calf muscles. Increased muscle pressure due to impaired venous outflow is usually the cause and this pain is not relieved quickly by rest.

Thigh and buttock claudication is different than calf claudication as the exertional pain is much less pronounced. Instead, patients typically complain of an exertional ache or discomfort that is associated with weakness. Patients might

acral portion of the foot and is not affected by gravity. The pain is usually diffuse and can extend above the ankle in severe cases. It is usually of sudden onset and may quickly increase in intensity when caused by arterial emboli (Fig. 6.1). Patients can describe the feeling as being struck in the limb after which they feel weak. In case of arterial thrombosis, the pain develops less rapidly, but patient is aware of some change in their baseline status. The rapid peak in pain intensity is also absent in arterial thrombosis. However, in the case of *massive* arterial thrombosis where the limb is threatened, the pain quickly and unexpectedly changes in intensity. The pain may subside in intensity after the initial vasospasm subsides and collateral flow is recruited. Finally, the discomfort may completely resolve if the collateral supply is able to meet the functional demands of the foot or it may convert into the pain typically seen in cCLI patients.

Pulses are usually difficult to palpate since the majority of this patient population have preexisting peripheral arterial occlusive disease.

The sensory deficit may be minimal and can easily be missed early in the course of presentation. Patients may lose sensation of light touch, the ability to differentiate two points, and experience altered vibratory perception and proprioception before deep pain ensues. Loss of motor function may present very late in the process as the majority of foot movements are produced by muscles originating below the knee. It can be challenging to test for the motor function of the foot as these muscle groups may not be developed at baseline in many PAD patients. The tests that are generally advocated in evaluating the intrinsic foot muscles are the paper grip test and intrinsic positive test:

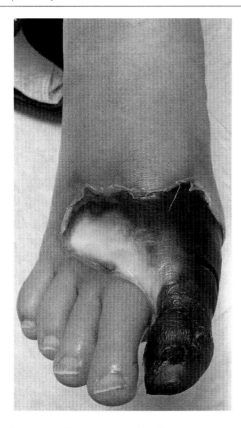

Fig. 6.2 Gangrene of the great toe and forefoot

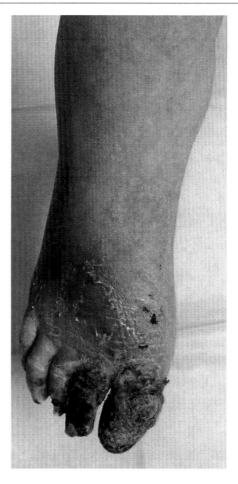

Fig. 6.3 Nonhealing ischemic ulceration

say that their hip or thigh "gives out" or "tires" after they have walked a stereotypical distance. Thigh and buttock claudication may be somewhat similar to the pain of hip osteoarthritis, but the amount of exercise that provokes discomfort in osteoarthritis is variable; the pain does not subside promptly upon cessation of activity, and there is considerable day-to-day pain variability. Neurospinal compression may also cause exertional buttock and thigh pain, but the main differentiating feature from claudication is associated limb numbness and that the symptom complex can also be produced by prolonged standing. Additionally, the pain and numbness of neurospinal compression can also involve the perineum. Affected patients often relate their symptoms are improved with truncal flexion such as when they shop in the supermarket and lean on the shopping cart. However, straightening of the lumbar spine is likely to exacerbate their symptoms. Since patients presenting with lumbar neuroforaminal compression are often elderly, coexistent PAD with claudication can confound the diagnosis and it is paramount that the predominant complaints be matched to the disease. Treating mild arterial occlusive disease in this patient will not relieve their symptoms. Thigh claudication can also be part of the postthrombotic syndrome that usually occurs when the patient has history of ilio-femoral deep vein thrombosis (DVT) and the collateral venous outflow fails to match the increased arterial inflow during exercise. The pain is often described as "bursting" or a severe tightness or heavy

sensation that is relieved by cessation of exercise, but the improvement is not as rapid as in arterial claudication.

Claudication involving the foot is uncommon and can occur independently or in association with calf claudication. Foot claudication is more common in the setting of thromboangiitis obliterans because of the distal distribution of occlusive arterial lesions. Foot claudication secondary to atherosclerotic occlusive disease is frequently associated with ischemic rest pain. There might be reference of acral numbness and/or cold sensation and patients may refer to feeling a "wooden foot." Inflammatory processes of the foot can cause similar focal pain but the variability of the discomfort with exercise that is not quickly relieved by exercise cessation helps differentiate the two (ischemic rest pain is not quickly relieved with exercise). Additionally, non vascular pain may not relate to activity level, may be affected by weight bearing.

cCLI occurs from severely reduced arterial blood flow resulting in ischemic rest pain, nonhealing ischemic ulceration(s), and/or gangrene (Figs. 6.2 and 6.3). The pain is usually located in the acral portion of the leg, toes, or heels, is severe, and is persistent. The feet may be insensitive to cold, the joints could be stiff, and/or patients may suffer from hyperesthesias. Patients note pain relief when feet are

Fig. 6.4 Buerger's sign with dependent rubor and elevation pallor. (**a**) Dependent rubor in critical limb ischemia due to impaired vasoconstriction. (**b**) Elevation pallor in critical limb ischemia

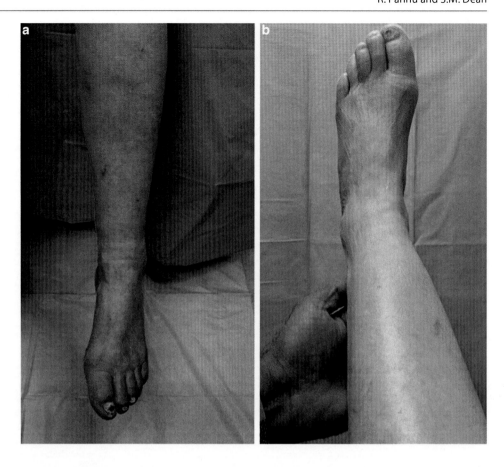

in dependent position and conversely an increase in pain if the feet are at or above the level of heart. Patients will often narrate how they have pain in the feet at night that improves when they hang their feet over the bedside. Thus, they eventually learn to sleep with their feet hanging down or in a chair with their feet dependent. A clinician may be deceived by pedal rubor, but it is important to stress that this "dependent rubor" (Fig. 6.4) is matched by "elevation pallor" (Buerger's sign) which is consistent with severe limb ischemia. Pain may be sharply localized to an ischemic ulcer or gangrenous toe. However, the initial presentation of cCLI may be acute gangrene or a minimally painful wound with associated advanced diabetes mellitus and peripheral neuropathy. It is very important to recognize that this particular patient subset is insensate and may not manifest rest pain. If cCLI is untreated, gangrene may ensue with the eventual loss of the limb (from amputation or mummification) and perhaps life (from sepsis).

Physical Examination

A comprehensive physical exam must include vital signs, including the blood pressure, heart rate, and respiratory rate. The blood pressure should be measured in both arms, with an

appropriately sized blood pressure cuff. The patient's overall appearance should be noted. The vascular examination includes inspection, auscultation of vascular structures, and palpation of axial pulses, and if the distal pedal pulses are not palpable, documentation of same should be completed with a handheld Doppler if available. A systemic approach is advocated and all the body systems should be examined. Examination of the abdomen should include more than palpation for an aortic aneurysm. Lower abdominal bruits may provide the sole clue to arterial occlusive disease in the patient with thigh and buttock claudication as there may be no sign of chronic ischemia and the femoral pulse exam maybe normal at rest. It is outside the scope of this chapter to detail the heart, lung, musculoskeletal, neurological, etc., examinations.

Visual Inspection

The limbs should be inspected carefully, assessing their appearance, symmetry, and color, and for evidence of edema or muscle wasting. Special attention should be given to any areas of discoloration, and if present, the patient should be interrogated about the timeline of discoloration appearance as this may clarify the acuity of presenting symptoms. Subtle

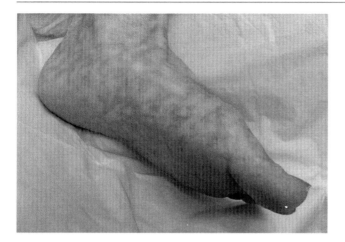

Fig. 6.5 Livedo reticularis is rash resembling fishnet pattern

findings of distal hair loss, trophic skin changes, and hypertrophic nails should be sought and may suggest severe underlying PAD. Patients presenting with lower extremity ulcerations suspected of having critical limb ischemia should be examined for the fishnet-like rash of livedo reticularis (Fig. 6.5). Also, the skin around the ulcerations should be inspected for changes in texture, color, elasticity, etc. It is important to visually inspect the base and margins of any presenting wound. In patients with neuropathy, the plantar foot surface should be inspected for the presence of unknown foreign bodies in the skin.

Arterial ulcers typically occur on the toes, heels, and bony prominences of the foot. They appear "punched out" with well-demarcated edges and a pale, nongranulating, and often necrotic base. The surrounding skin may be cool to touch and can exhibit dusky erythema. Examination of the arterial system demonstrates decreased or absent distal pedal pulses.

In contrast to the arterial ulceration, the majority of the venous leg ulcers develop in the gaiter area of the limb, usually around the malleoli (Fig. 6.6). The ulceration may be circumferential or discrete, and the ulcer bed is often covered with a fibrinous layer mixed with granulation tissue surrounded by irregular margins. Pitting-dependent edema is often present and may predate the ulcer. Extravasation of erythrocytes into the skin occurs, resulting in the deposition of hemosiderin within macrophages, which stimulates melanin production, pigmenting the skin brown.

Pulse Exam

The pulse exam of upper and lower extremities is a critical part of the vascular exam. The exam should be conducted in warm and well-lit room. Asymmetry, decreased intensity, or the absence of pulses suggests arterial occlusive disease and provides clues to the location of disease. There are two

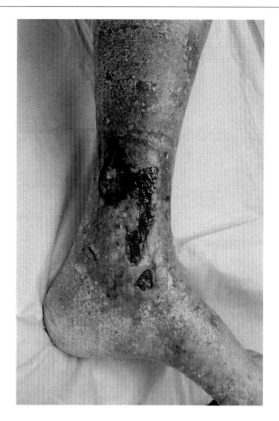

Fig. 6.6 Gaiter area venous ulcer

widely used numeric scales used to grade pulses ranging from 0 (absent) to 4 (aneurysmal). We recommend using a simpler 0 (absent), 1 (diminished), and 2 (normal) scale as there may be a substantial inter-user variability in grading pulses on 0–4 scale [6]. A bounding pulse may suggest aortic valvular insufficiency and an expansive pulse may suggest the presence of an arterial aneurysm.

Pulse exam of the lower extremity includes palpation of the femoral, popliteal, posterior tibial, and dorsalis pedis arteries and the examination should performed with the patient in supine position.

The femoral pulse is located below the inguinal ligament, approximately midway between the iliac spine and symphysis pubis. It may be challenging to palpate this pulse in muscular or obese patients. In order to facilitate femoral pulse detection, the hips should be externally rotated so the artery can be palpated over the pubic ramus of the ilium approximately 1–2 finger breadths lateral to the pubic tubercle where there is less fat.

Palpation of popliteal artery is often difficult and has led to premise that if the popliteal pulse is very easily palpable, it should raise suspicion for an aneurysm. The leg should be straight, slightly flexed at the knee joint. The leg should be relaxed enough that it "falls" on to the examiner's hands. The popliteal pulse is usually palpated with three fingers from each hand and the thumb applying a moderate opposing

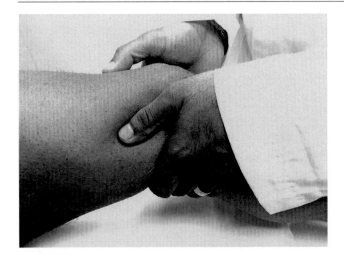

Fig. 6.7 Palpation of popliteal artery

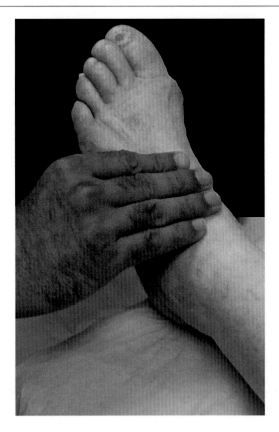

Fig. 6.9 Palpation of dorsalis pedis artery

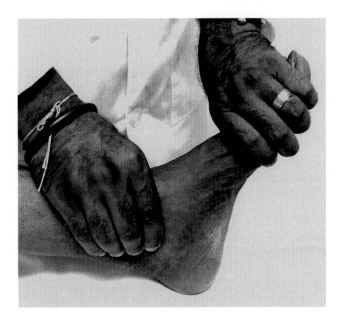

Fig. 6.8 Palpation of posterior tibial artery

force to the top of the knee (Fig. 6.7). The pulse can be felt at the junction of medial and lateral third of the popliteal fossa.

The posterior tibial pulse is located slightly behind the medial malleolus. The examiner should approach the depression behind the malleolus from the lateral side and apply their digits to the lower curvature. Passive dorsiflexion of the foot may aid the palpation of the posterior tibial pulse (Fig. 6.8). The absence of posterior tibial pulse is diagnostic for peripheral arterial disease.

The dorsalis pedis pulse is palpated along the dorsum of the foot between the first and second metatarsal bones. Ideally, arteries should be palpated with the sensitive palmer surface of fingers (Fig. 6.9). The dorsalis pedis artery may be absent in 5–10 % of the population. In such cases, the lateral tibial artery, the terminal branch of peroneal artery should be

sought. This artery can be palpated higher up in the foot, below the lateral ankle, and medial to fibular prominence.

With wide availability of handheld Doppler devices, it is imperative to document the presence of Doppler signals in the pedal arteries that are not palpable. This assumes increased significance in endovascular interventions below the knee and could help determine if pedal vessels could potentially be used as an access for complex interventions. To perform the Doppler exam, a copious amount of gel is applied to the medial malleolus area where the posterior tibial pulse is expected to be found and the Doppler probe is held between the index finger and thumb. It is important to apply minimal pressure with the probe as even slight compression can obliterate flow through a diseased artery (Fig. 6.10). The Doppler flow can be further documented as triphasic, biphasic, or monophasic. Similar maneuvers should be performed on dorsalis pedis artery (Fig. 6.11). Examiners can use the handheld Doppler along the course of dorsalis pedis artery toward the hollow between the first and second phalangeal bones to ascertain the patency of pedal plantar arch. If the dorsalis pedis artery is not audible, place the Doppler probe on the dorsum of the foot between the first and second phalangeal bones to evaluate for the presence of flow within deep plantar artery (Fig. 6.12); subsequently, try to follow its course back to the expected location of dorsalis pedis artery between the first and second metatarsal bones.

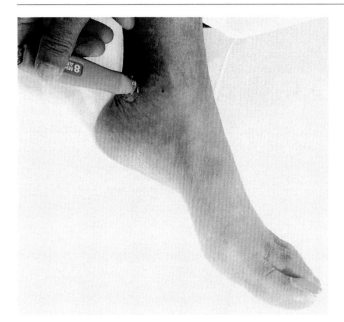

Fig. 6.10 Doppler of posterior tibial artery with liberal gel and slight pressure on the artery

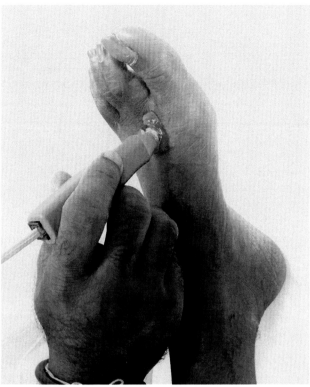

Fig. 6.12 Doppler of deep plantar artery

to intervention. Wounds secondary to thromboangiitis obliterans are not amenable to endovascular interventions.

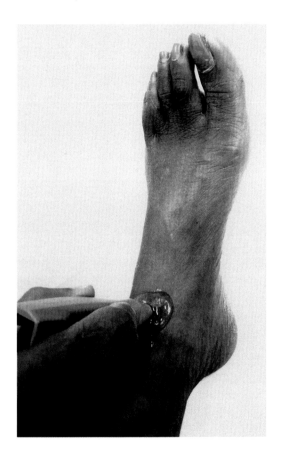

Fig. 6.11 Doppler of dorsalis pedis artery

The examiner should document the farthest point that the flow is detected. This aids in planning future interventions and may even help ascertain if the disease is even amenable

References

1. Ramani S. Promoting the art of history taking. Med Teach. 2004;26(4):374–6.
2. Rajagopalan S, Grossman PM. Management of chronic critical limb ischemia. Cardiol Clin. 2002;20(4):535–45.
3. de Win MM, et al. The paper grip test for screening on intrinsic muscle paralysis in the foot of leprosy patients. Int J Lepr Other Mycobact Dis. 2002;70(1):16–24.
4. Garth Jr WP, Miller ST. Evaluation of claw toe deformity, weakness of the foot intrinsics, and posteromedial shin pain. Am J Sports Med. 1989;17(6):821–7.
5. Spink MJ, et al. Foot and ankle strength assessment using hand-held dynamometry: reliability and age-related differences. Gerontology. 2010;56(6):525–32.
6. Hirsch AT et al. ACC/AHA 2005 Practice Guidelines for the management of patients with peripheral arterial disease (lower extremity, renal, mesenteric, and abdominal aortic): a collaborative report from the American Association for Vascular Surgery/Society for Vascular Surgery, Society for Cardiovascular Angiography and Interventions, Society for Vascular Medicine and Biology, Society of Interventional Radiology, and the ACC/AHA Task Force on Practice Guidelines (Writing Committee to Develop Guidelines for the Management of Patients With Peripheral Arterial Disease): endorsed by the American Association of Cardiovascular and Pulmonary Rehabilitation; National Heart, Lung, and Blood Institute; Society for Vascular Nursing; TransAtlantic Inter-Society Consensus; and Vascular Disease Foundation. Circulation 113(11):e463–654.

Rand S. Swenson, Norman J. Snow, and Brian Catlin

Vasculature of the Upper Limbs

The arterial circulation of the upper limb is depicted in Fig. 7.1. The subclavian arteries are the major arteries supplying the upper limbs. On the right side the subclavian artery is one of the terminal branches of the brachiocephalic trunk, while on the left it is one of the direct branches of the aortic arch. The subclavian artery passes immediately superior to the first rib and becomes the axillary artery at the lateral margin of this rib. The axillary artery, in turn, becomes the brachial artery as it reaches the inferolateral aspect of the teres major muscle. Although the brachial artery occasionally ends in its terminal division in the proximal arm, it usually continues to reach the neck of the radius, where it bifurcates into the radial and ulnar arteries just medial to the tendon of the biceps brachii muscle. The radial and ulnar arteries continue into the hand, ending as the deep and superficial palmar arterial arches, respectively (see Fig. 7.1).

Venous drainage occurs via both deep and superficial veins. The deep veins follow the course of the arteries. In the distal limb, paired veins are intimately associated with the arteries as venae comitantes. These veins are encased in the perivascular connective tissue sheath that surrounds both the artery and these deep veins. More proximally, the venae comitantes join to form a single deep vein paralleling the artery. The superficial veins (depicted in Fig. 7.2) include the cephalic (lateral) and basilic (medial). The superficial veins are connected to the deep system via venous connections with valves that limit retrograde flow from the deep to superficial systems. We will first discuss the arterial system before considering the veins.

R.S. Swenson, MD, PhD (✉)
Anatomy and Neurology, Geisel School of Medicine at Dartmouth, Dewey Field Rd. HB 7100, Hanover, NH 03755, USA

N.J. Snow, MD • B. Catlin, MD
Anatomy, Geisel School of Medicine at Dartmouth, Hanover, NH, USA

The Subclavian Artery

In addition to being the principal artery of the upper limb, the subclavian artery supplies many structures in the neck, the scapular region, and pectoral region, with branches reaching as far distally as the upper abdominal wall. The left subclavian artery is normally somewhat longer, arising directly from the aortic arch. This is distinct from the right subclavian, which is a terminal branch of the brachiocephalic trunk. Occasionally, the right subclavian artery takes origin directly from the aorta, in which case it passes posterior to the esophagus.

The subclavian artery has three portions (Fig. 7.3) with the first part extending from the artery's origin to the medial border of the anterior scalene muscle, which is directly anterior to the artery. This portion is somewhat longer on the left side since the left subclavian has a significant intrathoracic portion prior to reaching the anterior scalene muscle. On both sides, the first part of the subclavian is just posterior to the sternoclavicular joint and several muscles (the sternocleidomastoid, sternohyoid, and sternothyroid). It is also posterior to several vascular structures (including the internal jugular vein and, on the left, the thoracic duct) and neural structures (the phrenic nerve on the left side, the vagus nerve, parasympathetic and sympathetic cardiac nerves, and the ansa subclavia of the sympathetic chain, which encircles the subclavian artery). This first part of the subclavian artery is just anterior to the apex of the lung (and the associated pleural cupola and suprapleural membrane) and several neural structures (including the sympathetic trunk and inferior cervical ganglion as well as the right recurrent laryngeal nerve).

The second portion of the subclavian artery is quite short and it arches above the clavicle. This portion of the artery is immediately posterior to the anterior scalene muscle, which separates the artery from the sternocleidomastoid, right phrenic nerve, and subclavian vein. It is immediately anterior to the middle scalene muscle as well as the apex of the lung and associated membranes.

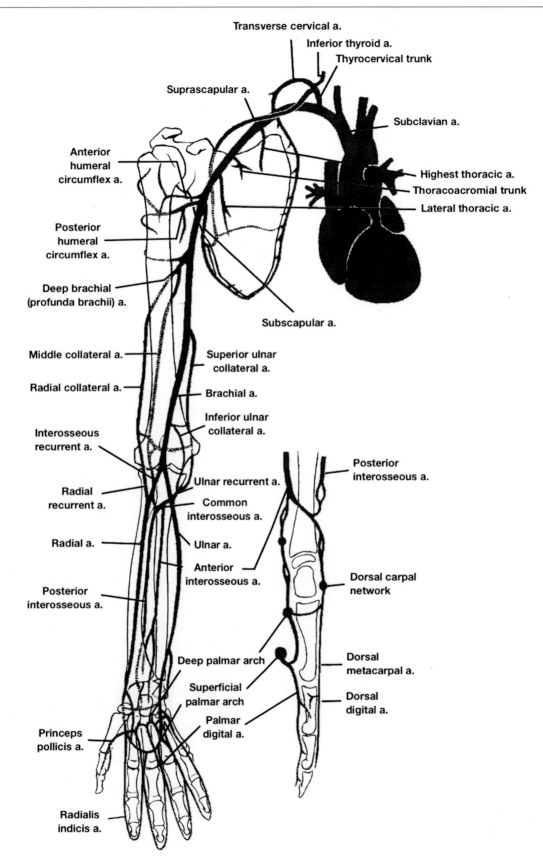

Fig. 7.1 Arteries of the upper limb. Figure by permission: Basic Human Anatomy. O'Rahilly, Müller, Carpenter & Swenson (http://www.dartmouth.edu/~humananatomy)

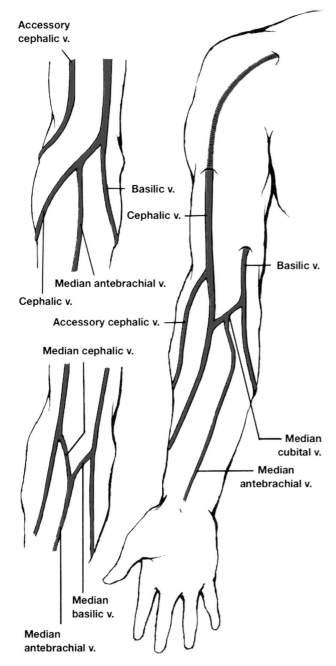

Fig. 7.2 Superficial veins of the upper limb with some common variations. Figure by permission: Basic Human Anatomy. O'Rahilly, Müller, Carpenter & Swenson (http://www.dartmouth.edu/~humananatomy)

The third part of the subclavian artery can be palpated within the supraclavicular triangle at the base of the neck, where it is immediately superior to the first rib. In this location it is posterior to the external jugular vein, the clavicle, and the subclavian vein. It is anterior to the lower trunk of the brachial plexus and middle scalene muscle.

The majority of the branches of the subclavian artery arise from the first part of the artery medial to the anterior scalene. The exceptions include the right costocervical trunk,

which usually arises from the second part, and the dorsal scapular artery (when present), which usually arises from the third part. The first three branches of the subclavian artery are the vertebral and internal thoracic arteries and the thyrocervical trunk.

The vertebral artery arises from the first part of the subclavian artery, although the left vertebral artery may branch from the aortic arch or the brachiocephalic trunk on rare occasions. This artery traverses the transverse foramina of the upper six cervical vertebrae, where it then turns to pass medially along the posterior arch of the atlas. It then penetrates the posterior atlanto-occipital membrane and passes though the foramen magnum. It joins with its mate of the other side to become the basilar artery forming the posterior circulation of the brain. The first part of the vertebral artery, the cervical part, passes posterior to the common carotid artery. The inferior thyroid artery crosses anterior to the vertebral artery, as does the thoracic duct on the left. The inferior cervical sympathetic ganglion is immediately anterior to the vertebral artery, as are the C7 and C8 roots of the brachial plexus. The cervical part of the vertebral artery gives muscular branches to the deep muscles of the neck.

The second part of the vertebral artery, the vertebral part, typically ascends through the transverse foramina from C6 to the atlas, although it rarely begins at C7 or C5. It is accompanied by a venous plexus and by sympathetic nerve fibers. Branches include variable spinal branches that include some radicular arteries that follow nerve roots to the spinal cord.

The internal thoracic (aka, internal mammary) artery is the second branch of the subclavian artery. This artery passes posterior to the subclavian and internal jugular veins and anterior to the cupola of the lung. The phrenic nerve crosses it obliquely, where the nerve can be damaged by procedures that use the internal thoracic artery for coronary bypass grafting. The internal thoracic artery passes posterior to the upper six costal cartilages immediately lateral to the sternum where it is held in place by the endothoracic fascia and slips of the transverse thoracic muscle intervene. Upon reaching the costal margin, the internal thoracic artery divides to become the superior epigastric and musculophrenic arteries.

The thyrocervical trunk (Fig. 7.3) divides into three branches almost immediately after arising from the first part of the subclavian artery. These are the inferior thyroid, transverse cervical, and suprascapular arteries.

The inferior thyroid artery (Fig. 7.1), which is occasionally absent, passes superior, immediately anterior to the anterior scalene muscle. It then arches medially to pass anterior to the vertebral vessels and posterior to the carotid sheath. In this location it is in very close proximity to the sympathetic chain, usually adjacent to the middle cervical sympathetic ganglion at the C6 vertebral level. The inferior thyroid artery passes anterior to the anterior scalene and longus coli muscles and to the vertebral artery. The inferior thyroid

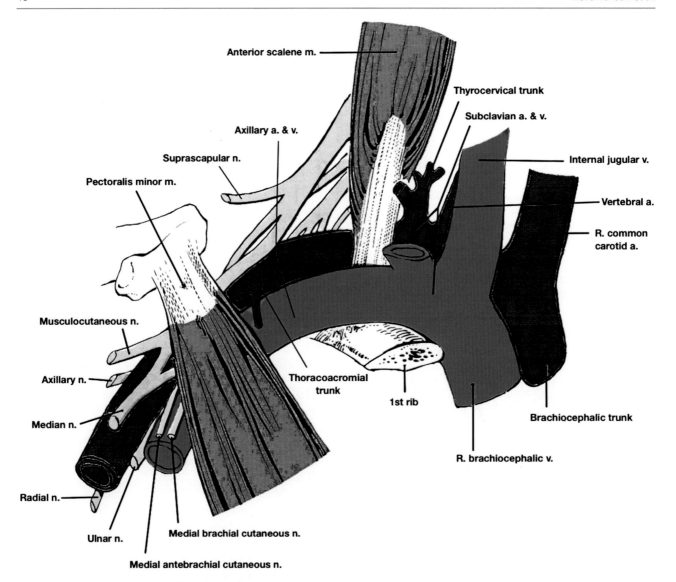

Anterior scalene m.

Thyrocervical trunk

Subclavian a. & v.

Axillary a. & v.

Suprascapular n.

Internal jugular v.

Pectoralis minor m.

Vertebral a.

R. common carotid a.

Musculocutaneous n.

Axillary n.

Thoracoacromial trunk

Median n.

1st rib

Brachiocephalic trunk

R. brachiocephalic v.

Radial n.

Ulnar n.

Medial brachial cutaneous n.

Medial antebrachial cutaneous n.

Fig. 7.3 The relationship of the subclavian and axillary artery and vein to the brachial plexus and major structures of the upper thorax. Figure by permission: Basic Human Anatomy. O'Rahilly, Müller, Carpenter & Swenson (http://www.dartmouth.edu/~humananatomy)

artery may pass posterior or anterior to the recurrent laryngeal nerve. This artery penetrates the fibrous capsule at the lower pole of the thyroid gland, dividing into several branches usually near the inferior parathyroid glands. These glandular branches anastomose with superior laryngeal artery branches and with its mate from the opposite side. In its course the inferior thyroid artery usually gives rise to visceral branches and a recurrent laryngeal branch that follows the nerve of the same name.

The suprascapular (or transverse scapular) artery (Fig. 7.1) is another branch of the thyrocervical trunk. It passes laterally, anterior to the anterior scalene and the phrenic nerve. Beyond the lateral border of the anterior scalene muscle it is anterior to the subclavian artery and the cords of the brachial plexus. More laterally it is posterior to the clavicle and subclavius muscle. It then passes superior to the transverse scap-

ular ligament to reach the posterior aspect of the scapula. The suprascapular artery has muscular branches in the supraspinous fossa and then passes lateral to the root of the spine of the scapula to enter the infraspinous fossa, where it ramifies widely, including muscular branches. Its branches anastomose with branches of other arteries including the dorsal scapular and subscapular to form an anastomosis around the scapula. Occasionally the suprascapular artery arises from the third part of the subclavian artery and very rarely from other arteries, including the axillary artery.

The transverse cervical artery usually is a branch of the thyrocervical trunk, often arising as a common stem with the suprascapular artery. It is somewhat superior to but otherwise parallels the suprascapular artery, crossing the anterior scalene muscle and phrenic nerve. It generally passes deep to the trapezius muscle as it exits the posterior aspect of the posterior triangle of the neck. Alternatively, it may divide into a superficial branch and a deep branch that pass on either side of the levator scapulae muscle. In this arrangement, the deep branch takes the place of the dorsal scapular artery (see below).

The ascending cervical artery may arise either directly from the thyrocervical trunk or from the transverse cervical artery. It ascends the cervical spine in close proximity to the lateral aspect of the spine and the longus colli muscles. It supplies deep paraspinal muscles and contributes to an arterial plexus in the spinal canal with some branches following nerve roots to the spinal cord.

The costocervical trunk arises from the posterior aspect of the first or second part of the subclavian artery with the right one being a little more distal than the left. It follows the first rib posteriorly toward its neck in close proximity to the cupola of the lung. There it ends by dividing into the highest (supreme) intercostal and the deep cervical arteries. The deep cervical artery courses posteriorly, immediately caudal to the transverse process of C7, to ascend in the neck surrounded by deep posterior neck muscles which it supplies. It also supplies a spinal branch to the vertebral canal. The highest (supreme) intercostal artery lies between the parietal pleura of the lung apex and the necks of the first two ribs where it gives rise to the posterior intercostal arteries to the first two intercostal spaces.

The dorsal scapular artery usually arises from the subclavian (second or third part) but may be the deep branch of the transverse cervical artery. When it arises directly from the subclavian, it typically passes between the upper and middle or, occasionally, the middle and lower trunks of the brachial plexus. This artery passes deep to the trapezius and levator scapulae muscles and follows the dorsal scapular nerve along the medial scapular border just deep to the rhomboid muscles. It provides blood supply to these muscles.

Axillary Artery

The axillary artery (Fig. 7.3) is the continuation of the subclavian artery, beginning lateral to the first rib. It is divided into three portions by the pectoralis minor muscle, which is immediately anterior to the mid-portion of the artery. The first part is superomedial to the muscle; the second is directly posterior to it; and the third is inferolateral to it. The axillary artery and vein, as well as lymphatics and the brachial plexus, are invested by dense connective tissue creating an axillary sheath (Fig. 7.4). This sheath is continuous

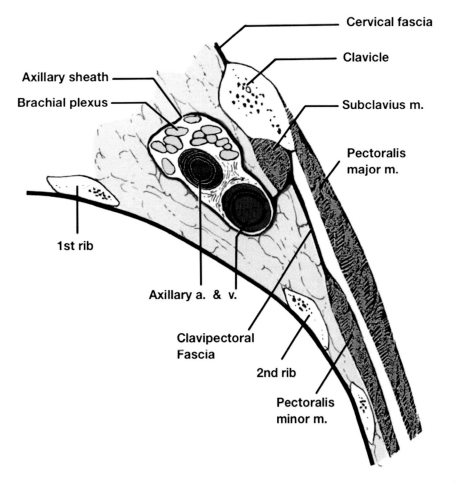

Fig. 7.4 Diagram of a sagittal section through the axillary sheath and clavipectoral region showing the relationship between the artery, vein and nerves. Figure by permission: Basic Human Anatomy. O'Rahilly, Müller, Carpenter & Swenson (http://www.dartmouth.edu/~humananatomy)

Cervical fascia

Clavicle

Subclavius m.

Pectoralis major m.

Axillary sheath

Brachial plexus

1st rib

Axillary a. & v.

Clavipectoral Fascia

2nd rib

Pectoralis minor m.

with the prevertebral layer of deep cervical fascia. The relative positions of these neurovascular structures are shown in Figs. 7.3 and 7.4.

As the axillary artery progresses inferolaterally it passes anterior to the long thoracic nerve and the muscles that form the posterior boundary of the axilla: the subscapular, latissimus dorsi, and teres major muscles. The lateral border of the teres major muscle is where the axillary artery changes its name to the brachial artery. The axillary artery is posterior to the pectoralis minor, the extent of which defines the second part of the axillary artery. The pectoralis major muscle covers the entire anterior aspect of the axillary artery.

The superior (or supreme) thoracic artery (Fig. 7.1) is the first branch, arising from the first part of the axillary artery. This is a small branch that supplies muscles in and around the first intercostal space.

The thoracoacromial artery (trunk) (Fig. 7.3) is the second branch. This arises very close to the superomedial border of the pectoralis minor muscle on either side of the transition from the first to second part of the axillary artery. It is a short trunk with four named branches, some of which may arise directly from the axillary artery. These branches pierce the clavipectoral fascia that stretches from the pectoralis minor muscle and coracoid process inferolaterally to the clavicle superiorly. The four branches are the acromial branch (which passes directly to the acromion process), the clavicular branch (to the subclavius muscle and the sternoclavicular joint), the pectoral branch (supplying the pectoralis major and minor and traveling with branches of the lateral pectoral nerve), and the deltoid branch (which travels with the cephalic vein in the groove between the deltoid and pectoralis major muscles).

The lateral thoracic artery (Fig. 7.1) is the third branch, which also arises from the second part of the axillary artery. It passes inferiorly on the chest wall just lateral to the pectoralis minor. It gives rise to lateral (external) mammary branches that supply the breast.

The subscapular artery (Fig. 7.1) is a large branch arising from the third part of the axillary artery near the lateral border of the pectoralis minor muscle at the level of the lateral border of the subscapularis muscle. It passes inferiorly along the lateral border of the scapula, ending by dividing into the circumflex scapular artery and the thoracodorsal artery. The thoracodorsal artery descends alongside the thoracodorsal nerve along the lateral border of the latissimus dorsi muscle where it anastomoses with lateral branches of intercostal arteries. The circumflex scapular artery (scapular circumflex artery) runs posteriorly across the triangular space (between the teres major and minor muscles and the long head of the triceps). It forms an anastomosis in the infraspinous fossa with branches of the transverse cervical and suprascapular arteries, forming a collateral pathway for blood to pass from the first part of the subclavian artery to the third part of the axillary in the event of intervening arterial obstruction.

The anterior humeral circumflex artery is a small artery that passes anteriorly around the surgical neck of the humerus deep to the deltoid muscle. It gives a branch that ascends in the intertubercular groove to the shoulder joint. The anterior and posterior circumflex arteries end by anastomosing with each other.

The posterior humeral circumflex artery is a larger branch that passes posteriorly around the surgical neck of the humerus through the quadrangular space along with the axillary nerve. It anastomoses with the anterior humeral circumflex artery deep to the deltoid muscle. This anastomosis connects with branches of the profunda brachii artery and supplies branches to muscles in the region and the shoulder joint. The circumflex arteries may arise from a common stem or occasionally from the subscapular artery.

Arteries of the Arm

The brachial artery (Fig. 7.1) begins where the axillary artery ends at the lower border of the teres major muscle. In the proximal arm the median nerve is immediately lateral to the artery, while the radial nerve is posterior, and the ulnar and medial antebrachial cutaneous nerves are medial (Fig. 7.5). The proximal brachial artery is easily palpated where it is medial to the humerus, although the more distal portion is anterior to the bone, where it can be damaged by supracondylar humeral fractures resulting in limb ischemia and subsequent contractures and disability. The posterior part of the artery is closely related to the triceps proximally, followed by the coracobrachialis, and brachialis muscles at more distal levels (Fig. 7.5). As the median nerve progresses from proximal to distal in the arm, the nerve gradually transitions from its lateral position to a medial one, usually passing anterior to the artery.

The brachial artery lies in the center of the cubital fossa, with the biceps tendon on its lateral side and the median nerve on its medial side (Fig. 7.6). The bicipital aponeurosis crosses anterior to it, separating the artery from the median cubital vein. The brachial artery ends by dividing into the radial and ulnar arteries at the level of the neck of the radius, although more proximal bifurcations, including divisions of the axillary artery into radial and ulnar arteries, are not uncommon.

In addition to a more proximal bifurcation, other common anomalies include persistence of a median artery (following the median nerve) or a superficial course for the ulnar artery (which more commonly occurs when there is a more proximal bifurcation of the brachial artery). More rarely the brachial artery may pass posterior to a supracondylar process on the medial aspect of the humerus, usually accompanied by the median nerve.

The brachial artery has a number of branches in the arm. These include muscular branches to arm muscles and a nutrient

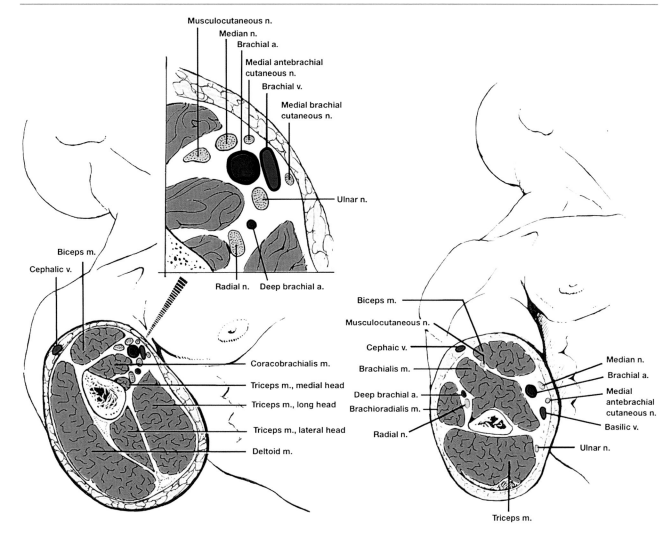

Fig. 7.5 Axial sections through the upper (*left*) and lower (*right*) parts of the arm. Figure by permission: Basic Human Anatomy. O'Rahilly, Müller, Carpenter & Swenson (http://www.dartmouth.edu/~humananatomy)

artery that enters the mid-shaft of the humerus. The most proximal named branch of the brachial artery is the deep brachial (profunda brachii) artery (Figs. 7.1 and 7.5). This generally arises from the posterior side of the brachial artery although it may on rare occasion arise from the subscapular artery. The deep brachial artery spirals around the posterior humerus in the spiral groove along with the radial nerve. A deltoid branch anastomoses with the posterior humeral circumflex artery. The deep brachial artery ends as it reaches the lateral aspect of the arm by bifurcating into a radial collateral artery, which accompanies the radial nerve, and a middle collateral artery (posterior descending branch), which ramifies posterior to the lateral epicondyle. These arteries contribute to the anastomoses around the elbow joint (Fig. 7.1).

The second named branch of the brachial artery is the superior ulnar collateral artery (Fig. 7.1). This begins approximately half way down the arm and travels with the ulnar nerve, passing posterior to the medial epicondyle and anastomosing mostly with the posterior ulnar recurrent artery.

The inferior ulnar collateral artery arises from the brachial artery just proximal to the elbow. It passes posteriorly to ramify both anterior and posterior to the medial epicondyle.

The anastomoses around the elbow joint occur both anterior and posterior to the medial and lateral epicondyles (Fig. 7.1). Anterior to the lateral epicondyle the radial collateral artery anastomoses with the radial recurrent artery (a branch of the radial artery in the proximal forearm). Posterior to the lateral epicondyle the middle collateral artery anastomoses with the interosseous recurrent artery, a branch of the interosseous branch of the ulnar artery. Anterior to the medial epicondyle the anterior branches of the inferior ulnar collateral artery anastomose with the anterior ulnar recurrent branch of the ulnar artery. And posterior to the medial epicondyle the superior ulnar collateral artery, along with posterior branches of the inferior ulnar collateral artery, anastomose with the posterior ulnar recurrent branch of the ulnar artery. All of these branches are highly variable in their size and ability to convey blood around obstructions of the distal brachial artery.

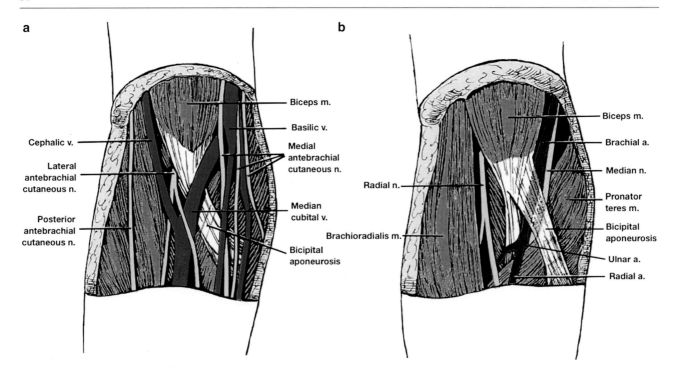

Fig. 7.6 The arteries and veins of the cubital fossa and their relationship with nerves. Figure by permission: Basic Human Anatomy. O'Rahilly, Müller, Carpenter & Swenson (http://www.dartmouth.edu/~humananatomy)

Arteries of the Forearm and Hand

The brachial artery terminates by dividing into a smaller and more superficial radial artery and a deeper and larger ulnar artery at the level of the neck of the radius (Figs. 7.1 and 7.6).

The radial artery travels deep to the brachioradialis muscle throughout the proximal forearm but becomes superficial in the distal part of the forearm, where it can be palpated immediately lateral to the flexor carpi radialis tendon. In its course it passes immediately medial to the biceps tendon and follows the line across the radius that defines the insertions of the pronator teres and the supinator muscles. It is medial to the superficial radial nerve through the mid portion of the forearm. At the wrist the radial artery passes dorsally under the tendons of the anatomical snuffbox, crossing the scaphoid bone in this location (Fig. 7.7). It passes into the hand between the first and second metacarpal bones.

The most dramatic anomaly of the radial artery is that it may be absent. The occurrence of a proximal origin in the arm has previously been described. Also, occasionally it remains superficial to the muscles of the lateral forearm.

In addition to muscular branches there are few named branches to the radial artery in the forearm. The radial recurrent artery passes superiorly to reach the anterior aspect of the lateral epicondyle under the cover of the brachioradialis muscle (Fig. 7.1). It approaches the radial nerve and anastomoses with the radial collateral branch of the deep brachial artery.

The distal part of the radial artery crosses the wrist by passing dorsally through the anatomical snuffbox (Fig. 7.7) in close proximity to the radial collateral ligament of the wrist and to the scaphoid and the trapezium bones. The tendons of the abductor pollicis longus, extensor pollicis brevis, and extensor pollicis longus muscles are superficial to it, as is the distal part of the superficial radial nerve. The most distal part of the radial artery passes between the first and second metacarpals and between the heads of the first dorsal interosseous muscle. It enters the palm between the heads of the adductor pollicis muscle to anastomose with the deep branch of the ulnar artery forming the deep palmar arch (Fig. 7.8).

There are several branches of the radial artery in the region of the hand. A superficial palmar branch (Figs. 7.8 and 7.9) arises above the wrist and passes superficial to the flexor retinaculum. It enters the thenar muscles and occasionally anastomoses with the distal part of the superficial palmar arch.

Palmar and dorsal carpal branches arise as the radial artery passes the wrist. They contribute to a network of small vessels on the palmar and dorsal aspect of the wrist. On the dorsal side the network gives rise to several dorsal metacarpal arteries that further divide into small dorsal digital arteries on either side of the ulnar fingers.

The radial digits, including the thumb and the radial side of the index finger, have dorsal digital branches that may arise directly from the radial artery or as a common trunk that is called the first dorsal metacarpal artery when present.

Fig. 7.7 The relationship between the radial artery at the wrist and other structures of the "anatomical snuffbox." Figure by permission: Basic Human Anatomy. O'Rahilly, Müller, Carpenter & Swenson (http://www.dartmouth. edu/~humananatomy)

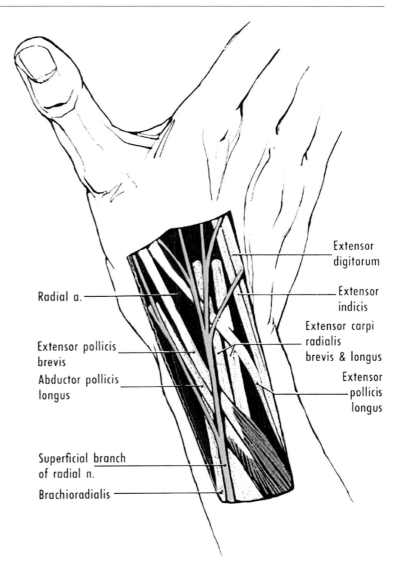

Radial a.

Extensor pollicis brevis

Abductor pollicis longus

Extensor digitorum

Extensor indicis

Extensor carpi radialis brevis & longus

Extensor pollicis longus

Superficial branch of radial n.

Brachioradialis

The remainder of the branches of the radial artery arise after it enters the palm of the hand (Fig. 7.8). The princeps pollicis artery passes distally along the first metacarpal and divides into palmar digital arteries for either side of the thumb. The radialis indicis artery, supplying the radial side of the index finger, is most often a branch of the princeps pollicis but may also arise from a first palmar metacarpal artery or as a branch from either the deep or superficial palmar arch. The radialis indicis divides to supply both sides of the index finger.

The ulnar artery is larger than the radial artery. As it leaves the cubital fossa, it passes inferomedially and deep to the pronator teres muscle. Throughout most of its subsequent course in the forearm, it is covered by the flexor carpi ulnaris muscle. Its origin is directed posterior and medially in the cubital fossa (Fig. 7.6) deep to the muscles arising from the medial epicondyle. The median nerve crosses this part of the artery, separated from it by the deep head of the pronator teres muscle. Once it reaches a position deep to the flexor carpi ulnaris muscle, it courses distally under the cover of this muscle in contact with the fascia of the flexor digitorum profundus muscle. The ulnar nerve travels along the medial side of the artery through the forearm. In the distal part of the forearm the ulnar artery and nerve emerge just lateral to the tendon of the flexor carpi ulnaris muscle where the ulnar pulse can be felt.

The ulnar artery enters the hand by passing anterior to the flexor retinaculum of the wrist, immediately lateral to the pisiform bone. In this location it gives off the deep palmar branch and continues as the superficial palmar arch (Fig. 7.9).

There are several branches of the ulnar artery in the forearm (Fig. 7.1). It gives rise to many muscular branches to adjacent muscles arising from the medial epicondyle. The first named branch is the ulnar recurrent artery, which arises deep to the flexor muscles and gives rise to anterior and posterior branches that contribute to the anastomosis around the elbow anterior and posterior to the medial epicondyle (previously described).

The common interosseous artery is usually the second named branch (Fig. 7.1). This is a short trunk that arises as

Fig. 7.8 The arterial supply
of the palm of the hand. Note:
the radial artery passes
dorsally after its superficial
palmar branch to contribute to
the deep arch after entering
the palm between the first and
second metacarpals. Figure by
permission: Basic Human
Anatomy. O'Rahilly, Müller,
Carpenter & Swenson (http://
www.dartmouth.
edu/~humananatomy)

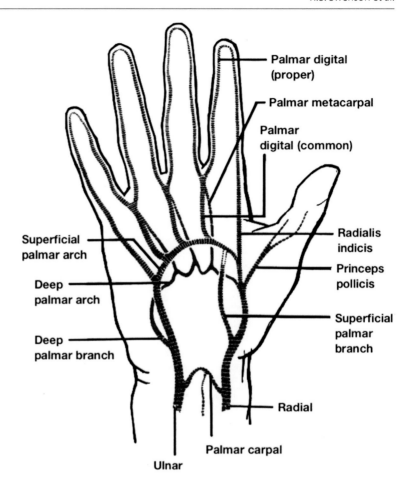

the ulnar artery passes deep to the pronator teres muscle. It quickly divides into anterior and posterior interosseous arteries.

The anterior interosseous artery courses distally immediately anterior to the interosseous membrane between the flexor pollicis longus and flexor digitorum profundus muscles. It travels with the anterior interosseous nerve branch of the median nerve. As the anterior interosseous artery approaches the pronator quadratus muscle, it passes through a hiatus in the interosseous membrane to join the dorsal carpal network (rete) of vessels (Fig. 7.1). It has several branches, including nutrient branches to the radius and ulna and also contributes to the palmar carpal network of vessels.

The median artery is a highly variable branch that usually arises from the interosseous artery system in the proximal forearm or directly from the ulnar artery. It accompanies the median nerve through the forearm into the hand. Although typically small or absent, at times it can be quite large and provide significant blood supply to the hand after passing through the carpal tunnel.

The posterior interosseous artery (Fig. 7.1) passes from the anterior to the posterior side of the forearm through a gap

immediately proximal to the superior border of the interosseous membrane. It emerges in the posterior forearm near the distal aspect of the supinator muscle where it joins with the posterior interosseous nerve. This neurovascular bundle is located between the superficial and deep extensor muscles. The artery terminates by anastomosing with the anterior interosseous artery in the distal forearm, joining the dorsal carpal network. The only named branch of the posterior interosseous artery, the interosseous recurrent artery, occurs near its origin. This branch courses to the posterior aspect of the lateral epicondyle under the cover of extensor muscles.

The ulnar artery enters the hand anterior to the flexor retinaculum, immediately lateral to the pisiform bone. It passes between that bone and the hook of the hamate (hamulus). Both the artery and the ulnar nerve, which is just medial to it, are covered by the pisohamate ligament and some superficial fibers of the flexor retinaculum (but not the main part of the flexor retinaculum nor the transverse carpal ligament). It then splits into terminal branches, the superficial palmar arch and the deep palmar branch.

As it approaches the wrist, the ulnar artery gives rise to a palmar (larger) and dorsal (smaller) carpal branch. These branches contribute to the palmar and dorsal carpal network,

Fig. 7.9 The formation of the superficial palmar arterial arch. Figure by permission: Basic Human Anatomy. O'Rahilly, Müller, Carpenter & Swenson (http://www. dartmouth. edu/~humananatomy)

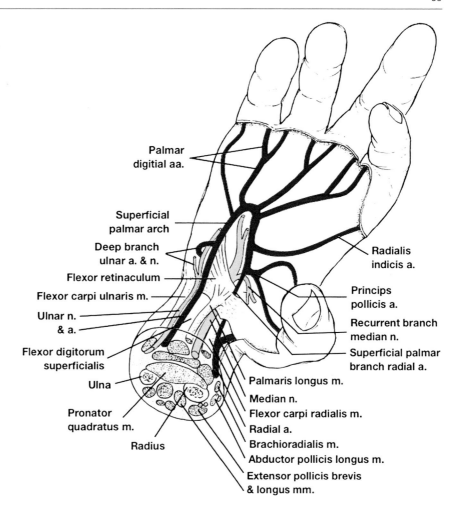

respectively, joining with corresponding branches of the radial artery. This network is deep to the tendons and adjacent to the wrist joint capsule.

The superficial palmar arch (Fig. 7.9) is the main continuation of the ulnar artery. After arching across the palm of the hand, it may anastomose with the radialis indicis, the superficial palmar branch of the radial or the princeps pollicis arteries to complete the arch. Less frequently, the median artery or an enlarged anterior interosseous artery may contribute to the formation of the arch, particularly in rare cases where the ulnar artery is absent. The distal extent of the superficial palmar arch typically reaches approximately the level of the two horizontal creases of the palm. The arch is superficial to the flexor tendons, the lumbrical muscles, and the branches of the median nerve but deep to the palmar aponeurosis and the palmaris brevis muscle.

The superficial palmar arch gives rise to a branch to the medial side of the fifth finger and three common palmar digital arteries. Each of these, in turn, divides to supply the adjacent sides of the fingers. In addition to supplying the tissues of the fingers the digital arteries have extensive arteriovenous anastomoses.

The deep palmar branch of the ulnar artery (Fig. 7.8) passes between the abductor digiti minimi and flexor digiti minimi brevis muscles accompanied by the deep branch of the ulnar nerve. It typically anastomoses with the distal end of the deep palmar arch, completing the arch. This arch is deep to the flexor tendons, immediately anterior to the metacarpal bones and interosseous muscles. It does not extend as far distal in the hand as the superficial arch. The deep palmar arch gives rise to three palmar metacarpal arteries, which course distally on the interosseous muscles, joining the palmar digital branches of the superficial arch and contributing to the blood supply of the fingers.

Veins of the Upper Limb

The drainage of the upper limb includes both a superficial and deep system of veins. In the upper extremity the deep venous system returns less of the blood than the superficial system. In the forearm the deep system consists of paired vena comitans that are ensheathed, along with the named arteries and often a nerve, within a neurovascular bundle.

This is the arrangement in the deep venous system around most arteries up to the diameter of the brachial artery.

In the distal arm, just proximal to the elbow, the brachial artery is accompanied by venae comitantes. More proximally these venae comitantes are joined by the basilic vein, which pierces the investing fascia of the arm, to form the axillary vein (Fig. 7.5).

The superficial and the deep venous systems are connected at irregular intervals through the forearm. These connections have valves that only permit flow from the superficial into the deep system of veins.

The superficial system of veins is a network of highly variable vessels residing within the superficial fascia (Fig. 7.2). These veins begin in the fingers and drain via a variable organization of palmar and dorsal digital veins. These are tributaries of a dorsal venous network or arch on the dorsum of the hand. There is a much finer superficial network in the palm. Blood from these networks passes into anastomosing channels in the forearm that roughly segregate into cephalic and basilic systems on the radial and ulnar sides of the forearm respectively. Each vein has several valves.

The cephalic system of veins extends from the dorsal aspect around the radial side of the forearm to reach the anterolateral part of the cubital region (Fig. 7.6). Most often one major trunk continues proximally along the lateral biceps. This continues in the groove between the deltoid and pectoralis major muscles. This branch then pierces the clavipectoral fascia to terminate by joining the axillary vein.

The basilic venous system continues from the veins on the dorsum of the hand around the ulnar aspect of the forearm to pass anterior to the medial epicondyle. From that position it continues proximally along the medial margin of the biceps. In the middle of the arm it pierces the deep fascia to travel with the brachial artery. Upon reaching the axilla it joins with the brachial vein or venae comitantes to become the axillary vein.

The cephalic and basilic veins are often connected anterior to the elbow by the median cubital vein. This vein classically courses superomedially from the cephalic to the basilic, crossing superficial to the bicipital aponeurosis which separates the vein from the deeper brachial artery and median nerve.

There is usually a significant communication between the superficial and deep venous system in the region of the cubital fossa, and there are also connections with superficial veins from the anterior aspect of the forearm. It must be kept in mind that the pattern of superficial veins anterior to the elbow is highly variable. There are often accessory connections between the cephalic and basilic systems. Nonetheless the median cubital or one of its tributaries is usually more prominent and therefore more useful for drawing blood or for catheterization.

The axillary vein begins at the lower border of the teres major as the continuation of the brachial vein. The axillary vein is located on the anterior and medial side of the axillary artery (Fig. 7.4), and it has one or more sets of valves. In its course it receives the cephalic vein and tributaries analogous to the branches of the axillary artery. The veins that parallel the branches of the thoracoacromial artery drain into the cephalic vein and then into the axillary vein.

The axillary vein commonly receives blood from the thoracoepigastric vein, which is actually an anastomotic pathway. This provides a collateral route for venous return in the event that the inferior vena cava becomes obstructed.

At the lateral border of the first rib the axillary vein continues as the subclavian vein (Fig. 7.3). The subclavian vein lies anterior to the subclavian artery and is separated from it by the anterior scalene muscle. It is also somewhat inferior to the artery but does reach the level of the clavicle. Posterior to the medial end of the clavicle it joins the internal jugular vein to form the brachiocephalic vein. The right and left brachiocephalic veins then join to form the superior vena cava which enters the heart.

Vascular Anatomy of the Lower Limbs

8

Rand S. Swenson, Norman J. Snow, and Brian Catlin

Vessels of the Lower Limb

This chapter describes the arterial and venous circulation of the lower limbs. The arterial circulation (Fig. 8.1) begins with the external and internal iliac arteries. The internal iliac artery mostly supplies the pelvic organs, although its branches also contribute to the arterial circulation of the gluteal region and proximal thigh. The external iliac artery continues as the femoral artery after it passes the inguinal ligament. A large proximal branch, the deep femoral artery, not only supplies deeper structures of the anterior thigh but is also the main blood supply of the posterior thigh and the anastomosis around the hip joint. The continuation of the femoral artery (often referred to clinically as the superficial femoral artery) transitions to the popliteal artery as it passes through the adductor hiatus. Branches of both the femoral and popliteal arteries contribute to the anastomosis around the knee. The popliteal artery ultimately gives rise to the three main arteries that supply the leg in a region sometimes called the "trifurcation." The posterior tibial artery is the continuation of the popliteal artery, beginning at the origin of the anterior tibial artery that branches from the anterior side of the popliteal. The anterior tibial passes between the tibia and fibula to supply the anterior leg. The fibular (peroneal) artery arises from the lateral aspect of the posterior tibial shortly after the origin of the anterior tibial. The fibular artery mostly supplies leg structures of the lateral compartment and some of the posterior compartment, and it ends by joining the anterior tibial in the distal anterior leg to contribute to the dorsalis pedis artery. Together, the fibular and anterior tibial arteries supply most of the dorsum of the foot, the lateral calcaneal region, and

the deep plantar arch. The posterior tibial arteries pass posterior to the medial malleolus to reach the plantar surface of the foot where they give rise to the medial and lateral plantar arteries and the medial calcaneal artery.

The vascular distribution of the foot has been conceptualized as having at least five "angiosomes," each with a relatively distinct arterial supply and restricted intercommunications through "choke vessels." These angiosomes include the distributions of the medial and lateral plantar and the dorsalis pedis arteries, as well as the medial and lateral calcaneal artery distributions. Similarly, the leg is conceptualized as having at least three angiosomes, one for each of the major vessels (the anterior and posterior tibial and the fibular arteries).

The venous system is divisible into deep and superficial systems with more blood traveling in the deep system. The deep system consists of venae comitantes distally in the limb, with single popliteal veins and femoral veins paralleling the arteries back to the iliac system. The superficial venous system (Fig. 8.2) is complex and includes great and small saphenous veins, with communications in between and also from the superficial system to the deep system at various points along its course.

Arterial Circulation

A discussion of the arterial supply of the lower extremities must begin with the iliac (formerly hypogastric) vessels. The newer terminology will be employed here, as will English (rather than Latin) nomenclature for vessels wherever possible. The description of lower limb arterial circulation will progress from proximal to distal in the limb, first with consideration of the gluteal region and thigh followed by the leg and foot.

Iliac Vessels

Lower limb circulation (Fig. 8.1) begins with the common iliac vessels, the terminal branches of the abdominal aorta.

R.S. Swenson, MD, PhD (✉)
Anatomy and Neurology, Geisel School of Medicine
at Dartmouth, Hanover, NH, USA

N.J. Snow, MD • B. Catlin, MD
Anatomy, Geisel School of Medicine at Dartmouth,
Hanover, NH, USA

© Springer International Publishing Switzerland 2017
R.S. Dieter et al. (eds.), *Critical Limb Ischemia*, DOI 10.1007/978-3-319-31991-9_8

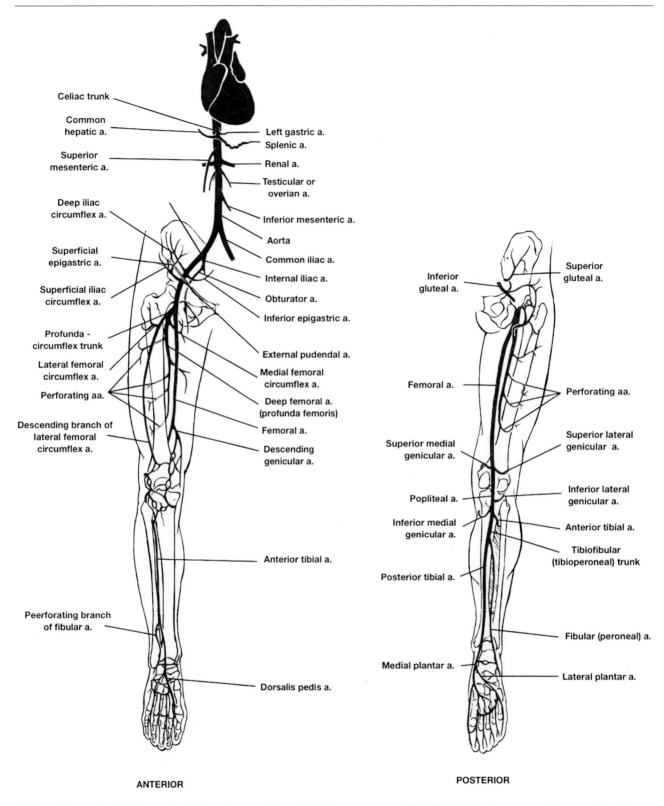

Fig. 8.1 The arteries of the lower limb. Figure by permission: Basic Human Anatomy. O'Rahilly, Müller, Carpenter and Swenson (http://www.dartmouth.edu/~humananatomy)

This bifurcation occurs anterior to the fourth lumbar vertebra slightly to the left of the midline. The common iliac arteries follow a course initially anteromedial and then medial to the psoas major muscles. They are usually around 4–5 cm long and end by dividing into internal and external iliac vessels. The external iliac vessels are the major supply to the lower limbs. They travel immediately medial to the psoas major muscle and give rise to two named branches immediately

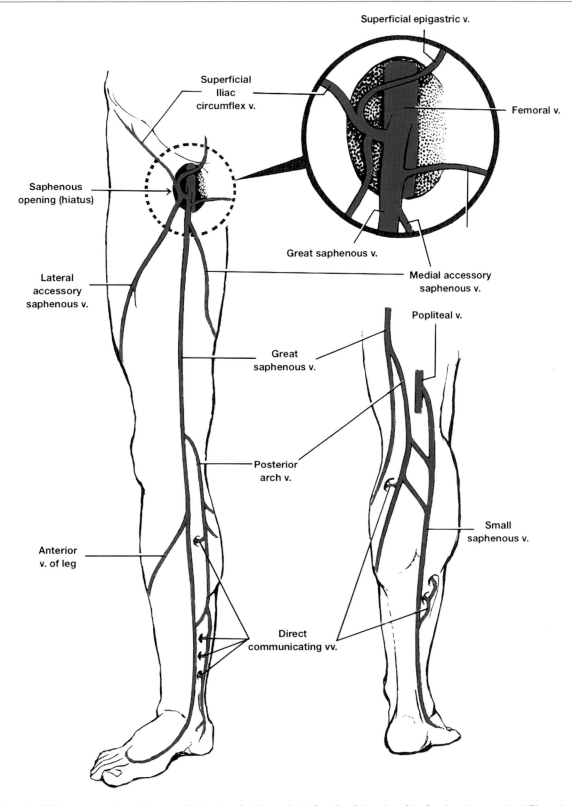

Fig. 8.2 A simplified representation of the superficial veins of the lower limb. Details of the veins of the foot have been omitted. Figure by permission: Basic Human Anatomy. O'Rahilly, Müller, Carpenter and Swenson (http://www.dartmouth.edu/~humananatomy)

prior to passing the inguinal ligament. The two consistent branches are the inferior epigastric artery to the anterior abdominal wall and the deep iliac circumflex artery that is directed toward the anterior superior iliac spine, supplying

some of the inguinal region. In as many as 20 % of cases, there is a major artery, usually called the accessory obturator artery, arising from either the distal external iliac or the inferior epigastric. This wraps around the superior pubic ramus

Fig. 8.3 *Above*: the branches
of the internal iliac artery,
medial aspect. *Below*: the
most frequent pattern of
branches of the internal iliac
artery. Figure by permission:
Basic Human Anatomy.
O'Rahilly, Müller, Carpenter
and Swenson (http://www.
dartmouth.
edu/~humananatomy)

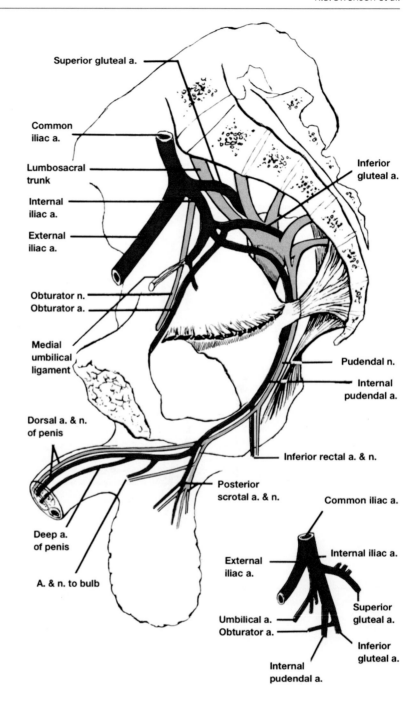

and usually anastomoses with the obturator artery but can entirely replace it.

The internal iliac artery (Fig. 8.3) supplies most of the blood to the pelvis and gluteal region. Here we will consider its branches that supply the gluteal region. Although the classic description of the internal iliac artery is that it has anterior and posterior divisions, variations are frequent.

The main branches extending into the gluteal and thigh regions are the obturator, the superior and inferior gluteal, and the internal pudendal arteries (Fig. 8.4). The obturator artery usually arises from the anterior division of the internal

iliac. It is crossed by the ureter on its course to the obturator foramen. As mentioned previously, it may be joined by or replaced by an accessory obturator artery arising from the external iliac system. The obturator artery divides into several branches. These include an anterior and posterior branch that ramifies around the obturator foramen and an acetabular branch to the ligament of the head of the femur.

The superior and inferior gluteal arteries (Fig. 8.4) classically arise from the anterior division of the internal iliac, but they may originate from the posterior. These arteries pass between roots of the sacral plexus, exiting the pelvis via the

Fig. 8.4 The relationship of the superior gluteal, inferior gluteal, and the internal pudendal arteries to other structures emerging into the gluteal region from the greater sciatic foramen. Figure by permission: Basic Human Anatomy. O'Rahilly, Müller, Carpenter and Swenson (http://www.dartmouth.edu/~humananatomy)

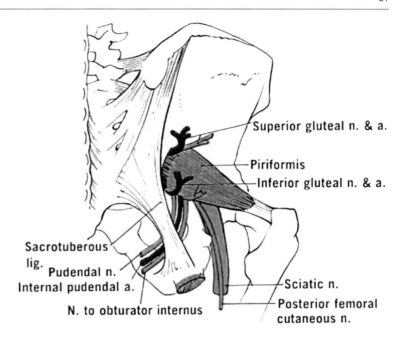

greater sciatic foramen immediately superior and inferior to the piriformis muscle, respectively.

The superior gluteal artery is the larger of the two gluteal arteries. Its entry to the gluteal region can be identified by a point one third of the way between the posterior superior iliac spine and the tip of the greater trochanter. It passes between the lumbosacral trunk and the first sacral nerve just prior to exiting the pelvis through the greater sciatic foramen superior to the piriformis muscle. It gives rise to muscular branches and a nutrient artery to the ilium prior to dividing into superficial and deep branches. The superficial branches enter the gluteus maximus muscle, while the deep branch passes between the gluteus maximus and medius muscles, supplying both. In its course, the deep branch is accompanied by the superior gluteal nerve.

The inferior gluteal artery is a branch of the internal iliac artery that leaves the pelvis by passing between two of the upper sacral nerves and exiting the greater sciatic foramen inferior to the piriformis muscle. Branches enter surrounding muscles, especially the gluteus maximus muscle, and it then joins the medial aspect of the sciatic nerve and then the posterior femoral cutaneous nerve. It gives branches to the deep external rotator muscles of the hip and the upper hamstrings. It provides cutaneous supply to the upper posterior thigh and, through coccygeal branches, the region around the coccyx. A branch passes laterally toward the greater trochanter of the femur, participating in the cruciate anastomosis posterior to the hip joint. There is usually a very small artery of the sciatic nerve. On occasion this artery can remain quite large (it is the remnant of a large axial artery in the embryo).

The internal pudendal artery (Fig. 8.3) also usually arises from the anterior division and exits the pelvis through the

greater sciatic foramen inferior to the piriformis muscle. It subsequently crosses the posterior aspect of the ischial spine and sacrospinous ligament and enters the lesser sciatic foramen to reach the perineum. It is accompanied by the pudendal nerve and is the source of the inferior rectal artery and vessels supplying the scrotum (or labia), perineum, bulb of the penis (or vestibule), and urethra.

The remainder of the visceral and parietal branches of the internal iliac system will not be described here.

Femoral Vessels

The main blood supply to the anterior thigh is the femoral artery (often referred to clinically as the common femoral artery). This is the continuation of the external iliac as it passes the inguinal ligament (Fig. 8.5). It is quite superficial in the upper thigh, but it becomes deep by passing posterior to the sartorius muscle in the adductor canal about a third of the way down the thigh. About 2/3–3/4 of the way down the thigh it passes through the adductor hiatus to leave the anterior thigh and assume a posterior position as the popliteal artery.

The initial (superior) parts of the femoral artery and vein are enclosed in a fascial investment called the femoral sheath. This is located medial to the iliopsoas muscle and anterior to the pectineus muscle (Fig. 8.5) and consists of fascial continuations from the transversalis fascia of the abdomen and the iliac fascia over the iliacus muscle. The sheath is a few centimeters long, tapering to fuse with the adventitia of the blood vessels. It is divided by connective tissue septae into three compartments with a lateral one for the artery, a middle one for the vein, and a medial, one called the femoral

Fig. 8.5 Structures entering
the thigh deep to the inguinal
ligament. Figure by
permission: Basic Human
Anatomy. O'Rahilly, Müller,
Carpenter and Swenson
(http://www.dartmouth.
edu/~humananatomy)

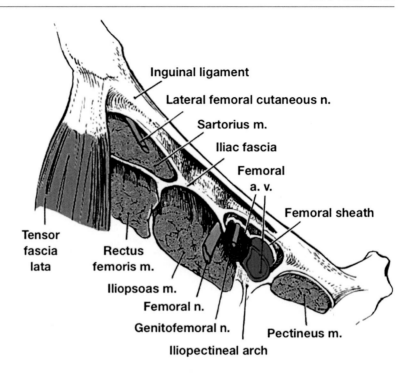

canal, containing fat and a few lymph vessels. Its superior end is termed the femoral ring and is normally closed by a condensation of connective tissue known as the femoral septum. There is a thickening of connective tissue, Henle's ligament, which borders the medial aspect of the femoral ring. Clinically, the femoral canal is the location of femoral hernias. The anterior aspect of the femoral sheath is pierced by small arteries and by the great saphenous vein.

The most proximal named branches of the femoral artery (Fig. 8.1) arise immediately after the femoral artery enters the femoral sheath by passing deep to the inguinal ligament. These arteries pierce the femoral sheath, entering the superficial fascia. They include the superficial epigastric artery, the superficial iliac circumflex artery, the superficial external pudendal artery, and the deep external pudendal artery. There are also several muscular and musculocutaneous branches. The superficial epigastric artery runs superiorly to enter the superficial fascia of the abdomen anterior to the inguinal ligament. It follows a course roughly toward the umbilicus, anastomosing with branches of the inferior epigastric artery. The superficial iliac circumflex artery passes superolaterally toward the anterior superior iliac spine, where it anastomoses with the deep iliac circumflex artery. The external pudendal arteries pass medial to the tissues over the medial part of the inguinal ligament and anterior structures of the pudendum (anterior scrotal/labial branches).

The superior 1/3 of the femoral artery is in the femoral triangle. This triangle is inferior to the inguinal ligament and is bounded on the lateral side by the medial border of the sartorius muscle and medially by the medial border of the adductor

longus muscle. The floor of the triangle is formed by the iliopsoas, pectineus, and adductor longus muscles from lateral to medial. Anteriorly, the triangle is covered by the fascia lata (the investing fascial layer of the thigh). Just inferior to the inguinal ligament, the fascia lata is perforated by the small anterior branches of the femoral artery and by the great saphenous vein. This perforated fascia has been termed the cribriform fascia, and the fascial gap has been called the saphenous hiatus. Within the more inferior portions of the femoral triangle, the femoral artery assumes a position anterior to the femoral vein, while the majority of the branches of the femoral nerve remain lateral to the artery in the triangle.

Approximately 1–5 cm distal to the inguinal ligament, the femoral artery gives off its largest branch, the deep femoral (profunda femoris) artery (Fig. 8.1). About half the time, this arises as a common trunk with the femoral circumflex arteries and can be called a profunda-circumflex trunk.

The deep femoral artery arises from the posterior side of the femoral artery and assumes a position deep and slightly medial to the femoral artery. Initially, it is anterior to the iliacus and pectineus muscles and subsequently passes posterior to the adductor longus muscle as it descends the thigh. At progressively more distal levels of the thigh, it is located medial to the femur and anterior to first the adductor brevis and then the adductor magnus muscles. In its course it gives rise to three perforating branches that pass through gaps in the insertion of the adductor magnus to reach the posterior thigh (Fig. 8.1). In that location they are the major arterial supply of the hamstrings and the vastus lateralis muscles. The deep femoral artery, itself, ends as a fourth perforating artery. The first perforating artery anastomoses with the inferior gluteal artery and with branches of the lateral and medial femoral circumflex arteries to form the cruciate anastomosis around the hip (Fig. 8.6). In addition to many muscular

branches, the deep femoral artery and its perforating branches supply nutrient arteries to the femur.

The lateral circumflex artery of the thigh (Fig. 8.1) takes a lateral course, passing between the iliacus muscle posteriorly and the sartorius and rectus femoris muscles on its anterior side. In its course, it passes between branches of the femoral nerve. It ends by dividing into ascending, transverse, and descending branches. The ascending branch passes anterior to the hip joint and between the gluteus medius and minimus muscles, anastomosing with the superior gluteal artery. The transverse branch extends laterally, piercing the insertion of the vastus lateralis as it reaches the posterior aspect of the thigh, anastomosing with the end of the medial circumflex artery (Fig. 8.6). The descending branch passes distally toward the knee. First it is posterior to the rectus femoris muscle, and later in its course it is deep to the vastus lateralis muscle.

The medial circumflex artery (Fig. 8.6) arises from the posterior aspect of the deep femoral artery. It courses posteriorly between the psoas major and pectineus muscles and then passes between the obturator externus and adductor brevis muscles. Ultimately, it divides into ascending and transverse branches after passing between the quadratus femoris and adductor magnus muscles. The ascending branch anastomoses with the gluteal arteries posterolateral to the hip joint. The transverse branch anastomoses with the end of the lateral circumflex artery. In its course, the medial circumflex artery has an acetabular branch that anastomoses with the obturator artery. This branch gives rise to an artery to the head of the femur as lateral epiphyseal arteries. These enter the neck of

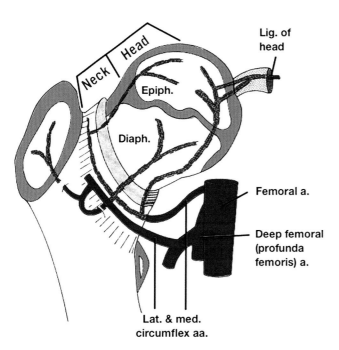

Fig. 8.6 The blood supply to the head and neck of the femur. Figure by permission: Basic Human Anatomy. O'Rahilly, Müller, Carpenter and Swenson (http://www.dartmouth.edu/~humananatomy)

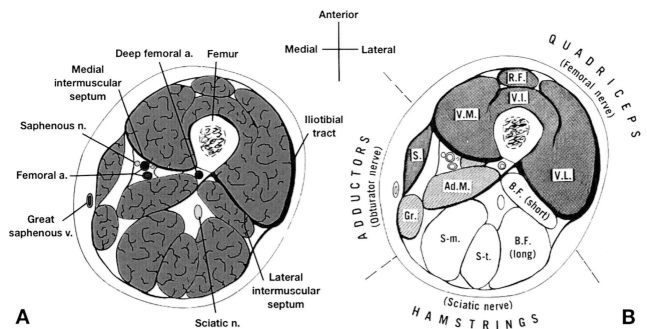

Fig. 8.7 Axial section through the middle of the thigh. (**a**) Depicts the relation of the vessels to surrounding structures. (**b**) Defines the location of the muscles of the thigh that relate to the vessels. *Ad.M.* adductor magnus, *B.F.* biceps femoris, *Gr.* gracilis, *R.F.* rectus femoris, *S.* sartorius,

S-m. semimembranosus, *S-t.* semitendinosus, *V.I.* vastus intermedius, *V.L.* vastus lateralis, *V.M.* vastus medialis. Figure by permission: Basic Human Anatomy. O'Rahilly, Müller, Carpenter and Swenson (http://www.dartmouth.edu/~humananatomy)

the femur and extend toward the head (Fig. 8.6). They can be disrupted by fractures of the neck of the femur or by procedures to repair such fractures.

Distal to the origin of the deep femoral branch, the femoral artery is usually referred to as the superficial femoral artery by clinicians. About a third of the way down the thigh, the artery enters the adductor canal (Fig. 8.7). In addition to the femoral artery and vein, the adductor (subsartorial) canal contains the saphenous nerve and usually a branch from the femoral nerve to the vastus medialis muscle. The canal is sometimes called the subsartorial canal because the sartorius muscle and subsartorial fascia form an anterior roof to the canal. At more distal levels of the thigh, the sartorius muscle becomes more medial (Fig. 8.7). In the canal, the femoral vein is immediately posterior to the artery. The femoral artery has a few muscular branches but only one named branch, the descending genicular artery (Fig. 8.1). This arises just above the adductor hiatus and divides immediately into saphenous and articular branches. The articular branches pass distally, entering the vastus medialis muscle and contributing to the anastomosis around the medial aspect of the knee joint. The saphenous branch joins the saphenous nerve medial to the knee. It contributes to the anastomosis around the knee by anastomosing with the inferomedial genicular artery after passing between the sartorius and gracilis muscles.

Popliteal Region

The popliteal artery is the continuation of the femoral artery after it passes through the adductor hiatus. This hiatus is the gap between the portion of the adductor magnus muscle that inserts on the adductor tubercle and the portion that inserts on the linea aspera. The popliteal artery is surrounded by fat but closely approximates the popliteal surface of the femur and the structures of the posterior knee joint, including the joint capsule and the popliteus muscle. The artery is anterior to the lateral portion of the semimembranosus muscle and the tibial nerve. More distally, the gastrocnemius and plantaris muscles are posterior to the artery. In the superior part of the popliteal fossa, the popliteal vein and tibial nerve are posterolateral to the artery. This relationship changes in the inferior part of the fossa, where the vein and nerve are posteromedial to the artery.

The popliteal artery has muscular branches to the muscles of the calf as well as cutaneous branches. One of these, the superficial sural artery, accompanies the small saphenous vein.

There are five named genicular arteries that arise from the popliteal and contribute to the anastomosis around the knee. Proximal to the knee, the superomedial and superolateral genicular arteries arise on the medial and lateral side of popliteal artery at the level of the femoral condyles and pass medially and laterally, respectively, above the corresponding femoral condyle and between the origins of the gastrocnemius muscles and inferior portions of the hamstring muscles. They anastomose with other genicular arteries within the substance of the vastus medialis and lateralis muscles, respectively. The middle genicular artery arises from the anterior aspect of the popliteal artery and pierces the oblique popliteal ligament to enter the knee joint. The inferomedial and inferolateral genicular arteries course deep to the medial and lateral heads of the gastrocnemius muscle and then to the medial and lateral collateral ligaments of the knee joint as they curve around the medial and lateral aspects of the knee, respectively. These branches also contribute to the anastomosis around the knee joint.

The popliteal artery ends by dividing into the anterior and posterior tibial arteries at the inferior border of the popliteus muscle (Fig. 8.8). This branching is misnamed the "trifurcation" since the third branch, the fibular (peroneal) artery, is a more distal branch of the posterior tibial artery. Between the origin of the anterior tibial artery and the origin of the fibular artery, the posterior tibial is sometimes called the tibioperoneal trunk.

In summary, the anastomoses around the knee joint include anastomoses between the two superior and the two inferior genicular arteries along with the descending genicular branch of the femoral artery and the descending branch of the lateral circumflex artery. There are also contributions from the fibular circumflex and anterior recurrent arteries of the anterior tibial artery. The medial and lateral arteries anastomose across the anterior side of the limb deep and superficial to the quadriceps muscle and deep to the patellar ligament.

Vessels of the Leg

The popliteal artery terminates by bifurcating into the anterior and posterior tibial arteries at the inferior border of the popliteus muscle (Fig. 8.8). The anterior tibial artery initially passes laterally between the fibrous origins of the tibial and fibular heads of the tibialis posterior muscle before turning anteriorly to pass the fibrous arch at the superior end of the interosseous membrane. As it reaches the anterior compartment, it occupies a position anterior to the interosseous membrane, where it runs distally in the anterior compartment of the leg. It joins the deep fibular (peroneal) nerve. In the inferior portion of the leg, it is directly anterior to the tibia, where it is accessible. On the dorsum of the foot, it continues into an arterial network usually via a well-defined direct continuation, the dorsalis pedis artery.

The anterior tibial artery has muscular and cutaneous branches that supply the adjacent muscles and skin of the anterior leg. Named branches include an occasional fibular circumflex branch, which more often arises from the poste-

Fig. 8.8 Structures in the right popliteal fossa (popliteal veins omitted). Figure by permission: Basic Human Anatomy. O'Rahilly, Müller, Carpenter and Swenson (http://www.dartmouth.edu/~humananatomy)

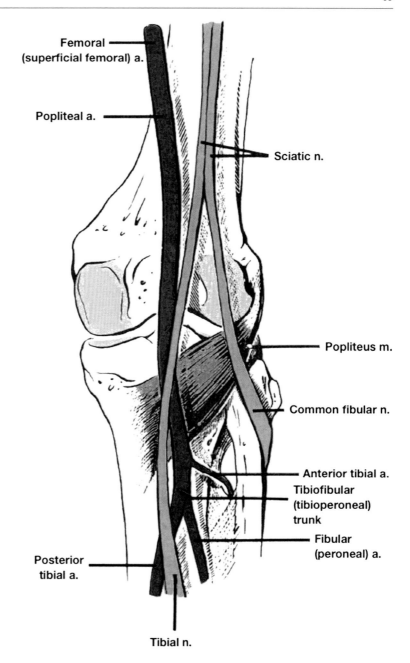

rior tibial artery. Additionally, there is a small and inconstant branch, the posterior tibial recurrent artery, which ascends deep to the popliteus muscle. The anterior tibial recurrent artery arises immediately after the anterior tibial artery passes the interosseous membrane. It courses superiorly toward the knee joint within the tibialis anterior muscle and joins the inferior part of the anastomosis around the knee.

Medial and lateral anterior malleolar arteries arise from the distal part of the anterior tibial artery, immediately proximal to the ankle joint (Fig. 8.9). These arteries contribute to an anastomosis around the ankle. The medial anterior malleolar artery passes posterior to the tendons of the extensor hallucis longus and tibialis anterior muscles, anastomosing with branches of

the posterior tibial and medial plantar arteries near the medial malleolus. The lateral anterior malleolar artery passes posterior to the extensor digitorum longus muscle to anastomose with the perforating branch of the fibular (peroneal) artery (Fig. 8.9). The contribution of the anterior tibial artery to the blood supply of the foot is described below.

The larger terminal division of the popliteal artery, which is essentially a continuation of its course, is the posterior tibial artery (Fig. 8.1). It is immediately anterior to the tibialis posterior muscle in the upper leg and then the flexor digitorum longus muscle and the posterior surface of the tibia at progressively distal levels. The artery is in the deep compartment of the posterior leg, just deep to the deep transverse

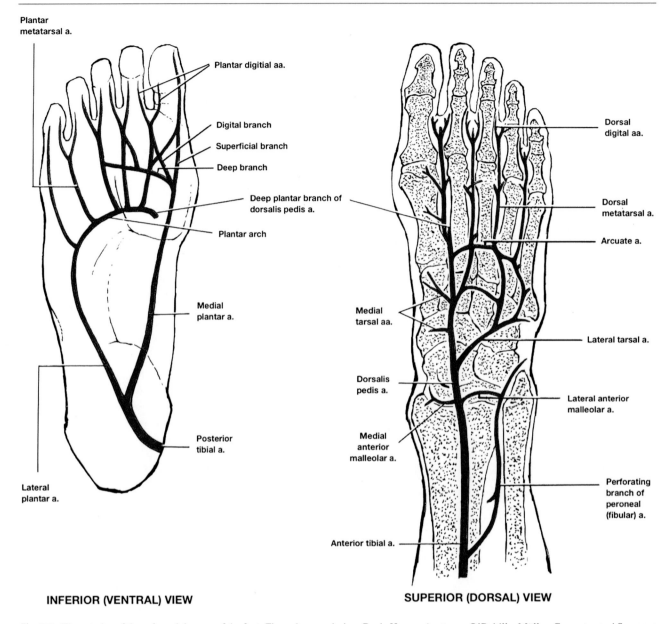

Fig. 8.9 The arteries of the sole and dorsum of the foot. Figure by permission: Basic Human Anatomy. O'Rahilly, Müller, Carpenter and Swenson (http://www.dartmouth.edu/~humananatomy)

fascia of the leg, which in turn is deep to the soleus and gastrocnemius muscles. It is more superficial distally as it passes the flexor retinaculum posterior to the medial malleolus and finally passes deep to the abductor hallucis muscle. It is closely related to the tibial nerve, which is medial to the artery in the upper leg and lateral in the lower leg after passing posterior to the artery in the mid leg.

There are several named branches of the posterior tibial artery. Shortly after its origin at the inferior border of the popliteus muscle, the circumflex fibular branch usually arises from the lateral aspect and passes laterally around the neck of the fibula under the cover of the origin of the fibularis (peroneus) longus muscle and contributes to the anastomosis around the knee joint.

The posterior tibial artery is the origin of a very large nutrient artery to the tibia that passes through the fibrous arch formed by the origin of the tibialis posterior muscle. In the proximal leg, one or more communicating branches with the fibular (peroneal) artery can be identified.

At the level of the ankle, the posterior tibial artery gives rise to medial malleolar branches that pass posterior to the medial malleolus. The medial calcaneal arteries may arise from these medial malleolar arteries or directly from the posterior tibial artery. There is a network of vessels that surround the heel that are contributed to by branches of the anterior tibial, posterior tibial, and fibular arteries. The fibular (peroneal) artery is the largest and most consistent branch of the posterior tibial artery, usually arising within a few centimeters of the origin of the posterior tibial artery. It is nearly as large as the posterior tibial artery in most cases. It crosses the tibialis posterior muscle to reach its fibular origin and passes distally following the medial aspect of the fibula (occasionally within the substance of the tibialis posterior muscle). Throughout its course in the leg, it remains in the posterolateral aspect of the posterior compartment.

The most important branches of the fibular arteries are the muscular branches (several) that pass through the membrane that separates the posterior compartment from the lateral compartment of the leg. These branches are the primary blood supply of the lateral compartment of the leg.

In the distal leg, the fibular (peroneal) artery ends by dividing into lateral calcaneal branches to the lateral aspect of the heel and lateral malleolar branches that contribute to a network of vessels around the lateral malleolus. There is also a variable interosseous branch that passes through the hiatus between the tibia and fibula distal to the interosseous membrane and proximal to the interosseous tibiofibular ligament of the ankle. This interosseous branch anastomoses with arteries anterior to the ankle. Occasionally, if the fibular artery is large and the anterior tibial artery is small, the interosseous branch replaces the anterior tibial artery in forming the dorsalis pedis artery. In most cases there is also a small anastomotic branch connecting the fibular artery with the posterior tibial in the distal leg.

Vessels of Foot

The main arterial supply of the foot is from the posterior tibial artery (Fig. 8.9). This artery passes posterior to the medial malleolus deep to the flexor retinaculum. It divides into medial and lateral planter arteries deep to the abductor hallucis muscle. The medial plantar artery, which is usually smaller than the lateral plantar, passes in the foot just deep to the abductor hallucis muscle between that muscle and the deeper-lying flexor digitorum brevis muscle. The medial side of the big toe is supplied by a consistent branch of this artery. There are cutaneous, muscular, and articular branches of the medial planter, and it usually gives rise to three superficial digital branches, which are usually joined by the medial three plantar metatarsal arteries. The medial plantar artery is accompanied by the artery of the same name on its lateral side.

The lateral plantar artery is usually substantially larger than the medial plantar artery. It originates on the medial side of the proximal foot and travels anterolaterally, deep to the flexor digitorum brevis and superficial to the quadratus plantae (flexor accessorius) muscle, as it progresses distally along the sole of the foot. Ultimately, it reaches a position between the flexor digitorum brevis and the abductor digiti minimi. Near the base of the fifth metatarsal, it turns medially contributing to the plantar arch, which has its major contribution

from the deep plantar branch of the dorsalis pedis artery. Prior to joining the deep plantar arch, the lateral plantar artery gives off calcaneal, muscular, and cutaneous branches.

The dorsalis pedis artery (Fig. 8.9) is usually the continuation of the anterior tibial artery. It arises at a point midway between the malleoli deep to the inferior extensor retinaculum. The origin of the extensor hallucis brevis muscle crosses and covers the initial part of this artery. It successively crosses the head of the talus, the navicular (which is a good landmark for palpation), and the intermediate cuneiform bones. It typically can be found between the extensor hallucis longus tendon and the extensor digitorum longus muscle. It ends after entering the upper part of the space between the first and second metatarsals by dividing into a metatarsal artery and then continues toward the space between the first and second toes and a deep plantar artery that passes between the first and second metatarsal to form the deep plantar arch. On the dorsum of the foot, the deep fibular nerve is immediately lateral to the dorsalis pedis artery.

The deep plantar branch of the dorsalis pedis artery forms the deep plantar arch, which is located deeply in the sole of the foot. The arch lies between the oblique head of the adductor hallucis muscle, which is part of the third layer of muscles of the sole of the foot and the interossei muscles, which comprise the fourth (deepest) layer of muscles. The deep plantar arch is usually completed by anastomosis with the terminal part of the lateral plantar artery near the medial aspect of the base of the fifth metatarsal. The deep branch of the lateral plantar nerve accompanies the arterial arch in the foot. The second, third, and fourth plantar metatarsal arteries are branches from the deep plantar arch and run toward the toes on the plantar aspect of the interossei muscles. Each of them divides into plantar digital arteries for adjacent aspects of successive toes. There is a single branch from the plantar arch that supplies the lateral side of the little toe. There are connections between the dorsal metatarsal arteries and the plantar metatarsal arteries via perforating branches.

The plantar arch (Fig. 8.9) gives rise to four plantar metatarsal arteries, the first of which arises just as the lateral plantar artery joins the dorsalis pedis in forming the plantar arch. The arch supplies plantar digital branches to the medial side of the big toe (anastomosing with the medial plantar artery) and to the adjacent sides of the first and second toes.

Angiosomes

The concept of angiosomes arose from anatomical investigations of the origin of the cutaneous vascular supply. In 1987, Taylor and Palmer used an injection technique on fresh cadavers to define the distribution of blood vessels to the skin and underlying tissues [1]. They found that the main feeding arteries to a region of skin also supply the underlying connective tissue and muscle tissue such that its distribution forms a three-dimensional network of arteries and veins. This organization they called an "angiosome." They also reported that adjacent angiosomes were connected by small arteries and arterioles that they termed "choke arteries."

Although they viewed the immediate ramification of their work as demonstrating the large number of potential skin flaps that might be used in reconstructive surgery, this concept has become heavily discussed and debated in revascularization since it implies that the vasculature of each angiosome must be attended to if tissue is to be preserved. However, it must be kept in mind that the original work did not assess the adequacy of potential collateral circulation through these "choke arteries" other than saying that many of these interconnections appeared to be through "spent terminal branches." Therefore, at this point in time, the angiosome concept is most controversial in terms of its implications for revascularization and is most discussed in terms of the circulation of the distal lower limbs. Additionally, angiosomes are most frequently discussed in the literature relating to diabetic vascular complication presumably because of compromise of whatever "choke arteries" might contribute to collateral supply from adjacent angiosomes.

In their original work, Taylor and Palmer [1] found that the skin and underlying tissues of the body are divisible into an average of 374 such regions, each supplied by a single source artery. They defined the foot and ankle as having five angiosomes (Fig. 8.10), including one each for the dorsalis pedis, medial plantar, and lateral plantar arteries and one each for the calcaneal branches of the posterior tibial artery and peroneal (fibular) artery (on the medial and lateral aspects of the heel, respectively). The leg was reported to have three angiosomes, one each for the anterior tibial, posterior tibial, and peroneal (fibular) artery. Several additional angiosomes have been suggested in the region of the ankle, including one at the anterior ankle from a branch of the anterior tibial artery and one on the anterolateral ankle arising from the peroneal (fibular) artery (see Attinger et al.[2]). Interestingly, these investigators also described the in vivo analysis of these angiosomes using Doppler ultrasound analysis.

There have been several recent systematic reviews and critical analyses of the clinical utility of angiosome-based revascularization versus more indirect revascularization procedures [3–5], and such analysis is beyond the scope of this chapter. However, there is strong anatomical evidence for distinct origins of vessels to defined cutaneous and subjacent subcutaneous tissues, termed "angiosomes," along with more tenuous interconnection between these adjacent regions.

Veins of the Lower Limb

The veins of the lower limb are divided into superficial and deep systems, similar to the two systems in the upper limb. However, in the lower limb, the majority of blood is returned through the deep venous system.

Superficial Veins

The superficial venous system (Fig. 8.2) resides in the superficial fascia of the lower limb. It has numerous valves that only allow unidirectional flow centrally, since the force of gravity on the blood column must be resisted and since these veins are not surrounded by compressing structures such as limb muscles. The superficial system of veins begins distally on the dorsal aspect of the toes as dorsal digital veins that mostly unite to form dorsal metacarpal veins. These are located between the metacarpals and end in a dorsal venous arch that is quite superficial and crosses the dorsal aspect of the metacarpals near their heads. This arch is part of a network of veins on the dorsum of the foot that receives communications from the plantar venous arch of the sole of the foot. The plantar arch receives plantar digital veins. The medial aspect of the dorsal venous arch continues as the great (large) saphenous vein traveling anterior to the medial

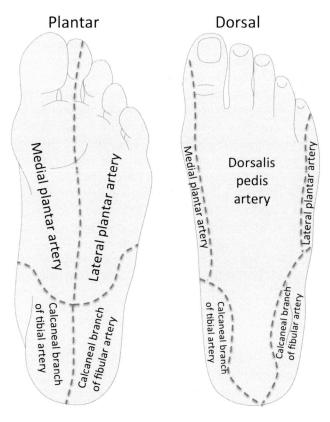

Fig. 8.10 An approximate representation of the original angiosomes of the foot as defined by Taylor and Palmer [1]

malleolus. Laterally the dorsal venous arch joins the lesser (small) saphenous vein.

The great saphenous vein, accompanied by the saphenous nerve, crosses the medial surface of the tibia from anterior to posterior in its course through the leg. More proximally in the leg, it is posterior to the medial border of the tibia and passes posterior to the medial femoral condyle, where it is closely related to the saphenous branch of the descending genicular artery.

It is located medially through most of the thigh, assuming a more anterior position over the upper part of the femoral triangle in the upper thigh. Its course can be approximated by a line connecting the adductor tubercle of the femur with the saphenous hiatus, the gap in the fascia lata through which the great saphenous vein passes to join the femoral vein. The center of this hiatus is about 4 cm inferolateral to the pubic tubercle. At the saphenous hiatus, the great saphenous vein pierces the cribriform fascia covering the hiatus. The great saphenous vein then pierces the anterior aspect of the femoral sheath to join the femoral vein.

There are a great number of unnamed tributaries of the great saphenous vein. These include perforating (communicating) veins that will be described below. In addition and despite a high degree of variability, there are several named vessels. In the proximal leg just below the knee, there is a posterior arch vein and anterior vein of the leg. In the thigh there are posterior medial (accessory saphenous vein) and anterior lateral veins that drain into the great saphenous vein at or near the saphenous hiatus. Near its termination in the femoral vein, the great saphenous is joined by the superficial circumflex iliac, superficial epigastric, and superficial external pudendal veins. These may either enter separately or, quite often, the superficial epigastric and superficial iliac circumflex vessels join prior to entering the great saphenous as a common trunk. The superficial epigastric vein anastomoses with tributaries of the lateral thoracic vein, an arrangement called the thoraco-epigastric vein. This collateral venous channel becomes dilated and important following obstruction of the superior or inferior vena cava.

The lesser (small) saphenous vein is continuous with the lateral end of the dorsal venous arch posterior to the lateral malleolus. It follows the lateral aspect of the Achilles tendon, continuing proximally in the superficial fascia over the gastrocnemius muscle along with the sural nerve. It pierces the deep fascia between the heads of the gastrocnemius muscle, entering the popliteal fossa. In more than half the cases it joins the popliteal vein. It can also end in deep veins in the lower thigh or join the great saphenous vein below the knee. Occasionally, it can end in muscular veins draining the gastrocnemius muscle. There are usually anastomoses with the great saphenous vein with blood flowing from the lesser to the great saphenous vein. In its course it has several valves (usually less than 10).

Deep Veins

Most blood in the lower limb is drained by deep veins. There are many connections between veins that permit drainage even with obstruction and ligation of major veins, including the femoral vein.

Distally up to the level of the popliteal vein, the deep venous system appears as venae comitantes encased in a common connective tissue sheath surrounding the arteries, including the anterior tibial, posterior tibial, and fibular (peroneal) arteries and their branches. The venae comitantes of the posterior tibial vein drain most of the blood from the plantar venous arch. They also receive the venae comitantes of the fibular (peroneal) arteries. These veins have many valves. Below the knee, the valves usually appear every few centimeters or so. It is noteworthy that the soleus muscle contains large venous sinuses lacking valves.

The popliteal vein (usually single) is formed by the union of the deep veins that are the venae comitantes of the anterior and posterior tibial arteries. This vein is tightly encased in a connective tissue sheath along with the popliteal artery. The vein crosses from posteromedial to the artery in the inferior part of the popliteal fossa, to a position posterolateral to the artery in the superior part of the fossa. The tibial nerve is lateral to the vein. In the superior aspect of the fossa, the vein is interposed between the artery and the more superficial nerve. The popliteal veins have several valves in their short course through the popliteal fossa. Tributaries include those corresponding to popliteal artery branches as well as (in most cases) the small saphenous vein. The popliteal vein (or veins) ends by passing through the adductor hiatus in the distal insertion of the adductor magnus muscle, becoming the femoral vein (or veins).

The femoral vein is often double in its lower extent. It accompanies the artery in the adductor canal lying posterolateral and then posterior to the artery. As it passes proximally through the femoral triangle, it becomes more medial, to assume its position in the femoral sheath. The main tributaries include the deep femoral (profunda femoris) vein, the medial and lateral circumflex veins, and the great saphenous vein. The femoral vein has a few valves, and usually there is no valve between the femoral vein and the right atrium of the heart.

The femoral vein becomes the external iliac vein as it passes deep to the inguinal ligament. This joins with the internal iliac (hypogastric) vein posterior to its corresponding artery, with tributaries corresponding mostly with the branches of the artery. It is noteworthy that this is the drainage of the superior and inferior gluteal veins, which are usually double. These veins communicate with tributaries of the femoral vein and can provide an important route for return of blood from the lower limb when flow is restricted in the femoral vein.

Perforating (Communicating) Veins

There are many perforating (communicating) veins that connect the superficial and deep venous systems of the lower limbs. The valves in these perforating veins permit blood to flow only from the superficial to deep veins. There are direct and indirect perforating veins. Direct perforating veins directly interconnect a superficial vein to one of the deep veins accompanying the arteries. These are more consistent with a major one in the thigh and another in the leg. There are several at the level of the ankle. Each of these perforating veins has a valve at its origin in the superficial vein and one at the end attached to the deep vein. Indirect perforating veins connect the superficial veins and muscular veins. The muscular veins then drain into the deep veins. These indirect connections are numerous, quite small, and inconsistent.

Venous Return

Up to 90 % of the blood of the lower limbs is returned through the deep venous system. The integrity of valves directing flow proximally and from the superficial to the deep system assures that blood flows in the proper direction.

Muscular action is a major factor driving venous return by providing external compressive force on the veins. This can be quite detrimentally affected by standing still.

Incompetence of the valves of the superficial veins results in dilated, tortuous (varicose) veins. Since the venous return in the superficial veins can easily be handled by the deep veins, the superficial veins can be obliterated without consequence to venous return.

References

1. Taylor GI, Palmer JH. The vascular territories (angiosomes) of the body: experimental study and clinical applications. Br J Plast Surg. 1987;40:113–41.
2. Attinger CE, Evans KK, Bulan E, Blume P, Cooper P. Angiosomes of the foot and ankle and clinical implications for limb salvage: reconstruction, incisions, and revascularization. Plast Reconst Surg. 2006;117(7 Suppl):261S–93.
3. Alexandrescu V, Söderström M, Venermo M. Angiosome theory: fact or fiction? Scand J Surg. 2012;101:125–31.
4. Sumpio BE, Forsythe RO, Kenneth R, Ziegler KR, van Baal JG, Lepantalo MJA, Hinchliffe RJ. Clinical implications of the angiosome model in peripheral vascular disease. J Vasc Surg. 2013; 58:814–26.
5. Biancari F, Juvonen T. Angiosome-targeted lower limb revascularization for ischemic foot wounds: systematic review and meta-analysis. Eur J Vasc Endovasc Surg. 2014;47:517–22.

Overlap of Atherosclerotic Disease

Natalie Gwilliam and Ross Milner

Introduction

The importance of identifying overlap disease aids not only in perioperative management but may explain the long-term success or failure of operative interventions. Arterial disease represents a systemic process; thus, isolated interventions may benefit regional symptoms but do not change the overall prognosis for patients. Mitigating these systemic risk factors would logically not only improve perioperative morbidity and mortality but also long-term survival.

Follow-up data from the REACH registry at 3 years demonstrated, similar to the 1-year follow-up, that patients with multivessel disease had nearly double the event rates (MI, vascular death, rehospitalization) compared to those with single disease (40.5 % vs 25.5 %) [1, 2]. Progression from uni- to poly-vascular disease varies based upon the initial location of disease. Not only progression to poly-vascular disease but event rates also vary based upon the primary vascular bed with PAD carrying the worst prognosis for both progression to multivessel disease and event rate [1].

CAD

Coronary artery disease (CAD) manifests as angina and may culminate as a myocardial infarction (MI) or progress to heart failure (HF). It may also be silent. It is estimated that in the USA alone, 620,000 people will have a new coronary attack, another 295,000 will have a recurrent attack, and 150,000 will have a silent event in 2014. Fatalities from

these events account for one out of every six deaths in the USA. This is despite a 39.2 % decrease in the number of deaths attributable to CAD from 2000 to 2010 [3].

Peripheral arterial diseases (PADs) of interest in relationship to CAD include lower extremity arterial disease (LEAD), renal artery stenosis (RAS), and carotid artery stenosis (CAS). Data out of the Cleveland Clinic in the 1980s indicated that patients with a primary diagnosis of PAD of any region carried a 21–41 % incidence of concomitant CAD [4]. Three decades later, a Japanese study of patients undergoing non-emergent CAG for suspicion of CAD found a similar incidence with 24 % of patients having one or more additional beds of disease (2 % CAS and RAS; 3 % CAS and PAD; 3.5 % RAS and PAD; 0.8 % CAS, RAS, PAD) [5].

The incidence of lower extremity arterial disease (LEAD) in CAD patients ranges from 10 to 40 %. Some lower estimates come from studies that use intermittent claudication (IC) as a surrogate for LEAD and thus underreport its prevalence [6–8]. Prevalence also depends on the geographical or ethnic population studied. The aforementioned Japanese study found that of patients undergoing CAG, 16 % had concomitant LEAD [5]. In a cross-sectional study of patients presenting to primary care physicians in France, over a quarter (26.6 %) of patients with CAD had undiagnosed LEAD based on ABIs [9]. At the higher end of the spectrum, Dieter et al. reported 40 % prevalence of PAD in patients hospitalized for stable CAD. The fact that a higher percentage of CAD patients ill enough for hospitalization have PAD is consistent with findings that PAD correlates with higher morbidity and mortality for CAD patients [10].

The coexistence of LEAD in CAD patients is associated with worse prognosis. This has been born out in multiple studies including REACH, GRACE, CASS, and PAMISCA [1, 11–14]. LEAD roughly doubles the morbidity and mortality for CAD patients. This is true for both symptomatic and asymptomatic CAD and symptomatic and asymptomatic LEAD and post-intervention [1, 14–17]. Furthermore, the presence of LEAD can predict the severity of CAD. A study of African-Americans undergoing cardiac catheterization

N. Gwilliam, MD
General Surgery, University of Chicago, Chicago, IL, USA

R. Milner, MD (✉)
Vascular Surgery, Center for Aortic Diseases,
University of Chicago, 5841 S. Maryland Ave.,
MC5028, Chicago, IL 60637, USA

© Springer International Publishing Switzerland 2017
R.S. Dieter et al. (eds.), *Critical Limb Ischemia*, DOI 10.1007/978-3-319-31991-9_9

with simultaneous ABIs found that 90 % of patients with ABI < 0.9 had CAD on angiography. Of those patients found to have severe CAD (three vessel or left main), 86 % had LEAD [18]. This study reinforces findings from larger, historical studies such as the Cardiovascular Health Study that demonstrated associations between ABI, MI, CHF, and angina [19].

The association between renal artery stenosis (RAS) and increased prevalence, severity, and mortality of CAD is well established [20–22]. Previous reports of renal artery stenosis (RAS) in patients with known CAD ranged from 22 to 89 % [23, 24]. These figures are significantly higher than recent studies which assess patients undergoing CAG to study prevalence of RAS in CAD. These studies report a range from 9 to 23 % RAS during CAG [5, 25–28]. In an Austrian study evaluating RAS in patients undergoing CAG, there was an overall rate of 10.7 % RAS, with 2.3 % demonstrating bilateral RAS, defined as ≥50 % luminal narrowing [26]. However, this study did not define what percentage of these patients demonstrated significant CAD. Based upon the authors' models, they did find that increasing numbers of stenotic coronary segments correlated with increased RAS frequency [26]. A Japanese study of similar design also found only 9 % prevalence [5] and a Korean study 9.4 % [29]. The Korean study reported only 26 % CAD in the entire cohort but did find CAD to be a statistically significant predictor of RAS with an odds ratio of 5.6 [29]. In a French study using CAG in patients with known CAD, a higher percentage (14.5 %) had significant unilateral disease of whom 3.1 % had bilateral disease [21]. A Polish study reiterated these findings with RAS ≥ 50 % found in 6 % of patients with one-vessel, 11 % with two-vessel, and 13.2 % in three-vessel CAD [30]. These studies also confirmed the correlation between the number of significant coronary lesions and RAS. Clinical interest in this relationship involves medical management of comorbid HTN. Pharmacological management of CHF and HTN must taken into account, primarily the need for an ACE inhibitor or ARB which may worsen renal function in bilateral renal artery stenosis.

Interest in overlap of CAS in known CAD has primarily been focused on perioperative screening and optimization to prevent incidence of stroke [15]. As a result, prevalence data comes from studies assessing CAS at the time of CAG as part of a preoperative workup. Estimates of CAS in patients with CAD range from 7 to 89 %, depending on imaging modalities and definitions of CAS [31]. For CAS defined as ≥70 % stenosis on ultrasound, there was 10.2 % prevalence. Rate of CAS increased with number of diseased coronary vessels: 1.3 % for one, 5.8 % for two, and 19 % for three vessels [31]. This is similar to older data defining stenosis as >75 % with an 8.7 % prevalence of CAS [32]. A Japanese study evaluated a population by ultrasound and angiography. Rates of CAS defined as >50 % on ultrasound by a number of diseased coro-

nary vessels (one, two, three) were 14.5 %, 21.4 %, and 36 %, respectively. When evaluated angiographically with CAS defined as >70 % luminal stenosis, these numbers decreased significantly to 3.4 %, 7.5 %, and 19.4 % [33]. A British study evaluating stress echo (SE) in new onset chest pain found that carotid intima-media thickness (CIMT) as a measure of CAS had better PPV for CAD than clinical stratification, and the addition of CIMT to SE improved the PPV of CAD from 56 to 70 %. Thirty-seven patients demonstrated CAD on CAG, of whom 33 had CAS based on CIMT (89 %) [34]. The disparity in prevalence between this and previous studies reflects different imaging modalities and definitions of CAS. However, as interest and use of CIMT increases, it will be important to understand how it relates to definitions based on percent stenosis and angiography.

LEAD

LEAD affects 3–10 % of the general population with rates rising with age, up to 12–22 % in those greater than 70, and twice as common in diabetics [35–38]. In the USA, rates increase in non-Hispanic blacks and Mexican Americans but are equivalent among non-Hispanic whites, Hispanics, and Asians [36, 39]. These numbers are relatively consistent in studies from multiple European and North American countries including the USA, England, Holland, Germany, and Italy [7, 38, 40–44]. As mentioned, LEAD, particularly symptomatic disease, correlates with two- to eightfold increase in cardiovascular events, including fatalities [1, 11–14]. Annual rate of death from combined CV etiologies (MI, CVA, vascular death) is 5–7 %, with rates corresponding to symptoms, severity, and a number of affected vascular beds [35, 42, 45]. Similar incidence rates were found in the Peripheral Arteriopathy and Cardiovascular Events (PACE) study, in which Brevetti et al. reported after 24 months of follow-up, 25 % of patients had a nonfatal CV event while 15 % of PAD patients died, 8 % from CV disease. PAD was associated with RR 4.03 for all-cause mortality, RR 7.77 for CV mortality, and RR 3.11 nonfatal CV [40].

Identifying those suffering from LEAD and, therefore, those at greater risk for CV complications, is not straightforward. At least two thirds of those with LEAD (ABI ≤ 0.9) are asymptomatic. Studies reporting only symptomatic LEAD represent more severe disease and thus worse outcomes. Early studies, such as the Whitehall study, had to rely on symptoms to diagnose disease and establish correlation between LEAD and mortality [44]. Later studies investigated both symptomatic and asymptomatic disease. In the Rotterdam study, out of 7715 males and females >55, there was a 19.1 % prevalence of PAD but only 6.3 % reported intermittent claudication (IC) [43]. Meijer et al. also found patients with PAD had an increased incidence of LVH, common carotid IMT, carotid plaques, and larger distal aortic diameter [43]. An Italian cross-sectional study of primary care patients 40–80 years old (4352 pts) demonstrated symptomatic LEAD in 1.6 % (0–6.4 % by sex and decade). Of those with LEAD, 34 % had CVD, 32 % had CAD, 12 % had previous MI, and 5 % had a previous stroke. In comparison, among controls for sex and age, only 11 % had CVD and 9 % CAD [7]. Other studies report higher rates ranging from 40 to 90 % for CAD and CVD and 50 % for CAS [35, 41, 46].

Incidence of RAS among LEAD patients varies by definition (>50 %, >60 %, >70 % stenosis) and means of identification (ultrasonography, arteriography, CT, MRI). Rates range from 9 to 60 % [5, 15, 24, 35, 43, 47–49]. For example, a single study found a 44.9 % overall rate for RS, but 17.3 % had mild disease, 15.7 % severe disease, and 11.8 % bilateral, where the severity of LEAD positively correlated with incidence of RAS [50]. A similar relationship was found in Japanese cohorts by Imori et al. [5]. They found LEAD to be an independent predictor of RAS in a Japanese population with an overall rate of 21 %. In a separate Japanese study, Endo et al. found 22.9 % had RAS >50 % and 11 % had RAS >75 %, demonstrating a positive correlation between RAS ≥ 50 % and critical limb ischemia (CLI) (HR 2.519) [48]. More proximal PAD also carries a higher prevalence of RAS, with 50 % of patients with aortic, bilateral iliac, femoral, and distal vessel disease having RAS [49].

Cerebrovascular disease is present in almost a quarter of patients with PAD. Incidence of CAS >50 % ranges from 25 to 33 %, while significant CAS >70 % ranges from 14 to 25 % [5, 46, 51, 52]. The shared pathophysiology of atherosclerosis explains the close link between PAD and CAS. In fact, an ABI <0.8 has been found to be an independent risk factor for CAS [51]. Furthermore, the presence of PAD is even a stronger predictor of CAS than CAD, AAA, and CBVD symptoms or carotid bruits [46]. As previously discussed, the presence of LEAD in addition to when ABI is used to predict stroke, the specificity is 92 % though sensitivity is low at 16 % with a likelihood ratio of 2.45 (95 % CI, 1.76–3.41) [53]. Adding ABI to the Framingham Risk Score (FRS) is an alternate means for predicting cardiovascular events and improved the overall performance of a risk calculator [54].

RAS

Prevalence of RAS varies by study from 4 to 18.4 % in the general public [55]. The majority will be unilateral with 12 % of cases bilateral in one study of people >65 years [56]. RAS may be due to atherosclerotic disease, fibromuscular dysplasia, or external compression of the vessels. Manifestations include onset and/or acceleration of renal failure, flash pulmonary edema, and difficult-to-control hypertension. Understanding the etiology of RAS, including

uni- vs bilaterality, alters treatment and ultimately outcome. When assessing overlap disease in other vascular beds, RAS relates in two ways. First, RAS may share an atherosclerotic etiology. Second, RAS may serve as the etiology of vascular bed disease. The second relationship is proposed to occur through activation of the RAAS pathway, though any of the numerous hormonal or metabolic pathways intimately associated with the kidneys may play a role [57, 58]. As eloquently discussed by Hostetter, the mechanism of action—and directionality—linking renal failure with cardiovascular disease is yet to be fully elucidated, but the renal vascular bed might actually serve as a canary in the coal mine for systemic vascular health [58]. Early recognition of renal demise allows for early intervention and prevention of progressive systemic vascular disease.

HTN is the most readily recognized symptom of RAS. Outside of essential HTN (EH), RAS is the most common cause of high blood pressure. RAS accounts for 12–27.8 % of patients with HTN [59]. Identifying patients with HTN due to RAS is important because mortality is increased by 23 % versus the general population and 7 % versus EH [60]. Related, there is also increased left ventricular hypertrophy (79 % vs 46 %) [15, 61–63]. Up to 54 % of patients with HF (EF <40 %) will have >50 % RAS, including those with preserved renal function [59]. These patients should be managed differently, as use of ACE inhibitors risks AKI [60]. Alternatively, procedure interventions with stenting were initially thought to decrease MAPs and LVH more than medications [64–66]. However, more recent trials such as CORAL found optimal medical therapy to be equivalent to stenting in regard to blood pressure and mortality [67, 68]. What is clear is that appropriate identification and management of RAS-HTN alters outcome for renal and systemic vascular beds [64]. Comparing to the general population, there are 194.5 adverse events per 1000 patient-years related to CHF compared to 56.3 in the general population [69].

CAD has an increased prevalence and severity among those with RAS [64–68, 70]. Rossi et al. found 58 % of patients with RAS >50 % had clinical evidence of CAD [71]. Multiple studies demonstrate a positive correlation between a number of atherosclerotic coronary arteries and RAS, with Safak et al. finding the following: 11.9 % RAS with one vessel, 25.3 % with two vessels, and 42.7 % with three vessels [59, 71–74]. Severity of CAD also correlates with RAS [26, 73]. Even when controlling for risk factors, RAS maintains an independent association with CAD [55]. Almost three fourths of RAS patients have clinical or subclinical symptoms, including angina [55]. With long-term follow-up at 10 years, more than a third of patients will have an AMI [72].

ESRD from RAS has been demonstrated to have even worse outcomes than ESRD from alternate etiologies. Fatica et al. found RAS-ESRD to have significantly higher rates of CAD (51 % vs 23 %), CVD (18 % vs 9 %), occlusive PAD

(44% vs 14%), HTN (75% vs 71%), CHF (47% vs 29%), and MI (21% vs 9%) [57]. The argument that these differences are the result of increased incidence of HTN—the most clinically recognizable effect of RAS—is less likely than a shared etiology of vascular disease. As noted above, RAS is an independent predictor of mortality compared to EH.

Up to 72.3% of RAS will have clinical and subclinical evidence of CVD, including increased prevalence of ICA stenosis and CIMT [55]. This increases to 83% if there is presence of HTN, compared to 43% for EH in one Japanese autopsy study [73]. Similar to CAD, severity of RAS correlates with severity of carotid disease [71, 74]. Symptomatic disease is also increased, with 175.5 CVA/TIA events for RAS vs 52.9 in the general population per 1000 patient-years [69]. During long-term follow-up, 5% of patients with RAS will suffer a stroke which increases to 18% for RAS-ESRD [57, 72].

PAD in any bed is found in 26–50% of those with RAS [49, 75–78]. One study found up to three fourths of patients with moderate to severe RAS have PAD, defined as ABI <0.95 [79]. Zierler et al. found a similar incidence of disease, with 41% mild LEAD (ABI <0.95), 38% moderate LEAD (ABI 0.5–0.95), and 21% severe LEAD (ABI <0.5) [74]. Of patients with severe RAS (≥60% bilateral or occluded unilateral), 66% had moderate to severe LEAD [74]. As discussed earlier, severity of RAS correlates with LEAD severity.

Mesenteric Artery Ischemia

Diagnosis of mesenteric artery disease is clinically challenging. Presence of mesenteric atherosclerosis is rarely clinically detected until two vessels are severely stenosed or even occluded due to the highly collateralized vasculature. One study found that in 18% of the general population >65, significant stenosis of the celiac artery or SMA is present without symptoms [80]. If symptoms are present, it is typically chronic mesenteric ischemia (CMI) with postprandial abdominal angina. Mesenteric atherosclerosis can present acutely and accounts for 25–30% of acute mesenteric ischemia cases [81]. As a result, mesenteric disease is important to identify but is typically silent and must be sought out based on comorbidities rather than primary symptoms.

Accurate prevalence estimates in the general population are challenging and range from 6 to 10% in older autopsy studies, 14–24% based on arteriography, and 17–18% on recent ultrasonographic studies [56, 80, 82]. Among patients with known atherosclerotic disease, reports range from 8 to 70% [80, 83–85]. Of patients undergoing elective surgical intervention for CMI, 85% are found to have coexistent arterial disease in other beds [86]. The rate for LEAD in this population was 78% [86]. CAD is present in 33–58% with CHF in 25% [86–89]. Atkins et al. found CAS in 13% of patients undergoing endovascular intervention versus 29% of open repairs [90].

AAA

Aortic abdominal aneurysms are increasing in incidence globally with the exception of Western Europe, where morbidity and mortality have been decreasing since the 1990s [91, 92]. Prevalence is related to increasing age, male sex, and smoking. For small AAAs, 2.9–4.9 cm in diameter, prevalence ranges from 1.3 to 12.5% in men and 0–5.2% in women, with increasing incidence in older cohorts [91]. Risk factors overlap between the two forms of atherosclerosis but biochemical marks and epidemiology are distinct [93]. Though grouped under atherosclerotic disease, the pathophysiology of AAA appears distinct from occlusive atherosclerosis. One group out of Norway found no correlation between size of AAA and atherosclerosis of other beds which may suggest that occlusive atherosclerosis and AAA are parallel rather than sequential processes [94].

Globally, CAD ranges from 25 to 60% in patients with AAA [4, 95–98]. An Italian study reported the incidence of CAD as 25% in AAA patients qualifying for surgery (AAA >4.5 cm) [93]. Of patients undergoing surgery for AAA, a study found serious cardiac events associated with 32% of operations and severe events with 24% [99]. Within the subgroup of AAA with CAD, 33–43% will have severe CAD amenable to operative intervention [100, 101].

Additional affected beds include the renal and mesenteric arteries. RAS >50% occurs in 22–38% [102]. A more recent report found 23.9% of patients with AAA had more severe RAS >75% [103]. In a meta-analysis of AAA and RAS, the pooled prevalence was 33.1%, demonstrating consistent finding across time and methods [59]. Mesenteric arterial stenosis occurs at a slightly higher rate of 40% [102]. CAS occurred in 27% of men with AAA though in a study directly comparing rates of CAS between AAA and CAD patients, CAS in AAA was only 9% [93, 104].

CAS

CAS accounts for approximately 20% of ischemic cerebral vascular accidents with a mortality rate of 10–30% [15]. For those who survive, they face an ever-increasing risk of recurrent cerebral events due to both progressive disease and age. Even asymptomatic patients with >60% stenosis have a 16% risk of stroke over 5 years [105]. As is obvious at this point, atherosclerotic disease in one bed correlates with increased rates in other regions resulting in increased morbidity and mortality, particularly cardiac pathologies. For CAS, the concomitant incidence of CAD is from 28 to 32% [106]. The incidence of LEAD is 43% and RAS 31% in a Japanese study [5]. Interestingly, patients with CAS and PAD had higher rates of stokes, MI, and death of cardiovascular etiology than those with CAS and CAD [107]. Nearly a quarter of those with TIA/stroke and symptomatic PAD were hospitalized or had another vascular event within 1 year [107].

References

1. Alberts MJ, et al. Three-year follow-up and event rates in the international REduction of Atherothrombosis for Continued Health Registry. Eur Heart J. 2009;30(19):2318–26. doi:10.1093/eurheartj/ehp355.

2. Steg P, Bhatt DL, Wilson PF, et al. One-year cardiovascular event rates in outpatients with atherothrombosis. JAMA. 2007;297:1197–206.

3. Ripa RS, Kjaer A, Hesse B. Non-invasive imaging for subclinical coronary atherosclerosis in patients with peripheral artery disease. Curr Atheroscler Rep. 2014;16:1–8.

4. Hertzer NR, et al. Coronary artery disease in peripheral vascular patients. A classification of 1000 coronary angiograms and results of surgical management. Ann Surg. 1984;199:223.

5. Imori Y, et al. Co-existence of carotid artery disease, renal artery stenosis, and lower extremity peripheral arterial disease in patients with coronary artery disease. Am J Cardiol. 2014;113:30–5.

6. Criqui MH. Peripheral arterial disease—epidemiological aspects. Vasc Med. 2001;6:3–7.

7. Brevetti G, Oliva G, Silvestro A, Scopacasa F, Chiariello M. Prevalence, risk factors and cardiovascular comorbidity of symptomatic peripheral arterial disease in Italy. Atherosclerosis. 2004;175:131–8.

8. Hirsch AT, Hiatt WR & PARTNERS Steering Committee. PAD awareness, risk, and treatment: new resources for survival—the USA PARTNERS program. Vasc Med. 2001;6:9–12.

9. Kownator S, et al. Prevalence of unknown peripheral arterial disease in patients with coronary artery disease: data in primary care from the IPSILON study. Arch Cardiovasc Dis. 2009;102:625–31.

10. Dieter RS, et al. Lower extremity peripheral arterial disease in hospitalized patients with coronary artery disease. Vasc Med. 2003;8:233–6.

11. Ohman EM, et al. The REduction of Atherothrombosis for Continued Health (REACH) Registry: an international, prospective, observational investigation in subjects at risk for atherothrombotic events-study design. Am Heart J. 2006;151:786–e1.

12. Bertomeu V, et al. Prevalence and prognostic influence of peripheral arterial disease in patients ≥40 years old admitted into hospital following an acute coronary event. Eur J Vasc Endovasc Surg. 2008;36:189–96.

13. Mukherjee D, et al. Impact of prior peripheral arterial disease and stroke on outcomes of acute coronary syndromes and effect of evidence-based therapies (from the Global Registry of Acute Coronary Events). Am J Cardiol. 2007;100:1–6.

14. Eagle KA, Rihal CS, Foster ED, Mickel MC, Gersh BJ. Long-term survival in patients with coronary artery disease: importance of peripheral vascular disease. J Am Coll Cardiol. 1994;23:1091–5.

15. Tendera M, et al. ESC guidelines on the diagnosis and treatment of peripheral artery diseases document covering atherosclerotic disease of extracranial carotid and vertebral, mesenteric, renal, upper and lower extremity arteries: the Task Force on the Diagnosis and Treatment of Peripheral Artery Diseases of the European Society of Cardiology (ESC). Eur Heart J. 2011;32:2851–906.

16. Saw J, et al. The influence of peripheral arterial disease on outcomes: a pooled analysis of mortality in eight large randomized percutaneous coronary intervention trials. J Am Coll Cardiol. 2006;48:1567–72.

17. Parikh SV, et al. Risk of death and myocardial infarction in patients with peripheral arterial disease undergoing percutaneous coronary intervention (from the National Heart, Lung and Blood Institute Dynamic Registry). Am J Cardiol. 2011;107:959–64.

18. Otah KE, et al. Usefulness of an abnormal ankle-brachial index to predict presence of coronary artery disease in African-Americans. Am J Cardiol. 2004;93:481–3.

19. Newman AB, et al. Ankle-arm index as a marker of atherosclerosis in the Cardiovascular Health Study. Cardiovascular Heart Study (CHS) Collaborative Research Group. Circulation. 1993;88:837–45.

20. Conlon PJ, Little MA, Pieper K, Mark DB. Severity of renal vascular disease predicts mortality in patients undergoing coronary angiography. Kidney Int. 2001;60:1490–7.

21. Ollivier R, et al. Frequency and predictors of renal artery stenosis in patients with coronary artery disease. Cardiovasc Revasc Med. 2009;10:23–9.

22. Amighi J, et al. Renal artery stenosis predicts adverse cardiovascular and renal outcome in patients with peripheral artery disease. Eur J Clin Invest. 2009;39:784–92.

23. Crowley JJ, et al. Progression of renal artery stenosis in patients undergoing cardiac catheterization. Am Heart J. 1998;136:913–8.

24. Jean WJ, et al. High incidence of renal artery stenosis in patients with coronary artery disease. Cathet Cardiovasc Diagn. 1994;32:8–10.

25. White CJ, et al. Indications for renal arteriography at the time of coronary arteriography: a science advisory from the American Heart Association Committee on Diagnostic and Interventional Cardiac Catheterization, Council on Clinical Cardiology, and the Councils on Cardiovascular Radiology and Intervention and on Kidney in Cardiovascular Disease. Circulation. 2006;114:1892–5.

26. Weber-Mzell D, Kotanko P, Schumacher M, Klein W, Skrabal F. Coronary anatomy predicts presence or absence of renal artery stenosis. A prospective study in patients undergoing cardiac catheterization for suspected coronary artery disease. Eur Heart J. 2002;23:1684–91.

27. Rihal CS, et al. Incidental renal artery stenosis among a prospective cohort of hypertensive patients undergoing coronary angiography. Mayo Clin Proc. 2002;77:309–16.

28. Vetrovec GW, Landwehr DM, Edwards VL. Incidence of renal artery stenosis in hypertensive patients undergoing coronary angiography. J Interv Cardiol. 1989;2:69–76.

29. Lee Y, Shin J-H, Park H-C, Kim SG, Choi S. A prediction model for renal artery stenosis using carotid ultrasonography measurements in patients undergoing coronary angiography. BMC Nephrol. 2014;15:60.

30. Przewlocki T, et al. Prevalence and prediction of renal artery stenosis in patients with coronary and supraaortic artery atherosclerotic disease. Nephrol Dial Transplant. 2008;23:580–5.

31. Kablak-Ziembicka A, et al. Association of increased carotid intima-media thickness with the extent of coronary artery disease. Heart. 2004;90:1286–90.

32. Faggioli GL, Curl GR, Ricotta JJ. The role of carotid screening before coronary artery bypass. J Vasc Surg. 1990;12:724–31.

33. Tanimoto S, et al. Prevalence of carotid artery stenosis in patients with coronary artery disease in Japanese population. Stroke. 2005;36:2094–8.

34. Ahmadvazir S, Zacharias K, Shah BN, Pabla JS, Senior R. Role of simultaneous carotid ultrasound in patients undergoing stress echocardiography for assessment of chest pain with no previous history of coronary artery disease. Am Heart J. 2014;168:229–36.

35. Norgren L, et al. Inter-society consensus for the management of peripheral arterial disease (TASC II). Eur J Vasc Endovasc Surg. 2007;33:S1–75.

36. Gregg EW, et al. Prevalence of lower-extremity disease in the U.S. adult population ≥40 years of age with and without diabetes 1999–2000 national health and nutrition examination survey. Diabetes Care. 2004;27:1591–7.

37. Criqui MH, et al. The prevalence of peripheral arterial disease in a defined population. Circulation. 1985;71:510–5.

38. Diehm C, et al. High prevalence of peripheral arterial disease and co-morbidity in 6880 primary care patients: cross-sectional study. Atherosclerosis. 2004;172:95–105.

39. Criqui MH, et al. Ethnicity and peripheral arterial disease the San Diego population study. Circulation. 2005;112:2703–7.

40. Brevetti G, et al. Peripheral arterial disease and cardiovascular risk in Italy. Results of the Peripheral Arteriopathy and Cardiovascular Events (PACE) study. J Cardiovasc Med. 2006;7:608–13.

41. Van Kuijk J-P, et al. Long-term prognosis of patients with peripheral arterial disease with or without polyvascular atherosclerotic disease. Eur Heart J. 2010;31:992–9.

42. Murabito JM, D'Agostino RB, Silbershatz H, Wilson PWF. Intermittent claudication: a risk profile from the Framingham Heart Study. Circulation. 1997;96:44–9.

43. Meijer WT, et al. Peripheral arterial disease in the elderly: the Rotterdam study. Arterioscler Thromb Vasc Biol. 1998;18:185–92.

44. Smith GD, Shipley MJ, Rose G. Intermittent claudication, heart disease risk factors, and mortality. The Whitehall study. Circulation. 1990;82:1925–31.

45. Criqui MH, et al. Mortality over a period of 10 years in patients with peripheral arterial disease. N Engl J Med. 1992;326:381–6.

46. Golomb BA, Dang TT, Criqui MH. Peripheral arterial disease morbidity and mortality implications. Circulation. 2006;114:688–99.

47. Ozkan U, Oguzkurt L, Tercan F, Nursal TZ. The prevalence and clinical predictors of incidental atherosclerotic renal artery stenosis. Eur J Radiol. 2009;69:550–4.

48. Endo M, et al. Prevalence and risk factors for renal artery stenosis and chronic kidney disease in Japanese patients with peripheral arterial disease. Hypertens Res. 2010;33:911–5.

49. Metcalfe W, Reid AW, Geddes CC. Prevalence of angiographic atherosclerotic renal artery disease and its relationship to the anatomical extent of peripheral vascular atherosclerosis. Nephrol Dial Transplant. 1999;14:105–8.

50. Missouris CG, Buckenham T, Cappuccio FP, MacGregor GA. Renal artery stenosis: a common and important problem in patients with peripheral vascular disease. Am J Med. 1994;96:10–4.

51. Cinà CS, Safar HA, Maggisano R, Bailey R, Clase CM. Prevalence and progression of internal carotid artery stenosis in patients with peripheral arterial occlusive disease. J Vasc Surg. 2002;36:75–82.

52. Ahmed B, Al-Khaffaf H. Prevalence of significant asymptomatic carotid artery disease in patients with peripheral vascular disease: a meta-analysis. Eur J Vasc Endovasc Surg. 2009;37:262–71.

53. Doobay AV, Anand SS. Sensitivity and specificity of the Ankle–Brachial index to predict future cardiovascular outcomes: a systematic review. Arterioscler Thromb Vasc Biol. 2005;25:1463–9.

54. Fowkes FGR, et al. Development and validation of an ankle brachial index risk model for the prediction of cardiovascular events. Eur J Prev Cardiol. 2014;21:310–20.

55. Edwards MS, et al. Associations between renovascular disease and prevalent cardiovascular disease in the elderly: a population-based study. Vasc Endovascular Surg. 2004;38:25–35.

56. Hansen KJ, et al. Prevalence of renovascular disease in the elderly: a population-based study. J Vasc Surg. 2002;36:443–51.

57. Fatica RA, Port FK, Young EW. Incidence trends and mortality in end-stage renal disease attributed to renovascular disease in the United States. Am J Kidney Dis. 2001;37:1184–90.

58. Hostetter TH. Chronic kidney disease predicts cardiovascular disease. N Engl J Med. 2004;351:1344–6.

59. De Mast Q, Beutler JJ. The prevalence of atherosclerotic renal artery stenosis in risk groups: a systematic literature review. J Hypertens. 2009;2009(27):1333–40.

60. Zoccali C, Mallamaci F, Finocchiaro P. Atherosclerotic renal artery stenosis: epidemiology, cardiovascular outcomes, and clinical prediction rules. J Am Soc Nephrol. 2002;13:S179–83.

61. Levy D, Garrison RJ, Savage DD, Kannel WB, Castelli WP. Left ventricular mass and incidence of coronary heart disease in an elderly cohort. Ann Intern Med. 1989;110:101–7.

62. Levy D, Garrison RJ, Savage DD, Kannel WB, Castelli WP. Prognostic implications of echocardiographically determined left ventricular mass in the Framingham Heart Study. N Engl J Med. 1990;322:1561–6.

63. Wright JR, et al. Left ventricular morphology and function in patients with atherosclerotic renovascular disease. J Am Soc Nephrol. 2005;16:2746–53.

64. Zeller T, et al. Regression of left ventricular hypertrophy following stenting of renal artery stenosis. J Endovasc Ther. 2007;14:189–97.

65. Van Jaarsveld B, et al. The Dutch Renal Artery Stenosis Intervention Cooperative (DRASTIC) Study: rationale, design and inclusion data. J Hypertens Suppl. 1998;16:S21–7.

66. Krijnen P, et al. A clinical prediction rule for renal artery stenosis. Ann Intern Med. 1998;129:705–11.

67. Cooper CJ, et al. Stent revascularization for the prevention of cardiovascular and renal events among patients with renal artery stenosis and systolic hypertension: rationale and design of the CORAL trial. Am Heart J. 2006;152:59–66.

68. Cooper CJ, et al. Stenting and medical therapy for atherosclerotic renal-artery stenosis. N Engl J Med. 2013;370:13–22.

69. Kalra PA, et al. Atherosclerotic renovascular disease in United States patients aged 67 years or older: risk factors, revascularization, and prognosis. Kidney Int. 2005;68:293–301.

70. MacDowall P, et al. Risk of morbidity from renovascular disease in elderly patients with congestive cardiac failure. Lancet. 1998;352:13–6.

71. Rossi G, et al. Excess prevalence of extracranial carotid artery lesions in renovascular hypertension. Am J Hypertens. 1992;5:8–15.

72. Safak E, et al. Long-term follow-up of patients with atherosclerotic renal artery disease. J Am Soc Hypertens. 2013;7:24–31.

73. Uzu T, et al. Prevalence and predictors of renal artery stenosis in patients with myocardial infarction. Am J Kidney Dis. 1997;29:733–8.

74. Zierler R, Bergelin RO, Polissar NL, et al. Carotid and lower extremity arterial disease in patients with renal artery atherosclerosis. Arch Intern Med. 1998;158:761–7.

75. Olin JW, Melia M, Young JR, Graor RA, Risius B. Prevalence of atherosclerotic renal artery stenosis in patients with atherosclerosis elsewhere. Am J Med. 1990;88:46N–51.

76. Harding MB, et al. Renal artery stenosis: prevalence and associated risk factors in patients undergoing routine cardiac catheterization. J Am Soc Nephrol. 1992;2:1608–16.

77. Valentine RJ, et al. The coronary risk of unsuspected renal artery stenosis. J Vasc Surg. 1993;18:433–40.

78. Wilms G, Marchal G, Peene P, Baert AL. The angiographic incidence of renal artery stenosis in the arteriosclerotic population. Eur J Radiol. 1990;10:195–7.

79. Tollefson DFJ, Ernst CB. Natural history of atherosclerotic renal artery stenosis associated with aortic disease. J Vasc Surg. 1991;14:327–31.

80. Wilson DB, et al. Clinical course of mesenteric artery stenosis in elderly Americans. Arch Intern Med. 2006;166:2095–100.

81. Cangemi JR, Picco MF. Intestinal Ischemia in the elderly. Gastroenterol Clin North Am. 2009;38:527–40.

82. Hirsch AT, et al. ACC/AHA 2005 guidelines for the management of patients with peripheral arterial disease (lower extremity, renal, mesenteric, and abdominal aortic): a collaborative report from the American Association for Vascular Surgery/Society for Vascular Surgery, Society for Cardiovascular Angiography and Interventions, Society for Vascular Medicine and Biology, Society of Interventional Radiology, and the ACC/AHA Task Force on Practice Guidelines (Writing Committee to Develop Guidelines for the Management of Patients with Peripheral Arterial Disease). J Am Coll Cardiol. 2006;47:e1–e192.

83. Ghosh S, Roberts N, Firmin RK, Jameson J, Spyt TJ. Risk factors for intestinal ischaemia in cardiac surgical patients. Eur J Cardiothorac Surg. 2002;21:411–6.
84. Mensink PBF, et al. Clinical significance of splanchnic artery stenosis. Br J Surg. 2006;93:1377–82.
85. Taylor Jr LM, Moneta GL. Intestinal ischemia. Ann Vasc Surg. 1991;5:403–6.
86. Mateo RB, et al. Elective surgical treatment of symptomatic chronic mesenteric occlusive disease: early results and late outcomes. J Vasc Surg. 1999;29:821–32.
87. Valentine RJ, Martin JD, Myers SI, Rossi MB, Clagett GP. Asymptomatic celiac and superior mesenteric artery stenoses are more prevalent among patients with unsuspected renal artery stenoses. J Vasc Surg. 1991;14:195–9.
88. Thomas JH, Blake K, Pierce GE, Hermreck AS, Seigel E. The clinical course of asymptomatic mesenteric arterial stenosis. J Vasc Surg. 1998;27:840–4.
89. Peck MA, et al. Intermediate-term outcomes of endovascular treatment for symptomatic chronic mesenteric ischemia. J Vasc Surg. 2010;51:140–147.e2.
90. Atkins MD, et al. Surgical revascularization versus endovascular therapy for chronic mesenteric ischemia: a comparative experience. J Vasc Surg. 2007;45:1162–71.
91. Go AS, et al. Heart disease and stroke statistics—2014 update a report from the American Heart Association. Circulation. 2014;129:e28–292.
92. Li X, Zhao G, Zhang J, Duan Z, Xin S. Prevalence and trends of the abdominal aortic aneurysms epidemic in general population—a meta-analysis. PLoS One. 2013;8.
93. Palazzuoli A, et al. Prevalence of risk factors, coronary and systemic atherosclerosis in abdominal aortic aneurysm: comparison with high cardiovascular risk population. Vasc Health Risk Manag. 2008;4:877–83.
94. Johnsen SH, Forsdahl SH, Singh K, Jacobsen BK. Atherosclerosis in abdominal aortic aneurysms: a causal event or a process running in parallel? The Tromsø study. Arterioscler Thromb Vasc Biol. 2010;30:1263–8.
95. Hollier LH, et al. Late survival after abdominal aortic aneurysm repair: influence of coronary artery disease. J Vasc Surg. 1984;1:290–9.
96. Roger VL, et al. Influence of coronary artery disease on morbidity and mortality after abdominal aortic aneurysmectomy: a population-based study, 1971–1987. J Am Coll Cardiol. 1989;14:1245–52.
97. Johnston KW. Multicenter prospective study of nonruptured abdominal aortic aneurysm. Part II variables predicting morbidity and mortality. J Vasc Surg. 1989;9:437–47.
98. Sakalihasan N, Limet R, Defawe O. Abdominal aortic aneurysm. Lancet. 2005;365:1577–89.
99. Kumar R, et al. Adverse cardiac events after surgery. J Gen Intern Med. 2001;16:507–18.
100. Hertzer NR, Young JR, Kramer JR, et al. Routine coronary angiography prior to elective aortic reconstruction: results of selective myocardial revascularization in patients with peripheral vascular disease. Arch Surg. 1979;114:1336–44.
101. Starr JE, et al. Influence of gender on cardiac risk and survival in patients with infrarenal aortic aneurysms. J Vasc Surg. 1996;23:870–80.
102. Valentine RJ, Myers SI, Miller GL, Lopez MA, Clagett GP. Detection of unsuspected renal artery stenoses in patients with abdominal aortic aneurysms: refined indications for preoperative aortography. Ann Vasc Surg. 1993;7:220–4.
103. Kuroda S, et al. Prevalence of renal artery stenosis in autopsy patients with stroke. Stroke. 2000;31:61–5.
104. Sukhija R, Aronow WS, Yalamanchili K, Sinha N, Babu S. Prevalence of coronary artery disease, lower extremity peripheral arterial disease, and cerebrovascular disease in 110 men with an abdominal aortic aneurysm. Am J Cardiol. 2004;94:1358–9.
105. Inzitari D, et al. The causes and risk of stroke in patients with asymptomatic internal-carotid-artery stenosis. N Engl J Med. 2000;342:1693–701.
106. Hertzer NR, et al. Coronary angiography in 506 patients with extracranial cerebrovascular disease. Arch Intern Med. 1985;145:849–52.
107. Banerjee A, Fowkes FG, Rothwell PM. Associations between peripheral artery disease and ischemic stroke implications for primary and secondary prevention. Stroke. 2010;41:2102–7.

Differential Diagnosis of Upper Extremity Ischemia

Laura Drudi and Kent MacKenzie

Introduction

This chapter will provide a general approach to a patient presenting with symptoms suggestive of acute and/or chronic upper extremity arterial insufficiency—claudication, ischemic rest pain, ulceration, digital gangrene, and Raynaud's phenomenon. We hope to provide the reader with an appreciation of the broad differential diagnosis of upper extremity arterial insufficiency, the appropriate conduct of a thorough clinical history and physical examination, as well as an understanding of appropriate diagnostic tools in the assessment of upper extremity arterial disease.

In sharp contrast to the lower extremity where atherosclerosis is by far the predominant cause of ischemia, non-atherosclerotic conditions play a much greater role than atherosclerosis in ischemia of the upper extremity. As such, classification of upper extremity arterial ischemia can be challenging. The overlap of pathologies in terms of etiology, anatomic location, size of the vessels, and natural history is significant. As an example, atherosclerosis of the upper extremity is most commonly seen in the proximal arteries after branching from the aortic arch and can result in ischemia from both occlusive disease and distal embolization. Atherosclerosis of the forearm vessels can be seen in isolation, as observed most commonly in diabetic patients with chronic kidney disease on dialysis, or in conjunction with proximal large-vessel atherosclerosis, and in either situation, may become clinically apparent only in the context of a low-flow state, with the use of vasopressors or after the creation of arteriovenous fistulae. Similarly, the proximal arterial lesions seen in arterial thoracic outlet syndrome (aTOS) may cause no proximal occlusive effect yet result in severe distal small-vessel occlusion secondary to embolization. For the purposes of this chapter, we have elected to classify the causes of upper extremity arterial ischemia based on both etiology and anatomic location (Fig. 10.1), recognizing that the actual ischemic insult occurring in the limb can be due to occlusive disease, embolic events, or vasospasm.

Differential Diagnosis

The causes of upper extremity arterial ischemia may be similarly classified based on the mechanism by which ischemia occurs.

Occlusive

Arterial occlusive disease may be further subdivided by anatomic location. Disorders that affect large-sized arteries, such as the aortic arch, the innominate, subclavian, axillary, and brachial artery include: atherosclerosis, arterial thoracic outlet syndrome, fibromuscular dysplasia, radiation-induced arteritis, trauma (including iatrogenic injuries), and vasculitis (primarily giant cell arteritis and Takayasu's arteritis). Small-sized arteries such as the radial, ulnar, and digital arteries may be affected by occlusive lesions from atherosclerosis, Buerger's disease, hypothenar hammer syndrome and other traumatic or occupational injuries, vasculopathies associated with connective tissue disorders, as well as injury from cold exposure, drugs, and toxins.

Embolic

Arterial embolic events in the upper extremity arise primarily from either cardiac embolism (from cardiac chambers or valvular vegetations) or embolic events from either

L. Drudi, MDCM
Division of Vascular Surgery, McGill University,
Montreal, QC, Canada

K. MacKenzie, MDCM (✉)
Program Director, Vascular Surgery Residency and Fellowship,
McGill University, McGill University Health Center – Royal
Victoria Hospital-Glen Site, 1001 Boulevard Decarie, CRC. 4208,
Montreal, QC, Canada H4A 3J1

© Springer International Publishing Switzerland 2017
R.S. Dieter et al. (eds.), *Critical Limb Ischemia*, DOI 10.1007/978-3-319-31991-9_10

Fig. 10.1 Differential
diagnosis for upper extremity
ischemia

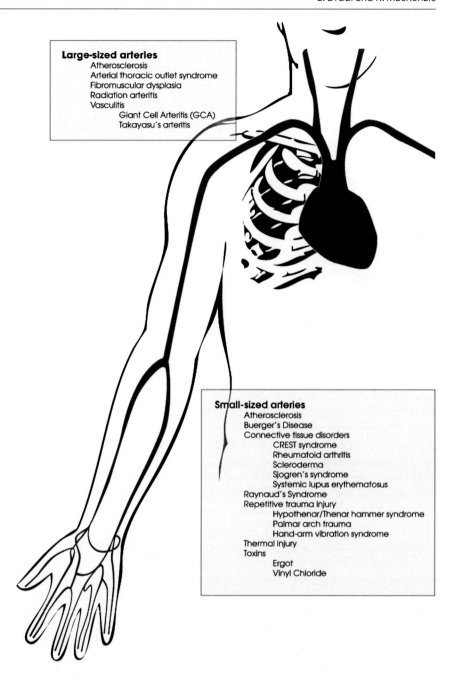

Large-sized arteries
Atherosclerosis
Arterial thoracic outlet syndrome
Fibromuscular dysplasia
Radiation arteritis
Vasculitis
Giant Cell Arteritis (GCA)
Takayasu's arteritis

Small-sized arteries
Atherosclerosis
Buerger's Disease
Connective tissue disorders
CREST syndrome
Rheumatoid arthritis
Scleroderma
Sjogren's syndrome
Systemic lupus erythematosus
Raynaud's Syndrome
Repetitive trauma injury
Hypothenar/Thenar hammer syndrome
Palmar arch trauma
Hand-arm vibration syndrome
Thermal injury
Toxins
Ergot
Vinyl Chloride

aneurysms or atherosclerotic lesions in arteries proximal to the affected vessel.

Vasospastic

Arterial vasospastic disorders may be a result of excessive systemic vasopressor use, trauma, toxin exposure (such as ergotamine and vinyl chloride), and Raynaud's syndrome. While vasospastic disorders typically affect the small-sized arteries of the hand and wrist, vasospasm can be seen in larger proximal arteries as had been described with ergotamine in the brachial artery. Raynaud's syndrome (or phenomenon)

results from vasospasm that is limited to the small digital arteries and in its most common idiopathic or primary form is not associated with other pathology proximal to the palmar arch. The causative and associated conditions of secondary Raynaud's syndrome are myriad and are discussed at greater length in another chapter.

Pathophysiology

Arterial ischemia is precipitated by disorders in which direct endothelial damage, stasis, and mural and/or luminal thrombus formation are at play. The common endpoint in all cases is reduced arterial perfusion of the limb, hand, or digits. What follows is a brief discussion of the pathophysiological pathways of the most common causes of upper extremity vascular ischemia seen by clinicians.

Atherosclerosis

The most common large-vessel arteriopathy is atherosclerosis. Clinical risk factors for atherosclerotic occlusive disease include tobacco use, hypertension, dyslipidemia, diabetes mellitus, male sex, and advanced age, although it must be recognized that many other conditional, predisposing, and novel associations are also recognized as being important in atherosclerosis development [1, 2]. Patients with diabetes mellitus are much more predisposed to cardiovascular disease and accelerated atherosclerosis compared to those with other atherosclerotic risk factors but without diabetes mellitus [1, 3]. Diabetes mellitus has been shown to promote the development and progression of aggressive atherosclerotic lesions through a variety of diabetic-specific mechanisms involving endothelial dysfunction, myeloid cells, reactive oxygen species, and insulin resistance [1]. This accelerated, aggressive atherosclerosis may affect the large and small-sized arteries of the upper extremity and lead to significant ischemia. The combination of end-stage renal disease with diabetes mellitus can result in dramatic examples of severe hand/digital ischemia from multilevel upper extremity occlusive disease (Fig. 10.2).

Buerger's Disease

Thromboangiitis obliterans (TAO), also known as Buerger's disease, is a syndrome characterized by segmental thrombotic occlusions of medium-and small-sized arteries of the upper extremities [4]. This clinical syndrome has been shown to be prevalent in young men (onset usually 45 to 50 years of age) who are excessive tobacco smokers. They typically present with signs of severe ischemia of hands and fingers, such as rest pain, trophic changes, digital ulceration, or gangrene [5]. Large-sized arteries such as the aortic arch and cerebral vessels are typically spared. The etiology of Buerger's disease is unknown; however, many investigators hypothesize an immune-mediated mechanism given that histopathologically the disease is characterized by vessel wall inflammation and linear deposition of immunoglobulins along the elastic lamina [5].

Arterial TOS

Arterial thoracic outlet syndrome (aTOS) is the least common form of TOS accounting for ~1% of all cases of TOS. The prevalence of arterial TOS is undefined in the general population; however, published literature suggests that most patients are young, active adults without gender discrepancies. Arterial TOS is associated with various anatomic abnormalities, the most common being a cervical rib. Other bone aberrations may be present, including anomalous

Fig. 10.2 Selective angiogram demonstrating occlusive disease in forearm ulnar artery (*solid black arrow, left panel*) and diffuse, severe occlusive disease in wrist and hand (*right panel*)

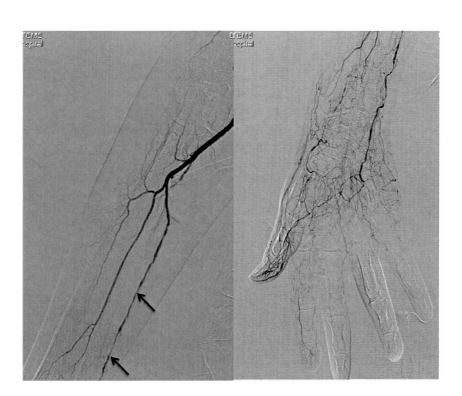

first ribs, fibrocartilaginous bands of the anterior scalene muscle, clavicular fractures, and enlarged C7 transverse processes [6]. These anatomic abnormalities may lead to extrinsic compression of the subclavian artery with associated post-stenotic dilatation from turbulent flow hemodynamics, aneurysmal degeneration, and subsequent distal embolization to digital, palmar, or interosseous arteries. Subclavian artery compression may further lead to intimal damage resulting in mural thrombus, embolization or thrombosis, and subsequent acute extremity ischemia. Variants of aTOS that may present with similar athletic, occupational, or repetitive movement risks also exist. Chronic injury of the second portion of the axillary artery injury can occur via compression by the pectoralis minor tendon [7]. Compression of the third portion of the axillary artery by the humeral head can similarly result in arterial injury and subsequent arterial degeneration leading to aneurysm and luminal thrombus formation.

Fibromuscular Dysplasia

Fibromuscular dysplasia (FMD) affects arterial vessels predominantly in Caucasian women between the ages of 40 and 50 years [8]. The etiology of fibromuscular dysplasia remains unknown, and it remains a distinct entity from atherosclerotic and inflammatory vascular disease. FMD typically affects medium- and small-sized arteries and has been reported most commonly in the renal, carotid, and cerebral arteries [9]. Given the rarity of upper extremity arterial ischemia, especially those affected by FMD, it is not surprising that only a handful of cases have documented FMD affecting the subclavian, axillary, brachial, radial, and ulnar arterial segments. Numerous potential etiologies have been proposed, including endocrine abnormalities, repetitive stress or trauma, as well as relative ischemia to the vasa vasorum. Despite these several hypothetical mechanisms, the final outcome results in medial fibrosis and smoother muscle cell hyperplasia with subsequent aneurysmal degeneration of the affected arterial segment [9]. Turbulent flow results in thrombus formation with the possibility of subsequent distal embolization. Patients with upper extremity fibromuscular dysplasia may present with upper extremity claudication from luminal narrowing or arterial ischemia secondary to distal embolization or thrombosis of the affected arterial segment.

Vasculitis

Giant cell arteritis (GCA) and Takayasu's arteritis (Fig. 10.3) are rare inflammatory arteriopathies affecting large arteries, such as the aorta and its major branches, predominantly affecting young women [10]. There is no clear consensus on

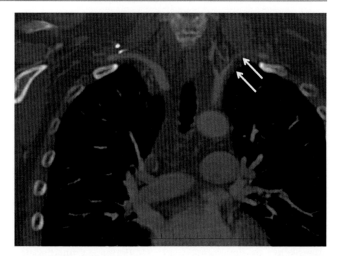

Fig. 10.3 Computed tomography (CT) demonstrating the diffuse smooth narrowing of the left subclavian artery (*solid white arrow*) typical of Takayasu's arteritis

the etiology of GCA and Takayasu's arteritis; however, hereditary, autoimmune and infectious causes have been suggested to be potential causes in the development of these arteriopathies [10]. It is suspected that an inflammatory process leads to stenoses and aneurysmal degeneration, and subsequent end-organ ischemia. Small-vessel vasculitidies, such as those seen with scleroderma, CREST syndrome, rheumatoid arthritis, and systemic lupus erythematosus (SLE) among others, result in varying degrees of digital ischemia from small-vessel vasculitis and immune-mediated fibrosis. These patients typically have continuous digital artery vasospasm and focal segmental occlusion resulting in Raynaud's phenomenon and digital ischemic lesions.

Raynaud's Phenomenon

Vasospastic arterial disorders, such as Raynaud's phenomenon, may be primary or secondary to other causes. Primary or idiopathic Raynaud's phenomenon has been shown to be prevalent in young women in cool climates with reports as high as 20–30 % in otherwise healthy women [11]. Secondary Raynaud's phenomenon occurs in the context of other local or systemic conditions [12]. A more detailed discussion of secondary Raynaud's syndrome will be found in Chap. 24. Raynaud's phenomenon is characterized by vasospastic attacks and is typically triggered by cold temperature exposure and emotional stress. The pathophysiologic mechanism of Raynaud's phenomenon is believed to be due to a disparity between the vasoconstriction and vasodilator mechanisms, including endothelial dysfunction, abnormalities in circulating mediators, and dysfunction of sympathetic vascular tone [13]. Attacks may involve both hands with discoloration of the digits but generally do not result in tissue necrosis.

The discoloration typically follows a classic pattern of pallor and cyanosis when exposed to cold and hyperemia when the attack subsides [13].

Trauma

Repetitive hand trauma can result in direct arterial injury with resultant digital ischemia from arterial thrombosis or embolization. The most commonly recognized of these rare entities is the hypothenar hammer syndrome (HHS). This rare vascular overuse condition affects predominantly men employed in physically demanding occupations and involving the dominant hand in the majority of cases. This clinical syndrome has been shown to be prevalent in individuals who use the hypothenar eminence in repetitive activities such as pushing, hammering, or squeezing objects [14]. Industrial workers are at particularly high risk for developing hypothenar hammer syndrome, with predisposed occupational hazards being carpenters, butchers, farmers, metal workers, mechanics, machinists, miners, and sawmill workers [15]. Furthermore, athletic and recreational activities at high risk for the development of hypothenar hammer syndrome include badminton, baseball, golf, hockey, tennis, volleyball, and weight lifting [15]. Given that many individuals participate in these occupations and recreational activities, the low prevalence of HHS may be explained by aberrant ulnar anatomy as well as likely asymptomatic and subclinical disease [16] or genetic abnormalities. While repetitive trauma is the most common setting for the development of hypothenar hammer syndrome, this clinical syndrome has been observed after a single severe blow to the hypothenar eminence [16]. Repetitive palmar trauma results in intimal layer injury of the ulnar artery, which leads to vasospasm, platelet aggregation, and ultimately formation of thrombus, which may lead to distal ischemia. Hemorrhage into the medial layer and medial fibrosis may lead to aneurysmal degeneration of the ulnar artery. Ulnar artery aneurysms may further lead to compressive symptoms such as paresthesias and pain given the proximity to the ulnar nerve [14]. Repetitive trauma injury in the hand is not limited to the ulnar artery at the hypothenar eminence. Repetitive injury has also been described in the radial artery, coined the thenar hammer syndrome [15, 17] as well as in the palmar arch of the hand [15].

Toxins

Exposure to certain toxins may result in upper extremity ischemia. Ergotamine is an alkaloid produced by a fungus (*Claviceps purpurea*) and is used for the treatment of severe migraine headaches [18]. Ergotamine-induced upper limb ischemia is an extremely rare occurrence. Ergotamine may cause a direct insult to the vascular endothelium and may further precipitate peripheral arterial vasoconstriction leading to ischemia and gangrene. Toxicity from ergotamine may result from (1) acute ingestion of normal doses in hypersensitive patients, (2) acute ingestion of an excessive dose, or (3) chronic use of therapeutic doses of ergotamine. Certain medications may be responsible for potentiating the effects of ergotamine, such as antibiotics interfering with hepatic metabolism, antiretroviral agents, oral contraceptives, and xanthine derivatives. Furthermore, a number of medical conditions may potentiate vasospasm in combination with the use of ergotamine. These conditions include coronary artery disease, hepatitis, hepatic dysfunction, malnutrition, peripheral arterial disease, pregnancy, renal dysfunction, sepsis, and thyrotoxicosis [18].

Environmental or occupational exposures to heavy metals and vinyl chloride may cause digital ischemia [19]. Vinyl chloride is a gas which is used during the production of polyvinyl chloride (PVC), a material found in numerous plastic products including pipes, wires, cable coatings, and packaging materials [20]. Some chemotherapeutic agents have been associated with the development of digital ischemia, with direct arterial injury and vasospasm thought to play a role [21].

Iatrogenic Injury

Iatrogenic injury may result in compartment syndrome or local tissue ischemia. A compartment syndrome in the upper extremity is rare but may be caused by trauma, burns, prolonged compression, and intravenous (IV) extravasation [22]. There are infrequent instances that IV infiltration will lead to compartment syndrome in the adult population, but there have been case reports in the pediatric population [23, 24]. Also, there have been documented cases of local tissue ischemia from peripheral administration of vasopressors secondary to vasoconstriction. In a recent systematic review, norepinephrine (80.4 %), dopamine (9.3 %), and vasopressin (6.9 %) were most commonly administered in instances of local tissue complications, resulting in skin necrosis, tissue necrosis, or gangrene [25]. Given the vasoconstrictive properties of these medications, they should be administered in a central venous catheter, but may be given peripherally in life-saving situations as a temporizing measure as a central venous access is being established.

Clinical History

The clinical endpoint of these various upper extremity pathologies is similar despite the differing etiologies. The most predominant presentation is digital cyanosis, although arm claudication, paresthesias, digital rest pain, and ulceration are observed as well. Patients' initial presentation may include signs of acute ischemia, with acute pain, pallor, paresthesias, paralysis, and poikilothermia. Upon further questioning in a patient with acute symptoms, a history of intermittent pain, waxing and waning cyanosis, or arm claudication is often elicited. Rarely, patients may present with an insidious history with symptoms of chronic arterial insufficiency [9].

For all patients it is essential to perform a thorough history, with a focus on previous similar symptoms, occupational history, and recreational activities as well as any known past medical history of atherosclerosis risk factors, collagen vascular disease, Raynaud's syndrome, and trauma. A complete medication list must be compiled. In many cases, the aggregate of symptoms, clinical risk factors, and past medical history may direct the clinician to an initial presumptive diagnosis, even before a physical examination and further testing have been performed.

For example, the presence of advanced age, diabetes mellitus, hypertension, chronic renal insufficiency, or history of smoking will direct the clinician to the likelihood of large or small-vessel atherosclerotic disease or perhaps Buerger's disease in the younger heavy smoker. Young, active individuals presenting with symptoms of digital ischemia or arm ischemia are most likely to have aTOS particularly when symptoms occur in the dominant arm. The vasculitides, connective tissue disorders, or fibromuscular dysplasia may also be suspected in a younger patient without atherosclerotic risk factors, particularly if a history of prodromal symptoms (fever, fatigue, malaise, weight loss, myalgias, and arthralgias) or another systemic connective tissue disorder is obtained. Any history of shoulder girdle trauma, clavicular fracture, or external beam radiation treatment of the head and neck, breast, or thorax must heighten the clinician's suspicion for occlusive lesions of the innominate, subclavian, and axillary arteries. The patient's past surgical history including arteriovenous fistula surgery or upper extremity arterial cannulation for diagnostic arteriography should be elicited. Any history of significant trauma to the thorax and upper extremity could be a signal to an underlying occult arterial lesion. Any individual with digital ischemia who has been exposed to chronic arm/hand trauma from either occupation or recreational activities should be investigated further for the possibility of repetitive trauma arterial injury.

Raynaud's phenomenon is a common complaint and may result in referral to a vascular specialist. A history of repeated episodes of digital color change, paresthesias, numbness, and pain when exposed to cold or stressful environments [26] in an otherwise healthy individual is typical for benign, primary Raynaud's syndrome. However, a complete history similar to the assessments noted above should be done for all patients presenting with new onset Raynaud's phenomenon in order to identify those patients who may have secondary Raynaud's syndrome from a potentially more serious underlying cause.

Physical Examination

Inspection

Evaluation of the hand may reveal signs suggestive of the underlying cause of arterial insufficiency. The identification of pallor and cyanosis is nonspecific but suggests the presence of severe distal ischemia. Atrophy of the intrinsic hand muscles is seen rarely but may indicate the presence of a chronic arterial lesion. Scars in the arm or hand may point to previous trauma and/or surgery, and the presence of visual callus on the hypothenar or thenar aspect of the palm may increase the suspicion of repetitive trauma injury [16]. The presence of frank digital ulceration or gangrene can be seen in severe arterial ischemia [14]. For patients with vasculitis, especially small-vessel variants, there may be signs of sclerodactyly and progressive fibrosis of the extremities, trunk, and face. Splinter hemorrhages in the nail bed may be indicative of embolic events.

Auscultation

Cardiac auscultation is an essential part of the evaluation of patients with upper extremity ischemia as an audible heart murmur may represent underlying embologenic cardiac abnormalities such as valvular disease or atrioventricular septal defects. Bruits may be detected with auscultation of the supraclavicular and infraclavicular fossae. The presence of a bruit in these locations, while nonspecific, indicates turbulent flow and may be a result of either severe arterial stenosis, aneurysm, or an arteriovenous communication [27]. Bilateral brachial blood pressures should be measured in all patients to rule out a proximal upper extremity pressure gradient.

Palpation

Palpation maneuvers should begin from proximal to distal in the affected extremity. Palpation in the neck and supraclavicular location may suggest the presence of a cervical rib or remote clavicular fracture callus. A pulsatile and/or expansile mass at any location, but in particular the supra- or infraclavicular space, is strongly suggestive of underlying aneurysm. The complete neurovascular exam should focus on the assessment of subclavian, axillary, brachial, radial, and ulnar pulses, as well as the motor and sensory function of the arm and hand. Tenderness over the hypothenar eminence with or without a palpable mass may be seen in acute presentations of hypothenar hammer syndrome. Other signs of acute or severe chronic arterial ischemia like cool extremity or digits with poor capillary refill may be seen [6].

Provocative Maneuvers

The Allen test is designed to assess patency of the superficial palmar arch. A positive Allen test suggests arterial stenosis, occlusion, or a congenital incomplete development of the superficial palmar arch [28]. An abnormal Allen test is not specific for a particular clinical syndrome, and thus further diagnostic imaging is warranted. However, a positive Allen test in a patient being evaluated for upper extremity ischemia may focus the clinician on the potential underlying causes as well as the expected underlying anatomical abnormality.

The role of arterial compression maneuvers in the context of evaluation of upper extremity ischemia is questionable. While these maneuvers can be helpful in the evaluation of patients with thoracic outlet syndrome, most patients presenting with clinically apparent upper extremity ischemia already have pulse deficits at rest without provocation. The clinician must also recognize that pulse obliteration with any of the maneuvers listed simply indicates compression of the artery, something seen commonly in normal, asymptomatic individuals, and not necessarily an underlying pathologic process [29]. This being said, the clinician evaluating patients with upper extremity ischemia should nonetheless be familiar with the physical examination maneuvers used to elicit arterial occlusion or compression in the thoracic outlet. A detailed discussion of positional compression maneuvers commonly utilized is beyond the scope of this chapter, but the reader is encouraged to familiarize himself or herself with the common maneuvers including the Adson maneuver, Wright maneuver, Roos test, and costoclavicular maneuver.

A cold immersion test is a functional test to determine the predisposition to vasospastic reactions and may have utility in the evaluation and diagnosis of selected patients with vasospastic disorders like Raynaud's. Variants of this test exist and can be conducted using Doppler-derived finger pressure and PPG measurements or with direct finger and hand temperature measurements. Baseline measurements of the warm hand are followed by measurements after immersion of the hand in water at 0 °C. In the temperature-derived test, temperature measurements at the level of the nail plate of D3 and at the wrist are recorded with a thermovisory camera at specified time intervals after cold immersion. Individuals with vasospastic disorders will demonstrate delayed return to initial temperature values [30]. It is important to understand that these tests are used primarily to confirm the diagnosis of vasospastic disorders, particularly if clinical features do not strongly support a presumptive diagnosis. Similar to the provocative compression tests discussed above, the role of these tests in the primary evaluation and diagnosis of patients with upper extremity ischemia, however, remains limited.

Diagnostics Evaluation

Laboratory Studies

For most upper extremity arterial pathologies, there is no specific laboratory testing. Standard laboratory tests may include a complete blood cell count (CBC), and coagulation profile. Further hypercoagulability investigations may be requested if there is a suspected hypercoagulable syndrome. An erythrocyte sedimentation rate (ESR), C-reactive protein (CRP) will be elevated in the majority of patients with active large-, medium-, and small-vessel vasculitis autoimmune disorders. However, in patients with quiescent disease, these tests may be normal. For patients with suspected connective tissue disorders, such as scleroderma, CREST syndrome, RA, or SLE, antinuclear antibody (ANA), antiphospholipid antibodies, and rheumatoid factor will often be positive [12].

Plain Radiographic Studies

Chest and neck radiography is done initially to identify bony abnormalities, such as elongated transverse process of C7, cervical ribs, anomalous first rib, and old clavicular fractures (Fig. 10.4). This is particularly important in patients where the clinical history and physical examination suggests a proximal arterial source or cause. The value of plain radiography in this context cannot be underestimated and can be very valuable at directing further investigation.

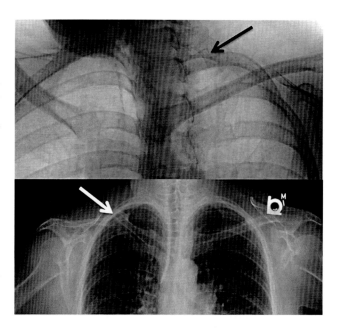

Fig. 10.4 Plain radiograph indicating left-sided cervical rib (*black arrow, top panel*) and bulky callus in healed right clavicular fracture (*white arrow, lower panel*)

Transthoracic Echocardiography

Patients presenting with upper extremity ischemia who have a history of atrial fibrillation or valvular heart disease or those patients who have physical examination findings suggesting a potential cardiac abnormality should be evaluated by echocardiography. Transthoracic echocardiography (TTE) is an essential screening tool for detecting a potential cardiac source for peripheral embolism [31]. Transesophageal echocardiography (TEE) may be employed in patients in whom the embolic source was not found through TTE [32] and is significantly better than conventional TTE at detecting cardiac sources of peripheral embolism [33].

Vascular Laboratory Evaluation

Doppler and Duplex Scanning

The diagnosis, severity, and extent and often the cause of arterial ischemia in the upper extremity can be determined in a noninvasive manner in the Vascular Laboratory using a combination of Doppler and duplex ultrasonography. These noninvasive tests should be the first-line diagnostic modalities utilized and will aid in directing further imaging of the arterial tree. Digital-brachial index (DBI), or wrist-brachial indices, and digital plethysmography will confirm the presence and severity of extremity ischemia [14]. Normal wrist-brachial indices range from 0.85 to 1.0, with an index below 0.85 considered abnormal. Segmental wave pressure measurements of the upper limb with photoplethysmography (PPG) studies of the digits with finger pressures should also be done [29] and may help to localize a segment of obstruction (Fig. 10.5).

Continuous-wave Doppler of selected arterial segments may allow the astute clinician to localize the level of arterial disease; however, color duplex ultrasonography better enables the direct assessment of the arterial segments, evaluation for intraluminal thrombus, and identification of stenoses or aneurysms. Color duplex ultrasonography may further visualize arterial segments in the thoracic outlet with assessment of blood flow during performance of positional compression maneuvers [29].

Contrast-Enhanced Imaging: CT and MR Angiography

Computed tomographic angiography (CTA) and magnetic resonance angiography (MRA) have both been shown to have good correlation with diagnostic angiography but can provide the added advantage of two-dimensional details of associated bony and soft tissue abnormalities [34]. CTA or MRA may more clearly demonstrate extensive atherosclerotic stenosis and post-stenotic aneurysmal dilation of the subclavian artery and may identify the associated cervical rib, anomalous first rib, and/or tendinous/cartilaginous bands that are missed by plain x-ray [6] (Fig. 10.6). High-quality multi-slice CTA may provide all the information necessary to diagnose as well as plan surgical intervention, and in many cases conventional arteriography may not be required.

Arteriography

While many feel arteriography to still be the gold standard to assess the arterial circulation in the upper extremities, as indicated above, the improved quality of CTA and MRA has in many cases supplanted arteriography as the primary or sole imaging method of the upper extremity. However, one cannot underestimate the value of good conventional angiography or digital subtraction angiography (DSA) in demonstrating in detail the characteristics of the offending lesion(s), the quality of the proximal and distal vessels as well as assessing the presence of collateralization [35]. In the authors' opinion, arteriography is of particular value in the assessment of the arteries beyond the elbow or brachial bifurcation as the imaging clarity and diagnostic specificity is much improved. Arteriography may also have the advantage of concurrent treatment with intraluminal intervention using angioplasty, stenting and infusion of intra-arterial vasodilators, or thrombolysis.

Specific angiographic findings are of course dependent on the underlying cause of ischemia as well as the duration and extent of disease. However, there are certain classic angiographic findings that may support a particular diagnosis. Angiography in arterial TOS typically demonstrates luminal irregularity and tortuosity of the subclavian artery with stenosis, post-stenotic dilatation, and distal occlusion (Fig. 10.7). Furthermore, an abducted upper extremity angiogram may show a positional stenosis or occlusion of the subclavian artery (Fig. 10.8). Embolic phenomenon, both acute and chronic, can be clearly identified on angiography (Fig. 10.9), and chronicity of occlusions can be strongly suggested via the presence of collaterals (Fig. 10.10).

Arteriography in the assessment of fibromuscular dysplasia (FMD) in the upper extremities may reveal the classic "string-of-beads" appearance in the affected arterial segment secondary to luminal narrowing and adjacent aneurysmal degeneration. In advanced cases of FMD where angiography of the arm shows only the segmental occlusions of the arteries of the forearm, angiography of other arterial segments commonly affected by FMD such as the contralateral limb, carotid arteries, and renal arteries may be the only evidence that supports the diagnosis of FMD.

Hypothenar or thenar hammer syndrome and other repetitive trauma syndromes are characterized by the corkscrew appearance of the artery with alternating areas of stenoses

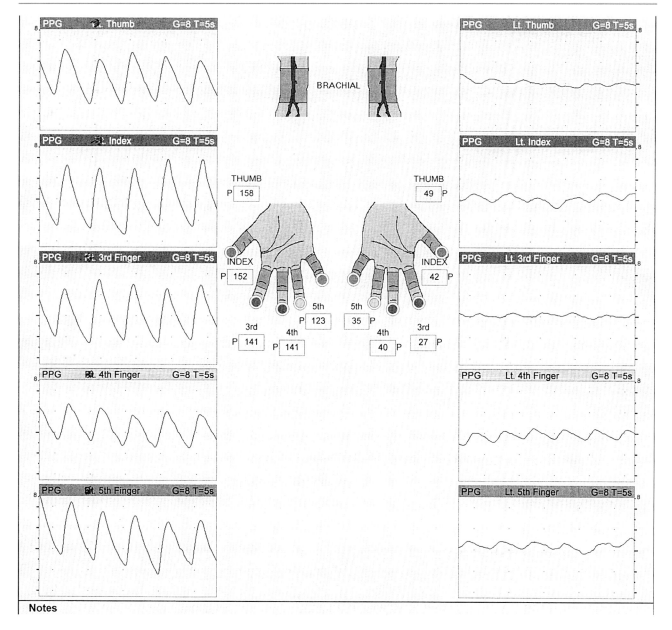

Fig. 10.5 Pulse volume recording and finger pressures measurements in patients with severe distal digital ischemia

and ecstasies, aneurysms, or occlusions (Fig. 10.11). There may be significant digital artery occlusions seen. Finally, the typical angiographic finding for ergotamine toxicity is a thin and threadlike smooth tapering of the brachial artery without opacification of the radial and ulnar arteries [18].

Treatment

Medical Treatment

Medical therapy depends on the underlying causative pathology as well as acuity and severity of ischemia. Examples of conservative treatments include risk factor modification,

smoking cessation, and counseling in patients with atherosclerosis and the avoidance of repetitive trauma and the use of padded protective gloves for those with occupational risk and hypothenar hammer syndrome. Cessation of medication or exposure to toxins and/or provocative factors, which are inducing ischemia, is critical. As an example, spontaneous reversal of ischemia in ergotism may be obtained by simple discontinuation of ergotamine in most circumstances [36]. Patients with non-atherosclerotic upper extremity ischemia, particularly those with vasospastic disease, who are also smokers, must be counseled on the importance of smoking cessation.

For patients requiring admission to hospital for acute or subacute ischemia, nonspecific initial measures including

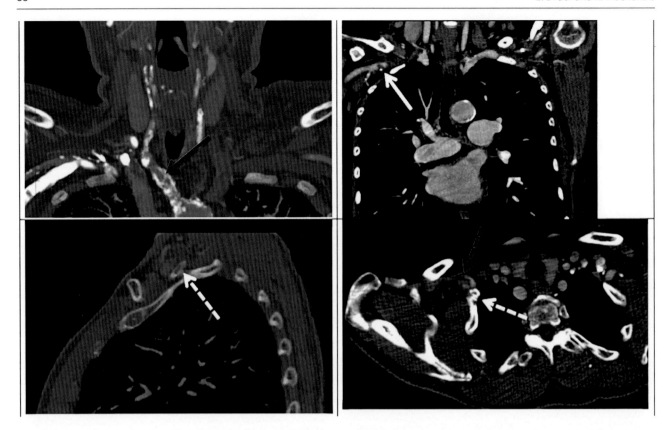

Fig. 10.6 Computed tomography images highlighting atherosclerosis of the innominate artery (*solid red arrow, upper left panel*), intraluminal filling defect of right subclavian artery (*solid white arrow, upper right* *panel*), articulation of right cervical rib with 1st rib (*dashed white arrow, lower right* and *left panel*) and resultant post-stenotic arterial dilatation with intraluminal thrombus (*dashed red arrow, lower right panel*)

Fig. 10.7 Nonselective angiogram illustrating the post-stenotic dilatation and luminal irregularity seen in arterial thoracic outlet syndrome

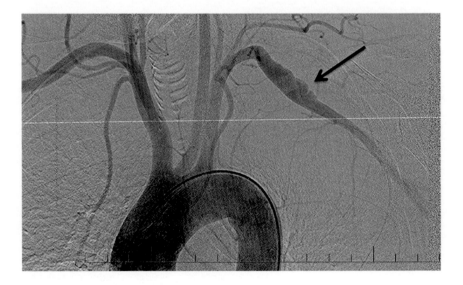

intravenous hydration, institution of antiplatelet therapy, and intravenous heparin will likely be appropriate in most cases. This may be definitive treatment in some patients whose ischemia improves rapidly; however, in the majority of patients, these treatments will be a bridge to further therapy.

It has been shown that for patients with acute coronary syndrome (ACS), lipid-lowering therapy with statin therapy reduces recurrent ischemic events in the first 16 weeks [37] and long-term outcomes in cardiovascular and cerebrovascular disease have improved with liberal use of statin therapy. The benefits of statin therapy seen in chronic cardiovascular disease management have been extrapolated to vascular surgery patients. In patients with symptomatic peripheral arterial disease, statin use resulted in an 18 % lower rate of

Fig. 10.8 Nonselective
angiogram illustrating
occlusion of left subclavian
artery (*solid black arrows*)
with arm in abduction

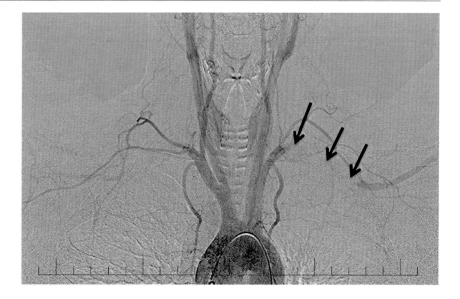

Fig. 10.9 Selective
angiogram demonstrating
embolic occlusion of the left
brachial bifurcation (*solid
black arrow*) as well as
emboli in mid-radial artery
(*dashed black arrow*)

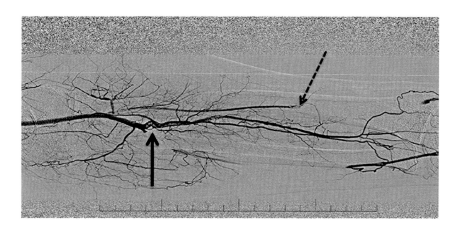

Fig. 10.10 Selective
angiogram demonstrating a
right subclavian artery
occlusion (*solid black arrow*)
with reconstitution to the
proximal brachial artery
(*dashed black arrow*) via
collaterals

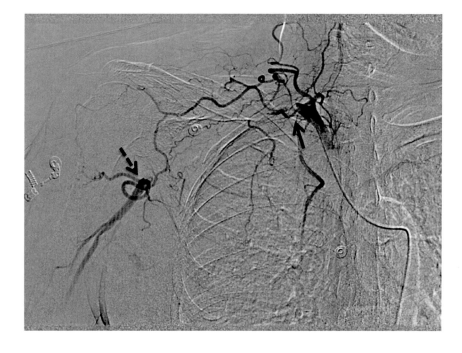

Fig. 10.11 Corkscrew appearance of artery at thenar eminence (*solid white arrow*) as a consequence of chronic repetitive trauma

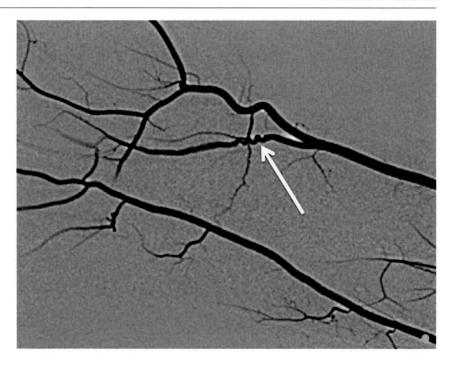

worsening symptoms, peripheral revascularization, and ischemic amputations, as well reducing adverse cardiovascular events [38]. Specifically for patients with chronic critical limb ischemia, statins are associated with an improved 5-year survival after revascularization with infrainguinal bypass [39]. There have been no studies investigating the benefits of statin use in patients with acute limb ischemia, although Baril et al. demonstrated that patients undergoing surgical revascularization for acute limb ischemia were less likely to be on a statin and therefore comprise a less medically optimized group of patients [40]. It seems reasonable to consider the addition of statin therapy for patients who are treated for chronic upper extremity arterial ischemia secondary to atherosclerosis as well as in patients with acute upper arm ischemia from embolic phenomenon who also have risk factors for atherosclerosis. The association of statin use (particularly simvastatin) with the development of systemic vasculitis [41] should probably deter the addition of statin therapy in patients being treated for upper extremity ischemia secondary to vasculitis and the connective tissue disorders.

For the small number of patients with vasospastic disorders who present with severe hand-threatening ischemia, initial intra-arterial vasodilator treatment with agents such as nitroglycerin, nitroprusside, or papavarine may be required. These treatments can be used only for short periods of time, and as such transition to oral therapy with calcium channel blockers and antiplatelet agents will be required to prevent vasospasm and reduce blood viscosity, respectively. Other treatments for vasospasm including prostaglandin E1 and tolazoline, which all have been demonstrated to produce

vasodilation [18], have been used to treat patients with other causes of severe distal ischemia, including ergotamine toxicity, Buerger's disease, and the advanced distal arterial occlusive disease seen in diabetic, end-stage renal failure patients. Nonsurgical sympathetic blockage with botulinum toxin A (Botox) and other agents has been described in the treatment of severe upper arterial vasospasm, although efficacy is not proven [16]. Assessing response to nonsurgical sympathectomy, however, may be an important step in selecting patients who are appropriately managed with surgical sympathectomy. In all patients treated for severe arm and hand ischemia, vigorous hand physiotherapy is crucial after restoration or improvement of arterial perfusion to optimize improvement of range of motion and strength.

For patients with large-vessel vasculitis, the progressive nature of this inflammatory disease has enabled success in conservative treatment and spontaneous resolution of ischemic symptoms with high-dose corticosteroids, typically greater than 40 mg/day for 6 weeks to 6 months with subsequent tapering thereafter [10].

Surgical Treatment

Selection of patients requiring immediate revascularization in the context of acute or subacute ischemia is critical to optimize outcomes. Rapid revascularization is the most appropriate initial measure in patients with evidence of neurologic compromise on presentation. The clinician must recognize that this initial revascularization may not constitute definitive

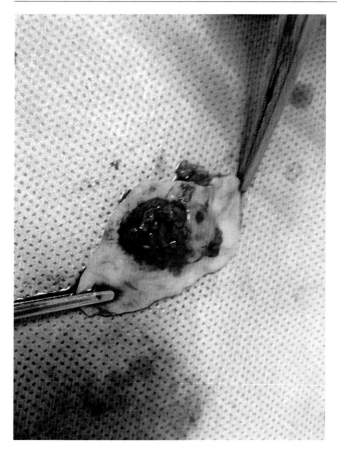

Fig. 10.12 Surgical specimen of aneurysmal subclavian artery secondary to aTOS with intimal ulcer and luminal thrombus

treatment of the underlying problem. Further investigation of the patient after initial surgical treatment for acute ischemia may pinpoint the underlying pathology and perhaps necessitate other interventions.

In cases of arterial TOS, definitive surgical management is directed at decompressing the thoracic outlet by removing the compressive element as well as reconstructing the diseased artery. This can be achieved through various approaches and may include resection of cervical ribs, anomalous first rib, normal first rib, fibrous bands, and the anterior/middle scalene muscles. Revascularization of the limb may involve resection of aneurysmal or diseased subclavian artery (Fig. 10.12) with either in-line arterial reconstruction or bypass from proximal normal artery to distal normal artery. Achieving appropriate decompression and revascularization in arterial TOS will almost always require either a supraclavicular or a combined supraclavicular/infraclavicular approach (Fig. 10.13). In the authors' opinion, the transaxillary approach to arterial TOS has extremely limited applicability. This approach could be considered in the rare case when the periclavicular region is hostile, no arterial reconstruction is required, and the subclavian/axillary artery can be decompressed via first rib resection alone.

Given that fibromuscular dysplasia of the upper extremities is such a rare condition, there is no consensus on the optimal surgical intervention for this disease. It has been described that sequential brachio-brachial exclusion bypass of the affected arteries with saphenous vein bypass may be ideal for a long length of brachial artery involvement.

Fig. 10.13 Reconstruction using supraclavicular and infraclavicular incision for arterial thoracic outlet syndrome with vein graft (*solid white arrow*)

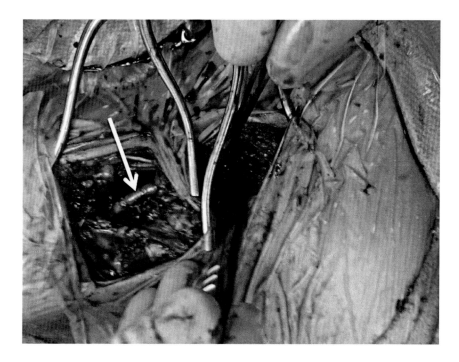

Arterial reconstructions are pursued if there are vascular abnormalities. The goal of vascular reconstruction is to bypass diseased arterial segments with the shortest possible conduits. First choice for conduits is saphenous vein conduits, with a second choice being polytetrafluoroethylene (PTFE) [35]. An abnormal subclavian artery is typically resected. A Fogarty balloon catheter is initially passed proximally and distally to remove residual thrombus. The reconstruction may be performed via a subclavian to axillary interposition vein graft or prosthetic graft, subclavian to carotid transposition, carotid to axillary bypass, or arterial end-to-end anastomosis. Overall, the patency of these vascular reconstructions is 67 % at 3 years, and the patency diminishes with the bypass distal to brachial artery [35].

Endovascular Treatment

The use of catheter-directed thrombolysis (CDT) for upper extremity ischemia is controversial, and there is no strong evidence supporting its use. Initial treatment with CDT for arterial thoracic outlet has been described but not extensively studied [6]. CDT has been described as a primary and adjunctive treatment for hypothenar hammer syndrome. A small retrospective study showed clinical improvement in four patients treated with intra-arterial urokinase [42], and the use of thrombolysis may be the most useful when thrombus is unorganized as opposed to chronic, organized thrombus.

The short- and long-term clinical data for the few patients who have been treated for endovascular repair for upper extremity arterial disease is certainly lacking. Balloon angioplasty has been widely used in the treatment of FMD affecting the renal arteries; however, the role of angioplasty in upper extremity FMD involvement has not been adequately studied given the small numbers of patients presenting with upper arterial ischemia secondary to FMD [9]. Balloon angioplasty and stenting of the large arteries in the area of the thoracic outlet and periclavicular region are problematic because of the risk of stent occlusion from fixed or dynamic compression. Angioplasty with or without stenting may be appropriate in this region, however, in patients who are high risk for surgical intervention because of systemic comorbidities or local factors that make surgery in this region hazardous.

Given the small size of the arteries as well as relatively straightforward surgical accessibility, balloon angioplasty of the brachial, radial, and ulnar artery is not the preferred treatment. However, in selected patients with good inflow and outflow and a short, isolated stenosis of either of these arteries, angioplasty can be considered, with reasonable outcomes [43]. In patients with severe occlusive disease of the forearm arteries which extends to the wrist and hand (Fig. 10.14), and in whom no adequate distal surgical target exists, balloon angioplasty is appropriate (Fig. 10.15).

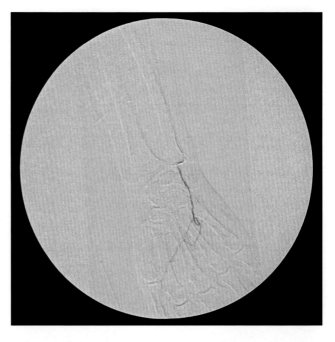

Fig. 10.14 Pre-angioplasty image of distal ulnar artery and palmar branches with both low-flow and diffuse occlusive disease

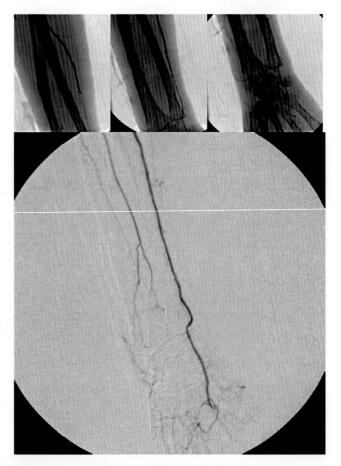

Fig. 10.15 Balloon angioplasty of ulnar artery from origin to the hand (*top panels*) with final arteriographic result post angioplasty (*bottom panel*)

References

1. Bornfeldt KE. 2013 Russell Ross memorial lecture in vascular biology: cellular and molecular mechanisms of diabetes mellitus-accelerated atherosclerosis. Arterioscler Thromb Vasc Biol. 2014;34:705–14.

2. Appelman Y, van Rijn BB, Ten Haaf ME, Boersma E, Peters SA. Sex differences in cardiovascular risk factors and disease prevention. Atherosclerosis. 2015;241:211–8.

3. Moreno G, Mangione CM. Management of cardiovascular disease risk factors in older adults with type 2 diabetes mellitus: 2002–2012 literature review. J Am Geriatr Soc. 2013;61:2027–37.

4. Mishima Y. Arterial insufficiency of the upper extremity with special reference to Takayasu's arteritis and Buerger's disease. J Cardiovasc Surg (Torino). 1982;23:105–8.

5. Mills Sr JL. Buerger's disease in the 21st century: diagnosis, clinical features, and therapy. Semin Vasc Surg. 2003;16:179–89.

6. Tan TW, Kenney R, Farber A. Left arterial thoracic outlet syndrome. Texas Heart Inst J. 2014;41:105–6.

7. Durham JR, Yao JS, Pearce WH, Nuber GM, McCarthy 3rd WJ. Arterial injuries in the thoracic outlet syndrome. J Vasc Surg. 1995;21:57–69. discussion 70.

8. Kolluri R, Ansel G. Fibromuscular dysplasia of bilateral brachial arteries--a case report and literature review. Angiology. 2004;55:685–9.

9. Reilly JM, McGraw DJ, Sicard GA. Bilateral brachial artery fibromuscular dysplasia. Ann Vasc Surg. 1993;7:483–7.

10. Weaver FA, Yellin AE, Campen DH, Oberg J, Foran J, Kitridou RC, Lee SE, Kohl RD. Surgical procedures in the management of Takayasu's arteritis. J Vasc Surg. 1990;12:429–37. discussion 438–429.

11. Coffman JD. Raynaud's phenomenon. Curr Treat Opt Cardiovasc Med. 2000;2:219–26.

12. Kallenberg CG, Wouda AA, Hoet MH, van Venrooij WJ. Development of connective tissue disease in patients presenting with Raynaud's phenomenon: a six year follow up with emphasis on the predictive value of antinuclear antibodies as detected by immunoblotting. Ann Rheum Dis. 1988;47:634–41.

13. Herrick AL. Pathogenesis of Raynaud's phenomenon. Rheumatology (Oxford). 2005;44:587–96.

14. Carter PM, Hollinshead PA, Desmond JS. Hypothenar hammer syndrome: case report and review. J Emerg Med. 2013;45:22–5.

15. Ablett CT, Hackett LA. Hypothenar hammer syndrome: case reports and brief review. Clin Med Res. 2008;6:3–8.

16. Swanson KE, Bartholomew JR, Paulson R. Hypothenar hammer syndrome: a case and brief review. Vasc Med. 2012;17:108–15.

17. Jousse-Joulin S, Plat E, Guias B, D'Agostino A, Bressollette ML, Saraux A. Bilateral thenar hammer syndrome. Joint Bone Spine. 2011;78:212–4.

18. Kim MD, Lee G, Shin SW. Ergotamine-induced upper extremity ischemia: a case report. Kor J Radiol. 2005;6:130–2.

19. Mills JL, Friedman EI, Taylor Jr LM, Porter JM. Upper extremity ischemia caused by small artery disease. Ann Surg. 1987;206:521–8.

20. Agency for Toxic Substances and Disease Registry, Vinyl Chloride. In: Toxic Substances, Agency for Toxic Substances and Disease Registry, Atlanta, FA, 2011.

21. Doll DC, Ringenberg QS, Yarbro JW. Vascular toxicity associated with antineoplastic agents. J Clin Oncol. 1986;4:1405–17.

22. Yamaguchi S, Viegas SF. Causes of upper extremity compartment syndrome. Hand Clin. 1998;14:365–70. viii.

23. Ibey A. Pediatric compartment syndrome caused by intravenous infiltration. Ann Plast Surg. 2012;69:340.

24. Schmit BM, Freshwater MF. Pediatric infiltration injury and compartment syndrome. J Craniofac Surg. 2009;20:1021–4.

25. O.M. Loubani, R.S. Green, A systematic review of extravasation and local tissue injury from administration of vasopressors through peripheral intravenous catheters and central venous catheters. J Crit Care 2015;30:653.e9–17

26. Cowen R, Richards T, Dharmadasa A, Handa A, Perkins JM. The acute blue finger: management and outcome. Ann R Coll Surg Engl. 2008;90:557–60.

27. Hill RD, Smith RB, Examination of the extremities: pulses, bruits, and phlebitis. In: Walker HK, Hall WD, Hurst JW, editors. Clinical methods: the history, physical, and laboratory examinations. Boston: Butterworth Publishers; 1990.

28. Bickley L, Szilagyi PG. Peripheral vascular system: techniques of examination, bates' guide to physical examination and history-taking. Philadelphia: Wolters Kluwer Health; 2013. p. 481–2.

29. Demondion X, Vidal C, Herbinet P, Gautier C, Duquesnoy B, Cotten A. Ultrasonographic assessment of arterial cross-sectional area in the thoracic outlet on postural maneuvers measured with power Doppler ultrasonography in both asymptomatic and symptomatic populations. J Ultrasound Med. 2006;25:217–24.

30. Stefanczyk L, Wozniakowski B, Pietrzak P, Majos A, Grzelak P. Comparison of thermography and Doppler sonography in the evaluation of the cold immersion test in women with excessive vasospastic reaction. Medical Sci Monit. 2007;13 Suppl 1:121–8.

31. Gossage JA, Ali T, Chambers J, Burnand KG. Peripheral arterial embolism: prevalence, outcome, and the role of echocardiography in management. Vasc Endovascular Surg. 2006;40:280–6.

32. Tofigh AM, Karvandi M, Coscas R. Current incidence of peripheral arterial embolism and role of echocardiography. Asian Cardiovasc Thorac Ann. 2008;16:439–43.

33. Lagattolla NR, Burnand KG, Stewart A. Role of transoesophageal echocardiography in determining the source of peripheral arterial embolism. Br J Surg. 1995;82:1651–4.

34. Anderson GB, Ashforth R, Steinke DE, Ferdinandy R, Findlay JM. CT angiography for the detection and characterization of carotid artery bifurcation disease. Stroke. 2000;31:2168–74.

35. McCarthy WJ, Flinn WR, Yao JS, Williams LR, Bergan JJ. Result of bypass grafting for upper limb ischemia. J Vasc Surg. 1986;3:741–6.

36. Henry LG, Blackwood JS, Conley JE, Bernhard VM. Ergotism. Arch Surg. 1975;110:929–32.

37. Schwartz GG, Olsson AG, Ezekowitz MD, Ganz P, Oliver MF, Waters D, Zeiher A, Chaitman BR, Leslie S, Stern T. I. Myocardial Ischemia Reduction with Aggressive Cholesterol Lowering Study. Effects of atorvastatin on early recurrent ischemic events in acute coronary syndromes: the MIRACL study: a randomized controlled trial. JAMA. 2001;285:1711–8.

38. Kumbhani DJ, Steg PG, Cannon CP, Eagle KA, Smith Jr SC, Goto S, Ohman EM, Elbez Y, Sritara P, Baumgartner I, Banerjee S, Creager MA, Bhatt DL, Investigators RR. Statin therapy and long-term adverse limb outcomes in patients with peripheral artery disease: insights from the REACH registry. Eur Heart J. 2014;35:2864–72.

39. Suckow BD, Kraiss LW, Schanzer A, Stone DH, Kalish J, DeMartino RR, Cronenwett JL, Goodney, PP, Vascular Study Group of New England. Statin therapy after infrainguinal bypass surgery for critical limb ischemia is associated with improved 5-year survival. J Vasc Surg. 2014;61:126–33e1.

40. Baril DT, Patel VI, Judelson DR, Goodney PP, McPhee JT, Hevelone ND, Cronenwett JL, Schanzer A, Vascular Study Group of New England. Outcomes of lower extremity bypass performed for acute limb ischemia. J Vasc Surg 2013; 58:949–56.

41. Sen D, Rosenstein ED, Kramer N. ANCA-positive vasculitis associated with simvastatin/ezetimibe: expanding the spectrum of statin-induced autoimmunity? Int J Rheum Dis. 2010;13:e29–31.

42. Wheatley MJ, Marx MV. The use of intra-arterial urokinase in the management of hand ischemia secondary to palmar and digital arterial occlusion. Ann Plast Surg. 1996;37:356–62. discussion 362–353.

43. Casserly I, Kapadia S. Upper extremity intervention. In: Bhatt D, editor. Guide to peripheral and cerebrovascular intervention. London: Remedica; 2004.

Differential Diagnosis for Lower Extremity Ischemia and Ulcerations: Focus on Non-atherosclerotic Etiologies

11

Sara E. Clark and Faisal Aziz

Arterial Causes of Lower Extremity Ischemia

Atherosclerosis is the most common cause of pain in the lower extremities. It can present as pain in the affected muscles upon exercise in initial stages of the disease or as rest pain and tissue loss in cases with advanced disease. Atherosclerotic plaques can be defined as a combination of changes in the intima of arteries including accumulation of lipids, complex carbohydrates, blood and blood products, fibrous tissue, and calcium deposits. Advanced plaques can invade the media and produce significant changes in the arterial wall including bulging or enlarged arteries. Advanced lesions are characterized by round cell infiltration, medial changes, and neovascularization.

The first stage of atherosclerosis is the "fatty streak" with minimally raised yellow lesions, containing lipids deposited intracellularly in macrophages and smooth muscle cells. This can then progress to form "foam cells" with LDL infiltration of macrophages that characterizes more advanced lesions. Oxidation of LDL causes further attraction of monocytes, which in turn become macrophages that produce cytokines that can initiate an inflammatory cascade. Lesions can then progress to fibrous plaques which are composed of large numbers of smooth muscle cells and connective tissue that forms a fibrous cap over an inner yellow (atheromatous) core. Fibrous plaques likely evolve from fatty streaks, with gelatinous plaques or injured arterial areas less commonly leading to plaque formation. Plaques can protrude into the arterial lumen causing compensatory remodeling of the arterial wall with dilatation. Plaque formation can also cause severe inflammatory reaction to promote inflammation, fibrosis, and lymphocytic infiltration. Neovascularization of the adventitia characterizes fibrofatty and fibrous plaque lesions. Fibrous plaques can further become complicated by calcification, ulceration, intraplaque hemorrhage, or necrosis. Later developments can cause the clinical complications of stroke, gangrene, and myocardial infarction. Alternatively, aneurysmal degeneration can develop secondary to severe atherosclerosis and may represent mechanical arterial response to the disease process.

There are several theories of the pathogenesis of atherosclerotic lesions. The lipid hypothesis proposed by Virchow states that atherosclerotic lesions are reactive responses to lipid infiltration. There has been an important epidemiologic link between hyperlipidemia and atherosclerosis, but this is not the only pathogenic factor. The thrombogenic hypothesis proposed in the mid-nineteenth century states that fibrinous substances are deposited on the arterial intimal surface as a result of abnormal hemostatic elements in the blood and undergo changes that result in atheromatous masses. Hemodynamic effects are also felt to play a role in the development of atherosclerotic disease. Pulsations associated with the cardiac cycle at branch points, unions, curvatures, and fusiform dilatations are responsible for fatigue failure, and atherosclerosis develops as a function of age. There is also a significant response-to-injury hypothesis in which the endothelium is injured either by migration of monocytes and macrophages in the setting of hypercholesterolemia or by outside insults including diabetes, cigarette smoking, or hypertension. Arterial trauma secondary to clamping or balloon injury can also produce stenoses either by myointimal hyperplasia or atheroma formation.

Atherosclerotic disease is a primary contributing etiology in the majority of cases of CLI. There is significant discussion of atherosclerotic disease throughout this textbook, and as such, this chapter will only highlight atherosclerotic lesions. Of patients with atherosclerotic lower extremity PAD, <5 % (1–3.3 %) will progress to CLI or amputation [1]. The incidence of new CLI is estimated at 220 new cases/year/million people [1]. Furthermore, it is important to recognize that above the ankle, most ulcer-

S.E. Clark, MD • F. Aziz, MD, RVT, RPVI (✉)
Heart and Vascular Institute, Penn State Hershey Medical Center, 500 University Drive, MC H053, Hershey, PA 17033, USA

© Springer International Publishing Switzerland 2017
R.S. Dieter et al. (eds.), *Critical Limb Ischemia*, DOI 10.1007/978-3-319-31991-9_11

ations are venous in etiology, whereas the majority of foot ulcers are arterial in nature [1]. It is important to note that many ulcers have multiple etiologies and each should be systematically addressed. Regardless of the arterial etiology (atherosclerotic or non-atherosclerotic), when the blood flow is insufficient to maintain tissue integrity, then an ulcer will develop; interestingly, cardiac dysfunction (low output states from congestive heart failure or valvular heart disease) may contribute to insufficient nutrient supply [1]. Typically, for CLI to develop, long-segment or multi-level disease is required.

While it is important to diagnose and appropriately classify the stage of peripheral arterial disease, the clinician must recognize the fact that there are multiple causes of lower extremity ischemia, which might not be related to atherosclerosis Table 11.1 [1]. Knowledge about non-atherosclerotic etiologies of lower extremity ischemia is crucial in making an accurate diagnosis and implementing appropriate treatment. The following text describes non-atherosclerotic conditions, associated with lower extremity ischemia.

Table 11.1 Non-atherosclerotic causes of peripheral vascular disease

Vasculitis
Takayasu's arteritis
Giant cell arteritis
Medium vessel (polyarteritis nodosa, Kawasaki's disease)
Small vessel (Wegener's granulomatosis, microscopic polyangiitis, Churg-Strauss syndrome)
Anatomic causes
Femoral and popliteal aneurysms
External iliac artery endofibrosis
Cystic adventitial disease
Popliteal artery entrapment
Congenital causes
Persistent sciatic artery
Mid-aortic syndrome
Ehlers-Danlos syndrome
Pseudoxanthoma elasticum
Immunologic
Thromboangiitis obliterans (Buerger's disease)
Raynaud's syndrome
Calciphylaxis
Drug related
Warfarin-induced skin necrosis
Heparin-induced skin necrosis
Ergot derivatives
Others
Atheroembolic episodes
Radiation
Brown recluse spider bite
Neurogenic claudication

Vasculitis

Systemic vasculitis, involving inflammation of the blood vessels, often is associated with necrosis and occlusive changes with diverse clinical manifestations. The most useful classification is based on the arterial size of affected arteries—large vessel vasculitides include giant cell (temporal) arteritis and Takayasu's arteritis; medium vessel vasculitides include polyarteritis nodosa and Kawasaki's disease; small vessel vasculitides include Wegener's granulomatosis, microscopic polyangiitis, and Churg-Strauss syndrome. The cause and pathogenesis of most vasculitides are complex and are currently incompletely understood. An immune-mediated injury is one of the basic mechanisms proposed that results in deposition of immune complexes in a vessel wall with complement activation and injury, deposition of antigen in a vessel wall, or a delayed hypersensitivity reaction. They are associated with cellular immunoreaction involving production of cytokines that results in neutrophilic, eosinophilic, monocytic, and lymphocytic interactions at the inflammatory site. The presentation of vasculitis is usually associated with subjective symptoms such as fever, malaise, myalgias, and arthralgias [2]. Patients also tend to have elevated inflammatory markers (erythrocyte sedimentation rate and C-reactive protein) in the acute phase, and chronically they can develop long segments of smooth narrowing or aneurysmal dilatation.

Treatment during acute stage involves administering anti-inflammatory agents with corticosteroids being the mainstay of therapy. Other immunosuppressant agents (methotrexate, azathioprine, and cyclophosphamide) have been described as well for refractory or recurrent symptoms. During the later fibrotic stage of the disease, patients may develop symptomatic ischemia with claudication, rest pain, or aneurysmal degeneration. Patients with symptomatic disease or aneurysm formation can be treated with general endovascular or open surgical procedures, if appropriate indications exist.

Takayasu's Arteritis

Takayasu's arteritis (TA) is a large vessel vasculitis that frequently affects the aorta and its major branches, in addition to the pulmonary artery. It typically affects young women of Asian or Latin descent, with a median age of onset of 25–41 years. There has been a reported prevalence of 0.8 per million in the United Kingdom database, compared with 3.3 per million in Japan. There are two recognized stages of the disease with the first characterized by fever, myalgias, and anorexia in two thirds of patients. In the second stage, the symptoms are followed by multiple arterial occlusive symptoms dependent on disease location. The areas of disease involvement have been characterized as types II, III, IV, and I.

Type I TA is limited to the aortic arch and arch vessels and occurs in 8.4 % of patients. Type II TA involves the descending thoracic and abdominal aorta and accounts for 11.2 % of patients. Type III TA involves the arch vessels and the abdominal aorta and its branches and accounts for 65.4 % of cases. Type IV TA is primary pulmonary artery involvement, with or without other vessels, and accounts for 15 % of patients.

Diagnosis is made based on history and physical exam, in addition to imaging modalities. Most lesions are stenotic, although localized aneurysms have been reported. On physical exam, diminished peripheral pulses may be seen in addition to hypertension (due to aortic coarctation or renal artery stenosis). Neurologic symptoms can result from hypertension or central nervous system ischemia associated with cerebrovascular stenosis. Coronary artery involvement in TA is rare, and any cardiac pathology associated with the disease is usually secondary to systemic and/or pulmonary hypertension. Arteriography has traditionally been the diagnostic modality of choice. Duplex ultrasonography, CT scan, and MRI have also recently emerged as alternatives to provide information affected vessels.

Medical therapy is the treatment of choice for the disease in the acute phase. Corticosteroids are the cornerstone of medical therapy, with cytotoxic agents (methotrexate), immunosuppressants (azathioprine, cyclosporine), and anti-tumor necrosis factor monoclonal antibody (infliximab) being used occasionally. Surgical intervention is generally reserved to treat symptomatic or aneurysmal lesions as a result of chronic Takayasu's arteritis. Surgical intervention is not recommended in the acute phase of the disease and is more likely to be successful in the quiescent state. Restenosis rates in the presence of active disease are as high as 45 %, compared with 12 % with the disease in remission. Surgical management may require bypass graft construction to disease-free arterial segments with continuation of corticosteroid therapy. Long-term survival rates are excellent with rates up to 75 % at 20 years.

Femoral and Popliteal Artery Aneurysms

Peripheral arterial aneurysms of the lower extremity are the second most common cause of arterial aneurysm after abdominal aortic aneurysm (AAA). Unlike AAA, however, the natural history of extremity arterial aneurysms is thromboembolism and not expansion and rupture. True aneurysms of the lower extremities are secondary to atherosclerosis and are degenerative in nature, unlike false aneurysms (pseudoaneurysms), which are often the result of access site complications from endovascular procedures. Both femoral and popliteal artery aneurysms are strongly associated with aneurysms of the contralateral extremity and those of the abdominal aorta, with as many as 50 % having concurrent AAA.

The diagnosis of lower extremity aneurysm mandates routine imaging evaluation to rule out disease in the contralateral extremity and the abdominal aorta.

Femoral Aneurysms

True degenerative aneurysms (including all three layers of the arterial wall) must be distinguished from false aneurysms or pseudoaneurysms. True degenerative aneurysms of the common femoral artery are relatively rare, with aneurysms of the superficial and deep femoral arteries being even less common. Femoral aneurysms are frequently asymptomatic and can be discovered incidentally as pulsatile masses or may present with localized pain or distal ischemia secondary to thromboembolic events. It is rare that a femoral aneurysm would rupture or bleed spontaneously. Once discovered, they should be evaluated with duplex ultrasound or contrast-enhanced CT scan with additional objective to evaluate for other concurrent aneurysms and the anatomic extent of the aneurysm. Contrast angiography and MRA can be used as adjunctive diagnostic tests to further provide information regarding the patency of outflow vessels if concern for thromboembolism exists.

All symptomatic femoral aneurysms regardless of etiology should be repaired. True aneurysms larger than 2.5 cm at presentation should be considered for repair; aneurysms less than 2.5 cm typically have a benign natural history and can be followed serially with duplex ultrasound. Open surgical repair for aneurysms isolated to the common femoral artery remains the gold standard of management with excellent early- and long-term results. Endovascular options are generally not recommended due to the flexion crease at the groin, which can subject endovascular prostheses to potential kinking, migration, and stent fatigue. Reconstruction depends on the extent of the aneurysm, the patency of the femoropopliteal segment, and the aneurysm patency. Type I femoral aneurysms (limited to the proximal common femoral artery) are often repaired with an interposition graft. Aneurysms that involve the origin of the deep femoral artery (type II) will require more complex reconstruction that involves revascularization of both the deep and superficial femoral arteries. Prosthetic grafts with 8–10 mm polyester or expanded polytetrafluoroethylene (ePTFE) can be used for most cases, although if concern for infected or mycotic aneurysms exists reversed saphenous vein graft would be the conduit of choice. Exposure can be achieved through a vertical groin incision to allow for proximal control of the common femoral artery as well as control of the superficial femoral artery and deep femoral artery branches. For aneurysms of the deeper branches of the deep femoral artery, ligation may be used or endovascular techniques with coil embolization can be utilized. Treatment of aneurysms of the superficial femoral artery depends on location with open surgical techniques preferred with interposition grafting of the proximal superficial femoral artery. Alternatively, bypass in conjunction with proximal and distal ligation of the aneurysmal segment is another viable option. Endovascular stent grafts have also been reported in the mid to distal superficial femoral artery.

Individual institution results have shown a 5-year patency rate of up to 85 % for open surgical repair of common femoral artery aneurysms, with choice of conduit not affecting results. Deep and superficial femoral artery aneurysms are rarer and do not have long-term results reported. Endovascular repairs have been recently reported with satisfactory short-term patency rates, but long-term patency remains unknown. Lack of adequate distal outflow appears to be negative prognostic factor when determining long-term patency.

Popliteal Aneurysms

Popliteal artery aneurysms are uncommon, with an estimated incidence of 1 % in the general population [3]. They account for almost 70 % of lower extremity aneurysms [4] and are most commonly true degenerative aneurysms. They can be bilateral in up to 50 % of patients and can be associated with abdominal aortic aneurysm in 30–50 % [4, 5]. They are frequently asymptomatic at time of presentation, with 25–50 % of popliteal artery aneurysms found incidentally. They can also present with symptoms from local compression, thromboembolism or acute limb ischemia, and ischemic rest pain or rarely rupture (less than 2 %). Symptoms from compression usually occur when the aneurysm reaches a size greater than 3 cm and can cause posterior knee fullness, nerve-related pain with paresthesias and foot drop, and congestive venous swelling from associated deep venous thrombosis. Diagnostic modalities are often dependent on initial presentation and will include physical exam findings, duplex ultrasound, and contrast-enhanced CT scans or MRI, which may assist in procedural planning. Vascular ultrasound can be used to evaluate the size of aneurysm, presence of mural thrombus and velocities through the vessel, as well as evidence of leg perfusion with ankle-brachial indices. Contrast angiography alone is limited by showing only luminal flow (when compared to 3D modalities of CT and MRI), but can be useful in demonstrating distal outflow, especially in cases in which there is evidence of distal thromboembolism or when endovascular intervention is considered.

Popliteal artery aneurysms can present as a limb-threatening event, usually caused by thrombosis of the aneurysm with concomitant loss of runoff vessels. From 40 to 50 % of patients present in this manner, an overall have the worst prognosis in respect to limb salvage. If patients present with symptomatic popliteal artery aneurysm or evidence of extremity ischemia, they should undergo urgent repair. In asymptomatic patients with aneurysms greater than 2 cm, elective repair is often recommended. The choice of repair is often dependent on patient-specific issues such as medical comorbidities, functional status, and life expectancy. Elective open repair can be accomplished via two different exposures: medial and posterior. The medial approach can be performed with non-tunneled saphenous vein graft with ligation of the intervening aneurysmal segment of artery. Although the medial approach allows greater ease at greater saphenous vein harvest, it permits the genicular branches to continue to feed the aneurysm sac and can lead to endotension and increased aneurysm size in few cases. The posterior approach with the patient in the prone position allows the surgeon to perform open repair of the aneurysm with ligation of geniculate branches—with complete aneurysm excision, ligation of all branches, and relief of compression symptoms by larger aneurysms. Vein harvest can be more challenging with the patient in the prone position, and the tibial nerve is at risk with a posterior approach.

Endovascular repair is an option for patient with suitable anatomy and adequate outflow vessels and may have a major role in patients with major medical comorbidities. As with any endograft, adequate proximal and distal seal zones are required with freedom from thrombus, excessive calcifications, or tortuosity. CT angiography is usually performed to assist in pre-procedural planning to determine diameter, length, and number of stent grafts necessary for the procedure. Access can be performed percutaneously in patients with normal-sized proximal and distal landing zones, but in patients with arteriomegaly and larger diameter landing zones requiring larger diameter devices, open arterial exposure may be required. When planning endovascular intervention that crosses the knee joint, proper stent graft overlapping can minimize graft slippage and kinking. After repair, patients should remain on dual antiplatelet therapy (clopidogrel and aspirin) with close follow-up with duplex ultrasonography or CT angiogram usually recommended. In patients with acute ischemia from thrombosis or distal embolism, mechanical thrombectomy and catheter-directed thrombolysis are recommended to restore distal runoff and are more likely to be successful with recent thromboembolic events. If there is severe limb ischemia at the time of diagnosis, then endovascular therapy would be contraindicated due to the increased amount of time required to establish distal perfusion, and surgical mechanical thrombectomy would instead be indicated.

Overall 30-day amputation rates are reported as 14.1 % with approximately 20 % of those amputations performed as the primary procedure without attempt at thrombectomy, thrombolysis, or surgical revascularization. Ruptured popliteal aneurysms tend to have higher risk of amputation, with rates as high as 50–75 %. Open operative therapy remains the gold standard for elective repair of popliteal artery aneurysms with long-term limb salvage rates of up to 90 % at 10 years for asymptomatic aneurysms. Success rates decrease significantly with symptomatic popliteal aneurysms, in particular those with acute limb ischemia. Endovascular repair is becoming a more popular option, especially in patients with significant comorbidities, and success rates are dependent on number of patent outflow vessels, with at least two vessels necessary for favorable short-term outcomes. Although patency rates tend to be similar to open repair, there is an increased incidence of interventions required to maintain patency.

External Iliac Artery Endofibrosis

Exercise-induced external iliac endofibrosis is a rare cause of arterial stenosis and is most commonly seen in high-functioning and competitive cyclists. Although it results from repetitive trauma of the external iliac artery, it is unclear why some individuals are affected and others are not. Histologically, the process is different from atherosclerosis, with loosely packed collagen, no calcification, and minimal cellularity causing narrowing of vessel lumen. Patients typically present with intermittent claudication and a sensation of swelling or paresthesias of the proximal lower limb at the time of exercise. Occasionally a bruit can be heard over the pelvic fossa or inguinal region. Diagnosis is made with pre-exercise and post-exercise ankle pressure determinations and duplex ultrasound. Contrast angiography can reveal concentric stenosis and lengthening of the external iliac artery, and intravascular ultrasound can also be used to aid in the diagnosis with measurement of intra-arterial trans-lesional pressure gradients. Conservative therapy should be the initial recommendation, as patients are typically only symptomatic with extreme levels of activity. If patients wish to continue with competitive athletics, there are surgical options available. Surgical treatment can be performed with endofibrosectomy with patch angioplasty or interposition graft replacement of the external iliac artery. Typically the external iliac artery needs to be treated because of the diffuse nature of the disease. Prosthetic bypass should be avoided in these predominantly young, healthy patients. Endovascular treatment has been described with angioplasty or stent placement across the lesion, with early recurrence of symptoms [6, 7].

Cystic Adventitial Disease

Cystic adventitial disease is a rare cause of claudication. Of the 400 described cases, 85 % have been reported in popliteal artery [8]. It is more prevalent in males as compared to females. It is caused by cysts that develop between the media and adventitia of the popliteal artery, which can be single or multiloculated. Theoretical etiologies including involvement of systemic disorders, repetitive trauma to the popliteal artery, and persistent embryonic synovial tract from the knee joint have been reported. Symptoms occur due to compression of the arterial lumen by the cystic collection of mucinous material that causes progressive narrowing of arterial lumen.

Most patients report a waxing and waning course with a sudden onset of calf cramps followed by intermittent claudication that is exacerbated by flexion of the knee. Rarely acute limb ischemia can be a presenting symptom due to compression and thrombosis of an already symptomatic artery. Diagnosis can be made with physical examination with reduced or absent pedal pulses on the affected side and a normal ipsilateral femoral pulses and on the asymptomatic leg. Symptoms are typically unilateral and are present at rest (distinguishing from popliteal artery entrapment which also causes claudication symptoms in young patients). Distal pulses can also be obliterated by sharp flexion of the knee (Ishikawa's sign), which can also distinguish from popliteal artery entrapment in which pulses disappear with knee extension due to contraction of the gastrocnemius. Traditionally the diagnosis of adventitial cystic disease was confirmed with arteriography with the intramural cyst causing a focal eccentric smooth stenosis (scimitar sign). Duplex ultrasound can also be used to combine arterial imaging with flow abnormalities and may be useful as an initial diagnostic modality. It may demonstrate an avascular, sonolucent arterial stenosis. CTA or MRA can be used to aid in the diagnosis, which can confirm narrowing of arterial lesion, by an intraluminal cystic structure.

There are no uniform recommendations regarding treatment. Image-guided aspiration of the cyst under ultrasound or CT guidance has been reported, but has a high recurrence rate. Endovascular therapy is typically successful for treatment of focal arterial stenosis, however; most attempts at endovascular treatment of adventitial cystic disease have not had durable success. Surgery remains the treatment of choice in popliteal adventitial cystic disease. Preoperative diagnosis with imaging techniques allows for selection of a posterior approach rather than the standard medial approach, and an S-shaped incision is made from medially above to lateral below the knee joint. In most patients, the cyst can be evacuated, and the artery can be reconstructed with patch angioplasty or interposition grafting. Arterial occlusion may require resection with interposition or bypass grafting. Endovascular angioplasty has not been very successful. Recurrence is 15 % after cyst evacuation and 6.7 % after cyst resection [9].

Popliteal Artery Entrapment

Popliteal artery entrapment is a rare anatomic abnormality that typically affects young men. Postmortem studies have shown an overall incidence of 3.5 % [10], but clinically the disease is even less prevalent with an incidence of 0.1 %. Median age at presentation is 32 years [11]. Symptoms result from pressure exerted on the popliteal artery by surrounding muscles and ligaments in the popliteal fossa. During the period of femoral maturation and sciatic artery regression as the popliteal artery develops, the heads of the gastrocnemius muscles also develop. As the muscle matures, it divides into larger medial and smaller lateral heads that gain their final attachments to the femoral epicondyles. The medial head of the gastrocnemius migrates from its lateral origin toward the medial epicondyle at the same stage as the mature popliteal artery develops from the femoral and sciatic arteries.

There are six different types of popliteal artery entrapment described, which are determined by which structures entrap the artery. Type I accounts for approximately 50 % of cases, in which the popliteal artery deviates medial to the normally placed medial head of the gastrocnemius. Type II occurs in 25 % of cases and involves an abnormal attachment of the medial head of the gastrocnemius with the popliteal artery passing medially with less deviation than type I. In type III (6 % of cases), the normally situated popliteal artery is compressed by muscle slips of the medial head of the gastrocnemius. Type IV entrapment has fibrous bands of the popliteus or plantaris muscles compressing the popliteal artery. Type V lesions occur with the popliteal vein accompanying the artery in it abnormal course, and type VI (or functional entrapment) occurs in symptomatic patients without identifiable anatomic abnormalities.

Majority of patients with popliteal entrapment syndrome present with intermittent claudication, but up to 10 % can present with acute limb ischemia. Symptoms are due to obstruction of the popliteal artery with gastrocnemius contraction, and repeated microtrauma to the vessel leads to inflammatory cell infiltration and vessel wall disruption. This ultimately causes fibrosis and collagen scar formation. Popliteal artery thrombosis, embolism, or aneurysm formation may then occur, and symptoms can progress to rest pain and tissue loss. The diagnosis of popliteal artery entrapment is difficult and can be made by physical examination by loss of distal pulses with active pedal plantar flexion against resistance, which causes popliteal artery compression. Adjunctive studies can include pulse volume recordings and segmental pressures measured at rest and with the ankle in neutral position, dorsiflexion, and plantar flexion. Exercise treadmill studies can also be useful to demonstrate decreased limb arterial pressure after exercise. Arterial duplex ultrasound may be able to demonstrate abnormalities in popliteal waveforms in those provocative positions as well. Dynamic

CTA or MRA is also used in order to confirm the diagnosis and describe anatomic abnormalities. Digital subtraction angiography may show evidence of medial deviation of the popliteal artery, segmental occlusions, or post-stenotic dilatations. MRI is currently considered the gold standard for defining the popliteal anatomy at rest and provides superior soft tissue definition. It is important to investigate both limbs regardless of whether symptoms are unilateral or bilateral due to high incidence of bilateral abnormalities.

Treatment of popliteal artery entrapment is aimed at relieving the compression through resection or translocation of the compression elements and restoring normal blood flow to the extremity. Early operation is advocated to prevent arterial occlusion or embolization. Medial or posterior approaches may be used for exposure and myotomy of the medial head of the gastrocnemius frees up the entrapped popliteal artery. Arterial reconstruction may be required in patients with significant arterial stenosis, occlusion, or aneurysm formation with autogenous vein being the favored conduit for bypasses across the knee joint. Long-term patency is reported as 94 % with early myotomy alone and 58–80 % patency with the need for concurrent revascularization. Functional popliteal entrapment (type VI) is a controversial topic with patients having clinical findings of popliteal entrapment with normal popliteal fossa anatomy. Proposed mechanisms include compression due to gastrocnemius hypertrophy and compression by the soleal sling or against the lateral condyle of the tibia.

Persistent Sciatic Artery

Persistent sciatic artery is a rare congenital anomaly that occurs as a result of the embryonic sciatic artery failing to regress during development. The reported incidence of this condition is 0.05 % in the general population [12]. During embryonic development, the sciatic artery serves as the main blood supply to the lower extremity, until it begins to regress during the sixth week of gestation. Its remnants will then serve to form the inferior gluteal, deep femoral, popliteal, peroneal, and pedal arteries. A complete sciatic artery, occurring in 63–79 % of cases, originates from the internal iliac artery, courses through the greater sciatic foramen, and runs along the adductor magnus muscle, joining the popliteal artery lateral to the insertion of the adductor magus. In this case, the superficial femoral artery is completely hypoplastic and ends in the thigh. An incomplete persistent sciatic artery is hypoplastic and ends in the thigh with the superficial femoral artery providing the main blood supply of the popliteal artery. They can be bilateral in up to 20 % of cases and can be associated with venous anomalies including persistent sciatic vein or large communicating veins between the deep femoral and popliteal vein.

Persistent sciatic arteries are asymptomatic in 40 % of patients, but can be prone to early atherosclerosis and aneurysm formation of the segment of the artery in the buttocks [13, 14]. This is thought to be secondary to congenital hypoplasia of the wall in addition to repetitive traumatic forces to the artery during sitting and hip flexion and extension. Patients can present with symptoms, most commonly buttock pain or mass that occur in 31 %. Claudication and gangrene are less common (25 and 11 %, respectively) and most commonly are secondary to distal embolization, thrombosis, or rupture. With larger aneurysms, the adjacent sciatic nerve can be compressed leading to sciatica, foot drop, or progressive loss of extremity function. Detection of a persistent sciatic artery by physical exam alone can be difficult, but should be suspected with the absence of femoral pulses and palpable popliteal and pedal pulses. In patients with aneurysmal degeneration, a palpable pulsatile mass can sometimes be felt over the buttock with an associated audible bruit. More commonly it is an incidental finding on arteriogram with selective internal iliac catheterization. Associated findings include enlargement of the internal iliac artery with or without a hypoplastic superficial femoral artery. The use of CTA and MRA has also been described for diagnostic use and surgical planning and allows visualization of surrounding structures, aneurysm size if present, intramural thrombus burden, and evaluation of the contralateral artery and demonstration of occluded vessels that may not be visualized on conventional arteriography.

Treatment for persistent sciatic artery is reserved for those patients who develop aneurysmal disease or complications. Even in the absence of symptoms, the presence of an aneurysm warrants treatment due to high rate of limb loss (up to 25 %) if left untreated. The goals of treatment are to prevent aneurysm rupture and distal embolization, and several methods have been described including arterial ligation, aneurysmorrhaphy, coil embolization, and covered stent placement. If there is an incomplete sciatic artery, embolization or ligation is often sufficient because it is not the main source of distal perfusion to the extremity. In the setting of a complete sciatic artery, the need for revascularization is more important to maintain lower extremity perfusion. Traditionally repair is performed with open surgical exposure of the sciatic artery through a retroperitoneal approach or high ligation by a transgluteal approach, with concurrent bypass procedure or interposition graft placement. If the common femoral artery is too diseased or hypoplastic to provide inflow, the sciatic artery proximal to the aneurysm can be approached through a posterolateral buttock curvilinear incision with splitting of the gluteus maximus muscle in the direction of its fibers. Careful dissection is necessary to avoid sciatic nerve injury, and proximal control can be difficult secondary to adjacent bony structures. A lower abdominal incision can aid in proximal control with common iliac artery exposure. Posterior interposition graft placement often results in graft thrombosis from repeated compression with sitting, and obturator or

standard iliofemoral-popliteal bypasses have been used with greater success to avoid transgluteal approaches. Endovascular approaches have also been described with covered stent placement to exclude aneurysm flow, but have been limited to few case reports and may be difficult secondary to vessel tortuosity or presence of bilateral sciatic arteries. Success rates are high for open repair with vein bypasses having technical success rates of up to 85 %.

Mid-aortic Syndrome

Mid-aortic syndrome is a form of coarctation that occurs during development in the subisthmic aorta. It is rare and accounts for only 2 % of all aortic coarctations with an incidence of 1:62,500 in autopsy studies. It can affect the suprarenal, renal, or infrarenal segments of the abdominal aorta and is usually diagnosed in children or young adults. The renal arteries are typically involved and will be diagnosed by patients developing renovascular hypertension, with claudication of the lower extremities being a much less described symptom. Other presenting symptoms include cardiac failure, abdominal bruit, and absent lower extremity pulses. 80 % of patients present with bilateral renal artery stenosis, 22 % with mesenteric stenosis, and up to 70 % with accessory renal arteries. The natural history of abdominal coarctation if untreated is severe hypertension, with death from either renal or cardiac failure within a few years of the onset of symptoms.

Diagnosis is usually made by duplex ultrasound, CT scan, or MRI to evaluate renovascular hypertension. Arteriography is generally necessary to define the extent of the lesion and plan treatment (either with traditional subtraction angiography or in combination with CT or MRI). Treatment usually is surgical resection with primary anastomosis or interposition grafting with renal artery reimplantation. Endovascular treatments with angioplasty usually have a high rate of recurrence due to extensive aortic involvement and elastic recoil, but may have a role as a bridge to surgery. Reports of high radial strength balloon-expandable stents have been made and may be an effective primary treatment modality. Outcomes are good with reported operative mortality of 0–8 %. Long-term outcomes are excellent with 89–100 % of patients being normotensive or with easily controlled hypertension. Patients usually can expect normal growth and development following repair with normal life span and long-term graft patency.

Thromboangiitis Obliterans (Buerger's Disease)

Thromboangiitis obliterans is a non-atherosclerotic, segmental inflammatory condition affecting small and medium arteries nerves and veins. It is generally seen in young patients (less than 50 years) with a history of tobacco abuse, with cigarette use being the most classically described. Other than tobacco, patients usually do not have other significant atherosclerotic risk factors. It has a worldwide distribution, but is more prevalent in the Mediterranean, the Middle East, and Asia. Recently the prevalence of disease has declined in the United States and Europe. The etiology of Buerger's disease is unknown, but it is strongly associated with heavy tobacco use, although a causal relationship has not been established. It is classified pathologically as a vasculitis but is distinguished from other forms of vasculitis in that it has highly inflammatory thrombus with relative sparing of the blood vessel wall, with normal acute phase reactants and no serum markers of immunoactivation.

Patients typically present with pain in their digits or extremity, with digital ischemia being the most common. The onset of symptoms usually occurs before the age of 40–45 years. Two or more limbs are always involved and all four limbs are affected in about 40 % of patients. Although Buerger's disease predominantly affects the vessels of the extremities, a few cases of aortic, cerebral, coronary, mesenteric, pulmonary, and renal involvement have been reported. Digital ischemia may progress to ulcerations and gangrene and may eventually require amputation. The risk of major amputation in patients with Buerger's disease is 4.4–11.8 %.

Diagnosis is typically made based on history and imaging. The physical exam often reveals cyanotic and erythematous extremities with sensory abnormalities due to ischemic neuropathy and cold sensitivity related to ischemia or increased muscle sympathetic nerve activity. Absent distal pulses in the presence of normal proximal pulses are typical, and ankle-brachial indices should be performed. Inflammatory markers and antibodies are usually absent; although anti-endothelial antibodies have been described, these are not routinely measured. In order to rule out other diseases that mimic TAO, often serologic studies are performed including complete blood count, electrolyte, renal and liver function tests, fasting blood glucose, urinalysis, sedimentation rate, C-reactive protein, and hypercoagulability workup including antiphospholipid antibodies. Other serologic markers that should be obtained include antinuclear antibodies, rheumatoid factor, complement measurements, and serologic markers for CREST syndrome and scleroderma (SCL-70 and anticentromere antibody). Imaging studies show normal proximal arteries with disease in distal small vessels. Noninvasive imaging methods such as magnetic resonance angiography (MRA) and computed tomography angiography (CTA) are alternatives for initial evaluation. Segmental arterial pressures and digital plethysmography are useful to documental distal occlusive disease. Proximal embolic sources should be considered with workup including echocardiogram and evaluation of the aorta with contrast studies (CTA). Digital subtraction angiography is typically performed to demonstrate involvement of medium to small arteries with absence of atherosclerotic lesions. Segmental arterial occlusions and corkscrew collaterals (Martorell's sign) are typical but not pathognomonic for Buerger's disease. A definitive diagnosis can only be made with vessel biopsy that demonstrates highly cellular thrombus with relative sparing of the vessel wall.

The mainstay of treatment is tobacco cessation, with complete abstinence being critical to prevent tissue necrosis and limb loss. Smoking is also closely related to exacerbation and remission of the disease, and a correlation has been found between continued smoking and limb loss. In patients with disease progression despite tobacco cessation, medical therapy may be started. Antiplatelet agents [15], therapeutic anticoagulation [16], pentoxifylline [17], calcium channel blockers, NSAIDs, and cyclophosphamide [18–22] have all been described with varying degrees of success. However, smoking cessation remains the cornerstone for any successful treatment plan [23, 24].

Raynaud's Syndrome

Raynaud's syndrome is a condition that occurs with an exaggerated vasoconstrictive response in the extremities that is triggered by cold or emotional stimuli. Characteristically a triphasic color progression is observed in the fingers and toes. Initially digital pallor occurs due to arterial spasm, followed by cyanosis as a consequence of reduced venous flow and pooling of deoxygenated blood, and finally a hyperemic response from warming reperfusion. Raynaud's is referred to as *primary Raynaud's syndrome* if there is no underlying disease process and is *Raynaud's disease* or *secondary Raynaud's syndrome* if there is an associated underlying disease such as systemic sclerosis or mixed connective tissue disease.

Raynaud's syndrome can occur at any age but typically has onset at younger ages, with overall incidence of 16 % among men and 21 % in women [25]. There is an increased prevalence in colder climates and increased frequency of attacks. Primary Raynaud's is the most common form in the general population and typically has a benign course with rare need for intervention. Secondary Raynaud's is less common and is associated with immune disorders and is characterized by episodes of intense pain that can eventually progress to ischemic ulceration and gangrene. Patients with secondary Raynaud's often need medical therapy and may progress to surgical intervention. It is unclear what is the underlying pathogenesis of Raynaud's syndrome with disruption of the vasoconstrictive and vasodilatory responses. Impaired endothelial productions of nitric oxide and prostacyclin, as well as endothelin-I and angiotensin II, have been theorized to contribute to impaired vasodilatory and vasoconstrictive responses. Hypercoagulable states with activated platelets and leukocytes as well as diminished fibrinolysis have been observed in both primary and secondary Raynaud's syndrome as well. Inflammatory responses that lead to structure changes including intimal fibrosis have been thought to be a result of abnormal expression of endothelial cytokines and growth factors. Impaired smooth muscle cell responses that lead to abnormal production of the vasodilator and calcitonin-related peptide or activation of the alpha-2 adrenergic receptor have also been thought to contribute to Raynaud's syndrome, as well as unopposed sympathetic vascular tone.

Diagnosis of Raynaud's syndrome is largely based on history, with episodes of pain with notable color variation. It is also important to note triggers that are related to the onset of symptoms and to exclude secondary causes with comprehensive occupational history, drug and medication use, family history, and current smoking status. Vascular exam should be performed to exclude underlying symptomatic aneurysmal or atherosclerotic arterial occlusive disease, thoracic outlet obstruction, as well as observation of scars or healed digital ulcerations, flexion deformities, skin pigmentation, or ulcers that can be associated with systemic diseases such as scleroderma or systemic lupus erythematosus. Blood work should include a complete blood count, immunologic and inflammatory markers for autoantibodies, antinuclear antibodies, Sjogren factors, rheumatoid factor, thyroid hormone levels, and an erythrocyte sedimentation rate. Temperature-dependent digital plethysmography can be obtained in noninvasive vascular laboratories. Angiography should be considered in the presence of severe hand ischemia or gangrene, particularly to exclude atherosclerotic occlusive disease or embolic sources.

It is important to distinguish between primary and secondary forms of Raynaud's disease to determine treatment plans. In primary Raynaud's, episodes are generally self-limited and respond to conservative supportive measures, changes in lifestyle, and avoidance of triggering factors. In secondary Raynaud's, it is important to treat the underlying systemic disease, and pharmacologic therapy is often required. Surgery may ultimately be required in the presence of digital ulceration and gangrene in addition to local wound care. Conservative therapies include avoidance of cold exposure and other triggers, discontinuation of smoking to reduce severity of symptoms, and reduction in stress with coping and relaxation techniques.

Surgery is generally reserved for those patients with severe and disabling symptoms that do not improved following conservative and pharmacologic interventions. Debridement and amputation may be necessary with progression to critical ischemia or digital ulcerations. Sympathectomy can be used to eliminate sympathetic tone to improve blood flow and reduce ischemic pain, improve oxygenation, and prevent further tissue damage. Injecting a regional anesthetic near the cervical or lumbar sympathetic ganglia or distally with a digital or wrist block can perform chemical sympathectomy. Interdigital injections of botulinum toxin have also been shown to be effective in decreasing pain, healing digital ulcers, and improving blood flow. Surgical sympathectomy is reserved for patients with refractory patients with digital ulceration and has more favorable outcomes in patients who have primary Raynaud's syndrome. Various methods are described, including chemical ablation, resection, and clipping and stripping of the thoracic sympathetic chain. Digital and palmar sympathectomy can also be performed with less of the major side effects associated with thoracotomy or thoracosopy, it may provide some symptomatic relief and enhance ulcer healing, but additional studies are needed to assess long-term benefit.

Calciphylaxis

Calciphylaxis is an uncommon necrotizing calcific ulcerative panniculitis that occurs in the setting of end-stage renal disease. Patients present with irregular livedo reticularis with subcutaneous nodules and plaques that can progress to painful large necrotic ulcerations. The lower extremities are most commonly involved, but the upper extremities, abdomen, and buttocks have also been reported. Patients may otherwise have a normal vascular exam with palpable distal pulses. Diagnosis is made with elevated parathyroid hormone and hyperphosphatemia, with decreased levels of protein C and S also reported. On x-ray one may be able to visualize calcified small and medium arteries, and pathologic examination shows calcium deposition within dermal-sized blood vessels (arterioles and venules) and subcutaneous tissues. Concurrent intimal hyperplasia, lymphohistiocytic infiltration and/or fibrin microthrombi can also be present. Treatment is aimed at treating the hyperparathyroidism, including medical treatment with decreasing dietary phosphate and calcium and substituting sevelamer hydrochloride for calcium-based phosphate binders. Parathyroidectomy is usually recommended, but its long-term value is controversial. Other treatment modalities described include hyperbaric oxygen, TPA, sodium thiosulfates, and bisphosphonates.

Warfarin-Induced Skin Necrosis

Warfarin-induced skin necrosis is a rare complication associated with warfarin therapy and most typically occurs in the first 10 days of anticoagulation therapy. It presents as a widespread, painful, full-thickness skin necrosis in fatty regions, typically in the buttocks and legs but can also be present on the abdominal wall, breasts, arms, and back. There may be periulcerative patchy erythema, petechiae, and hemorrhagic vesicles and bullae. There is a tendency toward female predisposition and an increased incidence with inherited or acquired protein C and protein S deficiency or can be associated with heparin-induced thrombocytopenia. Pathologically the dermis and subcutaneous tissues show evidence of necrosis and erythrocyte extravasation with microthrombosis in capillaries, venules, and small veins. Therapy is mostly supportive and conservative with discontinuation of warfarin therapy first and vitamin K or FFP reversal. Temporary anticoagulation can be achieved with LMWH or unfractionated heparin. Surgical intervention is often necessary for debridement, and wounds may ultimately require skin grafting or myocutaneous flaps. Warfarin therapy can occasionally be reinitiated in low doses and with long periods of overlapping heparin therapy.

Heparin-Induced Skin Necrosis

Similar to warfarin-induced skin necrosis, heparin can also be rarely associated with skin lesions, typically 6–12 days after exposure. Multiple painful erythematous nodules and plaques can progress to hemorrhagic bullae and full-thickness necrotic ulcerations, either at the site of heparin injection or at distant sites. It has been described to occur with both unfractionated and low molecular weight heparin therapies and may be a sign of heparin-induced thrombocytopenia, local trauma, or allergic reaction. It occurs as a result of an IgG antibody directed against the platelet factor 4 when heparin is present and histologically resembles warfarin-induced necrosis. Treatment is supportive with immediate discontinuation of heparin products (especially in the setting of heparin-induced thrombocytopenia) and treatment with direct thrombin inhibitors or fondaparinux. Surgical debridement with reconstruction may be necessary to treat wounds.

Atheroembolic Episodes

Arterial macroembolism can cause significant morbidity and also be associated with mortality. In the extremity, it can cause acute limb ischemia, which requires rapid diagnosis and restoration of blood flow to decrease limb loss. Typically it occurs in aged patients with significant medical comorbidities that can contribute to their mortality even after successful revascularizations. Arterial macroembolisms are most commonly from a cardiac source, typically in a patient with atrial fibrillation and left atrial thrombus or after myocardial infarction with left ventricular thrombus. Emboli tend to lodge at arterial bifurcations where the artery caliber changes, such as the aortic bifurcation (35%), femoral bifurcation (50%), or popliteal artery (12%). The diagnosis is typically made with history and physical with the typical symptoms of limb ischemia, the six "Ps": pain, pulselessness, poikilothermia, pallor, paresthesias, and paralysis. Often the level of the embolism can be determined by physical exam alone and may have complete normal pulses contralateral to the occlusion. Men and women are equally affected, and modern series have amputation rates as high as 13% with mortality approaching 10%.

Treatment should begin with fluid resuscitation and oral or rectal aspirin, and standard laboratory screening should be done. All patients with acute limb ischemia should receive rapid, full anticoagulation with heparin therapy (or direct thrombin inhibitors in the case of previously documented HIT or antithrombin deficiency). Open embolectomy is the most direct and quickest way to reestablish blood flow surgically and can be performed under local anesthesia if the patient is too critically ill to undergo more extensive surgery. Typical complications include infection, bleeding, and cardiac events with groin incision complications being the most common. Anticoagulation should be continued through the procedure and until the patient is fully anticoagulated with a vitamin K antagonist. An echocardiogram and CTA of the chest, abdomen, and pelvis should be performed to evaluate for a source. If the embolism occurs in a younger patient without known source, a thrombophilia workup should be performed in addition to scan for deep venous thrombosis (to rule out paradoxical embolism source).

Atheroembolism involves the process of embolization of atherosclerotic plaque debris into small arteries and arterioles. It can occur spontaneously, but can also occur after interventional procedures and anticoagulation, and multiple organ systems may be involved. A single embolic episode can occur with acute plaque rupture, but may also consist of multiple episodes of embolic showers. A fibrin layer that separates the underlying atheromatous debris from the bloodstream covers ulcerated plaques. The microdebris can be launched into the blood stream and traverse large- and medium-sized vessels to lodge in small arteries and arterioles. Cholesterol crystals can then cause an inflammatory reaction within the arteriolar wall causing patchy ischemia of affected organs and tissues leading to scarring, fibrosis, and infarction with tissue loss. The aorta, sometimes in its entirety (shaggy aorta), is most commonly involved, with the iliac and femoral popliteal segments less commonly the source.

Although spontaneous atheroembolism may not be silent and not clinically significant, there are several syndromes that can be present. The classic "blue toe syndrome" usually occurs secondary to lesions in the infrarenal aorta and branches. Patients present with painful cyanotic toe or toes with scattered petechiae and mottled reticular cyanosis of the soles of the lower extremities (livedo reticularis). This can extend to the thighs and buttocks, and calf muscle tenderness and skin infarcts can also occur. This typically occurs in the presence of palpable pulses. If occurring in other vascular beds, renal involvement can present as sudden kidney failure, hypertension, and eosinophilia; colon or small bowel involvement may present with GI bleeding. Patients usually have other signs of atherosclerosis with risk factor history including smoking, hypertension, and hyperlipidemia. Evaluation includes duplex ultrasound to evaluate the peripheral arterial supply as well as evaluation for a popliteal artery aneurysm as an embolic source. CTA should be performed of the chest, abdomen, and pelvis to evaluate for aortic and iliac sources (aneurysms and intramural thrombus). Echocardiogram is also indicated to evaluate for cardiac source of emboli. Arteriography is indicated even with distal pulses being present if there is a concern for a potentially treatable source.

Therapy is aimed at pain control and prevention of additional embolic events with antiplatelet agents, statin therapy, and potentially therapeutic anticoagulation. Surgical or endovascular procedures may be indicated to exclude, bypass, or replace involved arteries to prevent additional embolic events [2].

Radiation

Radiation therapy is commonly used to treat a variety of neoplastic processes including radiation to the lower abdomen and pelvis for cervical, ovarian, bladder, prostate, and testicular cancers. Acutely this results in injury to the endothelium with increased permeability to lipids. This is followed by platelet and fibrin deposition and in weeks leads to fibrosis and hemolytic necrosis of the media and adventitial layers of the artery. In months the intima and adventitia become thickened and periadventitial fibrosis results, leading to an increased incidence of large artery or aortoiliac occlusive disease. Most typically this results after significant radiation (dosages of 4125–7500 rads) at a mean interval of approximately 9 years following treatment. There is an unusually high incidence of carotid artery stenosis in patients following neck irradiation. In the lower extremities, iliac arteries are most typically involved, followed by femoral and then aorta, and most patients present with claudication or rest pain symptoms.

Diagnosis may be made by noninvasive methods including duplex ultrasonography showing evidence of stenosis without significant atherosclerotic disease present. CT and MRI may also be used to evaluate symptoms noninvasively. The gold standard in diagnosis is arteriogram which may demonstrate segmental occlusions or diffuse arterial involvement. Treatment may be accomplished with standard revascularization procedures or may require extra-anatomic bypass to avoid the radiated field. Thromboendarterectomy can be performed, but it may be preferable to avoid this technique due to inability to define the subadventitial planes. Successful treatment has also been described with endovascular techniques, which

avoid re-operative or irradiated fields. Increased incidence of late graft infections occurring 2–5 years after surgery has been shown [3].

Brown Recluse Spider Bite

Brown recluse spiders of the *Loxosceles* species group can cause dermonecrotic, ischemic-appearing wounds most commonly on the thigh. Initially they are painless but then can develop pruritis, swelling, and erythema and progress to vesicles or blebs and develop central necrosis with a "bull's-eye" appearance. Systemic manifestations include arthralgias, fever, vomiting, and widespread rash. Severe reactions can progress to disseminated intravascular coagulation, renal failure, hemolysis, hemoglobinuria, and myoglobinuria, although this is rare, occurring in 0.7–1.8 %. Treatment is usually supportive but may require debridement of necrotic tissues and reconstruction. Different pharmacotherapy may be used including colchicine, dapsone, corticosteroids, antihistamines, NSAIDS, and hyperbaric oxygen. Antibiotics are also frequently given for the soft tissue infection.

Ehlers-Danlos Syndrome

Ehlers-Danlos syndrome is a disorder of collagen synthesis and processing and has 11 described types. Clinically the disease is characterized by hyperextensible skin, hypermobile joints, fragile tissue, and a bleeding diathesis primarily related to fragile vessels. It is the most common of the heritable connective tissue disorders and occurs in autosomal dominant, autosomal recessive, and sex-linked patterns with an incidence of approximately 1 in 5000 live births. The extreme fragility of the tissues leads to problems with surgical repair with skin and soft tissues being easily disrupted and heal poorly. In additional to problems with any surgery, many patients with Ehlers-Danlos syndrome are prone to arterial disorders that may require intervention. Types I, III, and IV frequently have arterial complications. Type IV is a deficiency of type III collagen that is of major structural importance in vessels, viscera, and skin. It accounts for 4 % of Ehlers-Danlos patients but causes the most severe surgical complications. The mean age of presentation is 26 years of age, and it is often seen involving large and medium arteries including the aorta, visceral arteries, subclavian and axillary arteries, cerebrovascular arteries (carotid/vertebral), and lower extremity (iliac/femoral/popliteal) and coronary arteries. Patients are prone to spontaneous rupture of major vessels, aneurysm formation, and acute aortic dissections. Other complications include spontaneous lacerations, false aneurysms, and arteriovenous fistulas. Bleeding and easy bruising occur in two thirds of patients with type IV Ehlers-Danlos syndrome. Hemorrhage can be life-threatening despite normal platelet function and coagulation proteins.

Diagnosis is typically made by history and physical exam and arterial disease confirmed with duplex ultrasonography or CT scan. It is important to avoid arteriogram if possible as this can result in significant morbidity and mortality (67 and 17%, respectively) due to extremity vessel friability. Treatment of spontaneous arterial rupture in patients with Ehlers-Danlos syndrome should be nonoperative, consisting of compression and transfusion whenever possible. If operation for major arterial disruption is required, the objective should be ligation to control bleeding if it can be accomplished without tissue loss. Gentle dissection techniques with proximal vessel control with external tourniquets or internal balloon catheters and the use of carefully applied heavy ligatures reinforced with fine vascular sutures are keys to success. Overall mortality is high with up to 44% death before intervention, 29% operative mortality, and a 64–76% overall mortality. Long-term survival in these patients is poor with a 51% mortality before the age of 40 [4].

Pseudoxanthoma Elasticum

Pseudoxanthoma elasticum is an inherited disorder of elastic fibers with an unknown precise biochemical abnormality. It occurs in 1:160,000 persons with an equal distribution between males and females. Patients can present with vascular complications due to stenosis or occlusion of peripheral, cerebral, and coronary arteries. On pathology there is evidence of fragmentation and clumping of the elastic tissue, with medial calcification of muscular arteries and endocardium. Clinically, 18% of patients present with intermittent claudication and are often associated with additional symptoms including GI hemorrhage, visual impairment, hypertension, and angina. Diagnosis is made by physical exam (85% have apparent angioid streaks on fundoscopic exam) or skin biopsy showing fragmented, elastic elastin. Noninvasive studies and arteriography may demonstrate advanced marked calcification of arteries. Arterial occlusive disease occurs at an early age, usually presenting in the 20s or 30s. Treatment is performed with standard vascular procedures but may be complicated by presence of heavily calcified arteries. Overall the disease is progressive and patients can expect slightly deceased life expectancies. Outcomes from revascularization are not affected but the underlying disease process and are comparable to standard outcomes.

Ergot Derivatives

Ergot derivatives are used for treatment of migraine headaches, postparturition hemorrhage, or occasionally DVT prophylaxis. Very rarely, the use of these medications can result in ergotism (St. Anthony's fire) which presents as severe burning in the lower extremities due to a severe vasospastic reaction. This occurs in 0.001–0.002% of users and predominantly in young females. The vasospasm usually begins in the SFA and progresses more distally and can result in occlusion. Upper extremities and cerebrovascular vessels may also be involved. Patients typically develop acute onset of pain, pallor, and numbness of the legs, and arteriogram will demonstrate severe spasm, segmental narrowing, and rarely intravascular thrombosis. Treatment consists of discontinuing the offending agent and administration of intravenous nitroprusside with close hemodynamic monitoring. Intra-arterial nitroprusside and nifedipine have also been described. In severe cases, patients may need angioplasty to break the vasospasm, but its use is controversial. Limb ischemia may progress to gangrene and amputation if untreated.

Neurogenic Claudication

Neurogenic claudication is due to intrinsic disease of the spinal cord, cauda equina, or the nerve roots. This may result from tumors, arteriovenous malformations, amyloidosis, or rarely syphilis or may be due to extrinsic compression with degenerative change of the lumbar vertebrae. Patients present with back pain, paresthesias, and weakness (typically in high thigh with dermatomal distribution). Unlike vascular claudication, they experience relief with spinal flexion or recumbent positioning and worsening symptoms when standing. Diagnosis can be made with CT scan or MRI demonstrating compression or neurologic involvement. EMG can be performed but is variable and not reliable. Noninvasive vascular testing usually demonstrates a normal vascular exam. Treatment is generally conservative and consists of rest, analgesia, and spinal support. Surgical decompression with laminectomy or facetectomy or interruption of the AVM has good results (80–90% with relief) but overall 50% failure rates at 10 years.

References

1. Norgren L, Hiatt WR, Dormandy JA, et al. Inter-society consensus for the management of peripheral arterial disease (TASC II). J Vasc Surg. 2007;45 Suppl S:S5–67.
2. Lightfoot Jr RW, Michel BA, Bloch DA, et al. The American College of rheumatology 1990 criteria for the classification of polyarteritis nodosa. Arthritis Rheum. 1990;33:1088–93.
3. Trickett JP, Scott RA, Tilney HS. Screening and management of asymptomatic popliteal aneurysms. J Med Screen. 2002;9:92–3.
4. Lawrence PF, Lorenzo-Rivero S, Lyon JL. The incidence of iliac, femoral, and popliteal artery aneurysms in hospitalized patients. J Vasc Surg. 1995;22:409–15. discussion 15-6.
5. Huang Y, Gloviczki P, Noel AA, et al. Early complications and long-term outcome after open surgical treatment of popliteal artery aneurysms: is exclusion with saphenous vein bypass still the gold standard? J Vasc Surg. 2007;45:706–13. discussion 13-5.

6. Alimi YS, Accrocca F, Barthelemy P, Hartung O, Dubuc M, Boufi M. Comparison between duplex scanning and angiographic findings in the evaluation of functional iliac obstruction in top endurance athletes. Eur J Vasc Endovasc Surg. 2004;28:513–9.

7. Ford SJ, Rehman A, Bradbury AW. External iliac endofibrosis in endurance athletes: a novel case in an endurance runner and a review of the literature. Eur J Vasc Endovasc Surg. 2003;26: 629–34.

8. Tsilimparis N, Hanack U, Yousefi S, Alevizakos P, Ruckert RI. Cystic adventitial disease of the popliteal artery: an argument for the developmental theory. J Vasc Surg. 2007;45:1249–52.

9. Baxter AR, Garg K, Lamparello PJ, Mussa FF, Cayne NS, Berland T. Cystic adventitial disease of the popliteal artery: is there a consensus in management? Vascular. 2011;19:163–6.

10. Gibson MH, Mills JG, Johnson GE, Downs AR. Popliteal entrapment syndrome. Ann Surg. 1977;185:341–8.

11. Sinha S, Houghton J, Holt PJ, Thompson MM, Loftus IM, Hinchliffe RJ. Popliteal entrapment syndrome. J Vasc Surg. 2012;55:252–62. e30.

12. Mayschak DT, Flye MW. Treatment of the persistent sciatic artery. Ann Surg. 1984;199:69–74.

13. McLellan GL, Morettin LB. Persistent sciatic artery: clinical, surgical, and angiographic aspects. Arch Surg. 1982;117:817–22.

14. Brantley SK, Rigdon EE, Raju S. Persistent sciatic artery: embryology, pathology, and treatment. J Vasc Surg. 1993;18:242–8.

15. Olin JW. Management of patients with intermittent claudication. Int J Clin Pract. 2002;56:687–93.

16. Kawata E, Kuroda J, Wada K, et al. Hypereosinophilic syndrome accompanied by Buerger's disease-like femoral arterial occlusions. Intern Med. 2007;46:1919–22.

17. Agarwal P, Agrawal PK, Sharma D, Baghel KD. Intravenous infusion for the treatment of diabetic and ischaemic non-healing pedal ulcers. J Eur Acad Dermatol Venereol. 2005;19:158–62.

18. Gur'eva MS, Baranov AA, Bagrakova SV, Kurdiukov AA. Pulse-therapy with glucocorticoids and cyclophosphamide in the treatment of thromboangiitis obliterans. Klin Med. 2003;81:53–7.

19. Fiessinger JN. Juvenile arteritis revisited. Buerger's disease-Takayasu's disease. Pathophysiol Haemost Thromb. 2002;32:295–8.

20. Saha K, Chabra N, Gulati SM. Treatment of patients with thromboangiitis obliterans with cyclophosphamide. Angiology. 2001;52: 399–407.

21. Giacomelli R, Pizzuto F, Cucinelli F, Tonietti G. Immunosuppressive therapy of vasculitis: current aspects and perspectives. Recenti Prog Med. 1996;87:124–34.

22. Fauci AS, Haynes B, Katz P. The spectrum of vasculitis: clinical, pathologic, immunologic and therapeutic considerations. Ann Intern Med. 1978;89:660–76.

23. Olin JW, Shih A. Thromboangiitis obliterans (Buerger's disease). Curr Opin Rheumatol. 2006;18:18–24.

24. Olin JW. Thromboangiitis obliterans (Buerger's disease). N Engl J Med. 2000;343:864–9.

25. Silman A, Holligan S, Brennan P, Maddison P. Prevalence of symptoms of Raynaud's phenomenon in general practice. BMJ. 1990;301:590–2.

Raymond A. Dieter, III, Tjuan L. Overly, Madhur A. Roberts, and Juan J. Gallegos Jr.

Arterial occlusive disease is associated with many cardiac etiologies including atrial fibrillation (AF) or flutter, ventricular mural thrombus, valvular diseases (rheumatic or prosthetic valves and endocarditis), cardiac tumors, paradoxical emboli via patent foramen ovale or atrial septal defect, aortic dissection, and iatrogenic causes. Limb-threatening or critical limb ischemia may have a variable time course, acute or chronic, and is associated with high morbidity and mortality. Critical limb ischemia occurs when the blood flow is compromised to the point that the affected extremity or extremities will be lost without intervention [1]. Presenting symptoms of patients with critical limb ischemia include limb pain at rest, ulceration, gangrene, numbness, and/or paralysis.

Chronic limb ischemia is almost always a manifestation of peripheral arterial atherosclerotic disease. It progresses slowly over a period of time and eventually reaches the critical stage. Similar to coronary atherosclerosis, progression of peripheral atherosclerosis has been well linked to traditional risk factors such as smoking, diabetes, hypertension, hyperlipidemia, age, and chronic kidney disease [1, 2].

Acute limb ischemia occurs from an abrupt interruption of blood flow to an extremity, usually because of embolic or thrombotic vascular occlusion. It can also result from trauma and dissection. Thrombosis in situ mainly occurs in the setting of underlying atherosclerotic disease and accounts for about 85 % of the acute limb ischemia [3]. The gradual progression of atherosclerotic narrowing often stimulates the formation of collateral channels. Therefore, thrombosis in this setting may not exhibit severe symptoms. Embolism, on the other hand, results in a greater degree of ischemia than thrombosis, as the embolus characteristically lodges in a "virgin" vascular bed with no prior collateral development. Therefore, the symptomatology of an acute limb ischemia may vary depending on the degree of collateral flow if chronic disease is present. The classic pentad to look for in acute limb ischemia includes extreme lower extremity pain, pallor, pulselessness, paresthesia, and paralysis.

With an embolic occlusion, a cardiac origin is the source of emboli in about 80–90 % of cases, most commonly in the setting of atrial fibrillation/flutter or acute myocardial infarction [4]. The presence of rheumatic or prosthetic cardiac valves, endocarditis, and cardiac tumors (such as left atrial myxoma) is also associated with increased risk of embolic events. Furthermore, paradoxical embolism of venous thrombi through an intra-atrial communication (such as an atrial septal defect or patent foramen ovale), or less commonly an intraventricular communication, is also encountered in some patients.

Atrial Fibrillation

Atrial Fibrillation (AF) is the most common arrhythmia and affects about 1 % of the US population [5]. The lifetime incidence of atrial fibrillation is about 26 % for men and 23 % for women [6]. The prevalence of AF in a population increases with age, a correlation with the increased incidence of acute occlusive disease in our aging population.

Thromboembolic events, both central and peripheral, are increased and contribute to the high morbidity and mortality with atrial fibrillation. The most common destination of emboli from atrial fibrillation is the cerebral circulatory system leading to strokes and transient ischemic attacks. Although the incidence of peripheral embolism from AF is lower as compared to cerebral vasculature, about 30–80 % of

R.A. Dieter, III, MD (✉)
Division of Cardiothoracic Surgery, The University of Tennessee Medical Center, Knoxville, TN, USA

T.L. Overly, MD • M.A. Roberts, MD
Cardiovascular Disease, University Cardiology, The University of Tennessee Medical Center, Knoxville, TN, USA

J.J. Gallegos Jr., MD
General Surgery, University of Tennessee Medical Center, Knoxville, TN, USA

© Springer International Publishing Switzerland 2017
R.S. Dieter et al. (eds.), *Critical Limb Ischemia*, DOI 10.1007/978-3-319-31991-9_12

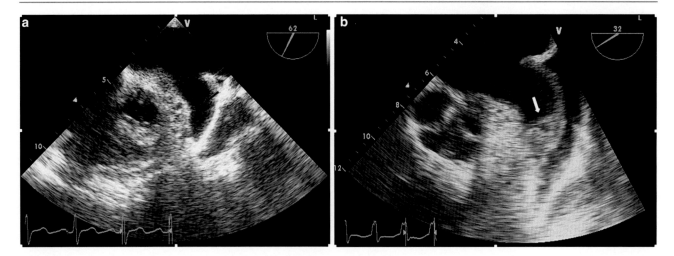

Fig. 12.1 (a) Left atrial appendage (*arrow*) without evidence of thrombus on transesophageal echocardiogram. (b) Left atrial appendage with thrombus (*arrow*) on transesophageal echocardiogram

patients with peripheral thromboembolic phenomenon have AF [7]. This makes AF one of the most significant risk factors in embolic peripheral ischemia. More specifically, the annual incidence of acute limb ischemia in AF is 0.4 % (lethality 16 %) [8]. Symptoms can vary depending on the degree of arterial luminal obstruction and extent of collateral flow caused by preexisting peripheral arterial disease.

Most thrombi associated with AF are formed in left atrial appendage. Echocardiography is an important diagnostic tool, with transesophageal echocardiography (TEE) significantly increasing the sensitivity of the detection of left atrial appendage thrombus (Fig. 12.1). Newer imaging technologies such as magnetic resonance imaging (MRI) or computerized tomography can also be utilized but are used less frequently in clinical practice.

The risk of thromboembolism varies widely across the population of patients with AF, according to the presence or absence of clinical risk factors. The rate of ischemic stroke or peripheral embolization (without antithrombotic therapy) also increases as the number of risk factors increase. This trend is the basis of the two major risk prediction models used in clinical practice to determine the need for anticoagulation—CHADS$_2$ score and more recently CHA$_2$DS$_2$-VASc score [9, 10]. Anticoagulation decreases the risk of thromboembolism (Tables 12.1, 12.2, and 12.3). The current American Heart Association guidelines recommend anticoagulation for patients with CHA$_2$DS$_2$-VASc score ≥2 [11].

Warfarin has been well established to reduce the risk of stroke or embolism in patients with atrial fibrillation, however requires regular blood level monitoring. Recently, new oral anticoagulants have been approved that do not require rigorous blood level monitoring of warfarin. These include dabigatran, apixaban, and rivaroxaban [11]. The major trials studying these novel oral anticoagulants did not separately analyze for peripheral embolism in their primary outcome. However, the overall

Table 12.1 CHADS$_2$ score [9]

CHADS$_2$ criteria		Score
C	Congestive heart failure	1
H	Hypertension	1
A	Age ≥75 years	1
D	Diabetes mellitus	1
S$_2$	Stroke/TIA	2

Maximum total score = 6 points
American College of Cardiology/American Heart Association/Heart Rhythm Society 2006 Anticoagulation Recommendations
Score = 0 aspirin. Score = 1 aspirin or oral anticoagulation. Score ≥ 2 Oral anticoagulation

Table 12.2 CHA$_2$DS$_2$-VASc score [10]

CHA$_2$DS$_2$-VASc criteria		Score
C	Congestive HF	1
H	HTN	1
A$_2$	Age ≥75 years	2
D	Diabetes mellitus	1
S$_2$	Stroke/TIA	2
V	Vascular disease (MI, PAD, aortic plaque)	1
A	Age 65–75	1
S	Female	1

Maximum total score = 9 points
American College of Cardiology/American Heart Association 2014 Anticoagulation Recommendations
Score = 0 no therapy or aspirin (no therapy preferred). Score = 1 aspirin or oral anticoagulation (oral anticoagulation preferred). Score ≥ 2 oral anticoagulation

rate of the combined primary outcome (i.e., stroke plus peripheral thromboembolism) has shown to be either non-inferior or significantly lower as compared to warfarin [12–14].

Furthermore, new devices to ligate, resect, or occlude the left atrial appendage, the most common location to form a

Table 12.3 Adjusted risk of stroke for CHADS₂ and CHA₂DS₂-VASc scores [9, 10]

Score	CHADS$_2$ (%/year)	CHA$_2$DS$_2$-VASc (%/year)
0	1.9	0
1	2.8	1.3
2	4	2.2
3	5.9	3.2
4	8.5	4.0
5	12.5	6.7
6	18.2	9.8
7		9.6
8		6.7
9		15.2

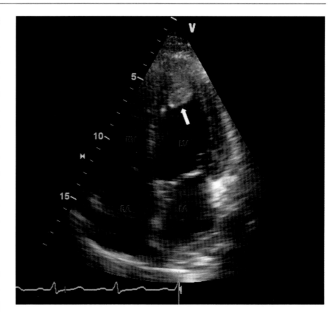

Fig. 12.2 Left ventricular protruding mural thrombus (*arrow*) on apical four-chamber view on transthoracic echocardiogram. *RV* right ventricle, *RA* right atrium, *LA* left atrium, *LV* left ventricle

thrombus, are under investigation. The Watchman device, manufactured by Boston Scientific, has shown superiority in primary outcome of stroke, cardiovascular death, and systemic embolism over warfarin [15]. In December 2013, Food and Drug Administration (FDA) advisors voted 13-1 that the benefits associated with the Boston Scientific Watchman device outweighed the risks in AF patients. The FDA approved the device in 2015.

Ventricular Mural Thrombus

Sluggish flow of the intracavitary blood in the ventricles predisposes to thrombus formation. As such, ventricular mural thrombus is most commonly associated with myocardial infarctions (MI), ventricular aneurysms, and dilated cardiomyopathies among other systemic diseases that affect the heart (e.g., amyloidosis, Chagas disease, systemic lupus erythematosus, carcinoid heart disease). Myocardial infarction can cause wall motion abnormality and/or systolic dysfunction, hence causing the sluggish flow. The likelihood of developing a left ventricular (LV) thrombus after an acute MI varies with infarct location and size. A large anterior myocardial infarction with anteroapical aneurysm formation has the highest rates of LV thrombus development, compared to other areas of infarction. Earlier studies, prior to the percutaneous coronary intervention (PCI) era, had reported the rates of up to 46 % in anterior MI [16–18]; however, more recent studies with PCI report an incidence of about 4 % [19]. Most LV mural thrombi develop within the first two weeks after MI [16, 20].

In the pre-thrombolytic era, the risk of embolization from a left ventricular thrombus has been reported to be anywhere from 10 to 20 % in patients not on anticoagulation [21–23]. Embolization from cardiomyopathies seems to occur more often than thrombus within an aneurysm, likely secondary to the thrombus surface exposure to the LV cavity [24]. The incidence

of systemic embolization of mural thrombus for left ventricular aneurysms, myocardial infarctions, and congestive cardiomyopathy are 0–36, 0–24, 11 %, respectively [25].

A number of diagnostic modalities can be used to diagnose ventricular mural thrombus. The most widely used modality in clinical practice is echocardiography (Fig. 12.2). Certain echocardiographic characteristics can predict the risk of embolization; the two most important ones associated with higher risk are thrombus mobility and protrusion into the left ventricular cavity [20–26]. Other diagnostic studies include angiography, radionuclide scintigraphy, indium II-labeled platelets, and computed tomography (CT). Once diagnosed, the recommended treatment is anticoagulation with warfarin or heparin products for at least three months.

Endocarditis

Endocarditis, whether acute or subacute, can be a source of emboli causing central nervous system injury, arteritis, and end-organ ischemia. Nearly 50 % of patients will develop an embolic event and often involve the coronary vessels, spleen, kidneys, brain, and extremities [27, 28]. The incidence of critical limb ischemia, however, is not very well defined. The risk of embolization is correlated with the size of the vegetation, location, and organism involved. Some studies have shown significantly greater rates of embolization with vegetation size >10 mm. This risk seems to be highest when mitral valve is involved [28–30]. Infective endocarditis (IE) caused by *Staphylococcus* or fungal organisms appears to carry a higher risk of embolization independent of the vegetation size [29].

Modified Duke's criterion is utilized to evaluate the patient with infective endocarditis (Table 12.4). The emphasis is given to the two more important diagnostic tests, the blood cultures and echocardiography. Echocardiography is fundamental in diagnosing endocarditis. The echocardiographic features included in the major classification of the Modified Duke's criteria are the evidence of an oscillating intracardiac mass or vegetation, an annular abscess, a prosthetic valve partial dehiscence, and a new valvular regurgitation [28].

Echocardiography should be done on all cases suspicious of infective endocarditis. In patients whom the clinical suspicion is low, and where it is likely to obtain good images, a transthoracic echocardiogram (TTE) is reasonable. On the other hand, if there are poor echocardiographic windows (e.g., in obese patients or patients with severe lung disease) or if there is high clinical suspicion of IE or its complications (prosthetic valve, staphylococcal bacteremia, or new atrioventricular block), then transesophageal echocardiogram should be performed first. This is because in these cases a negative TTE will not definitely rule out IE or its potential complications (Fig. 12.3).

There are no randomized controlled trials to assess the benefits of surgical intervention in infective endocarditis. However, observational data comparing the mortality risk of complications of IE with and without surgery have assisted in the development of certain indications for surgery in IE [28, 31, 32].The mainstay of treatment is medical management with antibiotics. Initial antimicrobial therapy is chosen based on clinical suspicion of the source bacteria. The risk of embolization drops significantly after 2–3 weeks of appropriate antibiotic therapy [29, 30].

Surgical intervention is mostly indicated in complicated IE [32]. Patients with IE should be evaluated for early surgery (during initial hospitalization before completion of a full therapeutic course of antibiotics) that develops heart failure or paravalvular complications such as heart block, annular or aortic abscess, or destructive penetrating lesions. It should also be considered in patients who have left-sided IE caused by *S. aureus* and fungal or other highly resistant organisms and in patients with evidence of persistent bacteremia or fever lasting longer than 5–7 days after onset of appropriate antimicrobial therapy [28].

To reduce the risk of embolic complications, it is also reasonable to consider surgical intervention in patients with recurrent emboli and persistent vegetations despite appropriate antibiotic therapy and in patients with native valve endocarditis who exhibit mobile vegetations greater than 10 mm in length (with or without clinical evidence of embolic phenomenon) [28].

Table 12.4 Definition of infective endocarditis (IE) according to the modified Duke criteria

Definite IE

Pathological criteria

Microorganisms (via culture or histology) in a vegetation, an embolized vegetation, or an intracardiac abscess specimen

Pathologic lesion; vegetation or intracardiac abscess on histologic examination showing active endocarditis

Clinical criteria

2 major criteria

1 major and 3 minor criteria

5 minor criteria

Possible IE

2 major criteria

1 major and 3 minor criteria

5 minor criteria

Rejected IE

Firm alternative diagnosis explaining evidence of IE

Resolution of IE syndrome with antibiotic therapy for ≤4 days

No pathological evidence of IE at surgery or autopsy, with antibiotic therapy for ≤4 days

Does not meet criteria for possible infective endocarditis as above

Definition of terms used in the modified Duke's criteria for the diagnosis of infective endocarditis

Major criteria

1. Blood culture positive for IE

   (a) Typical microorganisms consistent with IE from two separate blood cultures: viridans streptococci, *Streptococcus bovis*, HACEK group, *Staphylococcus aureus*; or community-acquired enterococci in the absence of a primary focus

   (b) Microorganisms consistent with IE from persistently positive blood cultures defined as follows: At least two positive cultures of blood samples drawn >12 h apart or all of three or a majority of ≥4 separate cultures of blood (with first and last sample drawn at least 1 h apart)

   (c) Single positive blood culture for *Coxiella burnetii* or anti-phase 1 IgG antibody titer >1:800

2. Evidence of endocardial involvement

   Echocardiogram positive for IE (TEE recommended for patients with prosthetic valves, rated at least "possible IE" by clinical criteria or complicated IE [paravalvular abscess]; TTE as first test in other patients) defined as follows: oscillating intracardiac mass on valve or supporting structures, in the path of regurgitant jets, or on implanted material in the absence of an alternative anatomic explanation; or abscess; or new partial dehiscence of prosthetic valve; new valvular regurgitation (worsening, changing, or preexisting murmur not sufficient)

Minor criteria

1. Predisposition, predisposing heart condition, or IDU

2. Fever, temperature >38 °C

3. Vascular phenomena, major arterial emboli, septic pulmonary infarcts, mycotic aneurysm, intracranial hemorrhage, conjunctival hemorrhages, and Janeway's lesions

4. Immunologic phenomena: glomerulonephritis, Osler's nodes, Roth's spots, and rheumatoid factor

5. Microbiological evidence: positive blood culture but does not meet a major criterion as noted above or serological evidence of active infection with organism consistent with IE

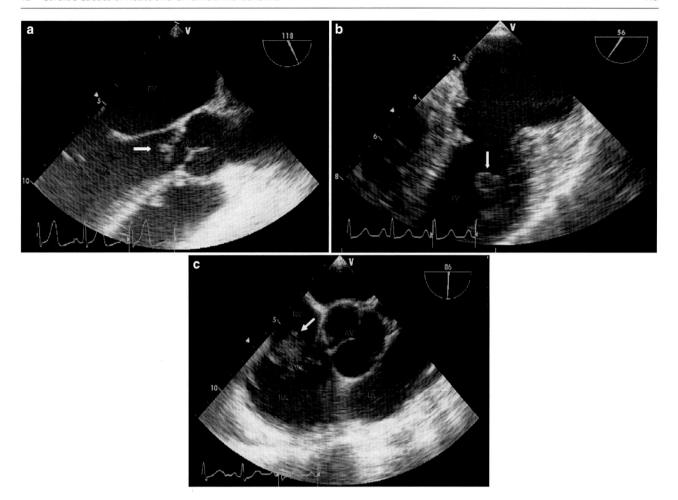

Fig. 12.3 (**a**) Aortic valve endocarditis (*arrow* pointing at the vegetation) on parasternal long-axis view of transthoracic echocardiogram. (**b**) Mitral valve endocarditis (*arrow* pointing at the vegetation) on transesophageal echocardiogram. (**c**) Tricuspid valve endocarditis (*arrow*) on a parasternal short-axis view on transthoracic echocardiogram. *RV* right ventricle, *RA* right atrium, *TV* tricuspid valve, *AV* aortic valve, *LA* left atrium, *LV* left ventricle

Cardiac Tumors

Primary cardiac tumors (Table 12.5) are extremely rare, whereas the metastatic involvement of heart is much more common. Up to around 80 % of primary cardiac tumors are benign. Among the primary benign tumors, atrial myxomas are the most common [33–35]. Although atrial myxoma is histologically benign, it can be catastrophic due to embolization. Embolization can occur in up to 30 % of patients with an atrial myxoma [36]. These tumors most commonly embolize to the central nervous system; however, peripheral embolization also occurs [37]. Large/saddle aortoiliac occlusions and acute limb ischemia have been documented in case reports as a result of myxoma embolization [38, 39].

Diagnosis is usually made on echocardiogram (Fig. 12.4); however, other imaging modalities can also be utilized. Patients with an unknown etiology of limb ischemia should undergo an echocardiogram. And vice versa, when a surgical intervention

Table 12.5 Cardiac tumors

Primary benign tumors	Primary benign or malignant
Myxomas	Paragangliomas
Papillary fibroblastoma	Mesotheliomas
Rhabdomyomas	
Fibromas	Primary malignant
Teratoma	Sarcomas
Purkinje cell tumors/hamartomas	
Lipomas	
Lipomatous hypertrophy of the interatrial septum	
Pseudoneoplasms	

is performed for critical limb ischemia, the embolism should be sent for pathological evaluation to determine its source. Most myxomas can be successfully treated with surgical resection, with low operative risk and low recurrence rate [40].

Other primary tumors of the heart have been reported in variable frequencies; however, papillary fibroelastomas are being reported more commonly. Papillary fibroelastomas are the most common tumors of the cardiac valves [41], although they can occur on the non-valvular surfaces as well. The most common valve involved is the aortic valve [42, 43]. Echocardiography can be utilized for diagnosis. They usually present as single, small, approximately 9 mm mean size, pedunculated, and mobile with a homogenous speckled pattern and a characteristic stippling along the edges [43, 44].

Because of their mobile and pedunculated nature, they most commonly present with an embolic event, whether of tumor itself or thrombus [42–44]. Because of their risk of embolization and associated morbidity, many suggest surgical excision as a curative treatment.

Paradoxical Embolism

Paradoxical embolism is an arterial embolism with an origin in the venous system, most common site being the lower extremity venous system. Although the thrombus is not cardiac in origin, these emboli usually occur in the presence of a patent foramen ovale (PFO) or an atrial septal defect (ASD). Foramen ovale is a flap between septum primum and septum secundum that is necessary in the fetus to bypass the immature lungs and transfer the oxygenated maternal blood to the fetal systemic circulation. After birth, expansion of the lungs lowers the right atrial pressure, and increased vascular resistance increases the left atrial pressure. This reversal of pressure gradient leads to the closure of the foramen flap

against the septum secundum. The contact between the septum primum flap and the septum secundum leads to fusion of these tissues with permanent closure of foramen ovale within the first year of life. The foramen ovale flap fails to fuse in approximately 20–30 % of the population [45, 46] (Fig. 12.5).

Less commonly, an open communication persists between the atria after septation, called atrial septal defect. This is due the abnormal development of the septum and the absence of sufficient tissue between the atria (Fig. 12.5).

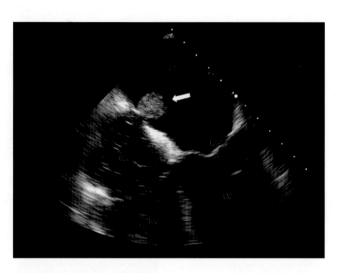

Fig. 12.4 Left atrial myxoma (*arrow*) attached to the left atrial septal wall on transesophageal echocardiogram. *LA* left atrium, *RA* right atrium, *MV* mitral valve, *TV* tricuspid valve, *RV* right ventricle, *LV* left ventricle

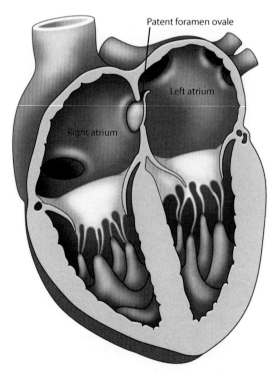
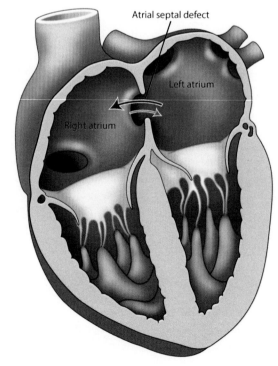

Fig. 12.5 *Left* patent foramen ovale; *right* atrial septal defect

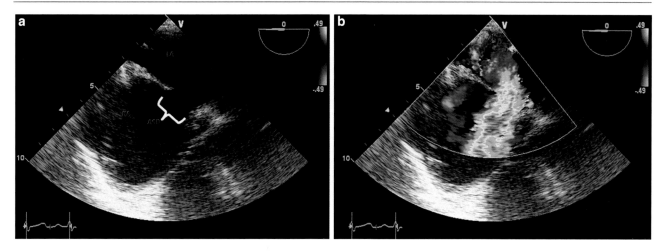

Fig. 12.6 (a) Large atrial septal defect (ASD) on transesophageal echocardiogram. *RA* right atrium, *LA* left atrium. (b) Color flow through the large ASD

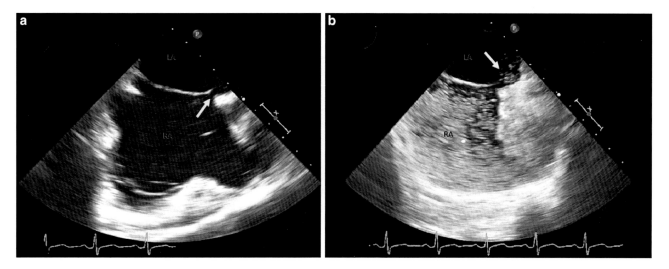

Fig 12.7 (a) Possible patent foramen ovale (*arrow*) on transesophageal echocardiogram. (b) Positive bubble study to confirm the patent foramen ovale (PFO) on transesophageal echocardiogram. The bubbles cross from right atrium to left atrium through the PFO (*arrow*). *RA* right atrium, *LA* left atrium

Patients with PFO or, much less often, with an ASD with right-to-left shunt are at a risk of paradoxical embolization. The two processes have different pathophysiology leading to different clinical presentations. ASD usually causes symptoms of right heart failure, dyspnea, and decreased exercise capacity, whereas a PFO usually presents with a transient ischemic attack or stroke due to paradoxical emboli to the cerebral circulation. While both ASD and PFO can cause paradoxical embolism to the peripheral circulation leading to limb ischemia, this is an infrequent occurrence [47, 48]. While considering paradoxical emboli, other constitutional symptoms should also be kept in mind such as lower extremity swelling (deep venous thrombosis) and shortness of breath (pulmonary embolism).

The diagnosis of paradoxical embolism is often a diagnosis of exclusion. The best imaging modality to identify intracardiac shunts is a transesophageal echocardiogram (Figs. 12.6 and 12.7), which is 100 % sensitive and 92 % sensitive [49].

The therapeutic interventions for intracardiac shunts in adults include surgical and catheter-based approaches. Catheter-based percutaneous interventions are still evolving and are being performed more often. The indications for ASD closure are well developed, whereas the indications for PFO closure are still being investigated. Currently the main indication for ASD closure is for the right-sided heart failure and symptoms. In PFO the consideration for closure is given for cryptogenic strokes or recurrent strokes.

Treatment modalities for secondary prevention of stroke in patients with a PFO include medical treatment (warfarin or antiplatelet agents) or closure of the PFO. A review of nonrandomized trials suggests that the rate of recurrence of stroke is at least as low or lower with PFO closure compared with medical treatment [50]. However, the results reported from the CLOSURE I trial [51], the first randomized clinical trial, which randomized 900 patients to either medical therapy or transcatheter closure of PFO with a CardioSEAL-STARFlex PFO device (NMT Medical, Inc., Boston, Massachusetts), showed no benefit in PFO closure over best medical management in preventing recurrence of stroke or transient ischemic attack.

There are two other percutaneous devices for PFO closure, namely, Amplatzer PFO/ASD occluder (St. Jude Medical, Plymouth, Minnesota), and Gore Helex occluder (W. L. Gore & Associates, Inc., Flagstaff, Arizona), that are currently being investigated in randomized clinical trials (RESPECT trial and REDUCE trail, respectively).

Iatrogenic Causes of Peripheral Ischemia

Cardiovascular devices and technologies are imperative in the treatment of cardiac disease. An understanding of complications associated with such devices is important in early diagnosis and treatment. Devices commonly used to support the cardiovascular system include intra-aortic balloon pumps (IABP), extracorporeal cardiopulmonary support during cardiac procedures, and extracorporeal membrane oxygenation (ECMO).

Intra-aortic balloon pumps use counterpulsion technology to increase coronary blood flow and decrease myocardial oxygen demand. Its use can be associated with thrombocytopenia, bleeding at insertion site, thromboembolism, and balloon entrapment-rupture [52, 53]. Along with these, lower extremity complication rates can be as high as 42–45 % [54, 55].

Extracorporeal membrane oxygenation is potentially a life-saving technique for patients with severe cardiopulmonary collapse. Among many other complications related to ECMO, it includes lower extremity ischemia from femoral artery cannulation. Arterial vascular complication rate varies from 3.2 to 28 % with venoarterial access [56, 57].

Percutaneous cardiac catheterizations usually result in digital ischemia due to cholesterol crystal emboli. However, critical limb ischemia has also been reported due to access site arterial thrombosis after a cardiac catheterization, including the radial artery access especially with underlying calcinosis or Raynaud's disease [58–60]. Now with the use of arterial closure devices, case reports have also described limb ischemia as a complication due to device embolization [61, 62].

Aortic or Arterial Dissection

Aortic dissection occurs after intimal rupture with hemorrhage into the arterial media. Medial degeneration is thought to predispose to dissection. The incidence of aortic dissection is 2–305/100,000. Overall mortality is 27.4 %. Stanford type A (Fig. 12.8) dissections are associated with mortality rates of 26 % in patients treated surgically versus 58 % if treated medically. Mortality rates for type B dissections are 31 % and 10.7 % for operative versus medical treatment, respectively [63].

Patients with dissection typically present with chest or back pain, hypotension, and/or renal failure. Isolated arterial dissections causing lower extremity ischemia are uncommon but can occur from iatrogenic, traumatic, or fibrodysplastic causes. Etiologies include aortic aneurysms, familial thoracic aortic aneurysms, Turner's syndrome, hypertension, hypercholesteremia, atherosclerosis, cardiac and vascular access-based interventions, aortic coarctation, inflammatory vasculitis, bicuspid aortic valves, trauma, and patients with connective tissue disorders. Cocaine abuse is a well-established association in aortic dissections in young patients. It is seen in 1 % of cocaine abusers [64]. Other contributors include tobacco and amphetamine abuse. Patient's most common presentation is pain from the dissection and can be variable but is located in the truncal region and a ventral or dorsal distribution. Pain is sudden and tearing or ripping in nature. Clinically, the patient may have discordant pulses, acute abdominal pain, peripheral pulselessness, pleural effusions, acute heart failure, acute mesenteric ischemia, acute renal failure, syncope, and various neurologic syndromes. Visceral infarction is a dismal sign [65]. Limb ischemia can be present in up to half of type A dissections and 25 % of type B dissections. When there is a clinical suspicion of a dissection, a prompt diagnosis is paramount [66–68].

The most accurate imaging modalities are computed tomography angiography (CTA), magnetic resonance imaging (MRI), aortography, and TEE. The most common used diagnostic modality is CT (Fig. 12.9). However, it is poor at identifying the origin of the intimal tear. Intimal tears are best visualized with MRI and TEE [65, 69]. Type A dissections are treated with surgical intervention unless there is a contraindication to therapy. The operative approach is through a median sternotomy with use of cardiopulmonary bypass. The origin of the intimal tear and aneurysm is typically replaced with a graft. Repair usually involves the ascending aorta but may also include the aortic root and arch.

Type B dissections are usually treated medically, controlling hypertension. Early repair of distal dissection is indicated with expanding aneurysm, impaired organ/limb perfusion, and impending rupture. Open surgical approach is via left posterolateral thoracotomy. Cardiopulmonary bypass may be required. Endovascular therapy is becoming more widely used in distal dissections. Successful treatment with endovascular therapy in type B aortic dissections is as high as 82 % with an overall survival at 5 years of 78 % and 30-day mortality of 8.5 %. Complications of endovascular therapy include retrograde type A dissections and endoleaks. Failure after endovascular therapy may require secondary endovascular intervention or open surgical therapy [70]. For uncomplicated

Fig. 12.8 Classification of
aortic dissection; DeBakey
and Stanford types

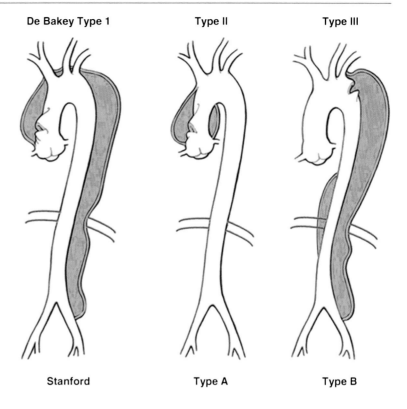

De Bakey

Type I   Originates in the ascending aorta, propagates at least to the
           aortic arch and often beyond it distally

Type II   Originates in and is confined to the ascending aorta

Type III   Originates in the descending aorta and extends distally
           down the aorta

Stanford

Type A   All dissections involving the ascending aorta

Type B   Involves the descending but not the ascending aorta

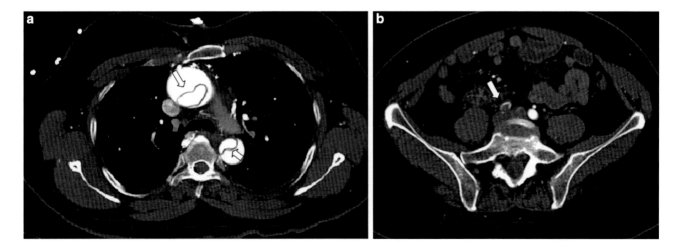

Fig. 12.9 (**a**) TT demonstrating acute aortic dissection involving ascending and descending aorta. *Arrow* depicts aortic flap. (**b**) Same patient near total occlusion of right iliac artery due to dissection flap on CT. *Arrow* depicts right iliac artery

type B dissections, medical management is still considered the treatment of choice. However, for complicated type B aortic dissections, thoracic endovascular repair (TEVAR) and open surgery may be considered. This is based on data from the International Registry of Acute Aortic Dissection (IRAD) and takes into account the INSTEAD-XL trial. Further studies are still underway to help better define the role of TEVAR in aortic dissection [71].

Lower limb ischemia that persists despite treatment may need to be addressed depending on the degree of malperfusion. A recent review of lower limb malperfusion in type B aortic dissections by Faggiola et al. compared medical, surgical, and endovascular treatment. Thirty-day morbidity and mortality for surgical versus endovascular treatment were 31%/14% and 46%/8%, respectively [72]. Endovascular treatment included stenting, fenestration, and TEVAR. Surgical treatment included open fenestration and extra anatomic bypass. Complications are high in both groups but mortality was lower in the endovascular group. Trimarchi also suggests that open fenestration be used as an option if endovascular procedures are contraindicated or fail for complicated type B dissections [73].

References

1. Hirsch AT, Haskal ZJ, Hertzer NR, Bakal CW, Creager MA, Halperin JL, et al. ACC/AHA 2005 guidelines for the management of patients with peripheral arterial disease (lower extremity, renal, mesenteric, and abdominal aortic). J Am Coll Cardiol. 2006;47(6):1239–312.
2. Falluji N, Mukherjee D. Critical and acute limb ischemia: an overview. Angiology. 2014;65(2):137–46.
3. Walker TG. Acute limb Ischemia. Tech Vasc Interv Rad 12:117–29.
4. O'Connell JB, Quiñones-Baldrich WJ. Proper evaluation and management of acute embolic versus thrombotic limb ischemia. Semin Vasc Surg. 2009;22(1):10–6.
5. Fuster V, Rydén LE, Cannom DS, et al. ACC/AHA/ESC 2006 Guidelines for the management of patients with atrial fibrillation: a report of the American College of Cardiology/American Heart Association Task Force on Practice Guidelines and the European Society of Cardiology Committee for Practice Guidelines (Writing Committee to Revise the 2001 Guidelines for the Management of Patients With Atrial Fibrillation): developed in collaboration with the European Heart Rhythm Association and the Heart Rhythm Society. Circulation. 114(7): e257–354.
6. Lloyd-Jones DM, Wang TJ, Leip EP, Larson MG, Levy D, Vasan RS, et al. Lifetime risk for development of atrial fibrillation: The Framingham Heart Study. Circulation. 2004;110:1042.
7. Frost L1, Engholm G, Johnsen S, Møller H, Henneberg EW, Husted S. Incident thromboembolism in the aorta and the renal, mesenteric, pelvic and extremity arteries after discharge from the hospital with a diagnosis of atrial fibrillation. Arch Intern Med. 2001;161: 272–6.
8. Menke J, Lüthje L, Kastrup A, Larsen J. Thromboembolism in atrial fibrillation. Am J Cardiol. 2010;105(4):502–10.
9. Gage BF, Waterman AD, Shannon W, Boechler M, Rich MW, Radford MJ. Validation of clinical classification schemes for predicting stroke: results from the National Registry of Atrial Fibrillation. JAMA. 2001;285(22):2864–70.
10. Lip GY, Nieuwlaat R, Pisters R, Lane DA, Crijns HJ. Refining clinical risk stratification for predicting stroke and thromboembolism in atrial fibrillation using a novel risk factor-based approach: the euro heart survey on atrial fibrillation. Chest. 2010;137(2):263–72.
11. January CT, Wann LS, Alpert JS, Calkins H, Cleveland JC Jr, Cigarroa JE, et al. 2014 AHA/ACC/HRS guideline for the management of patients with atrial fibrillation: a report of the American College of Cardiology/American Heart Association Task Force on Practice Guidelines and the Heart Rhythm Society. J Am Coll Cardiol. 2014;28. pii: S0735-1097(14)01740-9.
12. Connolly SJ, Ezekowitz MD, Yusuf S, Eikelboom J, Oldgren J, Parekh A, et al. Dabigatran versus warfarin in patients with atrial fibrillation. N Engl J Med. 2009;361(12):1139–51.
13. Granger CB, Alexander JH, McMurray JJ, Lopes RD, Hylek EM, Hanna M. Apixaban versus warfarin in patients with atrial fibrillation. N Engl J Med. 2011;365(11):981–92.
14. Patel MR, Mahaffey KW, Garg J, Pan G, Singer DE, Hacke W. Rivaroxaban versus warfarin in nonvalvular atrial fibrillation. N Engl J Med. 2011;365(10):883–91.
15. Holmes DR, Reddy VY, Turi ZG, Doshi SK, Sievert H, Buchbinder M. Percutaneous closure of the left atrial appendage versus warfarin therapy for prevention of stroke in patients with atrial fibrillation: a randomised non-inferiority trial. Lancet. 2009;374(9689):534–42.
16. Asinger RW, Mikell FL, Elsperger J, Hodges M. Incidence of left-ventricular thrombosis after acute transmural myocardial infarction. Serial evaluation by two-dimensional echocardiography. N Engl J Med. 1981;305(6):297–302.
17. Delewi R, Zijlstra F, Piek JJ. Left ventricular thrombus formation after acute myocardial infarction. Heart. 2012;98(23):1743–9.
18. Chiarella F, Santoro E, Domenicucci S, Maggioni A, Vecchio C. Predischarge two-dimensional echocardiographic evaluation of left ventricular thrombosis after acute myocardial infarction in the GISSI-3 study. Am J Cardiol. 1998;81(7):822–7.
19. Gianstefani S, Douiri A, Delithanasis I, Rogers T, Sen A, Kalra S, et al. Incidence and predictors of early left ventricular thrombus after ST-elevation myocardial infarction in the contemporary era of primary percutaneous coronary intervention. Am J Cardiol. 2014;113(7):1111–6.
20. Küpper AJ, Verheugt FW, Peels CH, Galema TW, Roos JP. Left ventricular thrombus incidence and behavior studied by serial two-dimensional echocardiography in acute anterior myocardial infarction: left ventricular wall motion, systemic embolism and oral anticoagulation. J Am Coll Cardiol. 1989;13(7):1514–20.
21. Stratton JR, Resnick AD. Increased embolic risk in patients with left ventricular thrombi. Circulation. 1987;75:1004.
22. Meltzer RS, Visser CA, Fuster V. Intracardiac thrombi and systemic embolization. Ann Intern Med. 1986;104(5):689–98.
23. Delewi R1, Zijlstra F, Piek JJ. Left ventricular thrombus formation after acute myocardial infarction. Heart. 2012;98(23):1743–49.
24. Cabin HS, Roberts WC. Left ventricular aneurysm, intraaneurysmal thrombus and systemic embolus in coronary heart disease. Chest. 1980;77(5):586–90.
25. Nixon JV. Left ventricular mural thrombus. Arch Intern Med. 1983;143(8):1567–71.
26. Jugdutt BI1, Sivaram CA. Prospective two-dimensional echocardiographic evaluation of left ventricular thrombus and embolism after acute myocardial infarction. J Am Coll Cardiol. 1989;13(3):554–64.
27. Weinstein L, Schlesinger JJ. Pathoanatomic, pathophysiologic and clinical correlations in endocarditis (second of two parts). N Engl J Med. 1974;291(21):1122–6.
28. Baddour LM, Wilson WR, Bayer AS, Fowler VG Jr, Bolger AF, Levison ME, et al. Infective endocarditis: diagnosis, antimicrobial therapy, and management of complications: a statement for healthcare professionals from the Committee on Rheumatic Fever,

Endocarditis, and Kawasaki Disease, Council on Cardiovascular Disease in the Young, and the Councils on Clinical Cardiology, Stroke, and Cardiovascular Surgery and Anesthesia, American Heart Association: endorsed by the Infectious Diseases Society of America. Circulation. 2005;111(23):e394–434.

29. Vilacosta I, Graupner C, San Román JA, Sarriá C, Ronderos R, Fernández C, et al. Risk of embolization after institution of antibiotic therapy for infective endocarditis. J Am Coll Cardiol. 2002;39(9):1489–95.

30. Mügge A, Daniel WG, Frank G, Lichtlen PR. Echocardiography in infective endocarditis: reassessment of prognostic implications of vegetation size determined by the transthoracic and the transesophageal approach. J Am Coll Cardiol. 1989;14(3):631–8.

31. Prendergast BD1, Tornos P. Surgery for infective endocarditis: who and when? Circulation. 2010;121(9):1141–52.

32. Nishimura RA, Otto CM, Bonow RO, Carabello BA, Erwin 3rd JP, Guyton RA, et al. 2014 AHA/ACC guideline for the management of patients with valvular heart disease: a report of the American College of Cardiology/American Heart Association Task Force on Practice Guidelines. J Am Coll Cardiol. 2014;63(22):e57–185.

33. Molina JE, Edwards JE, Ward HB. Primary cardiac tumors: experience at the University of Minnesota. Thorac Cardiovasc Surg. 1990;38 Suppl 2:183.

34. Tazelaar HD, Locke TJ, McGregor CG. Pathology of surgically excised primary cardiac tumors. Mayo Clin Proc. 1992;67(10):957.

35. Odim J, Reehal V, Laks H, Mehta U, Fishbein MC. Surgical pathology of cardiac tumors. Two decades at an urban institution. Cardiovasc Pathol. 2003;12(5):267.

36. Livi U, Bortolotti U, Milano A, Valente M, Prandi A, Frugoni C, et al. Cardiac myxomas: results of 14 years' experience. Thorac Cardiovasc Surg. 1984;32(3):143–7.

37. Reynen K. Cardiac myxomas. N Engl J Med. 1995;333(24):1610–7.

38. Coley C, Lee KR, Steiner M, Thompson CS. Complete embolization of a left atrial myxoma resulting in acute lower extremity ischemia. Tex Heart Inst J. 2005;32(2):238–40.

39. Chiba K, Abe H, Kitanaka Y, Makuuchi H. Left atrial myxoma complicated with an acute upper extremity embolism. Ann Thorac Cardiovasc Surg. 2012;18(4):391–4.

40. Bhan A, Mehrotra R, Choudhary SK, Sharma R, Prabhakar D, Airan B. Surgical experience with intracardiac myxomas: long-term follow-up. Ann Thorac Surg. 1998;66(3):810–3.

41. Edwards FH, Hale D, Cohen A, Thompson L, Pezzella AT, Virmani R. Primary cardiac valve tumors. Ann Thorac Surg. 1991;52(5):1127–31.

42. Gowda RM, Khan IA, Nair CK, Mehta NJ, Vasavada BC, Sacchi TJ. Cardiac papillary fibroelastoma: a comprehensive analysis of 725 cases. Am Heart J. 2003;146(3):404.

43. Sun JP, Asher CR, Yang XS, et al. Clinical and echocardiographic characteristics of papillary fibroelastomas: a retrospective and prospective study in 162 patients. Circulation. 2001;103:2687–93.

44. Klarich KW, Enriquez-Sarano M, Gura GM, Edwards WD, Tajik AJ, Seward JB. Papillary fibroelastoma: echocardiographic characteristics for diagnosis and pathologic correlation. J Am Coll Cardiol. 1997;30:784–90.

45. Kerut EK, Norfleet WT, Plotnick GD, Giles TD. Patent foramen ovale: a review of associated conditions and the impact of physiological size. J Am Coll Cardiol. 2001;38(3):613–23.

46. Hagen PT, Scholz DG, Edwards WD. Incidence and size of patent foramen ovale during the first 10 decades of life: an autopsy study of 965 normal hearts. Mayo Clin Proc. 1984;59(1):17–20.

47. Hugl B, Klein-Weigel P, Posch L, Greiner A, Fraedrich G. Peripheral ischemia caused by paradoxical embolization: an underestimated problem? Mt Sinai J Med. 2005;72(3):200–6.

48. Miller S, Causey MW, Schachter D, Andersen CA, Singh N. A case of limb ischemia secondary to paradoxical embolism. Vasc Endovascular Surg. 2010;44(7):604–8.

49. Chen WJ, Kuan P, Lien WP, Lin FY. Detection of patent foramen ovale by contrast transesophageal echocardiography. Chest. 1992;101(6):1515–20.

50. Tobis J, Shenoda M. Percutaneous treatment of patent foramen ovale and atrial septal defects. J Am Coll Cardiol. 2012;60(18):1722–32.

51. Furlan AJ, Reisman M, Massaro J, Mauri L, Adams H, Albers GW, et al. Closure or medical therapy for cryptogenic stroke with patent foramen ovale. N Engl J Med. 2012;366(11):991–9.

52. Parissis H, Soo A, Al-Alao B. Intra aortic balloon pump: literature review of risk factors related to complications of the intraaortic balloon pump. J Cardiothorac Surg. 2011;6:147.

53. Vales L, Kanei Y, Ephrem G, Misra D. Intra-aortic balloon pump use and outcomes with current therapies. J Invasive Cardiol. 2011;23(3):116–9.

54. Kantrowitz A, Wasfie T, Freed PS, Rubenfire M, Wajszczuk W, Schork MA. Intraaortic balloon pumping 1967 through 1982: analysis of complications in 733 patients. Am J Cardiol. 1986;57(11):976–83.

55. Alderman JD, Gabliani GI, McCabe CH, Brewer CC, Lorell BH, Pasternak RC, et al. Incidence and management of limb ischemia with percutaneous wire-guided intraaortic balloon catheters. J Am Coll Cardiol. 1987;9(3):524–30.

56. Al-Attar N, Roussel A, Khaliel F. Extracorporeal membrane oxygenation (ECMO). ESC Council Cardiol Pract. 2013;11(22).

57. Zangrillo A, Landoni G, Biondi-Zoccai G, Greco M, Greco T, Frati G, et al. A meta-analysis of complications and mortality of extracorporeal membrane oxygenation. Crit Care Resusc. 2013;15(3):172–8.

58. Taglieri N1, Galiè N, Marzocchi A. Acute hand ischemia after radial intervention in patient with CREST-associated pulmonary hypertension: successful treatment with manual thromboaspiration. J Invasive Cardiol. 2013;25(2):89–91.

59. Rose SH. Ischemic complications of radial artery cannulation: an association with a calcinosis, Raynaud's phenomenon, esophageal dysmotility, sclerodactyly, and telangiectasia variant of scleroderma. Anesthesiology. 1993;78(3):587–9.

60. Mangar D1, Laborde RS, Vu DN. Delayed ischaemia of the hand necessitating amputation after radial artery cannulation. Can J Anaesth. 1993;40(3):247–50.

61. Khakha RS, Ali T, Chong P, Gerrard D, Leopold P. Embolisation of Angio-Seal™ device: an unusual case of post-cardiac catheterisation limb ischaemia. Ann R Coll Surg Engl. 2011;93(5):e41–2.

62. Teso D, Karmy-Jones R. Distal embolism of percutaneous arterial closure device resulting in critical limb ischemia. J Vasc Interv Radiol. 2010;21(10):1487–8.

63. Hagan, P, Nienaber C, Isselbacher E, et al. The international registry of acute aortic dissection (IRAD) new insights into an old disease. JAMA. 2000;283(7):897–903.

64. Nusair M, Abuzetun J, Khaja A, Dohrmann M. A case of aortic dissection in a cocaine abuser: a case report and review of the literature. Cases J. 2008;1:369.

65. Fann JI, Sarris GE, Mitchell RS, Shumway NE, Stinson EB, Oyer PE, Miller DC. Treatment of patients with aortic dissection presenting with peripheral vascular complications. Ann Surg. 1990;212(6):705–13.

66. Sutton MS, Oldershaw PJ, Miller GA, Paneth M, Williams B, Braimbridge M. Dissection of the thoracic aorta. A comparison between medical and surgical treatment. J Cardiovasc Surg (Torino). 1981;22(3):195–202.

67. Slater EE, DeSanctis RW. The clinical recognition of dissecting aortic aneurysm. Am J Med. 1976;60(5):625–33.

68. Cambria RP, Brewster DC, Gertler J, Moncure AC, Gusberg R, Tilson MD, et al. Vascular complications associated with spontaneous aortic dissection. J Vasc Surg. 1988;7(2):199–209.

69. Steingruber I, Chemelli A, Glodny B, Hugl B, Bonatti J, Hiemetzbeger R, Jaschke W, Czermak B. Endovascular repair of

acute type B aortic dissections: midterm results. J Endovasc Ther. 2008;15(2):150–60.

70. Khan IA, Nair CK. Clinical, diagnostic, and management perspectives of aortic dissection. Chest. 2002;122(1):311–28.

71. Patel AY, Eagle KA, Vaishnava P. Acute type B aortic dissection: insights from the international registry of acute aortic dissection. Ann Cardiothorac Surg. 2014;3(4):368–74.

72. Gargiulo M, Massoni CB, Gallitto E, Freyrie A, Trimarchi S, Faggioli G, Stella A. Lower limb malperfusion in type B aortic dissection: a systematic review. Ann Cardiothorac Surg. 2014; 3(4):351–67.

73. Trimarchi S, Segreti S, Grassi V, Lomazzi C, Cova M, Piffaretti G, Rampoldi V. Open fenestration for complicated acute aortic B dissection. Ann Cardiothorac Surg. 2014;3(4):418–22.

Progression of Peripheral Artery Disease to Critical Limb Ischemia

13

Michael J. McArdle, Jay Giri, and Emile R. Mohler, III

Introduction

Critical limb ischemia (CLI), often considered the end stage of peripheral artery disease (PAD), is a tipping point in the balance between metabolic supply and demand of the lower extremity. This balance hinges on many factors, and the progression from stable PAD to CLI depends on the complex interplay of these variables. Despite the fact that PAD is classically categorized by disease severity, the natural history of PAD progression and general development of CLI does not follow a strictly linear path, a fact characterized by the often insidious clinical presentation of CLI. From a pathophysiologic perspective, CLI is the final result of the common atherogenic pathway that causes PAD. However, CLI manifests only in selected case largely due to a loss of compensatory mechanisms that leads to overt tissue ischemia. Many of the risk factors that contribute to the development of PAD are also responsible for its progression and ultimately for development of CLI, and important information can be gleaned from their modification both in PAD and CLI.

M.J. McArdle, MD
Department of Internal Medicine, University of Pennsylvania, Philadelphia, PA, USA

J. Giri, MD, MPH • E.R. Mohler, III, MD (✉)
Cardiovascular Division, Department of Medicine, Hospital of the University of Pennsylvania, Perelman School of Medicine, University of Pennsylvania, 3400 Civic Center Blvd 11-103, Philadelphia, PA 19104, USA

Pathophysiology

CLI clinically presents with rest pain and tissue ulceration that are a result of insufficient peripheral perfusion [1]. This presentation is gradual and chronic, unlike the sudden manifestations of acute limb ischemia [1]. The progression rom stable arterial narrowing to outright hemodynamic compromise in the lower extremity depends on many factors. From a pathophysiologic standpoint, CLI can be difficult to distinguish from stable PAD, and they are, in fact, part of the same spectrum [1]. In certain cases, CLI may develop in the setting of conditions such as atherothrombotic or embolic disease, in situ thrombosis, inflammation, or trauma [1, 2]. These situations, however, do not account for the vast majority of CLI cases, which ultimately stem from severe peripheral atherosclerotic disease [2]. Underlying disease progression to CLI is thus generally a progression of underlying atherosclerosis [3, 4], in contrast to acute limb ischemia where a defined perfusion-limiting event is culprit [1]. Atherosclerosis in the extremities occurs in the arterial intimal layer [3], specifically in regions of turbulent blood flow [5], and some evidence points to periods of rapid progression involving plaque ulceration and hemorrhage similar to that seen in coronary artery disease [3].

What separates CLI from stable PAD is the complex chronic regulation of macro-vascular and microvascular circulation that results in an inability of innate protective mechanisms to maintain capillary bed perfusion [6]. When blood flow is restricted to the point that tissue viability is compromised, compensatory mechanisms fail, and tissue ischemia leads to pain and poor wound healing [6]. This process occurs initially with macrocirculatory reduction in arterial lumen diameter as a result of severe atherosclerotic disease, a situation which reduces blood flow. The severe multi-segment arterial disease is compounded by vasomotor paralysis and vasogenic edema [1, 7]. Microcirculatory compensatory mechanisms ultimately cannot withstand this critical level of ischemia [6]. This leads to multisystem vascular dysfunction in CLI. Endothelial cell dysfunction and dysregulation, white blood cell activation and inflammation, impaired defense mechanisms, altered microvascular flow regulation, and significant oxidative stress, among others, contribute to the final clinical picture of CLI [6].

Epidemiology and Natural History

The epidemiologic burden of CLI varies per study, but general estimates put the prevalence at between one to two million in the United States [8, 9] with an annual incidence of 220–300 per million per year [10, 11]. One large Medicare cohort, including patients only over age 65, reported an overall prevalence and annual incidence of 0.23 and 0.20%, respectively, which is in line with prior estimates [8]. However, it was noted that with the aging population, this implies a potential increase in prevalence to 2.8–3.5 million by 2020 [8]. These numbers are significant given the high morbidity and mortality of this condition. Each decrease of ankle-brachial index (ABI) of 0.10 is associated with a 10% increase in relative risk for a major vascular event, primarily ischemic heart disease [1, 12], and there is a 20% mortality in the first year following presentation of CLI [1]. In fact, the 5-year mortality of CLI is estimated at 60% [13], greater than that of acute myocardial infarction, stroke, and prostate, breast, and colorectal cancers [6].

The natural history of PAD and development of CLI, especially in an era of treatment and intervention, is difficult to define but represents a combination of both progressive decline and less linear primary presentation [1]. Contemporarily, many patients with PAD progression are treated before their symptoms reach the critical tipping point [1]. In general, more than half of patients with PAD receive some form of medical or interventional treatment, with those not receiving treatment having generally stable symptoms [1]. Claudication symptoms remain stable in approximately 75% of patients throughout their lifetime, without evidence of progressive lower extremity deterioration [3, 14]. And when progression does occur, it is more common during the first year following diagnosis [15]. Between 6 and 9% of patients develop symptom worsening in this first year, compared to an annual rate of 2–3% thereafter [16]. There is evidence, however, that functional decline may not be readily recognized and may be more common than previously realized [3]. For example, in one cross-sectional study, diminished ABI was highly correlated to leg weakness and multiple functional outcomes, including reduced 6-min walk, even after adjustment for initial symptom score [16].

Longitudinal data support a progressive decline in PAD [6, 15, 17]. Of patients with claudication, approximately 15–20% will develop rest pain or gangrene within their lifetime [1, 2]. In one cohort with claudication, more severe claudication was reported in 60% of patients after 2.5 year follow-up, with a decline in ABI by at least 0.15 carrying a relative risk of 1.8 for severe claudication [18]. An additional longitudinal study of smokers with claudication reported an annual decrease in ABI by 21, 16, and 17% in the first three consecutive years of follow-up, with an overall 12.5% incidence of CLI during follow-up [19]. One 15-year outcome study of patients with claudication demonstrated gradual increase in need for major and minor amputations over time, though with a relative plateau after 2 years [17]. There remains a cohort of patients, however, who present initially with CLI without prior symptoms [6, 19–21]. This cohort represents 1–3% of patients with CLI and is particularly common in patients who present after minor trauma and subsequent development of a non-healing ulcer [22]. These patients are typically limited by multiple comorbidities and have impaired functional capacity, often attributing pain to other etiologies limiting detection of PAD until advanced stages [22].

Much additional information can be extrapolated from data on symptom development in PAD prior to reaching CLI. The vast majority of patients develop claudication subtly [3]. Using clinical and imaging data, several characteristics of this transition have been identified. In the landmark Edinburgh Artery Study, a large-scale cohort of 1592 subjects aged 55–74 years, the overall PAD incidence, as defined by development of claudication, was reported in 179 cases (11.2%) during 12-year follow-up [23]. Conversion to claudication is often a bilateral phenomenon, demonstrated in a small series assessing subjective symptom progression [3]. This was confirmed via angiographic data that demonstrated more rapid progression of arterial disease in superficial femoral arteries with concomitant contralateral superficial femoral artery occlusion [24]. Atherosclerotic disease may progress without significant change in symptoms in legs with higher ABIs [3]. In these patients, symptom development may lag behind imaging-based progression. In one small cohort with known PAD, claudication symptoms progressed in two extremities over a 5-year period, while angiographic disease progressed in 14 of the 19 assessed extremities (73%) [25]. In an additional cohort, those with known PAD developed new or progressive lesions in 17 of 48 extremities (35%), which correlated with development of claudication and functional impairment as a result of decreased 6-min walk distance [3]. These results indicate that PAD progression, while ultimately leading to increased symptoms, may often proceed unnoticed despite radiographic evidence of disease progression. Patients may subtly decrease their activity levels to compensate for increasing disease burden [26, 27], giving both patients and caregivers a false sense of security. Over time, as disease severity increases and tissue perfusion is compromised, CLI may emerge. And unfortunately, in many cases, patients die secondary to cardiovascular events before stable PAD progresses to CLI.

Table 13.1 Risk factors associated with the progression of PAD to CLI

Traditional, non-modifiable	Older age
	Race
Traditional, modifiable	Smoking
	Diabetes mellitus
	Hypertension
	Dyslipidemia
Nontraditional	Obesity
	Sedentary behavior
	Chronic renal insufficiency
	Hyperhomocysteinemia
	Elevated CRP and other inflammatory markers
	Hypothyroidism[a]
	Hyperviscosity[a]
	Acute illness[a]
	Reduced cardiac output[a]
	Peripheral neuropathy[a]

[a]Proposed but with limited evidence

Fig. 13.1 Risk factors, with corresponding approximate magnitude, for development of critical limb ischemia in patients with peripheral arterial disease [1]. From Norgren et al. Inter-society consensus for the management of peripheral arterial disease (TASC II). J Vasc Surg. Copyright © 2007;45 Suppl S:S5–67. Reprinted with permission from Elsevier Science and Technology Journals

Risk Factor Modification and Effect on CLI Development

Many of the same risk factors that give rise to PAD initially are also suspected in the development of CLI (Table 13.1 and Fig. 13.1). Early recognition and aggressive risk factor modification in PAD is thought to decrease symptom severity and reduce incidence of CLI [28], but data in this area is limited. Given the difficulty in identifying the transition between stable PAD and CLI, much of the recommendations for management and prevention of CLI are extrapolated from stable PAD and claudication data and management recommendations [28]. Additionally, since CLI is rarely studied in isolation, it is important to extract information from surgical and amputation-based studies where CLI, resulting in significant ischemia and gangrene, may prompt treatment necessity.

Non-modifiable risk factors, namely, age, race, and gender, all have associations with PAD and development of CLI. PAD develops in a longitudinal pattern with prevalence increasing linearly with age [1]. Both the seminal Framingham Study [29] and National Health and Nutrition Examination Survey (NHANES) report [30] document this increased prevalence. A large series of Medicare data in patients with CLI demonstrated that this longitudinal progression is also true of CLI. A progressive rise in prevalence and incidence was noted in patients between 65 and 85 years [8]. Though patients who first present at younger ages repre-

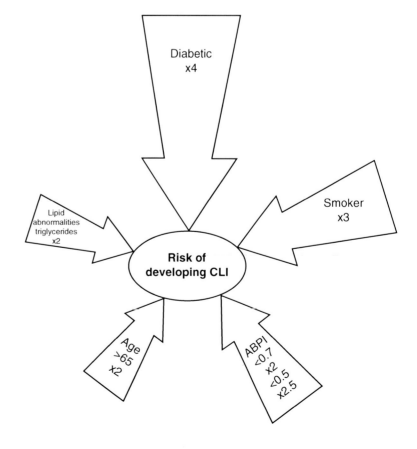

sent a small portion of the overall PAD cohort, they have overall poorer long-term outcomes [31]. This includes higher late amputation rate (17 versus 3.9%) [32] and increased rate of failed bypasses (92 versus 65%) [33]. Additionally, in a comparative series of contrasting patients younger than 49 years of age (mean age 43 years) and those between 60 and 75 years of age (mean age 67 years) who had PAD requiring amputation, though there was no overall difference in 5-year survival between the groups (62 versus 47%), the mean age of death in the younger cohort was greater than 20 years earlier than the older group (mean age of death 48 versus 69 years) [33].

Racial predispositions identified for PAD appear to be similar in CLI. In the aforementioned Medicare cohort, overall prevalence and incidence of CLI was highest in black patients (0.49 and 0.41%, respectively), while lowest in Asian patients (0.12 and 0.10%, respectively) [8]. Black patients, after risk factor adjustment, had a 2.3 times higher risk of CLI development than white patients [8]. This difference has important clinical applications, as black patients are also at 2–4 times higher risk of lower limb loss than white patients. Additionally, in the year following CLI diagnosis, black patients demonstrated the highest incidence of amputation and lowest rates of revascularization (27.8%, HR 0.87, respectively) in stark contrast to white patients who demonstrated the highest incidence of revascularization with lower rates of amputation (32.8%, HR 1.3, respectively) [8].

Gender differences may also have significant clinical impact in the progression of CLI. Women tend to have lower overall prevalence of symptomatic PAD, but are more likely to present with CLI [34]. This initial PAD prevalence gap narrows significantly with advancing age [34]. Sex-related differences have been reported in several vascular diseases, and a multitude of prior studies have demonstrated essentially equivocal rates of amputation and overall survival in PAD between men and women [34]. However, one recent study investigating gender differences in the era of intervention reports that women were on average 3.5 years older at the time of intervention and were more likely to present with CLI (OR 1.21) [34]. This study noted that women were more likely to present with more advanced disease, resulting in higher mortality in both intermittent claudication and CLI [34]. This was attributed, potentially, to relative underutilization of preventative care in women [35], with less consistent achievement of target outcomes (e.g., blood pressure, low-density lipoprotein, and hemoglobin A1c) [36], which may have resulted in increased perioperative cardiovascular events and death in this intervention-based study [34].

Tobacco use, specifically smoking, is the greatest modifiable contributor to PAD and is a well-defined driver of CLI development. Smoking increases the risk of PAD, with greater risk evident in heavy smokers (RR3.94) [23]. A direct correlation has been noted with number of cigarettes smoked

[37, 38]. In fact, the association between smoking and PAD is almost twice that of smoking and coronary artery disease [39]. Smoking also directly correlates with PAD progression [40, 41]. Smoking accelerates claudication onset by nearly 10 years compared to nonsmoking patients, and these patients are more than twice as likely to develop CLI [23, 31]. This has many important clinical implications, as smokers with PAD have greater disease severity, poorer survival rates, increased amputation risk, and reduced arterial bypass graft patency [31, 42]. In patients with claudication, continued smoking increases amputation risk [43, 44]. Smoking cessation, not surprisingly, leads to clinical benefit. Smoking cessation, even within just a few years, reduces risk of progression from PAD to CLI [1, 12], with improved ankle pressure and exercise tolerance and decreased risk of fatal vascular complications [37]. Smoking cessation also improves 10-year survival compared to continued smoking (82 versus 46%, respectively) [40]. Additionally, alternative vascular pathology associated with smoking, including thromboangiitis obliterans (Buerger's disease), increases risk of ulcer formation by limiting protective sensory mechanisms and increasing inflammation [1].

Diabetes mellitus (DM) similarly has a strong link to PAD and is a substantial contributor to CLI development, though minimal data is available to assess the effect of DM control in prevention of CLI. There is a high coincidence of these two diseases, with as many as 20–30% of patients with PAD having concomitant DM [40]. Annual CLI prevalence and incidence are remarkably higher in those with DM (1.03 and 0.86%, respectively) than in the general population [8]. Both the degree and duration of DM are linked to PAD development, and there are independent associations between PAD progression to CLI and diabetes [40, 45, 46]. Patients with diabetes are at least five times as likely as nondiabetics to develop CLI and have an overall mortality two times that of nondiabetics [45]. There are also increased rates of complications. In patients who have developed CLI, progression to gangrene is much greater in those with diabetes (40 versus 9%) [47]. In fact, greater than 50% of gangrenous lesions causing amputation occur in the diabetic population [48]. DM patients have lower limb salvage rates [49], with an overall 15–28 times greater likelihood of requiring amputation [8, 50]. This situation is compounded by increased interventional complication rates, including postoperative myocardial infarction, wound infection and need for additional surgical debridement, and increased hospital and long-term mortality [37, 51–53]. The etiology of this increased morbidity is unclear but likely multifactorial. Pathophysiologically, PAD in DM is similar to non-DM though with a greater predilection for the infrapopliteal vessels [40]. The altered metabolic milieu of DM is pro-inflammatory and pro-atherogenic, with increased vascular bed dysfunction [40]. Additionally, DM presents a host of increased clinical complications. These include peripheral neuropathy masking symptoms and delaying PAD diagnosis as well as the additional effect of diabetes and hyperglycemia in impairment of wound healing [40]. And among those with DM, risk of CLI development may be predicted by less traditional PAD risk factors, highlighting the large effect that DM plays on CLI development [54]. As demonstrated in a small survey of PAD and CLI patients, these less traditional risk factors include ABI less than 0.5 in the prior 1–3 years (OR 3.39), microvascular complications such as retinopathy (OR 12.98), heart failure (OR 1.91), and previous prostanoid treatment (OR 15.92) [54]. Overall, DM presents great risk for both the development and management of CLI, a situation of increasing concern as rates of DM continue to increase in the US population at large.

Hypertension is an independent risk factor for PAD but has unclear direct association to CLI. The NHANES and PAD Awareness, Risk and Treatment: New Resources for Survival (PARTNERS) reports both demonstrated a high prevalence of hypertension in patients with PAD (74 and 92 %, respectively), and patients in the Framingham Heart study demonstrated a 2.5–4 times rate of claudication in those with elevated blood pressure [4, 29]. In patients with DM and PAD, blood pressure lowering leads to reduced cardiovascular events [40, 55]. However, tight blood pressure control in the United Kingdom Prospective Diabetes Study (UKPDS), also assessing DM and PAD, did not have any effect on PAD development as assessed by amputation risk [56]. Traditional recommendations have followed general guidelines, with target blood pressure less than 140/90 mmHg in the absence of other comorbidities [1]. However, acute blood pressure reduction carries a potential risk of decreased limb perfusion [49]. Of note, initial concern that blood pressure control with nonselective beta-blockade (e.g., propranolol) may be detrimental through reduction of cardiac output and decreased skeletal muscle vasodilatation was not confirmed in two meta-analyses of mild-moderate lower limb ischemia, and beta-blockers are generally safe to use in this population [49]. In CLI, lower extremity perfusion is paramount and blood pressure control becomes a less clear goal. In one center, target blood pressure for CLI is recommended to be set above traditional guidelines until ulcer healing has occurred, though this approach has not been scientifically investigated [37, 57]. Interestingly, in one longitudinal study of claudication, systolic blood pressure in the middle tertile (153–170 mmHg) was the only variable which led to a reduced risk of ABI deterioration [19].

Dyslipidemia is a common vascular risk factor thought to significantly contribute to the progression of PAD to CLI. Elevated total cholesterol, low-density lipoprotein, triglycerides, and lipoprotein(a) all have independent associations with PAD, with a prevalence of hyperlipidemia in PAD patients as high as 77 % and a direct relationship to total cho-

lesterol [49]. Statin therapy, via both lipid lowering and pleiotropic effects, has been shown to decrease major vascular events in a PAD subgroup of the Heart Protection Study [58] as well as to reduce ischemic heart disease in patients with claudication in the Scandinavian Simvastatin Survival Study [59]. A Cochrane review of statin use in PAD demonstrated reduced coronary events, but unclear direct associations with lipid lowering [60]. Much of the benefit derived from statin therapy may be a result of beneficial effects on plaque stabilization, platelet adhesion, thrombosis, inflammation, increased endothelial progenitor cells, extracellular microvesicle modification, and endothelial function [37, 61, 62]. Statin therapy is associated with improved survival especially in patients with severe PAD and elevated inflammatory states and may improve objective measures of leg function [2, 63]. Statins additionally improve functional parameters and reduce longitudinal decline in PAD. High-intensity atorvastatin intervention was shown to improve ambulation from both a subjective quality of life perspective and more objective pain-free walking time 12 months following initiation of treatment in patients with stable PAD [64]. Statin use is associated with decreased lower extremity performance decline, including less annual decline in traditional and rapid walking velocity, overall 6-min walk performance, and summary performance score in a longitudinal study of functional outcomes in PAD with mean follow-up of 12.4 months [65]. Low high-density lipoprotein level [51] and elevated lipoprotein(a) levels, an independent inflammatory marker, are associated with increased mortality in CLI [37, 66]. The general inflammatory state of PAD and particularly CLI often leads to a negative acute phase reaction and falsely low lipid levels [67]. The best data available assessing the use of statin therapy in CLI comes from a subgroup analysis of PREVENT III, a study of lower extremity bypass grafts comparing edifoglide, a novel transcription regulator, to placebo [68]. Statin therapy in a cohort with CLI was associated with reduced 1-year mortality, whereas beta-blocker and antiplatelet medications had no effect on survival [69]. This analysis also reported that hypertriglyceridemia, among both lipid-specific and general variables, was the only risk factor independently associated with progression from claudication to CLI (RR 1.9) [19]. However, data is limited assessing the effects of statin therapy and lipid-lowering on development of CLI, and no data is available directly investigating the potential effect of reducing triglycerides in CLI progression [7].

Weight reduction and exercise are generally recommended in patients with PAD to improve functional capacity; however, the direct effect on progression of CLI and with CLI in general is less clear [1]. Overall higher daily physical activity, importantly, is associated with reduced 5-year mortality (HR 3.48) in patients with stable PAD [70]. An optimal exercise regimen in PAD consists of intermittent walking to near-maximal pain to improve claudication pain distance [43, 71]. Exercise has beneficial functional effects in stable PAD. In a randomized study of patients with PAD comparing supervised exercise to stent revascularization or optimal medical therapy, supervised exercise led to improved treadmill walking performance compared to both stent revascularization and optimal medical therapy at 6 months [72]. Self-directed walking exercises, likewise, are associated with decreased functional decline in PAD, as determined by 6-min walk distance in an observational study of stable PAD over a median 36-month follow-up [73]. These results are especially impactful in PAD, as these patients have a significantly lower baseline physical activity level compared to non-PAD patients [26, 27]. There is, however, no available data on the effect of PAD progression and development of CLI. Additionally complicating the picture, exercise is often contraindicated in CLI due to risk of causing or worsening ischemic lower extremity wounds [49].

The role of thrombosis in the development of CLI and subsequent prevention with antiplatelet agents has limited data with primary recommendations stemming from studies conducted in PAD. For example, both the Clopidogrel versus Aspirin in Patients at Risk of Ischemic Events (CAPRIE) trial and Antithrombotic Trialists' Collaboration report reduced vascular events with antiplatelet therapy in PAD [49]. However, one of the primary drivers of this effect is likely the prevention of vascular events in other related diseases such as myocardial infarction and stroke [2]. Some evidence exists linking antiplatelet therapy to improved outcomes following lower limb bypass and endovascular therapy [49], but this does not have direct implications for the natural progression of PAD or CLI.

Chronic renal insufficiency, and in particular end-stage renal disease, induces a strong inflammatory reaction and is associated with PAD [1]. In a secondary analysis of the Heart and Estrogen/Progestin Replacement Study (HERS) examining PAD development, renal insufficiency was associated with significant risk of PAD development (creatinine clearance less than 30 and 30–59 mL/kg/m^2, HR 1.63 and 3.24, respectively) [74]. While less data is available regarding the effect of renal disease on CLI and the development of CLI, one recent study from the Veteran Affairs National Surgical Quality Improvement Program (NSQIP) demonstrated an increased rate of limb loss following revascularization in CLI patients receiving dialysis compared to those with no or mild degrees of renal impairment [7]. This same group also reported dialysis dependence as the most important risk factor limiting amputation-free survival [7]. In an additional prospective single-center study of patients admitted to the hospital with CLI, elevated serum creatinine was an independent marker of mortality at 1 year [51].

Given the multifactorial nature of PAD progression, a host of additional variables may contribute to disease evolu-tion. These include elevation of C-reactive protein (CRP), hyperhomocysteinemia, hyperviscosity, hypothyroidism, acute illness, reduced cardiac output, and peripheral neuropathy [1, 75]. However, as previously noted, the transition from PAD to CLI is difficult to target, and there is currently limited data suggesting a definitive causal relationship among many of these variables. Elevated baseline levels of CRP, as demonstrated in the Physicians Health Survey, are predictive of future PAD development [76]. CRP also correlates to overall PAD severity, as determined by need for revascularization (highest quartile PAD RR 4.1) [76]. In addition to CRP, both fibrinogen and IL-6, additional important inflammatory markers, are correlated to PAD development [77]. Higher baseline markers of inflammation, namely, D-dimer, CRP, amyloid A, and fibrinogen, have also been associated with lower extremity functional decline in patients with PAD as determined by a physical performance test but not by 6-min walk performance [78]. Elevation of other inflammatory markers, including increased leukocyte count, interleukin-6, tumor necrosis factor-α, neopterin, and high-sensitivity CRP, have all been associated with increased mortality in patients with CLI [51]. Peripheral neuropathy in particular poses an increased risk for development of CLI. This has traditionally been thought secondary to loss of protective sensory mechanisms but may have direct circulatory effects [1]. For example, one recent meta-analysis of spinal cord stimulation in CLI, which is presumed to relieve pain through improved tissue microcirculation, demonstrated improved pain relief and an 11 % decrease in amputation rate [79]. But, again, limited data is available regarding the direct effect of these variables in progression to CLI. Table 13.1

Conclusions

The progression of PAD and ultimate development of CLI is a difficult and ill-defined area of study. Much of the current understanding of this transition stems from data available in PAD and in surrogate studies on need for intervention and amputation. However, these data together paints a picture of CLI development that is progressive yet insidious. Atherosclerosis builds until compensatory hemodynamics cannot overcome a critical obstruction. While some patients may present initially with CLI, it remains likely that their underlying arterial disease progressed in the same slowly building fashion as others. There are definite predispositions to CLI development, and a multitude of environmental risk factors play a role in increasing this predisposition and tipping the scale in the direction of ischemia. Among the most significant of these risk factors are smoking, diabetes, and hyperlipidemia. By creating a pro-atherogenic, pro-inflammatory environment, arterial disease flourishes and limb viability fades.

References

1. Norgren L, Hiatt WR, Dormandy JA, et al. Inter-society consensus for the management of peripheral arterial disease (TASC II). J Vasc Surg. 2007;45(Suppl S):S5–67.

2. Minar E. Critical limb ischaemia. Hamostaseologie. 2009;29(1): 102–9.

3. Mohler ER 3rd, Bundens W, Denenberg J, Medenilla E, Hiatt WR, Criqui MH. Progression of asymptomatic peripheral artery disease over 1 year. Vasc Med. 2012;17(1):10–16.

4. Hirsch AT, Criqui MH, Treat-Jacobson D, et al. Peripheral arterial disease detection, awareness, and treatment in primary care. JAMA. 2001;286(11):1317–24.

5. van der Feen C, Neijens FS, Kanters SD, Mali WP, Stolk RP, Banga JD. Angiographic distribution of lower extremity atherosclerosis in patients with and without diabetes. Diabet Med. 2002;19(5): 366–70.

6. Rogers R, Hiatt W. Pathophysiology and treatment of critical limb ischemia. http://www.vascularmed.org/clinical_archive/ Pathophysiology-Treatment-of-CLI_11Feb2013.pdf. Accessed 8 Apr 2014.

7. Varu VN, Hogg ME, Kibbe MR. Critical limb ischemia. J Vasc Surg. 2010;51(1):230–41.

8. Baser O, Verpillat P, Wang L. Prevalence, incidence, and outcomes of critical limb ischemia in the US medicare population. http:// www.vasculardiseasemanagement.com/content/prevalence-incidence-and-outcomes-critical-limb-ischemia-us-medicare-population. Updated 2013. Accessed 8 Apr 2014.

9. Goodney PP, Travis LL, Nallamothu BK, et al. Variation in the use of lower extremity vascular procedures for critical limb ischemia. Circ Cardiovasc Qual Outcomes. 2012;5(1):94–102.

10. Rothwell PM, Eliasziw M, Gutnikov SA, Warlow CP, Barnett HJ, Carotid Endarterectomy Trialists Collaboration. Endarterectomy for symptomatic carotid stenosis in relation to clinical subgroups and timing of surgery. Lancet. 2004;363(9413):915–24.

11. Weitz JI, Byrne J, Clagett GP, et al. Diagnosis and treatment of chronic arterial insufficiency of the lower extremities: a critical review. Circulation. 1996;94(11):3026–49.

12. Fowkes FG, Housley E, Cawood EH, Macintyre CC, Ruckley CV, Prescott RJ. Edinburgh artery study: prevalence of asymptomatic and symptomatic peripheral arterial disease in the general population. Int J Epidemiol. 1991;20(2):384–92.

13. Nehler MR, Peyton BD. Is revascularization and limb salvage always the treatment for critical limb ischemia? J Cardiovasc Surg (Torino). 2004;45(3):177–84.

14. Hirsch AT, Haskal ZJ, Hertzer NR, et al. ACC/AHA 2005 practice guidelines for the management of patients with peripheral arterial disease (lower extremity, renal, mesenteric, and abdominal aortic): A collaborative report from the american association for vascular Surgery/Society for vascular surgery, society for cardiovascular angiography and interventions, society for vascular medicine and biology, society of interventional radiology, and the ACC/AHA task force on practice guidelines (writing committee to develop guidelines for the management of patients with peripheral arterial disease): endorsed by the american association of cardiovascular and pulmonary rehabilitation; national heart, lung, and blood institute; society for vascular nursing; TransAtlantic inter-society consensus; and vascular discase foundation. Circulation. 2006;113(11):e463–654.

15. Dormandy J, Heeck L, Vig S. The natural history of claudication: risk to life and limb. Semin Vasc Surg. 1999;12(2):123–37.

16. McDermott MM, Criqui MH, Greenland P, et al. Leg strength in peripheral arterial disease: associations with disease severity and lower-extremity performance. J Vasc Surg. 2004;39(3):523–30.

17. Muluk SC, Muluk VS, Kelley ME, et al. Outcome events in patients with claudication: a 15-year study in 2777 patients. J Vasc Surg. 2001;33(2):251 7. discussion 257–8.

18. Cronenwett JL, Warner KG, Zelenock GB, et al. Intermittent claudication. current results of nonoperative management. Arch Surg. 1984;119(4):430–6.

19. Smith I, Franks PJ, Greenhalgh RM, Poulter NR, Powell JT. The influence of smoking cessation and hypertriglyceridaemia on the progression of peripheral arterial disease and the onset of critical ischaemia. Eur J Vasc Endovasc Surg. 1996;11(4):402–8.

20. Dormandy J, Belcher G, Broos P, et al. Prospective study of 713 below-knee amputations for ischaemia and the effect of a prostacyclin analogue on healing. Hawaii study group. Br J Surg. 1994;81(1):33–7.

21. Dormandy JA, Charbonnel B, Eckland DJ, et al. Secondary prevention of macrovascular events in patients with type 2 diabetes in the PROactive study (PROspective pioglitAzone clinical trial in macroVascular events): a randomised controlled trial. Lancet. 2005;366(9493):1279–89.

22. Falluji N, Mukherjee D. Critical and acute limb ischemia: an overview. Angiology. 2014;65(2):137–46.

23. Price JF, Mowbray PI, Lee AJ, Rumley A, Lowe GD, Fowkes FG. Relationship between smoking and cardiovascular risk factors in the development of peripheral arterial disease and coronary artery disease: Edinburgh artery study. Eur Heart J. 1999;20(5):344–53.

24. Walsh DB, Gilbertson JJ, Zwolak RM, et al. The natural history of superficial femoral artery stenoses. J Vasc Surg. 1991;14(3): 299–304.

25. Coran AG, Warren R. Arteriographic changes in femoropopliteal arteriosclerosis obliterans. A five-year follow-up study. N Engl J Med. 1966;274(12):643–7.

26. McDermott MM, Liu K, O'Brien E, Guralnik JM, Criqui MH, Martin GJ, et al. Measuring physical activity in peripheral arterial disease: a comparison of two physical activity questionnaires with an accelerometer. Angiology. 2000;51(2):91–100.

27. Sieminski DJ, Gardner AW. The relationship between free-living daily physical activity and the severity of peripheral arterial occlusive disease. Vasc Med. 1997;2(4):286–91.

28. Paraskevas KI, Hamilton G, Mikhailidis DP, Liapis CD. Optimal medical management of peripheral arterial disease. Vasc Endovascular Surg. 2007;41(1):87.

29. Murabito JM, D'Agostino RB, Silbershatz H, Wilson WF. Intermittent claudication. A risk profile from the framingham heart study. Circulation. 1997;96(1):44–9.

30. Selvin E, Erlinger TP. Prevalence of and risk factors for peripheral arterial disease in the united states: results from the national health and nutrition examination survey, 1999–2000. Circulation. 2004;110(6):738–43.

31. Bartholomew JR, Olin JW. Pathophysiology of peripheral arterial disease and risk factors for its development. Cleve Clin J Med. 2006;73 Suppl 4:S8–14.

32. Harris LM, Peer R, Curl GR, Pillai L, Upson J, Ricotta JJ. Long-term follow-up of patients with early atherosclerosis. J Vasc Surg. 1996;23(4):576–80. discussion 581.

33. Valentine RJ, Myers SI, Inman MH, Roberts JR, Clagett GP. Late outcome of amputees with premature atherosclerosis. Surgery. 1996;119(5):487–93.

34. Lo RC, Bensley RP, Dahlberg SE, et al. Presentation, treatment, and outcome differences between men and women undergoing revascularization or amputation for lower extremity peripheral arterial disease. J Vasc Surg. 2014;59(2):409–18.e3.

35. Miller M, Byington R, Hunninghake D, Pitt B, Furberg CD. Sex bias and underutilization of lipid-lowering therapy in patients with coronary artery disease at academic medical centers in the united states and canada. prospective randomized evaluation of the vascu-

lar effects of norvasc trial (PREVENT) investigators. Arch Intern Med. 2000;160(3):343–7.

36. Chou AF, Brown AF, Jensen RE, Shih S, Pawlson G, Scholle SH. Gender and racial disparities in the management of diabetes mellitus among medicare patients. Womens Health Issues. 2007;17(3):150–61.

37. Gottsater A. Managing risk factors for atherosclerosis in critical limb ischaemia. Eur J Vasc Endovasc Surg. 2006;32(5):478–83.

38. Dormandy JA, Rutherford RB. Management of peripheral arterial disease (PAD). TASC working group. TransAtlantic inter-society consensus (TASC). J Vasc Surg. 2000;31(1 Pt 2):S1–296.

39. Ingolfsson IO, Sigurdsson G, Sigvaldason H, Thorgeirsson G, Sigfusson N. A marked decline in the prevalence and incidence of intermittent claudication in icelandic men 1968–1986: a strong relationship to smoking and serum cholesterol–the reykjavik study. J Clin Epidemiol. 1994;47(11):1237–43.

40. Marso SP, Hiatt WR. Peripheral arterial disease in patients with diabetes. J Am Coll Cardiol. 2006;47(5):921–9.

41. Freund KM, Belanger AJ, D'Agostino RB, Kannel WB. The health risks of smoking. the framingham study: 34 years of follow-up. Ann Epidemiol. 1993;3(4):417–24.

42. Cimminiello C. PAD. epidemiology and pathophysiology. Thromb Res. 2002;106(6):V295–301.

43. Aronow WS. Peripheral arterial disease in women. Maturitas. 2009;64(4):204–11.

44. Juergens JL, Barker NW, Hines EA. Arteriosclerosis obliterans: review of 520 cases with special reference to pathogenic and prognostic factors. Circulation. 1960;21:188–95.

45. Jude EB, Oyibo SO, Chalmers N, Boulton AJ. Peripheral arterial disease in diabetic and nondiabetic patients: a comparison of severity and outcome. Diabetes Care. 2001;24(8):1433–7.

46. Faglia E, Favales F, Quarantiello A, et al. Angiographic evaluation of peripheral arterial occlusive disease and its role as a prognostic determinant for major amputation in diabetic subjects with foot ulcers. Diabetes Care. 1998;21(4):625–30.

47. Kannel WB. Risk factors for atherosclerotic cardiovascular outcomes in different arterial territories. J Cardiovasc Risk. 1994; 1(4):333–9.

48. Porth C. Pathophysiology: Concepts of Altered Health States. Philadelphia: Lippincott; 1995. p. 203–22.

49. Diehm N, Schmidli J, Setacci C, et al. Chapter III: Management of cardiovascular risk factors and medical therapy. Eur J Vasc Endovasc Surg. 2011;42 Suppl 2:S33–42.

50. Bild DE, Selby JV, Sinnock P, Browner WS, Braveman P, Showstack JA. Lower-extremity amputation in people with diabetes. epidemiology and prevention. Diabetes Care. 1989;12(1):24–31.

51. Barani J, Nilsson JA, Mattiasson I, Lindblad B, Gottsater A. Inflammatory mediators are associated with 1-year mortality in critical limb ischemia. J Vasc Surg. 2005;42(1):75–80.

52. Virkkunen J, Heikkinen M, Lepantalo M, Metsanoja R, Salenius JP, Finnvasc Study Group. Diabetes as an independent risk factor for early postoperative complications in critical limb ischemia. J Vasc Surg. 2004;40(4):761–7.

53. AhChong AK, Chiu KM, Wong MW, Hui HK, Yip AW. Diabetes and the outcome of infrainguinal bypass for critical limb ischaemia. ANZ J Surg. 2004;74(3):129–33.

54. Bosevski M, Meskovska S, Tosev S, Peovska I, Asikov I, Georgievska-Ismail LJ. Risk factors for development of critical limb ischemia – a survey of diabetic vs. nondiabetic population. Prilozi. 2006;27(2):89–96.

55. Mehler PS, Coll JR, Estacio R, Esler A, Schrier RW, Hiatt WR. Intensive blood pressure control reduces the risk of cardiovascular events in patients with peripheral arterial disease and type 2 diabetes. Circulation. 2003;107(5):753–6.

56. UK Prospective Diabetes Study Group. Tight blood pressure control and risk of macrovascular and microvascular complications in type 2 diabetes: UKPDS 38. BMJ. 1998;317(7160):703–13.

57. De Backer G, Ambrosioni E, Borch-Johnsen K, et al. European guidelines on cardiovascular disease prevention in clinical practice. third joint task force of european and other societies on cardiovascular disease prevention in clinical practice. Eur Heart J. 2003;24(17):1601–10.

58. Heart Protection Study Collaborative Group. MRC/BHF heart protection study of cholesterol lowering with simvastatin in 20,536 high-risk individuals: a randomised placebo-controlled trial. Lancet. 2002;360(9326):7–22.

59. The Scandinavian Simvastatin Survival Study (4S). Randomised trial of cholesterol lowering in 4444 patients with coronary heart disease. Lancet. 1994;344(8934):1383–89.

60. Aung PP, Maxwell HG, Jepson RG, Price JF, Leng GC. Lipid-lowering for peripheral arterial disease of the lower limb. Cochrane Database Syst Rev. 2007;(4):CD000123.

61. Takemoto M, Liao JK. Pleiotropic effects of 3-hydroxy-3-methylglutaryl coenzyme a reductase inhibitors. Arterioscler Thromb Vasc Biol. 2001;21(11):1712–9.

62. Curtis AM, Edelberg J, Jonas R, Rogers WT, Moore JS, Syed W, et al. Endothelial microparticles: sophisticated vesicles modulating vascular function. Vasc Med. 2013;18(4):204–14.

63. Schillinger M, Exner M, Mlekusch W, et al. Statin therapy improves cardiovascular outcome of patients with peripheral artery disease. Eur Heart J. 2004;25(9):742–8.

64. Mohler ER 3rd, Hiatt WR, Creager MA. Cholesterol reduction with atorvastatin improves walking distance in patients with peripheral arterial disease. Circulation. 2003;108(12):1481–6.

65. Giri J, McDermott MM, Greenland P, Guralnik JM, Criqui MH, Liu K, et al. Statin use and functional decline in patients with and without peripheral arterial disease. J Am Coll Cardiol. 2006; 47(5):998–1004.

66. Cheng SW, Ting AC. Lipoprotein (a) level and mortality in patients with critical lower limb ischaemia. Eur J Vasc Endovasc Surg. 2001;22(2):124–9.

67. Bismuth J, Kofoed SC, Jensen AS, Sethi A, Sillesen H. Serum lipids act as inverse acute phase reactants and are falsely low in patients with critical limb ischemia. J Vasc Surg. 2002;36(5): 1005–10.

68. Conte MS, Bandyk DF, Clowes AW, Moneta GL, Namini H, Seely L. Risk factors, medical therapies and perioperative events in limb salvage surgery: observations from the PREVENT III multicenter trial. J Vasc Surg. 2005;42(3):456–64. discussion 464–5.

69. Schanzer A, Hevelone N, Owens CD, Beckman JA, Belkin M, Conte MS. Statins are independently associated with reduced mortality in patients undergoing infrainguinal bypass graft surgery for critical limb ischemia. J Vasc Surg. 2008;47(4):774–81.

70. Garg PK, Tian L, Criqui MH, Liu K, Ferrucci L, Guralnik JM, et al. Physical activity during daily life and mortality in patients with peripheral arterial disease. Circulation. 2006;114(3):242–8.

71. Gardner AW, Poehlman ET. Exercise rehabilitation programs for the treatment of claudication pain. A meta-analysis. JAMA. 1995;274(12):975–80.

72. Murphy TP, Cutlip DE, Regensteiner JG, Mohler ER, Cohen DJ, Reynolds MR, et al. Supervised exercise versus primary stenting for claudication resulting from aortoiliac peripheral artery disease: six-month outcomes from the claudication: exercise versus endoluminal revascularization (CLEVER) study. Circulation. 2012; 125(1):130–9.

73. McDermott MM, Liu K, Ferrucci L, et al. Physical performance in peripheral arterial disease: a slower rate of decline in patients who walk more. Ann Intern Med. 2006;144(1):10–20.

74. O'Hare AM, Vittinghoff E, Hsia J, Shlipak MG. Renal insufficiency and the risk of lower extremity peripheral arterial disease: results from the heart and estrogen/progestin replacement study (HERS). J Am Soc Nephrol. 2004;15(4):1046–51.

75. Mya MM, Aronow WS. Increased prevalence of peripheral arterial disease in older men and women with subclinical hypothyroidism. J Gerontol A Biol Sci Med Sci. 2003;58(1):68–9.

76. Ridker PM, Cushman M, Stampfer MJ, Tracy RP, Hennekens CH. Plasma concentration of C-reactive protein and risk of developing peripheral vascular disease. Circulation. 1998;97(5): 425–8.

77. McDermott MM, Guralnik JM, Corsi A, Albay M, Macchi C, Bandinelli S, et al. Patterns of inflammation associated with peripheral arterial disease: The InCHIANTI study. Am Heart J. 2005; 150(2):276–81.

78. McDermott MM, Ferrucci L, Liu K, Criqui MH, Greenland P, Green D, et al. D-dimer and inflammatory markers as predictors of functional decline in men and women with and without peripheral arterial disease. J Am Geriatr Soc. 2005;53(10):1688–96.

79. Ubbink DT, Vermeulen H. Spinal cord stimulation for critical leg ischemia: a review of effectiveness and optimal patient selection. J Pain Symptom Manage. 2006;31(4 Suppl):S30–5.

Basic Science of Wound Healing

Stephanie R. Goldberg and Robert F. Diegelmann

Introduction

A wound can be defined as any disruption of the normal tissue architecture resulting in a loss of function [1]. Acute healing wounds "progress through an orderly and timely healing process so as to restore anatomic continuity and function." In contrast, chronic non-healing wounds such as seen in diabetic, venous stasis, and pressure ulcers "fail to proceed through an orderly and timely process to produce anatomic and functional integrity, or proceeded through the repair process without establishing a sustained anatomic and functional result" [1]. This review will analyze the various phases of wound healing with specific attention to the key elements responsible for normal repair as contrasted to the factors and influences responsible for delayed healing present in chronic ischemic limbs.

Phases of Wound Healing

Wound healing consists of a set of four highly coordinated phases in which specific cells interact with an extracellular matrix to provide a new architecture for collagen growth and deposition [2]. These phases include hemostasis, inflammation, proliferation, and remodeling (Fig. 14.1). The interaction between the cells and the extracellular matrix is driven by chemical mediators including growth factors, chemokines, and their inhibitors. One of the most critical growth factors required for normal wound repair is transforming

S.R. Goldberg, MD (✉)
Surgery Department, Virginia Commonwealth University
Medical Center, 1200 East Marshall Street, PO Box 980454,
Richmond, VA 23298, USA

R.F. Diegelmann, PhD
Biochemistry and Molecular Biology, Virginia Commonwealth
University Medical Center, Richmond, VA, USA

factor beta (TGF-β), and it functions throughout the healing response [3, 4]. Because of the central role of growth factors required for wound healing, many attempts have been made to apply them locally to chronic non-healing wounds to [5]. However, Robson points out "numerous clinical studies of recombinant growth factors used to treat chronic dermal wounds have generally reported disappointing results" [6].

Hemostasis Phase

The process of wound healing begins immediately after a tissue sustains an injury and mechanisms are triggered to control the bleeding. This initial process is called hemostasis and consists of vasoconstriction followed by platelet activation by binding to collagen on the extracellular matrix. Activated platelets release proteins including fibronectin, thrombospondin, sphingosine-1-phosphate, and von Willebrand factor that facilitate further platelet activation and subsequent aggregation and, in turn, enhance the clotting cascade [7–9]. Additionally, a "provisional matrix" of insoluble fibrin is formed; platelets aggregate to and become lodged in the matrix to form a plug or clot-like structure (Fig. 14.2) [10].

The hemostasis phase of wound healing is regulated by chemical mediators released by platelets. These substances are vital to the progression of wounds through the subsequent phases of wound healing. Abnormalities in these mediators can contribute to impaired wound healing at both extremes including excessive scarring and fibrosis or an overall lack of scar formation. Overproduction of TGF-β, released by platelets, has been associated with keloid formation, pulmonary fibrosis, and cirrhosis [11–14]. Conversely, the application of TGF-β in chronic venous stasis and pressure ulcers have been shown to improve wound healing [15, 16]. Platelet-derived growth factor (PDGF), produced by platelets as well as macrophages, appears to have a synergistic role with TGF-β by recruiting neutrophils and macrophages into the wound thus facilitating progression through the following wound healing phases [17]. PDGF also recruits

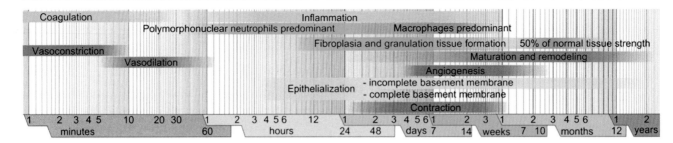

Fig. 14.1 Phases of normal wound healing. Cellular and molecular events during normal wound healing progress through four major, integrated, phases: hemostasis, inflammation, proliferation, and remodel-ing. Reprinted with permission: Häggström, Mikael (2014). "Medical gallery of Mikael Häggström 2014". Wikiversity Journal of Medicine 1

Fig. 14.2 Hemostasis phase. At the time of injury, the fibrin clot forms the provisional wound matrix, and platelets release multiple growth factors that initiate the repair process. Reprinted with permission from the Textbook of Surgery: Scientific Principles and Practice, J. B. Lippincott Co., Philadelphia, PA, 1992

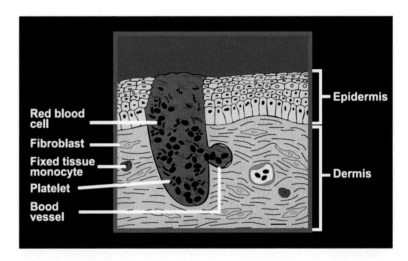

and stimulates proliferation of fibroblasts which are responsible for collagen deposition and formation of the extracellular matrix [10, 18, 19]. In addition, it has been reported recently in animal studies that a platelet neuropeptide (NPY) is critical for ischemic revascularization [20]. It remains to be determined if NPY is also active in human ischemic limbs as it is in stress-related diseases [21]. If it does play a role in human ischemic limb pathology, agonists may be beneficial to promote revascularization.

Inflammatory Phase

Following hemostasis and within the first 24 h post-injury, the wound progresses into a second phase of wound healing called inflammation. The purpose of this phase is twofold: to allow for removal of bacteria and necrotic and/or devitalized tissue components to create a "clean" canvas for collagen deposition and neovascularization in subsequent stages. Successfully progression beyond the inflammatory phase, which typically lasts to post-injury day 4, serves as a key determinant as to whether a wound will heal appropriately or progress to a chronic non-healing wound.

The inflammatory phase relies on mast cells, neutrophils, and macrophages to further prepare the injury site for repair

(Fig. 14.3). In this phase, mast cells release vasoactive amines and histamine-rich granules which cause blood vessels to vasodilate and leak allowing plasma-rich fluid and neutrophils to migrate to the wound bed. Clinically, these wounds are characterized by redness (rubor), swelling (tumor), warmth (calor), and pain (dolor), the cardinal signs of inflammation recognized since ancient times.

Neutrophils play a main role in the inflammatory phase as scavenger cells and are attracted to wound sites by binding to specialized cell adhesion molecules (CAMs) called selecting on nearby endothelial cells within blood vessels. Through a series of coordinated movements, the neutrophils are grabbed and bound to the endothelial cell surface ("pavementing"), roll along the endothelial lining, and then squeeze through leaky cell junctions into the interstitial space by a process termed diapedesis [22].

The process of neutrophil migration to the wound is called "chemotaxis" and is mediated by both the chemokine IL-8 and the breakdown products of the complement system activated by the presence of bacteria in a wound [23, 24]. Neutrophils release interleukin 1 and TNFα that activates fibroblasts and epithelial cells and transitions to the next stage of wound healing, the proliferative phase [25].

Once the neutrophils migrate to the site of injury, they release reactive oxygen species as a first line of defense

Fig. 14.3 Inflammatory phase. Within a day following injury, the inflammatory phase is initiated by neutrophils that attach to endothelial cells in the vessel walls surrounding the wound (margination), change shape and move through the cell junctions (diapedesis), and migrate to the wound site (chemotaxis). Reprinted with permission from the Textbook of Surgery: Scientific Principles and Practice, J. B. Lippincott Co., Philadelphia, PA, 1992

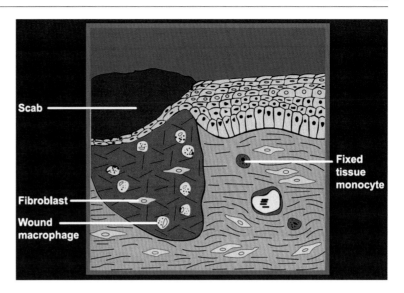

against bacteria and they also phagocytize foreign debris and nonfunctional cells. As neutrophils die, they release enzymes such as matrix metalloproteinases and elastase to further digest surrounding damaged tissue [26, 27]. Excessive amounts of these enzymes cause severe damage to the extracellular matrix and are responsible for much of the pathology seen in chronic, non-healing wounds [27].

On a basic science level, an overproduction of MMPs not only causes extensive tissue damage but also destruction of vital growth factors such as PDGF and TGF-β [28–30]. These wounds exhibit an unregulated, continuous inflammatory phase resulting in extensive loss of tissue and become chronic non-healing wounds [27]. In situations of chronic inflammation, macrophages and fibroblasts proliferate such that new tissue cannot be productively formed. Examples include repetitive trauma, the presence of foreign bodies, and the use of cytotoxic agents such as Betadine and hydrogen peroxide. In fact, a greater understanding of these factors which influence chronic inflammation has led to a shift in the standard of care for wound consisting of a wet to dry normal saline gauze mechanical debridement to gentler, cytotoxic, and trauma-free wound care in continued moist environments.

In addition to mast cells and neutrophils, macrophages are activated within the wound from chemokines, cytokines, growth factors, and digested extracellular matrix byproducts produced by proteolytic degradation of collagen and fibronectin [31]. Macrophages have incredible phagocytic function and are the most important inflammatory cell required for healing [32, 33]. Similar to neutrophils, macrophages remove residual foreign bodies, necrotic debris, and bacteria, yet their phagocytic abilities are enhanced by their release of protease inhibitors and resulting proteolytic destruction of injured tissue [34]. Furthermore, macrophages ingest and remove bacterial-laden neutrophils and secrete multiple growth factors and cytokines to recruit fibroblasts and endothelial

cells into the wound to enhance the repair process. These factors consist of PDGF, TGF-β, TNFα, FGF, IGF-1, and IL-6 and mediate progression from into the next stage of wound healing, the proliferative phase [32].

In contrast, many clinical conditions can impair the inflammatory phase such that minimal inflammation occurs and the normal repair process is impaired. These include patients with impaired immune systems resulting from autoimmune disorders and acquired immune system disorders, diabetes, and drug-induced immunosuppression from the consumption of high doses of steroids and/or nonsteroidal anti-inflammatory drugs [35]. Advanced age and poor nutritional status also lead to effective immunosuppression and prevent wounds from progressing through subsequent phases.

For inflammation to occur, there must be adequate vascularization and an absence of necrotic tissue such that neutrophils can migrate into the wounds. Some wounds lack enough MMPs to breakdown all necrotic debris or have such extensive devitalized tissue such that debridement is necessary. Excisional sharp debridement to vascularized tissue may be required. Other wounds with less necrotic debris have been shown to benefit from the use of topical bacterial collagenase which functions similar to the body's MMPs to facilitate degradation and removal of devitalized tissue but in a more controlled manner [36].

Proliferative Phase

The proliferative phase occurs typically between days 4 and 21 post-injury and is characterized by collagen deposition, cross-linking, and reestablishment of the extracellular matrix (Fig. 14.4). Fibroblasts proliferate and migrate in great numbers into the provisional fibrin matrix and begin to synthesize collagen, proteoglycans, and fibronectins which can

Fig. 14.4 Proliferation phase.
Fixed tissue monocytes
activate, move into the site of
injury, transform into
activated wound macrophages
that kill bacteria, release
proteases that remove
denatured ECM, and secrete
growth factors that stimulate
fibroblast, epidermal cells,
and endothelial cells to
proliferate and produce scar
tissue. Reprinted with
permission from the Textbook
of Surgery: Scientific
Principles and Practice, J. B.
Lippincott Co., Philadelphia,
PA, 1992

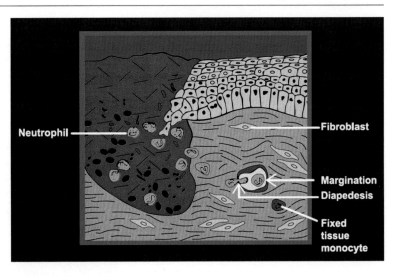

then serve as a scaffold for new tissue structure. Angiogenesis is driven by pericytes to regenerate capillaries and endothelial cells to produce the lining of the blood vessels [37]. This allows nourishment for the new wound matrix. Clinically, these wounds appear to have "beefy" red granulation tissue and easily bleed if mechanically agitated. Finally, specialized fibroblasts with tight junctions that have some cytoskeletal elements characteristic of smooth muscle cells such as SMA-actin have been termed "myofibroblasts" and are thought to facilitate wound contraction [38].

The proliferative phase of wound healing relies heavily on fibroblast migration into the wound bed and is mediated by the release of cytokines and growth factors from platelets and macrophages remaining in the wound site. Fibroblast movement through the extracellular matrix by the binding of their integrin transmembrane receptors a specific amino acid sequence (R-G-D or arginine-glycine-aspartic acid) on fibronectin, vitronectin, and fibrin already present as part of the hemostatic plus at the site of injury [39]. Further fibroblast movement through the wound matrix occurs from their release of MMPs to digest and facilitate further removal of damaged matrix components. The balance of MMP activity and regulation by tissue inhibitor of matrix metalloproteinases (TIMPs) is vital such that there is more tissue deposition rather than tissue destruction [40]. Fibroblasts then produce collagen, proteoglycans, adhesion glycoproteins, and other key components for the new extracellular matrix.

Fibroblast activity is mediated primarily by the growth factors platelet-derived growth factor (PDGF) and TGF-β. Specifically, PDGF is secreted by platelets and macrophages; stimulates fibroblast proliferation, migration, and angiogenesis; and is mediated in part by oxygen tension and thrombin within a wound along with other factors such as hypoxia-inducible factor alpha and vascular endothelial factor [41, 42].

Overexpression of PDGF has been associated with fibrotic diseases including pulmonary fibrosis, cirrhosis, and scleroderma [43]. These forms of fibrosis result from an initial insult and subsequent abnormal wound healing process.

Given the role of PDGF in myeloproliferation and fibrosis, PDGF receptors have emerged as a potential therapeutic target for anti-fibrotic drugs. Animal studies have shown some promise especially in the treatment of lung fibrosis [44].

Similar to PDGF, TGF-β has long been shown to play a key role in wound healing specifically in cell proliferation and differentiation. At least three isoforms of TGF-β exist including TGF-β1, TGF-β2, and TGF-β3. All 3 isoforms bind the same serine/threonine kinase cell receptor but activate different Smad cell signaling pathways leading to very different effects on wound healing [45]. Overexpression of TGF-β1 has been associated with pulmonary fibrosis and cirrhosis, whereas TGF-β3 has been associated with decreased fibrosis and scar formation [13, 14]. Mutations in fibrillin gene results in overexpression of TGF-β and has been linked to connective tissue disorders including Marfan's syndrome.

Interestingly, much of our understanding of the role of TGF-β in wound healing stems from research in fetal animal wounds [46]. Fetal wounds heal in a scarless fashion with very minimal TGF-β present [47, 48]. Midgestational fetal wounds in the rabbit model contract in the presence of TGF-β1 and TGF-β3. We have shown that midgestational wounds heal rapidly and are associated with an increase in TGF-β1 and TBR-2 expression compared with surrounding normal skin [49].

Remodeling Phase

Once the various components of granulation tissue have been deposited, the wound then undergoes the process of remodeling and evolves into a scar during the final phase of wound healing (Fig. 14.5). This phase can last for many years postinjury, and the maximum regain in tensile strength usually is only about 80 % of the original tissue strength prior to injury [50]. The ability to heal these wounds relies significantly on good nutrition and oxygen delivery to support a high metabolic rate [41, 51–53]. The role and use of hyperbaric oxy-

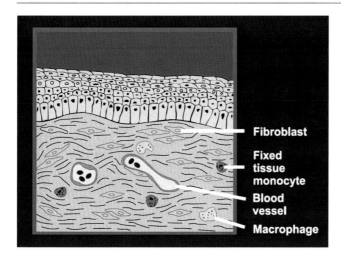

Fibroblast

Fixed tissue monocyte

Blood vessel

Macrophage

Fig. 14.5 Remodeling phase. The initial, disorganized scar tissue is slowly replaced by a matrix that more closely resembles the organized ECM of normal skin. Reprinted with permission from the Textbook of Surgery: Scientific Principles and Practice, J. B. Lippincott Co., Philadelphia, PA, 1992

gen for the treatment of chronic limb ischemia is the focus of Chap. 39 and therefore will not be discussed here.

The changes that occur within the wound during the remodeling phase result in a mature wound with a gradual replacement of the initial type III collagen by the stronger type I collagen cross-linked by the enzyme lysyl oxidase [54]. As the wound desiccates, small capillaries coalesce into larger blood vessels. The high metabolic rate that was necessary to support the proliferative phase decreases as the key components of the evolving wound are maturing. Grossly, the wound takes on less of a reddish hue and the neo-dermis begins to resemble normal, mature skin.

Critical Limb Ischemia and Wound Healing

Critical limb ischemia is often associated with tissue loss resulting from lack of adequate blood flow to limbs. Treatment efforts employing medical, endovascular, and surgical techniques have focused largely on reestablishing blood perfusion to distal blood vessels and risk factor modification to relieve pain, heal wounds, and preserve limbs [55]. For those patients who progress to amputation, they often face challenges in healing their surgical stump wounds due to chronic small vessel disease leading to high morbidity and wound complications of up to 30 % in these high-risk patients [56–60].

At-risk wounds in the setting of critical limb ischemia have been monitored using transcutaneous oximetry (PtCO2) to measure the partial pressure of oxygen on the skin surface [61, 62]. The challenge in using PtCO2 clinically is that PtCO2 levels represent an estimation; measurements in adjacent tissue may not adequately reflect oxygen tension within wounds. Consensus statements for the use of PtCO2 have

been used to qualitatively predict response rates to wound healing and hyperbaric oxygen therapy but further research is necessary to define a clinical role [63].

References

1. Lazarus GS, Cooper DM, Knighton DR, Margolis DJ, Pecoraro RE, Rodeheaver G, et al. Definitions and guidelines for assessment of wounds and evaluation of healing. Arch Dermatol. 1994;130:489–93.
2. Diegelmann RF, Evans MC. Wound healing: an overview of acute, fibrotic and delayed healing. Front Biosci. 2004;9:283–9.
3. Pakyari M, Farrokhi A, Maharlooei MK, Ghahary A. Critical role of transforming growth factor beta in different phases of wound healing. Adv Wound Care. 2013;2(5):215–24.
4. Finnson KW, McLean S, Di Guglielmo GM, Philip A. Dynamics of transforming growth factor beta signaling in wound healing and scarring. Adv Wound Care. 2013;2(5):195–214.
5. Barrientos S, Brem H, Stojadinovic O, Tomic-Canic M. Clinical application of growth factors and cytokines in wound healing. Wound Repair Regen. 2014;22(5):569–78.
6. Robson MC. The role of growth factors in the healing of chronic wounds. Wound Repair Regen. 1997;5(1):12–7.
7. Cho J, Mosher DF. Role of fibronectin assembly in platelet thrombus formation. J Thromb Haemost. 2006;4(7):1461–9.
8. Rabhi-Sabile S, de Romeuf C, Pidard D. On the mechanism of plasmin-induced aggregation of human platelets: implication of secreted von Willebrand factor. Thromb Haemost. 1998;79(6):1191–8.
9. Ono Y, Kurano M, Ohkawa R, Yokota H, Igarashi K, Aoki J, et al. Sphingosine 1-phosphate release from platelets during clot formation: close correlation between platelet count and serum sphingosine 1-phosphate concentration. Lipids Health Dis. 2013;12:20.
10. Gailit J, Clark RA. Wound repair in the context of extracellular matrix. Curr Opin Cell Biol. 1994;6(5):717–25.
11. Song C. Hypertrophic scars and keloids in surgery: current concepts. Ann Plast Surg. 2014;73 Suppl 1:S108–18.
12. Wolters PJ, Collard HR, Jones KD. Pathogenesis of idiopathic pulmonary fibrosis. Annu Rev Pathol. 2014;9:157–79.
13. Broekelmann TJ, Limper AH, Colby TV, McDonald JA. Transforming growth factor beta 1 is present at sites of extracellular matrix gene expression in human pulmonary fibrosis. Proc Natl Acad Sci U S A. 1991;88(15):6642–6.
14. Gressner AM, Weiskirchen R, Breitkopf K, Dooley S. Roles of TGF-beta in hepatic fibrosis. Front Biosci. 2002;7:d793–807.
15. Robson MC, Phillip LG, Cooper DM, Lyle WG, Robson LE, Odom L, et al. Safety and effect of transforming growth factor-beta(2) for treatment of venous stasis ulcers. Wound Repair Regen. 1995;3(2):157–67.
16. Hirshberg J, Coleman J, Marchant B, Rees RS. TGF-beta3 in the treatment of pressure ulcers: a preliminary report. Adv Skin Wound Care. 2001;14(2):91–5.
17. Pierce GF, Mustoe TA, Lingelbach J, Masakowski VR, Griffin GL, Senior RM, et al. Platelet-derived growth factor and transforming growth factor-beta enhance tissue repair activities by unique mechanisms. J Cell Biol. 1989;109(1):429–40.
18. Bennett NT, Schultz GS. Growth factors and wound healing: biochemical properties of growth factors and their receptors. Am J Surg. 1993;165(6):728–37.
19. Bennett NT, Schultz GS. Growth factors and wound healing: Part II. Role in normal and chronic wound healing. Am J Surg. 1993;166(1):74–81.
20. Tilan JU, Everhart LM, Abe K, Kuo-Bonde L, Chalothorn D, Kitlinska J, et al. Platelet neuropeptide Y is critical for ischemic revascularization in mice. FASEB J. 2013;27(6):2244–55.

21. Kuo LE, Zukowska Z. Stress, NPY and vascular remodeling: implications for stress-related diseases. Peptides. 2007;28(2): 435–40.

22. Kolaczkowska E, Kubes P. Neutrophil recruitment and function in health and inflammation. Nat Rev Immunol. 2013;13(3):159–75.

23. Guo R-F, Ward PA. Role of C5a in inflammatory responses. Annu Rev Immunol. 2005;23:821–52.

24. Tschaikowsky K, Sittl R, Braun GG, Hering W, Rügheimer E. Increased fMet-Leu-Phe receptor expression and altered superoxide production of neutrophil granulocytes in septic and posttraumatic patients. Clin Investig. 1993;72(1):18–25.

25. Matsukawa A, Yoshinaga M. Sequential generation of cytokines during the initiative phase of inflammation, with reference to neutrophils. Inflamm Res. 1998;47 Suppl 3:S137–44.

26. Moor AN, Vachon DJ, Gould LJ. Proteolytic activity in wound fluids and tissues derived from chronic venous leg ulcers. Wound Repair Regen. 2009;17(6):832–9.

27. Diegelmann RF. Excessive neutrophils characterize chronic pressure ulcers. Wound Repair Regen. 2003;11:490–5.

28. Nwomeh BC, Liang HX, Diegelmann RF, Cohen IK, Yager DR. Dynamics of the matrix metalloproteinases MMP-1 and MMP-8 in acute open human dermal wounds. Wound Repair Regen. 1998;6:127–34.

29. Nwomeh BC, Liang HX, Cohen IK, Yager DR. MMP-8 is the predominant collagenase in healing wounds and nonhealing ulcers. J Surg Res. 1999;81:189–95.

30. Yager DR, Zhang LY, Liang HX, Diegelmann RF, Cohen IK. Wound fluids from human pressure ulcers contain elevated matrix metalloproteinase levels and activity compared to surgical wound fluids. J Invest Dermatol. 1996;107:743–8.

31. Diegelmann RF, Cohen IK, Kaplan AM. The role of macrophages in wound repair: a review. Plast Reconstr Surg. 1981;68:107–13.

32. Ferrante CJ, Leibovich SJ. Regulation of macrophage polarization and wound healing. Adv Wound Care. 2012;1(1):10–6.

33. Novak ML, Koh TJ. Phenotypic transitions of macrophages orchestrate tissue repair. Am J Pathol. 2013;183(5):1352–63.

34. Laskin DL, Sunil VR, Gardner CR, Laskin JD. Macrophages and tissue injury: agents of defense or destruction? Annu Rev Pharmacol Toxicol. 2011;51:267–88.

35. Cruse JM, Lewis RE, Dilioglou S, Roe DL, Wallace WF, Chen RS. Review of immune function, healing of pressure ulcers, and nutritional status in patients with spinal cord injury. J Spinal Cord Med. 2000;23(2):129–35.

36. Shi L, Carson D. Collagenase Santyl ointment: a selective agent for wound debridement. J Wound Ostomy Continence Nurs. 2009;36(6 Suppl):S12–6.

37. Demidova-Rice TN, Durham JT, Herman IM. Wound healing angiogenesis: innovations and challenges in acute and chronic wound healing. Adv Wound Care. 2012;1(1):17–22.

38. Kendall RT, Feghali-Bostwick CA. Fibroblasts in fibrosis: novel roles and mediators. Front Pharmacol. 2014;5:123.

39. Clark RA, An JQ, Greiling D, Khan A, Schwarzbauer JE. Fibroblast migration on fibronectin requires three distinct functional domains. J Invest Dermatol. 2003;121:695–705.

40. Gill SE, Parks WC. Metalloproteinases and their inhibitors: regulators of wound healing. Int J Biochem Cell Biol. 2008;40(6–7): 1334–47.

41. Castilla DM, Liu Z-J, Velazquez OC. Oxygen: implications for wound healing. Adv Wound Care. 2012;1(6):225–30.

42. Chen L, Endler A, Shibasaki F. Hypoxia and angiogenesis: regulation of hypoxia-inducible factors via novel binding factors. Exp Mol Med. 2009;41(12):849–57.

43. Bonner JC. Regulation of PDGF and its receptors in fibrotic diseases. Cytokine Growth Factor Rev. 2004;15(4):255–73.

44. Wollin L, Maillet I, Quesniaux V, Holweg A, Ryffel B. Antifibrotic and anti-inflammatory activity of the tyrosine kinase inhibitor nintedanib in experimental models of lung fibrosis. J Pharmacol Exp Ther. 2014;349(2):209–20.

45. Ten Dijke P, Hill CS. New insights into TGF-beta-Smad signalling. Trends Biochem Sci. 2004;29(5):265–73.

46. Lanning DA, Nwomeh BC, Montante SJ, Yager DR, Diegelmann RF, Haynes JH. TGF-beta1 alters the healing of cutaneous fetal excisional wounds. J Pediatr Surg. 1999;34:695–700.

47. Mast BA, Diegelmann RF, Krummel TM, Cohen IK. Scarless wound healing in the mammalian fetus. Surg Gynecol Obstet. 1992;174(5):441–51.

48. Frantz FW, Diegelmann RF, Mast BA, Cohen IK. Biology of fetal wound healing: collagen biosynthesis during dermal repair. J Pediatr Surg. 1992;27:945–8. discussion 949.

49. Goldberg SR, McKinstry RP, Sykes V, Lanning DA. Rapid closure of midgestational excisional wounds in a fetal mouse model is associated with altered transforming growth factor-beta isoform and receptor expression. J Pediatr Surg. 2007;42(6):966–71. discussion 971–973.

50. Gamelli R, He L. Incisional wound healing: model and analysis of wound breaking strength. In: DiPietro LA, editor. Wound healing: methods and protocols. Totowa: Humana Press; 2003. p. 37–54.

51. Kavalukas SL, Barbul A. Nutrition and wound healing: an update. Plast Reconstr Surg. 2011;127 Suppl 1:38S–43.

52. Sen CK, Khanna S, Gordillo G, Bagchi D, Bagchi M, Roy S. Oxygen, oxidants, and antioxidants in wound healing: an emerging paradigm. Ann N Y Acad Sci. 2002;957:239–49.

53. Howard MA, Asmis R, Evans KK, Mustoe TA. Oxygen and wound care: a review of current therapeutic modalities and future direction. Wound Repair Regen. 2013;21(4):503–11.

54. Clore JN, Cohen IK, Diegelmann RF. Quantitation of collagen types I and III during wound healing in rat skin. Proc Soc Exp Biol Med. 1979;161:337–40.

55. Norgren L, Hiatt WR, Dormandy JA, Nehler MR, Harris KA, Fowkes FGR, et al. Inter-society consensus for the management of peripheral arterial disease (TASC II). J Vasc Surg. 2007;45 Suppl S:S5–67.

56. Mayfield JA, Reiber GE, Maynard C, Czerniecki JM, Caps MT, Sangeorzan BJ. Survival following lower-limb amputation in a veteran population. J Rehabil Res Dev. 2001;38(3):341–5.

57. Stone PA, Flaherty SK, Aburahma AF, Hass SM, Jackson JM, Hayes JD, et al. Factors affecting perioperative mortality and wound-related complications following major lower extremity amputations. Ann Vasc Surg. 2006;20(2):209–16.

58. Bates B, Stineman MG, Reker DM, Kurichi JE, Kwong PL. Risk factors associated with mortality in veteran population following transtibial or transfemoral amputation. J Rehabil Res Dev. 2006;43(7):917–28.

59. Cruz CP, Eidt JF, Capps C, Kirtley L, Moursi MM. Major lower extremity amputations at a Veterans Affairs hospital. Am J Surg. 2003;186(5):449–54.

60. Aulivola B, Hile CN, Hamdan AD, Sheahan MG, Veraldi JR, Skillman JJ, et al. Major lower extremity amputation: outcome of a modern series. Arch Surg Chic Ill 1960. 2004;139(4):395–9; discussion 399.

61. Niinikoski JHA. Clinical hyperbaric oxygen therapy, wound perfusion, and transcutaneous oximetry. World J Surg. 2004;28(3):307–11.

62. Rich K. Transcutaneous oxygen measurements: implications for nursing. J Vasc Nurs. 2001;19(2):55–9. quiz 60–61.

63. Fife CE, Smart DR, Sheffield PJ, Hopf HW, Hawkins G, Clarke D. Transcutaneous oximetry in clinical practice: consensus statements from an expert panel based on evidence. Undersea Hyperb Med. 2009;36(1):43–53.

Diagnostic Approach to Chronic Critical Limb Ischemia

15

Tadaki M. Tomita and Melina R. Kibbe

Introduction

Critical limb ischemia (CLI), if left untreated, is associated with a high risk of limb loss [1–3]. Before revascularization can be performed, a thorough but efficient diagnostic approach is warranted. The diagnostic process begins with an initial clinical evaluation to assess for the presence of peripheral artery disease (PAD). Any underlying comorbidities the patient has must be identified as they will influence decisions regarding the diagnostic evaluation. CLI is manifested by rest pain and/or tissue loss of the lower extremity but is also an indicator of atherosclerotic disease in other vascular beds that increases the patient's risk of cardiovascular events [4–8]; this along with other comorbidities will determine the patient's risk of revascularization. The process then proceeds to diagnostic studies to confirm the presence of PAD, localize the lesions that need treatment, and finally plan a revascularization procedure if indicated [1]. With the recent explosion of treatment modalities for PAD, there has been an equal development of imaging modalities available to delineate the patient's vascular anatomy prior to revascularization [9, 10]. Noninvasive vascular lab studies are used to determine the hemodynamic significance of the patient's vascular lesions [3]. Anatomic imaging by arterial duplex ultrasound, computed tomography angiography (CTA), magnetic resonance angiography (MRA), or catheter-based digital subtraction angiography (DSA) can then be used to plan a revascularization procedure [3, 10–13]. The best imaging study to obtain depends on the patient's underlying comorbidities, distribution of disease, and institution-specific imaging capabilities (Fig. 15.1).

T.M. Tomita, MD
Department of Surgery, Northwestern University Feinberg School of Medicine, 676 N. St. Clair Street, Suite #650, Chicago, IL 60611, USA

M.R. Kibbe, MD (✉)
Department of Surgery, University of North Corolina, Chapel Hill, NC, USA

Clinical Diagnosis

Each CLI patient should undergo a thorough history and physical examination to establish a clinical diagnosis of CLI, determine the etiology of CLI, and assess suitability for revascularization prior to proceeding with further diagnostic imaging [1, 3, 14, 15]. The clinical evaluation should focus on the patient's symptoms, cardiovascular risk factors, and comorbidities [1]. Patients with CLI will complain of rest pain or have tissue loss of their lower extremities [14]. The duration of symptoms and status of tissue loss are important indicators when determining the urgency of further workup and need for revascularization [2]. A time course of peripheral vascular symptoms can also be helpful in establishing a diagnosis of PAD or other etiologies for CLI such as embolic disease [1]. Patients with PAD will often (but not always) have pre-existing symptoms of claudication. These patients are at significant risk of having atherosclerotic disease in other vascular beds that contributes to cardiovascular morbidity and mortality. Furthermore, they often have other comorbidities that may require diagnostic consideration in tandem with the CLI workup [4–8]. Diabetes mellitus, renal insufficiency, decreased cardiac output, and a smoking history are commonly found in patients with CLI and also contribute to poor microvascular blood supply [1, 16]. This information is critical to determine the patient's ability to tolerate a revascularization procedure [1, 14]. These comorbidities will also influence which imaging modality is best suited to each patient individually. Lastly, the functional status of the patient should be assessed along with their living situation and ambulatory status to determine the risk/benefit ratio of open revascularization, endovascular revascularization, primary amputation, or best medical management [1, 3, 14].

On physical examination, CLI patients require an assessment of the cardiovascular system with a systematic examination of pulses and evaluation of tissue perfusion to establish the level of obstructive lesions. All pulses should be palpated and recorded, including the common femoral, popliteal,

Fig. 15.1 Diagnostic
decision tree for patients with
critical limb ischemia

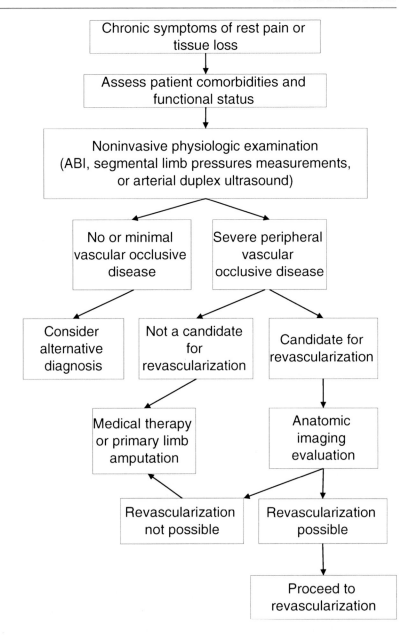

dorsalis pedis, and posterior tibial arteries. An ankle-brachial index (ABI) should be measured at the bedside even if a pulse is palpated as it is a much more objective measure that quantifies blood flow to the limb [14, 17–19]. Signs of severe chronic ischemia include dependent rubor, pallor of the extremity with elevation, reduced capillary refill, and a paucity of hair. The skin should be evaluated for signs of atheroembolization; the characteristic livedo reticularis is suggestive of an embolic source from the heart, proximal arterial aneurysm, atherosclerotic plaque, or hypercoagulable state that may require further diagnostic consideration [1]. The feet and legs should be meticulously inspected for wounds. When tissue loss is encountered, it is important to determine if the

underlying etiology is due to arterial disease, venous disease, or pressure-related problems or if it is multifactorial [1]. Careful attention must be paid to signs of infection, and the clinician must have a low threshold for administration of antibiotics and early debridement [14]. The extent of tissue loss and involvement of deep structures are an important factor in determining if the limb is salvageable [2]. If deemed a candidate for revascularization, patients with CLI should undergo an expedited evaluation for revascularization as this condition is associated with high risk of major limb amputation [1, 3]. Further diagnostic evaluation depends on the patient's comorbidities, characteristics of each imaging modality, and the technical expertise of the given institution [10].

Diagnostic Testing

The objective of diagnostic testing in patients with CLI is to confirm the presence of PAD, identify the distribution and hemodynamic significance of disease, and provide anatomic information to plan a revascularization procedure [1, 3, 14]. Diagnostic tests can be grouped into three broad categories: (1) hemodynamic/physiologic measurements, (2) tissue perfusion, and (3) anatomic imaging. Most patients with CLI should undergo a noninvasive physiologic vascular laboratory study and an anatomic imaging study prior to revascularization. Anatomic imaging of the vascular tree is required to plan a revascularization procedure. Catheter-based DSA has long been accepted as the gold standard for anatomic imaging in patients with PAD, but arterial duplex ultrasound, CTA, and MRA have emerged as excellent noninvasive alternatives [1, 3, 10, 12, 14]. With the increased utilization of endovascular interventions and broad spectrum of device options, preoperative noninvasive imaging is becoming utilized more frequently for device selection along with planning open bypass and hybrid operations [10]. Noninvasive imaging modalities can potentially reduce the operative risk to the patient by minimizing the contrast volume during the intervention and selecting the safest site for vascular access [20].

Noninvasive Physiologic Tests

Continuous Wave Doppler

The handheld continuous wave Doppler (CWD) is the most basic noninvasive diagnostic tool used in the assessment of arterial flow. The probe emits continuous ultrasound waves and is continuously listening for the reflection of these ultrasound waves to measure the velocity of blood flow. It can be used in a variety of clinical settings from the office, to the emergency department, to the operating room. The audible Doppler signal provides a qualitative assessment of the arterial flow in a vascular bed. In a high-resistance vascular bed, like the lower extremity, a normal Doppler signal is triphasic with forward flow in systole, reversal of flow in early diastole, and forward flow in late diastole (Fig. 15.2). As a vascular bed develops occlusive disease, the Doppler signal becomes biphasic losing the reversal of flow during early diastole and then becomes monophasic as the disease progresses further (Fig. 15.2) [21]. The diagnostic accuracy of CWD can be improved with waveform analysis; this is most commonly used in combination with other noninvasive diagnostic tools that will be discussed later in the chapter [22, 23]. The main limitation to the CWD is its qualitative nature, but its ease of use makes it a very helpful tool in the assessment of patients with CLI.

Ankle-Brachial Index

The ankle-brachial index (ABI) is a simple, noninvasive test that can be used in most clinical settings to establish a diagnosis of PAD [1, 3]. The ABI is a ratio of the ankle systolic blood pressure to the brachial blood pressure. Systolic blood pressure measurements are taken using a CWD ultrasound probe and a manual blood pressure cuff. To measure the ankle pressure, an appropriately sized blood pressure cuff is placed just proximal to the ankle; measurements are recorded for both the posterior tibial (PT) and dorsalis pedis (DP) arteries in each leg. The brachial artery pressure is measured in each arm, and the highest recorded systolic brachial pressure is used to calculate the ABI for both legs. The ratio of highest ankle systolic pressure in each leg to the highest brachial pressure in either arm is then recorded to two decimal points (Fig. 15.3). Normal systolic blood pressures at the ankle are 10–15 mmHg higher than the systolic blood pressure in the brachial artery. A normal range for the ABI is 0.91–1.29 [18, 24]. An ABI of 1.3 and greater is abnormal and considered to be falsely elevated or noncompressible, generally due to heavily calcified tibial vessels. In these patients, the ABI cannot be used as a diagnostic index. An ABI of 0.41–0.9 is consistent with mild to moderate PAD, and an ABI of less than 0.4 is consistent with severe PAD. Furthermore, patients with an ABI of less than 0.4 are more likely to have CLI with either rest pain or tissue loss [3, 18]. Several investigations have been conducted to evaluate the interobserver variability of the ABI. These studies have demonstrated a measurement difference of between 0.05 and 0.08 [25, 26]. These results have been interpreted to indicate a change in ABI of greater than 0.15 to be clinically significant [14, 27]. The ABI is a useful diagnostic tool and can also be used to monitor a patient over time and evaluate the quality of a therapeutic intervention [1].

In addition to being used as a diagnostic tool in PAD, a reduced ABI is also an indicator of the patient's overall health status [1, 14, 27]. Both a reduced ABI and a noncompressible ABI are predictors of cardiovascular events and premature mortality [6–8]. In a meta-analysis of almost 50,000 patients, an ABI of less than 0.9 was associated with a twofold increase of all-cause mortality, cardiovascular mortality, and major coronary events [6]. This demonstrates the systemic effects of atherosclerotic disease and the need to risk stratify these patients prior to proceeding to revascularization.

The ABI is a useful, quick, and simple test to determine the presence of PAD, but it is not without its limitations. Several studies have demonstrated a significant variability in the method in which the ABI is measured by clinicians [25]. The ABI may also be insensitive to detect disease progression over time [27]. The information obtained from the ABI can only establish the presence of an occlusive lesion

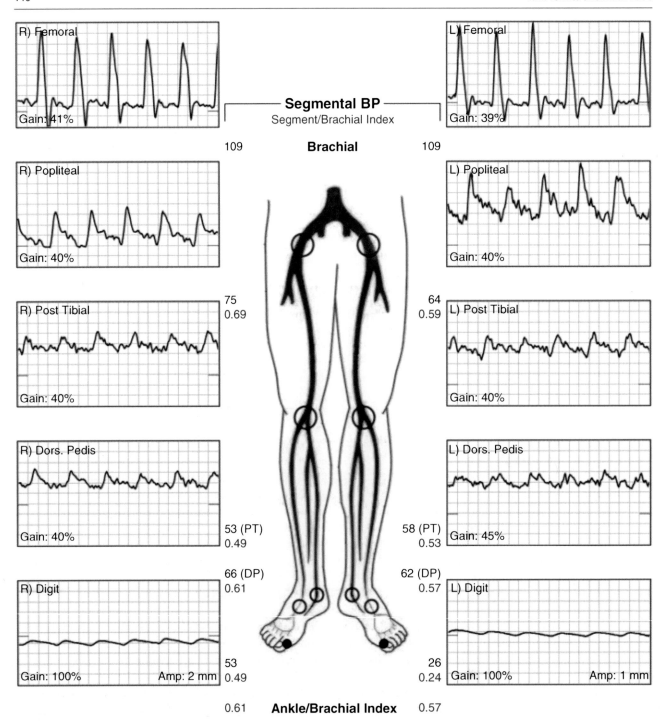

Fig. 15.2 Continuous Doppler waveforms and segmental limb pressures in a patient with bilateral superficial femoral artery occlusion. The femoral waveform is triphasic. The popliteal waveform is biphasic. The dorsalis pedis (DP) and posterior tibial (PT) waveforms are monophasic

but cannot localize the lesion. With slight differences in technique and insensitivity to early disease progression, the test may be less reliable when conducted over long periods of time and between institutions.

The ABI is of limited reliability in patient populations that have a falsely elevated ankle pressure. The result is the illusion of a normal ABI when there is actually significant

ischemia. Patients with diabetes, who have a high prevalence of medial arterial calcification, may have a falsely elevated ABI because of severely calcified tibial vessels [28–30]. Elderly patients, patients with very distal tibial lesions, and those with minor stenosis may also have a falsely elevated ABI (Fig. 15.4) [30]. Clinicians must have a high index of suspicion for PAD in these high-risk patient populations.

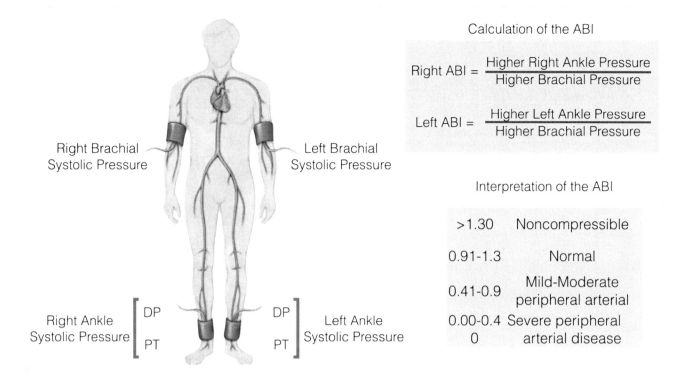

Calculation of the ABI

$$\text{Right ABI} = \frac{\text{Higher Right Ankle Pressure}}{\text{Higher Brachial Pressure}}$$

$$\text{Left ABI} = \frac{\text{Higher Left Ankle Pressure}}{\text{Higher Brachial Pressure}}$$

Interpretation of the ABI

>1.30	Noncompressible
0.91-1.3	Normal
0.41-0.9	Mild-Moderate peripheral arterial
0.00-0.4	Severe peripheral arterial disease
0	

Right Brachial Systolic Pressure

Left Brachial Systolic Pressure

Right Ankle Systolic Pressure [DP PT]

[DP PT] Left Ankle Systolic Pressure

Fig. 15.3 Ankle-brachial index. From Hiatt WR, Medical Treatment of Peripheral Arterial Disease and Claudication, NEJM, 344: p 21 [18]. Copyright (2001) Massachusetts Medical Society. Reprinted with permission from Massachusetts Medical Society

CWD waveform analyses, toe-brachial index, or tissue perfusion examinations can be used in these patients with a noncompressible ABI to evaluate and monitor over time [28, 31, 32]. Despite these limitations, the ABI is a simple noninvasive test that can be used to diagnose PAD, follow patients over time, and evaluate the quality of therapeutic interventions in the right patient population.

Segmental Limb Pressure

Similar to the ABI, measurement of segmental limb pressures is a noninvasive test that uses blood pressure cuffs and a CWD probe to assess the perfusion of the lower extremities. The arrangement of cuffs can vary by institution by using either two, three, or four cuffs. When using four cuffs, in addition to the brachial artery cuff, the lower extremity cuffs are typically placed on the high thigh, low thigh, calf, and ankle (Fig. 15.5) [33, 34]. Figure 15.2 shows the segmental pressures using a two-cuff method. This study shows a characteristic pressure gradient between the brachial artery pressure and the low thigh pressure along with changes in the CWD waveform from triphasic in the common femoral artery to biphasic in the popliteal artery. The cuff width should be 40 % greater than the diameter of the limb, as inappropriately small cuffs are associated with a falsely elevated pressure [35]. A gradient of over 20 mmHg between cuffs within the

same limb is indicative of a hemodynamically significant lesion in the intervening segment (Fig. 15.6) [1]. In contradistinction to the ABI that is not able to localize an occlusive lesion, having segmental cuffs distributed along the length of the leg gives the clinician a good idea of the level of disease especially when using the four-cuff system [34, 36–38]. Though there is some ability to localize the level of disease, this is still an indirect assessment of the vascular tree as there is no direct visualization of the diseased segment. Furthermore, the pressure gradient may be the result of a short occlusion or a long stenosis. As with the ABI, severely calcified arteries can falsely elevate the recorded pressures, making the study invalid [28, 29]. Despite these limitations, this remains a useful tool to establish a diagnosis of PAD and plan further imaging studies or as a means to survey patient before and after an intervention.

Pulse Volume Recording

Segmental air plethysmography or pulse volume recording (PVR) is another noninvasive technique to evaluate patients with PAD. This technique measures the subtle changes in limb volume with each arterial pulsation to obtain qualitative information regarding the nature of arterial flow to the extremity. Similar to segmental limb pressures, cuffs are placed on the thigh, calf, ankle, and forefoot to record the PVR.

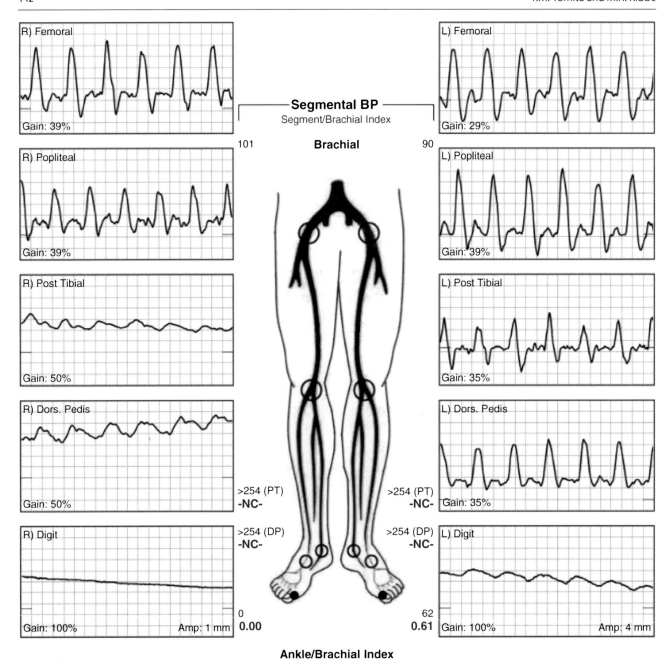

Ankle/Brachial Index

Fig. 15.4 Continuous Doppler waveforms in a patient with diabetes. Note the noncompressible ankle pressures with pressure measured >250 mmHg. The common femoral artery waveform is triphasic and the popliteal artery waveform is biphasic. The right leg has monophasic dorsalis pedis (DP) and posterior tibial (PT) waveforms and a toe pressure of 0. The left leg has preserved DP and PT waveforms with a toe pressure of 62. These findings are consistent with severe right tibial occlusive disease, often observed in patients with diabetes

A brachial cuff is also used to record a PVR in the upper extremity and is used as a comparison for the lower extremity waveforms. The cuffs are inflated to ~60–65 mmHg to record the waveform but not occlude the vessel being measured. The waveforms collected are similar but not identical to those recorded using the CWD for segmental limb pressure measurements. The normal PVR waveform has a quick and sharp upstroke with a rapid decline (Fig. 15.7) [39]. As arterial obstruction progresses, the PVR waveform flattens and widens [39, 40]. The PVR is more reliable in patients who have noncompressible vessels than the ABI [41]. Foot PVR waveforms have been shown to be an indicator of heeling potential of tissue loss and forefoot amputations. The major limitation of the PVR is its qualitative nature. PVR is also abnormal in patients with a diminished cardiac stroke volume, making the test less reliable in this patient population. In this situation, the brachial artery waveform is a helpful comparison to the lower extremity waveforms to determine if the abnormality is

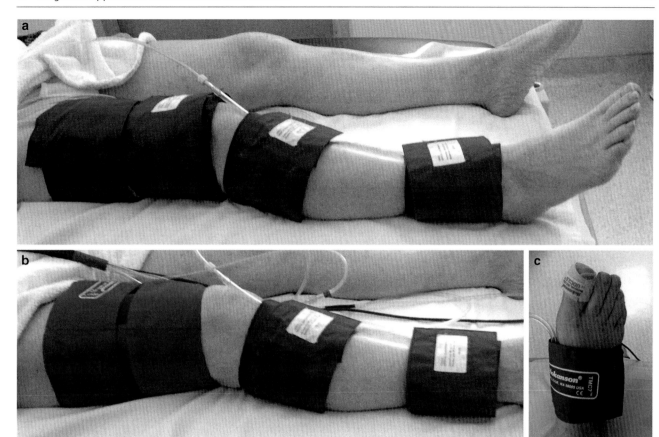

Fig. 15.5 Cuff position for segmental limb pressures. (**a**) Four-cuff technique with two thigh cuffs, a calf cuff, and an ankle cuff. (**b**) Three-cuff technique with a single wide thigh cuff, a calf cuff, and an ankle cuff. The two-cuff technique (not shown) uses a single thigh cuff and an ankle cuff. (**c**) Transmetatarsal cuff and great toe cuff

the result of PAD or poor cardiac function. Segmental limb pressures have better interobserver reliability than PVR [36, 38]. Currently, PVR is not widely used due to its qualitative nature and the development of arterial duplex ultrasound.

Toe Pressure

As mentioned previously, the ABI is not a valid diagnostic test to assess the degree of PAD in certain patient populations [28–30]. In patients that have noncompressible tibial vessels, the digital vessels are typically spared from significant calcification, making the toe systolic blood pressure a more reliable indicator of lower extremity perfusion [42]. Similar to the ABI, the toe-brachial index (TBI) is the ratio of the toe systolic blood pressure to the highest brachial systolic blood pressure. A normal toe systolic blood pressure is 30 mmHg less than that of the systolic ankle pressure making a normal TBI 0.7 or greater. A TBI of less than 0.25 is considered to be severe CLI. The TBI has been shown to be more reliable than the ABI when assessing lower extremity perfusion in diabetic patients who have noncompressible arteries [28]. The absolute toe systolic blood pressure is also

a useful clinical indicator. Diabetic patients with an absolute toe pressure of 55 mmHg or higher have been shown to have a better chance of healing their tissue loss [14]. One of the main limitations of measuring the toe pressure is that it cannot be used in patients that have painful tissue loss or inflammation of their digits. Measuring a toe pressure also requires specialized equipment that prevents it from being used in the variety of clinical settings that the ABI can be conducted (Fig. 15.4c). Lastly, the toe pressure will vary corresponding to the systolic pressure. For this reason, the TBI is often a better indicator. Despite these limitations, the TBI is a useful clinical index in patients that have a noncompressible ABI.

Evaluation of Tissue Profusion

Inadequate tissue perfusion is the underlying etiology of CLI and the goal of revascularization is to restore tissue perfusion to the meet the demands of the affected tissue. Several noninvasive techniques, such as transcutaneous oxygen pressure, skin perfusion pressure, and hyperspectral imaging, have been developed to assess the quality of tissue

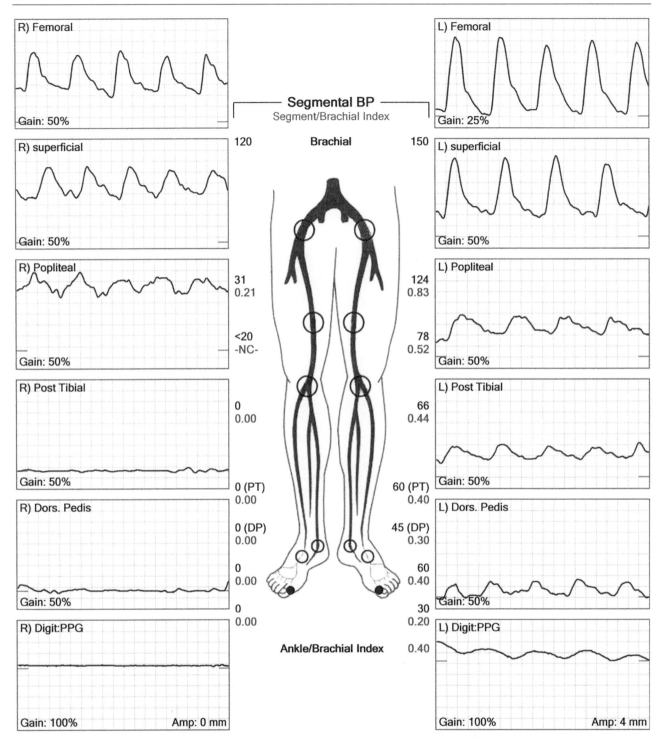

Fig. 15.6 Continuous Doppler waveforms and segmental limb pressures in a patient with bilateral aortoiliac disease as well as infrainguinal occlusive disease. The four-cuff technique is able to identify a pressure gradient across the left thigh suggesting a mid-superficial femoral artery (SFA) stenosis

perfusion in patients with CLI [31, 43, 44]. Unfortunately, due to limitations in their techniques, none of these diagnostic studies are widely used; though there are emerging technologies that may prove to be valuable in the evaluation of tissue perfusion.

Transcutaneous Oxygen Pressure

Transcutaneous partial pressure of oxygen (TcPO2) is a noninvasive test that measures the partial pressure of oxygen at the skin surface. Small probes are placed on the foot or leg.

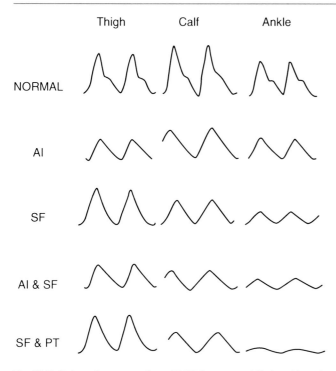

Fig. 15.7 Pulse volume recordings (PVR) from normal limbs with various combinations of peripheral vascular disease. *AI* aortoiliac, *SF* superficial femoral, *PT* popliteal-tibial. From Rutherford RB, Lowenstein DH, Klein MF: Combining segmental systolic pressures and plethysmography to diagnose arterial occlusive disease of the legs. Am J Surg 1979;138:p 216 [39]. Reprinted with permission from Elsevier Limited

A probe placed on the chest is used as a reference to standardize the test for each patient. The probes are constructed of a platinum cathode with a surrounding silver-silver chloride anode ring. Oxygen diffusing to the surface of the skin reacts with the cathode producing an electric current that is then used to measure the partial pressure of oxygen in the target tissue [45]. A normal TcPO2 is above 60 mmHg. A TcPO2 above 30 mmHg has been associated with wound healing in diabetic patients [32, 45]. Some have argued that the TcPO2 may be a better indicator for wound healing and resolution of rest pain compared to a palpable pulse because it is a direct measurement of tissue perfusion at the affected site. A TcPO2 less than 30 mmHg indicates severely reduced perfusion to the target tissue and that healing is less likely to occur [32]. TcPO2 has been shown to be a better indicator of wound healing with hyperbaric oxygen therapy than the TBI or ABI in diabetic patients [46]. Another benefit of the TcPO2 is that heavily calcified vessels do not influence the reliability of the test, and as such it is useful in diabetic patients with a noncompressible ABI [31, 32].

The measured TcPO2 is affected by the amount of arterial flow to the tissue, but it is also impacted by several other factors that may limit its clinical reliability. The measurements are affected by variables such as skin temperature, sympathetic tone, cellulitis, hyperkeratosis, obesity, edema, metabolic

activity, age, and probe position [47–49]. Additionally, an abnormal TcPO2 does not necessarily indicate poor perfusion to the tissue; a low TcPO2 can be found when oxygen consumption is increased in the target tissue [45]. The use of TcPO2 has not been shown to be superior to toe pressure measurement in the management of patients with CLI [49]. Because of the number of variables that impact the measurement of TcPO2, it is not routinely used by most vascular labs.

Skin Perfusion Pressure

Skin perfusion pressure is another noninvasive method of measuring tissue profusion that uses laser Doppler. The laser Doppler probe is placed on the target tissue and detects the motion of cutaneous red blood cells. The waveform generated by the laser Doppler corresponds to arterial flow, but due to the irregular geometry of the cutaneous capillary network, the actual arterial flow cannot be calculated. As laser Doppler detects flow within the skin, it is used in conjunction with a pressure cuff to measure the skin perfusion pressure [45]. A normal skin perfusion pressure is 50–70 mmHg, with skin perfusion pressures of less than 30 mmHg associated with CLI [50, 51]. The variables that impact the reliability of TcPO2 also impact the reliability of laser Doppler. This technique is not widely used among vascular labs because of the inability of laser Doppler to directly measure arterial flow and limitations on calibrating the instrumentation.

Hyperspectral Imaging

Hyperspectral imaging is an emerging noninvasive technique being used in patients with PAD to assess tissue perfusion. The test uses scanning spectroscopy to evaluate the relative cutaneous concentrations of oxyhemoglobin and deoxyhemoglobin. An image is captured with wavelengths of visual light between 500–660 nm; this includes the absorption peaks for oxyhemoglobin and deoxyhemoglobin. These wavelengths only penetrate 1–2 mm below the skin, so only the cutaneous concentrations of these molecules are being measured. A two-dimensional (2D) surface map is then constructed, giving a visual representation of differential oxygenation of the tissue being imaged [43, 52, 53]. Studies evaluating concentrations of deoxyhemoglobin concentrations have shown statistically different concentrations between patients with and without PAD [43]. Additionally there are statistically different concentrations of deoxyhemoglobin between angiosomes with monophasic, biphasic, and triphasic CWD waveforms [43]. This technique has been used to evaluate healing potential of diabetic foot ulcers at 6 months [54]. Although there have been several promising studies in patients that have tissue loss, there have been other studies that show no correlation between the ABI and hyperspectral imaging [52, 53].

Unlike the other noninvasive tests that require placement of probes on the skin or inflation of pressure cuffs to measure pressures, this technique does not require any physical contact with the patient. There is a clear benefit to using this technique for patients that have painful tissue loss in which the other tests may be poorly optimized. Additionally the other tests of tissue profusion can only take measurements at a single point, whereas hyperspectral imaging generates a 2D image of the perfusion to a larger surface area [53]. At this time there have been no large-scale studies involving patients with CLI. As this is an emerging diagnostic tool, more investigation is required before it can be widely implemented.

Noninvasive Anatomic Imaging

Arterial Duplex Ultrasound

Duplex ultrasonography is a noninvasive, inexpensive imaging modality that can provide both physiologic data and anatomic imaging in a variety of clinical settings. Duplex ultrasound equipment is now widely available and inexpensive. With the portability of modern equipment, this imaging modality can be utilized in a variety of clinical settings ranging from the office, to the emergency department, to the operating room. When B-mode imaging is combined with pulsed wave Doppler (PWD), this is commonly referred to as duplex ultrasonography. B-mode or gray-scale imaging produces 2D cross-sectional images of an arterial wall, the arterial lumen, and surrounding tissue. This provides anatomic information about the artery, characteristics of any atherosclerotic plaque within the wall of the artery, or other anatomic pathologies such as aneurysmal disease. As opposed to DSA and MRA, duplex ultrasound can provide useful information about the size and degree of calcification to help identify suitable targets for a distal bypass [12]. PWD gives the ultrasonographer the ability to obtain physiologic measurements within the arterial system [37]. The velocity of blood through an area of stenosis increases relative to the velocity of blood in the artery immediately proximal to the stenosis. Using this principle, the ultrasonographer can identify areas of stenosis in the arterial system by identifying segments with increased velocities. The velocity prior to the stenosis and highest velocity within the stenosis are recorded. A peak systolic velocity (PSV) within a lesion of greater than 200 cm/sec or a ratio of PSV prior to the lesion to the PSV within the lesion of greater than 2.5 is generally consistent with a 50 % or greater stenosis and is considered hemodynamically significant [55]. The combination of these imaging characteristics can give anatomic information about the location, length, and degree of stenosis [23, 56]. Figure 15.8 shows an example of a stenotic lesion in the native superficial femoral artery.

Though there are many benefits to duplex ultrasound in the assessment of patients with CLI, there are also some limitations. As with any ultrasound study, the accuracy and reliability of the results are operator dependent and require an experienced technician [23]. The entire leg must be scanned in a continuous systematic manor as to not miss a focal lesion. Ultrasound becomes less reliable the further away the target is from the probe, which can limit the utility in obese patients. This does not pose as much of a problem in the lower leg but can severely limit studies conducted on the aortoiliac segment. Ultrasound does not travel through air, making overlying bowel gas an additional challenge when imaging vessels in the abdomen and pelvis. Sound waves are also reflected off high-density surfaces, making heavily calcified lesion difficult to image and obtain reliable physiologic data. The patient must be positioned in a way for the technologist to evaluate the entire vascular tree. The patient's pain or wounds may make this challenging and limit the quality of the study. Imaging of pedal vessels may be conducted, but they are easily compressed with the probe and may invalidate the measured values.

The anatomic information obtained from duplex arterial ultrasound can be used to plan revascularization procedures in patients with CLI. This imaging modality has been used to select tibial targets for a distal bypass in place of DSA [11, 20]. Interestingly, one study showed no difference in patency or limb salvage of distal bypasses constructed using either duplex ultrasound versus other angiographic methods to determine the distal target [57]. An arterial duplex ultrasound done prior to an endovascular procedure allows for selective angiography, thereby minimizing the contrast dose during the procedure [20, 58].

Though there has been tremendous advancement in the resolution of modern ultrasound equipment, further advancements are on the horizon to further aid in the diagnostic evaluation of patients with CLI. The addition of intravenous contrast agents can be used to improve the assessment of the lower extremity vasculature [59, 60]. Contrast-enhanced ultrasound of the tibial vessels has been shown to improve the accuracy of arterial duplex ultrasound when compared to DSA [59]. The use of contrast agents may be able to assess the adequacy of muscle perfusion before and after revascularization, which may prove to be a superior means to assess the quality of revascularization compared to other noninvasive tests [61, 62]. The advancement of 3D ultrasound may aid in characterizing the anatomy of short segments of the arterial tree [63]. Robotic ultrasound systems are also being developed in the hopes of automating the study to eliminate some of the variability of the current ultrasound examina-

Fig. 15.8 Arterial duplex ultrasonography. (**a**) A normal triphasic waveform in the common femoral artery and (**b**) a superficial femoral artery stenosis with an increased peak systolic velocity and biphasic waveform with spectral broadening

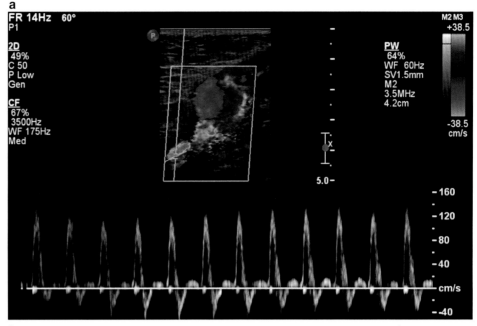

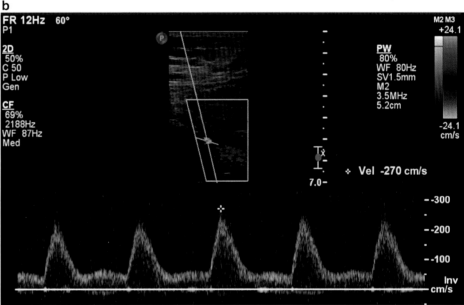

tions [63, 64]. With these advances, duplex ultrasound will become an even more powerful noninvasive tool in the evaluation of patients with CLI.

Computed Tomography Angiography

Computed tomography angiography (CTA) is a noninvasive imaging modality that has become widely accepted as a primary imaging technique in patients with CLI [9]. The CTA images are produced using an X-ray source and a series of detectors surrounding the patient. The data obtained by this technique is then processed by a computer to produce cross-sectional images of the patient for analysis. Modern multi-detector scanners allow for rapid image acquisition with high anatomic detail of the vascular tree and surrounding soft tissue [65–68]. CTA has a high accuracy to identify, characterize, and measure peripheral arterial occlusive disease with a sensitivity of 91–100 % and specificity of 93–96 % when compared to DSA [65, 69, 70]. The sensitivity of CTA to occlusive lesions is higher than that for stenotic lesions [69]. With a high negative predictive value, a CTA without significant stenosis is clinically important to rule out occlusive arterial disease as the cause of CLI [12]. As with duplex ultrasound, but in contrast to DSA and MRA, CTA gives morphologic characteristics of the arterial wall and surrounding structures that can be used to determine the quality of the artery as a target for distal bypass [12, 69]. This information can also be used to identify other nonatherosclerotic causes of limb ischemia such as peripheral aneurysmal disease [69]. This imaging modality is also faster and more comfortable to patients when compared to MRA that requires a long acquisition time in a confined space and the invasive catheter-based angiography [12]. CTA allows for imaging through previously stented arteries that appear as flow voids when imaged by MRA [71]. Using CTA as a primary imaging modality, though associated with the increased need for additional imaging, is more cost effective than primary DSA and MRA [65, 72].

Modern multi-detector scanners obtain axial images that can then be reformatted into other views that can aid in preoperative planning [69]. These reformats can be 2D multiplanar reformats, curved planar reformats perpendicular to the arterial centerline, or 3D renderings (Fig. 15.9) [68, 70]. Maximum intensity projection is a reformatting method that displays the highest attenuation value, preferentially displaying high-density structures such as arteries with intravenous contrast [65, 70]. Advances in software development have been helpful in increasing the speed at

which these reconstructions are produced and may improve the interpretation of the luminal characteristics within heavily calcified arteries. The quality of reformatted images depends on the type of scanner used to generate the axial images, the protocol used to obtain the axial images, and the software used to make the reconstructed images [66, 67]. Reformatted images give the clinician more information about the anatomic characteristics of the vascular tree that can be used to plan revascularization procedures [73].

CTA has some limitations when imaging the vasculature. Heavily calcified vessels, as seen in diabetic patients, with median calcinosis can make it difficult to determine if small vessels are patent [12]. The way the scanners are designed, the contrast bolus must be followed down the leg as it moves through the arterial tree. Poor timing or high-grade proximal obstruction may impact the quality of the contrast bolus within the distal vessels, limiting the diagnostic accuracy of the study [66]. Additional scans with or without additional contrast may be required to obtain diagnostic images of the tibial vessels. This comes with added radiation exposure and the risk associated with additional intravenous contrast administration. Modern scanners have reduced some of the issues encountered

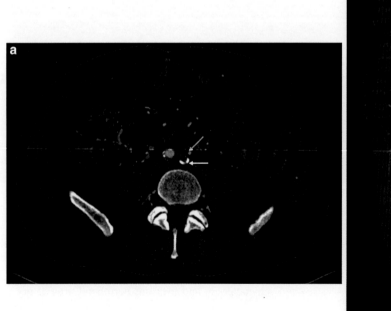
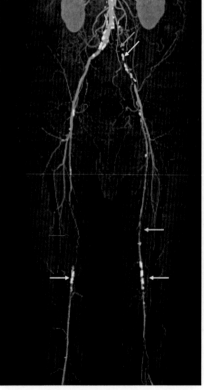

Fig. 15.9 Computed tomography angiography. (**a**) Axial image showing a left iliac occlusion (*green arrow*) and (**b**) 3D reformat showing left iliac occlusion (*green arrow*), right superficial femoral artery (SFA) occlusion (*red arrow*), and left SFA stenosis (*yellow arrow*). Calcifications are also depicted (*white arrows*)

with previous-generation scanners but have not eliminated the problem [66, 67].

Though there are some significant benefits of using CTA as a primary anatomic imaging modality in patients with CLI, there are also several drawbacks. CTA requires intravenous contrast to obtain clinically relevant information when planning a revascularization procedure. Iodinated contrast agents used for CTA are nephrotoxic and must therefore be used cautiously in patients with renal insufficiency [74–77]. Contrast-induced nephropathy (CIN) is defined as an increase in serum creatinine greater than 25 % or greater than 0.5 mg/dl above baseline within 3 days of contrast administration without another identifiable cause [74, 75]. All patients exposed to iodinated contrast are at risk of developing CIN, but patients with renal insufficiency are at an increased risk [78]. Diabetes is an independent risk factor for CIN, and diabetic patients with renal insufficiency are at the highest risk of developing CIN [76, 79]. The incidence of CIN ranges from 2.9 to 12.1 % and is largely dependent on the degree of renal insufficiency prior to the contrast exposure [76, 78, 79]. Fortunately, only about 1 % of patients will have a persistent change in renal function and only a small fraction of these patients will go on to require hemodialysis [76, 79]. However, the development of CIN is associated with an increased all-cause hospital mortality [75]. To prevent CIN, high-risk patients should be hydrated prior to and after exposure to intravenous contrast [80–83]. The administration of Mucomyst and/or sodium bicarbonate before and after exposure to iodinated contrast has been shown to reduce the risk of CIN in some studies [84, 85]. When used intravenously, as with CTA, there is no difference in the incidence of CIN between iso-osmolar and low-osmolar contrast agents; however, there is a decreased incidence of CIN when iso-osmolar contrast agents are used intra-arterially [86]. Nephrotoxic medications should be held around the time of contrast exposure to also reduce the risk of CIN [74, 75].

Another drawback to using CTA as a primary imaging modality is the exposure of patients to ionizing radiation. Most of the patients that have CLI are elderly with reduced life expectancy and will therefore be less likely to develop malignancy from repeated exposure [87]. Nevertheless, exposure to radiation should be considered. Though CTA does require radiation, the effective dose of radiation can be about half of what a patient is exposed to during catheter-based angiography depending on the technique [70]. Modern scanners allow for rapid image acquisition time, reducing the radiation exposure encountered with previous-generation scanners [67, 88]. This also allows for a reduction in contrast volume required to obtain the images. Despite these potential drawbacks, in the right patient population, CTA is a quick and inexpensive primary imaging modality for patients with CLI.

Magnetic Resonance Angiography

Magnetic resonance angiography (MRA) has emerged as another noninvasive imaging modality that provides high-resolution images of the aorta and peripheral vascular tree in patients with CLI [9]. MRA uses strong magnetic field and electromagnetic waves to produce cross-sectional images that do not require ionizing radiation [89]. Just as there has been a rapid development and deployment of advanced imaging technology for CTA, there has been an equal development of advanced imaging for MRA that has shortened the image acquisition time and improved image resolution [89–93]. MRA has been shown to have a sensitivity of 73–98 % and specificity 64–97 % for the detection of peripheral stenotic lesions greater than 50 % and occlusions [12, 90, 94, 95]. There is conflicting evidence, but some studies have suggested that MRA is superior to DSA when evaluating the outflow vessels as a target for distal bypass in patients with CLI [13, 90, 96–98]. This was also seen in a series of diabetic patients who had patent pedal vessels detected by MRA that were not visualized on DSA [96]. The large range in sensitivities reported in the literature and variability of results likely reflects the variety of methods available to perform MRA that are largely center specific [9, 89, 98].

However the MRA study is performed, image reformatting is required to create meaningful images for interpretation by the clinician (Fig. 15.10). As with CTA, maximum intensity projection images are generated and additional 3D images can be constructed. Some anatomic information of the arterial wall and surrounding structures can provide additional information regarding the extent of atherosclerosis or presence of peripheral aneurysmal disease [92, 94]. Information regarding the degree of calcification of vessels is not readily apparent on MRA [72]. The anatomic information acquired by MRA is much harder for the general clinician to interpret when compared to CTA.

As with CTA, MRA uses intravenous contrast to maximize the visualization of the arterial system when evaluating patients with CLI. Gadolinium-based contrast agents are the most commonly used contrast agents for MRA [89]. Until recently, these contrast agents were thought to be non-nephrotoxic and safe to use in patients with renal insufficiency. The use of MRA in patients with severe renal insufficiency was touted as one of the benefits of this imaging modality over CTA that carries a known risk of contrast-induced nephropathy. This is no longer the case, as the use of gadolinium in patients with severe renal insufficiency is now contraindicated because of both renal toxicity and the potential of systemic complications [99, 100]. Several studies have shown a risk of acute renal failure with standard MRA doses of gadolinium [99, 101]. Patients with diabetic nephropathy and low glomerular filtration rate are at the highest risk of

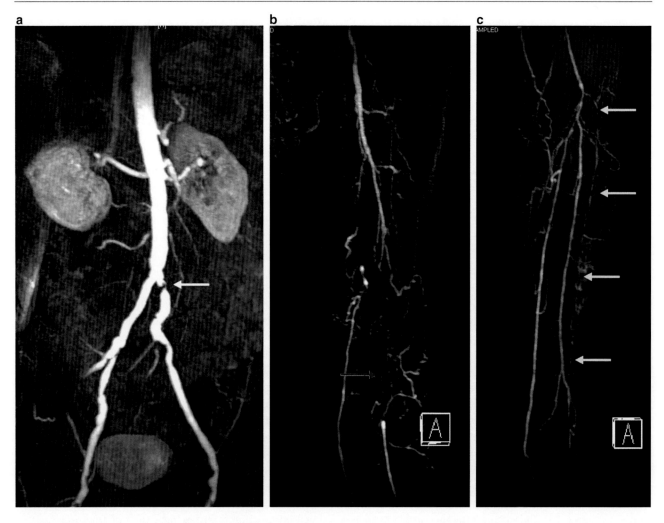

Fig. 15.10 Magnetic resonance angiography. (**a**) Left common iliac stenosis (*white arrow*), (**b**) left superficial femoral artery occlusion (*red arrow*), and (**c**) long segment left anterior tibial artery stenosis (*yellow arrows*)

developing acute renal failure from exposure to gadolinium [99, 101]. Nephrogenic systemic fibrosis (NSF) is the other complication of using gadolinium in patients with severe renal insufficiency [100, 102]. With just under 400 reported cases of NSF [103], it remains a rare but serious syndrome that causes severe systemic fibrosis in a number of organ systems. The disorder was originally called nephrogenic fibrosing dermopathy because of the characteristic skin lesions but was subsequently renamed because of the clear involvement of other organ systems including the cardiovascular, pulmonary, and musculoskeletal systems. Cases of NSF have only been reported in patients that have some element of renal insufficiency, so patients with normal renal function are thought to be safe from developing this devastating complication [100, 102].

Though contrast-enhanced MRA (CE-MRA) is contraindicated in patients with severe renal insufficiency, noncontrast-enhanced MRA (NC-MRA) can be performed safely in this patient population. The algorithms used to obtain the images are beyond the scope of this chapter, but several techniques have been developed that use arterial spin, electrocardiographic (ECG) gating, or a combination of the two to obtain angiographic images without the need of intravenous contrast [92, 104–107]. Older techniques of time of flight and phase contrast have been replaced with ECG-gated Fourier fast spin and balanced steady-state free precession. At our institution, we use ECG-gated quiescent-interval single-shot MRA (QISS-MRA) as our NC-MRA technique (Fig. 15.11). Regardless of imaging technique, NC-MRA requires longer acquisition times and suffers from poorer image resolution when compared to CE-MRA [92]. QISS-MRA has been shown to have superior detection of segmental stenosis in the tibial vessels when compared to CE-MRA; however, CE-MRA was superior for imaging the distal aorta, pelvic arteries, and femoral arteries [106]. Other studies have shown comparable results for the evaluation of these segments between NC-MRA and CE-MRA [105, 107]. Though NC-MRA has some limitations, it is a viable option for

Fig. 15.11 Electrocardiographic-gated quiescent-interval single-shot magnetic resonance angiography (QISS-MRA). (**a**) Patent aortoiliac segment and (**b**) tibial station. Occluded anterior tibial artery (*white arrow*). Occluded distal peroneal artery (*red arrow*). Occluded posterior tibial artery (*yellow arrow*)

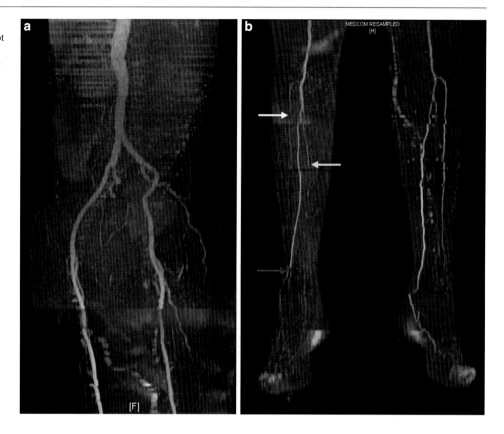

patients that cannot receive intravenous contrast because of severe renal insufficiency.

The major limitations of MRA are cost, duration of exam, and patient intolerance of the examination. Of the noninvasive imaging modalities used to assess patients with CLI, MRA is the most expensive. Patients with severe claustrophobia or inability to lay flat for extended periods of time frequently cannot tolerate the length of the study. Many patients are excluded from MRA because of metallic devices that cannot be exposed to high magnetic fields such as pacemakers, automatic implantable cardioverter-defibrillators, certain stent grafts, and other metal implants [12, 72]. More powerful 3 T magnets may also prevent some patients with certain types of intravascular stents from getting this study [93]. Though MRA-compatible, intravascular stents appear as a flow void within the artery and may be interpreted as an occlusion when one is not present [71]. Alternatively there may be a high-grade stenosis or occlusion within the stent that could be missed in these patients. Though MRA has many disadvantages in the evaluation of patients with CLI, it has been shown to have a higher sensitivity for the detection of occlusive lesions than duplex ultrasound, has better specificity than CTA, and is better tolerated than DSA [12]. MRA protocols are vendor specific so no single universal protocol has been standardized [89]. Characteristic of the machine used to acquire the MRA images, vendor-specific protocols used to obtain these images, and the software used to reconstruct these images make the quality of MRA center specific.

Venous contamination and short intra-arterial half-life of traditional gadolinium-based contrast agents are major limitations of MRA when used for the planning of lower extremity revascularization procedures in patients with CLI [89]. This is most problematic for the visualization of the tibial vessels and can make it difficult to identify a viable target for distal bypass. Venous contamination is seen in up to 43 % of studies in the infrapopliteal segment causing the images to be nondiagnostic (Fig. 15.12) [108]. Blood-pool contrast agents are a new class of intravenous contrast used for MRA that have a longer intravascular half-life. These contrast agents bind to circulating albumin keeping them intravascular, maximizing acquisition time compared to traditional contrast agents that quickly diffuse into the extracellular space [91, 109, 110]. When blood-pool contrast agents are used in the same manner as traditional gadolinium-based contrast agents, they have similar results in the identification of PAD [91, 109]. In this situation, first-pass MRA can overestimate the degree of an infrapopliteal stenosis. A study using gadofosveset, a blood-pool contrast agent, showed better concordance with DSA in the steady-state phase of the MRA than first-pass MRA [91]. The blood-pool contrast agent allows for longer acquisition times that results in better image quality.

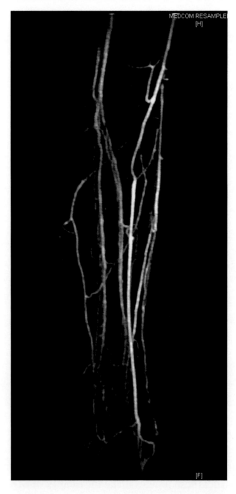

Fig. 15.12 Magnetic resonance angiography demonstrating venous contamination of the tibial station, making it hard to diagnose disease in the arterial system

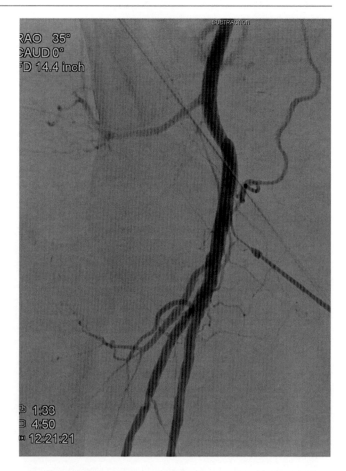

Fig. 15.13 Appropriate cannulation of the right common femoral artery at the mid-femoral head location (*arrow*)

Invasive Imaging

Digital Subtraction Angiography

Digital subtraction angiography is the gold standard imaging modality in patients with PAD and CLI. The use of DSA provides high-quality images of the arterial tree with the added benefit of simultaneous treatment of appropriate lesions. However, it is the most costly imaging strategy, requires nephrotoxic iodinated contrast, exposes the patient to radiation, and is invasive with potentially local and systemic complications [12]. DSA only provides images of the lumen of the artery and does not provide any images of the morphologic information regarding the arterial wall. Eccentric plaque may not be detected without orthogonal views. Long segment occlusion may limit the visualization of distal vessels preventing the characterization of these potential targets for distal bypass [96].

There are techniques that can be employed to minimize the risk to the patient associated with DSA. Contrast exposure and radiation exposure can be limited by selective visualization of the vascular bed. Other noninvasive imaging modalities may provide information that allows the clinician to perform a targeted angiogram, reducing the amount of contrast and radiation exposure [20, 58, 111]. The other risk associated with invasive imaging modalities is the possibility of access site complications such as a hematoma, pseudoaneurysm, arteriovenous fistula, dissection, and embolization [112–114]. Care should be taken to limit the risk of these complications by selecting appropriate vessels for arterial access, minimizing the sheath size, and using image-guided access [115–117]. At our institution, we confirm appropriate cannulation of the common femoral artery by performing an angiogram with a small micropuncture sheath in place prior to upsizing to a larger sheath (Fig. 15.13). Despite these limitations, in the right patient population, catheter-based DSA is a good primary anatomic imaging modality that has the added benefit of possible simultaneous revascularization.

Carbon Dioxide Angiography

Carbon dioxide (CO_2) angiography can be a useful tool when evaluating CLI patients that have renal insufficiency and a high risk of developing CIN [118]. To perform catheter-based CO_2 angiography, CO_2 gas is used in place of iodinated contrast. The CO_2 gas temporarily displaces blood from the artery being imaged. The gas is radiolucent relative to blood and the surrounding soft tissue, creating a void in the imaging (Fig. 15.14). This technique requires faster frame rates and special equipment to infuse the CO_2, thereby limiting its use [118]. Detailed tibial vessel imaging may be limited especially in the setting of long segment proximal occlusion. CO_2 angiography does not eliminate the need for contrast but can reduce the volume required [119, 120].

Intravascular Ultrasound

Intravascular ultrasound (IVUS) is an invasive imaging technique that uses a miniature ultrasound probe attached to the tip of a catheter. When used for patients with CLI, the catheter is inserted intra-arterially over a wire to image the artery from the lumenal surface. IVUS can accurately measure the diameter of the artery and can be used to determine the length of a lesion without using intravenous contrast [121]. The main benefit of IVUS is that it can replace the need for intravenous contrast used during an intervention [122], potentially reducing the risk of contrast-induced nephropathy. The anatomic information obtained by IVUS can be used to plan revascularization procedures and perform endovascular interventions [121, 123]. Newer IVUS catheters have more advanced imaging, providing improved characterization of atherosclerotic lesions and better assessment of how these lesions will respond to endovascular intervention [124–126]. The main limitation to wide adopting the use of IVUS for infrainguinal interventions is the high cost of the catheters.

Alternative Imaging Modalities

Positron Emission Tomography

Positron emission tomography (PET) is a nuclear medicine imaging modality that detects the metabolic activity of a variety of tissues and has been applied to patients with PAD. To produce the images, a positron emitting radionuclide is attached to glucose, water, or other biologically active molecules. When introduced to the body, the tagged molecule concentrates in areas of higher metabolic activity.

Fig. 15.14 Carbon dioxide angiography. (**a**) Carbon dioxide angiography demonstrating a right superficial artery stenosis (*green arrow*) and (**b**) digital subtraction angiography of the same lesion (higher magnification)

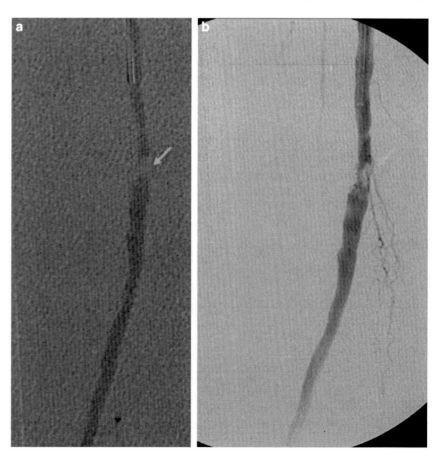

This technique is most commonly applied to cancer imaging in which the metabolically active cancer cells have higher concentrations of the tagged molecule [127, 128]. The molecules being used in the evaluation of patients with PAD are fluorodeoxyglucose (FDG) and oxygen-15-water ($H_2^{15}O$) [129–132]. Studies have evaluated this imaging modality in the assessment of PAD severity and tissue response to revascularization, but it has yet to be studied in the diagnosis of PAD [133]. Several studies have applied this technique to measure regional blood flow to lower extremity skeletal muscle tissue in patients with PAD [129, 130, 134]. In the future, FDG-PET could help differentiate viable and nonviable skeletal muscle based on the metabolic activity [130]. This would be useful in determining those patients with CLI that will benefit from revascularization from those that have a non-salvageable limb. $H_2^{15}O$-PET has not shown difference in signal uptake between healthy controls and patients with PAD but has shown a decrease in flow reserve among patients with PAD [129]. The main limitation to wide acceptance of implementing this imaging modality is the economic cost to the patient.

Molecular Imaging

Molecular imaging is an emerging technology that uses tagged molecules to visualize specific molecular processes in vivo [135]. Currently used imaging modalities focus on the structural components of an atherosclerotic plaque and the hemodynamic effects these lesions have on the circulation in order to determine the appropriate intervention. In contrast, molecular imaging focuses on specific molecular processes within the atherosclerotic plaque that could supplement the anatomic information when planning revascularization procedures in patients with CLI. Specialized algorithms and imaging strategies are being developed for currently available imaging systems like MRI, PET, CT, single-photon emission computed tomography, and optical imaging to conduct these molecular imaging studies [127, 133, 136–139]. Depending on what markers are visualized, this imaging technology could potentially identify what lesions are likely to rupture in the future or how they will respond to specific therapeutic interventions. This could allow for tailoring therapeutic interventions specifically to the needs of the patient, whether they be medical, interventional, or surgical.

Summary

Patients with CLI require an expedited but thorough diagnostic evaluation to plan the appropriate therapeutic strategy. If deemed to be a surgical candidate, most patients will undergo a physiologic study and an anatomic imaging study to plan a revascularization procedure with the goal of limb salvage. With advances in noninvasive anatomic imaging and potential cost saving associated with them, most patients will undergo either a CTA or a MRA prior to revascularization. The choice of which study is most appropriate depends on the patient's underlying comorbidities, presence and degree of renal insufficiency, presence of MRI-incompatible devices, ability to lay flat for an extended period of time, and expertise of the local imaging facility. As technology develops, newer imaging modalities will become available that may better aid the clinician in selecting patients who will benefit from revascularization as well as the means to accomplish that revascularization.

References

1. Hirsch AT, et al. ACC/AHA 2005 practice guidelines for the management of patients with peripheral arterial disease (lower extremity, renal, mesenteric, and abdominal aortic): a collaborative report from the American Association for Vascular Surgery/Society for Vascular Surgery, Society for Cardiovascular Angiography and Interventions, Society for Vascular Medicine and Biology, Society of Interventional Radiology, and the ACC/AHA Task Force on Practice Guidelines (Writing Committee to Develop Guidelines for the Management of Patients With Peripheral Arterial Disease): endorsed by the American Association of Cardiovascular and Pulmonary Rehabilitation; National Heart, Lung, and Blood Institute; Society for Vascular Nursing; TransAtlantic Inter-Society Consensus; and Vascular Disease Foundation. Circulation. 2006;113(11):e463–654.
2. Abou-Zamzam Jr AM, et al. A prospective analysis of critical limb ischemia: factors leading to major primary amputation versus revascularization. Ann Vasc Surg. 2007;21(4):458–63.
3. Anderson JL, et al. Management of patients with peripheral artery disease (compilation of 2005 and 2011 ACCF/AHA guideline recommendations): a report of the American College of Cardiology Foundation/American Heart Association Task Force on Practice Guidelines. Circulation. 2013;127(13):1425–43.
4. Criqui MH, Langer RD, Fronek A, Feigelson HS, Klauber MR, McCann TJ, Browner D. Mortality over a period of 10 years in patients with peripheral arterial disease. N Engl J Med. 1992;326:381–6.
5. Caro J, et al. The morbidity and mortality following a diagnosis of peripheral arterial disease: long-term follow-up of a large database. BMC Cardiovasc Disord. 2005;5:14.
6. Fowkes FGR, et al. Ankle brachial index combined with Framingham risk score to predict cardiovascular events and mortality – a meta-analysis. JAMA. 2008;300(2):197–208.
7. Resnick HE, et al. Relationship of high and low ankle brachial index to all-cause and cardiovascular disease mortality: the Strong Heart Study. Circulation. 2004;109(6):733–9.
8. Suominen V, et al. PAD as a risk factor for mortality among patients with elevated ABI--a clinical study. Eur J Vasc Endovasc Surg. 2010;39(3):316–22.
9. Harris TJ, Zafar AM, Murphy TP. Utilization of lower extremity arterial disease diagnostic and revascularization procedures in medicare beneficiaries 2000–2007. AJR Am J Roentgenol. 2011;197(2):W314–7.
10. de Vos MS, et al. National variation in the utilization of alternative imaging in peripheral arterial disease. J Vasc Surg. 2014;59(5):1315–22. e1.

11. Grassbaugh J. Blinded comparison of preoperative duplex ultrasound scanning and contrast arteriography for planning revascularization at the level of the tibia. J Vasc Surg. 2003;37(6):1186–90.

12. Collins R, et al. Duplex ultrasonography, magnetic resonance angiography, and computed tomography angiography for diagnosis and assessment of symptomatic, lower limb peripheral arterial disease: systematic review. BMJ. 2007;334(7606):1257.

13. Lowery AJ, et al. A prospective feasibility study of duplex ultrasound arterial mapping, digital-subtraction angiography, and magnetic resonance angiography in management of critical lower limb ischemia by endovascular revascularization. Ann Vasc Surg. 2007;21(4):443–51.

14. Norgren L, et al. Inter-society consensus for the management of peripheral arterial disease (TASC II). J Vasc Surg. 2007;45 Suppl S:S5–67.

15. Olin JW, et al. ACCF/AHA/ACR/SCAI/SIR/SVM/SVN/SVS 2010 performance measures for adults with peripheral artery disease. A report of the American College of Cardiology Foundation/American Heart Association Task Force on Performance Measures, the American College of Radiology, the Society for Cardiac Angiography and Interventions, the Society for Interventional Radiology, the Society for Vascular Medicine, the Society for Vascular Nursing, and the Society for Vascular Surgery (Writing Committee to Develop Clinical Performance Measures for Peripheral Artery Disease). Developed in collaboration with the American Association of Cardiovascular and Pulmonary Rehabilitation; the American Diabetes Association; the Society for Atherosclerosis Imaging and Prevention; the Society for Cardiovascular Magnetic Resonance; the Society of Cardiovascular Computed Tomography; and the PAD Coalition. Endorsed by the American Academy of Podiatric Practice Management. J Vasc Surg. 2010;52(6):1616–52.

16. Selvin E, Erlinger TP. Prevalence of and risk factors for peripheral arterial disease in the United States: results from the National Health and Nutrition Examination Survey, 1999–2000. Circulation. 2004;110(6):738–43.

17. Ouriel K, Zarins C. Doppler ankle pressure. Arch Surg. 1982;117:1297–300.

18. Hiatt WR. Medical treatment of peripheral arterial disease and claudication. N Engl J Med. 2001;344(21):1608–21.

19. Klein S, Hage JJ. Measurement, calculation, and normal range of the ankle-arm index: a bibliometric analysis and recommendation for standardization. Ann Vasc Surg. 2006;20(2):282–92.

20. Koelemay MJ, et al. Duplex scanning allows selective use of arteriography in the management of patients with severe lower leg arterial disease. J Vasc Surg. 2001;34(4):661–7.

21. Campbell WB, Fletcher EL, Hands LJ. Assessment of the distal lower limb arteries: a comparison of arteriography and Doppler ultrasound. Ann R Coll Surg Engl. 1986;68:37–9.

22. Stewart AHR, et al. Pre-operative hand-held doppler run-off score can be used to stratify risk prior to infra-inguinal bypass surgery. Eur J Vasc Endovasc Surg. 2002;23(6):500–4.

23. Eiberg JP, et al. Duplex ultrasound scanning of peripheral arterial disease of the lower limb. Eur J Vasc Endovasc Surg. 2010;40(4):507–12.

24. Lijmer JG, et al. ROC analysis of noninvasive tests for peripheral arterial disease. Ultrasound Med Biol. 1996;22(4):391–8.

25. Kaiser V, et al. The influence of experience on the reproducibility of the ankle-brachial systolic pressure ratio in peripheral arterial occlusive disease. Eur J Vasc Endovasc Surg. 1999;18(1):25–9.

26. Holland-Letz T, et al. Reproducibility and reliability of the ankle-brachial index as assessed by vascular experts, family physicians and nurses. Vasc Med. 2007;12(2):105–12.

27. McLafferty RB, et al. Ability of ankle-brachial index to detect lower-extremity atherosclerotic disease progression. Arch Surg. 1997;132:836–41.

28. Brooks B, et al. TBI or not TBI: that is the question. Is it better to measure toe pressure than ankle pressure in diabetic patients? Diabet Med. 2000;18:528–32.

29. Potier L, et al. Ankle-to-brachial ratio index underestimates the prevalence of peripheral occlusive disease in diabetic patients at high risk for arterial disease. Diabetes Care. 2009;32(4), e44.

30. Nam SC, et al. Factors affecting the validity of ankle-brachial index in the diagnosis of peripheral arterial obstructive disease. Angiology. 2010;61(4):392–6.

31. Hauser CJ, et al. Superiority of transcutaneous oximetry in noninvasive vascular diagnosis in patients with diabetes. Arch Surg. 1984;119(6):690–4.

32. Ballard JL, et al. A prospective evaluation of transcutaneous oxyen measurements in the management of diabetic foot problems. J Vasc Surg. 1995;22:485–92.

33. Bone GE, et al. Value of segmental limb blood pressures in predicting results of aortofemoral bypass. Am J Surg. 1976;132(6):733–8.

34. Lynch TG, et al. Interpretation of doppler segmental pressures in peripheral vascular occlusive disease. Arch Surg. 1983;119:465–7.

35. Pickering TG, et al. Recommendations for blood pressure measurement in humans and experimental animals: part 1: blood pressure measurement in humans: a statement for professionals from the Subcommittee of Professional and Public Education of the American Heart Association Council on High Blood Pressure Research. Circulation. 2005;111(5):697–716.

36. Symes JF, Graham AM, Mousseau M. Doppler waveform analysis versus segmental pressure and pulse-volume recording: assessment of occlusive disease in the lower extremity. Can J Surg. 1984;27(4):345–7.

37. Moneta GL, et al. Noninvasive localization of arterial occlusive disease: a comparison of segmental Doppler pressures and arterial duplex mapping. J Vasc Surg. 1993;17(3):578–82.

38. Eslahpazir BA, et al. Pulse volume recording does not enhance segmental pressure readings for peripheral arterial disease stratification. Ann Vasc Surg. 2014;28(1):18–27.

39. Rutherford RB, Lowenstein DH, Klein MF. Combining segmental systolic pressures and plethysmography to diagnose arterial occlusive disease of the legs. Am J Surg. 1979;138(2):211–8.

40. Allen J, et al. A prospective comparison of bilateral photoplethysmography versus the ankle-brachial pressure index for detecting and quantifying lower limb peripheral arterial disease. J Vasc Surg. 2008;47(4):794–802.

41. Khandanpour N, et al. The association between ankle brachial pressure index and pulse wave velocity: clinical implication of pulse wave velocity. Angiology. 2009;60(6):732–8.

42. Williams DT, Price P, Harding KG. The influence of diabetes and lower limb arterial disease on cutaneous foot perfusion. J Vasc Surg. 2006;44(4):770–5.

43. Chin JA, Wang EC, Kibbe MR. Evaluation of hyperspectral technology for assessing the presence and severity of peripheral artery disease. J Vasc Surg. 2011;54(6):1679–88.

44. Yamada T, et al. Clinical reliability and utility of skin perfusion pressure measurement in ischemic limbs--comparison with other noninvasive diagnostic methods. J Vasc Surg. 2008;47(2):318–23.

45. Andersen CA. Noninvasive assessment of lower extremity hemodynamics in individuals with diabetes mellitus. J Vasc Surg. 2010;52(3 Suppl):76S–80.

46. Londahl M, et al. Relationship between ulcer healing after hyperbaric oxygen therapy and transcutaneous oximetry, toe blood pressure and ankle-brachial index in patients with diabetes and chronic foot ulcers. Diabetologia. 2011;54(1):65–8.

47. Jorneskog G, Djavani K, Brismar K. Day-to-day variability of transcutaneous oxygen tension in patients with diabetes mellitus and peripheral arterial occlusive disease. J Vasc Surg. 2001;34(2):277–82.

48. de Meijer VE, et al. Reference value of transcutaneous oxygen measurement in diabetic patients compared with nondiabetic patients. J Vasc Surg. 2008;48(2):382–8.

49. de Graaff JC, et al. Evaluation of toe pressure and transcutaneous oxygen measurements in management of chronic critical leg ischemia: a diagnostic randomized clinical trial. J Vasc Surg. 2003;38(3):528–34.

50. Adera HM, et al. Prediction of amputation wound healing with skin perfusion pressure. J Vasc Surg. 1995;21(5):823–8. discussion 828–9.

51. Castronuovo Jr JJ, et al. Skin perfusion pressure measurement is valuable in the diagnosis of critical limb ischemia. J Vasc Surg. 1997;26(4):629–37.

52. Jafari-Saraf L, Gordon IL. Hyperspectral imaging and ankle: brachial indices in peripheral arterial disease. Ann Vasc Surg. 2010;24(6):741–6.

53. Jafari-Saraf L, Wilson SE, Gordon IL. Hyperspectral image measurements of skin hemoglobin compared with transcutaneous PO2 measurements. Ann Vasc Surg. 2012;26(4):537–48.

54. Khaodhiar L, et al. The use of medical hyperspectral technology to evaluate microcirculatory changes in diabetic foot ulcers and to predict clinical outcomes. Diabetes Care. 2007;30:903–10.

55. Cossman DV, et al. Comparison of contrast arteriography to arterial mapping with color-flow duplex imaging in the lower extremities. J Vasc Surg. 1989;10(5):0522–9.

56. Ernst CB, et al. Accuracy of lower extremity arterial duplex mapping. J Vasc Surg. 1992;15(2):0275–84.

57. Proia RR, et al. Early results of infragenicular revascularization based solely on duplex arteriography. J Vasc Surg. 2001;33(6):1165–70.

58. Kakkos SK, Tsolakis IA. Is duplex ultrasound scanning for peripheral arterial disease of the lower limb a non-invasive alternative or an adjunct to angiography? Eur J Vasc Endovasc Surg. 2010;40(4):513–4.

59. Ubbink DT, Legemate DA, Llull J-B. Color-flow duplex scanning of the leg arteries by use of a new echo-enhancing agent. J Vasc Surg. 2002;35(2):392–6.

60. Amarteifio E, et al. Dynamic contrast-enhanced ultrasound and transient arterial occlusion for quantification of arterial perfusion reserve in peripheral arterial disease. Eur J Radiol. 2012;81(11):3332–8.

61. Duerschmied D, et al. Success of arterial revascularization determined by contrast ultrasound muscle perfusion imaging. J Vasc Surg. 2010;52(6):1531–6.

62. Amarteifio E, et al. Dynamic contrast-enhanced ultrasound for assessment of therapy effects on skeletal muscle microcirculation in peripheral arterial disease: pilot study. Eur J Radiol. 2013;82(4):640–6.

63. Janvier MA, et al. A 3-D ultrasound imaging robotic system to detect and quantify lower limb arterial stenoses: in vivo feasibility. Ultrasound Med Biol. 2014;40(1):232–43.

64. Onogi S, et al. Robotic ultrasound guidance by B-scan plane positioning control. Procedia CIRP. 2013;5:100–3.

65. Kock MC, et al. DSA versus multi-detector row CT angiography in peripheral arterial disease: randomized controlled trial. Radiology. 2005;237(2):727–37.

66. Sommer WH, et al. Diagnostic value of time-resolved CT angiography for the lower leg. Eur Radiol. 2010;20(12):2876–81.

67. Utsunomiya D, et al. Comparison of standard- and low-tube voltage MDCT angiography in patients with peripheral arterial disease. Eur Radiol. 2010;20(11):2758–65.

68. Kayhan A, et al. Multidetector CT angiography versus arterial duplex USG in diagnosis of mild lower extremity peripheral arterial disease: is multidetector CT a valuable screening tool? Eur J Radiol. 2012;81(3):542–6.

69. Met R, et al. Diagnostic performance of computed tomography angiography in peripheral arterial disease a systematic review and meta-analysis. JAMA. 2009;301(4):415–24.

70. Duan Y, et al. Diagnostic efficiency of low-dose CT angiography compared with conventional angiography in peripheral arterial occlusions. AJR Am J Roentgenol. 2013;201(6):W906–14.

71. Bueno A, et al. Diagnostic accuracy of contrast-enhanced magnetic resonance angiography and duplex ultrasound in patients with peripheral vascular disease. Vasc Endovascular Surg. 2010;44(7):576–85.

72. Ouwendijk R, et al. Multicenter randomized controlled trial of the costs and effects of noninvasive diagnostic imaging in patients with peripheral arterial disease: the DIPAD trial. AJR Am J Roentgenol. 2008;190(5):1349–57.

73. de Vos MS, et al. Treatment planning for peripheral arterial disease based on duplex ultrasonography and computed tomography angiography: consistency, confidence and the value of additional imaging. Surgery. 2014;156(2):492–502.

74. Morkos SK, Thomsen HS, Webb JA. Contrast-media-induced nephrotoxicity: a consensus report. Eur Radiol. 1999;9:1602–13.

75. McCullough PA, et al. Epidemiology and prognostic implications of contrast-induced nephropathy. Am J Cardiol. 2006;98(6A):5K–13.

76. Kim SM, et al. Incidence and outcomes of contrast-induced nephropathy after computed tomography in patients with CKD: a quality improvement report. Am J Kidney Dis. 2010;55(6):1018–25.

77. Murakami R, et al. Contrast-induced nephropathy in patients with renal insufficiency undergoing contrast-enhanced MDCT. Eur Radiol. 2012;22(10):2147–52.

78. Herts BR, et al. Probability of reduced renal function after contrast-enhanced CT: a model based on serum creatinine level, patient age, and estimated glomerular filtration rate. AJR Am J Roentgenol. 2009;193(2):494–500.

79. Kooiman J, et al. Meta-analysis: serum creatinine changes following contrast enhanced CT imaging. Eur J Radiol. 2012;81(10):2554–61.

80. Zagler A, et al. N-acetylcysteine and contrast-induced nephropathy: a meta-analysis of 13 randomized trials. Am Heart J. 2006;151(1):140–5.

81. Ratcliffe JA, et al. Prevention of contrast-induced nephropathy: a randomized controlled trial of sodium bicarbonate and N-acetylcysteine. Int J Angiol. 2009;18(4):193–7.

82. Klima T, et al. Sodium chloride vs. sodium bicarbonate for the prevention of contrast medium-induced nephropathy: a randomized controlled trial. Eur Heart J. 2012;33(16):2071–9.

83. Traub SJ, et al. N-acetylcysteine plus intravenous fluids versus intravenous fluids alone to prevent contrast-induced nephropathy in emergency computed tomography. Ann Emerg Med. 2013;62(5):511–20. e25.

84. Briguori C, et al. Renal insufficiency following contrast media administration trial (REMEDIAL): a randomized comparison of 3 preventive strategies. Circulation. 2007;115(10):1211–7.

85. Chousterman BG, et al. Prevention of contrast-induced nephropathy by N-acetylcysteine in critically ill patients: different definitions, different results. J Crit Care. 2013;28(5):701–9.

86. Merten GJ, et al. Prevention of contrast-induced nephropathy with sodium bicarbonate. JAMA. 2004;291(19):2328–34.

87. de Gonzalez AB, et al. Projected cancer risks from computed tomographic scans performed in the United States in 2007. Arch Intern Med. 2009;169(22):2071–7.

88. Iessi R, et al. Low-dose multidetector cT angiography in the evaluation of infrarenal aorta and peripheral arterial occlusive disease. Radiology 2012;(263):287–98.

89. Josephs SC, et al. Atherosclerotic peripheral vascular disease symposium II: vascular magnetic resonance and computed tomographic imaging. Circulation. 2008;118(25):2837–44.

90. Mell M, et al. Clinical utility of time-resolved imaging of contrast kinetics (TRICKS) magnetic resonance angiography for infrageniculate arterial occlusive disease. J Vasc Surg. 2007;45(3):543–8.

91. Christie A, Chandramohan S, Roditi G. Comprehensive MRA of the lower limbs including high-resolution extended-phase infra-inguinal imaging with gadobenate dimeglumine: initial experience with inter-individual comparison to the blood-pool contrast agent gadofosveset trisodium. Clin Radiol. 2013;68(2):125–30.

92. Kassamali RH, et al. A comparative analysis of noncontrast flow-spoiled versus contrast-enhanced magnetic resonance angiography for evaluation of peripheral arterial disease. Diagn Interv Radiol. 2013;19(2):119–25.

93. van den Bosch HC, et al. Peripheral arterial occlusive disease: 3.0-T versus 1.5-T MR angiography compared with digital subtraction angiography. Radiology. 2013;266(1):337–46.

94. Visser K, Hunink MG. Peripheral arterial disease: gadolinium-enhanced MR angiography versus color-guided duplex US--a meta-analysis. Radiology. 2000;216(1):67–77.

95. Burbelko M, et al. Comparison of contrast-enhanced multi-station MR angiography and digital subtraction angiography of the lower extremity arterial disease. J Magn Reson Imaging. 2013; 37(6):1427–35.

96. Kreitner K, et al. Diabetes and peripheral arterial occlusive disease: prospective comparison of contrast-enhanced three-dimensional MR angiography with conventional digital subtraction angiography. Am J Roentol. 1999;174:171–9.

97. Owen AR, et al. Critical lower-limb ischemia: the diagnostic performance of dual-phase injection MR angiography (including high-resolution distal imaging) compared with digital subtraction angiography. J Vasc Interv Radiol. 2009;20(2):165–72.

98. Hansmann J, et al. Impact of time-resolved MRA on diagnostic accuracy in patients with symptomatic peripheral artery disease of the calf station. AJR Am J Roentgenol. 2013;201(6):1368–75.

99. Sam AD, et al. Safety of gadolinium contrast angiography in patients with chronic renal insufficiency. J Vasc Surg. 2003;38(2):313–8.

100. Kuo PH, et al. Gadolinium-based MR contrast agents and nephrogenic systemic fibrosis. Radiology. 2007;242(3):647–9.

101. Ledneva E, et al. Renal safety of gadolinium-based contrast media in patients with chronic renal insufficiency. Radiology. 2009;250(3):618–28.

102. Sandowski EA, et al. Nephrogenic systemic fibrosis: risk factors and incidence estimation. Radiology. 2007;243:148–57.

103. Cowper SE. Nephrogenic systemic fibrosis [ICNSFR Website], 2001–2013. Available at http://www.icnsfr.org. Accessed 09/01/2014.

104. Gutzeit A, et al. ECG-triggered non-contrast-enhanced MR angiography (TRANCE) versus digital subtraction angiography (DSA) in patients with peripheral arterial occlusive disease of the lower extremities. Eur Radiol. 2011;21(9):1979–87.

105. Hodnett PA, et al. Peripheral arterial disease in a symptomatic diabetic population: prospective comparison of rapid unenhanced MR angiography (MRA) with contrast-enhanced MRA. AJR Am J Roentgenol. 2011;197(6):1466–73.

106. Klasen J, et al. Nonenhanced ECG-gated quiescent-interval single-shot MRA (QISS-MRA) of the lower extremities: comparison with contrast-enhanced MRA. Clin Radiol. 2012;67(5): 441–6.

107. Diop AD, et al. Unenhanced 3D turbo spin-echo MR angiography of lower limbs in peripheral arterial disease: a comparative study with gadolinium-enhanced MR angiography. AJR Am J Roentgenol. 2013;200(5):1145–50.

108. von Kalle T, et al. Contrast-enhanced MR angiography (CEMRA) in peripheral arterial occlusive disease (PAOD): conventional moving table technique versus hybrid technique. RoFo. 2004;176(1):62–9.

109. Gerretsen SC, et al. Multicenter, double-blind, randomized, intra-individual crossover comparison of gadobenate dimeglumine and gadopentetate dimeglumine for MR angiography of peripheral arteries. Radiology. 2010;255(3):988–1000.

110. Galizia MS, et al. Improved characterization of popliteal aneurysms using gadofosveset-enhanced equilibrium phase magnetic resonance angiography. J Vasc Surg. 2013;57(3):837–41.

111. Tarvis DR, et al. Bleeding and vascular complications at the femoral access site following percutaneous coronary intervention (PCI): an evaluation of hemostasis strategies. J Invasive Cardiol. 2012;24(7):2–8.

112. Tiroch KA, et al. Risk predictors of retroperitoneal hemorrhage following percutaneous coronary intervention. Am J Cardiol. 2008;102(11):1473–6.

113. Alvarez-Tostado JA, et al. The brachial artery: a critical access for endovascular procedures. J Vasc Surg. 2009;49(2):378–85. discussion 385.

114. Wheatley BJ, et al. Complication rates for percutaneous lower extremity arterial antegrade access. Arch Surg. 2011;146(4): 432–5.

115. Fitts J, et al. Fluoroscopy-guided femoral artery puncture reduces the risk of PCI-related vascular complications. J Interv Cardiol. 2008;21(3):273–8.

116. Seto AH, et al. Real-time ultrasound guidance facilitates femoral arterial access and reduces vascular complications: FAUST (Femoral Arterial Access With Ultrasound Trial). JACC Cardiovasc Interv. 2010;3(7):751–8.

117. Weiner MM, Geldard P, Mittnacht AJ. Ultrasound-guided vascular access: a comprehensive review. J Cardiothorac Vasc Anesth. 2013;27(2):345–60.

118. Díaz LP, et al. Assessment of CO_2 arteriography in arterial occlusive disease of the lower extremities. J Vasc Interv Radiol. 2000;11(2):163–9.

119. Spinosa DJ, et al. Lower extremity arteriography with use of iodinated contrast material or gadodiamide to supplement CO_2 angiography in patients with renal insufficiency. J Vasc Interv Radiol. 2000;11(1):35–43.

120. Dowling K, et al. Safety of limited supplemental iodinated contrast administration in azotemic patients undergoing CO_2 angiography. J Endovasc Ther. 2003;10(2):312–6.

121. Arthurs ZM, et al. Evaluation of peripheral atherosclerosis: a comparative analysis of angiography and intravascular ultrasound imaging. J Vasc Surg. 2010;51(4):933–8. discussion 939.

122. Kusuyama T, Iida H, Mitsui H. Intravascular ultrasound complements the diagnostic capability of carbon dioxide digital subtraction angiography for patients with allergies to iodinated contrast medium. Catheter Cardiovasc Interv. 2012;80(6):E82–6.

123. Irshad K, et al. Early clinical experience with color three-dimensional intravascular ultrasound in peripheral interventions. J Endovasc Ther. 2001;8(4):329–38.

124. Ikeno F, et al. Mechanism of luminal gain with plaque excision in atherosclerotic coronary and peripheral arteries: assessment by histology and intravascular ultrasound. J Interv Cardiol. 2007;20(2):107–13.

125. Hassan AH, et al. Mechanism of lumen gain with a novel rotational aspiration atherectomy system for peripheral arterial disease: examination by intravascular ultrasound. Cardiovasc Revasc Med. 2010;11(3):155–8.

126. Niwamae N, et al. Intravascular ultrasound analysis of correlation between plaque-morphology and risk factors in peripheral arterial disease. Ann Vasc Dis. 2009;2(1):27–33.

127. van der Vaart MG, et al. Application of PET/SPECT imaging in vascular disease. Eur J Vasc Endovasc Surg. 2008;35(5):507–13.

128. Cavalcanti Filho JL, et al. PET/CT and vascular disease: current concepts. Eur J Radiol. 2011;80(1):60–7.

129. Burchert W, et al. Oxygen-15-water PET assessment of muscular blood flow in peripheral vascular disease. J Nucl Med. 1997;38(1):93–8.

130. Kalliokoski KK, et al. Perfusion heterogeneity in human skeletal muscle: fractal analysis of PET data. Eur J Nucl Med. 2001;28(4):450–6.

131. Rudd JH, et al. Atherosclerosis inflammation imaging with 18F-FDG PET: carotid, iliac, and femoral uptake reproducibility, quantification methods, and recommendations. J Nucl Med. 2008;49(6):871–8.

132. Rudd JH, et al. Relationships among regional arterial inflammation, calcification, risk factors, and biomarkers: a prospective fluorodeoxyglucose positron-emission tomography/computed tomography imaging study. Circ Cardiovasc Imaging. 2009;2(2):107–15.

133. Myers KS, et al. Correlation between arterial FDG uptake and biomarkers in peripheral artery disease. JACC Cardiovasc Imaging. 2012;5(1):38–45.

134. Pande RL, et al. Impaired skeletal muscle glucose uptake by [18F]fluorodeoxyglucose-positron emission tomography in patients with peripheral artery disease and intermittent claudication. Arterioscler Thromb Vasc Biol. 2011;31(1): 190–6.

135. Jaffer FA, Libby P, Weissleder R. Molecular and cellular imaging of atherosclerosis: emerging applications. J Am Coll Cardiol. 2006;47(7):1328–38.

136. Jaffer FA, et al. Optical visualization of cathepsin K activity in atherosclerosis with a novel, protease-activatable fluorescence sensor. Circulation. 2007;115(17):2292–8.

137. Roivainen A, et al. Whole-body distribution and metabolism of [N-methyl-11C](R)-1-(2-chlorophenyl)-N-(1-methylpropyl)-3-isoquinolinecarboxamide in humans; an imaging agent for in vivo assessment of peripheral benzodiazepine receptor activity with positron emission tomography. Eur J Nucl Med Mol Imaging. 2009;36(4):671–82.

138. Strauss HW, et al. PET and PET–CT imaging in the diagnosis and characterization of atheroma. Int Congr Ser. 2004;1264:95–104.

139. Winter PM, et al. Molecular imaging of angiogenic therapy in peripheral vascular disease with alphanubeta3-integrin-targeted nanoparticles. Magn Reson Med. 2010;64(2):369–76.

Carlo Setacci, Gianmarco de Donato,
Giuseppe Galzerano, Maria Pia Borrelli, Giulia Mazzitelli,
and Francesco Setacci

Introduction

Acute limb ischemia (ALI) is a serious medical emergency leading to high rate of complications, being not only limb but even life threatening, often despite early successful revascularization. The prognosis of this potentially devastating disease is mainly related to the rapidity and accuracy of diagnosis and treatment. However, timely recognition of signs and symptoms may be challenging, since clinical onset may range from sub-clinic and pauci-symptomatic to dramatic and irreversible ischemia.

Every specialist involved in the management of vascular diseases (preferably every physician) must be able to promptly recognize the singular signs and symptoms of ALI, avoiding any time loss to the establishment of the correct treatment.

This chapter focuses on epidemiology, natural history, etiology, clinical manifestation, classification, and noninvasive and invasive evaluation.

Definitions, Epidemiology, and Natural History

Acute limb ischemia (ALI) is defined as any sudden decrease in limb perfusion causing a potential threat to limb viability in patients who present within two weeks of the acute event [1]. The incidence of this condition is approximately 15 cases per 100,00 persons per year [2]. The prevalence is <0.1 % in

general population and about 5–10 % in patients with other risk factors for cardiovascular disease.

The lower limbs are more frequently involved, being caused by acute arterial thrombosis in the most of cases. The acute ischemia of upper limbs represents only 1/5 of all ALI events, with an incidence of 2.4 cases per 100.000 persons per year. The embolization from a cardiac source is the most common etiology (80 % of cases). Acute upper limb ischemia has a better prognosis quoad vitam and quoad valitudinem than ALI of lower limbs, even if the conservative treatment is associated to a higher risk of limb dysfunction.

Acute lower limb ischemia is still considered to be a dramatic event, carrying a risk of amputation between 15 and 30 % and a high perioperative morbidity and mortality (20–30 %) [3–8]. Concomitant underlying diseases, the metabolic derangement that seems as a result of the acute insult, and a possible reperfusion injury following revascularization may account for this severe prognosis [9–11].

The natural history of any ALI is characterized by the rapid onset of ischemia and by the tissue injuries when the ischemia persists. The sudden cessation of blood supply and nutrients to the metabolically active tissues of the limb, including the skin, muscles, and nerves, is responsible to tissue damage and cell death. Firstly energy metabolism shifts from aerobic to anaerobic process, and then established ischemia leads to cell dysfunction and death.

Nervous tissue cells are the most susceptible to ischemia, followed by muscle cells, the skin, and subcutaneous tissue. Peripheral nerves are perfused by arterioles that anastomosed themselves with a "T shape" along the nerve trunk. The longitudinal vessels that derive from these anastomoses are fundamental for the functionality of the nerve. So lesion of these vessels can lead to serious and irreversible alteration and can explain the failure of nerve resumption even after revascularization. In the pathogenesis of nerve injury, in addition to the ischemia, extrinsic compression due to edematous tissue is important. The prognosis of these lesions is variable: in general, the resumption of sensibility is more

C. Setacci, MD (✉) • G. de Donato, MD • G. Galzerano, MD
M.P. Borrelli, MD • G. Mazzitelli, MD
Department of Medicine, Surgery and Neuroscience,
Unit of Vascular Surgery, University of Siena, Viale Bracci 1,
Siena 53100, Italy

F. Setacci, MD
Department of Surgery "P. Valdoni", Sapienza University of Rome,
Rome, Italy

© Springer International Publishing Switzerland 2017
R.S. Dieter et al. (eds.), *Critical Limb Ischemia*, DOI 10.1007/978-3-319-31991-9_16

common than motility, depending on the time spent between the ischemic insult and revascularization.

Muscle is also sensitive to anoxia due to its high oxygen consumption. Intramuscular edema causes the dissociation of the fibers and the loss of their syncytium feature, instead becomes more evident the transverse streak and starts Bowman degeneration with loss of muscle contractility [12]. The last stage of muscle necrosis is characterized by Zenker's degeneration in which fibers become swollen and homogeneous and lose their streak. The time of ischemia that a muscle can endure it's difficult to determine; it seems that within 6 h lesions are still reversible, instead after 12 h they can't regress [13, 14]. Muscle necrosis can be massive or circumscribed and in the same muscle may coexist different degrees of cell degeneration.

Sequential modifications of the skin are related to the time of ischemia: after 10 h modifications of the nucleus and homogenization of the deep layers are evident, while after 20 h the detachment of basal layers of the papillae occurs. These alterations are still reversible after 48 h. Skin phlyctena, which results from an increased capillary permeability and extravasation of plasma fluid, comes just before gangrene and carries a very high negative prognostic significance.

After ischemia onset, a series of compensatory mechanisms are activated in order to ensure adequate perfusion, including vasodilatation and perfusion through collateral vessels. If these mechanisms are unsatisfactory, secondary thrombosis of distal and smaller vessels may occur.

The rapidity of evolution of any ALI event is related to general and local factors. Systemic hemodynamic conditions are really crucial, since an acute arterial occlusion could be almost completely compensated if systemic blood pressure is satisfactory. On the other hand, extension of thrombosis can occur in case of hypercoagulable concomitant acute episode or real thrombophilic states [15]. Local factors influencing natural history of ALI include the site of occlusion (i.e., more proximal location of clot causes a severe ischemia due to the lower possibility of compensation by the collateral circulation) and a preexisting chronic ischemia, which typically promotes formation of collateral circulation that can ensure distal compensation during an acute event. However, an acute occlusion of these collaterals can determine rapid secondary thrombosis of the whole arterial tree.

Etiology

The etiology of ALI can be roughly distinguished in two large categories: thrombosis and embolism. Distinction of these two conditions is important because treatment and prognosis are different.

Table 16.1 Etiology of acute limb ischemia

1. Embolus
Cardiac source
Atrial fibrillation
Valvular heart disease
Endocarditis
Myocardial infarction (with mural thrombus)
Atrial myxoma
Cardiomyopathy
Arterial source
Aortic and peripheral arterial aneurysms
Ulcerated atherosclerotic plaque with intraplaque hemorrhage
Venous source
Venous embolism in the presence of inter-atrium or inter-ventricle abnormal communication
2. Thrombosis
On pathologic artery
Atherosclerotic occlusive disease
Aortic and peripheral arterial aneurysms
Intraplaque hemorrhage with arterial stenosis and occlusion
Buerger disease
Vasculities
Adventitial cystic disease
Post-actinic arteritis
On healthy artery
Hypercoagulable states (C or S protein deficiencies)
Entrapment syndromes
Stasis/low-flow states
Drugs of abuse
Heparin-induced thrombosis
3. Trauma
Penetrating
Blunt
Interventional vascular procedures
4. Distal progression of aortic dissection
5. Ischemic thrombophlebitis (phlegmasia cerulea dolens)

Basically any ALI should be distinguished as consequence of embolism or thrombosis [16, 17] and more specifically as occurring on a pathologic or healthy artery or related to other less common conditions (Table 16.1).

Embolism

The embolic disease is characterized by the presence of a mass (embolus) that travels in the bloodstream and lodges in a blood vessel. The etiology of embolism is changing; before 1950, the majority of ALI ($\approx 60\%$) was caused by rheumatic heart disease; today that figure is about 8%. Nowadays cardiac emboli are commonly associated with atrial fibrillation or mural thrombus after a myocardial infarction. Rarely, the embolus arises from valve vegetation or from an atrial myxoma. Emboli may also arise from aneurysms, so the abdomen and popliteal fossa should be palpated carefully. Atheromatous arteries may also cause distal emboli in case of plaque rupture.

Embolism on Healthy Artery

Embolism on healthy artery may have a cardiac, arterial, and venous origin.

Approximately 80–90 % of all embolisms are associated with heart disease and predisposing conditions as atrial fibrillation, valvular disease, severe cardiac failure, aneurysms of left ventricle, myocardial infarction, thrombus endocarditic vegetation, and valve replacements [18–20]. Clinical onset generally occurs in case of sudden rhythm and frequency modifications, which may occur spontaneously or after drug administration.

Embolism of arterial generally arises from aortic or peripheral (femoral, popliteal) aneurysms but may also be the consequence of atheromatous plaque ulceration or rupture, iatrogenic lesions secondary to invasive diagnostic or interventional procedures, and other lesions of the arterial wall (bruises, compressions, inflammatory processes) [21]. The propulsive element is represented by abrupt modifications of pressure or direct trauma on the artery, especially in the presence of aneurysm.

The circumstance of "paradoxical embolism" (also called "crossed embolism") is a rare condition when a venous thromboembolism may reach the arterial circulation through inter-atrium or inter-ventricle abnormal communication, potentially causing arterial ischemia of any tissue.

Other possible causes of embolism on healthy artery include lipid embolism (i.e., trauma, fractures), neoplastic/septic embolism, and air embolism (decompression in divers).

Embolism on Pathologic Artery

In some cases embolism may occur on pathologic artery. This condition is typical of elderly patient with a cardiac source of emboli (i.e., atrial fibrillation) and asymptomatic femoropopliteal artery disease. The embolism causes the acute blood flow blockage at the level of stenotic segment, with consequent thrombosis of collateral vessels causing a severe acute limb ischemia. This kind of embolism should be considered and treated as arterial thrombosis.

Thrombosis

Thrombosis generally occurs in the setting of preexisting vascular lesion. Clinical presentation in case of thrombosis on atherosclerotic stenosis (so-called acute-on-chronic ischemia) may be less severe than in patients with embolic occlusion, as with the former, there may be sufficient collaterals present.

It's essential to obtain information about any history of claudication or rest pain, to look for the changes associated with chronic ischemia such as atrophy of skin appendages, and to examine the opposite leg for loss of pulses and the presence of bruits.

Thrombosis on Atherosclerotic Plaque

More frequently thrombosis occurs on a pathologic artery for the presence of an atherosclerotic lesion. It is characterized by a referred history of intermittent claudication and cardiovascular disease, and it is generally associated by a less severe limb dysfunction.

Thrombosis of peripheral aneurysm is the second cause of ALI on pathologic artery. The sudden interruption of the blood flow may occur at the level of popliteal aneurysm, but also iliac or femoral aneurysms may occlude acutely. The thrombosis is generally related to an increase of peripheral artery resistances. Emboli can depart from the aneurysmal sac causing an acute occlusion of more distal vessels (blue toe syndrome).

Thrombosis on Non-atheromatous Pathological Artery

This situation may occur in patients with Buerger disease, vasculitis, adventitial cystic disease, and post-actinic arteritis [22, 23]. Thrombosis is the result of the presence of a chronic narrowing in the bloodstream, and clinical presentation is similar to ALI that occurs in patients with atherosclerotic plaques.

Thrombosis on Healthy Artery

Thrombosis may also occur on a healthy artery. This is a less frequent cause of ALI that may be secondary to an ab-estrinseco compression (i.e., popliteal entrapment), to hyperviscosity (hemoconcentration in great dehydrations, thrombophilia, severe hypotension, hemoglobinopathies), to systemic coagulation disorder (congenital anomalies such as protein C or S and antithrombin III deficiencies, malignancy), or to drugs (oestroprogestative, ergotism, drug addiction, chemotherapy). Heparin-induced thrombosis is another important cause of ALI on healthy artery; it is generally recognized by a significant decrease in the platelet count during heparin therapy and the manifestation of the thrombosis.

Extreme low-flow states can produce ALI in patients with hypovolemic shock or cardiac failure, especially when chronic peripheral arterial disease (PAD) is already evident.

Post-traumatic Thrombosis

Trauma may cause acute thrombosis, rupture, or embolism of the artery. Penetrating trauma may directly damage the artery, while blunt trauma may cause indirect injury including spasm, arterial rupture, mural hematoma or intimal dissection, and consequent thrombosis. Blunt trauma may also cause fracture with associated arterial injury.

In case of partial arterial rupture, the natural evolution is represented by pseudoaneurysm formation, vessel occlusion, or artero-venous fistula.

Distal Progression of Aortic Dissection

Occasionally ALI represents the clinical presentation of acute aortic dissection. Patients are typically hypertensive and complain intensive chest and back pain. If aortic dissection is misdiagnosed and patient is treated for ALI by thromboembolectomy, Fogarty catheter passage beyond the occlusion generally fails, carrying the risk of vessel damage and disconnecting part of the dissected intima rather than removing the clot. Of course, failure to determine the correct diagnosis may be fatal.

Ischemic Thrombophlebitis (Phlegmasia Cerulea Dolens)

Infrequent cause of ALI occurs in the setting of massive deep venous thrombosis that causes severe soft tissue swelling of sufficient magnitude to impede arterial inflow to the extremity. Usually, phlegmasia cerulea dolens occurs in those afflicted by a life-threatening illness (underlying malignancy in 50 % of cases).

Clinical Presentation

Clinical Manifestation

When acute limb ischemia occurs, it represents an emergency in which restoration of perfusion through early intervention can lead to limb salvage, whereas delay may results in significant morbidity, including limb loss and, potentially, death. In many ways, this kind of acute vascular disease in the leg may be considered similar to that in the heart. The risk factors, underlying conditions, and pathogenic process are the same, and in many cases, patients have both conditions. And just as cardiologist has learned that in acute myocardial infarction "time is muscle," the vascular community is coming to recognize that in cases of limb ischemia, "time is tissue." In fact, as we know, any sudden decrease in limb perfusion—because of either embolic or in situ thrombotic vascular occlusion—can lead a potential threat to limb viability [11, 24].

The rapid onset of limb ischemia results from a sudden cessation of blood supply and nutrients to the metabolically active tissues of the limb, including the skin, muscle, and nerves. The severity of symptoms depends on the level of the obstruction and, most important, the presence of adequate collateral vessels.

Table 16.2 Clinical features of embolic and thrombotic ALI

	Acute embolic occlusion	Thrombotic occlusion
Symptom onset	Abrupt and severe	More gradual, less severe initially
Prior PAD	Infrequent	Common
Contralateral limb	Often normal	Frequent evidence of coexistent PAD
Coexistent cardiac disease	Frequent (especially AF)	May or may not be present

PAD peripheral arterial disease, *AF* atrial fibrillation

The clinical presentation is considered to be acute if it occurs within 2 weeks after symptom onset: symptoms can develop over a period of hours to days. Patients with cardiac embolism, trauma, and aneurysms responsible for peripheral embolization or occlusion of vascular reconstruction tend to present early (hours) due to the severity of symptoms related to the lack of collaterals, the extension of thrombus to arterial outflow, or a combination of both. On the other hand, later presentation—within days—tends to be restricted to those patients with a native thrombosis ("acute-on-chronic ischemia").

The clinical evaluation of acute limb ischemia should include both a physical examination and an investigation of patient's medical history: these factors, combined together, could provide clues to the origin of ALI. The collection of medical records should focus on history of claudication, previous ischemic symptoms, and previous vascular reconstruction or diagnostic cardiac catheterization and heart disease. Moreover, any potential risk factor and/or disease contributing to the genesis of the ALI should be carefully investigated (i.e., hypertension, diabetes, smoking, hypercholesterolemia, blood clots, arterial aneurysms as possible embolic sources, family history of cardiovascular disease, hematologic disorders). A correct diagnosis should carefully assess the onset of pain, its abruptness, the location, and the intensity, as well as its change over time and the presence of any motor or sensory deficit. A concomitant examination of the contralateral lower limb provides important suspicions regarding the pre-ischemic status of the involved limb (Table 16.2).

ALI typically presents a clinical manifestation of pain, paresthesia, paralysis, pallor, pulselessness, and poikilothermia (so-called six Ps):

> **The "Six Ps" of ALI Clinical Presentation**
> Pain
>   Paresthesia
>   Paralysis
>   Pallor
>   Pulselessness
>   Poikilothermia

Pain It is usually severe and progressive, with major localization at most distal part of the extremity. Although pain is generally always present, in diabetic and elderly patients, it may be more vague. The pain of acute ischemia is usually also at the level of the ischemic muscle, which may be tender on palpation or on passive movement of the toes or foot. At the beginning pain is confined and after it became crampy (muscular ischemia). Finally when ischemia continues and sensory deficits appear, they may mask the pain, making diagnosis more complex.

Paresthesia Nerves are generally very sensitive to ischemia and are rapidly damaged when blood perfusion is interrupted. Fibers responsible for touch impulse are the most sensitive, while pain fibers are less ischemia sensitive. This explains why paresthesia is so frequent in patients with ALI, and it is associated to numbness and tingling in more than half of patients. Because of underlying neuropathy, diabetic patients may already have a sensory deficit that masks the change. When ischemia persists, paresthesia leads to anesthesia.

Paralysis Motor nerve fibers are more resistant to ischemia. However, when ischemia persists for hours, loss of motor function occurs due to motor nerve fiber injury firstly and because of ischemic injury direct on the muscular issue subsequently. Asking the patient to move and spread the toes generally allows collection of information about the evolution of motor deficit. The degree of motor deficit can vary from mild paresis of toes to complete paralysis of leg, whose prognostic value is really unfavorable. At physical examination muscles injured by ischemia are tender, and this rigid paralysis may simulate consequence of cerebral stroke.

Pallor Change of skin color is a very common finding in ALI. Acute arterial occlusion is associated with intense spasm in the distal arterial tree, and initially the limb appears "marble" (Fig. 16.1a). Typically the obstruction is one joint above the level of pallor demarcation. In the following hours, the spasm typically decreases, and the skin fills with deoxygenated blood leading to mottling that is light blue or purple, having a fine reticular pattern, and blanches on pressure (Fig. 16.1b). As ischemia endures, stagnant blood coagulates leading to mottling that is darker in color, is gross in pattern, and does not blanch. Finally, large patches of fixed staining progress to blistering and liquefaction.

Pulselessness Physical examination should always include the research of palpable pulse at different level of the lower extremity (i.e., femoral, popliteal, anterior and posterior tibial pulses). A palpable pulse means that the flow at that

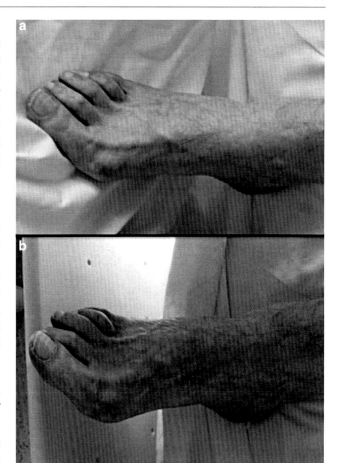

Fig. 16.1 Clinical findings of ALI: at early inspection the foot is typically pale (**a**), later spasm typically decreases, and the skin fills with deoxygenated blood leading to mottling that blanches on pressure to cyanosed (**b**)

level is sufficient and that ischemia is located at a more distal level. A particular circumstance is when the palpation is performed exactly at the level of the beginning of the occlusion: in such a case pulse may be appreciated even as stronger than normal, representing the stump flow at the level of vessel blockage. So the general principle that a palpable pulse rejects the hypothesis of occlusion at that level should be applied with caution. In all cases it is a good recommendation to measure blood pressure by CW Doppler at different level to confirm data obtained by pulse palpation. Ankle/brachial index is then crucial to determine the severity of ALI and to estimate the prognosis.

Poikilothermia This is the inability to regulate temperature of the affected limb that generally compares immediately after flow interruption. At palpation, the skin is cold, and the level of temperature change is an important parameter of occlusion estimation.

All findings at physical examination of the affected leg are most important when different from the contralateral limb.

Two particular clinical manifestations of ALI are the blue toe syndrome and the phlegmasia cerulea dolens. The first is typically caused by microembolization from plaque or thrombi located in aorta and iliac/femoral or popliteal artery. It leads to the occlusion of small vessels of the toes; lesions are small in size, multiple, painful, and cyanotic [25] (Fig. 16.2).

The phlegmasia cerulea dolens is an infrequent cause of ALI. It occurs in the setting of massive deep venous thrombosis that causes severe soft tissue swelling of sufficient magnitude to impede arterial inflow to the extremity (see also *Ischemic Thrombophlebitis (Phlegmasia Cerulea Dolens)*.

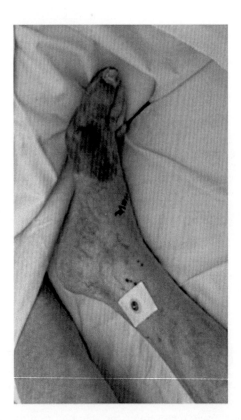

Fig. 16.2 Occlusion of small vessels of the big toe due to microembolization from popliteal aneurysm (blue toe syndrome)

Clinical Classification

When ALI is diagnosed, the determination of its severity is crucial to evaluate the prognosis of the event. A classification of ALI that reflects patient's complaints, objective findings, and prognosis has been offered by the Society for Vascular Surgery/International Society for Cardiovascular Surgery (Table 16.3).

Patients with a viable limb (class I) don't generally complain persevering pain, lower limb extremity is not cyanotic, and they are able to voluntarily move the toes. The flow at the level of dorsalis pedis or posterior tibial artery can be appreciated by CW Doppler examination. Generally a threshold of 30 mmHg for the ankle pressure is the applied limit to make sure that the insonated flow, which may be very slow, is from the artery and not from the vein.

Patients in class IIa present limbs that are marginally threatened. Sensibility is impaired, and there is no audible Doppler signal. When ischemic pain persists, sensory deficit increases, and there are initial signs of motor deficit, ischemia is classified as class IIb, and limb has to be considered as immediately threatened. The threatened leg differs from the irreversibly damaged leg by the presence of venous Doppler signal. In class III ALI sensory and motor deficits are profound, venous flow is stagnant, and any tissue changes are basically irreversible.

According to the classification of ALI severity, a viable leg does not need immediate intervention and a careful diagnostic workout can be performed; a class II threatened leg requires urgent revascularization, minimizing any lose of time before intervention especially for marginally threatened limb (class IIb).

Noninvasive Instrumental Diagnostics

Although diagnosis of acute limb ischemia is essentially based on clinical examination, instrumental investigations may allow a better evaluation of the level of obstruction and severity of ischemia. In case of immediately threatened

Table 16.3 Classification system by the society of vascular surgery and international society of cardiovascular surgery

Category	Description/prognosis	Findings		Doppler signals	
		Sensory loss	Muscle weakness	Arterial	Venous
I. Viable	Not immediately threatened	None	None	Audible	Audible
IIa. Marginally threatened	Salvageable if promptly treated	Minimal (toes) or none	None	(Often) inaudible	Audible
IIb. Immediately threatened	Salvageable with immediate revascularization	More than toes, associated with rest pain	Mild, moderate	(Usually) inaudible	Audible
III. Irreversible	Major tissue loss or permanent nerve damage inevitable	Profound, anesthetic	Profound, paralysis (rigor)	Inaudible	Inaudible

Obtaining an ankle pressure is very important. However, in severe ALI, blood flow velocity in the affected arteries may be so slow that Doppler signals are absent. Differentiating between arterial and venous flow signals is vital: arterial flow signals will have a rhythmic sound (synchronous with cardiac rhythm), whereas venous signals are more constant and may be affected by respiratory movements or be augmented by distal compression (caution needs to be taken not to compress the vessels with the transducer)

limbs, any further radiologic or vascular laboratory tests may be unnecessary and should not be performed to avoid any delay of treatment. When the ischemic limb is still viable or marginally threatened, there is room for a more precise diagnostic evaluation.

In recent years, noninvasive imaging of the peripheral arteries has had a great development. Technological improvements that have increased the performance of CT angiography and MRA have widely extended the indication of use of these methods for the preliminary study of PAD [26–30]. The quality and completeness of images may assist the specialist in the choice of a therapeutic option (conventional or endovascular surgery, palliative or medical), as well as in the selection of the best level for surgical access.

First-Level Noninvasive Diagnostic Examination: Duplex Ultrasound

The advantages of duplex ultrasound (DUS) investigation are well known; in particular the noninvasiveness, the low cost, and the repeatability of this examination make it a widely used first-level diagnostic approach in all centers of vascular surgery for the diagnosis of ALI. It has been shown that DUS in experienced hands for the study of hemodynamic arterial lesions in the vascularization of the lower extremities may offer quality data as high as coming from the angiography [31–34].

The B-mode investigation provides the ability to display important morphological details. It is possible to observe the thromboembolism which is characterized by an echogenicity equal to that of the blood, appearing almost completely anechoic in the acute phase and gradually increasing in echogenicity in a later phase (thrombus organization). The echogenicity of the thrombus is therefore a key parameter by which is possible to hypothesize the onset of the disease, which results to be a key point for the choice of treatment.

Not only thrombus echogenicity but also vessel wall status are important findings that a DUS examination may offer. The embolus tends to localize at sites of bifurcation, and the vessel walls appear healthy, with regular profile and lumen and no signs of atherosclerotic lesion. In thrombotic disease DUS may show signs of chronic arteriopathy: the vessel profile is irregular, and calcifications appear as hyperechoic thickening of the vessel wall (Fig. 16.3). Occasionally calcified plaque causes intense shadowing that may mask the thrombosis.

For a proper performance of the test, it's important that the environment is at a suitable temperature (>20 °C) to prevent peripheral vasoconstriction that could affect the velocity pattern. The combined use of the three main functions: B-mode, power/color, and Doppler, is essential for a complete evaluation.

Fig. 16.3 Duplex ultrasound findings at different limb levels: (**a**) Doppler spectral analysis above the acute occlusion ("stump" signal). (**b**) The vessel profile is irregular, some calcifications appear as hyperechoic thickening of the vessel wall, and hypoechoic material is present intraluminally at the level of thrombotic occlusion. (**c**) Downstream to the occlusion a monophasic flowmetry (reduced PSV and significant systolic phase prolongation) with low resistance patterns may be appreciated

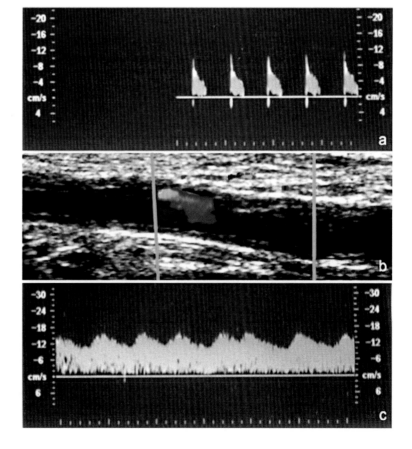

Modulation of PRF (pulse repetition frequency) and color gain is an indispensable element for the assessment of low-speed pathological flows. The Doppler spectral analysis and the calculation of the speed should always be performed with an angle of 60°, positioning the cursor along the main axis of the vessel, which coincides with the direction of flow.

The "color" mode allows deriving direct and indirect signs of thromboembolic disease. The direct sign is the absence of flow within the vessel (this finding is purchasing the highest sensitivity after reducing the PRF, increasing the color gain, or even using the function power Doppler). An indirect sign quite characteristic is the presence of a downstream indirect flow at low speed, which is characterized by the need to reduce the PRF or having to use the power Doppler for proper viewing. The display of an indirect flow downstream of the disease is also an index of the presence of collateral circulation and therefore of capacity of hemodynamic compensation, but this can only occur in case of thrombosis where the underlying atherosclerotic disease had made possible the establishment of collateral circulation during time. Sometimes is possible to see the collateral circulation upstream of the obstruction and circles back to the valley, whose flows are hyperdynamic (high-speed Doppler aliasing) and can be mistaken for stenosis.

The Doppler spectral analysis provides information on the type of flow inside the vessel. Direct sign of thromboembolic occlusion is the lack of flow within the vessel lumen (also in this case, the use of Doppler gain may be useful to increase the sensitivity of the procedure, especially in the case of pathological arteries). Upstream of the occlusion, the Doppler signal is often physiological, preserving the typical triphasic morphology. As flow analysis gets closer to the occlusion, the Doppler signal acquires the characteristic findings due to the obstacle encountered by the flow. Typical is the monophasic or biphasic "stump" signal (Fig. 16.3a) in which the lack of antegrade flow during diastole expresses the effective difficulty of unloading that the flow meets immediately upstream occlusion. This sign can however be absent in case of abundant collateral circulation, as in the case of thrombosis on pathological artery; in fact a well-developed collateral circulation can ensure a discharge sufficient to render the Doppler signal almost normal (as in the case of complete occlusion of the superficial femoral artery with deep femoral artery disease-free and able to ensure the metabolic demand of the periphery).

Other signs of downstream occlusion are the progressive reduction of the PSV (peak systolic velocity) that expresses the difficulty of unloading flow and the prolongation of the systolic descent of the signal that is due to the reflection of the pressure wave immediately upstream of the obstacle.

The situation downstream of the occlusive disease is always dependent on the timing and type of disease. In acute occlusion, as in the case of embolic occlusion, the hemodynamic status downstream is often characterized by the absence of flow, contrary to what happens in the case of thrombotic disease, in which, thanks to the development of collateral circulation, we will have downstream to the occlusion a reentrant indirect flowmetry (monophasic, with reduced PSV and with significant prolongation of systole) with low resistance patterns typical of low amplitude (parvus) and a slowing of systolic rise time (tardus) of spectrum analytical wave (Fig. 16.3c).

Second-Level Noninvasive Diagnostic Examination: CT Angiography and MR Angiography

Both CT angiography and MR angiography (MRA) allow an accurate analysis of the location, extent, and grading of steno-obstructive disease with high overall sensitivity and specificity [35]. CT angiography has a sensitivity of 92 % and a specificity of 93 %, while the MRA with 3D technique has a sensitivity between 75 and 100 % and a specificity between 85 and 100 % [36–38].

Images acquired by CT and MR angiography may be post-processed, offering a two-/three-dimensional reconstructions using VR (volume rendering), MIPs (maximum intensity projections), and MPR (multiplanar reconstruction) algorithms, which offer an overview of the disease and a documentation of synthesis (Fig. 16.4). Undoubted advantages of CT angiography are linked to the higher spatial resolution and to the higher speed of acquisition, plus the ability to display also the arterial wall. In contrast, CT angiography has disadvantages associated with the use of ionizing radiation, to the nephrotoxicity of iodinated contrast media and to the difficult analysis of small and calcified vessels. In fact, the most important limitation of CT angiography is in fact determined by the "blooming artifact," which affects the evaluation of the lumen of diffusely calcified vessels and increases with the reduction of the caliber of the vessels in question (in particular at the level of below-the-knee vessels).

The disadvantages of MRA include reduced availability and higher costs compared with CT angiography, the largest number of artifacts, and the inability to perform the investigation in claustrophobic patients or in patients with contraindications to exposure to the magnetic field [39, 40].

In general, CT angiography and MRA offer significant advantages compared to angiography in terms of preliminary treatment planning, less invasiveness, and a more precise assessment of the actual length of the segments affected by vascular occlusive disease due to improved visualization of collateral circulation and to the good visualization of the arteries of the foot, often obtainable in a comparable manner only with a selective catheterization during angiography. Furthermore, the multiplanar reconstruction allows a more

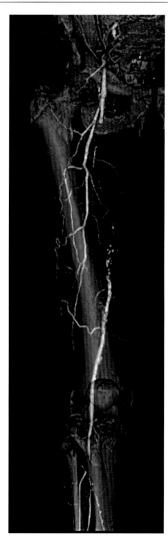

Fig. 16.4 CT angiography: overview of thrombotic occlusion of the femoropopliteal arterial segment

Invasive Instrumental Diagnostics

In addition to medical history and physical examination, angiography has been considered the only diagnostic method to assess arterial disease including ALI for a long time. However, the role of angiography has profoundly changed in recent years, and the reasons are related to the evolution of both diagnostic and therapeutic approaches to ALI. The etiology of the disease has changed, and the treatment has evolved from embolectomy under local anesthesia to the current hybrid revascularization procedures that include the use of surgical and endovascular techniques [43]. Then there has been a considerable development of noninvasive diagnostic methods, which are useful to confirm the clinical diagnosis.

As a result, the use of angiography as pure diagnostic tool has diminished. It is still practiced occasionally as a diagnostic test in cases of clinical signs not well defined and with not diriment hemodynamic tests, being able to document accurately the type and the level of the occlusion and the eventual coexistence and extension of parietal lesions and to ensure an appropriate treatment planning.

Actually the development of less-invasive imaging methods has questioned the role of arteriography in the preoperative diagnosis; currently it is no longer the gold standard in diagnosis of acute arterial disease. Actually angiography has a more defined role as part of endovascular treatment of ALI that now is considered more and more as therapeutic option complementary, supplementary, or alternative to the conventional surgical technique.

Angiography may still offer detailed and accurate information regarding the etiology, the location of the obstruction, and the extent of the insult that has caused ALI and may allow a catheter-based treatment in some patients. On the other hand, angiography has to be considered as an invasive diagnostic test that exposes patient both to radiation, to potentially nephrotoxic contrast medium, and to the risk of post-procedural access complications. Nevertheless it is quite time consuming and often related to the availability of a radiology staff.

Different angiographic pictures may be very useful in the discrimination of etiology (emboli or thrombus): embolus may appear as squashing of contrastive material just above the blocked place ("abrupt interruption"), with identification of a crescent-shaped occlusion (meniscus sign) in an otherwise normal artery (Fig. 16.5a); in case of acute thrombosis on plaque, the break of contrastive material in the shape of diagonal cloth line shape may be evident, and a typical collateral arterial circulation is present (Fig. 16.5b), as well as atherosclerotic signs in other arterial segments. The location of the occlusion may also be helpful, with emboli tending to lodge in areas of bifurcations. However, this distinction can be less clear in case of clot propagation, which may occur both after an embolic and a thrombotic event.

precise grading of eccentric stenotic lesions that in some cases are underestimated by angiography [41, 42].

In the case of acute occlusive disease with thrombotic etiology (i.e., thrombosis on plaque or bypass thrombosis), these methods are efficient for the detection of location, extension, and type of lesion and for the visualization of any collateral circulation or vessel upstream and downstream the lesion. CT angiography has become a determinant gold standard in the polytrauma patient, where very often the acute ischemic lesions may overlap with musculoskeletal limb lesions, with respect to which the vascular "timing" is predominant.

In conclusion, CT angiography and MRA are currently reliable and complementary methods in the evaluation of patients with acute occlusive disease. The availability and accessibility of these methods, as well as the organization of dedicated staff, are essential requirements for the management of vascular disease (see also section "Summary of Diagnostic Algorithm for Acute Leg Ischemia").

Fig. 16.5 (a) Typical angiographic picture of embolic acute limb ischemia. (b) Angiographic aspect of acute thrombosis on chronic atherosclerotic plaque. To note differences on clot line shape and collateral arterial circulation, see text

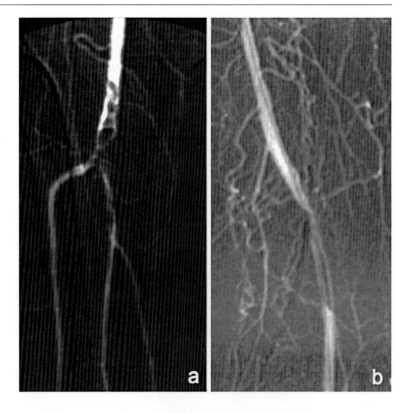

Nowadays intraoperative arteriography may have a role during arterial thromboembolectomy as a guide for extension of the procedure to ensure complete clearance of the arterial tree and distal patency and for the evaluation of immediate results after surgical treatment [44]. When intraoperative arteriography shows inadequate clearance of the distal tree, further attempts to remove the distal clot should be undertaken. Moreover, in patients with preexisting arteriosclerotic disease, angiography provides objective information about the collateral circulation and outflow. In such cases further treatments may be evaluated as possible or required (i.e., "on-table" fibrinolysis, transluminal angioplasty, or bypass surgery).

It is still a matter of debate if intraoperative angiography should be routinely performed in all cases or only in selected cases, depending on operative findings, when the surgeon suspects an incomplete revascularization after clot removal.

Summary of Diagnostic Algorithm for Acute Leg Ischemia

Prompt recognition of signs and symptoms of ALI is clearly the key point for the management of ALI (Fig. 16.6). The morbidity and mortality of this acute event are deeply related to the overall medical condition of the patients, to the severity of ischemia at presentation, and to the promptness of diagnosis and management.

Physical examination should be focused on the presence of one or more of the "six Ps" (pain, pallor, paralysis, paresthesia, pulselessness, poikilothermia). At the same time, the history of the status of lower limb before the acute event should be collected, since it can reveal important clinical clues about the etiology of the current event. Patients with a clear source of emboli and with no history of intermittent claudication or previous vascular intervention and with normal contralateral limb are probably suffering from embolization; patients with history of PAD, claudication, or previous vascular intervention, with contralateral limb suggestive of PAD, and with no identifiable source of emboli are probably suffering from thrombosis.

At the time of presentation, ALI patients should also be evaluated for general condition, since acute myocardial infarction, heart failure, and arrhythmias may occur simultaneously. In such cases stabilization of hemodynamics, replenishment of circulating volume, and an adequate urine output are mandatory before any further investigation. In the meantime, heparinization of patients with ALI is a well-established recommendation to limit proximal and distal propagation of thrombus (at least 10,000 UI of intravenous heparin to achieve immediate and complete anticoagulation). A patient with a history of heparin-induced thrombosis or with associated injuries is not a candidate for systemic heparinization.

When hemodynamics has been stabilized, and adequate clinical examination of the limb is completed, a duplex ultrasound examination should be rapidly performed to obtain

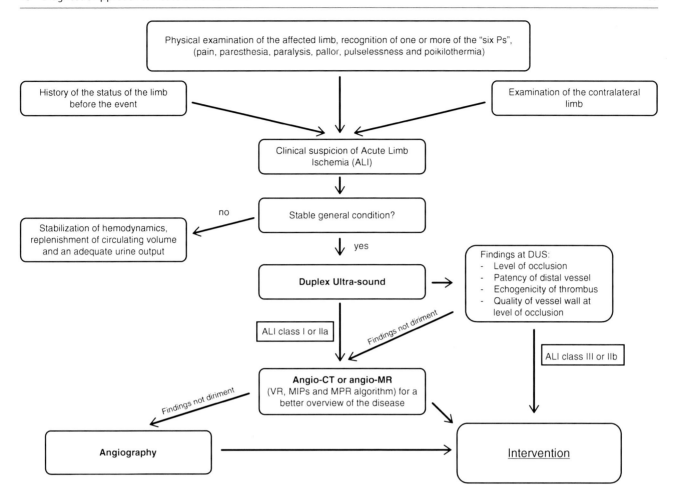

Fig. 16.6 Diagnostic algorithm for acute limb ischemia

details regarding the level of the occlusion and the patency of distal vessels. Other important findings at duplex ultrasound examination are the echogenicity of the thrombus (which can reveal data about the onset of the disease) and the quality of vessel walls (which can suggest an etiology of acute-on-chronic atherosclerotic disease). DUS examination is not time consuming in experienced hands, and it is recommendable as first-line diagnostic strategy for any kind of ALI.

While any further loss of time should be avoided for immediately threatened ALI (class IIb), in case of marginally threatened (class IIa) or viable (class I) ALI, a second-level instrumental examination as CT and RM angiography may have a role, especially when findings at DUS are not diriment. CT angiography offers a higher spatial resolution of vascular lesions with two-/three-dimensional reconstructions (VR, MIPs, and MPR algorithms) for an overview of the disease and a documentation of synthesis but has disadvantages associated with the use of ionizing radiation (nephrotoxicity). MR angiography has similar advantages but is not easily available because of costs and may be affected by several artifacts, although being not appropriate in claustrophobic patients.

Finally angiography, which has been considered the gold standard for ALI diagnosis for decades, has now a limited role as diagnostic test, mainly in cases of clinical signs not well defined and with not diriment hemodynamic tests. Nowadays arteriography has a limited role as preoperative test, while it has an expanding role as intraoperative test during surgical, endovascular, or hybrid procedure.

References

1. Norgren L, Hiatt WR, Dormandy JA, Nehler MR, Harris KA, Fowkes FG. Inter-society consensus for the management of peripheral arterial disease (TASC II). J Vasc Surg. 2007;45(Suppl):S5–67.
2. Creager MA, Kaufman JA, Conte MS. Clinical practice. Acute limb ischemia. N Engl J Med. 2012;366:2198–206.
3. de Donato G, Gussoni G, de Donato G, Andreozzi GM, Bonizzoni E, Mazzone A, et al. The ILAILL study: iloprost as adjuvant to surgery for acute ischemia of lower limbs: a randomized, placebo-controlled, double-blind study by the Italian society for vascular and endovascular surgery. Ann Surg. 2006;244:185–93.
4. The STILE Investigators. Results of a prospective randomized trial evaluating surgery versus thrombolysis for ischaemia of the lower extremity. Ann Surg. 1994;220:251–8.

5. Aune S, Trippestad A. Operative mortality and long-term survival of patients operated on for acute lower extremity ischaemia. Eur J Vasc Endovasc Surg. 1998;15:143–6.

6. Nypaver TJ, White BR, Endean ED, Schwarcz TH, Hyde GL. Non traumatic lower-extremity acute arterial ischaemia. Am J Surg. 1998;176:147–52.

7. Pemberton M, Varty K, Nydahl S, Bell PR. The surgical management of acute limb ischaemia due to native vessel occlusion. Eur J Vasc Endovasc Surg. 1999;17:72–6.

8. Ouriel K, Veith FJ, Sasahara AA, for the Thrombolysis Or Peripheral Arterial Surgery (TOPAS) Investigators. A comparison of recombinant urokinase with vascular surgery as initial treatment for acute arterial occlusion of the legs. N Engl J Med. 1998;338:1105–11.

9. Blaisdell FW. The pathophysiology of skeletal muscle ischemia and the reperfusion syndrome: a review. Cardiovasc Surg. 2002;10:620–30.

10. Falluji N, Mukherijee D. Critical and acute limb ischemia: an overview. Vascular. 2012;20:174–7.

11. Shishehbor MH. Acute and critical limb ischemia: when time is limb. MJ Case Rep. 2014;15.

12. McGuigan MR, Bronks R, Newton RU, Sharman MJ, Graham JC, Cody DV, et al. Muscle fiber characteristics in patients with peripheral arterial disease. Med Sci Sports Exerc. 2001;33:2016–21.

13. Manojlović V, Popović V, Nikolić D, Milosević D, Pasternak J, Kaćanski M. Analysis of associated diseases in patients with acute critical lower limb ischemia. Med Pregl. 2013;66:41–5.

14. Tang GL, Chang DS, Sarkar R, Wang R, Messina LM. The effect of gradual or acute arterial occlusion on skeletal muscle blood flow, arteriogenesis, and inflammation in rat hindlimb ischemia. J Vas Surg. 2005;41:312–20.

15. Burns PJ, Mosquera DA, Bradbury AW. Prevalence and significance of thrombophilia in peripheral arterial disease. Eur J Vasc Endovasc Surg. 2001;22:98–106.

16. O'Connell JB, Quiñones-Baldrich WJ. Proper evaluation and management of acute embolic versus thrombotic limb ischemia. Semin Vasc Surg. 2009;22:10–6.

17. Cambria RP, Abbott WM. Acute thrombosis of the lower extremity. Arch Surg. 1984;119:784–91.

18. Kossuth I, Lewandowski M, Modrzejewski A, Gorący J. Acute limb ischaemia during myocardial infarction. Kardiol Pol. 2014;72:757.

19. Patel A, Almuti W, Polenakovik H. Acute limb ischemia due to Candida lusitaniae aortic valve endocarditis. Heart Lung. 2014;43:338–40.

20. Dormandy J, Heeck L, Vig S. Acute limb ischemia. Semin Vasc Surg. 1999;12:148–53.

21. Patel SD, Guessoum M, Matheiken S. Cystic adventitial disease of the common femoral artery presenting with acute limb ischaemia. Ann Vasc Surg. 2014;28:1937.e9–1937.e11.

22. Olin JW, Shih A. Thromboangiitis obliterans (Buerger's disease). Curr Opin Rheumatol. 2006;18:18–24.

23. Carlson JA. The histological assessment of cutaneous vasculitis. Histopathology. 2010;56:3–23.

24. Setacci C. Time is tissue. J Endovasc Ther. 2012;19(4):515–6.

25. Hirschmann JV, Raugi GJ. Blue (or purple) toe syndrome. J Am Acad Dermatol. 2009;60:1–20.

26. Willmann JK, Baumert B, Schertler T, Wildermuth S, Pfmmatter T, Verdun FR, et al. Aortoiliac and lower extremity arteries assessed with 16-detector row CT angiography: prospective comparison with digital subtraction angiography. Radiology. 2005;236:1083–93.

27. Lin PH, Bechara C, Kougias P, Huynh TT, LeMaire SA, Coselli JS. Assessment of aortic pathology and peripheral arterial disease using multidetector computed tomographic angiography. Vasc Endovascular Surg. 2008/2009;42:583–98.

28. Ersoy H, Rybicki FJ. MR angiography of the lower extremity. AJR. 2008;190:1675–84.

29. Heijenbrok-Kal MH, Kock MC, Hunink MG. Lower extremity arterial disease: multidetector CT-angiography meta-analysis. Radiology. 2007;245:433–9.

30. Laswed T, Rizzo E, Guntern D, Doenz F, Denys A, Schnyder P, et al. Assessment of occlusive arterial disease of abdominal aorta and lower extremities arteries: value of multidetector CT angiography using an adaptive acquisition method. Eur Radiol. 2008;18:263–72.

31. Lewis DR, Baird RN, Irvine CD, Lamont PM. Color flow duplex imaging of occlusive arterial disease of the lower limb. Br J Surg. 1997;84:1625–31.

32. Elmahdy MF, Ghareeb Mahdy S, Baligh Ewiss E, Said K, Kassem HH, Ammar W. Value of duplex scanning in differentiating embolic from thrombotic arterial occlusion in acute limb ischemia. Cardiovasc Revasc Med. 2010;11:223–6.

33. El-Gengehe AT, Ammar WA, Ewiss EB, Mahdy SG, Osama D. Acute limb ischemia: role of preoperative and postoperative duplex in differentiating acute embolic from thrombotic ischemia. Cardiovasc Revasc Med. 2013;14:197–202.

34. Elmahdy MF, Ghareeb Mahdy S, Baligh Ewiss E, Sid K, Kssem HH, Ammar W. Value of duplex scanning in differentiating embolic from thrombotic arterial occlusion in acute limb ischaemia. Cardiovasc Revasc Med. 2010;11:223–6.

35. Ouwendijk R, de Vries M, Stijnen T, Pattynama PM, van Sambeek MR, Buth J, et al. Multicenter randomized controlled trial of the costs and effects of non-invasive diagnostic imaging in patients with peripheral arterial disease: the DIPAD trial. AJR. 2008;190:1349–57.

36. Kock MC, Adriaensen ME, Pattynama PM, van Sambeek, van Urk H, Stijnen T, et al. DSA versus multi-detector row CT angiography in peripheral arterial disease: randomized controlled trial. Radiology. 2005;237:727–37.

37. Deutschmann HA, Schoellnast H, Portugaller HR, Preieller KW, Reittner P, Tillich M, et al. Routine use of three-dimensional contrast-enhanced moving-table MR angiography in patients with peripheral arterial occlusive disease: comparison with selective digital subtraction angiography. Cardiovasc Intervent Radiol. 2006;29:762–70.

38. Levin DC, Rao VM, Parker L, Frangos AJ, Sunshine JH. The effect of the introduction of MR and CT angiography on the utilization of catheter angiography for peripheral arterial disease. J Am Coll Radiol. 2007;4:457–60.

39. Vogt FM, Zenge MO, Ladd ME, Herborn CU, Brauck K, Luboldt W, et al. Peripheral vascular disease: comparison of continuous MR angiography and conventional MR angiography-pilot study. Radiology. 2007;243:229–38.

40. Andreisek G, Pfammatter T, Goepfert K, Nanz D, Hervo P, Koppensteinr R, et al. Peripheral arteries in diabetic patients: standard bolus-chase and time-resolved MR angiography. Radiology. 2007;242:610–20.

41. Schertler T, Wildermuth S, Alkadhi H, Kruppa M, Marincek B, Boehm T. Sixteen-detector row CT angiography for lower-leg arterial occlusive disease: analysis of section width. Radiology. 2005;237:649–56.

42. Zhang HL, Khilnani NM, Prince MR, Winchester PA, Golia P, Veit P, et al. Diagnostic accuracy of time-resolved 2D projection MR for symptomatic infrapopliteal arterial occlusive disease. AJR. 2005;184:938–47.

43. de Donato G, Setacci F, Sirignano P, Galzerano G, Raucci A, Palasciano G, et al. Hybrid procedures for acute limb ischemia. J Cardiovasc Surg. 2010;51:845–53.

44. de Donato G, Setacci F, Sirignano P, Galzerano G, Massaroni R, Setacci C. The combination of surgical embolectomy and endovascular techniques may improve outcomes of patients with acute lower limb ischemia. J Vasc Surg. 2014;59:729–36.

CT Evaluation of Critical Limb Ischemia

17

Suraj Rao, Shankho Ganguli, and Mark G. Rabbat

Introduction

Since the advent of multi-detector CT scanners, much progress has been made in the evaluation of peripheral arterial disease. Spiral CT was introduced in the early 1990s providing basic assessment of vasculature during contrast injection studies. However, it was multichannel CT that provided the resolution required to confidently elucidate vascular disease. Multi-slice CT emerged in the late 1990s and allowed for better volume coverage with shorter scan times, as multiple slices could be captured during one gantry rotation with decreased gantry rotation time. Overlapping image slices during reconstruction add to the improved longitudinal resolution, and post-processing techniques using submillimeter slices allow for superior two and three-dimensional rendering (Fig. 17.1). Table 17.1 provides a list of key terms to better understand the literature.

In a meta-analysis published in JAMA in 2009, 20 diagnostic cohort studies analyzed with 957 patients predominately presenting with intermittent claudication (68%) showed that the overall sensitivity for CTA detecting more than 50% stenosis or occlusion was 95% (95% CI, 92–97%) and specificity was 96% (95% CI, 93–97%), when compared to intra-arterial DSA [1] (Fig. 17.2). Understaging (underestimation of disease severity) occurred in 9% of segments and overstaging (a significant stenosis was diagnosed by CTA as an occlusion) occurred in 4% of segments. However, this meta-analysis only included one study with critical limb ischemia (CLI) patients, identifying the need for further evaluation in this population. In addition to lesion severity, CTA is also highly accurate in identifying length and number of lesions [2], as are required for correct treatment decisions per TASC guidelines, making CTA a valuable tool for therapeutic planning. More recent data with 64 slice CT scanning echoes previous studies, with 98% accuracy for CT angiography detecting greater than 70% stenosis, in a prospective cohort of 212 symptomatic PAD patients (acute CLI excluded) [3] (Fig. 17.3). It further suggested that results could be used to effectively guide clinical management, as therapy recommendations based on CT angiographic findings alone were identical to those based on DSA findings in all but one patient. Similar results can be found in a cohort of 41 patients with critical limb ischemia and severe claudication [4], making CTA a useful tool in treatment planning.

CT Angiogram: Protocol Basics

Typical CT angiography scanning protocols include a digital radiograph called the "scout image," a non-enhanced scan, a test bolus or bolus triggering, the contrast-enhanced CT angiogram, and an optional delayed-phase acquisition to capture late opacification of distal vessels. The delayed-phase acquisition may be necessary in conditions of slow moving contrast, due to severe vascular disease, low cardiac output states, or significant aneurysms. Popliteal artery aneurysms can be well visualized by CTA (Fig. 17.4).

Patients are positioned supine, arms overhead to reduce contributing artifact, and legs close together with slight internal rotation of the feet. Proper positioning is important. For example, plantar extension of the foot can cause compression of the popliteal artery by the gastrocnemius muscle in popliteal artery entrapment syndrome and can be misinterpreted as atherosclerotic steno-occlusive disease. Only a

S. Rao, MD
Department of Cardiology, Scripps, San Diego, CA, USA

S. Ganguli, MD
Cardiology, Aurora St. Luke's Medical Center,
Milwaukee, WI, USA

Cardiology, Aurora Sinai Medical Center, Milwaukee, WI, USA

M.G. Rabbat, MD (✉)
Department of Cardiology, Loyola University Chicago,
2160 S. 1st Avenue, Building 110, Maywood, IL 60153, USA

© Springer International Publishing Switzerland 2017
R.S. Dieter et al. (eds.), *Critical Limb Ischemia*, DOI 10.1007/978-3-319-31991-9_17

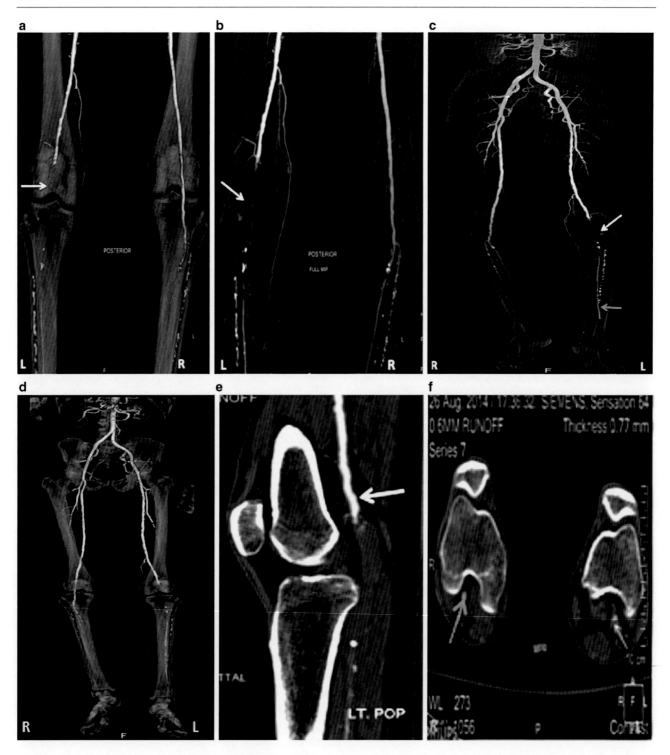

Fig. 17.1 A 67-year-old male who presented, with LLE ischemic pain, found to have left popliteal artery occlusion, and seen in a–f. (**a**) Zoomed 3D VR with transparent bone for visual landmarks. (**b**) MIP, posterior view, with abrupt interruption of luminal enhancement at the L popliteal artery (*arrow*). (**c**) 3D full MIP showing L popliteal occlusion (*white arrow*) with faint distal reconstitution of the peroneal artery (*green arrow*) due to collateral flow. (**d**) 3D VR with transparent bone to better appreciate the vascular anatomy in relation to adjacent bony structures. (**e**) Sagittal MIP with contrast proximal to occlusion highlighted (*arrow*). (**f**) Axial image showing R popliteal artery with normal enhancement (*green arrow*) as compared to diseased L popliteal artery (*white arrow*)

single breath-hold is necessary (during abdominal acquisitions), and scan times can be as short as 15–40 s. The entire study can involve less than 15 min of room time, making CTA useful when rapid assessment of critical limb ischemia is required, as opposed to more time-consuming modalities such as ultrasound or MRI. Table 17.2 contains a CTA runoff

Table 17.1 Key terms

Pitch	Table feed per rotation in a spiral scan divided by the total width of the collimated beam. Pitch, $p < 1$ signifies data acquisition with overlap in the longitudinal direction
Gantry rotation	The gantry is the spherical portion of the CT that houses the X-ray tube and the detector. One gantry rotation is one 360-degree rotation around the patient over a period of time
Voxel	Each CT image has a defined thickness. The smallest distinguishable matrix in a CT image is known as voxel, which is a pixel with a defined thickness
Attenuation	The loss of X-ray beam strength as it passes through an object. Usually highly attenuating structures are denser, making it harder for X-rays to pass through, allowing for stronger reflection and brighter appearance on CT imaging
Dual-source CT	Makes use of two X-ray and detector sources perpendicular to each other. This increases temporal resolution, reduces radiation, and increases the speed of image acquisition
Kernels	Post-processing filter or algorithm applied to the raw CT images to specifically select for desired structures. For example, a "sharper" kernel will increase the image contrast but will also introduce more noise
Hounsfield Unit	A unit of measurement to quantify radiodensity. A more radiopaque structure has a higher value. A HU of 0 is calibrated to the radiodensity of distilled water at standard pressure and temperature (STP)
Detector rows	The area across from the X-ray beam within the gantry. It receives the X-ray beam after it passes through an object. Multiple detector rows allow the acquisition of images from slightly different angles resulting in greater volume coverage and scan speed

protocol utilized at Loyola University Medical Center, adopted from D. Fleischmann at Stanford University.

Basic Principles of Image Acquisition

The scout image is typically a coronal topogram from below the diaphragm (to include the renal arteries) to the tip of the feet, roughly 130 cm. Contrast is injected through an established peripheral IV typically no smaller than 20G. The amount of time needed for contrast to appear in the abdominal aorta, the contrast transit time, can be accounted for via test bolus or bolus-triggering protocols. This is important as it determines when to start image acquisition. For bolus triggering, a region of interest is identified in the abdominal aorta typically at a level above the renal arteries, and an attenuation threshold is set (e.g., 130 HU). The scan is started when a desired attenuating threshold is met. A test bolus (typically 20 cc) can allow for correct timing of scan initiation; however, table speed and overall scan times should be carefully selected as to not allow image acquisition to "outrun" the contrast. Low flow states, such as with cardiomyopathy, and severe atherosclerotic disease should be accounted for. Additionally, aortic aneurysms can have turbulent blood flow with dilution of contrast media and cause delay in transit. Another approach is to calculate aortic and popliteal transit times via the use of two test boluses. Of note, prolonged scan times may also result in venous opacification, which can be adjusted for in post-processing. Contrast flow

Fig. 17.2 A 65-year-old male with known peripheral arterial disease, with a history of acute-on-chronic left lower extremity claudication, found to have stenosis of the right superficial femoral artery. (**a**) Magnified CTA-MIP showing severe stenosis of SFA mid-thigh with atherosclerotic plaque along its course. (**b**) DSA showing the same SFA stenosis

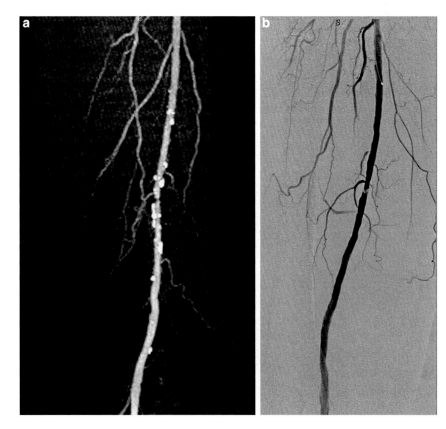

Fig. 17.3 A 65-year-old male with HTN, DM, HLD presenting with LLE claudication and L common iliac stenosis. (**a**) CTA-MIP showing calcified plaque causing high-grade stenosis at the origin of L common iliac artery (*inferior arrow*). Also, note the presence of mural thrombus with calcification (*superior arrow*) in the distal abdominal aorta just above the bifurcation. (**b**) DSA demonstrating the same severe L common iliac stenosis (*arrow*)

Fig. 17.4 A 58-year-old heavy smoker, who presents with LLE pain, found to have a popliteal aneurysm containing thrombus. (**a**) Full MIP showing bilateral fem-pop circulation with L popliteal aneurysm (starred). (**b**) MPR-left sagittal view of popliteal aneurysm with thrombus. (**c**) MPR-axial images of the left popliteal aneurysm. Note the normal right popliteal artery for comparison in axial view. *Arrows* in b and c outline the aneurysm containing thrombus

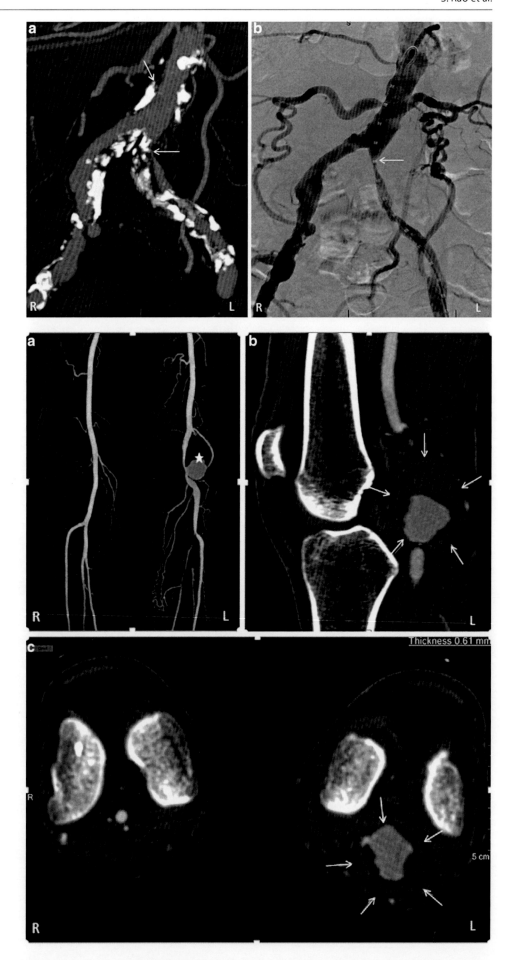

Table 17.2 Scanning protocol; adapted from D. Fleischmann, Stanford University Medical Center

Lower extremity runoff, Siemens S 64	
Topogram	1500 mm AP; feet first, arms up; feet still and relaxed; support with cushions/tape
Range 1 + 2	Bolus tracking, ROI in the abdominal aorta at the level of the celiac artery
Range 3	Runoff: from above the celiac trunk (D12 vertebral body) through the toes 120 kV/Care dose 4D w. 250 ref-mAs (voltage weight adjusted)
	64×0.6 mm, 0.5 s gantry rotation
	40 s scan time (will result in a pitch <1)
	Set scan range first and then change scan time to 40 s
Range 4	Runoff: Preprogrammed optional second CTA acquisition to cover popliteal and crural territories. This range is only initiated if there is no contrast medium opacification seen in the popliteal/crural vascular territories
Breath-hold	At inspiration
Scan direction	Cranio-caudal
Injection	20–22G IV line, Isovue (iopamidol) 370
Protocol	Bolus tracking with ROI in the abdominal aorta (beginning of scan range)
	Minimum delay (3 s including automated breath-hold command)
	Use biphasic injection protocol with 35 s injection duration
	Injection rates and volumes (adjusted to patient size)

	Weight (kg)	Vol1 (mL)	Flow1 (mL/s)	Vol2 (mL)	Flow2 (mL/s)
XS	<55	20	4	96	3.2
S	<65	23	4.5	108	3.6
Avg	75	25	5	120	4
L	>85	28	5.5	132	4.4
XL	>95	30	6	144	4.8

	Saline flush: 40 mL volume, flow rate equal to "Flow2"
Reconstruction (STh/RI)	
Range 3	2/1.0, B25f (patients w. Fontaine IIb)
	1/0.7, B25f (patients w. Fontaine III/IV)
	5/5, B31f Abd/Pel only
Range 4	1/0.7, B25f

rate and volume can be adjusted for body weight/size and delivered via a power injector. Typical flow rates are between 3 and 6 mL/s of iodinated contrast media, resulting in approximately 1.5 g of iodine per second depending on media concentration selected and total contrast volume around 130 mL. Biphasic injections are often used to provide steady delivery over time.

Radiation Exposure

Tube voltage, collimation, and pitch can be adjusted to reduce radiation exposure and maintain adequate resolution, with lower voltage for patients with lower BMI. Protocols have been developed lowering the tube voltage from commonly used 120–80 kVp, showing significant reductions in radiation exposure [5]. Using a 64 channel multi-detector CT, Iezzi et al. demonstrated a weighted CT dose index of 12.96 mGy for their 120-kVp moderate noise reduction protocol, 6.34 mGy for their 80-kVp moderate noise reduction protocol, and 5.89 mGy for their 80-kVp high noise reduction protocol, with an effective calculated dose of 29.32, 14.64, and 11.43 mSv, respectively. These protocols combined with a high iodine concentration media allowed for significant radiation reduction, up to 61%, without sacrificing image quality. Low radiation doses and good diagnostic performance have also recently been demonstrated with 128 slice dual-source CT using 80 kVp with high pitch [6]. For a point of reference, a chest X-ray gives a radiation dose of 0.01 mSv, and annual background radiation is 3.0 mSv [1]. Preserving scan quality with decreasing radiation remains an active area of research.

Post-processing Techniques

Post-processing techniques have dramatically advanced our ability to detect steno-occlusive disease, aiding in identification of lesion severity, length, and number along the course of any given vessel. Stacks of two-dimensional axial slices can be assimilated into three-dimensional volumetric data sets. From these data sets, maximum intensity projections (MIPs), multiplanar reformatted (MPR) images, curved multiplanar (CPR) images, and volume-rendered images can be created to aid in pathological analysis (Fig. 17.5). A maximal intensity projection (MIP) provides a layout that most

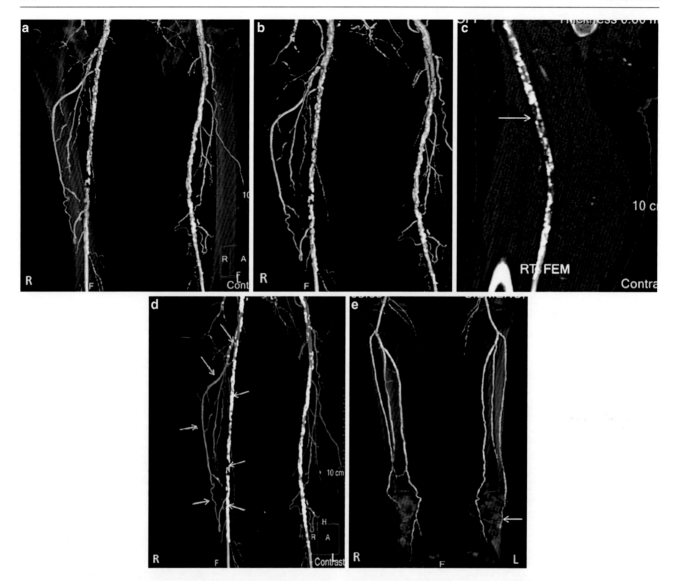

Fig. 17.5 A 50-year-old female with known PAD and RLE claudication, found to have severe right SFA stenosis with collateralization. (**a**) and (**b**) show VR images with transparent bone and bone removed, respectively, that help visualize the vasculature in relation to adjacent structures. (**c**) Coronal CPR of R SFA highlighting atherosclerotic disease (*arrow*). (**d**) MIP showing diseased R SFA (*white arrows*) and well-developed collateralization via the deep femoral artery (*yellow arrows*). (**e**) VR with transparent bone showing extent of vasculature to pedal arteries (*arrow*)

closely resembles an invasive angiogram and is very useful in providing a road map view of the course of peripheral vessels. MIPs are created by displaying the brightest voxel in every ray or line of sight. This ensures that high attenuation structures such as contrast-filled vessels and calcification/bone are prominently displayed. The bone is typically removed by automated or semiautomated programs, leaving the arterial tree. One should be aware that this can be a source of artifact (editing misregistration, Fig. 17.6). MIPs however do not provide adequate depth information and can pose a problem defining relationships to anatomic structures. Volume-rendered images however provide color and three-

dimensional displays of the vasculature in relation to organs and bone, which can additionally be edited. The MIP and VR image alone is not sufficient for evaluating vessel stenosis in the presence of dense calcifications or stents, because the brightness of these elements can obscure interpretation of the vessel lumen. Thin-slab MIPs and multiplanar reformations allow better visualization of steno-occlusive disease in the presence of calcifications and stents (Fig. 17.7). The most basic MPRs are transverse cuts such as sagittal and coronal images. However, because peripheral vessels can be tortuous, they may cut in and out of the MPR plane, thus allowing only short segments of the vessel of interest to be

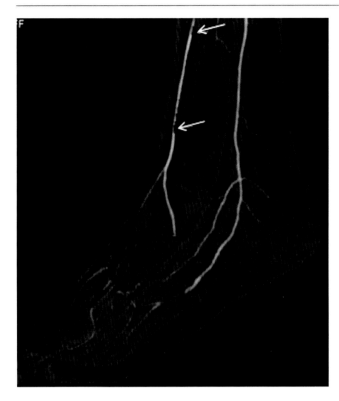

Fig. 17.6 Editing artifact secondary to bone removal misregistration, leading to inadvertent removal of adjacent vasculature (*arrows*)

istered and removed as the bone. Alternatively, misregistration can cause part of the bone to be left in mimicking pathological disease. Stents can also provide streak artifacts known as beam hardening. Multiple view MPR and CPR images are paramount for further analysis. However, inaccurately drawn center lines when constructing CPR images can overestimate steno-occlusive disease.

CTA Evaluation of Vascular Stents

Stent evaluation has made progress in the era of 64 slice multi-detector CT scanning with improved resolution and image reconstruction. Despite this, there are still challenges, such as metallic (gold) markers at bilateral stent edges providing artifact that can hinder interpretation [7]. When stents are overlapped, the artifact can extend to the stent body. In a study using 64 slice MDCT to evaluate 41 patients with a total of 81 stents, Li et al. found that 19 stents (23.5%) had uninterpretable segments due to artifact. Protocol parameters included collimation width 64 mm×0.6 mm, pitch 1.1, rotation time 0.33 s, table speed 63 mm/s, tube voltage 120 kV, and tube current 250 mAs. They determined that specificity remained high despite sensitivity being somewhat lower due to un-evaluable stents and concluded that overall accuracy for detecting in-stent stenosis was still acceptably good [7]. Multiple cross-sectional views using multiplanar reformatted images should be used for stent lumen evaluation. Furthermore, contrast enhancement of distal runoff vessels alone was found not to be a reliable indicator of stent patency, due to the presence of collateral vessels. Collateralization can be well appreciated by CT angiography (Fig. 17.9).

In order to evaluate stent restenosis, not only must one visualize the lack of contrast within the lumen in a sagittal or coronal section but also look at specific axial sections to truly evaluate stent patency. Manipulation of raw CTA is needed to help enhance spatial resolution. Spatial resolution can be improved by decreasing slice thickness and by manipulating reconstruction kernels or filters.

Kohler et al. used dual-source CT (DSCT) to evaluate stent characteristics by analyzing lumen diameter, intraluminal density, and noise of 22 peripheral stents in a vessel phantom [8]. The vessel phantoms that were used were made of plastic tubes of different diameters filled with contrast material and then submersed in vegetable oil diluted to 250 HU and then in a larger plastic container, which was then diluted to −70 HU to simulate perivascular fat. Each of the 22 stents of different luminal size and length then underwent DSCT with four different types of image acquisitions that were obtained by different reconstruction kernels. It was found that visualized stent lumen diameter varied depending on the type of stents. Visibility of the lumen diameter could

viewed. In this case, the vessel path can be traced along its center line using multiple MPR (coronal, sagittal, oblique) and axial images to create a curved planar reformatted image (CPR) which can delineate an entire vessel's course, in one image. CPR images are essential in evaluating eccentric lesions, since multiple cross-sectional views are obtained to adequately visualize the vessel lumen and construct the CPR image. MPR/CPR slices can be thickened as needed for full vessel view.

Imaging Artifacts

With calcifications, endovascular stents and automated image processing, certain artifacts, and misrepresentations may arise, which are summarized in Table 17.3. In the setting of a narrow viewing window, calcifications or stent struts can display overly bright and appear artificially larger in size giving the appearance of more severe steno-occlusive disease and thus overestimation of disease severity. This is known as blooming artifact (Fig. 17.8). Window level/width should be increased for better grayscale differentiation to diminish brightness of calcification/stents and allow visualization of vessel lumen when possible. Editing artifacts, perhaps during automated bone removal, may lead to false vessel narrowing or occlusion if part of the vessel is misreg-

Fig. 17.7 A 64-year-old female
with history of PAD status-post
RLE bypass, presenting with LE
ischemic pain found to have left
common iliac stent stenosis. (**a**)
DSA with selective engagement of
the L iliac artery showing in-stent
stenosis. (**b**) CTA-MIP reveals
in-stent stenosis (*arrows*). (**c**)
Sagittal CPR and (**d**) coronal CPR
are used to delineate vessel course
along with stenotic disease
(*arrows*)

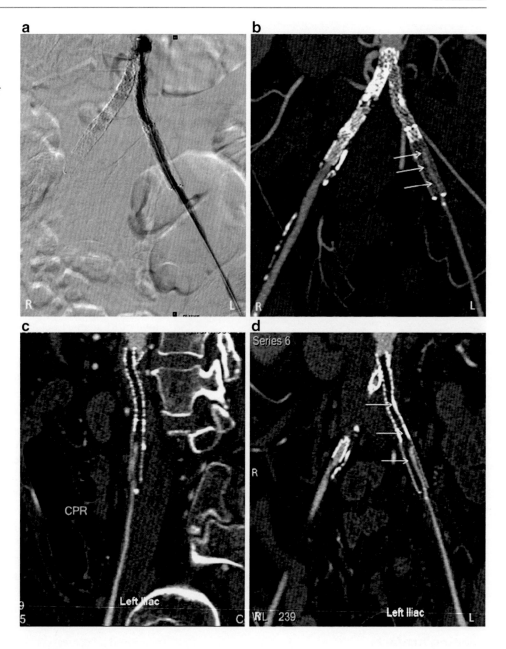

Table 17.3 Common artifacts [13]

Beam hardening	Artificial darkening of the center of an object compared to its edges. This happens secondary to the polychromatic nature of the X-ray beam with different attenuation rates as it passes through an object
Blooming	This artifact is caused by the CT software's averaging of signal intensity from a given imaging region. This is common to see in images with high-attenuating structures adjacent to low attenuating structures. For example, vessel stenosis severity may be overestimated secondary to blooming from adjacent calcified plaque
Streaking	Dark streaks that appear between highly attenuating structures. It can be reduced by increasing the kV of the X-ray, with risk of compromising the contrast of the image
Cone beam artifact	With MDCT, the X-ray beam is detected at an angle from the individual detector source. Thus if there is a high contrast edge, it can lead to dark streaks on the image

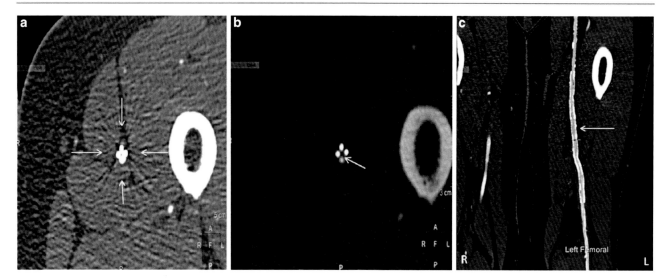

Fig. 17.8 (**a**) Cross-sectional image of a femoral stent shows streaking artifact (radial lines emanating from the center) and blooming artifact (inappropriate radiodensity of stent struts leading to concealment of vessel lumen). (**b**) Blooming artifact reduced by manual changes in window/level allows for the vessel lumen to be visualized (*arrow*). (**c**) Femoral stent in a and b, in curved planar reconstruction, providing visualization of the lumen throughout the vessel's course. The *green line* represents the constructed "center line." Arrow approximates the half-way point of the femoral stent

Fig. 17.9 A 53-year-old patient with history of bilateral lower extremity PAD status-post L fem-peroneal bypass and multiple peripheral stents, with bilateral femoral stent occlusion and patent LLE bypass graft (*green arrow*) and patent RLE collaterals. (**a**) MPR image showing bilateral stents that are occluded (*arrows*). (**b**) 3D MIP showing the patency of LLE bypass graft (*green arrow*) and RLE collateral vessels (*white arrow*) which provide adequate distal flow in the setting of occluded femoral stents

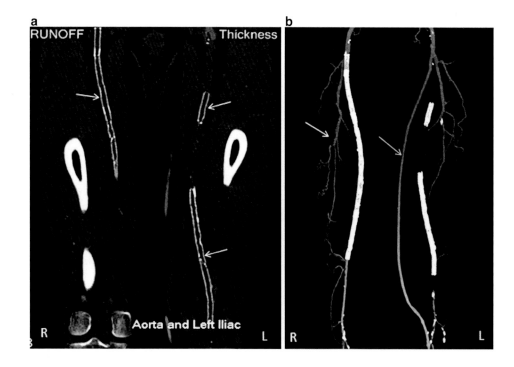

Fig. 17.10 An example of
the level of detail of the
infra-popliteal system that can
be achieved by CTA with
distal runoff and bolus
tracking

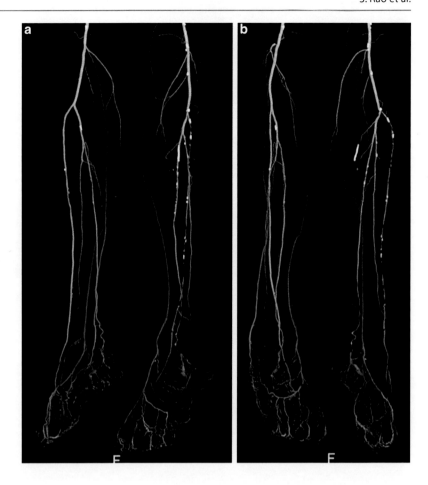

be increased with increasing the sharpness of reconstruction kernel, whereas smoothening of the reconstruction kernel resulted in more realistic intraluminal density measurement with less intraluminal noise. It is important to note that while assessing for stent restenosis, the CTA protocol may need to be tailored based on the type of stent being evaluated [8].

Imaging of Infra-popliteal Vasculature

In patients with extensive arterial wall calcification or atherosclerosis, imaging of infra-iliac and specifically infra-popliteal arteries can be difficult due to slower flow of contrast through these areas and resulting CT image acquisition "outrunning" the contrast. To compensate, a test run is done from below the diaphragm to the toes. Next, the delay time between the initiation of contrast administration and the initiation of scanning for optimal intraluminal contrast enhancement is calculated. Those with poor cardiac output or slow

distal runoffs can undergo delayed imaging, for example, 90 s delay from contrast initiation. This technique is not always necessary and should only be employed when the poor enhancement of the distal arteries is noticed after the initial scan (Fig. 17.10).

Digital Subtraction Angiography (DSA) and CTA

Although DSA is used as a reference standard against which noninvasive imaging is compared, it has downsides as well, one limitation being two-dimensional imaging of a three-dimensional structure. The severity of an occlusion may be over- or underestimated depending on the angle from which the vessel's image is acquired [9]. In a study comparing pre-amputation angiogram vs. post-amputation pathology, DSA tended to underestimate the severity of stenosis, plaque concentricity, and grading of calcification even in normal-

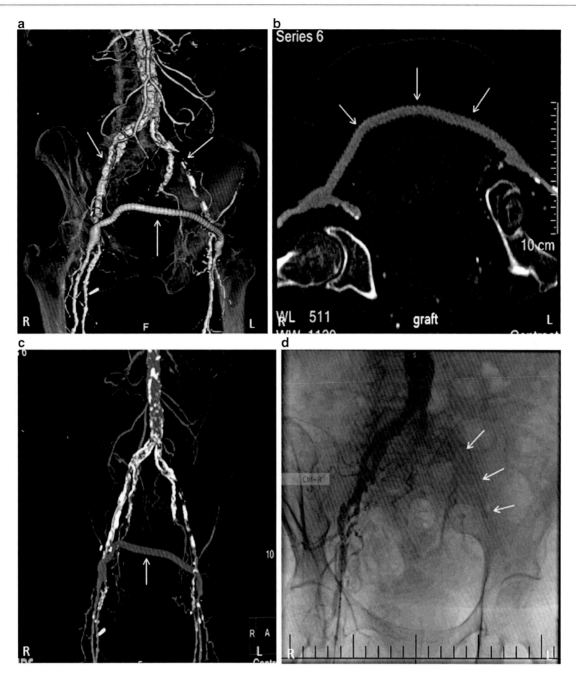

Fig. 17.11 A 68-year-old female with CAD status-post CABG, ESRD, DM who underwent fem-fem bypass grafting after DSA revealed occluded L iliac artery. (**a**) 3D VR shows severe steno-occlusive disease of the left iliac artery (*superior arrows* depict L and R external iliac arteries, *inferior* *arrow* depicts bypass graft). (**b**) CPR showing patency of the fem-fem bypass graft. (**c**) 3D full MIP again showing calcified atherosclerotic disease burden with patent fem-fem bypass graft (*arrow*). (**d**) DSA performed pre-bypass grafting showing occlusion of the L iliac artery

appearing vessels [10]. Another drawback is DSA's need for good contrast timing for visualization of the vasculature in satisfactory detail. This task may be difficult in assessing different bypass grafts given complex anatomy leading to poor contrast timing and suboptimal vessel opacification (Fig. 17.11). Compared with conventional DSA, the sensitivity and specificity of multi-detector row CT (MDCT)

angiography in the detection of significant stenosis, aneurysmal changes, and arteriovenous fistulas of arterial bypass grafts were more than 95 % [11] (Fig. 17.12). Advances in MDCT and post-processing techniques make CT angiography a valuable tool in the assessment of critical limb ischemia, acute and chronic [12].

Fig. 17.12 A 28-year-old male with history significant for a gunshot wound to his RLE, status-post fempopliteal bypass, who presents with LE pain. (**a**) CTA-MIP showing femoral-popliteal bypass (*arrow*) and its distal touchdown site. (**b**) DSA in comparison. Note the similar angiographic findings

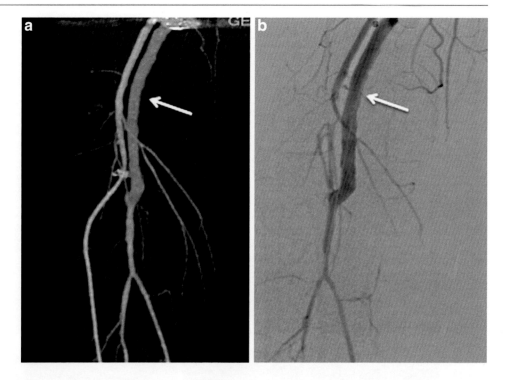

Acknowledgment Mr. Vasilios "Bill" Vasilopoulos, AA, AAS, R.T.(R), 3D Technologist in Radiology at Loyola Medical Center for post-processed images, annotated vascular anatomy, adjusted the colors of the indicator arrows for homogeneity, and anonymized for exporting.

References

 1. Met R, et al. Diagnostic performance of computed tomography angiography in peripheral arterial disease. A systematic review and meta-analysis. JAMA. 2009;301(4):415–24.
 2. Schernthaner R, et al. Multidetector CT angiography in the assessment of peripheral arterial occlusive disease: accuracy in detecting the severity, number, and length of stenosis. Eur Radiol. 2008;18:665–71.
 3. Napoli A, et al. Peripheral arterial occlusive disease: diagnostic performance and effect on therapeutic management of 64-section CT angiography. Radiology. 2011;261(3):976–86.
 4. Fotiadis N, et al. 64-section CT angiography in patients with critical limb ischemia and severe claudication: comparison with digital subtractive angiography. Clin Radiol. 2011;66:945–52.
 5. Iezzi R, Santoro M, Marano R, Di Stasi C, Dattesi R, Kirchin M, Tinelli G, Snider F, Bonomo L. Low-dose multidetector CT angiography in the evaluation of infrarenal aorta and peripheral arterial occlusive disease. Radiology. 2012;263(1):287–98. doi:10.1148/radiol.11110700.
 6. K.S. Choo, et al. Diagnostic performance and radiation dose of lower extremity CT angiography with 128-slice dual source CT using 80 kVp plus high pitch. ECR. 2014;Poster C-1372.
 7. Li XM, et al. Evaluation of peripheral artery stent with 64-slice multi-detector row CT angiography: prospective comparison with digital subtraction angiography. Eur J Radiol. 2010;75:98–103.
 8. Kohler M, et al. Dual-source CT angiography of peripheral arterial stents: in vitro evaluation of 22 different stent types. Radiol Res Pract. 2011;2011: Article ID 103873, 7 p. doi:10.1155/2011/103873.
 9. Duran C, Bismuth J. Advanced imaging in limb salvage. Methodist Debakey Cardiovasc J. 2012;8:28–34.
10. Kashyap VS, Pavkov ML, Bishop PD, et al. Angiography underestimates peripheral atherosclerosis: lumenography revisited. J Endovasc Ther. 2008;15(1):117–25. doi:10.1583/07-2249R.1.
11. Willmann JK, Mayer D, Banyai M, Desbiolles LM, Verdun FR, Seifert B, Marincek B, Weishaupt D. Evaluation of peripheral arterial bypass grafts with multi–detector row CT angiography: comparison with duplex US and digital subtraction angiography. Radiology. 2003;229(2):465–74.
12. Fleischmann D, Hallett RL, Rubin GD. CT angiography of peripheral arterial disease. J Vasc Interv Radiol. 2006;17(1):3–26. Review.
13. Boas E, Fleischmann D. CT artifacts: Causes and reduction techniques. Imaging Med. 2012;4(2):229–40. http://www.edboas.com/science/CT/0012.pdf.

Rajeev R. Fernando, Lara Bakhos, and Mushabbar A. Syed

Introduction

Cardiovascular magnetic resonance imaging (CMR) is routinely used in the evaluation of a wide variety of cardiovascular diseases. CMR is a noninvasive imaging modality and is widely regarded as the reference standard in the assessment of cardiovascular morphology and function. A combination of function, morphology, stress imaging for perfusion and wall motion, and late gadolinium enhancement for infarct or fibrosis imaging provides a comprehensive diagnostic evaluation by CMR. Appropriate indications for CMR have been published by the American College of Cardiology, Society of Cardiovascular Magnetic Resonance, American College of Radiology, and other relevant societies [1]. These include evaluation of LV function in heart failure or after myocardial infarction, determining viability prior to revascularization, evaluation of specific cardiomyopathies (amyloid, sarcoid, hypertrophic cardiomyopathy, arrhythmogenic right ventricular cardiomyopathy, etc.), evaluation of myocarditis or myocardial infarction with normal coronary arteries, pericardial diseases, cardiac masses, and complex congenital heart disease. There is significant ongoing research and development in CMR leading to new acquisition methods, image processing and viewing tools, and novel applications. The high spatial and temporal resolution of CMR has made it possible to investigate myocardial tissue in more detail with imaging of extracellular matrix and biologic processes at the cellular or subcellular level (molecular imaging).

R.R. Fernando, MD • L. Bakhos, MD
Division of Cardiology, Department of Medicine, Loyola University Medical Center, Maywood, IL, USA

M.A. Syed, MD (✉)
Departments of Medicine (Cardiology), Radiology and Cell and Molecular Physiology, Loyola University Medical Center, 2160 S. First Avenue, Maywood, IL 60153, USA

Magnetic resonance angiography (MRA) of central and peripheral arteries and veins with the use of gadolinium contrast is a well-established method. Appropriate indications for vascular imaging include pulmonary vein imaging prior to radiofrequency ablation for atrial fibrillation, pulmonary artery imaging in congenital heart disease, evaluation for aortic dissection or aneurysm, diagnosis of peripheral arterial disease (PAD), selecting patients for endovascular intervention or surgical bypass of lower extremity PAD, and post-revascularization surveillance of lower extremity PAD [1–3]. ACC/AHA 2005 Practice Guidelines for the Management of Patients with Peripheral Arterial Disease recommends that MRA of the extremities should be performed with gadolinium enhancement (class I recommendation); however, there is significant ongoing development in the field of non-contrast MRA due to the cost and safety risk of gadolinium-based contrast agents, which has shown initial promising results (see below).

CMR of heart and blood vessels is performed on clinical MRI scanners with some additional equipment. MRI scanner is a large cylindrical structure that house a powerful superconducting magnet whose magnetic field strength is measured in Tesla (T). Commercially available MRI scanners suitable for CMR are 1.5 T or 3.0 T. Generally 3.0 T scanner provides better spatial resolution and faster acquisition speed compared to 1.5 T but may have more artifacts related to the higher field strength. Due to the technical requirements of CMR, the so-called open MRI machines are not at present suitable for cardiovascular applications. MRI images the hydrogen nuclei (^{1}H protons) which are in high concentration in the body. Radiofrequency signals from the MRI scanner excite the ^{1}H protons which leads to image signal generation. Special surface coils are placed over the area of interest to receive the generated signal. Images are processed and displayed on dedicated workstations. A power injector is needed to inject contrast for MRA and certain cardiac applications. A moving patient table is required to chase the contrast bolus after injection for extremity imaging. MRI-compatible patient monitoring system and infusion pump (for delivering drugs) is needed for imaging critically ill patients.

CMR has several advantages in imaging of cardiovascular system compared to other modalities. CMR provides high spatial and temporal resolution and images can be acquired in any tomographic plane without body habitus limitations. There is no ionizing radiation which makes this modality ideal for serial follow-up imaging particularly in younger patients whose radiation-related risk may be higher due to accumulated lifetime exposure. MRA is inherently three-dimensional; hence, eccentric lesions or complex vascular anatomy is better characterized to aid in procedural planning. A variety of CMR methods are used for evaluating vascular pathology. Black-blood imaging with T1-and T2-weighted techniques is used for vessel wall imaging. Vascular blood flow is evaluated by phase contrast imaging, and more recently introduced time-resolved MRA allows direct visualization of blood flow dynamics which is useful in the assessment of shunts, dissections, and conduits. There are also several specialized sequences used for non-contrast MRA that are discussed below.

This chapter provides a concise overview of contrast-enhanced and non-contrast MRA in patients with PAD. A review of MRI contrast agents and MRA techniques is also provided. For more information, readers are directed to articles referenced in bibliography and dedicated textbooks on this subject.

MRI Contrast Agents

Image contrast refers to the relative difference in signal intensity between two adjacent tissues and forms the basis for visual perception to differentiate between the two tissues in MRI. Contrast media is frequently used to enhance these differences by modifying the amplitude of the signal generated by ^{1}H protons [4]. Gadolinium, a lanthanide metal element, is currently the most commonly used contrast agent in clinical practice. In its free form, Gd^{3+} is highly toxic and therefore must be complexed to a ligand or chelate before intravenous (IV) administration [5]. The chelate encapsulates the gadolinium, resulting in a thermodynamically stable and biologically inert complex.

There are currently nine available gadolinium-based contrast agents (GBCAs) approved for clinical use by the FDA in the United States. GBCAs can be further classified into categories based on their biodistribution, which is determined by the chemical structure of the chelate. The two most clinically relevant categories are the extracellular and intravascular/blood pool contrast agents.

Extracellular Contrast Agents

The first approved GBCAs were extracellular contrast agents (ECCAs). ECCAs distribute rapidly into both intravascular and extracellular spaces. After IV injection, the water-soluble contrast agent initially distributes into the intravascular space. Peak intravascular enhancement occurs over a short period, the arterial phase typically lasting less than 20 s in duration, followed by rapid extravasation into the interstitial space. This makes the timing of arrival of the contrast bolus with image acquisition critical. Therefore, although extracellular contrast agents are frequently used for MRA, they are not the ideal agents for this because of their pharmacokinetic profile.

Intravascular/Blood Pool Contrast Agents

Intravascular or blood pool contrast agents were specifically designed to overcome this limitation of ECCAs through deliberate confinement to the intravascular space. This was achieved by modifying the size, charge, and molecular shape of the ligand relative to the permeability of the capillary bed, resulting in a longer plasma half-life with prolonged intravascular enhancement on the order of tens of minutes as compared to seconds with ECCAs [6]. Blood pool agents therefore eliminate the need for bolus timing and allow for the imaging of multiple vascular beds, both arterial and venous phase imaging, and covering a larger anatomic area without the need for reinjection. The commercially available intravascular contrast agent is gadofosveset (Ablavar) which is FDA approved for imaging of aortoiliac disease in adults.

Novel/Experimental Contrast Agents

Ferumoxytol (Feraheme, AMAG Pharmaceuticals, Cambridge, MA) is a ultrasmall paramagnetic iron oxide nanoparticle which is FDA approved as an IV iron replacement therapy for the treatment of iron deficiency anemia in adult patients with chronic kidney disease (CKD). More recently, ferumoxytol has been investigated for use as a contrast agent in MRI [7]. Ferumoxytol has a long half-life of 14–15 h and behaves as a blood pool agent, distributing only in the intravascular compartment. Because ferumoxytol is made of iron oxide particles, it carries no risk of nephrogenic systemic fibrosis (NSF) as seen with GBCAs. Ferumoxytol has been used off-label as a MRA blood pool agent, in the imaging of the carotid arteries, thoracic and abdominal aorta, renal arteries, and peripheral arteries and veins. The main advantage is likely to be in patients with end-stage renal disease where GBCA use is contraindicated.

Safety of Gadolinium-Based Contrast Agents

GBCAs are generally considered safe with an exceptionally low incidence of adverse reactions occurring with a frequency of 0.07–2.4 % [8]. The vast majority of reactions are considered mild as defined by the American College of Radiology (ACR). The largest assessment of GBCA safety came in 2013 in 120 million administrations which reported an incidence of severe reactions of only 0.003 % [9].

Nephrogenic Systemic Fibrosis (NSF)

NSF is a rare disorder characterized by fibrosis, most often involving the skin. In its more severe form, NSF can result in systemic fibrosis of the connective tissue, lungs, liver, and heart leading to debilitating contractures, multi-organ dysfunction, and occasionally death [10]. Treatment options are limited. In 2006, the link between GBCA exposure to this rare but potentially fatal disease was recognized [11].

The incidence of NSF primarily varies with the degree of renal insufficiency. It is estimated that patients with stage 4–5 CKD (eGFR <30 mL/min/1.73 m^2) have a 1–7 % risk of developing NSF after exposure to GBCAs [8]. There have been no reported cases of NSF in patients with normal renal function to date. Other identified risk factors include acute kidney injury (AKI) accounting for 12–20 % of confirmed NSF cases, high dose GBCA [12], and multiple GBCA exposures [13].

Although the link between NSF and the exposure to GBCAs in the setting of severe renal impairment is widely recognized, the exact pathogenesis remains unknown. The leading hypothesis relates to the dissociation of gadolinium from its chelate due to prolonged elimination times in patients with impaired renal function. This has been supported by the finding that the agents most associated with NSF are the least thermodynamically stable contrast agent [14]. The data for the intravascular contrast agent gadofosveset (Ablavar) is limited.

Based on the current level of understanding, there are several measures that should be taken to minimize the risk of NSF. First and foremost, a screening method should be instituted to identify those patients at risk for NSF prior to GBCA exposure. Once a patient at risk is identified, alternative diagnostic testing should be considered. If there is no acceptable alternative and the clinical indication is compelling enough, a GBCA with a lower incidence of NSF should be used and at the lowest possible dose necessary. The institution of such simple precautions has already resulted in a profound reduction in the incidence of NSF with a near elimination of new cases [15].

Special Populations

Pregnancy

In animal models, GBCAs have been shown to cross the placenta within minutes of IV administration and, when administered at high and/or repeated doses, result in several adverse effects including fetal growth retardation, fetal loss, and teratogenicity [16]. In the limited human studies, there have been no known adverse human fetal effects after giving clinically recommended doses of GBCAs during pregnancy [17]. However, given the findings in animal studies, all FDA-approved gadolinium chelates are classified as "Pregnancy Category C" and should only be used during pregnancy when the benefits outweigh the potential fetal risks. In that event, a GBCA considered low risk for the development of NSF should be used and at the lowest possible dose necessary.

Breastfeeding

It has been shown that <0.04 % of the maternal dose is excreted into the breast milk in the first 24 h and estimated that <1 % of the contrast medium is subsequently absorbed from the infant's gastrointestinal tract [18]. This would result in an expected systemic dose absorbed by the infant of <0.0004 % of the maternal dose, an amount far less than the permissible dose in neonates [8]. Accordingly, the current ACR position is that it is likely safe for a mother to continue breastfeeding after receiving GBCAs. Ultimately, an informed decision to abstain from breastfeeding should be left up to the mother, although there is no benefit in doing so beyond 24 h.

MRA Techniques

Contrast-Enhanced MRA (CE-MRA)

CE-MRA was first introduced in the early 1990s and represents the workhorse MR technique for imaging peripheral vasculature. CE-MRA uses GBCA, which shortens the T1 of spins in blood and is independent of flow pattern, direction, or velocity [19]. Because the arterial phase of GBCA is only 20 s, the images are acquired rapidly by arterial first pass imaging; however, newer blood pool gadolinium-based agents are available for steady-state imaging as discussed above.

CE-MRA Technique
Patient Preparation
MRA procedure must be explained to the patient in detail. If a patient has rest pain or skin ulcerations, appropriate care must be taken of the affected limb and analgesics provided if

necessary. Patients must remain still during the scan, as movement will affect image quality. A 1.5 T MRI machine with high-performance gradient strength is adequate for peripheral MRA. Incremental gains in study quality can be obtained with higher gradient strengths, multichannel phased array coil, and a 3 T scanner. Dedicated bilateral lower extremity phased array coils are ideal for peripheral MRA image quality. Additional body coils will often be placed over the lower abdomen just above the extremity coil assembly to image the abdominal aorta and iliofemoral vessels. Patients are placed feet first with their arms by their sides and are forewarned that the table will move during the study and compression devices may be placed about the thighs to minimize venous contamination [20]. Care must be taken not to compress any regions especially the calves because this may result in pseudo stenosis. For lower extremity MRA, a 20 gauge venous access must be obtained in either antecubital fossa. Lower limb venous access is not recommended due to significant venous contamination of the region of interest. A multiphase MR-compatible injector pump is important in attaining consistency in injection timing and flow rates [21]. Extension tubing flushed with normal saline is required to reach the pump injector. Once a patient is appropriately positioned, large field of view localizers are obtained. In obese patients and crossover bypass grafts, it is important to ensure that relevant vascular anatomy is not excluded from the imaging volume. Rapid scout images in axial, coronal, and sagittal orientations are obtained. These initial images are useful to define the vascular territory to plan the eventual MRA examination. Individual 3D volumes oriented in the coronal plane are acquired sequentially in multiple stations (abdomen, pelvis, legs, and calves) chasing a gadolinium-based contrast agent as it flows down into the peripheral vessels (Fig. 18.1). Subtraction of the post-contrast images from the pre-contrast images is performed and the data is transmitted to a 3D workstation.

MRA Acquisition

To maximize tissue contrast, the sequences are heavily T1 weighted, and acquisition is timed to the maximum intravascular concentration of gadolinium. Typically a fast 3D gradient echo sequence is used for imaging acquisition. Images are acquired first without contrast (mask images) and then same acquisition is repeated with contrast. Subtraction of mask images from the contrast-enhanced images suppresses the background tissue signal. The major limitation with this method is patient movement and breathing between the mask and contrasted portions of the scan and different table positions between stations, which may result in misregistration artifacts. Image acquisition (both mask and actual CE-MRA) must be obtained with breath holding, which significantly improves image quality [22].

Fig. 18.1 Peripheral multi-station 3D contrast-enhanced MRA. The sketches show a longitudinal cross section of a scanner. The patient, with RF surface coils on top, is firstly positioned with the thorax in the isocenter of the scanner (**a**). The coronal 3D acquisition volume [three-dimensional (3D) slab] is positioned within the isocenter. During the course of the examination, the patient platform, together with the patient, is advanced stepwise toward the feet (**b–d**). Given the appropriate synchronization between the contrast agent bolus and the imaging time per station, the contrast agent bolus is followed along its path from the aorta via the pelvis-leg vessels to the feet. This also allows vessels to be depicted whose dimensions exceed the size of a conventional FOV (MRA in Fig. 18.2). From Kramer H et al. Eur Radiol 2008; 18:1925–1936. Reprinted with permission from Springer

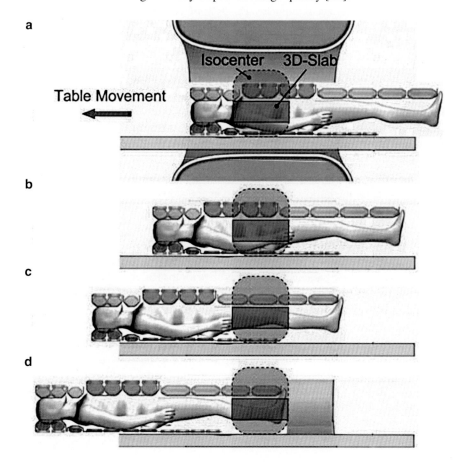

In CE-MRA the synchronization of image acquisition to intra-arterial GBCA concentration is extremely important, and data acquisition must coincide with the arrival of the contrast in the vessel of interest. The GBCA dose volume is small, and since the acquisition time for MRA is long, the contrast bolus must encompass 40–60 % of the duration of acquisition for optimum image contrast. Improper timing of acquisition results in image artifacts that can be especially problematic with bolus chase MRA of extremities, in which multiple stations are acquired with one contrast bolus. On average, the contrast material requires 24 s to reach the femoral artery but only 5 more seconds to reach the popliteal artery and additional 7 s to reach the ankle artery [23]. The rapid transit of contrast makes it especially difficult for first pass CE-MRA as table movement and imaging time needs to be fast enough to keep up with the bolus transit. In recent years, parallel imaging (SENSE, SMASH, GRAPPA) has emerged as powerful method to decrease acquisition time without degrading spatial resolution. In parallel imaging, data are acquired simultaneously using multiple surface coils with different spatial sensitivities. The disadvantage of parallel imaging is reduced signal to noise ratio (SNR) in proportion to the acceleration factor. Due to intrinsically higher SNR, higher acceleration factors can be achieved with 3 T MRI scanners.

We typically use 0.1–0.2 mmol/kg dose of intravenous GBCA for CE-MRA at the infusion rate of 2 cc/s using a power injector followed by a saline flush of 20 cc to ensure that the contrast material does not pool within the tubing or peripheral veins and is delivered to the central veins. Since the time to peak arterial enhancement is dependent on multiple variables such as contrast injection volume and rate, saline flush volume and rate and cardiac output, it is not possible to predict the scan delay reliably; a "test bolus method" or "bolus-tracking method" should be used to assess the peak-enhancement time.

- The test bolus method measures the time taken for a small amount of contrast agent (1–2 mL) to travel from the injection site to the vessel of interest. After injection of 1–2 mL contrast, serial images of the target vessel are sequentially acquired at the rate of 1 image/s for 40–60 s. Signal intensity in the vessel is then graphically plotted against time and the time to peak enhancement is calculated. However, physiological changes in heart rate, cardiac output, and depth of breath hold may vary between the test bolus and the full bolus.
- Real time bolus-tracking method: With this method visualizing contrast arrival in the vessel of interest triggers the acquisition of CE-MRA. This technique is especially useful for imaging vessels below the knees. Repetitive low resolution, background suppressed 2D images are acquired until contrast arrival and CE-MRA acquisition is triggered manually or automatically.

An important factor in achieving high diagnostic accuracy in peripheral MRA is the spatial resolution. Reliable diagnosis of arterial stenosis in MRA requires at least 3 pixels to be present across the arterial lumen. In the lower leg, this can be challenging, as the vessel diameters are 2–3 mm in this area. 3D computer workstations are used for image post-processing and viewing. The post-processing techniques used are multiplanar reformations (MPR), curved MPR, maximum intensity projections (MIP), and volume rendering (VR). MPR allows viewing anatomy in all planes and the image resolution is improved if the acquisition voxels are isotropic. Curved MPR allows reformation along tortuous vessels. MIPs produce images comparable to digital subtraction angiography and can provide a quick preview of the peripheral vasculature, but diagnosis must always be confirmed by looking at thin MPR images. Volume-rendered images allow excellent display of surface-rendered 3D images but are not useful for stenosis quantitation.

Types of CE-MRA
First Pass CE-MRA

There are several types of first pass CE-MRA acquisitions based on region of interest. Single-station MRA is used to acquire a single field of view when the area of interest is limited such as the abdominal aorta, carotid arteries, and renal arteries. Multi-station MRA is used to image the peripheral vasculature from the abdominal aorta to the feet by acquiring multiple overlapping fields of views. In multi-injection MRA, contiguous overlapping stations are acquired with separate injection of GBCA at each station but are limited by the total volume of GBCA that can be administered and by the effects of residual contrast in the blood pool from the previous injections. In moving table MRA, the entire region of interest is acquired by moving the scanner table through the center of the magnet in a stepwise fashion chasing a single contrast bolus through multiple discrete stations (Figs. 18.1 and 18.2). Typically three discrete stations are imaged in peripheral MRA: aortic bifurcation and the iliac arteries, femoral arteries, and the runoff vessels (Fig. 18.3). Image acquisition must be fast enough to keep up with the arterial bolus. Failure to do so will result in incomplete arterial opacification and venous contamination that can further degrade image quality. The sequential bolus chase acquisition images the lower leg region last and is most likely to suffer from venous contamination. The most common cause of venous contamination is timing problems but may also occur as a result of inflammatory hyperemia in cellulitis or spontaneous or iatrogenic formation of arteriovenous shunts in patients with diabetes and prior surgical or endovascular interventions. Faster acquisition times decrease the likelihood of venous contamination. Biphasic contrast administration with the initial rate of 1.5 mL/s followed by 0.5 mL/s prolongs the arterial phase.

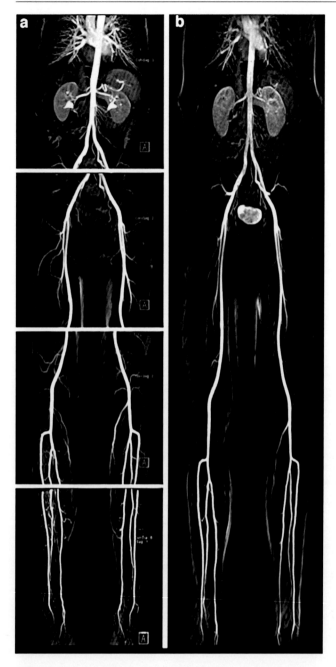

Fig. 18.2 Contrast-enhanced peripheral MRA acquired with the multi-station technique (**a**) compared with the "move during scan"(MDS) technique (**b**), with which continuous data acquisition takes place during patient table movement. The multi-station technique requires acquisition from several discrete, easy-to-overlap FOVs (**a**), whereas the MDS technique delivers a large, seamless FOV. From Kramer H et al. Eur Radiol 2008; 18:1925–1936. Reprinted with permission from Springer

of thrombosis. In patients with bypass grafts, hybrid protocols in which the leg station is imaged first followed by abdomen and thigh result in lesser venous contamination.

Steady-State MRA

Blood pool contrast agents allow us to image the peripheral vasculature beyond the short arterial first-pass phase [25]. Because there is no time constraint, MRA with very high spatial resolution can be achieved. Steady-state MRA (SS-MRA) provides images of both arteries and veins, but the excellent spatial resolution allows separation of arteries and veins. Combined first-pass and SS-MRA approach of the peripheral arteries improves results as compared to first-pass imaging alone [26].

Time-Resolved MRA

Time-resolved MRA is based on rapid repeated acquisitions of 3D images at the same location over time. Due to the rapidity of image acquisition, there is no need for appropriate contrast timing, and it provides both arterial and venous phase information in a dynamic fashion. Time-resolved acquisition techniques when used with parallel imaging can efficiently improve temporal resolution but degrade spatial resolution. Time-resolved MRA is more reliable than first-pass MRA and digital subtraction MRA for the leg station, especially in patients with arteriovenous malformations and diabetics with small vessel disease.

Advantages of CE-MRA

CE-MRA is a noninvasive imaging technique that does not require arterial access such as digital subtraction angiography. Unlike CT angiography and DSA, CE-MRA does not expose patients to the deleterious effects of ionizing radiation or iodinated contrast agents. Since it is unobstructed by the bone and has excellent tissue characterization, protocols can be tailored to the tissue type and clinical question. Unlike ultrasound, MRI has the unique ability to acquire images in numerous planes without repositioning the patient and generate excellent three-dimensional recreations of anatomic structures.

CE-MRA has >90 % sensitivity and specificity as compared with DSA. Table 18.1 summarizes studies reporting diagnostic accuracy of CE-MRA for the detection of significant stenosis in patients with known or suspected PAD [27]. CE-MRA performs similar to CT in the evaluation of the aorta and renal arteries but is superior to CT in vessel segments with extensive calcifications as calcium tends to bloom on CT limiting lumen evaluation.

Disadvantages of CE-MR

CE-MRA conventionally has longer acquisition times compared to CT. Although moving table ensures coverage from the mid-abdomen to the foot, covering a large volume over several vascular territories with sufficient intra-arterial contrast without venous overlay can be difficult. Since MRA

The latter phase equals tissue extraction and reduces venous filling [24]. Venous compression techniques using blood pressure cuffs inflated to 50–60 mmHg around the thigh or calf have proven effective in reducing venous contamination [20]. However, cuff compression should not be used in patients with superficial vascular bypass grafts due to the risk

Fig. 18.3 Peripheral CE-MRA in a patient with peripheral arterial disease. Note: occlusion of the left superficial femoral artery (*arrow*). In this patient, bolus-acquisition timing was successful with resulting good arterial contrast and no venous overlay. From Nielsen YW, et al. Acta Radiologica 2012;53:769–77. Reprinted with permission from Sage Publications

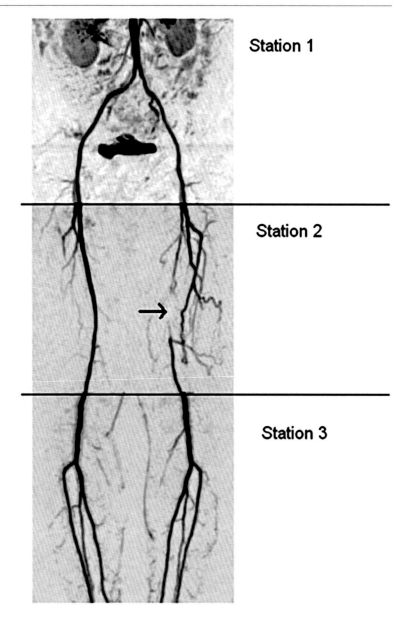

has lower spatial resolution when compared to CT, evaluating vessels with smaller diameters can be problematic. Total examination times for CE-MRA is longer (average 35 vs 24 min for CT [28].

CE-MRA depends upon optimal timing of data acquisition relative to peak arterial enhancement. Early data acquisition results in incomplete arterial opacification and may cause a ringing artifact that mimics a dissection [29]. Delayed acquisitions will have reduced signal to noise ratio and artifacts from venous and soft tissue enhancement that will obscure the visualization of arteries [30]. Metallic clips and intravascular stents can cause artifacts that may mimic stenosis on CE-MRA images but can be clarified by reviewing the source images and patient's clinical history (Fig. 18.4). Prosthetic joint replacements can cause extensive signal loss that cannot be resolved. Inappropriate positioning of the acquisition slices may result in exclusion of the vessel of

interest, in which case the acquisition must be repeated with appropriate positioning. Vessel segments near the edge of coils can appear to have stenosis due to decreased coil sensitivity near the edges, which can be avoided by overlapping slices between contiguous stations. Patient movement between the unenhanced and enhanced images can result in misregistration artifacts, when severe may require a repeat study. It's essential to review the source images in order to confirm a finding seen on processed images.

Non-Contrast-Enhanced MRA (NC-MRA)

CE-MRA is considered the standard method of acquiring MRA with high spatial resolution and accuracy. However, due to safety issues with GBCA particularly the risk of NSF in patients with advanced renal disease, there is increased interest

Table 18.1 Diagnostic accuracy of contrast-enhanced magnetic resonance angiography for the detection of significant stenosis in patients with known or suspected peripheral arterial disease

Study (year)[a]	Number of patients	Sensitivity (%)	Specificity (%)
Rofsky et al. (1997)	15	97	96
Yamashita et al. (1998)	20	96	83
Ho et al. (1998)	28	93	98
Sueyoshi et al. (1999)	23	97	99
Meaney et al. (1999)	20	81–89[b]	91–95[b]
Winterer et al. (1999)	76	100	98
Ruehm et al. (2000)	61	91	97
Huber et al. (2000)	24	100	96
Ruehm et al. (2001)	11	91–94[b]	93–90[b,c]
Loewe et al. (2002)	106	97	96
Goyen et al. (2002)	13	95[c]	95[c]
Hentsch et al. (2003)	186	90+91[d]	90+97[d]
Leiner et al. (2004)	23	86–90[b]	76–76[b]
Herborn et al. (2004)	51	92–93[b,c]	89–88[b,c]
Krause et al. (2005)	26	79	93
Leiner et al. (2005)	152	84	97
Janka et al. (2005)	25	94–91[b]	91–91[b]
Gjonnaess et al. (2006)	58	94	95
Fenchel et al. (2006)	34	95[b,e]	95[b,e]

From Dellegrottaglie S, Sanz J, Macaluso F, et al. Technology insight: magnetic resonance angiography for the evaluation of patients with peripheral artery disease. Nature Clinical Practice Cardiovascular Medicine 2007;4:677–87. Reprinted with permission from Nature Publishing Group
[a]For consistency, study selection was conducted on the basis of the following criteria: publication period (1996–2006), reference test (invasive angiography), definition of lesion significance (luminal stenosis >50 %), and evaluation of the entire arterial tree in the lower extremities (aortoiliac, femoropopliteal, and infrapopliteal levels)
[b]Values refer to two independent readers
[c]Values are cumulative for multiple territories, as detected by whole-body magnetic resonance angiography
[d]Values refer to the detection of stenoses and occlusions, respectively
[e]Values obtained with lesion significance defined as >70 % luminal stenosis

in non-contrast MRA (NC-MRA) techniques. NC-MRA was first described 30 years ago, but recent improvements in MRI hardware technology have made it clinically feasible. There are several techniques of acquiring NC-MRA, most of which are used in specialized centers and may not be available on commercial scanners; the detailed description of each technique is beyond the scope of this chapter.

- Time of flight MRA (TOF-MRA)—This technique is perhaps the most well-described non-contrast technique for MRA and is primarily used in neurovascular imaging including assessment of extracranial carotid and vertebral arteries [31]. TOF images are acquired by a 3D or 2D technique with better spatial resolution with 3D technique. Both techniques are time consuming and susceptible to motion artifacts that limit their use in peripheral MRA.

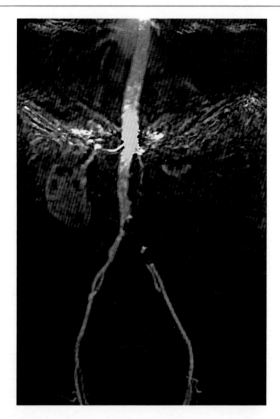

Fig. 18.4 Coronal gadolinium-enhanced MR angiographic MIP image of the iliac arteries in a 57-year-old female patient with two metallic stents in the left internal iliac artery. The MIP image shows the absence of signal in the lumen of both stents due to susceptibility artifact. Both stents were patent on ultrasound examination. Also note susceptibility artifact over aorta at origin of renal arteries due to metal in patients' bra. From Ho K, et al. Eur Radiol 1999;1765–74. Reprinted with permission from Springer

- Phase contrast angiography—This technique provides information about blood flow, velocities, and an estimation of pressure gradients across stenosis. Clinical applications include neurovascular imaging (intracranial, carotid, and vertebral arteries), aortic imaging for dissection (may demonstrate entry and exit sites between true and false lumens) or coarctation, and evaluating intra- or extracardiac shunts. It has not found widespread use in peripheral angiography.

- Flow-spoiled fresh blood imaging (FS-FBI)—This technique was first described in 1985 but has only recently become clinically feasible due to significant improvements in MRI technology [32]. FBI is a 3D, ECG-gated technique that relies on the physiological signal intensity changes in blood vessels due to differential arterial and venous flow velocities during the cardiac cycle. In fast flow vessels, diastolic-triggered images show bright-blood arteries due to maintained flow, but in systolic-triggered images, fast arterial flow causes signal void resulting in black-blood arteries. Because venous flow is slow and nonpulsatile, it will appear bright in both systolic- and

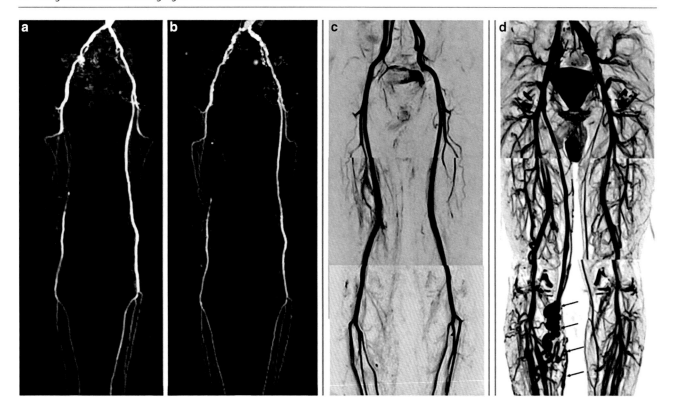

Fig. 18.5 (**a**) Three-station FBI runoff image on a 66-year-old patient with occlusions of the right superficial femoral artery and the right anterior tibial artery. (**b**) A 16-row CTA image. Good agreement between the two modalities for depicting normal to occlusion regions with collateral branches. (**c**) Arterial MIP images of three-station peripheral runoffs on a patient acquired using FS-FBI. (**d**) The additional subtraction of arterial images from systolic images provides venous images. Note that varicose veins (*arrows*) are unambiguously depicted in the popliteal station. Because of double subtraction, fluid is depicted in (**d**). From Miyazaki M & Akahane M. J Magn Reson Imaging 2012;35:1–19. Reprinted with permission from John Wiley and Sons

diastolic-triggered images. A bright-blood arteriogram without venous overlay is produced after subtracting the systolic images from the diastolic images [33]. Continuous acquisition of both systolic and diastolic images during a single scan minimizes motion-related misregistration artifacts. However, in peripheral vessels due to slower flow and smaller flow velocity differences between systole and diastole, all vessels are depicted in bright blood even in systolic triggering making it difficult to separate arteries from veins. The system is usually preset to subtract the systolic from diastolic-triggered source images, which generates the arteriogram after MIP processing (Fig. 18.5). Because the MIP images represent flow difference between systole and diastole, evaluation of the diastolic source image is important especially to prevent overestimation of the severity and length of stenosis. Fresh blood imaging is faster than TOF, 10 min for a whole-leg examination versus 25 min with fewer artifacts and better vessel to background contrast resolution [34]. Lim et al. compared FBI with bolus chase and time-resolved CE-MRA for imaging peripheral runoff vessels in 36 patients. Serious artifacts led to poor diagnostic imaging in 47 % patients and a reported sensitivity of 85.4 %, specificity of 75.8 %, and a

negative predictive value of 92.3 % [35]. Gutzeit et al. reported excellent overall image quality for FBI in the thigh and calf regions, yet insufficient diagnostic quality in the pedal arteries [36]. Tachycardia and atrial fibrillation pose a challenge as the technique relies on the prescription of fixed trigger delays. In patients with severely reduced left ventricular systolic dysfunction, due to the narrow pulse pressures, differentiation of arteries and veins may be difficult. Patients with critical limb ischemia may have rest pain and resultant involuntary twitching which can degrade image quality, as fresh blood imaging is exquisitely sensitive to motion.

- Arterial spin labeling angiography—Arterial spin labeling (ASL) acquires two sets of images followed by subtraction which displays the arteries and provides complete suppression of background signal. ASL is used in neurovascular imaging and can have potential applications in imaging of small vessels of hands and feet, where CE-MRA can be challenging due to slow arterial flow and venous contamination.

- Flow-dependent non-contrast MRA—These techniques include quiescent-inflow single-shot (QISS) angiography, inflow inversion recovery angiography, and velocity

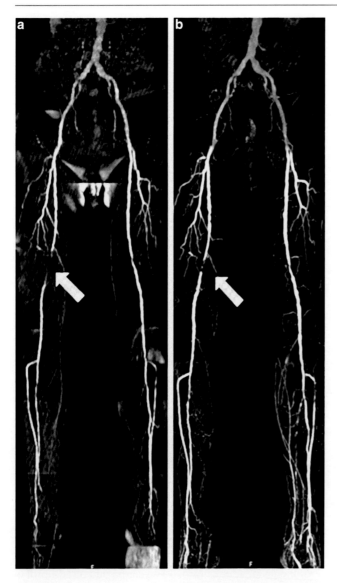

Fig. 18.6 A 77-year-old male patient with occlusion of the right superficial femoral artery (*thick arrow*) and severe arteriosclerosis of the lower leg. The length of the occlusion is overestimated with QISS-MRA (**a**) as compared to CE-MRA (**b**). From Klasen J et al. Clinical Radiology 2012;67:441–446. Reprinted with permission from Elsevier Limited

selective angiography. QISS is an emerging technique for imaging the peripheral arteries and can provide static images of blood vessels (conventional QISS) or cine images of blood flow patterns (cine QISS). In a pilot study of this technique using CE-MRA as the reference standard, the sensitivity and specificity of QISS-MRA for detecting arterial occlusion or stenosis $\geq 50\%$ were 87% and 95%, respectively [37]. The positive predictive value and negative predictive value were 84% and 96%, respectively (Fig. 18.6). Further large studies are needed to assess the clinical value of this technique.

NC-MRA has other advantages besides reducing costs and eliminating the risk of NSF. Unlike CE-MRA, which usually can only be acquired once in each exam, NC-MRA can be repeated in the case of technical error. NC-MRA acquired before CE-MRA can also serve as a backup examination if CE-MRA images are nondiagnostic due to patient motion or technical error.

Clinical Applications of MRA

MRA of peripheral arteries has become a routine application for a variety of established and evolving indications [38]. Most common indication of peripheral MRA is symptomatic peripheral vascular disease. Dellegrottaglie et al. suggested an algorithm for diagnostic evaluation of patients with known or suspected PAD as shown in Fig. 18.7 [27]. Clinical history, physical examination, and ankle-brachial index remain the cornerstone of initial evaluation of patients with known or suspected PAD. Noninvasive angiography of peripheral arteries with MRA or CTA is indicated for patients who are diagnosed with moderate to severe disease on initial evaluation. MRA is useful in treatment planning particularly when revascularization option is being considered. In these patients, MRA can help with decision making between percutaneous or surgical revascularization by characterizing the degree and extent of stenosis or occlusion and the site of reconstitution of native circulation. Suboptimal filling of small, diffusely diseased vessels or early venous filling affecting image interpretation can complicate the evaluation of below knee PAD. There are dedicated protocols to address these issues that have been described above and include rapid acquisition on a bolus chase MRA, use of time-resolved MRA, steady-state MRA, acquiring leg station first, or a combination of these methods. If imaging of pedal arteries is required, then it's best to acquire a dedicated high-resolution CE-MRA as a separate station.

Evaluation of bypass grafts usually does not pose a problem for MRA image quality (Fig. 18.8). Occasionally a metallic clip at the anastomotic site may cause an artifact. Due to 3D nature of MRA acquisition and ability to do multiplanar reformatting that allows for viewing the dataset from different angles, a detailed evaluation of grafts and anastomotic sites can be performed. Visualization of lumen inside the stent can be challenging particularly in stainless steel stents, which causes a signal void mimicking stenosis; however, the artifact is minimal in nitinol stents (Fig. 18.4). Stent grafts for abdominal aortic aneurysms have been well studied using MRA (Fig. 18.9). Both in vitro and in vivo studies of 3D CE-MRA of stent grafts have not only documented safety of MR imaging but also accuracy of lumen diameter measurements and stent patency [39, 40]. In a small study, CE-MRA was compared with CTA for follow-up evaluation of patients with thoracic aortic stent graft [41]. MRA was comparable to CTA for stent-graft morphology evaluation;

Fig. 18.7 Suggested diagnostic algorithm in patients with known or suspected peripheral artery disease. From Dellegrottaglie S et al. Nat Clin Pract Cardiovasc Med 2007; 4: 677–87. Reprinted with permission from Nature Publishing Group

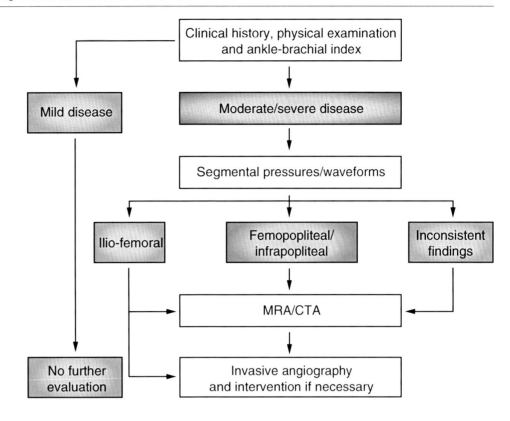

however, arterial phase leak assessment (endoleak) was less evident on CE-MRA compared to CTA. In this setting, delayed imaging of the aorta is necessary and is best performed with a VIBE technique (3D, T1 weighted with fat saturation).

The role of MRA is limited in patients with acute critical limb ischemia primarily due to the need for urgent diagnosis and intervention that can readily be achieved with invasive angiography. However, in these patients CE-MRA can detect a clot in the peripheral arteries in the form of filling defect (Fig. 18.10). In patients with peripheral embolism, CMR is an excellent modality to evaluate the heart and proximal aorta to assess for source of embolism and is superior to echocardiography for the detection of ventricular thrombi. Spontaneous dissection of iliofemoral arteries is less common than propagation of dissection in thoracic aorta. MRA is a useful technique for the initial assessment and subsequent follow-up of patients with aortic dissection (Fig. 18.11). Short- or long-term complications of dissection can be readily identified, e.g., arterial supply to abdominal or pelvic organs from false lumen, aneurysm formation, etc.

MRI Safety

MRI is an established and safe imaging modality with millions of diagnostic studies performed worldwide. MRI itself does not have short- or long-term adverse effects unlike radiation-based imaging modalities. However, there are certain precautions and safety consideration that are critical to understand before using this methodology. These safety considerations are similar to all cardiovascular or non-cardiovascular MR imaging. The sources of patient risk are the electromagnetic field of the MRI scanner and the contrast agents used for MRI. MRI generates a strong static magnetic field and is always "on" whether or not actual patient scanning is taking place. The static magnetic field generated by MRI is 30, 000 (1.5 T scanner) to 60, 000 (3 T scanner) times the earth magnetic field (0.00005 T). In addition to the static magnetic field that is present all the time, MRI scanner also generates gradient field and radiofrequency field during scanning. The risk of these electromagnetic fields is significantly higher when a ferromagnetic material is present. The ferromagnetic material may be implanted inside the patient in the form of medical devices (pacemakers, insulin pumps, neurostimulators, aneurysm clips) or introduced from external sources in the form of non-MRI-compatible equipment (oxygen tanks, wheelchairs, infusion pumps, monitoring devices, IV poles, etc.).

There are few reported cases of deaths associated with MRI scanning in the presence of ferromagnetic materials. All these deaths were related to poor screening procedures, lack of patient monitoring during the scan, and unfamiliarity with established safety precautions. There are also reported cases of burns next to ferromagnetic implants from radiofrequency waves [42]. Gradient field causes loud

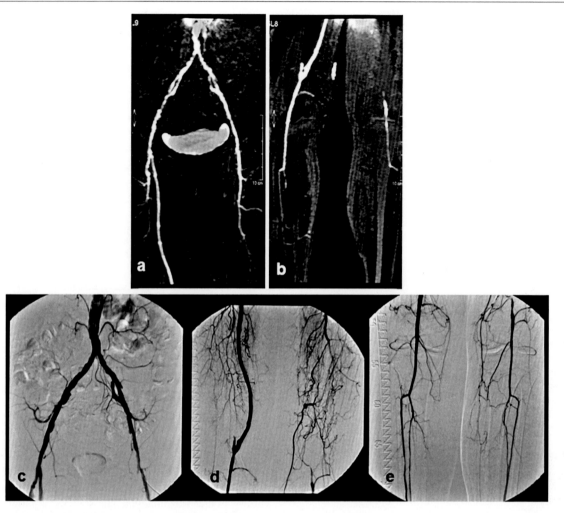

Fig. 18.8 A 65-year-old female patient with a femoropopliteal bypass graft. (**a**) Coronal MIP of the upper leg shows patent proximal portion of the femoropopliteal bypass graft on the right leg. Note moderate stenoses in both external iliac arteries and occlusions of both superficial femoral arteries. (**b**) Coronal MIP of the calf shows patent distal portion of the bypass graft and a 50 % stenosis distal to the anastomosis. Insufficient opacification of the calf arteries. (**c**) Corresponding DSA image of the pelvis confirms moderate stenoses of both external iliac arteries (inflow vessels) and patency of the proximal portion of the bypass part. (**d**) DSA image at the level of the thigh shows a patent right bypass graft and a 50 % stenosis distal to the anastomosis. (**e**) Calf arteries are better visualized on the DSA. From Loewe C, et al. Eur Radiol 2000;10:725–32. Reprinted with permission from Springer

noise which necessitates use of ear protection by ear plugs and/or MRI compatible headphones. Other adverse effects may include peripheral nerve stimulation causing muscle twitching and body heating particularly in patients with impaired thermoregulation (elderly, obesity, diabetes). There are no deleterious effects noted in pregnant patients; however, the safety of MR during pregnancy has not been proven [43]. MRI in pregnant patients can be considered if other diagnostic imaging is inadequate or to avoid radiation-based imaging.

All patients should be screened by the MRI staff before the patient enters the scanner area. There are standard screening questionnaire forms available that patients complete before their scan. It's absolutely essential that no external ferromagnetic device enters the MRI room unless previously tested. All patients with implanted metallic devices should be evaluated on case by case basis. All patients should also be evaluated for the risk of nephrogenic systemic fibrosis associated with gadolinium-based contrast agents as outlined above.

Common contraindications for MRI include:

- Cardiac pacemakers and defibrillators (relative contraindication)
- Implanted infusion pumps
- Neurostimulator/spinal stimulator
- Ferromagnetic aneurysm clips (most are nonmagnetic)
- Metal in the eyes (e.g., from machining)
- Cochlear implants
- Metal fragments in the body (shrapnel, bullets)

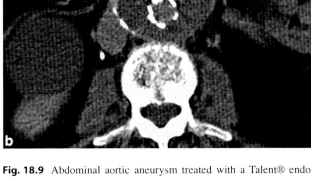

Fig. 18.9 Abdominal aortic aneurysm treated with a Talent® endograft. Enhancement of the perigraft thrombus in a central location at arterial (**a**) and delayed (**b**) CT angiogram precluded its classification. (**c**) MRA clearly shows a posteriorly located leak, close to a lumbar enhanced artery (the most probably implicated vessel). From Ayuso JR, et al. J Magn Reson Imaging 2004;20:803–10. Reprinted with permission from John Wiley and Sons

For patients with biomedical implants, it's important to identify the manufacturer, type or model, material, serial number, or other pertinent information to identify the specific type and their suitability for MRI. Devices with non-ferromagnetic materials (titanium, titanium alloy, Elgiloy, Phynox, MP35N, tantalum, nitinol) may undergo MRI immediately after implantation. Devices with weakly ferromagnetic materials (coils, filters) may need a waiting period of 6–8 weeks for endothelialization. Most prosthetic heart valves including Starr-Edwards model Pre-6000 pose no hazard in the MR environment [43]. The presence of a cardiac pacemaker or defibrillator was considered an absolute contraindication for MRI; however, more recent reports show that in selected and closely monitored patients, MRI can be performed on 1.5 T systems without adverse effects [44]. In our center CMR is routinely performed in patients with cardiac devices under close monitoring, pre and post scan device interrogation and adjustment of device parameters. Most of currently implanted coronary stents are weakly ferromagnetic and can undergo MRI any time after implantation [45]. A comprehensive list of MR safe, conditional, or unsafe devices is available at www.MRIsafety.com.

Conclusions

MRA of peripheral arteries is an established technique using 3D CE-MRA with high sensitivity and specificity when compared to digital subtraction angiography as reference standard. This is a highly reproducible and robust technique without the use of radiation or nephrotoxic contrast agents. Appropriate indications of peripheral MRA include evaluation for arterial dissection, diagnosis of peripheral arterial disease (PAD), selecting patients for endovascular intervention or surgical bypass of lower extremity PAD, and post-revascularization surveillance of lower extremity PAD.

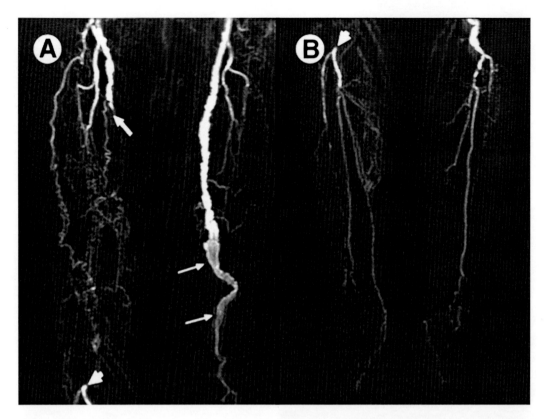

Fig. 18.10 MIP images from MRA obtained in a patient with acute right lower extremity ischemia (**a**) show a left popliteal artery aneurysm (*small arrows*) and occlusion of the midportion of the right superficial femoral artery (*large arrow*) and the entire right popliteal artery with distal reconstitution (**b**) at the anterior tibial arterial level (*arrowhead*). There is relatively intact infrapopliteal runoff present bilaterally. The right-sided occlusion is most likely secondary to thrombosis of a popliteal artery aneurysm, given the high incidence of bilateralism. From Walker TG. Tech Vasc Interventional Rad 2009;12:117–29. Reprinted with permission from Elsevier Limited

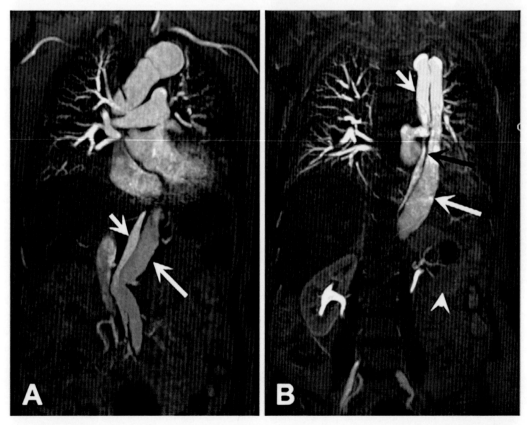

Fig. 18.11 A 58-year-old woman with type A aortic dissection post repair. High-resolution CE-MRA shows dissection flap (**b**, *black arrow*) between the true (**a** and **b**, *small white arrows*) and false lumens (**a** and **b**, *large white arrows*) and decreased left renal parenchymal enhancement (**b**, *arrowhead*). From Krishnam MS, et al. Clinical Radiology 2008;63:744–55. Reprinted with permission from Elsevier Limited

In patients suitable for revascularization procedure, MRA can assist in deciding between percutaneous or surgical intervention. Due to safety concerns of gadolinium-based contrast agents, there is an increasing interest in the development of non-contrast MRA with several evolving techniques that have shown promising results in initial studies. Further ongoing development in MRA hardware and software has the potential for improvement in spatial resolution and diagnostic accuracy.

References

1. Patel MR, Spertus JA, Brindis RG, et al. ACCF proposed method for evaluating the appropriateness of cardiovascular imaging. J Am Coll Cardiol. 2005;46:1606–13.
2. Hirsch AT, Haskal ZJ, Hertzer NR, et al. ACC/AHA 2005 practice guidelines for the management of patients with peripheral arterial disease (lower extremity, renal, mesenteric, and abdominal aortic): a collaborative report from the American Association for Vascular Surgery/Society for Vascular Surgery, Society for Cardiovascular Angiography and Interventions, Society for Vascular Medicine and Biology, Society of Interventional Radiology, and the ACC/AHA Task Force on Practice Guidelines (Writing Committee to Develop Guidelines for the Management of Patients With Peripheral Arterial Disease). J Am Coll Cardiol. 2006;47:e1–192.
3. Sacks D, Bettmann M, Casciani T, et al. Expert panel on cardiovascular imaging: claudication appropriateness criteria. 2005. Available at: http://www.acr.org/ac. Accessed 21 Jan 2015.
4. Ni Y. MR contrast agents for cardiac imaging. In: Bogaert J, Dymarkowski S, Taylor AM, Muthurangu V, editors. Clinical cardiac MRI. 2nd ed. Berlin: Springer; 2012. p. 31–51.
5. Bellin MF, Vasile M, Morel-Precetti S. Currently used non-specific extracellular MR contrast media. Eur Radiol. 2003;13:2688–98.
6. Edelman RR. Contrast-enhanced MR, imaging of the heart: overview of the literature. Radiology. 2004;232:653–68.
7. Bashir MR, Bhatti L, Marin D, Nelson RC. Emerging applications of ferumoxytol as a contrast agent in MRI. J Magn Reson Imaging. 2015;41:884–98.
8. ACR Manual on Contrast Media. Version 9. 2013. http://www.acr.org/~/media/ACR/Documents/PDF/QualitySafety/Resources/Contrast Manual/2013_Contrast_Media.pdf.
9. Matsumura T, Hayakawa M, Shimada F, et al. Safety of gadopentetate dimeglumine after 120 million administrations over 25 years of clinical use. Magn Reson Med Sci. 2013;12:297–304.
10. Cowper SE. Nephrogenic systemic fibrosis: an overview. J Am Coll Radiol. 2008;5:23–8.
11. Grobner T. Gadolinium–a specific trigger for the development of nephrogenic fibrosing dermopathy and nephrogenic systemic fibrosis? Nephrol Dial Transplant. 2006;21:1104–8.
12. Prince MR, Zhang H, Morris M, et al. Incidence of nephrogenic systemic fibrosis at two large medical centers. Radiology. 2008; 248:807–16.
13. Sadowski EA, Bennett LK, Chan MR, et al. Nephrogenic systemic fibrosis: risk factors and incidence estimation. Radiology. 2007;243:148–57.
14. High WA, Ayers RA, Chandler J, Zito G, Cowper SE. Gadolinium is detectable within the tissue of patients with nephrogenic systemic fibrosis. J Am Acad Dermatol. 2007;56:21–6.
15. Martin DR, Krishnamoorthy SK, Kalb B, et al. Decreased incidence of NSF in patients on dialysis after changing gadolinium contrast-enhanced MRI protocols. J Magn Reson Imaging. 2010;31:440–6.

16. Mühler MR, Clément O, Salomon LJ, et al. Maternofetal pharmacokinetics of a gadolinium chelate contrast agent in mice. Radiology. 2011;258:455–60.
17. De Santis M, Straface AF, Cavaliere B, et al. Gadolinium periconceptional exposure: pregnancy and neonatal outcome. Acta Obstet Gynecol. 2007;86:99–101.
18. Wang PI, Chong ST, Kielar AZ. Imaging of pregnant and lactating patients: Part 1. evidence-based review and recommendations. AJR Am J Roentgenol. 2012;198:778–84.
19. Neimatallah MA, Ho VB, Dong Q, et al. Gadolinium-enhanced 3D magnetic resonance angiography of the thoracic vessels. J Magn Reson Imaging. 1999;10:758–70.
20. Zhang HL, Ho BY, Chao M, et al. Decreased venous contamination on 3D gadolinium-enhanced bolus chase peripheral MR angiography using thigh compression. AJR Am J Roentgenol. 2004;183:1041–7.
21. Earls JP, Rofsky NM, DeCorato DR, Krinsky GA, Weinreb JC. Breath-hold single-dose gadolinium enhanced three-dimensional MR aortography: usefulness of a timing examination and MR power injector. Radiology. 1996;201:705–10.
22. Marks B, Mitchell DG, Simelaro JP. Breath-holding in healthy and pulmonary-compromised populations: effects of hyperventilation and oxygen inspiration. J Magn Reson Imaging. 1997;7:595–7.
23. Prince MR, Chabra SG, Watts R, et al. Contrast material travel times in patients undergoing peripheral MR angiography. Radiology. 2002;224:55–61.
24. Meissner OA, Rieger J, Weber C, et al. Critical limb ischemia: hybrid MR angiography compared with DSA. Radiology. 2005; 235:308–18.
25. Goyen M, Edelman M, Perreault P, et al. MR angiography of aortoiliac occlusive disease: a phase III study of the safety and effectiveness of the blood-pool contrast agent MS-325. Radiology. 2005;236:825–33.
26. Rapp JH, Wolff SD, Quinn SF, et al. Aortoiliac occlusive disease in patients with known or suspected peripheral vascular disease: safety and efficacy of gadofosveset-enhanced MR angiography–multicenter comparative phase III study. Radiology. 2005;236:71–8.
27. Dellegrottaglie S, Sanz J, Macaluso F, et al. Technology insight: magnetic resonance angiography for the evaluation of patients with peripheral artery disease. Nat Clin Pract Cardiovasc Med. 2007; 4:677–87.
28. Willmann JK, Wildermuth S, Pfammatter T, et al. Aortoiliac and renal arteries: prospective intraindividual comparison of contrast-enhanced three-dimensional MR angiography and multi-detector row CT angiography. Radiology. 2003;226(3):798–811.
29. Svensson J, Petersson JS, Stahlberg F, et al. Image artifacts due to a time-varying contrast medium concentration in 3D contrast-enhanced MRA. J Magn Reson Imaging. 1999;10:919–28.
30. Maki JH, Prince MR, Londy FJ, Chenevert TL. The effects of time varying intravascular signal intensity and k-space acquisition order on three-dimensional MR angiography image quality. J Magn Reson Imaging. 1996;6:642–51.
31. Laub GA. Time-of-flight method of MR angiography. Magn Reson Imaging Clin N Am. 1995;3:391–98.
32. Wedeen VJ, Meuli RA, Edelman RR, et al. Projective imaging of pulsatile flow with magnetic resonance. Science. 1985;230:946–48.
33. Miyazaki M, Takai H, Sugiura S, et al. Peripheral MRA: separation of arteries from veins with flow-spoiled gradient pulses in electrocardiography-triggered three-dimensional half-Fourier fast spin-echo imaging. Radiology. 2003;227:890–96.
34. Wong P, Graves MJ, Lomas DJ. Interactive two-dimensional fresh blood imaging: a feasibility study. Eur Radiol. 2009;19:904–11.
35. Lim RP, Hecht EM, Xu J, et al. 3D Nongadolinium-enhanced ECG-gated MRA of the distal lower extremities: preliminary clinical experience. J Magn Reson Imaging. 2008;28:181–89.

36. Gutzeit A, Stutter R, Froehlich JM, et al. ECG-triggered non-contrast-enhanced MR angiography (TRANCE) versus digital sub-traction (DSA) in patients with peripheral arterial occlusive disease of the lower extremities. Eur Radiol. 2011;21:1979–87.

37. Edelman RR, Sheehan JJ, Dunkle E, et al. Quiescent-interval single-shot unenhanced magnetic resonance angiography of periph-eral vascular disease: technical considerations and clinical feasibil-ity. Magn Reson Med. 2010;63:951–58.

38. Grizzard J, Shah DJ, Klem I, Kim RJ. MR angiography of the lower extremity circulation with protocols. In: Mukherjee D, Rajagopalan S, editors. CT and MR angiography of the peripheral circulation, 1st ed. London: Informa Healthcare; 2007.

39. Hilfiker PR, Quick HH, Pfammatter T, Schmidt M, Debatin JF. Three-dimensional MR angiography of a nitinol-based abdomi-nal aortic stent graft: assessment of heating and imaging character-istics. Eur Radiol. 1999;9:1775–80.

40. Engellau L, Olsrud J, Brockstedt S, et al. MR evaluation ex vivo and in vivo of a covered stent-graft for abdominal aortic aneurysm: ferromagnetism, heating, artifacts and velocity mapping. J Magn Reson Imaging. 2000;12:112–21.

41. Weigel S, Tombach B, Maintz D, et al. Thoracic aortic stent graft: comparison of contrast-enhanced MR angiography and CT angiogra-phy in the follow-up: initial results. Eur Radiol. 2003;13:1628–34.

42. Hardy 2nd PT, Weil KM. A review of thermal MR injuries. Radiol Technol. 2010;8:606–9.

43. Shellock FG, Kanal E. Magnetic resonance: bioeffects, safety, and patient management. 1st ed. New York: Lippincott-Raven; 1996.

44. Nazarian S, Roguin A, Menekhem ZM, et al. Clinical utility and safety of a protocol for noncardiac and cardiac magnetic resonance imaging of patients with permanent pacemakers and implantable-cardioverter defibrillators at 1.5 Tesla. Circulation. 2006;114: 1277–84.

45. Syed MA, Carlson K, Murphy M, et al. Long-term safety of cardiac magnetic resonance imaging performed in the first few days after bare-metal stent implantation. J Magn Reson Imaging. 2006;24: 1056–61.

Noninvasive Imaging in Critical Limb Ischemia

19

John H. Fish, III and Teresa L. Carman

Introduction

The noninvasive assessment of the critically ischemic limb has evolved from air plethysmography for pulse volume wave recordings and quantitative pressure evaluation to imaging of occlusive arterial lesions utilizing duplex color ultrasonography which produces highly reliable and reproducible data. These physiologic and anatomic data have practical implications for pre-interventional planning, operative guidance, and post-interventional surveillance in critical limb ischemia (CLI). Adjunctive diagnostic measures have become available with the advances in technology over the past decades to determine oxygen tension and microvascular pressures for poorly perfused distal extremities and feet which utilize transcutaneous oximetry, laser Doppler, and near-infrared spectroscopy. Fluorescence angiography is also now among the newest of the commercially available modalities that can be offered at the bedside for both qualitative and quantitative evaluation of skin perfusion in ischemic distal extremities.

The noninvasive laboratory provides invaluable information for the evaluation of critical limb ischemia (CLI) in acute, subacute, and chronic management settings. A multitude of tests are available for the rapid assessment of limb-threatening ischemia, to assess foot and skin perfusion, to help predict wound healing, or to determine the level of amputation. These inexpensive tests provide information to confirm peripheral artery disease (PAD) and aid in assessing the anatomic level of disease and a quantifiable extent of

J.H. Fish, III, MD (✉)
Anticoagulation Services, Aurora Cardiovascular, Vascular Medicine, Aurora St. Luke's Medical Center,
Milwaukee, WI, USA

T.L. Carman, MD
Vascular Medicine, University Hospitals Case Medical Center,
Cleveland, OH, USA

arterial obstruction along with helping to plan or even guide intervention. In cases of acute limb ischemia, ultrasound is helpful in not only identifying and quantifying arterial occlusion but also identifying and characterizing a potential artery-to-artery source of embolization such as an infrarenal aortic aneurysm or a popliteal aneurysm. Following revascularization, these modalities are fundamental to any post-interventional surveillance program.

A typical vascular laboratory will provide segmental limb pressures with pulse volume wave recordings (commonly via air and photo plethysmography), continuous wave Doppler tracings, exercise treadmill testing, and duplex ultrasonography. More advanced labs or wound care centers may additionally offer testing which is more geared toward measuring microvascular (skin) perfusion to assess more specific angiosome surface perfusion. These testing modalities include transcutaneous oximetry (tcPO$_2$), laser Doppler flowmetry, near-infrared spectroscopy (NIRS), and fluorescence angiography.

Plethysmography and Segmental Pressures

The most basic assessment of PAD severity can be performed outside the vascular lab in the office setting utilizing appropriately sized blood pressure cuffs and a handheld continuous wave Doppler ultrasound device (4–8 MHz) for ankle/brachial index (ABI) determination. This gives both acoustic real-time flow dynamics of the tibial, peroneal, and pedal arteries along with quantitative data of the cumulative severity of PAD at the level of the ankle. The normal flow pattern has a triphasic characteristic with initial forward flow produced by cardiac systole, a brief phase of reversal in early diastole, and a second low-velocity forward phase in late diastole produced by vascular recoil. This triphasic flow pattern can be affected by decreased peripheral vascular resistance (vasodilation) which abolishes the second phase of flow reversal. Stenosis or occlusion will exhibit downstream changes to the pattern where a single forward phase is observed and the peak systolic flow velocity is blunted with a flattened, rounded waveform morphology.

In addition to the ankle cuff pressure, segmental pressures with pulse volume wave recordings of the lower limbs can be performed with a standard 4-cuff method in a noninvasive vascular laboratory utilizing high and low thigh cuffs along with calf and ankle cuffs. In a normal patient, a high thigh/brachial index is usually greater than 1.2. An index of 0.8–1.2 indicates aortoiliac stenosis, whereas an index <0.8 indicates occlusion [1]. The difference in systolic pressures between two adjacent levels should be no more than 20 mmHg, and elevated gradients in pressure between levels correspond with occlusive disease within the intervening segment. In addition to the 4-cuff method, a transmetatarsal cuff can be employed, and frequently a great toe pressure and pulse volume wave recording will also be obtained. A normal toe/brachial index is commonly defined as >0.65. Furthermore, the 2007 Trans-Atlantic Inter-Society Consensus II (TASC II) further defined CLI as an absolute ankle pressure of <50 mmHg or a toe pressure <30 mmHg. These pressures correspond to the threshold for impairment of normal repair mechanisms for cellular regeneration in dermal ischemia. Others have suggested an ABI cutoff for CLI defined as <0.35, but this does not take into account the degree of collateralization which may not reflect well in the ABI determination [1].

Alongside pressure recordings, segmental cuffs provide pulse volume wave recordings (PVRs) to detect volume changes at a particular level. These air plethysmographic recordings should not be confused with Doppler waveform patterns, however. A normal PVR should have a short rise time (<160 ms) and a dicrotic notch (Table 19.1) and differences in amplitude observed from the contralateral side (delta usually of >40 %) indicate pathology assuming that the gain is not adjusted. Exercise testing on a treadmill at a standard 2 mph and 12 % grade can be employed to stress the lower extremity arterial circulation in patients with claudication but in CLI, however, this is usually not necessary [1].

Arterial Duplex Ultrasonography

While PVR and segmental pressure measurements are helpful for identifying patients with advanced limb ischemia, reliable arterial mapping is required in patients with critical limb ischemia or acute limb ischemia who are considered for intervention or surgery for limb salvage. Imaging should provide an assessment of the anatomic location, morphology of the lesions, and the overall extent of the stenosis or occlusive disease. Digital subtraction angiography is considered the gold standard for arterial imaging. However, computed tomography angiography (CTA), magnetic resonance angi-

Table 19.1 Pulse volume waveform morphologies

Normal pulse waveform		Rapid ascent (<160 ms)
		Dicrotic notch
		Ascent <30 % descent time
Vasospastic pulse waveform		Saw tooth oscillations in the descending waveform
Difference in time to peak		Pathologic prolongation of the time to peak (>40 ms)
Difference in amplitude		Difference >40 % indicates probable pathologic cause
Mild pathologic change		Slowed ascent >160 ms
		Loss of dicrotic notch
Severe pathologic change		Slowed ascent >180 ms
		Loss dicrotic notch
		Symmetric appearing ascent and descent
Chaotic pulse waveform		Severe or indeterminate pathology
Flatline waveform		No pulsation with maximum amplification

Adapted from Kappert [36]

ography (MRA), and duplex ultrasound (DU) have similar ability to assist with procedural planning and are frequently the initial mapping tools used in many centers. Duplex ultrasound (DU) combines B-mode ultrasound imaging and pulsed Doppler spectral analysis. It has the ability to provide both anatomic information and hemodynamic information. In carotid stenosis, duplex ultrasound is used for diagnosis as well as preoperative planning and has largely obviated the need for advanced imaging using digital subtraction angiography (DSA), CTA, or MRA. In peripheral arterial imaging, DU has been validated as a planning and procedural tool and may have advantages over other imaging modalities. DU is routinely used for post-procedural surveillance of venous conduit bypass grafts, and despite the apparent advantages of DU compared to other modalities, DU is not as widely employed for peripheral interventional or surgical planning or as an intervention imaging modality as its more expensive and attractive arteriography counterparts.

More than three decades ago, noninvasive lower extremity arterial duplex mapping was described and validated by Jager and colleagues [2]. Using a mechanically oscillated transducer, they acquired B-mode and Doppler spectral data from the groin to the popliteal artery. Based on the acquired B-mode and Doppler information, waveform contour, peak systolic velocity, and spectral broadening, they described five categories of arterial occlusive disease (Table 19.2). Compared to angiography, duplex had an overall sensitivity of 96 % and a specificity of 81 % for identifying normal

Table 19.2 Arterial duplex ultrasound interpretation for peripheral arterial disease

Normal	Triphasic waveforms without spectral broadening. Waveforms may be biphasic lacking diastolic forward flow in the elderly
0–19% stenosis	Normal triphasic waveform contour in the presence of spectral broadening and noted arterial wall abnormalities
20–49% stenosis	Biphasic waveforms are noted. Peak systolic velocity (PSV) is increased by >30% compared to the proximal vessel. The presence of spectral broadening
50–99% stenosis	Monophasic flow (loss of the diastolic reversal). Peak systolic velocity shift >100% compared to the proximal vessel (PSV ratio >2:1). Extensive spectral broadening is noted
>75% stenosis	Suggested by PSV ratio >4:1
>90% stenosis	Suggested by PSV >7:1
Occlusion	No flow is detected in the arterial segment

Data from Jager et al. [1] and Gerhard-Herman et al. [8]

versus abnormal segments and a 70% agreement with regard to the degree of stenosis [2]. In many laboratories, these criteria are still used. Over the next decade, there was a marked improvement in ultrasound technology including the introduction of color-flow Doppler and mechanical transducers. During this time, there was widespread adoption of DU for surgical planning in carotid stenosis and other vascular surgery planning, yet DU was not widely used for evaluation in lower extremity PAD. In 1992, Moneta et al. systematically validated the use of DU in 150 patients, including 96 with limb-threatening ischemia [3]. The overall sensitivity for detecting stenosis >50% was 89% in the iliac vessels and 67% at the level of the popliteal artery. Ultrasound equipment has continued to evolve since the early studies that validated the use of DU for imaging and planning intervention. Despite the improvement in ultrasound technology, in many centers, DU continues to be less commonly utilized than other imaging modalities. In 2005, the ACC/AHA published guidelines on the management of patients with peripheral arterial disease. These guidelines were a collaborative effort and were endorsed by many vascular, interventional radiology and interventional cardiology societies. Using a standardized evaluation of the current literature, they provided classification of the available literature and level of evidence (LoE) available. These guidelines recognized duplex ultrasound as useful to diagnose anatomic location and the degree of stenosis in PAD (class I, LoE: A) and recommended DU for routine surveillance of venous conduits after femoral-popliteal or femoral-tibial-pedal bypass (class I, level of evidence: A) [4]. Recommendations for the use of DU to select patients for endovascular intervention, surgical bypass, and

the site of surgical anastomosis carried a class II, LoE: B recommendation. More contemporary data suggests that DU may be used as the sole imaging modality for planning bypass or endovascular revascularization in patients with critical limb ischemia with excellent technical success and long-term outcomes [5]. This study by Sultan et al. reported on 520 patients with CLI undergoing endovascular or bypass revascularization. Although approximately 20% required adjunctive MRA imaging, DU demonstrated a sensitivity of 97% and a specificity of 98% compared to intraoperative DSA for lesion identification. Immediate clinical improvement and 6-year freedom from restenosis, TLR, and amputation-free survival were the same between groups. Using DU for preoperative planning was also estimated to result in cost savings over MRA [5]. Another trial compared the outcome of surgical planning based on DU compared to DSA. Compared to the surgical outcome, the DU-identified surgical plan was correct in 77% of cases, and arteriography did not change planning for 97% of procedures. This was similar to the surgical planning based on arteriography in which 79% of procedures were performed as planned and DU did not change planning in 98% of cases [6].

While there is an expanding body of literature regarding the use of DU in chronic PAD and critical limb ischemia, the body of knowledge in acute limb ischemia (ALI) is more limited. One retrospective study examined DU for evaluation of 68 patients with ALI where DU was able to successfully identify the most distal patent inflow vessel and the most proximal patent outflow vessel in 99% of cases [7]. DU was able to identify 100% of cases that were amendable to thromboembolectomy alone and 94% of those that required bypass or hybrid procedures. Given the limited literature available, however, it is difficult to ascertain whether DU may play as strong a role in managing ALI as it does in CLI.

Peripheral arterial imaging with DU may be time-consuming when done properly, requiring up to 90 min for a complete bilateral lower extremity examination. The examination should include all arterial segments from the aorta to the ankle or even pedal vessels. In patients with a palpable femoral artery pulse, beginning at the inguinal crease with the common femoral artery may be sufficient. To optimize imaging of the aorta and the iliac arteries, the examination should be performed after an overnight fast in order to avoid signal dropout from overlying bowel gas. B-mode imaging should be performed in longitudinal and transverse orientation to allow adequate imaging of the vessel wall. The addition of color-flow Doppler will allow for identification of areas of turbulence. Power Doppler may be added in areas with slow flow to aid in identifying the lumen. Pulsed Doppler waveform and spectral analysis should be performed systematically at all vessel segments with special attention to areas where B-mode and color or power Doppler identify abnormalities. As described previously, normal peripheral artery Doppler waveforms are triphasic. In the presence of plaque or stenosis, spectral broadening and altered waveforms are noted (Fig. 19.1). Many labs identify stenosis >50 % by a peak systolic velocity (PSV) ratio greater than 2:1 when comparing the velocity at or just beyond the stenotic lesion to the preceding segment (Fig. 19.2). This is in addition to using spectral analysis, the presence or absence of turbulence, and waveform analysis. Some authors have advocated further stratifying the degree of stenosis by using a PSV ratio greater than 4:1 to identify >75 % stenosis and using a PSV ratio greater than 7:1 to identify >90 % stenosis [8, 9]. Other ratio stratification schemes have also been described but are not widely accepted; this may be regarded as a limitation when trying to analyze studies utilizing DU for evaluation and accuracy compared to other imaging modalities.

There are numerous advantages of DU imaging when compared to other arteriographic imaging modalities. In general, it is widely available, is noninvasive, does not require nephrotoxic contrast, and is relatively inexpensive compared to other imaging techniques. DU is readily portable and can be used at the bedside, in the intensive care unit, or in the surgical or endovascular suite to assist with planning and intervention. While DSA allows for imaging of only the lumen of the vessel, duplex ultrasound additionally offers visualization of the arterial wall, a property that is especially useful when arteritis is present. There are no known harmful side effects from DU, and studies can be readily repeated without concern for harm.

It is clear from the variability in the literature that peripheral DU requires experience and commitment to acquire the expertise for consistent and reliable imaging. Peripheral artery DU is highly operator dependent, and suitable training and credentialing is required [10, 11]. As with all vascular ultrasound imaging, there are limitations to applying the technology that must be understood and respected. However, many of the limitations can be overcome with experience [10]. DU of the aorta and iliac vessels may be limited in some patients by body habitus, tortuosity, or the presence of bowel gas. The femoral artery may be difficult to visualize as it passes through the adductor canal, which may be further hampered in patients who are obese or edematous. Slow flow (<20 cm/s) in DU is likely unreliable, and additional imaging may be required. Extensive vascular calcification may attenuate the ultrasound beam and limit optimal imaging, especially if the arterial flow is scant and slow. The hemodynamic significance of long segmental stenosis may also be overestimated due to slow flow, and the significance of tandem stenoses may be underestimated because of collaterals as well as the inability to rely on velocity ratios. While DU is generally well tolerated, one study compared patient preferences for MRA versus DU and found that 50 % of patient had no

preference between tests, of the remaining 50 %, 41 % preferred MRA over DU. The main discomforts experienced with DU were pain with the examination and fasting before the procedure [12].

Few studies have directly compared CTA imaging to DU for planning revascularization. In 2014, de Vos et al. published a study looking at 12 patients with PAD (three with CLI) and compared the preoperative planning from three operators based on DU results and then evaluated the impact of added CTA. Of the 36 DU-planned procedures, 75 % (27/36) did not change after the addition of CTA [13]. When asked to assess their confidence of DU planning compared to CTA, all operators felt less confident in the diagnostic quality of DU compared to CTA and less confident in therapeutic planning using DU compared to CTA.

Studies comparing DU and contrast-enhanced (CE) MRA have yielded mixed results. Earlier studies suggested that MRA may provide better imaging and a higher degree of accuracy for predicting stenosis [14] with DU showing a sensitivity of 76 %, specificity 93 %, and accuracy 89 % compared to CE-MRA with a sensitivity of 84 %, specificity 97 %, and accuracy 94 %. However, a more contemporary study by Bueno et al. suggests that DU and MRA are similar in sensitivity, specificity, and accuracy in predicting >50 % stenosis compared to DSA imaging [15] (DU sensitivity 81 % and specificity 99 %, compared to CE-MRA, 91 % and 99 %, respectively). Compared to operative decision-making using DSA, DU accurately identified all target arterial lesions requiring intervention in patients with critical limb ischemia, while MRA overestimated lesion severity in 14 % of lesions. Both cost and hospital length of stay were significantly less with DU compared to DSA or MRA [16].

Suboptimal scans in low-flow states are one limitation of DU. The use of echo-enhancing contrast agents may help overcome this limitation. While not yet clinically approved for peripheral ultrasound, contrast agents are widely employed in echocardiography and have been evaluated in peripheral arterial disease, endograft surveillance, renal artery stenosis, and other clinical settings. Limited studies have evaluated the use of ultrasound contrast for peripheral artery DU. While it appears that there may be some utility for contrast-enhanced (CE) ultrasound in patients with CLI, this has not been widely investigated or utilized [17, 18]. In addition to using CE ultrasound for macrovascular endoluminal visualization, there are expanding reports in the literature investigating the use of CE ultrasound to evaluate the microcirculation and skeletal muscle perfusion in patients with PAD. To date no studies have investigated patients with CLI using this technology [19].

With current ultrasound technology, DU has the ability to provide imaging information suitable for use with planning both endovascular and bypass grafting procedures. In addition, studies utilizing DU for procedural imaging have been pub-

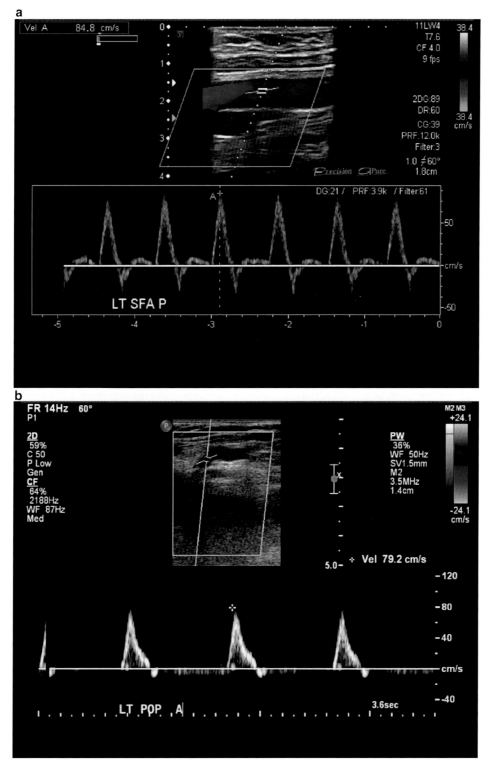

Fig. 19.1 (**a**) Normal triphasic waveform without significant spectral broadening. (**b**) Biphasic waveform with associated spectral broadening consistent with some flow disturbance and arterial irregularity. (**c**) Monophasic waveform with persistent forward diastolic flow and marked spectral broadening. (**d**) Preocclusive "thump" precedes vessel occlusion

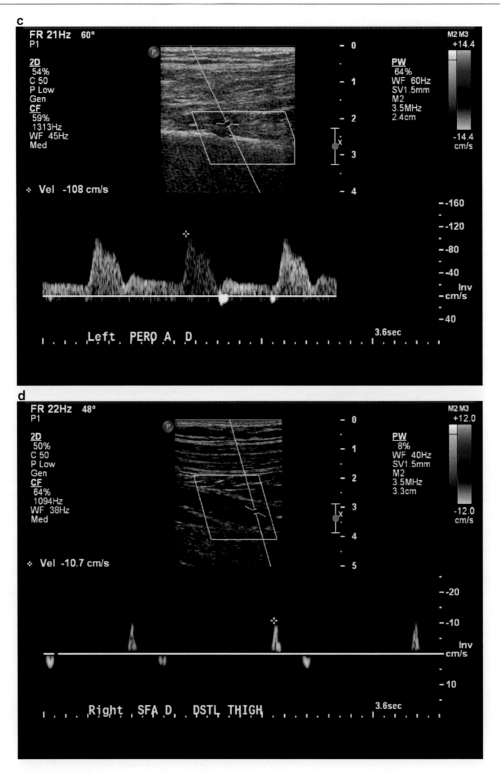

Fig. 19.1 (continued)

lished. Ascher et al. published early experience using DU for preoperative planning. In 466 patients undergoing preoperative evaluation, DU was able to identify optimal inflow and outflow anastomosis sites in 449 procedures without the addition of preoperative DSA [20]. These same authors have since published numerous reports on the use of DU-guided peripheral intervention for occlusive and stenotic disease in the infrainguinal arteries [21–24]. Overall, their reported

Fig. 19.2 (**a** and **b**) Example
of a typical 50–99 % stenosis
in a superficial femoral artery
due to calcified atheromatous
plaque. Note the more than
tripling of velocity, the loss of
diastolic flow reversal, and the
broadening of the acoustic
spectrum all caused by
disturbed flow from vessel
stenosis

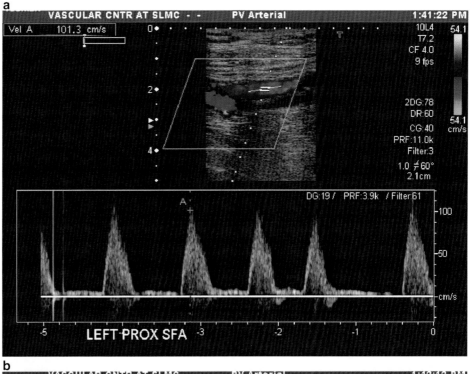

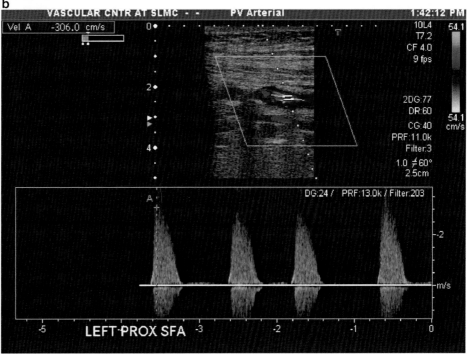

technical success rate is >90 % for patients with CLI and
claudication who were treated with a variety of interventions
including balloon angioplasty and stent placement as well as
subintimal procedures. Reported limb-salvage rates and
12-month patency rates were consistent with those in the literature for similar TASC classifications. The authors

acknowledge the potential benefits related to DU use including avoiding contrast and radiation exposure [21–24].

The use of DU-guided intervention for iliac arteries may be
more challenging because of less accessible anatomic imaging
due to the depth of the vessel, body habitus, and overlying
bowel gas. Krasznai et al. reported their experience using

DU-guided angioplasty and stenting in 35 iliac artery lesions. They reported technical success and clinical improvement in 94 % of treated lesions. The only reported complication was dislodgment of one balloon-mounted stent [25].

Taken in aggregate, the literature suggests that while DU may not be perfectly accurate, when combined with clinical information, the operator should have adequate information to plan and execute an endovascular or bypass procedure in select patients. DU planning and intraoperative use will decrease radiation exposure to the patient and the operator. In patients with contrast allergies or renal disease where avoiding iodinated contrast is necessary, this provides another option for preoperative evaluation and intraoperative imaging for the interventionalist.

Transcutaneous Oximetry

Transcutaneous partial pressure of oxygen (tcPO$_2$) measurement is one method of assessing microvascular perfusion. TcPO$_2$ measures the excess tissue space oxygen that has diffused from the capillary bed into the interstitial space and is not consumed during cellular metabolism. It is a noninvasive measurement of the oxygen delivered to the tissues. The examination is performed using a heated probe (44 °C) which liquefies the crystalline structure of the stratum corneum, allowing for rapid gas diffusion. For wound healing, this should be placed over normal intact skin and as close to the wound as possible, taking care to avoid bony prominences and heavily callused tissue. In most centers, a reference measurement is performed over the anterior chest wall to serve as a baseline. A normal tcPO$_2$ value will usually range from 50–70 mmHg. Studies differ in findings regarding absolute values for wound healing [26]. Most studies suggest measurements >40 mmHg support wound healing while values <20 mmHg are associated with lower rates of wound healing [27, 28]. Additional assessment may be performed using inhaled oxygen to help predict healing [29, 30].

Skin Perfusion Pressure, Near-Infrared Spectroscopy, and Fluorescein Angiography

There are some limitations to the assessment of both macro- and microvascular perfusion at the level of the ankle and foot with the aforementioned noninvasive methods, namely, ankle and toe pressures, PVR, duplex ultrasound, and tcPO$_2$. Calcified vessels do not lend themselves well to occlusion when compressed (the so-called "noncompressible" vessel) which is common to diabetics, the elderly, and patients with chronic kidney disease. Calcification can also limit the visualization of flow within vessels on DU, especially in the infr-

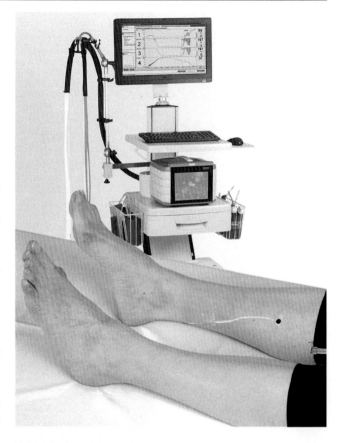

Fig. 19.3 Skin perfusion pressure (SPP) cuff and laser Doppler probe setup. Provided by Perimed Inc., Stockholm, Sweden

apopliteal runoff. Skin lesions and digital amputation can limit the use of toe pressure assessment. Transcutaneous oxygen pressure may be affected by ambient and skin temperature, movement, and patient comfort due to the need to lay flat for long periods of time.

Skin perfusion pressure (SPP) has been well studied and calibrated through multiple studies to provide an indication of the status of the more proximal arterial system of a limb without being effected by arterial wall calcification. Typically, it is calculated using laser Doppler technology which penetrates to a subcutaneous depth of about only 1.5 mm along with inflatable cuffs to determine the capillary opening pressure, most frequently on the dorsal surface of the foot. The laser Doppler probe is conventionally placed below the inflatable cuff where the movement of red blood cells is to be monitored after deflation to assess reactive hyperemia (Fig. 19.3). A retrospective analysis of this technique in 211 patients showed excellent correlation with toe pressure ($r=0.690$) and can be used as a surrogate for the toe pressure [31]. These authors suggested a threshold perfusion pressure of 40 mmHg (which was equivalent to a corresponding great toe pressure of 30 mmHg) as being a significant predictive pressure above which healing could be more accurately predicted. A receiver operating characteristic

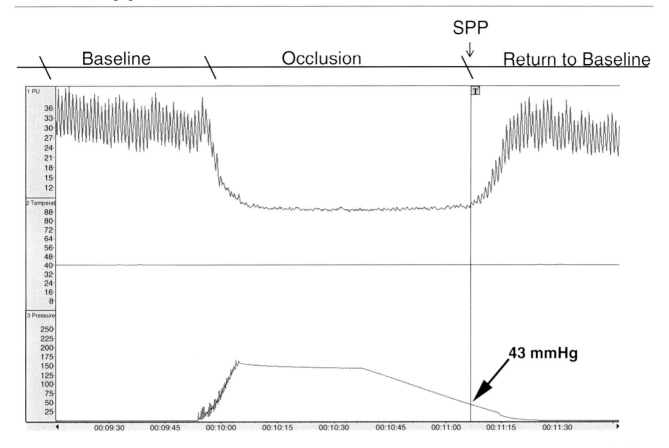

Fig. 19.4 Basic SPP curve showing flux (PU, perfusion units, *blue curve*) which changes with inflation and deflation of the cuff. The SPP is calculated at around 4.5–6 PU (which is 1.5 times the biologic zero flux of 3–4 PU) during the deflation portion of the exam (mmHg, *black curve*). Provided by Perimed Inc., Stockholm, Sweden

(ROC) analysis for predicting wound healing of SPP, ankle pressure, toe pressure, and tcPO₂ showed the greatest area under the curve with SPP and therefore was the most reliable of the four modalities. In a prospective study with 100 patients in 2009, Lo demonstrated that SPP was significantly more accurate in predicting wound healing than tcPO₂ [32]. Technology that supports SPP will often graph other information such as percentage perfusion increase above baseline, total response time, perfusion reappearance time, and perfusion contour (Fig. 19.4).

Near-infrared spectroscopy (NIRS) monitors tissue oxygen delivery, a pathophysiological determinate of the severity of downstream effects of severe PAD and CLI. The percentage of hemoglobin saturated with oxygen can be determined by measuring the pattern of absorption of various near-infrared wavelengths when the light is passed through blood since oxygenated and deoxygenated blood have distinctly different patterns of absorption. Muscle or subcutaneous tissue oxygenation can be determined to estimate blood flow, and several parameters can be followed objectively and have been shown to be significantly different in PAD patients versus controls. For example, in a systematic review of 21 prospective studies, Vardi and Nini outlined eight separate parameters that have been studied with NIRS which can assist in demonstrating the severity of occlusive disease and response to treatment [33]. These parameters can be summarized as those which reflect oxygen consumption and those which measure tissue post-hypoxia re-saturation. Although NIRS is a promising technique to reflect tissue blood flow dynamics, there are no widely agreed-upon parameters or threshold values that reflect correlation to wound healing or reversal of ischemia; therefore, in the words of the review authors, "its utilization is still awaiting refinement."

More recently, fluorescein angiography using indocyanine green (ICG) has been marketed to be available at the bedside in clinics and during surgery which appears to be particularly sensitive to microvascular anatomy (LUNA™ Fluorescence Microangiography System). This modality was studied alongside distal arterial pressure in a study by Wallin et al. in 1989 showing good correlation between the optical density measured over time (slope of the fluorescence density over time curve) and corresponding ankle and toes pressures [34]. In conclusion, the authors postulated that this

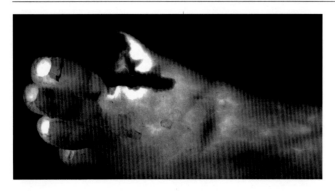

Fig. 19.5 Fluorescein angiogram of an ischemic hallux that resulted in amputation. Note the complete lack of ICG uptake in the hallux. Courtesy of Christopher Attinger and Paul Kim, Georgetown University

modality is particularly useful in patients where ankle or toe pressures are unobtainable or unreliable and the images confer valuable information about the overall anatomic distribution of capillary blood flow to the skin of the foot not obtainable by any other method, including tcPO$_2$ and SPP. The newly marketed LUNA™ technology (Novadaq, USA) utilizes a near-infrared laser and a charge-coupled camera. The clinically safe ICG imaging agent is intravenously injected and bound by plasma protein and distributed throughout the intravascular space. As ICG arrives at the wound area within 3–5 mm of the skin surface, the molecule is excited by near-infrared light emitted from the imaging head. The resulting fluorescence is captured by the camera with real-time imaging along with a quantitative graph of the uptake intensity based on pixel strength (ingress and egress). Since its peripheral vascular debut in 2012, fluorescence angiography use has been mostly in wound care and limb salvage clinics to provide quantitative data and visual information regarding angiosome foot perfusion in order to enhance diagnosis and treatment strategies (Fig. 19.5). A pilot evaluation of the technique in 2013 was studied in 24 CLI patients showing evidence for statistically significant improvement in multiple LUNA™ parameters such as ingress and egress when comparing pre- and post-interventional imaging along with good correlation with ABI and toe pressures [35].

In conclusion, the noninvasive lab can provide rapid, cost-effective valuable information regarding macro- and microvascular perfusion of the critically ischemic limb. This data can be used to assist prediction of healing, to help determine the level of amputation, and to assess the success of revascularization by comparing quantitative and qualitative improvements in post-procedural testing when compared to baseline values. Duplex ultrasound in particular has been shown to offer numerous advantages over other arteriographic modalities in a multitude of applications. Of the modalities mentioned in this chapter, plethysmography, ankle and toe pressures, and duplex ultrasonography have firmly established themselves within the noninvasive vascu-

lar lab and are widely available. Adjunctive data regarding microvascular perfusion and tissue oxygenation has traditionally been quantitatively assessed with transcutaneous oximetry, but given problems with reproducibility, other technologies have emerged to fill this void including laser Doppler, NIRS, and fluorescence angiography. These latter modalities have shown promise in various scenarios for helping to manage patients with ischemic distal limbs and feet and have proven to be particularly effective in diabetics, in patients with extensive vessel calcification, and in those with prior amputation.

References

1. Zierler RE. Nonimaging physiologic tests for assessment of lower extremity arterial occlusive disease. In: Zwiebel WJ, Pellerito JS, editors. Introduction to vascular ultrasonography. 5th ed. Philadelphia: Elsevier; 2005. p. 275–95.
2. Ka J, Martin PRL, Hanson C, Roederer GO, Langlois YE, et al. Noninvasive mapping of lower limb arterial lesions. Ultrasound Med Biol. 1985;11:515–21.
3. Moneta GL, Yeager RA, Antonovic R, Hall LD, Caster JD, et al. Accuracy of lower extremity arterial duplex mapping. J Vasc Surg. 1992;15:275–84.
4. Hirsch AT, Haskal ZJ, Hertzer NR, Bakal CW, Creager MA, et al. ACC/AHA 2005 practice guidelines for the management of patients with peripheral arterial disease (lower extremity, renal, mesenteric, and abdominal aortic): a collaborative report from the American Association for Vascular Surgery/Society for Vascular Surgery, Society for Cardiovascular Angiography and Interventions, Society for Vascular Medicine and Biology, Society for Interventional Radiology, and the ACC/AHA Task Force on Practice Guidelines (Writing committee to develop guidelines for the management of patients with peripheral arterial disease): endorsed by the American Association of Cardiovascular and Pulmonary Rehabilitation; National Heart, Lung, and Blood Institute; Society for Vascular Nursing; TransAtlantic Inter-Society Consensus; and Vascular Disease Foundation. Circulation 2006;113:e463–654.
5. Sultan S, Tawfick W, Hynes N. Ten-year technical and clinical outcomes in TransAtlantic Inter-Society Consensus II infrainguinal C/D lesions using duplex ultrasound arterial mapping as the sole imaging modality for critical lower limb ischemia. J Vasc Surg. 2013;57:1038–45.
6. Lujan S, Criado E, Puras E, Izquierdo LM. Duplex scanning or arteriography for preoperative planning of lower limb revascularization. Eur J Vasc Endovasc Surg. 2002;24:31–6.
7. Ascher E, Hingorani A, Markevich N, Schutzer R, Kallakuri S. Acute lower limb ischemia: the value of duplex ultrasound arterial mapping (DUAM) as the sole preoperative imaging technique. Ann Vasc Surg. 2003;17:284–9.
8. Cao P, Eckstein HH, DeRango P, Setacci C, Ricco JB, et al. Chapter II: diagnostic methods. Eur J Vasc Endovasc Surg. 2011; 42(S2):S13–32.
9. Gerhard-Herman M, Gardin JM, Jaff M, Mohler E, Roman M, et al. Guidelines for noninvasive vascular laboratory testing: a report from the American society of echocardiography and the society for vascular medicine and biology. J Am Soc Echocardiogr. 2006;19:955–72.
10. Hingorani AP, Ascher E, Marks N. Duplex arteriography for lower extremity revascularization. Perspect Vasc Surg Endovasc Ther. 2007;19:6–20.

11. Eiberg JP, Hansen MA, Gronvall Rasmussen JB, Schroeder TV. Minimum training requirement in ultrasound imaging of peripheral arterial disease. Eur J Vasc Endovasc Surg. 2008;36:325–30.

12. Visser K, Bosch JL, Leiner T, van Engelshoven JMA, Passchier J, et al. Patients' preferences for MR angiography and duplex US in the work-up of peripheral arterial disease. Eur J Vasc Endovasc Surg. 2003;26:537–43.

13. De Vos MS, Bol BJ, Gravereaux EC, Hamming JF, Nguyen LL. Treatment planning for peripheral arterial disease based on duplex ultrasonography and computed tomography angiography: consistency confidence and the value of additional imaging. Surgery. 2014;156:492–502.

14. Leiner T, Kessels AGH, Nelemans PJ, Vasbinder GBC, de Haan MW, et al. Peripheral arterial disease: comparison of color duplex US and contrast-enhanced MR angiography for diagnosis. Radiology. 2005;235:699–708.

15. Bueno A, Acin F, Canibano C, Fernandez-Casado JL, Castillo E. Diagnostic accuracy of contrast-enhanced magnetic resonance angiography and duplex ultrasound in patients with peripheral vascular disease. Vasc Endovasc Surg. 2010;44:576–85.

16. Lowery AJ, Hynes N, Manning BJ, Mahendran M, Tawfik S, et al. A prospective feasibility study of duplex ultrasound arterial mapping, digital-subtraction angiography, and magnetic resonance angiography in management of critical lower limb ischemia by endovascular revascularization. Ann Vasc Surg. 2007;21:443–51.

17. Sidhu PS, Allan PL, Cattin F, Cosgrove DO, Davies AH, et al. Diagnostic efficacy of SonoVue, a second generation contrast agent, in the assessment of extracranial carotid or peripheral arteries using colour and spectral doppler ultrasound: a multicenter study. Br J Radiol. 2006;79:44–51.

18. Eiberg JP, Hansen MA, Jensen F, Gronvall Rasmussen JB, Schroder TV. Ultrasound contrast-agent improves imaging of lower limb occlusive disease. Eur J Vasc Endovasc Surg. 2003;25:23–8.

19. Aschwanden M, Partovi S, Jacobi B, Fergus N, Schulte AC, et al. Assessing the end-organ in peripheral arterial occlusive disease – from contrast-enhanced ultrasound to blood-oxygen-level-dependent MR imaging. Cardiovasc Diagn Ther. 2014;4:165–72.

20. Ascher E, Hingorani A, Markevich N, Costa T, Kallakuri S, et al. Lower extremity revascularization without preoperative contrast angiography: experience with duplex ultrasound arterial mapping in 485 cases. Ann Vasc Surg. 2002;16:108–14.

21. Ascher E, Marks N, Schutzer RW, Hingorani AP. Duplex-guided balloon angioplasty and stenting for femoropopliteal arterial occlusive disease: an alternative in patients with renal insufficiency. J Vasc Surg. 2005;42:1108–13.

22. Ascher E, Marks N, Hingorani AP, Schutzer RW, Nahata S. Duplex-guided balloon angioplasty and subintimal dissection of infrapopliteal arteries: early results with a new approach to avoid radiation exposure and contrast material. J Vasc Surg. 2005;42:1114–21.

23. Ascher E, Marks N, Hingorani AP, Schutzer RW, Mutyala M. Duplex-guided endovascular treatment for occlusive and stenotic lesions of the femoral-popliteal arterial segment: a comparative study in the first 253 cases. J Vasc Surg. 2006;44:1230–8.

24. Ascher E, Hingorani AP, Marks N. Duplex-guided balloon angioplasty of lower extremity arteries. Perspect Vasc Surg Endovasc Ther. 2007;19:23–31.

25. Krasznai AG, Sigterman TA, Welten RJ, Heijboer R, Sikkink CJJM, et al. Duplex-guided percutaneous transluminal angioplasty in iliac arterial occlusive disease. Eur J Vasc Endovasc Surg. 2013;46:583–7.

26. Arsenault KA, McDonald J, Devereaux PJ, Thorlund K, Tittley JG, et al. The use of transcutaneous oximetry to predict complications of chronic wound healing: a systematic review and meta-analysis. Wound Repair Regen. 2011;19:657–83.

27. Ladurner R, Kuper M, Konigsrainer I, Lob S, Wichmann D, et al. Predictive value of routine transcutaneous tissue oxygen tension ($tcpO_2$) measurement for the risk of non-healing and amputation in diabetic foot ulcer patients with non-palpable pedal pulses. Med Sci Monit. 2010;16:CR273–7.

28. Ruangsetakit C, Chinsakchai K, Mahawongkajit P, Wongwanit C, Mutirangura P. Transcutaneous oxygen tension: a useful predictor of ulcer healing in critical limb ischemia. J Wound Care. 2010;19:202–6.

29. Fife CE, Buyukcakir C, Otto GH, Sheffield PJ, Warriner RA, et al. The predictive value of transcutaneous oxygen tension measurement in diabetic lower extremity ulcers treated with hyperbaric oxygen therapy: a retrospective analysis of 1144 patients. Wound Repair Regen. 2002;10:198–207.

30. Fife CE, Smart DR, Sheffield PJ, Hopf HW, Hawkins G, et al. Transcutaneous oximetry in clinical practice: consensus statements from an expert panel based on evidence. Undersea Hyperb Med. 2009;36:43–53.

31. Yamada T, Ohta T, Ishibashi H, et al. Clinical reliability and utility of skin perfusion pressure measurement in ischemic limbs – comparison with other noninvasive diagnostic methods. J Vasc Surg. 2008;47:318–23.

32. Lo T, Sample R, Moore P, Gold P. Prediction of wound healing outcome using skin perfusion pressure and transcutaneous oximetry: a single center experience in 100 patients. Wounds. 2009; 21:310.

33. Vardi M, Nini A. Near-infrared spectroscopy for evaluation of peripheral vascular disease. A systematic review of literature. Eur J Endovasc Surg. 2008;35:68–74.

34. Wallin L, Lund F, Westling H. Fluorescein angiography and distal arterial pressure in patients with arterial disease of the legs. Clin Pysiol. 1989;9:467–80.

35. Braun JD, Trinidad-Hernandez M, Perry D, Armstrong DG, Mills JL. Early quantitative evaluation of indocyanine green angiography in patients with critical limb ischemia. J Vasc Surg 2013;57: 1213–8.

36. Kappert A. Lehrbuch und Atlas der Angiologie. 10th ed. Bern: Huber; 1998.

Sohail Ikram and Prafull Raheja

Critical Limb Ischemia

Critical limb ischemia (CLI) refers to a condition due to severe obstruction of the peripheral arteries which markedly reduces blood flow to the extremities characterized by chronic ischemic at-rest pain, ulcers, or gangrene in one or both extremities and objectively proven arterial occlusive disease. Critical limb ischemia implies chronicity and is to be distinguished from acute limb ischemia. The incidence of CLI is approximately 500–1000 per million years, with the highest rates among older subjects, smokers, and diabetics. The rate of primary amputation has been reported to be in the range of 10–40 % and was performed only when there were no distal vessels for grafting or in patients with neurologic impairment [1].

In a study with a population of age more than 65 years with intermittent claudication followed over 5 years, 5–10 % subjects developed CLI, out of which approximately 5 % required amputation [2].

CLI, the most severe form of peripheral arterial disease (PAD), does not always follow a systematic progression from asymptomatic phase to exercise pain to rest pain and finally to tissue damage. It can present anytime during these various clinical stages.

Patients with critical limb ischemia have an elevated risk of cardiovascular events, stroke, and vascular death. In a study comprising of patients with PAD from Mayo Clinic, survival rate was 75 % at 5 years and 50 % at 10 years, and three fourths of deaths were attributed to cardiovascular causes [3].

CLI is a major public health issue due to the significant impact it has on the quality of life and the grim prognosis it carries both in terms of limb salvage and survival.

Invasive Imaging Modalities in Critical Limb Ischemia

Angiography

Invasive angiography remains the gold standard for the diagnosis of critical limb ischemia. Noninvasive vascular imaging studies, e.g., duplex ultrasonography, computed tomographic angiography, and magnetic resonance angiography, are also frequently utilized. Angiography with concomitant potential for ad hoc endovascular intervention offers an attractive option with reduced morbidity, especially in high-risk patients with coexisting coronary artery disease. Endovascular intervention can restore antegrade flow and aids in the healing of ischemic ulcers. It can also move the level of amputations more distally resulting in less morbidity.

Invasive angiography can be performed using small 4–6 F catheters with adequate visualization. To assess the lower extremities, access can be obtained from contralateral common femoral artery (CFA) (Fig. 20.1), antegrade ipsilateral CFA, radial artery, brachial artery, and rarely axillary artery. Contralateral arterial access and crossover remains the most utilized technique. In CLI patients, depending on the site of obstruction, catheter should be placed proximal to the lesion in order to visualize the collaterals, followed by selective stepwise angiogram (Figs. 20.2 and 20.3). Contralateral 30° angle during angiography will help visualize the iliac bifurcations, and ipsilateral 30° will open up the vessel below the external iliac artery.

Access can usually be obtained by feeling the femoral pulsations against the femoral head. If the pulse is not palpable due to severe disease or morbid obesity, access can be

S. Ikram, MBBS (✉)
Invasive and Interventional Cardiology and Peripheral Vascular Interventions, School of Medicine, University of Louisville, 550 South Jackson St., Ambulatory Care Building, Louisville, KY 40202, USA

P. Raheja, MBBS
Interventional Cardiology, Department of Medicine, School of Medicine, University of Louisville, Louisville, KY, USA

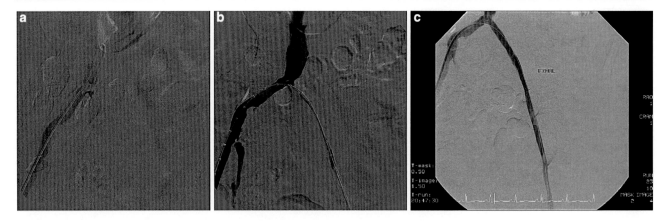

Fig. 20.1 Example of peripheral angiography in CLI: (**a**) Iliac occlusion, (**b**) sizing after first stent deployment, (**c**) final result after stent

achieved under fluoroscopy using the bony land marks. The use of ultrasound has also been suggested in identifying the femoral artery, especially for antegrade access. A recent study comparing the time for antegrade common femoral artery access and safety between the ultrasound-guided access versus fluoroscopy-guided access showed that ultrasound-directed common femoral artery access was faster and safer [4]. Also, in a recent multicenter randomized controlled trial, routine real-time ultrasound-guided access improved common femoral artery cannulation in patients with high CFA bifurcations and also showed reduced number of attempts, less time to access, decreased risk of venipunctures, and less vascular complications [5]. During antegrade CFA access, ultrasound-guided technique is faster and safer compared to fluoroscopic technique.

In addition to defining the arterial anatomy, angiography can usually distinguish between two most common causes for CLI, i.e., atherothrombosis and embolism. Thrombus usually appears as sharp or tapered but not a rounded cutoff on angiography. Diffuse atherosclerosis along with collateral circulation is generally visualized too. An embolus usually has a sharp cutoff with a rounded reverse meniscus sign. An embolus may also be visible as an intraluminal filling defect if the vessel is not completely occluded. The presence of otherwise normal vessels, the absence of collateral circulation, and the presence of multiple filling defects are also signs of embolic phenomenon.

Carbon Dioxide (CO₂)-Mediated Angiography

Iodinated contrast is most commonly used for angiography. Carbon dioxide (CO_2)-mediated angiography is utilized when there is coexistent chronic kidney disease in patients with PAD to decrease the risk of contrast induced nephropathy (CIN). CO_2 angiography can also be utilized in patients with iodine contrast allergy. Due to a risk of embolism related to CO_2, it should be utilized with caution, especially

if used for vessels above the diaphragm. In a recent prospective multicenter registry, the safety and efficacy of CO_2 angiography-guided endovascular therapy for renal and iliofemoral artery disease was assessed. Patients with an estimated glomerular filtration rate (eGFR) of <60 mL/min/ and stage 3 CKD were enrolled. Incomplete CO_2 angiograms were supplemented by intravascular ultrasound, pressure wire, and/or minimal iodinated contrast media. The primary endpoint was a composite of freedom from renal events and freedom from major CO_2 angiography-related complications. The study included 98 patients with 109 lesions. The mean eGFR at baseline was 35.2 ± 12.7 mL/min. The technical success rate was 97.9%. The primary endpoint was achieved in 92.8% (91/98) patients. Incidence of CIN was 5.1%, and CO_2 angiography-related total complications occurred in 17.3% patients including leg pain, abdominal pain, and diarrhea, and two patients developed severe, fatal, nonocclusive mesenteric ischemia.

CO_2 angiography-guided angioplasty was effective for preventing CIN; however, CO_2 angiography-related complications are high [6]. All patients undergoing CO_2 angiography should be monitored with ECG and pulse oximetry; blood pressure, respiratory rate, and heart rate should also be monitored. Capnograms should be obtained if the patient is intubated.

Intravascular Ultrasound (IVUS)

Intravascular ultrasound is a well-established invasive imaging modality in vascular imaging and interventions; however, its use is much more commonplace in coronary vasculature.

Standard angiography is limited in providing information only about the contour of the vascular lumen. Hazy angiographic lesions observed during standard angiography could represent an irregular plaque, distorted lumen, thrombus, calcification, or a dissection. IVUS is helpful in differen-

Fig. 20.2 Example of peripheral angiography in CLI. (**a, b**) SFA long occlusion, (**c**) angioplasty/ stenting with filter, (**d**) final result

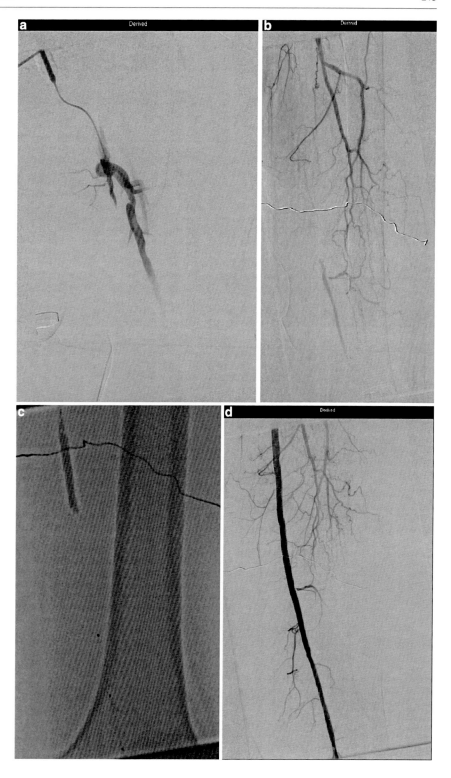

tiating in these ambiguous situations [7]. Plaque morphology, components of the vascular wall, sizing of the vessel, and extent of disease are accurately visualized with IVUS. IVUS can also differentiate between a ruptured plaque, in-stent thrombosis, and in-stent restenosis [8]. IVUS is therefore helpful in diagnosing, planning, and optimizing interventional strategies.

The frequencies of IVUS catheters used in peripheral imaging are chosen depending on the vessel involved. 10–40 MHz transducers are available for peripheral imaging. Low-frequency transducers (usually around 15 MHz) are used for aortoiliac disease, and 30 MHz are used for femoral, SFA, and infrapopliteal vessels. Low-frequency transducers usually require 8 F sheaths, while the high frequency transducers are

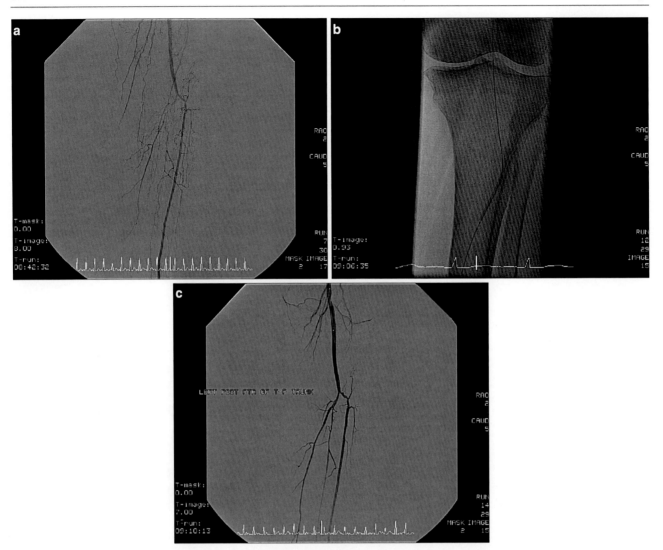

Fig. 20.3 Example of peripheral angiography in CLI. (**a**) Tibioperoneal trunk occlusion, (**b**) angioplasty and, (**c**) final result after angioplasty

similar to coronary system and can be accommodated in 6 F sheaths. During IVUS image acquisition, moving blood appears black with occasional white speckles from the red blood cells. Calcified plaque and stagnated blood will appear bright white. Darker gray color represents tissue with more water or lipid content, while lighter shades represent fibrous tissue. IVUS has higher resolution and provides cross-sectional images of both plaque and lumen. Calcification and ulceration are readily observed during IVUS. The ability of IVUS to delineate plaque morphology helps in CLI, as it can differentiate between thrombus and dissection. Thrombus appears as an echogenicity in the lumen, which is usually layered, but can be of different shapes. Dissection appears as disruption in the vessel wall [9]. In CLI with layered thrombus, it becomes relatively difficult to size the vessel with standard angiography alone. IVUS aids in planning the intervention with lumen sizing, lesion morphology, and length. IVUS helps to define extensive calcification in a lesion causing CLI, thus aiding in

the best strategy of revascularization. Also post-intervention, IVUS in many studies has been proven to detect inapparent dissections, stent under-expansion, residual lesions, and thrombus that are further treated as required [10–12]. IVUS-aided interventions have shown to have better patency rates compared to angiography alone [13].

Optical Coherence Tomography (OCT)

OCT works on the reflection of light in the infrared wavelength zone to obtain cross-sectional images of the tissue. Its use in coronary vasculature is increasing and has indications similar to the ones established for IVUS [9]. The resolution of OCT is higher than IVUS as the bandwidth of the infrared light and the wave velocity used are of higher magnitude than in ultrasound. OCT images are displayed similar to IVUS as cross-sectional views of the vessel. Majority of the OCT work has been done in coronary vasculature, and relatively fewer studies have used OCT in peripheral vasculature.

Intracoronary OCT is performed by introducing a small (2.7 French) imaging catheter over a guide wire (0.014 in.) distally into the vessel of interest using standard guide catheters (6 F or larger). The pullback speed is around 20 mm/s with a frame rate of 100 frames per second or higher. During OCT imaging, it is prudent to temporarily clear the blood within the vessel, as otherwise it causes scattering of the OCT signal. An injection of X-ray contrast medium during the duration of the OCT pullback is used to clear the blood. A variety of solutions, warmed to 37 °C, have been used alternatively as flush medium, including Lactated Ringer's and mixtures of Lactated Ringer's and contrast media or low molecular weight dextrose. OCT is limited in assessing ostial disease as it is difficult to clear the vessel from blood with a nonselective guide catheter position, required for complete visualization of the ostium. OCT can detect early atherosclerosis, necrotic core or lipid-rich tissues, thrombi, and calcifications. OCT, with its high resolution, allows one to visualize stented vessels in greater detail than IVUS [14]. In a prospective study comparing OCT and IVUS in 112 popliteal and infrapopliteal arterial segments, OCT imaging of infrapopliteal arteries was feasible and safe, and accurate assessment of vessel lumen, wall, and plaque was achieved [15]. OCT has been reported as a safe and feasible imaging modality during femoropopliteal angioplasty procedures [16].

Summary

Invasive angiography remains the gold standard for the diagnosis of CLI. Noninvasive modalities, e.g., CT angiography and MRI, are very useful in situations where comorbid conditions outweigh the benefits of invasive approach. Sophisticated imaging modalities, e.g., IVUs and OCT, are more useful in delineating ambiguous lesions and in aiding optimal endovascular interventions.

References

1. Novo S, Coppola G, Milio G. Critical limb ischemia: definition and natural history. Curr Drug Targets Cardiovasc Haematol Disord. 2004;4(3):219–25.

2. Meru AV, Mittra S, Thyagarajan B, et al. Intermittent claudication: an overview. Atherosclerosis. 2006;187:231–7.

3. Juergens JE, Parker NW, Hines EA. Arteriosclerosis obliterans: review of 520 cases with special references to pathogenic and prognostic factors. Circulation. 1960;21:188–95.

4. Slattery MM, Goh GS, Power S, Given MF, McGrath FP, Lee MJ. Comparison of ultrasound-guided and fluoroscopy-assisted antegrade common femoral artery puncture techniques. Cardiovascular Intervent Radiol. 2015;38(3):579–82.

5. Seto AH, Abu-Fadel MS, Sparling JM, et al. Real-time ultrasound guidance facilitates femoral arterial access and reduces vascular complications: FAUST (femoral arterial access with ultrasound trial). JACC Cardiovasc Interv. 2010;3(7):751–8. doi:10.1016/j.jcin.2010.04.015.

6. Fujihara MI, Kawasaki D, Shintani Y, et al. on behalf of the CO_2 Angiography Investigators. Endovascular therapy by CO_2 angiography to prevent contrast-induced nephropathy in patients with chronic kidney disease: a prospective multicenter trial of CO_2 angiography registry. Catheter Cardiovasc Interv. 2014. doi:10.1002/ccd.25722. [Epub ahead of print]

7. Ziada KM, Tuzcu EM, De Franco AC, et al. Intravascular ultrasound assessment of the prevalence and causes of angiographic "haziness" following high-pressure coronary stenting. Am J Cardiol. 1997;80:116.

8. Di Mario C, Gorge G, Peters R, et al. Clinical application and image interpretation in intracoronary ultrasound. Euro Heart J. 1998;19:207–29.

9. Mintz GS, Pichard AD, Kovach JA, et al. American college of cardiology clinical expert consensus document on standards for acquisition, measurement and reporting of IVUS. J Am Coll Cardiol. 2001;37:1478–92.

10. Arko F, McCollough R, Manning L, et al. Use of Intravascular ultrasound in the endovascular management of atherosclerotic aortoiliac occlusive disease. Am J Surg. 1996;172:546–9.

11. Buckely CJ, Arko FR, Lee S, et al. Intravascular ultrasound scanning improves long tern patency of iliac lesions treated with balloon angioplasty and primary stenting. J Vasc Surg. 2002;35:316–23.

12. Navarro F, Sullivan TM, Bacharach JM. Intravascular ultrasound assessment of iliac stent procedures. J Endovasc Ther. 2000;7:315–9.

13. Iida O, Takahara M, Soga Y, et al. Efficacy of intravascular ultrasound in femoropopliteal stenting for peripheral artery disease with TASC II class A to C lesions. J Endovasc Ther. 2014;21(4):485–92. doi:10.1583/14-4721R.1.

14. Bouma BE, Tearney GJ, Yabushita H, et al. Evaluation of intracoronary stenting by intravascular optical coherence tomography. Heart. 2003;89:317.

15. Eberhardt KM, Treitl M, Boesenecker K, et al. Prospective evaluation of optical coherence tomography in lower limb arteries compared with intravascular ultrasound. J Vasc Interv Radiol. 2013;24(10):1499–508.

16. Karnabatidis D, Katsanos K, Paraskevopoulos I, et al. Frequency-domain intravascular optical coherence tomography of the femoropopliteal artery. Cardiovasc Intervent Radiol. 2011;34(6):1172–81.

Vascular Trauma to the Extremity: Diagnosis and Management

Julia M. Boll, Andrew J. Dennis, and Elizabeth Gwinn

Introduction

The management of vascular injury is a common component in trauma care. Prior to the 1950s, the acute management of peripheral vascular injury largely centered on arterial and venous ligation primarily due to high rates of infection and secondary hemorrhage that often followed attempts at complex vascular repairs. Poor outcomes were common with amputation rates being very high. With the advent of improved suture material, blood banking, antibiotics, anticoagulation, and advanced vascular surgery techniques, primary repair of injured vessels became more common, and surgeons began to explore the possibility of arterial reconstruction in the face of limb trauma. Following the Korean and Vietnam wars, continued advances and improved techniques in the treatment of traumatic limb ischemia reduced amputation rates to less than 10–15 % [1]. Due to the advances in body armor and the commonality of improvised explosive devices, the rate of vascular injury in both the Afghanistan and Iraqi Freedom wars has been estimated to be five times the frequency seen in previously reported combat situations [2]. This increase in pathology has led to significant advances in the way surgeons approach vascular trauma, the most notable of which being the introduction of endovascular therapies into the arsenal of treatment techniques. This chapter reviews current management of critical limb ischemia secondary to trauma, including presentation concerns, diagnostic modalities, and treatment strategies.

Mechanism of Injury

Peripheral vascular injury secondary to trauma predominantly occurs in males between the ages of 20–40 years old. Overall, civilian trauma causes more upper extremity vascular injuries than lower, in contrast to military trauma, which predominantly affects the lower extremities. An important initial step in the treatment of extremity vascular trauma is to identify the mechanism of injury. The mechanism, be it blunt, low- or high-velocity penetrating, or explosive, is critical to not only planning the initial method of reconstruction, but can also impact and predict the subsequent secondary injuries that frequently accompany limb trauma. The overwhelming majority of peripheral vascular traumatic injuries are secondary to penetrating and explosive trauma both in the civilian and military sectors. However, blunt mechanisms occur in greater proportion in civilians, especially in rural areas [1]. In the civilian sector, gunshot wounds account for 64 % of penetrating trauma, knife wounds 24 %, and shotguns 12 %. Vascular injury in the setting of bullet trauma can occur from blast effect, fragmentation by the projectile or by damaged bone, or from massive disruption of soft tissues. Blunt injury to the peripheral vasculature typically occurs secondary to major extremity trauma and fractures from motor vehicle crashes or falls.

Blunt trauma most commonly injures the iliac, internal carotid, and brachial arteries as well as the thoracic aorta. Penetrating trauma most commonly injures the brachial arteries or the superficial femoral arteries [3]. Mortality is more common with injuries to the common femoral or superficial femoral arteries, and mortality rate decreases as injuries occur more distally. Penetrating injuries are associated with a higher rate of mortality than blunt injuries; however, blunt injuries are associated with a 9.1 % amputation rate, while penetrating injuries carry a lower 5.1 % amputation rate [4].

J.M. Boll, MD (✉)
Department of General Surgery, John H. Stroger Hospital
of Cook County, Rush University Medical Center,
Chicago, IL 60611, USA

A.J. Dennis, DO
Surgery, Division of Pre-Hospital and Emergency Trauma
Services, Department of Trauma and Burn, JSH Cook County
Hospital, Rush Medical College, Chicago, IL, USA

E. Gwinn, MD
Department of Trauma and Burn, JSH Cook County Hospital,
Chicago, IL, USA

© Springer International Publishing Switzerland 2017
R.S. Dieter et al. (eds.), *Critical Limb Ischemia*, DOI 10.1007/978-3-319-31991-9_21

Prehospital Evaluation

Prehospital evaluation of vascular injuries is important, as delay in diagnosis and time to revascularization are recognized as the two most critical factors in determining outcomes. The National Trauma Data Bank reports a 2.8 % mortality rate for patients with isolated lower extremity traumatic arterial injuries, and this group of patients has a 6.5 % risk of lower extremity amputation secondary to their injuries [4]. Although civilian trauma statistics do not provide exact numbers for prehospital mortalities caused by extremity exsanguination, case and anecdotal reports indicate that a small percentage of people die each year from isolated extremity trauma, although fatalities from extremity trauma are much more common in military settings [1, 5]. Optimal management of patients in the field requires triage skills and planning to prevent hemorrhagic death. Immediate airway control needs to be obtained, as well as good vascular access. The patient must be fully examined to determine the site of external hemorrhage, and this should be controlled by direct pressure, pressure dressing, or tourniquet when possible.

Tourniquet Use

Prehospital tourniquet use is one of the more controversial topics in the trauma community. Despite the potential advantages of using tourniquets in a prehospital setting to control extremity hemorrhage, their use has been debated due to their potential complications. The debate over tourniquet use began in the Civil War as surgeons started seeing ischemic complications secondary to their placement. Conversely, many argue that tourniquets still confer the benefit of saving lives that may otherwise have been lost from uncontrolled hemorrhage [6].

Controversy exists because the use of tourniquets has long been feared in the civilian world due to concern over improper use. Serious complications can arise if tourniquets are left in place too long, resulting in limb ischemia, muscle injury, nerve deficits, gangrene, and even amputation (Table 21.1).

These unfortunate side effects are inherent in the physiology behind how and why a tourniquet works. They function by radially compressing muscle and soft tissues that surround extremity artery and veins. This then compresses the lumens

of these vessels to completely arrest distal flow both into and out of the extremity. Generally, the risks increase in limbs with larger circumference, given that this correlates with a higher tension required to stop arterial flow.

Prolonged tourniquet application more than 1.5–2 h can result in tourniquet palsy or tourniquet paralysis from injury to extremity muscles or nerves. Overall tourniquet time is important because it has been shown in animal studies that while after 1 h, little to no muscle damage was seen, 2 h of tourniquet time led to elevated levels of lactic acid and CPK, suggesting some degree of muscle damage, and 3 h or more led to myonecrosis of the muscles directly beneath the tourniquet. Nerve injuries have been reported after only 30 min of tourniquet time. Irreversible ischemic damage occurs after 6 h of tourniquet placement, and in this case, amputation of a limb above the level of tourniquet placement is routinely recommended. The less severe phenomenon known as post-tourniquet syndrome is a clinical entity comprised of extremity weakness, paresthesias, pallor, and stiffness. This constellation of symptoms is common after any length of tourniquet placement but seems to resolve in around 3 weeks [7].

Tourniquets are also associated with venous complications. They are a known cause of venous thromboembolism due to the venous stasis that occurs during their use, and these clots have the potential to embolize once the tourniquet is removed. Paradoxically, inappropriate usage when arterial injury does not exist can actually increase extremity bleeding by occluding venous return while not completely arresting arterial flow [8].

Despite this seemingly daunting list of complications, the military success and lives saved attributed to tourniquets are noteworthy as limb loss and limb trauma due to explosive injuries are so common. In this setting, military individuals, who are well trained in tourniquet use, demonstrate an associated complication rate less than 2 % [9]. Hence, contemporary EMS training now embraces the use of tourniquets in the right circumstances. Tourniquet use also has application in the use of mass casualty triage where EMS personnel can stop extremity hemorrhage in patients quickly and effectively and then move on to other victims who also require prompt attention. Guidelines regarding proper tourniquet application are evolving and vary among regions (Table 21.2). The pervasive rule,

Table 21.1 Complications of tourniquets

Local	Systemic
Postoperative swelling/stiffness	Hypertension
Neuropraxia	Increased central venous pressure
Muscle injury/paralysis	Venous thrombosis
Direct vascular injury	Changes in acid–base status
Soft tissue necrosis	Rhabdomyolysis
Compartment syndrome	Fibrinolysis

Table 21.2 Principles of tourniquet application

1. Set at the lowest effective pressure to stop hemorrhage
2. Minimize the tourniquet time to ideally <2 h
3. Apply the tourniquet early to minimize hemorrhage
4. Closely monitor hemorrhage control and extremity viability
5. Keep record of tourniquet time
6. Wider tourniquets or side-by-side tourniquets minimize tissue damage

Modified from Sambasivan CN, Schreiber MA. Emerging therapies in traumatic hemorrhage control. *Curr Opin Crit Care.* 2009;15(6):560–8

however, remains that tourniquet time should be minimized whenever possible and that total application time should not exceed more than 2 h [6–9]. In the civilian setting where transport times are typically short, prolonged placement of a tourniquet should be of little issue. On the contrary, in rural settings where transport times can be prolonged, the use of tourniquets remains controversial due to increased associated risks and guidelines must be established.

The safest tourniquets are made of uniform, smooth material with rounded, rather than sharp, edges, and wider devices are more effective. Pneumatic tourniquets such as blood pressure cuffs provide a more uniform pressure over a wide area, but their use is limited by their inability to maintain high pressures for long periods of time. The pneumatic tourniquet used by many surgeons today was developed in 1904 and has the advantage over previous versions of providing more uniform pressure around a limb, as well as being easier to place and remove. Surgical tourniquets should be placed over the thickest portion of the affected limb in order to maximize the amount of tissue through which pressure is exerted. This is contrary to military and EMS tourniquets which should be placed in close proximity to the wound as to preserve maximal limb length in the event limb loss occurs at the level of the tourniquet. Proximal placement of tourniquets allows for speed of application, minimization of pressure injury, and better hemorrhage control in the event that multiple distal bleeding sites exist [7–10].

In 2014, the American College of Surgeons Committee on Trauma convened a panel of nationally recognized experts in prehospital trauma care to develop an algorithm for prehospital external hemorrhage control recommendations (Fig. 21.1). Generally, based on the evidence for survival benefits, they strongly recommended the use of tourniquets in the prehospital setting when direct pressure is ineffective or impractical. The panel also suggested against releasing a tourniquet properly applied in the field before the patient reaches definitive care; however, the evidence for this recommendation was less strong [10].

It has been common teaching that once a tourniquet is placed, it should be left in place until assessment by a physician, regardless of the "tourniquet time." This is due to the relatively short transport times seen with most emergency medical services; however, it is also acceptable for reassessment and possible de-escalation to a pressure dressing, should circumstances permit. This has significant relevance in the tactical and triage arena where an extreme early intervention was chosen but when circumstances permit may, in fact, be medically excessive [7]. Typically "reperfusion intervals" wherein the tourniquet is released are not effective at reducing complications unless perfusion is restored for a full 30 min or more. However, this could potentially lead to life-threatening exsanguination, so proposed algorithms have been created that can help determine the ongoing need for a tourniquet or if removal is a possibility (Fig. 21.2) [11].

In general, safe prehospital tourniquet use depends on a number of factors, including tourniquet design, placement location, tourniquet tightness, and tourniquet time. Fundamentally, for tourniquet use to gain more widespread acceptance, specific protocols need to be set in place, and regular training on these protocols for prehospital providers is required.

Fig. 21.1 Prehospital external hemorrhage control algorithm

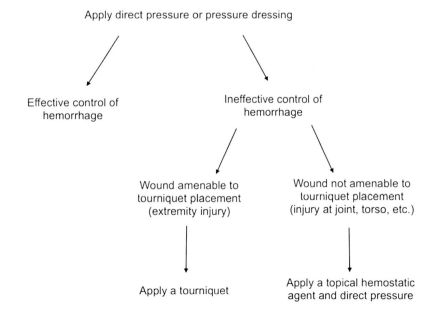

PRE-HOSPITAL EXTERNAL HEMORRHAGE CONTROL

Apply direct pressure or pressure dressing

Effective control of hemorrhage

Ineffective control of hemorrhage

Wound amenable to tourniquet placement (extremity injury)

Wound not amenable to tourniquet placement (injury at joint, torso, etc.)

Apply a tourniquet

Apply a topical hemostatic agent and direct pressure

PRE-HOSPITAL TOURNIQUET USE ALGORITHM

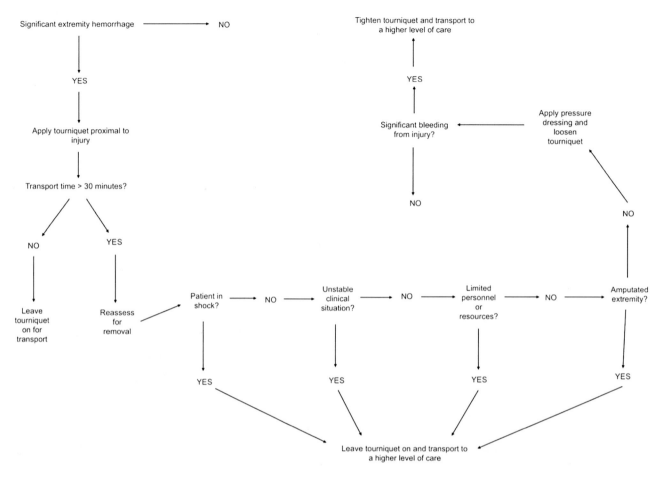

Fig. 21.2 Prehospital tourniquet use algorithm

Presentation of Injury

When a patient arrives to the trauma unit with suspected extremity vascular trauma, it is of utmost importance to first address any airway compromise or breathing difficulties and implement resuscitation in accordance with Advanced Trauma Life Support (ATLS). Simultaneously, active ongoing life-threatening hemorrhage must be addressed. Hemorrhagic shock is a common consequence of any extremity vascular trauma, making resuscitation and support of organ perfusion of vital importance. Following this assessment, physical exam should be performed to assess for hard signs of arterial injury, such as obvious pulsatile bleeding, absent peripheral pulses, a rapidly enlarging hematoma, or a clearly cold pulseless ischemic limb (Table 21.3). Patients who present with any of these hard signs of arterial injury demand immediate operative exploration with no need for further diagnostic testing. On occasion, if a patient is stable, the surgeon may perform preoperative diagnostic imaging or

Table 21.3 Signs of traumatic vascular injury

Hard signs
Pulsatile bleeding
Palpable thrill
Bruit over area of injury
Absent peripheral pulses
Expanding hematoma
Soft signs
Significant hemorrhage at scene of injury
Neurologic deficits
Diminished pulses compared to unaffected extremity
Waxing or waning pulses
ABIs <0.9 in otherwise healthy patients
Proximity of bony or penetrating injury to vessel

an intraoperative angiogram in order to better identify the exact location and extent of the injury so as to more efficiently plan the operation [1, 3, 12].

Soft signs, such as altered ankle-brachial indices, diminished pulse exam, neurologic compromise, and extensive

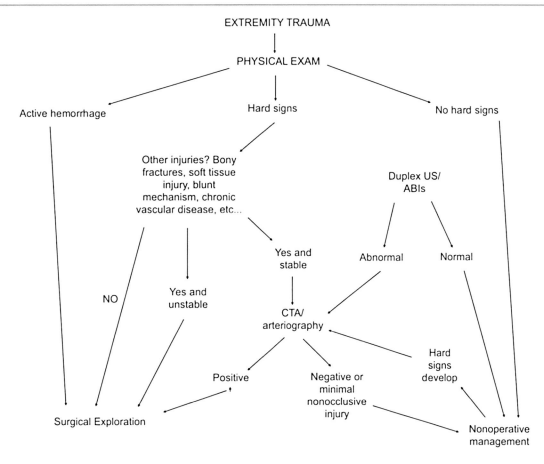

Fig. 21.3 Extremity trauma

fractures were once operative triggers. As a large majority of traumatic injuries present with only soft signs and can be harder to diagnose, these patients were commonly taken to the operating room and often underwent nontherapeutic operations where normal, intact vessels were found [1, 13]. This common occurrence changed the diagnostic approach for patients who do not present with hard signs of vascular injury, in that most patients with soft signs or isolated vessel proximity on presentation undergo preoperative imaging. Additionally, any subsequent presence of hard signs mandates arteriography (Fig. 21.3) [1, 3, 14].

Physical examination must focus on establishing whether or not distal vascular integrity exists while simultaneously addressing bony fractures and soft tissue injuries. A thorough neurovascular exam often cannot be accomplished without reducing fractures, as comminuted distorted limbs can offer a falsely compromised vascular exam. Distal circulation is evaluated by the presence of pallor in the skin, skin temperature, and rate of capillary refill, which is assessed by blanching a small area of skin with digital pressure. Findings on the injured limb should be compared to those on an uninjured limb to determine if concerning differences exist between the two. Disruptive arterial injuries cause a pale, cool limb with prolonged or absent capillary refill. Prolonged

ischemia can lead to a loss of skin turgor and paresthesias or paralysis [1, 3]. Motor and sensory deficits are typically the first manifestation of tissue ischemia because peripheral nerves have a high basal energy requirement and no glycogen stores, making them extremely susceptible to ischemic damage. In contrast, an isolated venous injury will cause a purple, congested, edematous limb [3].

The Six Ps of Tissue Ischemia
Pulselessness
Pain
Pallor
Paralysis
Paresthesia
Poikilothermy (coolness)

Open wounds should not be blindly probed or clamped, as this can lead to more damage; however, extension of the incision and clamping or ligation of visible bleeding can be lifesaving, especially in areas such as the groin where direct compressibility is difficult. Any obviously ischemic limbs require systemic anticoagulation to be started, as long as no contraindications such as intracranial trauma exist.

Ideally, diagnostic efforts should be completed and definitive treatment undertaken within 6 h, as this provides successful results in greater than 95 % of cases [1, 15].

Diagnostic Modalities

Angiography

The implementation of arteriography gives surgeons the best chance to avoid negative traumatic wound explorations in the case of extremity trauma. Given the cost, time, invasive nature of angiography, and potential nephrotoxicity from the contrast dye, routine contrast imaging of all patients presenting with extremity trauma has been abandoned, due to the large percentage of normal studies that resulted. Now it is the practice in most trauma centers to perform selective arteriography on patients who present with increased suspicion for extremity arterial injury, often based on proximity of the injury to the neurovascular bundle. Suspicion in these patients arises based on "soft signs" of vascular injury noted on physical exam or Doppler ankle-brachial indices (ABI) of less than 0.9, both of which are considered indications to pursue arteriography [16]. Other indications for angiography include complex soft tissue injuries and fractures, large hematomas in proximity to the injury, any subjective neurological or vascular compromise, chronic vascular disease, multiple potential sites of injury, and thoracic outlet injuries. Based on the results of the angiogram, those with no signs of vascular injury may be observed, those with minimal vascular injury may be observed or serial angiograms can be performed, while those with major arterial injuries require either an operative exploration or endovascular intervention [1, 16].

Drawbacks to angiography include its costliness, potential for suboptimal and useless studies, and the high rate of negative studies that result from overuse. Additionally, obtaining this imaging can cost valuable time in the event of an ischemic limb. Arteriography can cause a delay of up to 3 h prior to definitive repair, which can translate to critical time lost and contribute to prognosis and limb salvage [17].

Doppler Indices

Handheld Doppler flow detectors screen for arterial injury by determining the phasic Doppler signals in a potentially injured vessel and can be used to determine the ABI in an extremity. This modality is useful to objectively establish the absence of flow in a vessel deemed to be pulseless on physical exam or if the exam is asymmetric. However, the presence of Doppler signals in the absence of a palpable pulse does not exclude a vascular injury, as signals can occur from collateral flow or from flow around or through a transected, partially transected, or thrombosed vessel [1]. Regardless, Doppler flow is an inexpensive, noninvasive, and easy method of confirming physical exam, as well a useful tool for serially monitoring any vascular reconstruction postoperatively. If ABIs are performed, a result of less 0.9 in otherwise healthy patients is considered abnormal and warrants further imaging [18].

Duplex Ultrasonography

The technology and diagnostic utility of duplex ultrasonography continues to improve. Ultrasound as a technique for extremity vascular trauma has several advantages in that it is noninvasive, painless, portable, and relatively inexpensive while still screening for extremity arterial injury with similar accuracy as arteriography [1]. Ultrasound can be used to follow exams serially and can be done at bedside by a nonphysician. Additionally, the direction of blood flow within a vessel can be assessed by color flow Doppler. The sensitivity of ultrasound for a traumatic vascular injury has been reported to be 67–95 %, while its specificity and accuracy are more than 98 % [3, 19]. The primary limitation to its use is operator dependency. Accuracy is thus reflected at institutions with well-trained vascular technologists and interpretations by physicians [3, 20].

Computed Tomographic Arteriography

The advent of computer tomographic arteriography (CTA) is quickly making it the diagnostic test of choice over conventional angiography to evaluate vascular trauma. Improved technology that allows for multiplanar and three-dimensional reformatting allows for simultaneous imaging of vasculature and adjacent body structures, allowing for the diagnosis of multiple consequences of any trauma with one single examination [21]. This can provide the surgeon with a priority guide for perioperative planning in the setting of other injuries. This can also eliminate any delays associated with calling in a team to perform conventional angiography. CTA has the advantages of being readily available in most hospitals and of being easy to interpret. It requires the administration of contrast material, which carries nephrotoxic risks, making subsequent need for contrast in the setting of endovascular interventions a consideration. Sensitivity and specificity are reported to be more than 90 % and equivocal to that of conventional angiography [22]. One critical limitation that must be mentioned relative to CTA revolves around penetrating trauma with retained metallic foreign body or patients with metallic surgical implants. In this setting the CTA can be difficult or impossible to interpret, especially when the associated metallic scatter is in proximity to the vascular area in question. This can severely limit the value of CTA and must be considered, as traditional angiography would then be the preferred test of choice [3, 21, 22].

Magnetic Resonance Arteriography

Although magnetic resonance arteriography (MRA) has increased in popularity as a diagnostic tool for vascular diseases in the general public, in acute traumatic situations, it is infrequently utilized. While MRA has the advantage of being specific, noninvasive, and not requiring contrast agents, its price, lack of accessibility in many hospitals, and contraindication in patients with metallic orthopedic implants make it impractical for use in acute extremity vascular trauma [3]. Artifacts due to metallic foreign bodies may interfere with interpretation of MRA images; however, of more concern is the risk of movement of the foreign object once placed in a high magnetic field. While magnetic deflection of various bullets and shotgun pellets is uncommon, the probability of migration cannot be predicted due to ferromagnetic contaminants that are commonly present in ballistics. Generally, MR imaging of patients with retained ballistic fragments is considered safe, but the indication for imaging, possible types of bullet present, and location of bullet fragments should all be considered. If the fragments are not associated with a vital organ such as brain, spinal cord, eye, or heart, or if the metallic fragments are clearly nonferromagnetic, MRA can be considered [23].

Operative Principles

Categories of Vascular Injury

Vessels can be injured in a number of ways secondary to trauma (Fig. 21.4). The most common forms of injuries sustained are lacerations or transections. A laceration is a full-thickness tear in a vessel where part of the wall remains intact, thus preserving vessel continuity. Mild lacerations involve less than 25 % of the wall, moderate lacerations involve 25–50 % of the wall, and severe lacerations involve more than 50 % of the wall. Oftentimes distal pulses persist in the case of lacerations. A transection is complete division of a vessel with a loss of continuity. This injury can be more difficult to approach and require a more extensive exploration, as the transected ends of the vessels tend to retract and constrict. This frequently causes thrombosis and cessation of hemorrhage, making diagnosing and identifying these injuries more complex. Most complete transections are coupled with loss of pulses, pain, pallor, paralysis, and paresthesias of the affected limb given the development of ongoing tissue ischemia [1].

Fig. 21.4 Vessel injuries

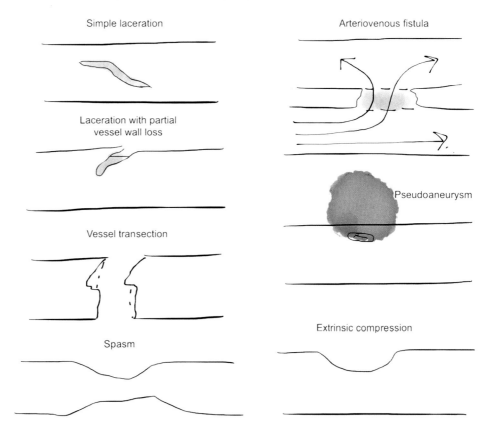

Arteriovenous fistulas develop when concomitant injuries occur to a neighboring artery and vein and an abnormal connection is created between the two. This can pressurize the vein and can lead to rupture of affected vessels, thrombosis, embolization, high-output cardiac failure, and impingement on surrounding nerves and soft tissues. Physical examination can reveal a bruit, murmur, or a thrill over the site of injury. However, diagnosis is often missed if physical findings are not present, in which case arteriovenous fistula can be picked up on angiography, CTA, or ultrasound [1, 24].

Vascular contusions are bruises of the arterial wall. Contusions can be mild and involve only the adventitia, causing no consequences of injury, or they can extend into the intima, causing constriction, occlusion of vessel lumen, or intimal rupture and subsequent thrombosis. Large contusions can cause full-thickness weakening of the arterial wall and create true arterial aneurysms [1, 25]. Alternatively, a false or pseudoaneurysm occurs when bleeding from injured vessels is contained within the vessel, muscles, or fascial compartments. Arterial spasm occurs as a myogenic reflex response to surrounding injury. This manifests as an area of narrowing seen either on angiography or on arterial exposure [1].

Nonoperative Management

Nonoperative management of traumatic vascular injuries is a controversial subject. While many surgeons insist that all arterial injuries require repair, there are many who believe that clinically asymptomatic injuries found to be minimal and nonocclusive by angiography may be managed without exploration [3]. A nonoperative approach can typically be employed when the vascular injury is of low-velocity mechanism and associated with intact distal circulation, has no active hemorrhage, and has less than 5 mm of arterial wall disruption in the event of intimal defects and/or pseudoaneurysms [14]. A large majority of nonocclusive arterial injuries have a self-limiting course and can resolve spontaneously in about 3 months. A small percentage may form false aneurysms and require surgical intervention, but no adverse sequelae seem to occur related to treatment delay. In the event of nonoperative management, it is typically recommended that the patient undergo some form of repeat imaging to confirm stability of the lesion and rule out acute thrombosis or distal embolization [26].

Endovascular Management

Endovascular interventions have grown in popularity over the last decade for the management of acute traumatic vascular injuries. Over a 9-year time span, the National Trauma Data Bank reports that the use of endovascular techniques to repair vascular traumas jumped from 2.1 % of procedures in 1994 to 8.1 % in 2003 [27]. While angiography was once strictly used for diagnostic purposes, the advent of stent grafts and coil embolization techniques has helped transform angiography into a therapeutic modality. Often, select catheter-based endovascular techniques are associated with decreased morbidity and mortality compared with open vascular reconstructive procedures. Endovascular interventions have been shown to decrease operating room times, blood losses, and iatrogenic injuries. The primary disadvantage of endovascular technology is the need to call in dedicated teams, the need for operating rooms or angiography suites adapted for endovascular interventions, and the need for hospital personnel with sufficient experience. Associated costs can vary depending on the institution. Failure of endovascular repair often revolves around the inability to cross the lesion with a wire. A relative contraindication is uncontrolled hemorrhage and hemodynamic instability, although this holds true only in the setting of an operating room not equipped to employ prompt and effective endovascular control of an injury. Other relative contraindications include the inability to use systemic anticoagulation such as multisystem trauma or closed-head injuries. Additional limitations include the possible need to cover major arterial branches with stents and the need to place stents in areas of mobility such as the popliteal artery, common femoral artery, or axillary artery [27–29].

Patient selection is an important concept in choosing when endovascular therapy for traumatic vascular injuries may be most effective. Endovascular intervention is best suited for difficult anatomic areas where obtaining operative exposure prolongs operating or ischemic time or increases the risk of bleeding. Additionally, if the anatomic region carries a risk of iatrogenic nerve injury, such as injuries involving the subclavian artery or internal carotid artery, endovascular therapies can eliminate the need to dissect in those areas [29]. Low-velocity penetrating traumatic injuries are the most easily repaired with endovascular techniques. Conversely, high-velocity, large cavitating injuries cause more damaging injuries and typically pose a need for definitive open repair due to associated contamination requiring debridement, fasciotomy for compartment syndrome, or embolectomy. Alternatively, larger injuries can be approached with proximal balloon occlusion to control hemorrhage and decrease blood loss during open exposure for definitive repair. Active hemorrhage from smaller, noncritical arteries can be embolized to permanently occlude bleeding. Perhaps the most widely accepted use of endovascular intervention is in single-vessel injuries below the trifurcation, where anterior tibial or tibioperoneal injuries are simply embolized, with no repair required [28–30].

Associated vascular injuries have also been managed with endovascular techniques. Pseudoaneurysms and arteriovenous fistulas caused by traumatic injury to vessels have been successfully treated both with the use of covered stents and coil embolization [31]. For fistulas, coils are deployed to occlude the arterial side, usually by isolating the fistula with proximal and distal coils. When utilizing coils, it is important to approximate the coil size to the diameter of the artery being embolized, as inappropriately sized coils have the potential to dislodge and embolize elsewhere. Dissections have also been treated with balloon dilation and stenting [3, 32].

Endovascular therapies are also being employed as temporary measures to control hemorrhaging vascular injuries in the event of other life-threatening injuries that require prompt attention by the trauma team prior to definitive repair of vasculature [32]. One such adjunct to primary trauma resuscitation is the development of resuscitative endovascular balloon occlusion of the aorta, or REBOA, which is a technique that provides the physiological benefit of aortic occlusion without the morbidity of emergency thoracotomy and aortic cross clamping. This technique was initially described as early as the 1950s during the Korean War; however, its use has been limited secondary to lack of skill set and/or concern over the ineffectiveness of the technique. Now with the advent of endovascular training courses for trauma surgeons that teach even the most basic of skill sets, REBOA is being revisited as a feasible and effective manner of aortic control in patients that present in profound hemorrhagic shock [33].

Operative Principles

In the case of an actively hemorrhaging traumatic extremity injury, the patient should be brought to the operating room promptly. Since the need for prosthetic grafting is a possibility, typically antibiotics with gram-positive coverage are administered to protect against skin flora; however, antibiotics with additional gram-negative coverage may be given if there is concern for bony injury and need for manipulation or hardware. For planning purposes, the entire injured extremity should be prepped and draped, and an uninjured extremity should be included in the operative field in the event that autologous vein needs to be harvested for grafting. Vein harvesting is avoided in the injured extremity to prevent further venous injury and worsened postoperative swelling.

The first goal of any operative intervention in the case of extremity vascular injury is to obtain proximal control of the injured vessels. To do so requires a widely prepped operative field, with incisions oriented longitudinally. Incisions should be placed directly over the injured vessel and in this manner may be extended proximally or distally as needed for adequate exposure. Proximal control of an uninjured segment of the vessel is obtained, and once this is secured, the same is done distally to obtain control over potential retrograde bleeding. Only after proximal and distal controls have been achieved should the injured portions of the vessels be exposed and explored.

When exposure of a vessel is difficult, either because of active hemorrhage, difficult anatomy, or associated injuries, endovascular techniques may be employed to achieve balloon occlusion proximal to the injury. Alternatively, a proximally placed tourniquet or blood pressure cuff can help to achieve control of the hemorrhage.

All arterial injuries must be properly explored and evaluated, and any associated venous or nerve injuries should also be identified. It is important to remember that in all types of traumatic injuries, the extent of injury to the intima can extend beyond the apparent area of injured vessel. Any soft tissue in the area that is contaminated, contused, or grossly defunctionalized should be debrided. Any intraluminal thrombus that is present needs to be removed in order to decrease risk of embolization as well as to assess patency of repair at the end of the operation. Fogarty catheters can be used both proximally and distally from an injury to achieve this goal, and both the proximal and distal lumens should be flushed with heparinized saline. Commonly, patients also receive systemic heparin to prevent thrombosis, unless anticoagulation is contraindicated [1, 3].

Occasionally circumstances exist where definitive repair of an arterial injury cannot be performed and ligation or shunting may be required. If a patient is hemodynamically unstable, acidotic, hypothermic, or coagulopathic, ligation or shunting is recommended as a damage control act to allow time for adequate resuscitation, warming, and stabilization of the patient. A formal revascularization can then be performed under more stable and controlled conditions at a later date [34].

The type of definitive arterial repair indicated is directed by the extent of arterial damage incurred. Injured vessels can be repaired by patch angioplasty if the defect is small but encompasses more than 50 % the diameter of a vessel. Alternatively, if the segment injured is short without a diameter defect and a reasonable anastomosis can be made under no tension, an end-to-end primary repair can be attempted. When the injured segment is too long to come together without tension, an interposition graft should be placed [3]. An extra-anatomic bypass graft may be required in the setting of severe soft tissue injury or sepsis and can increase limb salvage rates in this high-risk population [35].

Choosing between autologous vein grafting and prosthetic graft material typically depends on the availability of suitable veins in the setting of associated traumatic injuries, as well as how grossly contaminated the surgical field is. Autologous vein grafting was first used by Spanish surgeon Goyanes in 1906 to treat a popliteal artery aneurysm. It was popularized during the Korean War and, since that time, has been performed most often using a reversed greater saphenous vein graft from a contralateral uninjured extremity [36].

Patency rates for autologous vein grafts are typically reported to be around 80% over a 5-year period of time. Expanded polytetrafluoroethylene (ePTFE) or Dacron grafts are now used in place of autologous vein grafts when those are not available, if a large size mismatch is present between a vein graft and the native artery, or in patients with varicosities, dilations, or stenosis in the saphenous vein [37, 38]. ePTFE is the most often used prosthetic graft material in traumatic extremity injuries as it has been shown to be more highly resistant to infection than other prosthetic materials. Graft infection most often occurs in the setting of adjacent osteomyelitis or large soft tissue injuries causing exposed graft. ePTFE and autologous vein grafts have similar patency rates when used to repair above knee arterial injuries in the iliac, common femoral, or superficial femoral arteries. However a significant difference in patency occurs below the knee, where graft failure is much more common when ePTFE grafts are used [38, 39].

Repairs are typically performed using 5-0 or 6-0 monofilament sutures, and repairs are most commonly performed in a running fashion; however, this is dependent on the preference of the operating surgeon. Interrupted sutures may be used in smaller vessels in order to decrease the likelihood of stenosis at the anastomosis. Repairs must be performed in a tension-free manner, and covering any graft with soft tissue is recommended, even if it requires performing an additional muscle flap procedure.

Postoperatively, repairs are generally interrogated using arteriography or duplex scanning, and this can be done either intraoperatively or immediately following. This interrogation is mandatory to visualize the vascular reconstruction, arterial runoff, and any potentially missed distal thrombi [1, 3].

Assessment of Associated Injuries

While traumatic vascular injuries can occur in isolation, patients often present with severely compromised extremities. Associated injuries must also be addressed during the exploration and repair of traumatic vascular injuries. Blunt vascular injuries are associated with a wider application of force and greater damage to extremity vessels and surrounding structures than penetrating vascular injuries, which are typically clean, isolated, and easier to diagnose and repair. High-velocity gunshot wounds, shotgun wounds, and blunt trauma are typically associated with higher degrees of tissue disruption and thus have higher rates of amputation and severe dysfunction leading to limb loss [1].

Certain orthopedic injuries, by sheer virtue of their location, carry a high risk of vascular injury (Table 21.4), and in cases of vascular trauma, orthopedic bony injuries have been shown to occur simultaneously in 10–70% of cases [40]. Occasionally in the setting of a fracture or dislocation, if no hard signs are present on exam but pulses are absent, simply reducing the bony injury can lead to regaining a pulse on

Table 21.4 Orthopedic injuries associated with vascular injuries

Posterior knee dislocation	Popliteal artery
Tibial plateau fracture	
Femur fracture	Superficial femoral artery
Shoulder dislocation	Axillary artery
Supracondylar humerus fracture	Brachial artery

Modified from Callcut RA, Mell MW. Modern Advances in Vascular Trauma. *Surg Clin N Am.* 2013: 93: 941–961

repeat physical exam [32]. Alternatively, if concomitant bony and vascular injuries that require definitive repair exist, it is important to repair arterial injuries first in order to restore circulation to the affected limb. It is also frequently recommended that comminuted unstable fractures undergo rapid external fixation prior to vascular repair as to minimize the risk to the revascularization. If vascular reconstruction is done first, it is imperative that vascular surgeons reassess and confirm the vessel reconstruction and repair patency prior to wound closure [3].

Related soft tissue injuries must be debrided to remove any nonviable tissues from around a vascular reconstruction to prevent a potential nidus for infection. Extensive soft tissue damage can disrupt collateral flow and make coverage of vascular repairs difficult. Frequent return trips to the operating room may be required to adequately debride any necrotic tissue. Large wound defects may require coverage with rotational flaps or free tissue transfer once concerns for soft tissue infection are reduced.

Vascular injuries are accompanied by nerve injuries approximately 50% of the time in the upper extremity and 25% of the time in the lower extremity [41]. Associated nerve injuries and their consequences can be more predicative of long-term limb function than bony or soft tissue injuries. In the case of major nerve disruptions, primary repair is pursued if the transection is clean and can be done promptly at the time of vascular repair. Oftentimes, however, immediate repair is impossible given the extent of the injury. In such cases, it is recommended to tag both ends of the nerve, which can be reassessed at a later time for repair or grafting [1, 3].

Limb Loss

Patients that present with devastating mangled extremity trauma force the surgeon to decide on primary amputation versus total limb reconstruction. While life always prevails over limb in traumatic injury decision-making algorithms, functional outcome also remains a primary objective when faced with such circumstances. While every effort should be made to preserve and restore function if possible, some severe extremity injuries are better served with amputation and prosthetic replacement rather than a protracted convalescence with a poor outcome and limited quality of life.

Extremity salvage rates dramatically decrease as ischemia time increases. With fewer than 6 h of ischemia, 90% of limbs can be salvaged, while 12–18 h of ischemia is associated with a 50 % salvage rate, and greater than 24 h of ischemia portends a less than 20 % limb salvage rate [42]. Although in many of these prolonged ischemia cases vascular reconstruction is still a technically feasible option, restoring distal flow does not revitalize a limb to functionality. Therefore, the decision to proceed with amputation cannot be based solely on vascular injuries but must be approached from a multidisciplinary standpoint. Currently primary amputation is advocated for limbs with massive bony, soft tissue, vascular, and nerve injuries, as even those who undergo complex reconstructions are commonly left with permanent limb disabilities ultimately requiring amputation [43]. Blunt trauma is associated with a higher graft failure rate than penetrating trauma, and in the case of any graft failure, the need for amputation is much more likely [39]. Other risk factors for amputation following traumatic arterial injury repairs are occluded bypass grafts, concomitant above and below knee injuries, and associated bony compound fractures [44].

Amputation is generally considered as a primary treatment in patients that are hemodynamically unstable at presentation, making a complex revascularization a risk to their survival. These cases are approached with a guillotine-style amputation. Efforts to preserve as much length and soft tissue as possible should be a priority as better coverage of the stump will allow for the best outcome. In the event that there is not enough soft tissue salvaged, multiple reconstructive options exist such as free tissue transfers, rotational flaps, and skin grafts to provide durable and useful stumps. Length of the stump is important, as the level of amputation greatly impacts future function and survival. The more proximal an amputation is performed, the greater the functional impairment, the greater degree of energy required to ambulate, and the less attractive the prosthetic options. The most ideal amputation level is at least 10 cm below the knee to preserve the joint and enough proximal tibia to provide for a good prosthetic fit [41, 43, 45].

Multiple scoring systems exist to aid decisions about limb salvage, all of which require consideration of multiple factors. Systemic factors that need to be assessed are the severity and duration of shock, the degree and extent of other bodily injuries, and the patient's age and comorbidities. Local factors included in the determination are duration and extent of ischemia, mechanism of injury, associated fractures, neurologic function, and muscle viability [3, 41]. One such scoring system is the Mangled Extremity Severity Score (MESS), which is calculated based on the sum of four parameters: skeletal and soft tissue injury, ischemia, shock, and age (Table 21.5). A total MESS score of 7 or more suggests the need for primary amputation.

While MESS is the most commonly used scoring system due to its simplicity, all scoring systems are more than 15 years old, and advances in orthopedic, vascular, and plastic surgery have changed dramatically in that time frame.

Table 21.5 Mangled extremity severity score (MESS)

Parameters	Points
Skeletal/soft tissue injury	
Low-energy mechanism (stab, low velocity penetrating)	1
Medium-energy mechanism (multiple fractures, dislocation)	2
High-energy mechanism (high-velocity penetrating, decelerating injuries)	3
Very high-energy mechanism (high-speed trauma with soft tissue avulsion)	4
Ischemia (time >6 h doubles ischemia score)	
Pulse reduced or absent; normal capillary refill	1
Pulseless, paresthesias, reduced capillary refill	2
Cool limb, paralysis, insensate, numb	3
Shock	
Normotension	0
Transient hypotension	1
Persistent hypotension	2
Age	
<30 years old	0
30–50 years old	1
>50 years old	2

Consequently, neither MESS nor any other scoring system has been proven to effectively predict the need for amputation or the functional outcome of a patient; thus, they are mostly used simply as guides for decision-making [46]. In cases where rapid revascularization can be performed in less than 5 h with liberal use of fasciotomies, limb salvage rates greater than 50 % have been achieved, thus challenging the cutoff score of 7 and giving new thought to selective salvage attempts in ideal patients [47].

Management of Specific Injuries

External Iliac Injuries

The external iliac arteries bifurcate off the common iliac arteries and proceed anteriorly and inferiorly along the medial border of the psoas major. They exit the pelvis posterior and inferior to the inguinal ligament at which point they become the femoral arteries [48].

For isolated lower limb trauma, a retroperitoneal approach is typically employed in order to gain proximal control of the external iliac artery (Fig. 21.5). This can be done by either extending a femoral incision proximally through the inguinal ligament or by making a separate incision 2 cm cranial to the inguinal ligament that is parallel to the lateral border of the rectus muscle. Either incision necessitates retracting the peritoneum and its contents medially in order to enter the retroperitoneal space and expose the distal aorta and iliac vessels. Iliac artery injury is associated with an approximate 40 % mortality rate [28], but mortality exceeds 50 % if combined with an aortic or iliac venous injury [49].

Fig. 21.5 Retroperitoneal
iliac vessel exposure

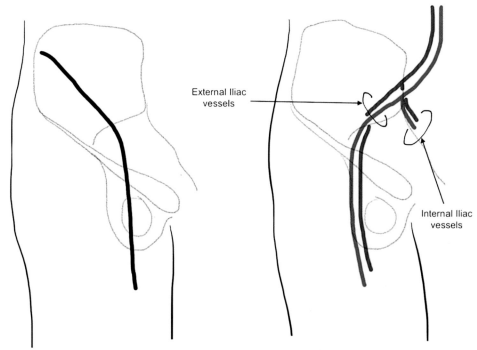

External Iliac
vessels

Internal Iliac
vessels

RETROPERITONEAL EXPOSURE
OF THE ILIAC VESSELS

The iliac vessels are often suitable for endovascular intervention when injured given their otherwise difficult exposure. The risk of disrupting a retroperitoneal hematoma or causing iatrogenic injury to ureters or iliac veins can dramatically compound the risks and complications. The use of angiographic embolization in the case of bleeding pelvic arterial vessels in the face of pelvic trauma and associated fracture has also been widely accepted [29].

Femoral Artery Injuries

The femoral artery is a continuation of the external iliac artery that begins at the inguinal ligament as the common femoral artery (CFA). As it proceeds distally in the thigh, it gives off the deep (profunda) femoral artery, and after that branching, it becomes the superficial femoral artery (SFA). It continues along the femur to provide blood to the geniculate arteries that encircle the knee and then enters the adductor canal. After it emerges from the adductor canal, it becomes the popliteal artery. Within the femoral sheath, the femoral nerve is lateral to the artery, while the femoral vein is medial to the artery [48]. Dissection in this area must be meticulous to avoid injury to those structures, as well as the deep femoral artery, in the event that they were unharmed by the inciting trauma.

The SFA is the most common peripheral vessel to be injured in trauma [28]. Both blunt and penetrating injuries are common. Exposure to the CFA, proximal deep femoral artery, and proximal SFA can all be obtained through a longitudinal thigh incision oriented over the femoral triangle, and this can be extended proximally through the inguinal ligament or distally as needed to explore the entire vessel (Fig. 21.6). This approach allows complete exposure and mobilization of the CFA and its bifurcation [50].

The femoral artery is easily accessible so endovascular options are usually not required unless in the setting of concomitant orthopedic injuries requiring hardware that makes exposure difficult or if the injury is discovered by angiography and can be easily treated with endovascular stenting. Blunt SFA trauma can lead to a dissection or thrombosis that could compromise other injuries such as a femur fracture, and oftentimes endovascular stenting is used in these cases to combat any potential flow limitations [28].

Popliteal Artery Injuries

The popliteal artery is the continuation of the SFA after it passes through the adductor canal. It continues distally posterior to the knee until its bifurcation into the anterior and posterior tibial arteries [48]. Popliteal artery injuries are challenging traumatic injuries to treat, as those that are penetrating are usually accompanied by soft tissue trauma and septic consequences. Penetrating popliteal arterial injuries have a mortality rate of 10.5 %, while blunt injuries portend a mortality rate of 27.5 % [28]. Popliteal artery injuries carry the highest risk of limb loss of any other peripheral artery injury [32]. Amputation rates for more destructive penetrating injuries to the popliteal artery approach 20 %, while stab

Fig. 21.6 Femoral vessels
exposure

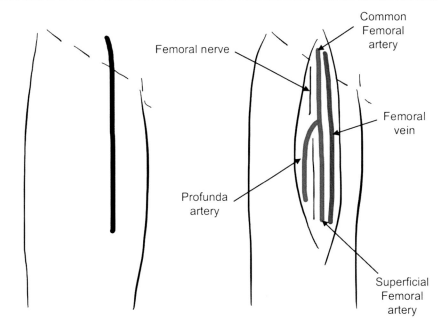

EXPOSURE OF FEMORAL VESSELS

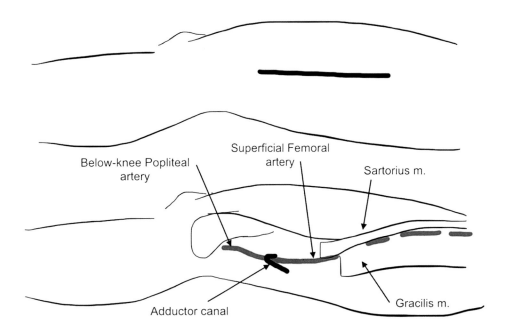

wounds and smaller missile injuries are associated with a lower rate [3].

Numerous different approaches can be utilized to access a popliteal artery injury. Injuries that occur above the knee are best accessed through a medial thigh incision, while below knee injuries are exposed through a medial leg incision (Fig. 21.7). Injuries isolated to behind the knee can be repaired through a posterior approach (Fig. 21.8) [50].

Endovascular interventions have been described when faced with popliteal artery injuries given the difficult surgical exposure and associated risk of injury to the veins, peroneal nerve, muscles, and tendons in the popliteal fossa; however, they are generally avoided as stent placement can limit mobility across joints [51].

Tibial Artery Injuries

The anterior tibial artery is the anterior continuation of the popliteal artery that courses down the front of the leg to the dorsum of the foot where it becomes the dorsalis pedis artery. The posterior tibial artery is the second branch of the popliteal

Fig. 21.7 Popliteal artery exposure

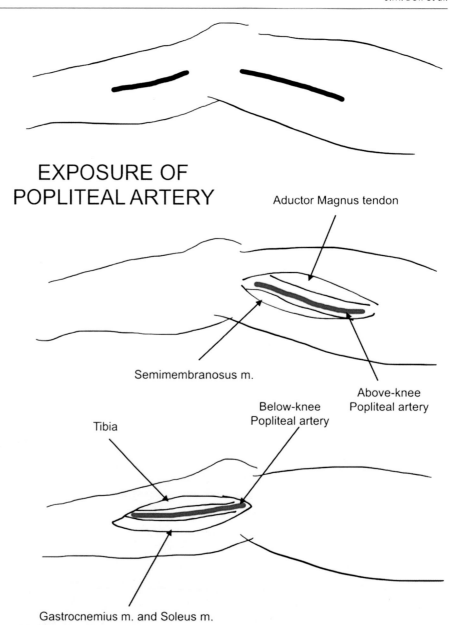

EXPOSURE OF
POPLITEAL ARTERY

Aductor Magnus tendon

Semimembranosus m.

Above-knee
Popliteal artery

Below-knee
Popliteal artery

Tibia

Gastrocnemius m. and Soleus m.

artery and supplies the posterior compartment of the leg down to the plantar surface of the foot. It gives off the peroneal artery, which supplies the lateral compartment of the leg [48].

Tibial artery injuries are associated with a 38 % amputation rate [28]. As with popliteal injuries, associated nerve, bone, and soft tissue trauma predict a lower rate of limb salvage. Isolated injury to one of the three infrapopliteal vessels rarely results in limb ischemia due to the robust collateral flow that exists in the system. Because of this, single artery injuries do not necessarily require operative intervention and can be treated by simple ligation or angiographic embolization. In the event of an injury to the tibioperoneal trunk injury or to two or more infrapopliteal arteries, definitive repair should be considered, if feasible, but it is also acceptable to accept single-vessel flow to the foot. This can be of particular importance when

distal fractures are associated with the vascular injury, as definitive vascular repair acts to ensure the best perfusion to heal the fractures and minimize bony nonunion [52].

The posterior tibial and peroneal arteries are usually approached medially, although the distal third of the peroneal is best exposed using a lateral leg incision directly over the distal fibula. The trifurcation and distal popliteal artery can also be exposed through a posterior approach by separating and retracting both heads of the gastrocnemius and releasing the soleus muscle from the tibia (Fig. 21.9) [50].

Axillary Artery Injuries

The axillary artery begins when the subclavian artery passes the lateral border of the first rib and it extends to the lateral border of the teres major muscle [48]. Injury to the axillary

Fig. 21.8 Posterior popliteal approach

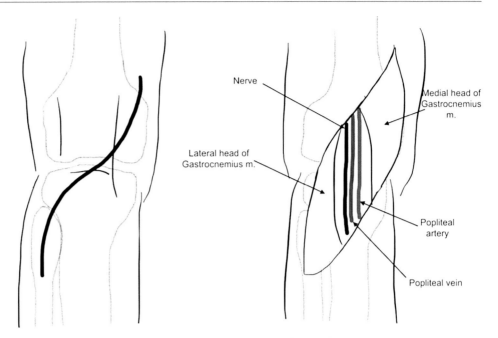

Nerve

Medial head of Gastrocnemius m.

Lateral head of Gastrocnemius m.

Popliteal artery

Popliteal vein

POSTERIOR APPROACH TO POPLITEAL ARTERY

artery is more common than injury to the subclavian artery. It is most common secondary to penetrating trauma, although anterior shoulder dislocation or humeral head fractures can also result in injury [3].

Critical ischemia following axillary artery injury is rare given the abundant collateral circulation around the shoulder; however, this can lead to diagnostic difficulties as, consequently, finding decreased or absent distal pulses with an axillary artery injury is rare. A high clinical suspicion is required, and oftentimes Doppler, ABIs, and arteriography must be used for diagnosis of these injuries. Morbidity from an axillary artery injury can be significant, given the associated brachial plexus injury rate of 20–43 % [3, 28].

The open surgical approach to the axillary artery is through a horizontal infraclavicular incision or an axillary incision with the arm abducted 90° (Fig. 21.10). It is important to keep in mind that proximal control of the distal subclavian artery may need to be obtained at the thoracic outlet. Some injuries require resection of part of the clavicle, and oftentimes multiple incisions must be used in order to gain proper control and exposure of the arterial injury [3, 28, 53].

Endovascular techniques are often employed in the case of axillary artery injury, as surgical exposure in this area raises concern for potential injury to neurovascular structures and prolonged operative times with large intraoperative blood losses. Obtaining proximal surgical control can potentially involve a median sternotomy or clavicle resection, making endovascular remote access to this area an attractive option. Additionally, many injuries in this location evolve into contained hematomas, allowing for a window of

time with which to use endovascular techniques to achieve definitive diagnosis and possible treatment [28]. At the very least, endovascular balloon occlusion of injuries in this area can control hemorrhage and serve to decrease risk of mortality from blood loss in the event an open approach is more appropriate [54].

Brachial Artery Injuries

The brachial artery is the major blood vessel of the upper arm and is the continuation of the axillary artery beyond the lateral border of teres major muscle. It continues down the ventral surface of the arm until it reaches the cubital fossa and divides into the radial and ulnar arteries at the elbow [48]. Injuries to the brachial artery are typically penetrating in nature, although there has recently been an increased incidence of iatrogenic trauma to this vessel secondary to endovascular access procedures. Blunt brachial injury most commonly results from supracondylar fractures of the humerus [3].

Much like the axillary artery, there exists a network of collaterals below the origin of the profunda brachii artery, so signs of ischemia may not be overtly present, and clinical suspicion is essential to diagnose these injuries. Morbidity from a brachial artery injury can be significant given its association with the brachial plexus. Therefore, endovascular treatment or proximal control can be advantageous to avoid extensive dissection in this area [29].

The proximal through middle third of the brachial artery is best approached openly through a medial incision located over the bicipital groove (Figs. 21.11 and 21.12). The median

Fig. 21.9 Calf vessels

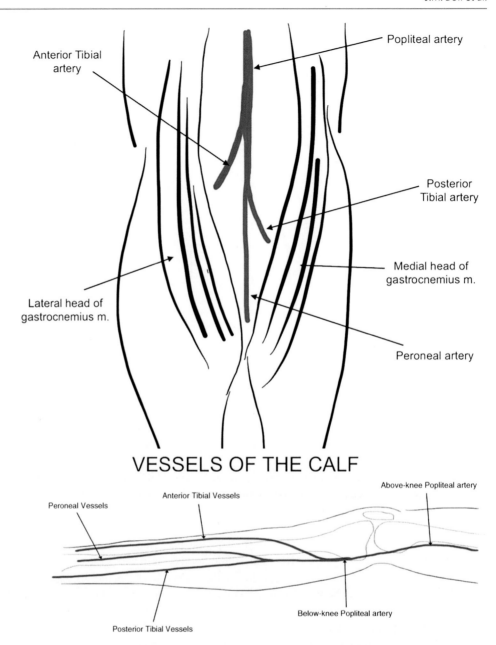

nerve is typically the first structure encountered once the brachial sheath is opened, and it is important to gently mobilize and retract it to avoid damage. The distal third of the brachial artery and its bifurcation are best exposed through an S-shaped incision at the antecubital fossa [53].

Distal Arm Injuries

Both the radial and ulnar arteries arise from the bifurcation of the brachial artery in the antecubital fossa. The radial artery runs distally on the anterolateral part of the forearm, while the ulnar artery runs medially down the forearm. The radial artery winds laterally around the wrist and becomes the superficial and deep palmar arch. The ulnar artery is the larger of the two terminal branches of the brachial artery and

in the wrist divides into a superficial and deep branch, joining the radial artery to complete the superficial and deep palmar arches [48]. The radial artery is superficial, and exposure is straightforward through a lateral longitudinal incision. The ulnar artery is relatively deeper than the radial artery, both proximally as it lies beneath the deep fascia of the forearm and distally at the wrist; however, both are accessed through a medially placed longitudinal incision [53] (Figs. 21.12 and 21.13).

Single-vessel injury to either the radial or ulnar artery in the distal arm may be ligated or embolized as long as good flow is present through the palmar arches, confirmed with bedside Doppler or manual Allen's test. Ten to fifteen percent of the population has an incomplete palmar arch, so determining its

EXPOSURE OF AXILLARY VESSELS

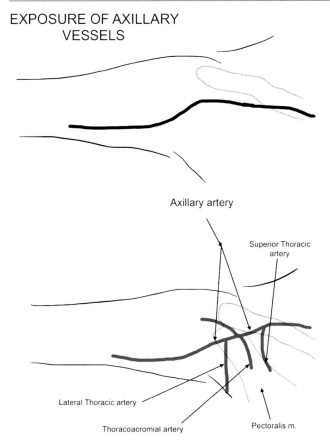

Fig. 21.10 Axillary exposure

EXPOSURE OF BRACHIAL VESSELS

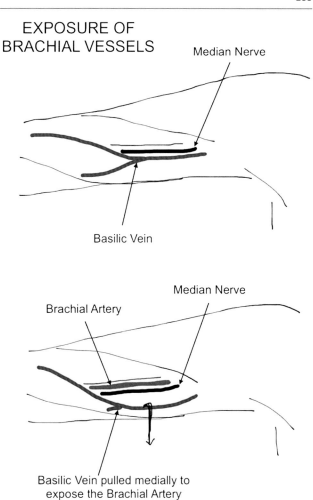

Fig. 21.11 Exposure brachial artery

patency is of utmost importance if ligation of either the radial or ulnar artery is planned. Repair becomes essential if the non-injured vessel had previously been traumatized or ligated, making the palmar arch incomplete. If both the radial and ulnar arteries are injured, the ulnar artery is preferentially repaired, as it is the dominant vessel to the forearm [55]. Endovascular techniques are typically only employed in event of embolization for single-vessel transections, pseudoaneurysms, or arteriovenous fistulas [29].

Venous Injuries

Traumatic injuries to extremity veins most commonly involve the superficial femoral vein, popliteal vein, and common femoral vein. If a patient is hemodynamically stable and a venous injury is identified, it should be definitively repaired. A small injury that can be repaired primarily is typically done so with an end-to-end or lateral venorrhaphy. More extensive venous injuries may require an interposition or spiral venous graft [56]. The largest risk with venorrhaphy is venous thrombosis, and this risk is approximately 60 % in the cases where an interposition repair must be performed, while ePTFE grafts are associated with an almost 100 % rate of stenosis or occlusion following repair [36, 38]. However, repair of venous injury in stable patients remains a reasonable decision, given that

venous repair is associated with decreased blood loss from soft tissue defects and fasciotomy sites in the postoperative period. Simple venous ligation is appropriate in hemodynamically unstable patients or if the venous repair that would need to be performed is complex and deemed unnecessary. Venous repairs should be studied and monitored postoperatively using Doppler or ultrasonography.

Complications

Reperfusion Injury

Restoration of arterial flow to an extremity after it has been devascularized for a period of time can lead to reperfusion injury. This phenomenon is a complex process that results in metabolic, thrombotic, and inflammatory damage throughout the body. Paradoxical tissue injury occurs following restoration of blood flow to ischemic tissues due to a complex combination of metabolic and inflammatory pathways. Simply put, at the time of reperfusion, a variety of inflammatory

Fig. 21.12 Upper extremity exposure

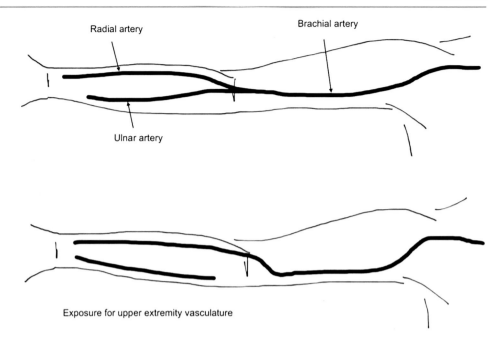

Radial artery

Brachial artery

Ulnar artery

Exposure for upper extremity vasculature

Fig. 21.13 Radial and ulnar exposure

EXPOSURE OF RADIAL AND ULNAR VESSELS

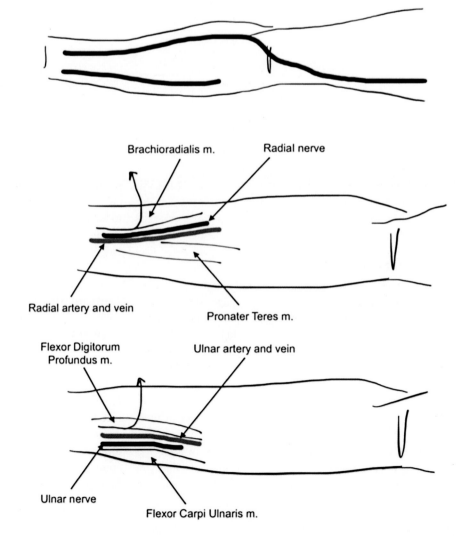

Brachioradialis m.

Radial nerve

Radial artery and vein

Pronater Teres m.

Flexor Digitorum Profundus m.

Ulnar artery and vein

Ulnar nerve

Flexor Carpi Ulnaris m.

mediators are delivered to previously ischemic tissues by macrophages, lymphocytes, neutrophils, and other cells. The complement system, reactive oxygen species, nitric oxide, and cytokines all then modulate a complex environment of inflammation and subsequent tissue injury [57].

Clinically, the patient's extremity will have marked edema, and necrosis can also be seen, culminating in compartment syndrome. As edema and intracompartmental pressures increase, the veins are compressed, and venous pressure increases, decreasing the arteriovenous gradient and resulting in diminished local perfusion. Additionally, the reduced venous drainage exacerbates the edema to a point that arteriolar compression develops and irreversible ischemia of both nerve and muscle tissue can occur. With restoration of flow, the toxic oxygen free radicals created by necrotic tissue are released into the circulation and can go on to damage other organs, specifically the heart and brain [57–59].

Injecting heparin into the lumen of an injured vessel prior to repair and administering systemic anticoagulation are both thought to mitigate some reperfusion injury effects and have the additional benefit of preventing thrombosis of distal vessels [60]. Limb loss has been shown to be significantly higher in patients who did not receive perioperative anticoagulation; thus, it remains important to consider in ischemic injuries in order to combat the detrimental effects of potential reperfusion injury. Ongoing research is being performed in the administration of enzyme scavengers such as superoxide dismutase or catalase, or mannitol or allopurinol to interrupt the reperfusion injury cascade. Animal models pretreated with these agents have displayed decreased oxygen free radical formation and subsequently less muscle edema and necrosis [61–63].

Compartment Syndrome

The most devastating consequence of reperfusion injury is compartment syndrome, which is documented to complicate up to 21% of acute ischemia cases. It is not limited to the lower extremity and can occur in various muscle groups, the most common areas being the calf and forearm. Even following successful revascularization, compartment syndrome can lead to limb loss as the increased pressure within fascial compartments compromises capillary perfusion. Potential for compartment syndrome is dependent on the size and perfusion extent of the vessel injured, with injury to the popliteal artery being the highest risk [64]. Risk of compartment syndrome is also increased in younger patients, with combined arterial and venous injuries, if one or more associated venous, bony, or soft tissue injuries exist, and if the time from injury to completion of repair lasts more than 6 h. Reperfusion of ischemic tissue is the most common cause of compartment

syndrome, although ligation of a major vein, hemorrhage into a compartment, and crush injuries can also be causes [65].

Muscle necrosis from compartment syndrome eventually culminates in rhabdomyolysis, which releases myoglobin, potassium, phosphate, and creatinine phosphokinase into the systemic circulation. Hyperkalemia can cause arrhythmias, myocardial stunning, and even cardiac arrest [66]. Myoglobinuria can cause renal failure by inducing renal vasoconstriction, tubular cast formation, and direct cytotoxicity. Progression to acute renal failure can be prevented with aggressive intravenous fluid resuscitation, diuresis, and alkalinization of the urine with bicarbonate [67].

Compartment syndrome often occurs quietly, in which case tissue damage occurs without obvious signs and symptoms. Classically the phenomenon of pain out of proportion to injury is described, along with increased pain on passive stretch, sensory and motor deficits, and tenseness and swelling of the limb. Unfortunately by the time many of these signs arise, irreversible ischemic necrosis has already occurred. It is important to remember that palpable distal pulses do not rule out compartment syndrome, as muscle and nerve necrosis often occurs before complete arterial occlusion from increased pressure gradients [68].

The most effective way to correctly diagnose and treat compartment syndrome is to have a high index of suspicion. Physical exam can be unreliable, so diagnosis requires knowledge of the patient's clinical situation and recognition of risk factors as described above. It is also possible to measure compartment pressures using manometers or handheld needle transducer devices. This is typically pursued in equivocal cases and is not required if clinical suspicion is high. Normal compartment pressures are defined to be less than 10 mmHg, while pressures above 25 mmHg require fasciotomy [64, 69].

The definitive treatment of compartment syndrome is decompression through fasciotomy. The most commonly used technique in the lower extremity is the two-incision, four-compartment fasciotomy (Fig. 21.14), whereby all four compartments in the lower leg can be decompressed and visualized to assess the degree of damage or need for debridement. A 12–20 cm lateral longitudinal incision is made 2 cm anterior to the fibula extending the length of the lower leg, and both the anterior and lateral compartments are accessed. A similar medial skin incision is made 2 cm posterior to the tibia, and both the superficial and deep posterior compartments are released. The deep posterior compartment must not be overlooked, as it contains the tibial nerve and both the peroneal and posterior tibial arteries [3, 64, 70].

The thigh is less commonly affected by compartment syndrome, but should the need for decompression arise, a single-incision, two-compartment fasciotomy can be performed. Although there are three compartments in the thigh (Fig. 21.15), the medial compartment rarely requires decom-

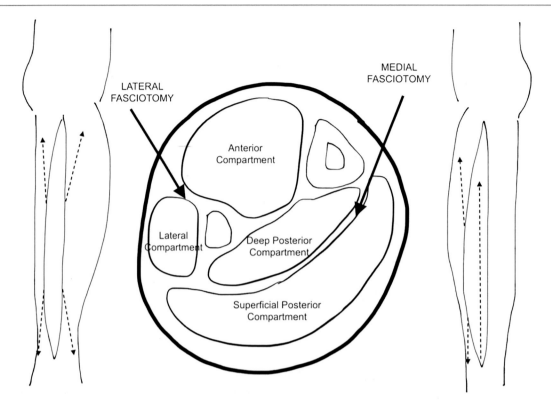

Fig. 21.14 Lower extremity fasciotomy

Fig. 21.15 Thigh
compartments

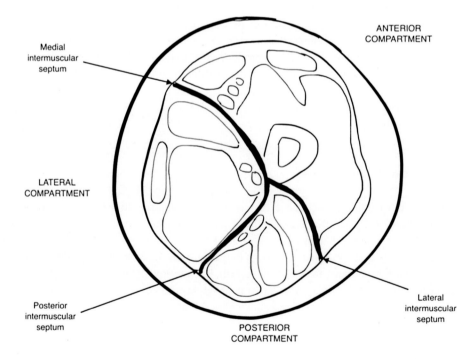

pression. The anterior and posterior compartments can be accessed through an incision along the lateral thigh that extends from the intertrochanteric line through the lateral epicondyle. The posterior compartment is then released by incising the lateral intermuscular septum [64, 71].

The forearm is the most common site of upper extremity compartment syndrome. Three compartments make up the forearm: superficial and deep volar compartments and an extensor dorsal compartment. These are decompressed through a volar curvilinear incision beginning proximal to

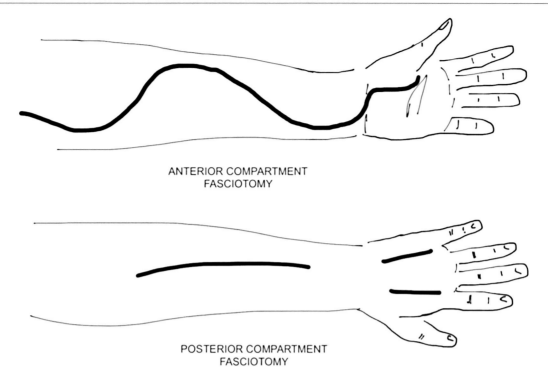

Fig. 21.16 Forearm fasciotomy

the antecubital fossa and medial to the biceps tendon. It then extends distally along the medial border of the brachioradialis muscle and crosses the carpal tunnel to extend onto the palm in the thenar crease (Fig. 21.16). The fascia overlying both the superficial compartment and the deep flexor compartment must be opened. If the dorsal compartment is also affected, an incision that extends from the lateral epicondyle to the wrist is used [72].

Early prophylactic fasciotomies are also commonly performed in high-risk situations. This can be done prior to any revascularization procedure to avoid potentially deleterious complications. High-risk patients include those with severely injured extremities (MESS greater than 7), those that required significant resuscitation or transfusion, those with complex orthopedic fractures, and those with repairs that were not complete within 6 h of injury [46, 73]. Delaying or missing the opportunity to perform fasciotomy can have devastating consequences such as significant neuropathy, contracture, or amputation.

Functionality/Mortality

Vascular repairs are performed with such success that it is rarely ischemia that leads to long-term complications with extremity function. Typically the associated orthopedic, soft tissue, and nervous injuries more accurately predict limb function outcomes. The salvage of a vascularly intact limb does not necessarily mean it is functional, and loss of neurologic,

muscular, or skeletal function can significantly impact a patient's quality of life. While many adverse long-term effects from severe extremity vascular trauma exist, advances in diagnosis and treatment have greatly improved many aspects of long-term survival, leading to successes in maintaining both life and limb in this patient population [15, 36, 74, 75].

In summary, given the advances in prehospital, resuscitative, and surgical management of major extremity vascular trauma, the associated mortality is becoming progressively infrequent. While it remains a common injury seen in combat, in the civilian sector vascular extremity trauma remains rare. Regardless of the cause, every surgeon should be familiar with recommended management and contemporary options available when faced with this injury.

References

1. Frykberg ER, Schinco MA. Peripheral vascular injury. In: Feliciano DV, Mattox KL, Moore EE, editors. Trauma. 6th ed. New York: McGraw-Hill; 2008. p. 941–71.
2. White JM, Stannard A, Burkhardt GE, Eastridge BJ, Blackbourne LH, Rasmussen TE. The epidemiology of vascular injury in the wars in Iraq and Afghanistan. Ann Surg. 2011;253(6):1184–9.
3. Patel KR, Rowe VL. Vascular trauma: extremity. In: Cronenwett JL, Johnston KW, et al., editors. Rutherford's vascular surgery. 7th ed. Philadelphia: Elsevier; 2010. p. 2361–73.
4. Kauvar DS, Sarfati MR, Kraiss LW. National trauma databank analysis of mortality and limb loss in isolated lower extremity vascular trauma. J Vasc Surg. 2011;53:1598–603.
5. Dorlac WC, DeBakey ME, Holcomb JB, Fagan SP, Kwong KL, Dorlac GR, Schreiber MA, Persse DE, Moore FA, Mattox

KL. Mortality from isolated civilian penetrating extremity injury. J Trauma. 2005;59(1):217–22.

6. Mabry RL. Tourniquet use on the battlefield. Mil Med. 2006;171(5):352–6.

7. Doyle GS, Taillac PP. Tourniquets: a review of current use with proposals for expanded prehospital use. Prehosp Emerg Care. 2008;12:241–56.

8. Sambasivan CN, Schreiber MA. Emerging therapies in traumatic hemorrhage control. Curr Opin Crit Care. 2009;15(6):560–8.

9. D'Alleyrand JC, Dutton RP, Pollak AN. Extrapolation of battlefield resuscitative care to the civilian setting. J Surg Orthop Adv. 2010;19(1):1–7.

10. Bulger EM, Snyder D, Schoelles K, Gotschall C, Dawson D, Lang E, Sanddal ND, Butler FK, Fallat M, Taillac P, White L, Salomone JP, Seifarth W, Betzner MJ, Johannigman J, McSwain N. An evidence-based prehospital guideline for external hemorrhage control: American College of Surgeons Committee on Trauma. Prehosp Emerg Care. 2014;18:163–73.

11. Horlocker TT, Hebl JR, Gali B, Jankowski CJ, Burkle CM, Berry DJ, Zepeda FA, Stevens SR, Schroeder DR. Anesthetic, patient, and surgical risk factors for neurologic complications after prolonged total tourniquet time during total knee arthroplasty. Anesth Analg. 2006;102(3):950–5.

12. Dennis JW, Frykberg ER, Crump JM, Vines FS, Alexander RH. New perspectives on the management of penetrating trauma in proximity to major limb arteries. J Vasc Surg. 1990;11:84–92.

13. Guede JW, Hobson RW, Padberg FT, Lynch TG, Lee BC, Jamil Z. The role of contrast arteriography in suspected arterial injuries of the extremities. Am Surg. 1985;51(2):89–93.

14. Frykberg ER. Advances in the diagnosis and treatment of extremity vascular trauma. Surg Clin North Am. 1995;75(2):207–23.

15. Pasch AR, Bishara RA, Lim LT, Meyer JP, Schuler JJ, Flanigan DP. Optimal limb salvage in penetrating civilian vascular trauma. J Vasc Surg. 1986;3(2):189–95.

16. Schwartz MR, Weaver FA, Bauer M, Siegel A, Yellin AE. Refining the indications for arteriography in penetrating extremity trauma: a prospective analysis. J Vasc Surg. 1993;17(1):116–22.

17. Frykberg ER, Crump JM, Vines FS, McLellan GL, Dennis JW, Brunner RG. A reassessment of the role of arteriography in penetrating proximity extremity trauma: a prospective study. J Trauma. 1989;29(8):1041–50.

18. Johansen K, Lynch K, Paun M, Copass M. Non-invasive vascular tests reliably exclude occult arterial trauma in injured extremities. J Trauma. 1991;31(4):515–9.

19. Bynoe RP, Miles WS, Bell RM, Greenwold DR, Sessions G, Haynes JL, Rush DS. Noninvasive diagnosis of vascular trauma by duplex ultrasonography. J Vasc Surg. 1991;14(3):346–52.

20. Schwartz M, Weaver F, Yellin A, Ralls P. The utility of color flow doppler examination in penetrating extremity arterial trauma. Am Surg. 1993;59(6):375–8.

21. Peng PD, Spain DA, Tataria M, Hellinger JC, Rubin GD, Brundage SI. CT angiography effectively evaluates extremity vascular trauma. Am Surg. 2008;74(2):103–7.

22. Busquéts AR, Acosta JA, Colón E, Alejandro KV, Rodriguez P. Helical computed tomographic angiography for the diagnosis of traumatic arterial injuries of the extremities. J Trauma. 2004;56(3):625–8.

23. Teitelbaum GP, Yee CA, Van Horn DD, Kim HS, Colletti PM. Metallic ballistic fragments: MR imaging safety and artifacts. Radiology. 1990;175:855–9.

24. Kollmeyer KR, Hunt JL, Ellman BA, Fry WJ. Acute and chronic traumatic arteriovenous fistulae in civilians. Arch Surg. 1981;116:697–702.

25. Smith RF, Szilagyi DE, Pfeifer JR. Arterial trauma. Arch Surg. 1963;86:825–35.

26. Dennis JW, Frykberg ER, Veldenz HC, Huffman S, Menawat SS. Validation of nonoperative management of occult vascular injuries and accuracy of physical examination alone in penetrating extremity trauma: 5- to 10-year follow up. J Trauma. 1998;44(2):243–52.

27. Reuben BC, Whitten MG, Sarfati M, Kraiss LW. Increasing use of endovascular therapy in acute arterial injuries: analysis of the National Trauma Databank. J Vasc Surg. 2007;46:1222–6.

28. Johnson CA. Endovascular management of peripheral vascular trauma. Semin Intervent Radiol. 2010;27:38–43.

29. Starnes BW, Arthurs ZM. Endovascular management of vascular trauma. Perspect Vasc Surg Endovasc Ther. 2006;18:114–29.

30. Feliciano DV, Moore FA, Moore EE, West MA, Davis JW, Cocanour CS, Kozar RA, McIntyre RC. Evaluation and management of peripheral vascular injury. Part 1. Western Trauma Association/critical decisions in trauma. J Trauma. 2011;70:1551–6.

31. Stecco K, Meier A, Seiver A, Dake M, Zarins C. Endovascular stent-graft placement for treatment of traumatic penetrating subclavian artery injury. J Trauma. 2000;48(5):948–50.

32. Callcut RA, Mell MW. Modern advances in vascular trauma. Surg Clin North Am. 2013;93(4):941–61.

33. Stannard A, Eliason JL, Rasmussen TE. Resuscitative endovascular balloon occlusion of the aorta (REBOA) as an adjunct for hemorrhagic shock. J Trauma. 2011;71(6):1869–72.

34. Rasmussen TE, Clouse WD, Jenkins DH, Peck MA, Eliason JL, Smith DL. The use of temporary vascular shunts as a damage control adjunct in the management of wartime vascular injury. J Trauma. 2006;61(1):8–12.

35. Stain SC, Weaver FA, Yellin AE. Extra-anatomical bypass of failed traumatic arterial repairs. J Trauma. 1991;31(4):575–8.

36. Feliciano DV. Management of peripheral arterial injury. Trauma. 2010;16:602–8.

37. Dorweiler B, Neufang A, Schmiedt W, Hessmann MH, Rudig L, Rommens PM, Oelert H. Limb trauma with arterial injury: long-term performance of venous interpositions grafts. Thorac Cardiovasc Surg. 2003;51(2):67–72.

38. Feliciano DV, Mattox K, Graham JM, Bitondo CG. Five year experience with PTFE grafts in vascular wounds. J Trauma. 1985;25(1):71–82.

39. Martin LC, McKenney MG, Sossa JL, Ginzburg E, Puente I, Sleeman D, Zeppa R. Management of lower extremity arterial trauma. J Trauma. 1994;37(4):591–8.

40. Bishara RA, Pasch AR, Lim LT, Meyer JP, Schuler JJ, Hall RF, Flanigan DP. Improved results in the treatment of civilian vascular injuries associated with fractures and dislocations. J Vasc Surg. 1986;3(5):707–11.

41. Howe HH, Poole GV, Hansen KJ, Clark T, Plonk GW, Koman LA, Pennell TC. Salvage of lower extremities following combined orthopedic and vascular trauma: a predictive salvage index. Ann Surg. 1987;53(4):205–8.

42. Miller HH, Welch CS. Quantitative studies on the time factor in arterial injuries. Ann Surg. 1949;130(3):428–38.

43. Weaver FA, Rosenthal RE, Waterhouse G, Adkins RB. Combined vascular and skeletal injuries of the lower extremities. Am Surg. 1984;50(4):189–97.

44. Hafez HM, Woolgar J, Robbs JV. Lower extremity arterial injury: results of 550 cases and review of risk factors associated with limb loss. J Vasc Surg. 2001;33(6):1212–9.

45. Smith WR, Stahel PF, Morgan SJ, Trafton PG. Lower extremity. In: Feliciano DV, Mattox KL, Moore EE, editors. Trauma. 6th ed. New York: McGraw-Hill; 2008. p. 907–39.

46. Johansen K, Daines M, Howey T, Helfet D, Hansen ST. Objective criteria accurately predict amputation following lower extremity trauma. J Trauma. 1990;30(5):568–72.

47. Callcut RA, Acher CW, Hoch J, Tefera G, Turnipseed W, Mell MW. Impact of intraoperative arteriography on limb salvage for traumatic popliteal artery injury. J Trauma. 2009;67(2):252–7.
48. Lower limb. In: Drake R, Vogl AW, Mitchell AWM, editors. Gray's anatomy for students. 2nd ed. Philadelphia: Elsevier; 2010. p. 512–649.
49. Carrillo EH, Spain DA, Wilson MA, Miller FB, Richardson JD. Alternatives in the management of penetrating injuries to the iliac vessels. J Trauma. 1998;44(6):1024–9.
50. Mills JL. Infrainguinal disease: surgical treatment. In: Cronenwett JL, Johnston KW, et al., editors. Rutherford's vascular surgery. 7th ed. Philadelphia: Elsevier; 2010. p. 1682–703.
51. Parodi JC, Schonholz C, Ferreira LM, Bergan J. Endovascular stent-graft treatment of traumatic arterial lesions. Ann Vasc Surg. 1999;13(2):121–9.
52. Shah DM, Corson JD, Karmody AM, Fortune JB, Leather RP. Optimal management of tibial arterial trauma. J Trauma. 1988;28(2):228–34.
53. Roddy SP, Darling RC. Upper extremity arterial disease: revascularization. In: Cronenwett JL, Johnston KW, et al., editors. Rutherford's vascular surgery. 7th ed. Philadelphia: Elsevier; 2010. p. 1798–806.
54. Becker GJ, Benenati JF, Zemel G, Sallee DS, Suarez CA, Roeren TK, Katzen BT. Percutaneous placement of a balloon-expandable intraluminal graft for life-threatening subclavian arterial hemorrhage. J Vasc Interv Radiol. 1991;2(2):225–9.
55. Johnson M, Ford M, Johansen K. Radial or ulnar artery laceration. Repair or ligate? Arch Surg. 1993;128(9):971–4.
56. Timberlake GA, Kerstein MD. Venous injury: to repair or ligate, the dilemma revisited. Am Surg. 1995;61(2):139–45.
57. Crawford RS, Watkins MT. Ischemia - reperfusion. In: Cronenwett JL, Johnston KW, et al., editors. Rutherford's vascular surgery. 7th ed. Philadelphia: Elsevier; 2010. p. 89–100.
58. Cambria RA, Anderson RJ, Dikdan G, Teehan EP, Hernandez-Maldonado JJ, Hobson RW. Leukocyte activation in ischemia – reperfusion injury of skeletal muscle. J Surg Res. 1991;51(1):13–7.
59. Blaisdell F. The pathophysiology of skeletal muscle ischemia and the reperfusion syndrome: a review. Cardiovasc Surg. 2002; 10:620–30.
60. Wright JG, Kerr JC, Valeri CR, Hobson RW. Heparin decreases ischemia-reperfusion injury in isolated canine gracilis model. Arch Surg. 1988;123(4):470–2.
61. Odeh M. Mechanisms of disease: the role of reperfusion-induced injury in the pathogenesis of the crush syndrome. N Engl J Med. 1991;324(20):1417–22.
62. Brown CV, Rhee P, Chan L, Evans K, Demetriades D, Velmahos GC. Preventing renal failure in patients with rhabdomyolysis: do bicarbonate and mannitol make a difference? J Trauma. 2004; 56(6):1191–6.
63. Ricci MA, Graham AM, Corbisiero R, Baffour R, Mohamed F, Symes JF. Are free radial scavengers beneficial in the treatment of compartment syndrome after acute arterial ischemia? J Vasc Surg. 1989;9(2):244–50.
64. Modrall JG. Compartment syndrome. In: Cronenwett JL, Johnston KW, et al., editors. Rutherford's vascular surgery. 7th ed. Philadelphia: Elsevier; 2010. p. 2412–21.
65. Papalambros EL, Panayiotopoulos YP, Bastounis E, Zavos G, Balas P. Prophylactic fasciotomy of the legs following acute arterial occlusion procedures. Int Angiol. 1989;8(3):120–4.
66. Frank A, Bonney M, Bonney S, Weitzel L, Koeppen M, Eckle T. Myocardial ischemia reperfusion injury: from basic science to clinical bedside. Semin Cardiothorac Vasc Anesth. 2012;16(3): 123–32.
67. Zager R. Rhabdomyolysis and myohemoglobinuric acute renal failure. Kidney Int. 1996;49:314–26.
68. Jensen SL, Sandermann J. Compartment syndrome and fasciotomy in vascular surgery. A review of 57 cases. Eur J Vasc Endovasc Surg. 1997;13:48–53.
69. McQueen MM, Court-Brown CM. Compartment monitoring in tibial fractures. The pressure threshold for decompression. J Bone Joint Surg Br. 1996;78:99–104.
70. Janzing H, Broos P, Rommens P. Compartment syndrome as a complication of skin traction in children with femoral fractures. J Trauma. 1996;41(1):156–8.
71. Tarlow SD, Achterman CA, Hayhurst J, Ovadia DN. Acute compartment syndrome in the thigh complicating fracture of the femur. J Bone Joint Surg Am. 1986;68(9):1439–43.
72. Gelberman RH, Garfin SR, Hergenroeder PT, Mubarak SJ, Menon J. Compartment syndromes of the forearm: diagnosis and treatment. Clin Orthop. 1981;161:252–61.
73. Williams AB, Luchette FA, Papconstantinou HT, Lim E, Hurst JM, Johannigman JA, Davis K. The effect of early versus late fasciotomy in the management of extremity trauma. Surgery. 1997; 122(4):861–6.
74. Fern KT, Smith JT, Zee B, Lee A, Borschneck D, Pichora DR. Trauma patients with multiple extremity injuries: resource utilization and long-term outcome in relation to injury severity scores. J Trauma. 1998;45:489–94.
75. Lin CH, Wei FC, Levin LS, Su JI, Yeh WL. The functional outcome of lower-extremity fractures with vascular injury. J Trauma. 1997;43:480–5.

Iatrogenic Extremity Ischemia with the Potential for Amputation

22

Raymond A. Dieter, Jr., George B. Kuzycz, Raymond A. Dieter, III , and Dwight W. Morrow

Introduction

Multiple causes are noted as to the etiology of extremity ischemia. Each of these etiologies may lead to significant and serious complications—particularly involving the upper and lower extremity. As one consults for a medical condition which is creating difficulty for the individual patient, one must be aware of the disease and its ramifications. When diagnostic or therapeutic regimens are suggested and then initiated, the potential benefit or benefits must outweigh the potential harm or secondary complications as a result of the diagnostic and therapeutic approach being planned for the individual patient and his or her symptomatology. We have seen a large number of patients with upper and lower extremity ischemia. Most of these patients and their affliction had ongoing and difficult concerns requiring intervention considerations of different modalities. The chance for complications and for potential life- or limb-threatening adversities must be evaluated in each individual in order to select the most appropriate diagnostic, therapeutic, and operative approach to be taken.

R.A. Dieter, Jr., MD, MS (✉)
Northwestern Medicine, At Central DuPage Hospital,
Winfield, IL, USA

International College of Surgeons, Cardiothoracic and Vascular Surgery, Glen Ellyn, IL, USA

G.B. Kuzycz, MD
Thoracic and Cardiovascular Surgery, Cadence Hospital of Northwestern System, Winfield, IL, USA

R.A. Dieter, III , MD
Division of Cardiothoracic Surgery, The University of Tennessee Medical Center, Knoxville, TN, USA

D.W. Morrow, MD
Pathology, Edward Hospital, Naperville, IL, USA

History

Limb amputation remains one of the more feared results of disease and interventional therapy. Over the years and centuries, a number of ritualistic, punitive, legal, and iatrogenic causes of limb loss have been delineated by Kirkup [1] (Table 22.1). A history of human mutilation and amputation has been documented in prehistoric caves from France and Spain with partial amputation of fingers and thumbs dating back 25,000 years. This procedure has even been performed more recently in the 1960s in the New Guinea Dugum Dani tribe. Such was also the case in the Moendan tribe in India. In the Assiniboine and Crow Indians of North America, using a sharp knife or a tomahawk, amputation was done in mourning. More recently in 2005, a South Korean physician was arrested for assisting in a self-inflicted finger amputation [1].

Punitive thumb and great toe amputations were performed on prisoners according to the *Book of Judges*. And, in 1314, three English soldiers under the king's service had punitive

Table 22.1 Historic causes of limb loss

Partial or total
Prehistoric: Spain/France
1960s New Guinea tribe
Moendan in India
Mourning—North American Crow Indians
Ritualistic
Punitive
Legal
Prisoners per *Book of Judges*
1600s arm or hand—infringement on tribal laws
2000 bc: loss one or both hands of a physician
Iatrogenic
Inappropriate splint application
Tourniquets misplaced
Seton complication
Wound infection or inappropriate surgical incision
Lack of knowledge/poor advice

R.S. Dieter et al. (eds.), *Critical Limb Ischemia*, DOI 10.1007/978-3-319-31991-9_22

hand amputations after the Battle of Bannockburn. In Peru, during the sixteenth century, infringement on tribal laws was punished by amputation of the hand for theft or a foot for laziness or both arms for rebellion. In 2000 BC, in Babylon, a physician could lose both hands if an operation on an eye failed.

Iatrogenic causes for amputation of an extremity have been known for centuries. Tourniquets have long been known to cause ischemia of the extremity upon which they were applied. Misapplied fracture splints and bandages and the consequent result were known by Hippocrates. In 1798, Folly—a Danish surgeon—reported on the death of 19 of 20 individuals from gangrene as a result of inappropriately placed splints and bandages for fractures. Unfortunately, these gangrenous results have more recently been noted in Ethiopia and with misapplied tourniquets placed on the battlefield during World War I. The problem was reportedly reduced after instructional programs.

Other iatrogenic or self-inflicted causes of extremity loss followed such items as seton treatment of wound infection or accidental scratching or cutting oneself in an operating room, prior to sterile techniques, knowledge, and antibiotics. Lack of understanding and thus appropriate advice by uninformed physicians has been known to lead to ischemia or loss of an extremity. We have been requested to assist in the treatment of such patient complications to avoid progressive ischemia or amputations, including accidental self-induced amputation of the upper extremity.

Current Experience

Over the past few decades, vascular surgery and vascular interventional procedures have escalated in both numbers and complexity. We have seen a large number of individuals with vascular complaints both electively and urgently, as well as in emergency situations [2]. These problems have included the outpatient as well as the inpatient situation. When evaluating patients, a complete history and physical exam are required in order to provide the most appropriate recommendation and therapy program for the individual. Initially, in the elective situation, when possible, noninvasive or minimally invasive procedures and testing are first utilized. Moreover, in the urgent or more emergent situation, such as a ruptured aneurysm, direct invasive and therapeutic procedures are usually required—time permitting. In these life or limb situations, the frequency and risk for complications are much greater. Immediate ambulance or ER to the OR may be the best approach with no intervening delays.

However, as the physician intervenes with more complicated and innovative procedures, the risk of side effects from the potential beneficial therapy also increases. Life and death situations, as well as limb salvage, must be balanced against the potential for complications. When the patient has severe ischemia or is in a shocklike situation, the treating team

utilizes the most appropriate therapy for the situation and the patient—even though in many instances the treatment is risky and highly complicated. Such intervention may lead to successful results for the patient, no improvement, continued deterioration, or to adverse side effects and complications—including loss of an extremity or life.

Over the years, we have seen a number of patients with multiple medical disorders who required intervention to save a life or an extremity. Many of these patients have had successful therapeutic approaches including vascular intervention utilizing either the open surgical approach or the percutaneous catheter system. Unfortunately, a number of these individuals required extensive intervention and/or multiple interventional procedures. Thus, the chance for vascular compromise and major vascular complications has developed during the course of treatment in a few patients. The causes of significant extremity ischemia or premorbid situations may present a difficult treatment challenge—especially when one is simultaneously working to salvage a life.

Listed above are a number of etiologies for iatrogenic ischemia of the extremities (Table 22.2). The most common

Table 22.2 Some iatrogenic causes of extremity ischemia

Shower emboli
Aortic or aneurysm surgery
Catheter induced
Vascular occlusion
Graft failure
Arterial compression occlusion
Prolonged aortic cross-clamping
Inappropriate cast application
Prolonged malposition of extremity
Diagnostic pressure line
Arterial—especially radial
Medication
Intra-arterial: especially epinephrine
HIPA/HIT syndrome
Prolonged ergot usage
Catheter manipulation
Guidewire vessel perforation
Balloon fracture
Hydrophilic catheter emboli
Vascular closure device embolization
Diagnostic or therapeutic catheterization—e.g., TAVR
Surgical injury
Operative—e.g., popliteal artery transection
Vessel penetration or laceration
Pediatrics
Tiny vessels
Arterial catheters
Diagnostic
Dislodged tumor
Cardiac—especially benign
Pulmonary—especially intracardiac extension

Table 22.3 Critical extremity ischemic due to occluded vessel

Occluded vessel	Ischemic structure
Radial artery	Hand/arm
Brachial artery	Lower arm
Subclavian artery	Arm
Posterior tibial artery	Foot
Popliteal artery	Lower leg
Femoral artery	Leg
Iliac artery	Entire leg
Aorta	Both legs

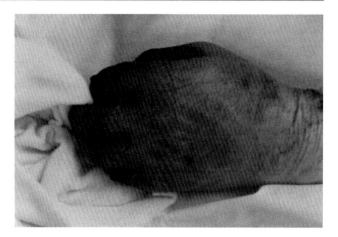

Fig. 22.1 Ischemic hand subsequent to arterial monitoring line placement

causes of ischemic compromise of an extremity occur after other treatment modalities result in either embolic (single or shower emboli) or vascular thrombotic occlusion during treatment, guidewire perforation of the vessel or plaque, plaque disruption and embolization, and inadvertent transection of vessels or clot disruption at the time of treatment of aneurysms. Most of the time, the source of significant embolic clot originates in the larger vessels during clamping or circumferential dissection about the clot-containing aorta. Other ischemic causes include inadvertent intra-arterial epinephrine, arterial pressure lines, large-bore catheters in small or tiny pediatric vessels, and prolonged clamp or tourniquet time. Almost any artery may inadvertently be involved in an iatrogenic injury or vascular occlusion. The more common vessels which might be occluded and lead to significant extremity complications or loss are delineated in Table 22.3.

Upper Extremity Ischemia

Fortunately, most patients have adequate circulation and a competent collateral circulatory system. This is well demonstrated by the large number of patients, in whom the radial artery is utilized for arteriovenous dialysis fistula creation, cardiac catheterization studies, and placement of arterial pressure monitoring lines [3]. Most of these patients tolerate the procedure well and require no further treatment at the completion of the radial or brachial artery procedure. Unfortunately, the occasional procedure will not proceed as planned. We have seen several patients with hand or arm ischemia, including one with blackened gangrene of the arm to above the elbow, following arterial monitoring line placement (Fig. 22.1). We have also seen patients lose digits after AV fistula creation for dialysis. Volkmann's contracture and persistent limb ischemia have resulted in upper extremity amputation after a brachial artery catheterization for hemodynamic monitoring [4]. Radial artery harvest for coronary surgery or catheterization for monitoring has also led to ischemia or amputation [5, 6]. Thus, radial artery pressure monitors as well as arteriovenous shunt creation for hemodialysis require careful consideration of the col-

Table 22.4 Arterial line guidelines

Identify patient with informed consent
Assess circulation to extremity/Allen's test
Insertion techniques
Check allergy and coagulation history—universal protocol
Sterile technique
Prepare line and fluids
On insertion of arterial catheter, secure zero level
Stabilize arm and set alarm parameters
Do baseline recording
Elevate hand
Maintenance/monitor
Periodic evaluation of hand and monitor wave form
Check tubing and connections frequently
Follow aspiration, flushing, and sterility guidelines
Always aspirate before flushing
Watch for bubbles or clots
Medications
None per A-line except heparin
Only IV flush fluid per line with bag pressure 300 mmHg
Chlorhexidine-based skin antiseptic—unless allergy
Removal
Assess ongoing necessity
Turn off arterial alarms
Remove catheter if coagulation profile is acceptable
Apply pressure with sterile dressing to avoid bleeding
Reassess the hand and site periodically

lateral circulation as well as pressure monitoring policies [7]. Irrigation techniques, anticoagulation, and pressure cuff application programs need constant awareness and compliance. Enclosed is an example of a monitoring program to minimize the risk of radial artery thrombosis, digital or upper extremity ischemia, and gangrene—especially in the low cardiac output patient (Table 22.4).

Another concern is the occasional patient who requires diagnostic interventional studies or therapeutic procedures while simultaneously requiring anticoagulation. This presents the therapeutic or diagnostic team a challenging situation. Should the anticoagulation therapy be discontinued and appropriate time allowed for hematologic correction to occur? Or, rather, should the team proceed with intervention despite the increased associated risks when delay may be felt inappropriate and more risky than intervention? If intervention is chosen, the increased risks are discussed with the patient/family, and the least risky (or safest of the high-risk options) approach is utilized.

Many times this will lead to an upper extremity and radial artery procedure. When this approach is utilized, pressure via hand or site-specific pressure dressings or apparatus may be used to occlude the access puncture site to prevent bleeding after completion of the procedure and removal of the intra-arterial line. Close nursing observation and monitoring of the extremity and the specific access area are then required. If the extremity becomes tense and upper arm compartment syndrome is suspected, surgery may be recommended when vascular compromise is a concern. Such a condition may also develop consequent to inadvertent intravenous fluid extravasation. It may be difficult to differentiate the cause for the compartment concerns however until actual surgical fascial release intervention occurs. Patient symptomatology may be of assistance in these situations, but not always definitive in the diagnosis and prevention of surgery.

Hydrophilic Polymer Emboli and Their Sequela: A Case Report

With the use of more catheter techniques for vascular diagnosis and therapy, a new and possibly underrecognized result of these catheter procedures is being reported [8]. An example of this was an 89-year-old female who presented with three painful purple toes on her left foot and new onset atrial fibrillation with slow capture. Initial evaluation suggested embolic events to the toes. Angiographic evaluation showed extensive peripheral vascular disease, with various occlusions of the left tibial-peroneal trunk and distal anterior tibial artery. Subsequent interventional procedures using wiring of the anterior tibial, peroneal, and posterior tibial arteries, laser atherectomy, AngioJet thrombectomy, balloon angioplasty, and tPA resulted in much greater patency of the anterior tibial and tibial-peroneal trunk. A repeat angiographic procedure was then performed for additional balloon angioplasty and stenting of several vessels. She now had more discrete areas of increasingly black toes and some beginning demarcation. She was maintained on Coumadin and Plavix.

Over the next few weeks, her toes showed increasing demarcation of black dry ischemic regions. Transcutaneous oxygen testing around the base of the toes and across the metatarsal arch was markedly abnormal. Two months after

her original presentation, she had a resurgence of pain in the left foot. Another vascular catheterization was performed, showing recurrent blockages in the anterior tibial and tibioperoneal trunk, which were unable to be resolved by additional atherectomy and PTA. She then had an arterial bypass procedure, which did not yield significant improvement.

As the angiographic presentation made it unlikely that she would be able to heal either a toe amputation or a transmetatarsal amputation, she underwent a below-knee amputation. The resected leg showed the expected vascular changes in the major vessels. What was a surprise finding was the presence of numerous diffuse hydrophilic polymer emboli in the arterial vessels in the metatarsal arch region from the base of the toes through the midfoot. This material presents microscopically, as a folded or coiled foreign body material in the arterial lumen, associated with blood clot and/or vascular wall reaction (Figs. 22.2, 22.3, and 22.4). In this patient, this material provided significant additional impediment to the reestablishment of adequate microcirculation and as it was felt may explain some of the initial difficulty in obtaining good transcutaneous oxygen values after the first three endovascular procedures.

This patient presents the findings of a developing technology to provide a catheter which is small in diameter and yet has a characteristic that permits easy slippage into and within a vessel to avoid clot formation. However, in having the needed quality or lumen to permit passage of drugs, dye, or blood, the catheter has some potential limitations. During the attempt to provide an optimal small-diameter catheter, which is both flexible and steerable and through which radiopaque contrast may be injected, the catheter wall is formulated with a substance which may break or flake off and embolize. Other authors have also noted this difficulty of iatrogenic ischemia and secondary infarction resulting from the hydrophilic polymer emboli [9, 10]. These emboli may cause a number of consequences ranging from no significant abnormalities to development of a stroke, pulmonary infarction, nonhealing catheter sites, and death (see Table 22.5). Microscopic examination of the embolized site may demonstrate the foreign body material (hydrophilic polymer) as well as microthrombus. With time, the polymer may eventually decompose or biodegrade in vivo, but this requires a long time period for dissolution.

Our first experience of catheter-induced ischemia occurred in 1967, when the embolectomy balloon ruptured and embolized during a balloon catheter embolectomy of the lower extremity. This balloon fragment was not retrievable and the patient experienced continued leg deterioration. Since that time, other authors have reported their complications with catheter-induced ischemia. More recently the hydrophilic polymer emboli have gained increasing attention, but other catheter complications including vessel rupture, plaque disruption, and vessel disruption or occlusion remain a concern.

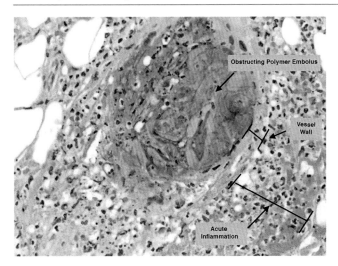

Fig. 22.2 Hydrophilic polymer embolus, with surrounding acute inflammation involving lower extremity

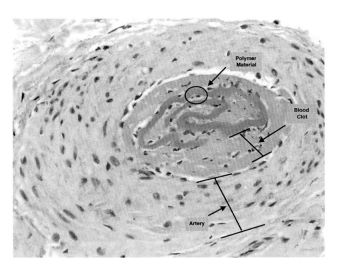

Fig. 22.3 Hydrophilic polymer material in arterial blood clot

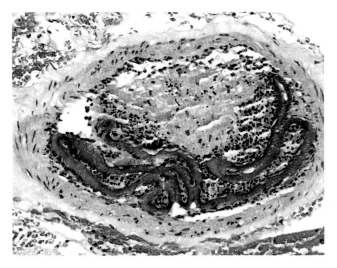

Fig. 22.4 Microscopic examination of endovascular hydrophilic polymer embolus with secondary occlusion of vessel

Table 22.5 Potential hydrophilic polymer emboli sequela

None
Pulmonary infarct or cavity
Central nervous system
CVA/stroke
Aseptic meningitis
Ongoing gangrene
Nonhealing catheter site
Death

Iatrogenic Arterial Injury

Arterial injury as a result of penetrating and blunt surgical trauma is seen on occasion. This usually requires intervention to avoid more serious complications, including false aneurysm formation, profound ischemia, or morbid deterioration of the extremity. Arterial injury including vascular transection may occur in the operating room, as well as in the community. Percutaneous iatrogenic injuries to the larger vessels, such as the femoral, subclavian, carotid, brachial, and popliteal arteries have all stimulated consultations with us. Massive bleeding, hematoma formation, and tissue compression by a false aneurysm as well as the ischemic concerns may develop from these injuries. Moramarco et al. demonstrated the endograft therapy for an iatrogenic popliteal artery arteriovenous fistula and an iatrogenic brachial artery transection after endovascular aneurysm repair [11].

Orthopedic surgery has led to transection, perforation, or ligation of major arteries, including the iliac, femoral, and popliteal arteries. Disruption of the iliac artery during hip surgery has been seen and repaired a number of times. The thin acetabulum may lend itself to perforation and arterial damage. When the patient has had previous hip surgery, they seem to be more susceptible to this type of injury with perforation or disruption of the iliac vessel. Simple suture repair or grafting may be utilized for leg salvage and to control bleeding. This may present a major concern when the hip surgery is for infection of the hip/prosthesis. Added to the problem is the occasional colonic perforation also found at exploration to control the bleeding and preserve the limb. Immediate operative repair or bypass procedures have been utilized to correct these injuries and avoid major bleeding or limb and organ ischemia. Primary repair has been our preferred choice, but saphenous vein or synthetic graft bypass, as well as endovascular repair, may be utilized in the specific case situation. Other large and small vessels that have been injured and required consultation and emergent surgical correction include the superior mesenteric, celiac, axillary, and renal arteries. Each of these, as with the extremities, may have profound side effects when not corrected.

Corrective procedures for iatrogenic arterial injuries to the upper and lower extremities have required diligence and

Table 22.6 Types of treatment or repair for iatrogenic limb ischemia

Primary suture
Ligation
Graft—patch or bypass
Tissue
Vein
Saphenous
Adjoining
Bovine
Homograft
Graft—synthetic
Dacron
Gore-Tex
Endograft
Vessel coverage
Omentum
Muscle
Resection
Amputation
Morbid tissue
Observation
Medications
Anticoagulation
Antibiotics
Specific diseases—e.g., diabetes
Analgesics
Autoamputation
Digits—especially
Endovascular
Vascular dilation/stent
Embolectomy
Enzymatic

innovation—particularly when there was infectious sequela to be considered. Demonstrated below are the various primary or secondary repair techniques which we have utilized (Table 22.6). On occasion, when the injury is more proximal and if there is any consideration for infection, the wound has been left open or the injured vessel is covered, when possible, with viable muscle or omentum. The use of various grafts, including the synthetic Dacron or Gore-Tex, the saphenous vein, bovine graft, or homograft, is individualized for the specific situation.

Lower Extremity Incidents

A large number of individuals have peripheral vascular symptoms referable to aortoiliac or femoropopliteal occlusive disease. These patients may be severely limited or only mildly disabled. Presence or absence of pulsation and noninvasive studies may define the location and severity of the disease. Questioning of the patient as to limitation on effort will assist in defining the need for intervention—both diagnostically and

therapeutically. It has always been our approach in the elective situation to use noninterventional therapy unless the working individual was unable to perform his duties and earn a satisfactory living. If the individual was not working and could ambulate to self-care for basic self-care functions, we did not encourage intervention—angiographic, percutaneous catheter, or open surgical. The basis for this approach revolves around the fact that any interventional procedure on a vessel—especially a smaller one—has the potential for a complication, including the loss of a portion or the entire extremity. Whether the intervention is an open, surgical endarterectomy, angiography, or a drug-eluting stent, complications and amputation may ensue [12, 13]. However, most authors report excellent salvage results of the limb with critical ischemia and few amputations or treatment failures upon initiation of treatment or intervention [14].

Tumor Emboli

On occasion, when dissecting major tumors—especially cardiothoracic—the vessel or heart may be involved by the tumor. Dissection or retraction techniques may initiate embolization of the tumor with subsequent leg, gastrointestinal, or CNS (central nervous system) symptoms, such as migraine, headaches, or stroke. Particularly, when one is unaware of the potential complicating situation, dissection of these malignancies and the area surrounding the involved tissues may disrupt the tumor, a portion of the tumor, or an adherent clot causing an embolic phenomenon—such as an atrial clot due to a benign or malignant mediastinal tumor compressing the atrium. These tumors may then embolize to the cerebral, gastrointestinal, or extremity vascularity. Such embolization almost always creates an acute ischemic situation, which usually is recognized in either the operating or recovery room. Depending on the situation and the patient's condition, the patient may be returned to the operating room for embolectomy and for removal of the tumor to avoid embolic ischemia, amputation, or stroke.

Miscellaneous

Other causes of iatrogenic ischemia of the extremities include medications related to prescribed therapy for migraine headaches and anticoagulants for treatment of coagulopathy—such as Coumadin, Coumadin necrosis, and other severe vasoconstrictor medications. Heparin antibodies may lead to peripheral or central clotting syndromes with myocardial infarction, peripheral thrombosis, ischemia, and/or amputation. Thus, a previous history of heparin therapy and possible heparin-induced thrombosis (HIT) may be a warning to the treatment team. In our experience, major or minor venous iatrogenic injury has not led to critical limb ischemia in the majority of patients but may, on occasion, lead to massive edema and fluid sequestration.

Whatever the situation, realization of the possibility of complications or side effects of vascular intervention—especially involving the arterial system—one must be alert to this potential for adverse events to occur. This is further emphasized by Gaudino et al. in reviewing the issues for usage of the radial artery as a conduit in coronary artery bypass surgery [15, 16]. Conservative and appropriate vascular testing for flow characteristics in the event of adverse results may minimize the potential for major complications when approaching the arterial system.

A recent technology has been associated with major vascular complications. Transcatheter aortic valve replacement (TAVR) has been associated with major vascular complications (MVC) including dissection, disruption, occlusion, and hematoma. The Partner Trial had an MVC rate of 15.3 % [17]. This has improved with smaller delivery devices as seen in the US Pivotal Trial with a MVC of approximately 6 %. Careful preoperative evaluation of access sites must be considered. Some complications may be treated with endovascular procedures and stents.

Newer procedures that may be less invasive, and yet therapeutic, continue to be employed by the practicing physician. Thinking "out of the box" may be beneficial, but also will have inherent side effects. Such is exemplified by the ischemia produced after the inadvertent embolization of an Angio-Seal (Vascular Closure) device to the superficial femoral artery and subsequent removal via the opposite common femoral artery utilizing a SpiderFX embolic protection device and sheath [18].

Acknowledgments A special thank you to Diane Paulini, Library Coordinator, Elmhurst Memorial Healthcare, Elmhurst, Illinois, Soukup Herter Library and Resource Center, for her assistance in locating the appropriate reference articles and to Lynn Murawski for typing and the preparation of the chapter.

References

1. Kirkup, J. A history of limb amputation. Ritual, punitive, legal and iatrogenic causes. London: Springer; 2007. pp. 35–44.
2. Dieter Jr RA, Asselmeier GH, McCray RM. Complications of arterial puncture and catheterization. Med Trial Tech Q. 1973;19:432–8.
3. Handlogten KS, Wilson GA, Clifford L, Nuttal CA, Kor DJ. Brachial artery catheterization: an assessment of use patterns and associated complications. Anesth Analg. 2014;118(2): 288–95.
4. Bagga V, Palmer M, Sadasivan R, Raghuraman G. Volkman's contracture, persistent limb ischemia, and amputation: a complication of brachial artery catheterisation for haemodynamic monitoring using PiCCo. Case Rep Crit Care. 2013;2013:474358. doi:10.1155/2013/474358.
5. Nunco-Mensah J. An unexpected complication after harvesting of the radial artery for coronary artery bypass grafting. Ann Thorac Surg. 1998;66(3):929–31.
6. Baker RJ, Chunprapaph B, Nyhus LM. Severe Ischemia of the hand following radial artery catheterization. Surgery. 1976;80(4): 449–57.
7. Garland A. Arterial lines in the ICU. Chest. 2014;146(5):1155–8.
8. Mehta RI, Mehta RI, Solis OE, Jahan R, Salamon N, Tobis JM, Yong WH, Vinters HV, Fishbein MC. Hydrophilic Polymer Emboli: an underrecognized iatrogenic cause of ischemia and infarct. Mod Pathol. 2010;23:921–30.
9. Fealy ME, Edwards WD, Giannini C, et al. Complications of endovascular polymers associated with vascular introducers sheaths and metallic coils in 3 patients, with literature review. Am J Surg Pathol. 2008;32:1310–6.
10. Allan RW, Alnuaimat H, Edwards WD, et al. Embolization of hydrophilic catheter coating to the lungs; report of a case mimicking granulomatous vasculitis. Am J Clin Pathol. 2009;132:794–7.
11. Moramarco LP, Fiorina I, Quaretti P. Endovascular management of upper and lower extremity vascular trauma. Endovasc Today. 2014;13:53–8
12. Giswold ME, Landry GJ, Taylor LM, Moneta GI. Iatrogenic arterial injury is an increasingly important cause of arterial trauma. Am J Surg. 2004;187:590–3.
13. Fukuda K, Higashimori A, Fujihara M, Jokoi Y. The breakage of a drug elevating stent delivery system leading to limb amputation. Cardiovasc Interv Ther. 2014;29:60–4.
14. Bosiers M, Scheinert D, Peeters P, Torsello G, Zeller T, Deloose K, Schmidt A, Tessarek J, Vinck E, Schwartz LB. Randomized comparison of everolimus: eluting versus bare-metal stents in patients with critical limb Ischemia and infrapopliteal arterial occlusive disease. J Vasc Surg. 2012;55(2):390–8.
15. Gaudino M, Crea F, Commertoni F, Mazza A, Tocsa A, Massetti M. Technical issues in the use of the radical artery as a coronary artery bypass conduct. Ann Thorac Surg. 2014;98(6):2247–54.
16. Gaudino M, Crea F, Cammertoni F, Massetti M. The radical artery: a forgotten conduct. Ann Thorac Surg. 2015;99: 1479–85.
17. Genereux P, et al. Vascular complications after transcatheter aortic valve replacement. J Am Coll Cardiol. 2012;60(12): 1043–52.
18. Suri S, Nagarsheth KH, Goraya S, Sengh K. A novel technique to retrieve a maldeployed vascular closure device. J Endovasc Ther. 2015;22(1):71–3.

Federico Bucci, Francesco Sangrigoli, and Leslie Fiengo

Introduction

Thromboangiitis obliterans (TAO) was first described in 1879, when Felix von Winiwarter, an Austrian surgeon who was an associate of Theodor Billroth, reported in the German Archives of Clinical Surgery a single case of what he described as presenile spontaneous gangrene [1]. In 1908, Leo Buerger, a physician at Mount Sinai Hospital (New York, NY, USA), noticed the same condition in 11 amputated limbs of patients of Jewish descent, describing the absence of large vessel involvement and termed the disease 'thromboangiitis obliterans' and in 1924 briefly reported a possible relationship with tobacco [2]. In 1922, Allen and Brown reported 200 cases of TAO from 1922 to 1926 and noticed that all were male smokers [3]. TAO or Buerger's disease (BD) is a segmental inflammatory arteriopathy affecting mostly medium- and small-sized vessels both arterial and venous in the lower and upper extremity. In some Eastern countries, this vasculitis can represent up to 40–60 % of all peripheral vascular diseases (PVD) [4, 5]. The disease affects mostly young male smokers and tends to present with rest pain and tissue loss. Tobacco exposure is strongly associated with initiation and progression of the disease even if the real mechanism remains still unclear. Since atherosclerotic risk factors other than smoking are commonly absent, smoking cessation is the only way to stop the disease progression. Clinical features, patient's history and angiographic findings are the basis of early diagnosis of TAO.

Epidemiology

TAO is a rare disease with differing worldwide prevalence. Reportedly, annual prevalence is 12.6 per 100,000, representing only 0.5 % of all PVD [6]. It is more frequent in East Europe, the Middle East and Asia with a high prevalence as 80 % among the Ashkenazi Jew population. Genetic influences are suggested by different prevalence in certain ethnic groups like in Israelis, some Indian groups, the Japanese, Southeast Asians and Middle Eastern groups and rarely in African-Americans. Buerger's disease is now increasing in prevalence among women owing to changing patterns in smoking with an incidence between 11 and 23 % in the most recent studies [6–8].

Etiopathogenesis

The precise cause of TAO is still unknown and different hypotheses are suggested but the most important is tobacco smoking. Because 95 % of the patients are smokers, it is suggested that the factor of initiation, progression and prognosis of this disease is a reaction to the constituents of cigarettes. TAO is probably a process of self-aggression triggered by nicotine or an idiosyncratic immune response to some agents present in tobacco such as arsenic. Other addictions such as cannabis and cocaine may be co-responsible for Buerger's disease, accelerating its clinical presentation and aggravating its extension. Since 1960, several case reports or case series, mainly from French authors, have reported distal arteritis mimicking TAO in cannabis users, suggesting a link with cannabis use [9–17]. Some authors suggest even the existence

F. Bucci, MD (✉)
Vascular Surgery Department, Polyclinique Bordeaux Rive Droite, Bordeaux, France

F. Sangrigoli, MD
Vascular Department, King's College Hospital, Hambleden West Wing, Second Floor, Denmark Hill, London SE5 9RS, UK

L. Fiengo, MD, PhD
Department of Surgery, La Sapienza University of Rome, Viale Regina Elena 324, Rome 00161, Italy

of a 'cannabis arteritis' [18], while others need more convincing scientific evidence [19]. However, if cannabis-associated arteritis is a distinct clinical entity, a subtype of TAO or a fortuitous association between a widely used drug and a rare disease, it remains controversial. Recurrent periodontal infections could play a role as well: polymerase chain reaction analysis demonstrated DNA fragments from anaerobic bacteria in both arterial lesions and oral cavities of patients with thromboangiitis obliterans but not in arterial samples from healthy controls [20]. Possibly, genetic modifications or autoimmune disorders are implicated [21]. Peripheral endothelium-dependent vasodilation is impaired in the no diseased limbs of patients with TAO, and this type of vascular dysfunction may contribute to such characteristics as segmental proliferative lesions or thrombus formation in the peripheral vessels [22]. Genetic influences are suggested by different prevalences in certain ethnic groups. In fact, TAO occurs frequently in Israelis, some Indian groups, the Japanese, Southeast Asians and Middle Eastern groups and rarely in African-Americans [23, 24]. Mutations in prothrombin 20210 G-A have also been the object of research [25, 26]. Studies have shown a possible relationship of TAO with hypercoagulable states, although its details are presently unknown. There are cases associated with protein S and protein C deficiencies [27, 28], antiphospholipid antibodies [29] and hyperhomocysteinemia [30, 31]. A recently published study showed that high concentrations of anticardiolipin antibodies were correlated with an early and more severe form of disease, including higher rates of amputation [32, 33].

Histology

Although TAO is a type of vasculitis, it is distinct from other vasculitis. There are two important distinctions: the absence of positive serological markers of inflammation and the nonexistence of autoantibodies. Acute-phase reactants such as erythrocyte sedimentation rate (ESR) and C-reactive protein (CRP), circulating immune complexes and autoantibodies such as antinuclear antibody, rheumatoid factor and complement levels are usually normal or negative.

Histologically, in the acute phase, preservation of the internal elastic lamina distinguishes it from the true necrotizing forms of arteritis. The artery or vein is modestly swollen, and there is a moderate infiltrate of the adventitia and media. The initial injuries are immune reactions associated with activation of lymphocytes, macrophages and dendritic cells in the arterial wall, followed by deposition of antiendothelial cell antibodies [4, 22, 23]. Pathologically, the thrombus in TAO is highly cellular, with much less intense cellular activity in the wall of the blood vessel. Lymphocytes exceed neutrophils, and occasional giant cells, and some eosinophils may be seen. In the chronic phase, cellularity of the vessel wall and thrombus decreases, microabscesses disappear and recanalization may begin.

Diagnosis and Differential Diagnosis

Buerger's disease is a clinical diagnosis that requires a compatible history, supportive physical findings and diagnostic vascular abnormalities on imaging studies [34–37]. Several different diagnostic criteria have been offered for the diagnosis of TAO (Table 23.1). The traditional diagnosis of TAO is based on the five criteria of Shionoya [34, 35], which are smoking history, onset before 50 years of age, infrapopliteal arterial occlusive disease, either upper limb involvement or phlebitis migrans and absence of atherosclerotic risk factors other than smoking, or based on the Olin criteria [6, 36], which are onset before 45 years of age; current tobacco use; distal extremity ischemia (infrapopliteal and/or infrabrachial) such as claudication, rest pain, ischemic ulcers or gangrene documented with noninvasive testing; laboratory tests to exclude autoimmune or connective tissue diseases and diabetes mellitus; exclusion of a proximal source of emboli with echocardiography and arteriography; and demonstration of consistent arteriographic findings in the involved and clinically noninvolved limbs.

Clinical manifestations of TAO may include painful digital ischemia, distal digital ulcerations, superficial thrombophlebitis and extremity claudication (Fig. 23.1). Raynaud's phenomenon is present in greater than 40 % of patients with TAO and may be asymmetric. As BD progresses, it may lead to gangrene and amputation. Commonly, two extremities are involved. Beacuse the disease affects the distal vessels, gangrene usually precedes claudication, which is not frequent and, whenever present, is confined to the foot. Sometimes, this pathology may be presented in asymptomatic patients as occlusive lesions and demonstrated in angiograms in the small arteries of the foot or hand. It may remain unnoticed until the involvement of arteries in the calf or forearm. Although most common in the extremities, TAO may also involve the cerebral, coronary, renal, mesenteric and pulmonary arteries.

The differential diagnosis of TAO is quite simple in the presence of a typical clinic pathological picture. There are situations in which diagnosis can be difficult, such as early onset arteriosclerosis in young male smokers and collagen and autoimmune diseases in young people associated with digital cyanosis, pain and gangrene. The literature has demonstrated that ischemia induced by cocaine and cannabis consumption can mimic BD [9–19, 38]. Superficial thrombophlebitis differentiates TAO from other vasculitides and atherosclerosis, though it may also be observed in Behçet's disease. In fact, patients may describe a migratory pattern of tender nodules that follow a venous distribution. Differential

Table 23.1 Diagnostic criteria

Shionoya criteria	Olin criteria
Smoking	Current or recent smoking
>50 years	>45 years
Infrapopliteal arterial occlusions, upper limb involvement or phlebitis migrans	Infrapopliteal arterial occlusions, upper limb involvement or phlebitis migrans
Absence of atherosclerotic risk factors other than smoking	Laboratory tests to exclude autoimmune or connective tissue diseases and diabetes mellitus
	Laboratory tests to exclude autoimmune or connective tissue diseases and diabetes mellitus
	Demonstrate consistent arteriographic findings in the involved and clinically noninvolved limbs

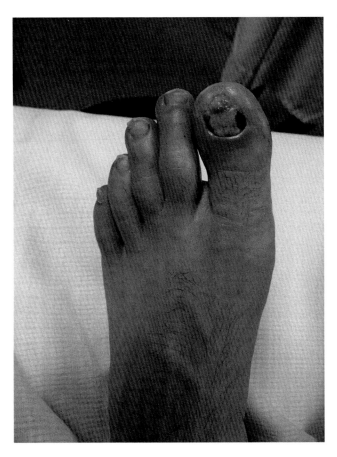

Fig. 23.1 Buerger's disease in the acute phase before initiation of treatment

diagnosis must be done also with other arteritis such as Takayasu's arteritis, in which larger elastic arteries such as the aorta and its branches are affected and where most of the patients are female in their second and third decade. With giant cell arteritis (temporal arteritis) which is a granulomatous vasculitis affecting large- and medium-sized arteries, cranial vessels are mostly affected. Polyarteritis nodosa is a necrotising vasculitis affecting small- and medium-sized artery vessels. Gastrointestinal and renal involvement is common, and males are mostly affected in middle age.

Connective tissue disorders have to be kept in mind in patients with digital ulceration without typical findings of atherosclerosis. Differential diagnosis includes atherosclerosis, thromboembolism, CREST syndrome, systemic lupus erythematosus, rheumatoid arthritis, connective tissue disease and antiphospholipid antibody syndrome [39]. Drugs induced such as sulphonamide, cocaine and penicillins must be kept in mind. In the presence of lower extremity involvement, the possibility of popliteal artery entrapment syndrome or cystic adventitial disease should be considered, both of which should be readily apparent on arteriography, computed tomography or magnetic resonance imaging. If there is isolated involvement of the upper extremity, thoracic outlet syndrome and occupational hazards such as use of vibratory tools and hypothenar hammer syndrome should be considered as well.

Diagnostic Workup

Physical examination must include a thorough vascular examination with particular attention to pulses, bruits and assessment of the ankle brachial index. An Allen test should be performed to demonstrate arterial involvement of the upper extremities even if asymptomatic. Laboratory testing in patients with suspected BD is used to exclude alternative diagnoses. Initial laboratory studies should include a complete blood count, metabolic panel, liver function tests, fasting blood glucose, inflammatory markers such as erythrocyte sedimentation rate and C-reactive protein, cold agglutinins and cryoglobulins. In addition, serological markers of autoimmune disease including antinuclear antibody (ANA), anticentromere antibody and anti-SCL-70 antibody should be obtained and are typically negative in thromboangiitis obliterans. Lupus anticoagulant and anticardiolipin antibodies are detected in some patients with thromboangiitis obliterans but may also indicate an isolated thrombophilia. Echocardiography may be indicated in certain cases when acute arterial occlusion due to thromboembolism is suspected, in order to detect a cardiac source of embolism. Computed tomography

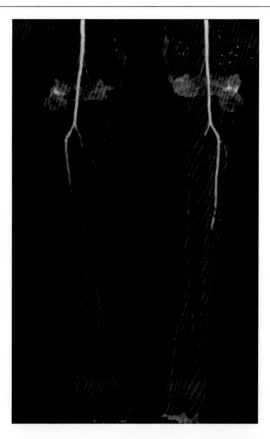

Fig. 23.2 Computerized tomography (CT) angiography of the lower limbs showing distal posterior and anterior tibial artery occlusion of the left side and three-vessel occlusion of the right side (Courtesy of Hindawi Publishing Corporation Case Reports in Vascular Medicine Volume 2013, Article ID 830540. Copyright © 2013 Federico Bucci et al. This is an open access article distributed under the Creative Commons Attribution License)

(Fig. 23.2), magnetic resonance or invasive contrast angiography may be performed to exclude a proximal arterial source of embolism and to define the anatomy and extent of disease. Although advances in computed tomographic and magnetic resonance angiography show promise for imaging distal vessels, most patients require invasive contrast angiography to provide the spatial resolution necessary to detect the distal arteriopathy (Fig. 23.3). The most important arteriographic features of the disease include segmental occlusive lesions of small- or medium-sized vessels (tibial, peroneal, plantar, palmar or digital arteries) interspersed with healthy-appearing segments; abundant collaterals described as 'corkscrew', 'spider legs' or 'tree roots'; and normal proximal arteries free of atherosclerosis or aneurysms [37]. Biopsy is rarely indicated, but is most likely to be diagnostic in a vein with superficial thrombophlebitis during the acute phase of the disease.

The angiographic findings in patients with TAO, although considered by some investigators to be pathognomonic, are not adequate to make a diagnosis, and their sensitivity and specificity are not high enough to be considered the gold standard. In fact, corkscrew collaterals are not pathognomonic and may be present in any connective tissue disease, such as scleroderma; calcinosis, Raynaud's phenomenon, esophageal dysmotility, sclerodactyly and telangiectasia (CREST) syndrome; lupus; or any other small-vessel obstructive disorder such as diabetes.

Treatment

It's well established that the severity of clinical manifestations of TAO is closely related to tobacco consumption. A specific treatment doesn't exist yet, and s*moking cessation* represents still nowadays the only effective treatment. To achieve that, in some countries you can find the so-called tobaccologists, who are licensed specialists that help you to get rid of your smoking addiction. A psychological support may be needed as well for these young and severely addicted patients, especially if there is a high risk of limb amputation [40].

Acute and Chronic Phase

We can distinguish an acute and a chronic phase of the disease: patients in the *acute phase*, which is limb threatening with severe symptoms mainly represented by critical limb ischemia (rest pain and tissue loss), should be treated on an *inpatient basis*. Patients in the chronic phase, should be encouraged to walk at least 30 min twice a day and don't need to stay at the hospital. The transition between the two phases is usually strictly related on the amount of tobacco consumption. Thus, patients who continue smoking are at risk of amputation of fingers and toes. The patients in the *chronic phase* can present with intermittent claudication, Raynaud's phenomenon or can be even totally asymptomatic. They should avoid any foot trauma, wear comfortable shoes, be very careful to prevent infections of the extremities and walk regularly.

Even if the cornerstone of treatment is tobacco cessation, we can consider several adjuvant medical and surgical therapies, especially during the acute phase.

Iloprost and Aspirin

A prospective randomised trial comparing intravenous infusion, on an inpatient basis, of a prostacyclin analogue (iloprost), with acetylsalicylic acid (aspirin), during the acute phase of Buerger's disease, showed that this drug was superior to aspirin alone for relief of ischemic symptoms and achieves healing [41]. Nevertheless, in another double-blind randomised placebo-controlled trial, the results of the oral analogue of iloprost were less satisfactory [42].

Other Oral Medications

Cilostazol, a phosphodiesterase III inhibitor, with both a vasodilator and an antiplatelet action, *pentoxifylline* through an unknown action over the red blood cell membrane, decreases

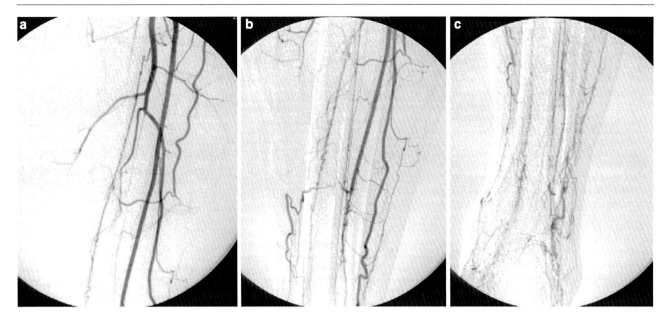

Fig. 23.3 (**a–c**) Intraoperative arteriography: occlusion of the left distal tibial and peroneal arteries, with the typical 'corkscrew' collateral arteries suggestive of a vasculitis

the viscosity of blood and thereby improves its flow through arteries, and calcium channel antagonists such as *amlodipine* are often prescribed to patients with TAO [43, 44]. However, the benefit of these orally administered anticlotting agents or vasodilators has not been evaluated by controlled studies.

Bosentan

Bosentan is an orally administered dual endothelin receptor antagonist used in the treatment of pulmonary artery hypertension. It has been recently used in a clinical pilot study to treat BD with encouraging short- and midterm results [45, 46]. Larger studies are required to confirm these results.

Thrombolysis

Intra-arterial thrombolytic agents such as streptokinase or recombinant tissue plasminogen activator (rtPA) may occasionally be used in the acute phase of the disease whenever there is evidence of fresh thrombus. A pilot study showed some benefit in BD patients suffering from acute exacerbations or thrombotic episodes with resulting variable degrees of gangrene or pre-gangrene of toes or feet [47].

Peripheral Sympathectomy and Spinal Cord Stimulation

Sympathectomy and spinal cord stimulation may be helpful in the short term for pain relief and ulcer healing, decreasing arterial spasm [48, 49]. A laparoscopic approach for sympathectomy can also be performed. Long-term benefit in patients with Buerger's disease should be confirmed with further studies.

Hyperbaric Oxygen Therapy

In a Japanese small cohort study, hyperbaric oxygen therapy was associated to autologous implantation of bone marrow mononuclear cells in seven patients affected with BD, showing good results for the achievement of therapeutic angiogenesis [50].

Bypass Surgery

The presence of a poor distal vascular bed doesn't allow performing a bypass in most BD patients. The benefit of arterial revascularization remains controversial because of the high rate of failure. However, in case of critical limb ischemia, and in the rare cases where a distal target vessel is present, bypass surgery with the use of an autologous vein could be theoretically feasible with acceptable results. In a retrospective study, primary and secondary patency rates at 5 years of a venous distal bypass were 48.8 and 62.5 %, respectively, with a satisfactory limb salvage rate of 82 % as long as patients stop smoking [51].

Endovascular Therapy

As for bypass surgery, percutaneous endoluminal interventions could play a role for limb salvage [52]. However, because of the diffuse inflammatory involvement of distal vessels, this can be rarely feasible, and midterm results are still unclear. A recent retrospective study demonstrated that percutaneous transluminal angioplasty (PTA) is safe and effective for the treatment of atypical (above the knee arterial occlusions) thromboangiitis obliterans [53].

Amputations

Amputation even of just a toe can be dramatic for this young population. The overall amputation rate (any and mayor) is about 25 % at 5 years, 38 % at 10 and 46 % at 20 years, whereas the risk of only major amputations is about 11 % at 5 years, 21 % at 10 and 23 % at 20 years [54].

Foot Care

Foot care and wound dressings are extremely important in order to prevent secondary infection. The patient must be encouraged to rest at bed to avoid any trauma; the wound should be kept clean and the skin lubricated with a moisturiser [55].

Further Researches

Some experimental studies have shown that vascular endothelial growth factor gene therapy can be very promising in patients with Buerger's disease, but results still remain controversial. Bone marrow mononuclear cell transplantation seems to promote significantly neoangiogenesis. In 1998, a first small cohort study demonstrated that intramuscular injection of endothelial growth factors (VEGF 165) was safe and effective for limb salvage in TAO patients [56]. Encouraging results were achieved by Japanese researchers for limb salvage in patients affected by critical limb ischemia due both to atherosclerosis and BD [50, 57–59]. Nevertheless, an unblinded and uncontrolled pilot study observed long-term adverse events, including death and unfavourable angiogenesis, in half of the patients receiving bone marrow mononuclear cell transplantation [60]. Given the current incomplete knowledge of the safety and efficacy of this strategy, careful long-term monitoring is required for future patients receiving these treatments.

References

1. Lie JT, Mann RJ, Ludwig J. The brothers von Winiwarter, Alexander (1848–1917) and Felix (1852–1931), and thromboangiitis obliterans. Mayo Clin Proc. 1979;54(12):802–7.
2. Buerger L. The circulatory disturbances of the extremities. Philadelphia, PA: WB Saunders; 1924.
3. Mills JL, Taylor Jr LM, Porter JM. Buerger's disease in the modern era. Am J Surg. 1987;154(1):123–9.
4. Joviliano EE, Dellalibera-Joviliano D, Dalio M, Evora PR, Piccinato CE. Etiopathogenesis, clinical diagnosis and treatment of thromboangiitis obliterans—current practices. Int J Angiol. 2009;18(3):119–25.
5. Weinberg I, Jaff M. Nonatherosclerotic arterial disorders of the lower extremities. Circulation. 2012;126:213–22.
6. Olin JW. Thromboangiitis obliterans (Buerger's disease). N Engl J Med. 2000;343(12):864–9.
7. Kobayashi M, Nishikimi N, Komori K. Current pathological and clinical aspects of Buerger's disease in Japan. Ann Vasc Surg. 2006;20(1):148–56.
8. Parvizi N, Shalhoub J, Davies AH. Buerger's disease: a multidisciplinary diagnostic and therapeutic challenge. JRSM Short. 2010;1(1):10.
9. Cazalets C, Laurat E, Cador B, et al. Cannabis arteritis: four new cases. Rev Med Interne. 2003;24(2):127–30.
10. Combemale P, Consort T, Denis-Thelis L, et al. Cannabis arteritis. Br J Dermatol. 2005;152(1):166–9.
11. Constans J. Cannabis-related arterial diseases. J Mal Vasc. 2002; 27(1):6.
12. Disdier P, Granel B, Serratrice J, et al. Cannabis arteritis revisited-ten new case reports. Angiology. 2001;52(1):1–5.
13. Karila L, Danel T, Coscas S, et al. Progressive cannabis-induced arteritis: a clinical thromboangiitis obliterans sub-group? Presse Med. 2004;33(18 Suppl):21–3.
14. Leithauser B, Langheinrich AC, Rau WS, et al. A 22-year old woman with lower limb arteriopathy. Buerger's disease, or methamphetamine- or cannabis-induced arteritis? Heart Vessels. 2005;20:39–43.
15. Noel B, Ruf I, Panizzon RG. Cannabis arteritis. J Am Acad Dermatol. 2008;58(5 Suppl 1):S65–7.
16. Peyrot I, Garsaud AM, Saint-Cyr I, et al. Cannabis arteritis: a new case report and a review of literature. J Eur Acad Dermatol Venereol. 2007;21(3):388–91.
17. Schneider HJ, Jha S, Burnand KG. Progressive arteritis associated with cannabis use. Eur J Vasc Endovasc Surg. 1999;18(4):366–7.
18. Martin-Blondel G, Koskas F, Cacoub P, Sne D. Is thromboangiitis obliterans presentation influenced by cannabis addiction? Ann Vasc Surg. 2011;25(4):469–73.
19. Grotenhermen F. Cannabis-associated arteritis. Vasa. 2010;39(1): 43–53.
20. Iwai T, Inoue Y, Umeda M. Oral bacteria in the occluded arteries of patients with Buerger disease. J Vasc Surg. 2005;42(1):107–15.
21. Tanaka K. Pathology and pathogenesis of Buerger's disease. Int J Cardiol. 1998;66 Suppl 1:S237–42.
22. Makita S, Nakamura M, Murakami H, Komoda K, Kawazoe K, Hiramori K. Impaired endothelium-dependent vasorelaxation in peripheral vasculature of patients with thromboangiitis obliterans (Buerger's disease). Circulation. 1996;94(9 Suppl):II211–5.
23. Numano F, Sasazuki T, Koyama T, et al. HLA in Buerger's disease. Exp Clin Immunogenet. 1996;3:195–200.
24. Chen Z, Takahashi M, Naruse T, et al. Synergistic contribution of CD14 and HLA loci in the susceptibility to Buerger's disease. Hum Genet. 2007;122:367–72.
25. Avcu F, Akar E, Demirkiliç U, Yilmaz E, Akar N, Yalçin A. The role of prothrombotic mutations in patients with Buerger's disease. Thromb Res. 2000;100:143–7.
26. Butt C, Zheng H, Randell E, Robb D, Parfrey P, Xie YG. Combined carrier status of prothrombin 20210A and factor XIII-A Leu34 alleles as a strong risk factor for myocardial infarction: evidence of a gene-gene interaction. Blood. 2003;101:3037–41.
27. Cailleux N, Guegan-Massardier E, Borg JY, et al. Pseudothromboangéite oblitérante et déficit qualitatif en protéine C: Á propos d'un cas. J Mal Vasc. 1996;21:47–9.
28. Feal Cortizas C, Abajo Blanco P, Aragüés Montañés M, Fernández Herrera J, García Diez A. Tromboangeitis obliterante (enfermedad de Buerger) y déficit de proteína C. Actas Dermosifiliogr. 1999;90:235–9.
29. Doko S, Katsumura T, Fujiwara T, Inada H, Masaka H. Antiphospholipid antibody syndrome and vasoocclusive diseases. Int J Angiol. 1995;4:55–60.
30. Stammler F, Diehm C, Hsu E, Stockinger K, Amendt K. The prevalence of hyperhomocysteinemia in thromboangiitis obliterans.

Does homocysteine play a role pathogenetically. Dtsch Med Wochenschr. 1996;121:1417–23.

31. Adar R, Papa MZ, Schneiderman J. Thromboangiitis obliterans: an old disease in need of a new look. Int J Cardiol. 2000;75:S167–70.

32. De Godoy JM, Braile DM, Godoy MF. Buerger's disease and anticardiolipin antibodies: a worse prognosis? Clin Appl Thromb Hemost. 2002;8:85–6.

33. Barbour SE, Nakashima K, Zhang JB, et al. Tobacco and smoking: environment factors that modify the host response (immune system) and have an impact on periodontal health. Crit Rev Oral Biol Med. 1997;8:437–60.

34. Shionoya S. What is Buerger's disease? World J Surg. 1983;7:544–51.

35. Shionoya S. Diagnostic criteria of Buerger's disease. Int J Cardiol. 1998;66(Suppl):243–5.

36. Olin JW, Young JR, Graor RA, Ruschhaupt WF, Bartholomew JR. The changing clinical spectrum of thromboangiitis obliterans (Buerger's disease). Circulation. 1990;825(Suppl):IV3–8.

37. Lambeth JT, Yong NK. Arteriographic findings in thromboangiitis obliterans with emphasis on femoropopliteal involvement. Am J Roentgenol Radium Ther Nucl Med. 1970;109:553–62.

38. Marder VJ, Mellinghoff IK. Cocaine and Buerger's disease: is there a pathogenetic association? Arch Intern Med. 2000;160(13):2057–60.

39. Pipitone N, Versari A, Salvarani C. Role of imaging studies in the diagnosis and follow-up of large vessel vasculitis: an update. Rheumatology. 2008;47:403–8.

40. Mills JL, Porter JM. Buerger's disease: a review and update. Semin Vasc Surg. 1993;6:14–23.

41. Fiessinger JN, Schafer M. Trial of iloprost versus aspirin treatment for critical limb ischaemia of thromboangiitis obliterans. The TAO Study. Lancet. 1990;335:555–7.

42. The European TAO Study Group. Oral iloprost in the treatment of thromboangiitis obliterans (Buerger's disease): a double-blind, randomised, placebo-controlled trial. Eur J Vasc Endovasc Surg. 1998;15:300–7.

43. Jorge VC, Araújo AC, Noronha C, Panarra A, Riso N, Vaz Riscado M. Buerger's disease (thromboangiitis obliterans): a diagnostic challenge. BMJ Case Rep. 2011;13:2011.

44. Dean SM. Pharmacologic treatment for intermittent claudication. Vasc Med. 2002;7(4):301–9. Review.

45. Todoli Parra JA, Hernandez MM, Arrebola Lopez MA. Efficacy of bosentan in digital ischemic ulcers. Ann Vasc Surg. 2010;24:690.e1–e4.

46. De Haro J, Acin F, Bleda S, Varela C, Esparza L. Treatment of thromboangiitis obliterans (Buerger's disease) with bosentan. BMC Cardiovasc Disord. 2012;12:5.

47. Hussein EA, el Dorri A. Intra-arterial streptokinase as adjuvant therapy for complicated Buerger's disease: early trials. Int Surg. 1993;78:54–8.

48. Ates A, Yekeler I, Ceviz M, Erkut B, Pac M, Basoglu A, Kocak H. One of the most frequent vascular diseases in northeastern of Turkey: thromboangiitis obliterans or Buerger's disease (experience with 344 cases). Int J Cardiol. 2006;28(111):147–53.

49. Donas KP, Schulte S, Ktenidis K, Horsch S. The role of epidural spinal cord stimulation in the treatment of Buerger's disease. J Vasc Surg. 2005;41:830–6.

50. Saito S, Nishikawa K, Obata H, Goto F. Autologous bone marrow transplantation and hyperbaric oxygen therapy for patients with thromboangiitis obliterans. Angiology. 2007;58:429–34.

51. Sasajima T, Kubo Y, Inaba M, Goh K, Azuma N. Role of infrainguinal bypass in Buerger's disease: an eighteen-year experience. Eur J Vasc Endovasc Surg. 1997;13:186–92.

52. Graziani L, Morelli L, Parini F, Franceschini L, Spano P, Calza S, Sigala S. Clinical outcome after extended endovascular recanalization in Buerger's disease in 20 consecutive cases. Ann Vasc Surg. 2012;26:387–95.

53. Yuan L, Bao J, Zhao Z, Lu Q, Feng X, Jing Z. Clinical results of percutaneous transluminal angioplasty for thromboangiitis obliterans in arteries above the knee. Atherosclerosis. 2014;235:110–5.

54. Cooper LT, Tse TS, Mikhail MA, et al. Long-term survival and amputation risk in thromboangiitis obliterans (Buerger's disease). J Am Coll Cardiol. 2004;44:2410–1.

55. O'Connor H. The treatment of Buerger's disease. J Wound Care. 1996;5:462–3.

56. Isner JM, Baumgartner I, Rauh G, Schainfeld R, Blair R, Manor O, Razvi S, Symes JF. Treatment of thromboangiitis obliterans (Buerger's disease) by intramuscular gene transfer of vascular endothelial growth factor: preliminary clinical results. J Vasc Surg. 1998;28:964–73.

57. Franz R, Shah K, Johnson J, Pin R, Parks A, Hankins T, Hartman J, Wright M. Short- to mid-term results using autologous bonemarrow mononuclear cell implantation therapy as a limb salvage procedure in patients with severe peripheral arterial disease. Vasc Endovasc Surg. 2011;45:398–406.

58. Matoba S, Tatsumi T, Murohara T, Imaizumi T, Katsuda Y, Ito M, Saito Y, Uemura S, Suzuki H, Fukumoto S, Yamamoto Y, Onodera R, Teramukai S, Fukushima M, Matsubara H, TACT Follow-up Study Investigators. Long-term clinical outcome after intramuscular implantation of bone marrow mononuclear cells (Therapeutic Angiogenesis by Cell Transplantation [TACT] trial) in patients with chronic limb ischemia. Am Heart J. 2008;156:1010–8.

59. Nishida T, Ueno Y, Kimura T, Ogawa R, Joo K, Tominaga R. Early and long-term effects of the autologous peripheral stem cell implantation for critical limb ischemia. Ann Vasc Dis. 2011;4:319–24.

60. Miyamoto K, Nishigami K, Nagaya N, Akutsu K, Chiku M, Kamei M, Soma T, Miyata S, Higashi M, Tanaka R, Nakatani T, Nonogi H, Takeshita S. Unblinded pilot study of autologous transplantation of bone marrow mononuclear cells in patients with thromboangiitis obliterans. Circulation. 2006;114:2679–84.

Critical Ischemia in Patients with Raynaud's Phenomenon

Michael Hughes, Ariane Herrick, and Lindsay Muir

Introduction

Raynaud's phenomenon (RP) is an episodic phenomenon in which the skin of the extremities undergoes a classical color change of white (the physiological basis for which is ischemia), blue (cyanosis), and red (hyperemia). The condition may be associated with significant discomfort and pain [1, 2]. RP is usually idiopathic (primary RP), but may occur due to a driving etiology (secondary RP). Primary RP does not progress to digital ulceration or critical ischemia. Classification criteria for primary RP have been proposed and are widely used by clinicians [3, 4]. There is a wide range of causes of secondary RP, which may (albeit rarely) progress to critical digital ischemia with potential gangrenous progression requiring amputation. The distinction between primary and secondary RP is important as both the prognosis and management may differ significantly. The aim of this chapter is to describe the background, clinical evaluation, and treatment of the patient with RP who then presents with critical digital ischemia. Most of our review applies especially to patients with systemic sclerosis (SSc) because this is where the (limited) evidence base is the strongest.

The first section of the chapter deals with general principles of assessment and treatment, initially in the patient in whom the cause of secondary RP is unknown, and then in the patient with a known diagnosis of SSc. Although critical ischemia is a relatively rare complication of RP, nonetheless a significant proportion of affected patients require surgery: the surgical approach to management is described in the second section.

General Approach to the Patient with RP and Critical Ischemia

Classification criteria for primary RP (listed below) have been proposed (adapted from the proposed LeRoy and Medsger criteria [3]). Patients who have abnormality in any one of these domains require further investigation.

- Episodic attacks of acral pallor or cyanosis
- Strong and symmetrical peripheral pulses
- Absence of ischemic tissue loss (digital pitting, ulceration, or gangrene)
- Negative anti-nuclear antibody
- Normal ESR

The Patient Presenting with RP and Critical Ischemia in Whom the Diagnosis is Unknown

The clinician must perform a comprehensive clinical assessment in patients with RP presenting with critical ischemia without a known diagnosis in order to identify any of the secondary causes of RP (Table 24.1). It is important to recognize that many of the secondary causes of RP, in particular SSc [5] and cancer-associated [6], are not uncommonly associated with severe digital vascular disease, including critical digital ischemia and necrosis. Establishing the diagnosis is of upmost importance as treating the underlying cause of patient's secondary RP may improve critical digital ischemia.

M. Hughes, MSc(Hons), MSc, MBBS
A. Herrick, MD (✉)
Centre for Musculoskeletal Research, The University
of Manchester and Salford Royal NHS Foundation Trust,
Stopford Building, Oxford Road, Manchester M13 9PT, UK

L. Muir, MB, MChOrth
Hand Surgery, Salford Royal NHS Foundation Trust,
Salford, Lancashire M6 8HD, UK

© Springer International Publishing Switzerland 2017
R.S. Dieter et al. (eds.), *Critical Limb Ischemia*, DOI 10.1007/978-3-319-31991-9_24

History and Physical Examination

Because the differential diagnosis of secondary RP is so diverse, a detailed medical history with full review of systems should be undertaken, including asking about symptoms suggestive of a connective tissue disease, in particular of SSc (e.g., skin changes and gastrointestinal motility issues). The duration of the patient's RP should be ascertained and whether this has historically proceeded to digital ulceration and/or critical ischemia. The patient's current drug treatments (both prescribed and "over the counter") should be scrutinized to detect any of the medications associated with secondary RP (as described in Table 24.1).

Table 24.1 The secondary causes of Raynaud's phenomenon, many of these can be associated with critical digital ischemia (note this is not an exhaustive list)

Rheumatological	Connective tissue diseases: Systemic sclerosis and systemic sclerosis–spectrum disorders, systemic lupus erythematous, Sjogren's syndrome, idiopathic inflammatory myopathies (dermatomyositis and polymyositis), mixed connective tissue disease, overlap conditions
	Vasculitis
Hand arm vibration syndrome (vibration white finger)	Developing in (some) individuals who have been exposed to vibrating tools
Drugs and toxins	Immunosuppressive agents (e.g., cyclosporine A and interferons)
	Chemotherapeutic agents (e.g., bleomycin and cisplatin)
	Drugs used in the treatment of hypertension (e.g., beta blockers and clonidine)
	Drug used in the treatment of anxiety and headache syndromes (e.g., ergots and methysergide)
	Toxins including occupational exposure (e.g., cocaine and vinyl chloride)
Endocrine/ metabolic	Hypothyroidism
	Rarer endocrinological conditions: Carcinoid syndrome, pheochromocytoma and POEMS (polyneuropathy, organomegaly, endocrinopathy, monoclonal protein, and skin changes) syndrome
Hematological	Abnormal blood components: Cold agglutinin disease, cryoglobulinemia, cryofibrinogenemia, and paraproteinemia
	Abnormal cellular constituents: Leukemia and lymphoma, polycythemia, and thrombocythemia
	Coagulopathy: Inherited and acquired (e.g., anti-phospholipid [Hughes] syndrome
Malignancy	Solid tumors: Most tumors have been implicated (in particular: lung, ovary, stomach, breast, and uterus)
	Hematological (e.g., leukemia and lymphoma)
	Paraneoplastic

In addition, the patient's family and occupational histories should be documented. For example, is there a history of vinyl chloride exposure?

Investigations

Initial blood investigations in all patients include routine hematology and biochemistry (± thyroid function) and coagulation studies (e.g., internal normalized ratio [INR] and activated partial thromboplastin time [APTT]). Doppler ultrasound examination of the vascular tree of the upper limbs should be obtained early to exclude significant large (proximal) obstructive disease, in particular when symptoms are asymmetric.

Additional coagulation studies may be indicated (e.g., testing for the presence of the lupus anticoagulant and anti-phospholipid serology) in patients with a suspected connective tissue disease or a history suggestive of anti-phospholipid (Hughes) syndrome (e.g., previous thrombotic events and/or pregnancy morbidity/mortality) [7]. Immunology should be performed where there is a clinical suspicion of an underlying autoimmune disease: anti-nuclear antibody, complements and also anti-neutrophilic cytoplasmic antibody (ANCA) if the clinical features are suggestive of a vasculitic illness. The urine should be examined (in particular if there is a clinical suspicion of systemic vasculitis or a connective tissue disease) to exclude an active renal sediment, initially by dipstick. If positive for blood and/or protein, then microscopy (e.g., to detect red cell casts indicative of glomerulonephritis) and/or the quantification of proteinuria are indicated. Blood cultures should be performed if there is concern as to systemic infection. Other blood investigations (e.g., cryoglobulins) should be performed if clinically indicated.

A chest radiograph/thoracic outlet view should be performed to exclude a cervical obstructive lesion (i.e., a bony cervical rib). Other investigations (where indicated) include angiography (either magnetic resonance or conventional digital subtraction X-ray angiography) and transthoracic echocardiography (if there is a clinical suspicion of a central embolic source from infective endocarditis).

Specialist investigations for RP include capillaroscopy (a non-invasive microscope examination of the nailfold capillaries in situ) and thermography (cold challenge testing with examination of temperature response using a thermal camera), in particular in the assessment of patients with possible SSc (Fig. 24.1).

Management

Irrespective of the cause of RP, critical ischemia in RP is always a medical emergency and the patient requires urgent hospitalization as the critical ischemia may rapidly progress to irreversible gangrene, with potential loss of the digit. The aim of treatment is to improve perfusion to the ischemic digit and to identify and treat (if appropriate) any underlying

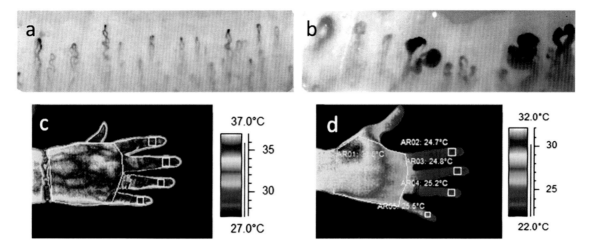

Fig. 24.1 Nailfold capillaroscopy and thermography. Capillaroscopy. (**a**) Normal nailfold capillaroscopy. The capillaries are regular in appearance (albeit slightly tortuous) and capillary density is preserved. (**b**) Capillaroscopy from a patient with systemic sclerosis. Several capillaries are grossly enlarged, and the capillaries are disordered in shape and arrangement. Thermography (measure of skin temperature) after cold challenge testing. (**c**) Healthy control. Normal thermographic appearance at 23 °C with no significant temperature gradient between the distal fingers and the dorsum of the hand. (**d**) Secondary Raynaud's phenomenon (in a patient with systemic sclerosis). Temperature gradient persists even after warming at a room temperature of 30 °C

Table 24.2 Contributory (and potentially modifiable) causes to the development and/or progression of critical digital ischemia

In all patients	Smoking
	Drug treatment that reduces digital perfusion, e.g., beta blockers
	Large (proximal) vessel disease
	Pro-thrombotic coagulopathy, e.g., anti-phospholipid syndrome
	Thromboembolic disease
Mainly in patients with SSc or other connective tissue diseases	Cryoglobulinemia
	Vasculitis

secondary cause of RP (Table 24.1) and/or potentially modifiable factors (Table 24.2).

Patients who smoke should be counseled as to the upmost importance of smoking cessation and given all possible support in their efforts to stop smoking. Analgesia must be optimized early, as critical ischemia is very often excruciatingly painful. Patients should receive intravenous prostanoid therapy (e.g., iloprost) unless contraindicated; however, it is often poorly tolerated (due to systemic vasodilation) and/or not effective. Critically ischemic digits are often secondarily infected and require treatment with appropriate intravenous antibiotic therapy. As described below under "surgical management" vascular intervention may be required (e.g., angioplasty) if there is a significant large (proximal) vascular disease. Many clinicians will also prescribe anti-platelet therapy and/or short-term anticoagulation in an attempt to save the digit; however, there is no good evidence base to support either of these interventions. Short-term statin therapy

may also be considered (the rationale being that statin therapy is often used in the management of patients with acute coronary syndromes) [8] but again there is no good evidence base for this approach.

Once critical ischemia is established it is often too late to save the digit, and therefore debridement and/or amputation of necrotic tissue (including the whole of the digit) may be indicated, in particular, if the area of necrosis has become established. The gangrenous tissue may autoamputate spontaneously. Digital (palmar) sympathectomy should also be considered, especially if the critical ischemia is progressing and/or involving the other digits. These surgical options are described in detail below.

The Patient Presenting with Known SSc and Critical Ischemia

Systemic Sclerosis

SSc is a complex autoimmune connective tissue disease that is characterized by vascular abnormalities, immune system activation, and a dramatic fibrotic response [9–11]. Vascular abnormalities (often referred to as the "vasculopathy") are postulated to have a key role in the pathogenesis of SSc (including the earliest events in the initiation of disease) and are responsible for many of the later complications of the disease (e.g., digital ulceration/critical ischemia and pulmonary arterial hypertension) [9–11]. An increased risk of macrovascular (including myocardial infarction, stroke, and peripheral vascular) disease has been reported in patients with SSc [12, 13] including at the level of the digital artery

[14, 15] and with selective involvement of the ulnar artery [14, 16–18] which is associated with more severe digital vascular disease, including digital ulceration [18].

There is an increasing emphasis internationally toward the earlier diagnosis of SSc, in part, due to the number of effective treatments that are available for the internal organ involvement (e.g., phosphodiesterase inhibition and endothelin receptor antagonism for pulmonary hypertension as well as for digital ulceration) [19–21]. The American College of Rheumatology and the European League Against Rheumatism classification criteria for SSc (although not intended for diagnostic purposes) are a useful clinical tool when assessing patients with possible SSc [22, 23].

Critical Digital Ischemia in Patients with SSc

Critical digital ischemia although uncommon represents the most severe end of the spectrum of digital vascular disease in patients with SSc. In a large (n = 1168) prospective cohort study from the United Kingdom, the authors reported that 1.4 % of patients with SSc developed critical digital ischemia within an 18-month period [5]. Critical ischemia may involve multiple digits and/or require amputation [24]. Positive associations with severe digital ischemia and anti-centromere antibody [24, 25] and anti-beta2-glycoprotein I [26] have been reported.

The management of critical digital ischemia in patients with SSc is very similar to those patients in whom the underlying diagnosis is unknown, with a few caveats to the approach to treatment. Again, critical digital ischemia is a medical emergency and requires prompt clinical assessment and hospitalization. All patients with SSc should be counseled to seek urgent medical device if any of the digits becomes permanently discolored. Smoking cessation is again of upmost importance. In a retrospective study that included 101 patients with SSc, those who were current smokers were more likely than never smokers to require debridement (odds ratio 4.5, 95 % confidence interval 1.1, 18.3) [27]. Any co-existing secondary causes of RP (Table 24.1) and/or contributory cause/s, although rare (e.g., cryoglobulins, systemic vasculitis, and anti-phospholipid syndrome) (Table 24.2) should be identified early and treated appropriately. Figs. 24.2 and 24.3 describe two cases of critical digital ischemia in patients with SSc.

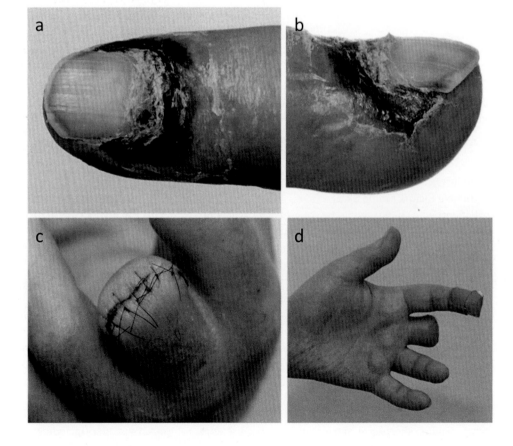

Fig. 24.2 A 59-year-old male with limited cutaneous SSc presented with a progressive area of ischemia and infection of the left middle terminal phalanx and was promptly admitted for intravenous antibiotic therapy. Despite intervention, he developed critical digital ischemia with a well-demarcated area of necrosis at the fingertip (**a, b**). He was known to have circulating cryoglobulins but this had never necessitated treatment (e.g., preserved complements with no features of cryoglobulinemic vasculitis). Urgent sympathectomy, botulinum injection (at the level of the digital nerve), and amputation of the tip of the digit was performed. Subsequently he required further surgery (**c**) to extend the level of his amputation due to progressive necrosis. He subsequently made a good recovery (**d**) and his hand function has been maintained. Copyright Salford Royal NHS Foundation Trust. Reproduced with permission

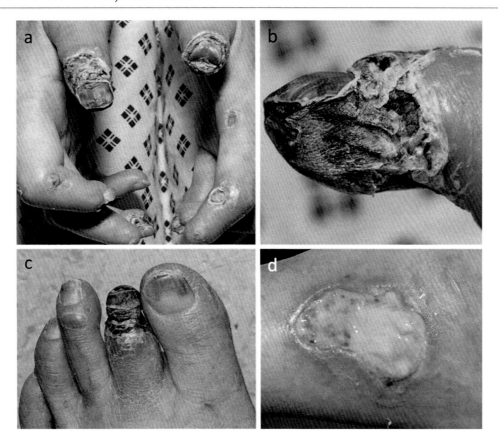

Fig. 24.3 A 37-year-old female with SSc/systemic lupus erythematosus overlap (anti-RNP antibody positive) with pulmonary hypertension and pulmonary fibrosis presented with a several month history of critical ischemia of multiple digits of the hands and feet (**a–c**) and areas of digital ulceration (over the small joints of the hands). She was thought to have a vasculitic component to her illness because of a large vasculitic looking ankle ulcer (**d**), and had previously received steroid therapy, cyclophosphamide, and rituximab (therapies used in the treatment of systemic vasculitis). There was no evidence of an associated coagu-

lopathy (in particular secondary anti-phospholipid syndrome). Surprisingly, she only reported minimal associated pain with the areas of critical ischemia (and digital ulceration). She had previously been treated with intravenous (IV) prostanoid therapy, but there were concerns about giving further IV prostanoid prior to further investigation of her pulmonary hypertension. Surgical debridement is planned, but it is likely that her hand function will remain severely compromised. Copyright Salford Royal NHS Foundation Trust. Reproduced with permission

Intravenous prostanoid therapy should be commenced, unless contraindicated (e.g., because of severe cardiorespiratory involvement). Many clinicians will also prescribe antiplatelet therapy and/or anticoagulation (although there is no evidence base to support either of these interventions). When prescribing anti-platelet therapy, in particular aspirin, it is important to consider carefully the risk: benefit ratio because many patients with SSc have gastrointestinal involvement, for example, gastric antral vascular ectasia which may predispose to (potentially life threatening) gastric bleeding. Again, statin therapy may be considered. Regardless of the outcome of the critically ischemic digit/s, a key point is to try and prevent the recurrence of future critical digital ischemia (and/or ulceration) by educating patients how to keep the fingers warm, supporting patients' efforts in smoking cessation, optimizing oral vasodilator therapy, and treating any contributory factor/s.

Surgical Approach to the Patient with RP and Critical Ischemia

Acute Ischemia

Patients with RP rarely present with acute critical ischemia. A consideration of the conditions linked to the phenomenon will demonstrate that they are primarily conditions that develop over a medium to long term. These patients, and in particular patients with SSc, are thus unlikely to present with the acute ischemia of say an arterial embolism.

Nonetheless, some patients will present with a rapid progression of their condition and an ischemic finger. The rest of this section will concentrate on the surgical management of the more chronic onset ischemia, and the management strategy for both groups follows the same principles.

Chronic Critical Ischemia

Firstly, it should be noted that patients with critical ischemia secondary to SSc-related RP should be managed in conjunction with the rheumatologists. In general, as with all unusual conditions, management in a center that has a specialist interest in the condition may be beneficial. For the surgeon attached to such a unit, the normal and usual method of referral will in any case be from the rheumatology team with an interest. It is very helpful to the rheumatology team to have easy access to the surgical team. In our institution the rheumatologists have open access to the hand clinic, with referrals accepted from all levels of doctor, so that time is not wasted on complex referral processes.

Assessment by the Surgical Team

By the time patients reach our hand surgery department, they have normally had an extensive workup in the rheumatology department (Table 24.3).

Treatment Options

The available surgical treatment tools (Table 24.4) for critical ischemia will now be discussed individually.

Preparation for Surgery

Patients with SSc presenting to the hand clinic often have additional comorbidities. They may, for instance, have pulmonary hypertension (Fig. 24.3). The anesthetic risk may

Table 24.3 Clinical assessment of critical ischemia by the surgical team

History taking
We focus on the following aspects:
Duration and evolution of symptoms
Pain
Smoking (it does no harm to reiterate the exhortation to give up, if appropriate)
Treatment to date
Examination
We look at the presence of ulcers, areas of ischemia, and general function of the hand. Some patients with SSc have stiff joints, sometimes with exposed PIP joints. By the time patients present with ischemia, up to 50 % will have an occluded ulnar artery [28]
Investigations
Doppler ultrasound is readily available in the clinic. Angiography, whether by digital subtraction or MR, may guide the reconstructive prospects. Plain radiology may show evidence of osteomyelitis. MR scanning of the fingers may help differentiate between acrolysis and secondary infection of this nature [29]

Table 24.4 The surgical therapeutic tools available for critical ischemia

• Wound debridement
• Botulinum toxin injection
• Sympathectomy
• Arterial reconstruction
• Arterialization of the venous system
• Amputation

thus be increased. It is possible to perform some surgery under metacarpal block or regional anesthesia. Although we originally feared that this would compromise blood supply, this has not yet proved to be the case. We avoid the use of epinephrine in this circumstance, however.

Wound Débridement

Patients with ischemic ulcers may find the simple expedient of curetting the ulcer provides some pain relief. This may be done simply by excising the necrotic tissue and curetting the base with a 15 blade. Sometimes a bead of pus will be found. In doing this it is important to remember that the underlying problem has not been addressed by this measure, and consideration should additionally be given to improving the blood supply by means of one of the procedures described below.

One should not expect to see brisk bleeding after débridement, and one should resist the temptation to resect tissue until such bleeding is encountered (see the section "Amputation").

Botulinum Toxin Injection

Botulinum A toxin is produced by the bacterium *Clostridium botulinum*. It blocks neurotransmitter response across the neuromuscular endplate by inhibiting the release of acetylcholine vesicles at the motor endplate terminals [30]. The exact mechanism of action is, however, as yet unclear and is probably multifactorial. The current theories are alternatively of an effective sympathetic blockade by modulation of abnormal adrenergic innervation, leading to a decrease in blood shunting and increased nutritional flow [31] or of a reduction of pain through antinociceptive pathways; the toxin can theoretically reduce glutamate, substance P, and calcitonin gene related peptide levels [32].

The toxin is injected adjacent to the neurovascular bundles at the level of bifurcation of the common digital arteries [33] at the level of the superficial palmar arch, or on either side of the base of the finger [34].

Iorio [30] found five studies detailing the use of Botulinum toxin. They concluded that the initial results were promising but that the studies had significant limitations and recommended a larger more careful study. Further, longer-term evaluation is required to better establish the role of botulinum toxin in the patient with severe RP.

In patients with critical ischemia we would use Botulinum toxin only if the patient was not fit for more major surgery, or as a temporizing measure. We do, however, consider the use of Botulinum toxin in conjunction with debridement of ulcers.

Periarterial (Digital, Radial, and Ulnar) Sympathectomy

Digital sympathectomy was first described by Adrian Flatt [35]. He postulated that a peripheral interruption of the sympathetic supply to the hand would intercept the pathways that arose from sources other than the sympathetic chain. Morgan and Wilgis [36] demonstrated that sympathetic fibers in the adventitia have limited capacity for regeneration even after 1 year in a rabbit ear model.

In a systematic review of the literature on peripheral sympathectomy, Kotsis and Chung [37] found that only 16 papers met their inclusion criteria. The majority of the patients studied had SSc. The reported ulcer healing times varied between 2 weeks and 7 months. Fifteen percent of patients required later amputation even after the sympathectomy, 16 % had a recurrence of ischemia and incomplete healing. The postoperative complication rate was 37 %. In the light of these findings the authors counseled that long-term prospective studies are still required in this field, and that patients should be warned of the uncertain success rate.

Koman [38] studied the microvascular physiology in seven hands with refractory pain and ulceration undergoing digital sympathectomy. In addition to symptomatic assessment the authors performed isolated cold stress testing, digital pulp temperature evaluation, and laser Doppler flowmetry. Following surgery all seven hands had diminished pain. The ulcers healed in six hands and improved in the remaining one. After sympathectomy, fingertip temperature did not increase (contrary to some other writers' experiences), suggesting that total blood flow was unaffected. Microvascular perfusion and vasomotion increased. On this basis, the authors postulated a preferential increase in flow in nutritional rather than in thermoregulatory vessels as the likely mechanism for the clinical effectiveness of sympathectomy.

Flatt's original series [35] was of eight patients with a variety of underlying pathologies. Flatt described the difficulty in assessing objectively the results of treatment. Hartzell et al. [39] studied 28 patients with a mixture of autoimmune and arteriosclerotic disease at an average follow-up of 96 months (minimum 23 months). Their technique was tailored to each patient's pattern of disease and involved surgery at any of the levels thought appropriate. Twenty of these patients had autoimmune disease. Of these, 11 saw complete healing of ulcers, with 15 experiencing some improvement.

However, 7 eventually underwent amputation (these are included in the unhealed ulcer group).

Kim et al. [40] undertook a combination of digital sympathectomy of the common digital vessels alone and radical sympathectomy including the proper digital vessels for their patients with type IV (all levels of vessel stenotic) and V (global ischemia) disease. Sixty-seven percent of patients with type IV and 53 % of patients with type V disease saw an improvement in symptoms. Twenty-three percent and 33 % had no change and 10 and 13 %, respectively, experienced a deterioration.

Technique

We perform palmar sympathectomy at the level of the common digital arteries. Some authors describe a more extensive approach, addressing also the ulnar and radial arteries. Koman [38] describes performing a sympathectomy on the superficial palmar arch and the three volar common digital vessels together with a section of the deep branch of the radial artery and the origin of the deep palmar arch through a fourth incision in the anatomic snuffbox. O'Brien et al. [41] describe an extensive sympathectomy of the ulnar artery, superficial palmar arch, and proper digital arteries.

We recommend general or regional anesthesia and an exsanguinating tourniquet. The use of loupe magnification or of an operating microscope is advisable. The common digital artery is approached through a Bruner incision. A 2-cm stretch of the artery is stripped of adventitia. Under the microscope this is a long stretch, and we always measure the extent with a ruler. Care must be taken not to damage the underlying vessel wall. No drain is required. If there is a transverse component to the wound, this may safely be left open. If desired, the radial and ulnar arteries are approached via a straight 3-cm incision. Again, the adventitia is stripped over a 2-cm stretch of artery.

Balloon Angioplasty

Kim et al. [40] describe the use of balloon angioplasty in patients with type II stenosis of the ulnar and radial arteries and narrowing in the palmar arch, common digital, and digital vessels. The procedure was performed using a balloon catheter with a 2.0-mm diameter and 14-mm length, inserted into the ulnar artery, and advanced as far as the common digital arteries. They reported overall improvement in 79 % of this group with 16 % no better and 4 % worse. There was one case of rupture of the ulnar artery.

Arterial Reconstruction

Arterial reconstruction is well described in the management of peripheral vascular disease. In the hand, reconstruction of the ulnar or radial arteries is relatively straightforward. Arterial grafting of the finger vessels represents a greater challenge because of the small size of the vessels and because of the complexity of the superficial palmar arch. Tomaino [42] described reconstruction of the radial digital artery to the middle finger. Kim et al. [40] described excision and grafting of a thrombosed radial or ulnar artery. In the case of an involved superficial palmar arch and spared common digital vessels, Kim advocates reconstruction of the arch with a deep inferior epigastric artery graft anastomosed to the common digital arteries. They note that the deep inferior epigastric artery has numerous branches and can thus be used to construct a new palmar arch, connecting the branches end to end to the common digital arteries. Higgins and McClinton [28] reported that patients can experience substantial and long-term improvement in the vascular status of their hands with arterial bypass procedures.

The choice of graft is varied. Kim et al. use either vein graft or use as their preferred donor artery the deep inferior epigastric artery. Alternative donor arteries, including the thoracodorsal artery and the descending branch of the lateral circumflex femoral artery, have also been described. Trocchia and Hammert [43] argue, in the light of the experience of higher patency rates in coronary artery surgery, arterial grafts should be studied in more detail in the hand. Kryger et al. [44] describe a series of six patients treated with a reversed lesser saphenous vein graft anastomosed end to side to the radial artery and tunneled to the common digital artery. No patient had any further ischemia leading to tissue loss after a follow-up of 4–40 months.

Technique

After careful preoperative planning with angiography, this surgery may be performed under general or regional anesthesia. Standard techniques of venous or arterial grafting are recommended, with careful attention to resection of all diseased artery until normal vessel is found and meticulous microsurgical technique. As described above, the exact pattern of the reconstruction depends on the extent of the disease. The role of postoperative anticoagulation is not yet clearly established. Aspirin and low molecular weight heparin are the commonest agents, but the ideal duration of treatment has not been established, and the use of these agents does run the risk of bleeding. Tomaino [42] recommends oral aspirin for 6 weeks postoperatively. The efficacy of Dextran has been questioned [45].

Revascularization of the Hand by Retrograde Venous Flow

If arterial reconstruction is not feasible, or has failed, consideration may, as a last resort, be given to arterialization of the venous tree. The surgical technique is described in detail by Matarrese and Hammert [46]. The cephalic vein is identified and the side branches ligated. The valves of the cephalic vein need to be divided with a valvulotome. The vein is then transected and joined end to side to the parent artery. If the radial artery is patent, the vein may be anastomosed directly. Matarrese and Hammert [46] describe anastomosing the vein to the brachial artery. The authors emphasize that this is a last chance solution and that the long-term results are not clear. Kind [47] reported a series of revascularization of five chronically ischemic hands in three patients by means of arteriovenous anastomosis. He describes good results in all five hands at a follow-up of 8–16 months. Pederson and Neumeister [48] caution against arterialization in the presence of severe infection.

Amputation

In cases refractory to treatment, amputation may be inevitable.

Before considering amputation, it is important to consider whether the perfusion of the rest of the hand can be improved by one or more of the above-listed procedures.

In a patient with a pain free, noninfected mummified tip it is reasonable to allow the digit to autoamputate. This may cause relatively little pain, although often some surgical help is necessary when the necrotic portion is almost detached. If patients are distressed by the appearance surgery may be reasonable, although allowing the finger to epithelialize under the biological dressing, that is, the necrotic end will leave a reasonable scar.

In the case of an ischemic, necrotic, and painful fingertip that has not improved with the preceding treatments, or in the case of refractory ulceration, amputation is likely to help the pain. Amputation may be performed at any level. In the case of patients with SSc-related RP we do not follow the standard surgical levels of amputation. It must be remembered that a cosmetically pleasing ray amputation of a first ischemic finger may lead to a more difficult decision making when the next finger is affected. We thus tend toward conservative resection, as some patients lose multiple fingertips. As indicated in the assessment section above, the function of the fingers may not be normal, and in this patient group cosmesis is seldom the main priority, whereas retention of as much function as possible and relief of pain are. General hand surgical procedures should be used, but we amputate at the level that is going to leave maximum length.

Table 24.5 Summary of surgical management of critical ischemia in RP

- Surgery has a role to play in critical ischemia secondary to secondary RP
- It should be performed in conjunction and in close cooperation with the medical team
- Initial consideration should be given to whether it is feasible to improve the blood flow to the hand
- The means of doing this are primarily botulinum toxin injection, sympathectomy, and revascularization by means of graft or balloon dilatation
- Amputation has a role to play in unsalvageable cases
- The normal surgical principles of amputation levels may not be applicable in this group of patients

It is rare to see the usual profuse bleeding one might anticipate in an operation on the hand until the metacarpophalangeal joint is reached. As discussed previously in this section, a rather lesser degree of bleeding of the skin edges may be accepted.

Summary of Surgical Management (Table 24.5)

Conclusion

In conclusion, critical digital ischemia in the patient with RP is uncommon, but when it does occur is a medical emergency that requires prompt recognition, assessment, and treatment, in an attempt to save the digit. There is a limited evidence base to guide clinicians as to the management of critical digital ischemia, most of which applies to the SSc population. Surgery is often required, and a number of different surgical procedures have been advocated.

Substantial research effort is still required to define the optimal management of critical digital ischemia in patients with RP. Such research endeavors represent a considerable challenge given the relative rarity of the problem and the heterogeneity of presentation between patients.

References

1. Block JA, Sequeira W. Raynaud's phenomenon. Lancet. 2001;357(9273):2042–8.
2. Wigley FM. Clinical practice. Raynaud's Phenomenon. N Engl J Med. 2002;347:1001–8.
3. LeRoy E, Medsger TA. Raynaud's phenomenon: a proposal for classification. Clin Exp Rheumatol. 1992;10:485–8.
4. Maverakis E, Patel F, Kronenberg DG, et al. International consensus criteria for the diagnosis of Raynaud's phenomenon. J Autoimmun. 2014;48–49:60–5.
5. Nihtyanova SI, Brough GM, Black CM, Denton CP. Clinical burden of digital vasculopathy in limited and diffuse cutaneous systemic sclerosis. Ann Rheum Dis. 2008;67(1):120–3.
6. Poszepczynska-Guigné E, Viguier M, Chosidow O, Orcel B, Emmerich J, Dubertret L. Paraneoplastic acral vascular syndrome: epidemiologic features, clinical manifestations, and disease sequelae. J Am Acad Dermatol. 2002;47(1):47–52.
7. Miyakis S, Lockshin MD, Atsumi T, et al. International consensus statement on an update of the classification criteria for definite antiphospholipid syndrome (APS). J Thromb Haemost. 2006; 4(2):295–306.
8. Kim JS, Kim J, Choi D, et al. Efficacy of high-dose atorvastatin loading before primary percutaneous coronary intervention in ST-segment elevation myocardial infarction: the STATIN STEMI trial. JACC Cardiovasc Interv. 2010;3:332–9.
9. Gabrielli A, Avvedimento EV, Krieg T. Scleroderma. N Engl J Med. 2009;360(19):1989–2003.
10. Katsumoto TR, Whitfield ML, Connolly MK. The pathogenesis of systemic sclerosis. Annu Rev Pathol. 2011;6:509–37.
11. Matucci-Cerinic M, Kahaleh B, Wigley FM. Review: evidence that systemic sclerosis is a vascular disease. Arthritis Rheum. 2013;65:1953–62.
12. Ho M, Veale D, Eastmond C, Nuki G, Belch J. Macrovascular disease and systemic sclerosis. Ann Rheum Dis. 2000;59(1):39–43.
13. Man A, Zhu Y, Zhang Y, et al. The risk of cardiovascular disease in systemic sclerosis: a population-based cohort study. Ann Rheum Dis. 2013;72:1188–93.
14. Hasegawa M, Nagai Y, Tamura A, Ishikawa O. Arteriographic evaluation of vascular changes of the extremities in patients with systemic sclerosis. Br J Dermatol. 2006;155(6):1159–64.
15. Allanore Y, Seror R, Chevrot A, Kahan A, Drapé JL. Hand vascular involvement assessed by magnetic resonance angiography in systemic sclerosis. Arthritis Rheum. 2007;56(8):2747–54.
16. Taylor MH, McFadden JA, Bolster MB, Silver RM. Ulnar artery involvement in systemic sclerosis (scleroderma). J Rheumatol. 2002;29(1):102–6.
17. Park JH, Sung YK, Bae SC, Song SY, Seo HS, Jun JB. Ulnar artery vasculopathy in systemic sclerosis. Rheumatol Int. 2009; 29(9):1081–6.
18. Frerix M, Stegbauer J, Dragun D, Kreuter A, Weiner SM. Ulnar artery occlusion is predictive of digital ulcers in SSc: a duplex sonography study. Rheumatology (Oxford). 2012;51(4):735–42.
19. Matucci-Cerinic M, Denton CP, Furst DE, Mayes MD, Hsu VM, Carpentier P, et al. Bosentan treatment of digital ulcers related to systemic sclerosis: results from the RAPIDS-2 randomised, double-blind, placebo-controlled trial. Ann Rheum Dis. 2011;70(1):32–8.
20. Badesch DB, Hill NS, Burgess G, et al. Sildenafil for pulmonary arterial hypertension associated with connective tissue disease. J Rheumatol. 2007;34(12):2417–22.
21. Pulido T, Adzerikho I, Channick RN, et al. Macitentan and morbidity and mortality in pulmonary arterial hypertension. N Engl J Med. 2013;369(9):809–18.
22. van den Hoogen F, Khanna D, Fransen J, et al. 2013 classification criteria for systemic sclerosis: an American college of rheumatology/European league against rheumatism collaborative initiative. Ann Rheum Dis. 2013;72:1747–55.
23. van den Hoogen F, Khanna D, Fransen J, et al. 2013 classification criteria for systemic sclerosis: an American college of rheumatology/European league against rheumatism collaborative initiative. Arthritis Rheum. 2013;65:2737–47.
24. Wigley FM, Wise RA, Miller R, Needleman BW, Spence RJ. Anti-centromere antibody as a predictor of digital ischemic loss in patients with systemic sclerosis. Arthritis Rheum. 1992;35(6):688–93.
25. Herrick AL, Heaney M, Hollis S, Jayson MIV. Anti-cardiolipin, anti-centromere and anti-Scl-70 antibodies in patients with systemic sclerosis and severe digital ischaemia. Ann Rheum Dis. 1994;53(8):540–2.

26. Boin F, Franchini S, Colantuoni E, Rosen A, Wigley FM, Casciola-Rosen L. Independent association of anti-β2-glycoprotein I antibodies with macrovascular disease and mortality in scleroderma patients. Arthritis Rheum. 2009;60(8):2480–9.

27. Harrison BJ, Silman AJ, Hider SL, Herrick AL. Cigarette smoking as a significant risk factor for digital vascular disease in patients with systemic sclerosis. Arthritis Rheum. 2002;46(12):3312–6.

28. Higgins JP, McClinton MA. Vascular insufficiency of the upper extremity. J Hand Surg [Am]. 2010;35(9):1545–53.

29. Zhou AY, Muir L, Harris J, Herrick AL. The impact of magnetic resonance imaging in early diagnosis of hand osteomyelitis in patients with systemic sclerosis. Clin Exp Rheumatol. 2014;32(6 Suppl 86):232.

30. Iorio ML, Masden DL, Higgins JP. Botulinum toxin A treatment of Raynaud's phenomenon: a review. Semin Arthritis Rheum. 2012;41(4):599–603.

31. Stone AV, Koman LA, Callahan MF, et al. The effect of botulinum neurotoxin-A on blood flow in rats: a potential mechanism for treatment of Raynaud phenomenon. J Hand Surg [Am]. 2012;37(4): 795–802.

32. Mannava S, Plate JF, Stone AV, et al. Recent advances for the management of Raynaud phenomenon using botulinum neurotoxin A. J Hand Surg [Am]. 2011;36(10):1708–10.

33. Neumeister MW. Botulinum toxin type A in the treatment of Raynaud's phenomenon. J Hand Surg [Am]. 2010;35(12):2085–92.

34. Fregene A, Ditmars D, Siddiqui A. Botulinum toxin type A: a treatment option for patients with digital ischemia in patients with Raynaud's phenomenon. J Hand Surg [Am]. 2009;34:446–52.

35. Flatt AE. Digital artery sympathectomy. J Hand Surg [Am]. 1980;5(6):550–6.

36. Morgan RF, Wilgis EF. Thermal changes in a rabbit ear model after sympathectomy. J Hand Surg [Am]. 1986;11(1):120–4.

37. Kotsis SV, Chung KC. A systematic review of the outcomes of digital sympathectomy for treatment of chronic digital ischemia. J Rheumatol. 2003;30(8):1788–92.

38. Koman LA, Smith BP, Pollock Jr FE, Smith TL, Pollock D, Russell GB. The microcirculatory effects of peripheral sympathectomy. J Hand Surg [Am]. 1995;20(5):709–17.

39. Hartzell TL, Makhni EC, Sampson C. Long-term results of periarterial sympathectomy. J Hand Surg [Am]. 2009;34(8):1454–60.

40. Kim YH, Ng SW, Seo HS, Chang AH. Classification of Raynaud's disease based on angiographic features. J Plast Reconstr Aesthet Surg. 2011;64(11):1503–11.

41. O'Brien BM, Kumar PA, Mellow CG, Oliver TV. Radical microarteriolysis in the treatment of vasospastic disorders of the hand, especially scleroderma. J Hand Surg (Br). 1992;17(4):447–52.

42. Tomaino MM. Digital arterial occlusion in scleroderma: is there a role for digital arterial reconstruction? J Hand Surg (Br). 2000;25(6):611–3.

43. Trocchia AM, Hammert WC. Arterial grafts for vascular reconstruction in the upper extremity. J Hand Surg [Am]. 2011;36(9):1534–6.

44. Kryger ZB, Rawlani V, Dumanian GA. Treatment of chronic digital ischemia with direct microsurgical revascularization. J Hand Surg [Am]. 2007;32(9):1466–70.

45. Froemel D, Fitzsimons SJ, Frank J, Sauerbier M, Meurer A, Barker JH. A review of thrombosis and antithrombotic therapy in microvascular surgery. Eur Surg Res. 2013;50(1):32–43.

46. Matarrese MR, Hammert WC. Revascularization of the ischemic hand with arterialization of the venous system. J Hand Surg [Am]. 2011;36(12):2047–51.

47. Kind GM. Arterialization of the venous system of the hand. Plast Reconstr Surg. 2006;118(2):421–8.

48. Pederson WC, Neumeister MW. Reconstruction of the ischemic hand. Clin Plast Surg. 2011;38(4):739–50.

25

Arjun Jayaraj, Waldemar E. Wysokinski,
and Robert D. McBane

Introduction

Acute arterial occlusion can be a limb-threatening condition characterized by acute severe restriction of blood flow to the involved extremity. This arises most commonly from either thromboembolism or in situ thrombosis at the site of a ruptured atherosclerotic plaque. Other less frequent mechanisms include arterial dissection, transection, surgical ligation, arteritis, tumor in situ, invasion or embolization, foreign body embolization, and vasospasm (sepsis, vasopressor use, shock).

"Thrombophilia" was coined to describe a group of congenital and acquired risk factors which increase the individual's propensity for thrombus formation. These factors are blood born and in general increase the risk of venous thrombosis. While often considered in the evaluation of patients presenting with limb ischemia, only a minority of these factors augment the risk of arterial thrombotic events including bypass graft thrombosis. In general, arterial thrombosis stems from disease of the affected artery. In contrast, venous thrombosis is often due to abnormalities of the blood such that the hemostatic homeostasis becomes unbalanced favoring thrombus formation. For the majority of vascular patients with acute arterial occlusion, a search for an underlying thrombophilia will therefore either be unfruitful or misleading if incidentally found to be abnormal. This chapter will review several conditions to consider in the evaluation of those patients suffering thrombotic arterial occlusion without an underlying diseased arterial substrate or obvious thromboembolic mechanism. Thrombophilic entities relevant to acute arterial occlusion will be reviewed including clinical clues which should alert the provider to suspect these diseases.

Antiphospholipid Antibody Syndrome

The diagnosis of antiphospholipid antibody syndrome requires clinical thrombosis combined with confirmatory laboratory testing [1]. The current definition includes arterial and venous thromboembolism or pregnancy complications (idiopathic fetal loss beyond the 10th week of gestation, birth prior to 34 weeks of gestation due to eclampsia or placental insufficiency, or three or more consecutive, idiopathic, spontaneous abortions before 10 weeks of gestation). Laboratory testing must include positive test results for either lupus anticoagulant (clot-based assays) or antiphospholipid antibodies (IgG, IgM ELISA) at medium to high titers (greater than 40 units) [2]. If positive, these assays must be repeated to establish persistence at least 12 weeks later . More recently, a testing for β2-glycoprotein-I antibodies has been added to the testing repertoire.

Pathogenesis

This autoimmune disorder is characterized by antibodies directed against specific glycoproteins (β2-glycoprotein-I antibodies) within the cellular phospholipid bilayer [3]. Specifically implicated is the oxidized form of β2GPI, a complement control protein which may be antigenic in selected individuals. The proposed pathogenesis involves a two-hit process of endothelial injury followed by thrombotic response to oxidative stress injury. Several additional interrelated mechanisms include activation of coagulation factors, monocytes, endothelial cells, and platelets. Antibodies directed against annexin II on endothelial cells may lead to both activation and local injury, thus promoting a procoagulant environment.

A. Jayaraj, MBBS, MPH, RPVI
Division of Vascular and Endovascular Surgery, Mayo Clinic, Rochester, MN, USA

W.E. Wysokinski, MD, PhD • R.D. McBane, MD (✉)
Department of Cardiovascular Diseases, Gonda Vascular Center, Mayo Clinic, Rochester, MN 55905, USA

Recurrent fetal loss and increased thrombogenicity have been linked to complement C5a-mediated inflammation [4, 5].

Clinical Presentation

Antiphospholipid antibody syndrome has been associated with both arterial and venous thromboembolism. Venous thrombosis is three times more prevalent compared to arterial events. Arterial events however must be promptly recognized due to their potentially devastating presentation as part of the so-called catastrophic antiphospholipid antibody syndrome. This syndrome requires multisystem organ failure (≥ 3 organs) occurring within 1 week combined with histopathologic evidence of arterial occlusion. When identified, patients should be screened by transesophageal echocardiography for nonbacterial thrombotic endocarditis (Libman–Sacks endocarditis) which may serve as a potential source for recurrent embolism [6]. This form of endocarditis may occur in up to one third of patients with primary antiphospholipid syndrome and half of patients with secondary antiphospholipid syndrome in the setting of systemic lupus erythematosus.

Venous thrombosis may present as the typical lower extremity deep vein thrombosis with pulmonary embolism or may involve atypical venous locations such as the cerebral, splanchnic, renal, or gonadal venous circulations. Prompt anticoagulation is a necessity whereby risk of propagation and recurrence in the absence of anticoagulation can be as high as eightfold [7, 8]. Epidemiologic data supports a differential risk relationship between the presence of lupus anticoagulant, antiphospholipid antibodies, and risk of thrombosis [9]. The Leiden Thrombophilia Study reported a 3.6-fold increased risk for deep vein thrombosis in individuals positive for lupus anticoagulant (LA), while this risk increase to 10.1 for patients positive for both LA and either antiprothrombin or anti-β2-glycoprotein-1 antibodies [10]. Patients who are "triple positive" for lupus anticoagulant, antiphospholipid antibodies, and β2-glycoprotein-1 antibodies are at the highest thrombotic risk.

Laboratory Evaluation

Laboratory testing for antiphospholipid antibody syndrome is broadly based on the use of clot-based assays for lupus anticoagulant and enzyme-linked immunosorbent assay (ELISA)-based assays for antiphospholipid or β2-glycoprotein-1 antibodies [5]. For lupus anticoagulant testing, the general approach includes multiple clot-based assays. This approach balances the desire to maximize case identification yield without compromising specificity. The general test repertoire includes the dilute Russell Viper Venom Time (dRVVT), aPTT with platelet neutralization procedure, and Staclot aPTT. The thrombin time and reptilase time are used to search for heparin or direct thrombin inhibitors which degrade test accuracy. Each assay combines the use of mixing studies to differentiate between assay inhibition (which would point to a lupus inhibitor) and factor deficiency. "Assay inhibition" is defined as clotting times which remain prolonged despite equal volume mixing with pooled donor plasma. If the equal volume mixing study normalizes the clotting time, then a "factor deficiency" is considered. When the assay shows inhibition, then the final step involves adding excess phospholipid to form a "sink" for the antibody. This final step results in a significant shortening of the clotting time and implies a phospholipid-dependent mechanism for clotting assay time prolongation consistent with a lupus anticoagulant. Our approach to this testing is to perform each step in the process including the screening, mixing, and confirmatory steps for consistency and quality assurance. If the confirmatory step is negative, then a specific factor inhibitor is sought. "Factor inhibitors" however present clinically with a bleeding phenotype in contrast to the thrombosis phenotype associated with a lupus anticoagulant. In general, all of the anticoagulants (heparins, warfarin, and direct factor inhibitors) have the potential for degrading test sensitivity and specificity and should be avoided if feasible at the time of testing.

To establish the diagnosis of antiphospholipid antibody syndrome, positive testing for either a lupus anticoagulant or antiphospholipid antibody is sufficient. Between 30 and 40 % of patients will have both a lupus anticoagulant and antiphospholipid antibody (by ELISA). If positive, both the clotting assays and the ELISA must be repeated to establish persistence at least 12 weeks or later [2]. An important caveat for ELISA testing of antiphospholipid antibodies (IgG, IgM) and β2-glycoprotein-I antibodies is that modest titers of these antibodies do not constitute a firm diagnosis. To support the diagnosis of antiphospholipid antibody syndrome, confirmatory titers must exceed 40 units. It has been our experience that providers often accept a weakly positive titer (<40 units) as diagnostic of this syndrome. Due to the lifelong implications of this diagnosis, we recommend strict application of the diagnostic criteria so as not to mislabel individuals.

If confirmed, the next step is to determine whether the patient has primary or secondary antiphospholipid syndrome. Patients with primary disease are more likely female with a mean age of 40 years [11]. For older patients with a new diagnosis of antiphospholipid antibody syndrome, a search for secondary causes is important. Relevant secondary causes include connective tissue diseases, both solid tumors and hematologic malignancies, medications, and infections particularly viral. Most viral-induced antibodies are not thought to carry a thrombotic propensity.

Management

Given high risk of recurrence, anticoagulant therapy is required. Warfarin therapy remains the cornerstone of management. Randomized warfarin trials comparing INR targets of standard intensity (2.0–3.0) to high intensity (3.0–4.0 or 3.0–4.5) resulted in similar or improved efficacy for those patients randomized to the standard intensity INR targets [12, 13]. Higher-intensity nomograms have the limitation of greater bleeding outcomes. Therefore, current clinical practice is to use the standard INR goal for most patients. An important point is that these trials included a minority of patients with arterial thrombosis (24 and 11 %, respectively). Whether a higher target for those patients with arterial thrombosis would be beneficial is not known. We would typically recommend aspirin therapy added to warfarin therapy.

For patients with a baseline prolongation of the prothrombin time, this assay cannot be reliably used to monitor warfarin therapy. Fortunately, only 5–10 % of patients have this baseline abnormality. For those rare patients with baseline prothrombin time inhibition, we favor monitoring with factor Xa or factor IIa (thrombin) assays aiming for a therapeutic target of between 20 and 30 % protein activity. It would be attractive to use novel anticoagulants, including factor Xa inhibitors and direct thrombin inhibitors, as an alternative to warfarin particularly in this setting. The use of these agents has not been well studied, and recommendations regarding their use must be tempered by concerns regarding potential failures. We have recently identified three consecutive patients with antiphospholipid antibody syndrome suffering arterial events who failed these direct factor inhibitor therapy [14]. Since the publication of this small cohort, we have identified two additional patients who failed novel anticoagulant therapy.

For patients suffering acute arterial occlusion in the setting of antiphospholipid antibody syndrome, we recommend fibrinolytic therapy over immediate bypass grafting whenever feasible. In this setting of acute arterial occlusion, bypass grafting has a high likelihood of early thrombotic failure regardless of the type of conduit used. We further recommend aggressive anticoagulant therapy during the acute and convalescent time frame. Prolonged use of subcutaneous low-molecular weight heparin at the twice-daily therapeutic dose has been quite useful in such patients. This form of therapy is advantageous due to immediate therapeutic levels, lack of monitoring in the setting of an inhibited aPTT (lupus anticoagulant), and generally low rate of major bleeding. Conversion to warfarin requires clinical judgment and does not need to be done promptly. For example, we often continue outpatient therapeutic low-molecular weight heparin for several months after an acute event before entertaining this conversion.

Heparin-Induced Thrombocytopenia

Heparin-induced thrombocytopenia (HIT) is an immune-mediated disorder with increased risk for both arterial and venous thrombosis [15]. The paradox of this entity is that thrombosis ensues despite anticoagulant therapy and despite falling platelet counts. The condition represents one of the strongest prothrombotic states.

Pathogenesis

HIT is characterized by the development of platelet-activating, noncomplement-fixing IgG antibodies directed against heparin–platelet factor 4 (H-PF4) complex [16]. Heparin is a negatively charged polysaccharide which complexes with PF4 unfolding and exposing neoepitopes within the protein. These neoepitopes may be highly antigenic and induce antibody formation in a small subset of patients receiving heparin. The degree of antigenicity corresponds to the net negative charge of the complex which is directly related to the size of the heparin molecule exposure. As such, unfractionated heparin carries a much higher risk of developing HIT (5 %) compared to low-molecular weight heparin (<1 %) or pentasaccharide therapy (fondaparinux—negligible risk) [17, 18]. Once formed, the heparin-PF4 antibody complex binds and activates platelets through interaction with the Fc receptor domain on the platelet surface. Platelet activation results in the release of procoagulant microparticles, platelet aggregation, leukocyte binding through platelet P-selectin expression, and coagulation factor activation. Tissue factor expression with cytokine release from monocytes and macrophages has also been reported [19]. This process ultimately leads to platelet sequestration and thrombocytopenia. Whereas endothelial cells are decorated with heparan sulfate and platelet factor 4, direct antibody-mediated vascular injury further promotes thrombus formation.

Clinical Presentation

The incidence of HIT ranges between 1 and 5 %, depending on the type of heparin used, the route of administration, associated comorbidities, and clinical settings [15]. Patients undergoing major joint replacement surgery appear to be at particular risk [20]. Vascular surgeons may be consulted by orthopedic colleagues for acute limb ischemia postoperatively and should keep this entity in mind. Up to 20 % of patients who undergo vascular surgical procedures develop heparin-associated antibodies, which are associated with a greater than twofold increased risk for thrombotic complications [21]. By comparison, outpatient LMWH therapy carries such a low risk that regular platelet monitoring is not recommended.

Table 25.1 Determining pretest probability of HIT

	2	1	0
Thrombocytopenia	>50% fall Nadir 20–100	30–50% fall Nadir 10–19	<30% fall Nadir <10
Timing	5–10 days <1 day (prior heparin)	>10 days	<5 days (no prior heparin)
Thrombosis	New event Skin necrosis	Progressive event Recurrent event	None
Other cause for thrombocytopenia	None	Possible	Definite
Pretest score	High 6–8	Intermediate 4–5	Low 0–3

From Warkentin TE. An overview of the heparin-induced thrombocytopenia syndrome. Semin Thromb Hemost. 2004 Jun;30(3):273–83. Reprinted with permission from Thieme

Laboratory Evaluation

When considering the diagnosis of HIT, it is important to define the pretest probability of disease [15]. The Warkentin "4 T" probability assessment tool for HIT is well validated and quite useful for this purpose. This tool includes an assessment of platelet counts relative to baseline, timing of thrombocytopenia in relation to heparin initiation, thrombosis assessment, and exclusion of other causes (Table 25.1). Each of these variables is given a weighted score which is then summed. Depending on the summed score, patients are deemed low, intermediate, or high pretest probability of having HIT. For those patients at low risk (score ≤ 3), the clinician should search for other causes of thrombocytopenia. These patients have <5% probability of having HIT such that testing for the heparin-PF4 antibody will be of low yield. The use of heparin in such patients may be pursued unless the degree of platelet decrement precludes its use. For patients at intermediate to high risk of HIT, heparin must be discontinued and confirmatory testing with ELISA for heparin-PF4 antibodies pursued. While waiting for these test results, most patients should receive a direct thrombin inhibitor such as argatroban. For patients with negative assay results, we recommend careful clinical reevaluation and request for hematology consultation. The heparin-PF4 ELISA carries a high negative predictive value approaching 90% for the exclusion of clinical HIT. For equivocal test results, we recommend repeat testing and if still equivocal, obtaining a serotonin release assay. The serotonin release assay carries high specificity but lower sensitivity compared to the heparin-PF4 ELISA. If the serotonin release assay is negative, the clinical diagnosis is effectively excluded. In the setting of intermediate to high pretest probability of disease, a positive assay result confirms the diagnosis of HIT.

In the clinical assessment of HIT, there are several caveats worth noting. First, there is an entity termed "nonimmune HIT" or type I HIT which occurs within 4 days of heparin exposure and results in only a modest and temporary platelet count decline (100–150,000). Patients with this type of HIT are not at risk of thrombosis, and the key is that platelet counts recover despite continued heparin exposure. This is the most common cause of heparin-associated platelet count decline but is harmless. The mechanism may include platelet "agglutination" from heparin–platelet binding. Second, it is important to scrutinize the platelet counts in total whereby a 50% decline may still be a normal platelet count if the baseline counts were ≥300. Third, thrombocytopenia will include a 50% drop from baseline but only rarely results in severely reduced platelet counts. The mean platelet count from published cohorts is approximately 60,000 (range 20,000–100,000). For patients with platelet counts less than 20,000, other causes should be sought particularly drug-induced thrombocytopenia due to non-heparin drugs. Exclusion of pseudothrombocytopenia is accomplished by simply repeating the phlebotomy using citrate in place of EDTA.

HIT may present as an isolated asymptomatic fall in platelet counts ("isolated HIT") without further difficulties [15, 22]. However up to 50% of patients developing HIT will suffer a thrombotic complication within the ensuing 30 days ("HIT with thrombosis, HITT"). The risk of thrombosis persists long after heparin is discontinued whereby heparin-PF4 antibodies may circulate for 100 days or longer postheparin discontinuation. With heparin reexposure during this time window, abrupt thrombocytopenia with thrombosis may occur ("rapid onset HIT"). This clinical presentation accounts for up to 30% of HIT cases and does not represent an amnestic response but rather is due to persistently circulating antibodies. For this reason, it is important to draw a baseline and follow up CBC within the first 24 h of starting heparin in all patients exposed to heparin within the past 100 days. "Delayed onset HIT" is an infrequent (3–5%) but uncomfortable subtype of HIT which occurs several days after stopping heparin typically when the patient may have already been discharged from the hospital. It is important to recognize this entity whereby treating a new thrombus with heparin in such patients can have devastating consequences.

Venous thrombosis exceeds arterial thrombotic by nearly 4:1. Phlegmasia cerulea dolens with associated digital gangrene may mimic arterial occlusion and must be kept in the differential diagnosis. Other thrombotic complications reported in patients with HIT include overt disseminated intravascular coagulation with hypofibrinogenemia, bilateral adrenal hemorrhage and necrosis, and cutaneous necrosis at sites of heparin injection (heparin skin necrosis) [10, 11, 23–25].

Appropriate platelet monitoring is essential for early diagnosis of HIT [15, 26]. A baseline platelet count should be obtained prior to heparin initiation. In heparin-naïve patients, the platelet count should be monitored every other day beginning 5 days after starting heparin and continued for 14 days or until heparin is discontinued whichever is shorter [15]. In patients with previous heparin exposure, platelets should be monitored with the start of unfractionated heparin use and continued as for heparin-naïve patients.

Management

Prompt recognition of HIT, immediate cessation of all forms of heparin, and rapid initiation of a direct thrombin inhibitor are essential to reduce morbidity and mortality [22]. Approximately 50 % of patients with HIT characterized by thrombocytopenia alone ("isolated HIT") will experience thrombosis within the ensuing 30 days if a direct thrombin inhibitor is not initiated [27]. The use of warfarin alone in these patients is not protective, and warfarin loading after a diagnosis of HIT can result in severe thrombotic complications including acute arterial occlusion [27, 28]. Parenteral direct thrombin inhibitor therapy is the cornerstone of initial treatment. There are currently three available agents for this purpose: argatroban, bivalirudin, and desirudin. Of these only argatroban is FDA approved for this indication. For patients with renal disease, argatroban is an ideal agent whereby it is cleared by the liver. For patients with liver disease, bivalirudin would be preferred. Both of these agents are attractive given their relatively short half-life. These agents are managed by monitoring the aPTT. Both agents to some degree also prolong the PT. Therefore, with concordant warfarin initiation, we recommend aiming for International normalized ratio (INR) values of 4–6 before stopping the direct thrombin inhibitor. The INR can then be reassessed 4 h later to insure that a therapeutic target has been achieved (INR 2.0–3.0). We recommend continued anticoagulation for a minimum of 3 months depending on the clinical situation. This will allow complete clearance of the circulating antibody. Warfarin initiation should be delayed until the platelet count rebounds to values exceeding 150,000, and large initiating doses should be avoided. Alternative agents which may be useful include fondaparinux (parenteral indirect factor Xa inhibitor), dabigatran (oral direct thrombin inhibitor), rivaroxaban, and apixaban (oral direct factor Xa inhibitors). Clinical experience with the novel anticoagulants in this setting is limited, and they are not FDA approved for such indications.

For many patients with vascular disease, heparin reexposure is required for additional procedures particularly cardiopulmonary bypass [29]. In our published experience, this can be safely accomplished once the patient has cleared the heparin-PF4 antibodies. In this case, a brief isolated rechallenge for purposes of the bypass run has been safe. We recommend restarting a direct thrombin inhibitor as soon as feasible postoperatively to avoid prolonged heparin reexposure.

Myeloproliferative Disorders

For any patient with an acute thrombotic event, a simple complete blood count (CBC) is an essential part of the initiation evaluation. Elevated red cell or platelet counts should alert the provider to a potential diagnosis of a myeloproliferative neoplasm. These diseases which include polycythemia vera, essential thrombocythemia, and primary myelofibrosis represent a stem cell-derived clonal myeloproliferation [30]. Polycythemia vera is recognized by an increased red cell, white cell, and platelet counts. Essential thrombocythemia involves platelet count expansion with normal or near normal white cell and red cell counts. Primary myelofibrosis is characterized by progressive fibrosis of the bone marrow with anemia, splenomegaly, extramedullary hematopoiesis, constitutional symptoms, cachexia, and ultimately leukemic transformation. This may result from progressive evolution of polycythemia vera and essential thrombocythemia and significantly shortens survival. Each of these disorders may transform to myeloid leukemia. Yet the most common cause of death in these patients remains thrombosis related [31].

These disorders are frequently associated with an acquired mutation of JAK2 resulting from a replacement of valine for phenylalanine in position 617 (V617F). JAK2, a member of the Janus kinase family of cytoplasmic tyrosine kinases, is associated with growth factor receptors and therefore results in growth factor-independent proliferation of bone marrow-derived cell lines. This mutation is found in over 90 % of patients with polycythemia vera and 50 % of patients with essential thrombocythemia [32]. Screening for this mutation is therefore indicated in the evaluation of patients with acute arterial occlusion and abnormal CBC with either elevated red cell or platelet counts [33]. Other clinical presentations may include erythromelalgia or a variety of neurologic or visual symptoms [34].

Essential thrombocythemia should be considered in any patient with a persistently elevated platelet count (>450,000). Other causes of thrombocytosis should be excluded. Several entities relevant to vascular surgery include postsplenectomy, elevated ferritin levels, or systemic inflammation. These patients should be referred for subspecialty consultation in hematology and if indicated, a bone marrow biopsy. For confirmed essential thrombocythemia, the thrombosis risk depends on patient age (>60 years), prior history of thrombosis, cardiovascular risk factors, and JAK2 mutation status. Hydroxyurea is the mainstay for treating this disorder [35]. Anagrelide is an alternative. Novel therapies targeting the JAK2 pathway show promise to inhibit cell proliferation in myeloproliferative neoplasms [36]. Regardless of therapeutic regimen, until the underlying disease is adequately treated, antithrombotic therapy may be associated with a high risk of failure.

Polycythemia rubra vera is a rare condition with an incidence of approximately 2 per 100,000 and often occurs in middle-aged individuals with a slight male predominance [37]. An important clinical clue is the history of pruritus following a warm bath or shower. Laboratory features which should prompt consideration of this disease is the finding of elevated hemoglobin (>18.5 g/dL in men or >16.5 g/dL in women) with a subnormal erythropoietin level [38]. As with essential thrombocythemia, these patients should be referred for hematology consultation and bone marrow biopsy. Treatment goals include maintaining adequate suppression of the hematocrit. For patients younger than age 60 without a thrombosis history, serial phlebotomy remains the mainstay of treatment [39]. For patients at increased risk of thrombosis including those with prior thrombosis, hydroxyurea is used [40]. Low-dose aspirin is recommended for all patients unless contraindicated due to a prior major hemorrhage [41]. For patients suffering arterial thrombotic events, in addition to treating the underlying neoplasm, we recommend warfarin at a goal INR of 2.0–3.0 in addition to low-dose aspirin. Treatment however may be complicated in these patients whereby there is also a propensity for major bleeding.

Paradoxic Embolism

A number of congenital thrombophilic risk factorswhich augment the propensity for venous thrombosis have been identified.

In general, these factors have not been convincingly shown to augment the risk of arterial thrombotic events. One caveat to this general rule is paradoxic embolism where an embolized venous thrombosis gains access to the arterial circulation through a septal defect in the heart. The contribution of paradoxic embolism to the spectrum of acute arterial occlusion however is unclear largely due to the difficulty in ascribing causality in patients with patent foramen ovale (PFO) or more rarely, septal defects (atrial or ventricular) (Fig. 25.1). The prevalence of patent foramen ovale is 25–35 % in the general population [42]. Variables associated with an increased risk of thromboembolism in the setting of PFO include large defects, large right-to-left shunts, spontaneous right-to-left shunts, atrial septal aneurysms, and large Eustachian valves [43, 44].

The relationship between PFO and arterial thromboembolism including stroke has been thoroughly studied including

Table 25.2 Comprehensive thrombophilia panel

Protein C activity
Protein C antigen*
Protein S total antigen
Protein S free antigen
Protein S activity*
Antithrombin activity
Plasminogen activity
Lupus anticoagulant
Activated protein C resistance
Factor V Leiden mutation*
Prothrombin G20210A mutation
Dysfibrinogenemia
Fibrinogen
Fibrin D-dimer
Anticardiolipin (IgG and IgM) antibodies
Homocysteine (fasting)

*Performed reflectively when the primary assay is abnormal

case-control studies, prospective population-based studies, and randomized controlled trials. In order to digest this topic, each of these bodies of evidence should be scrutinized. For patients suffering cryptogenic stroke, case-control studies have shown an increased prevalence of PFO among cases arguing that this mechanism is relevant in the evaluation of patients under the age of 55 years [45]. For older patients, the association is less clear.

There have been two important prospective population-based studies assessing the risk of ischemic stroke in patients with PFO. The multiethnic "NOMAS" study assessed the prevalence of PFO by transthoracic echocardiography and the risk of future stroke in 1100 stroke-free subjects older than 39 years [46]. At baseline, 14.9 % of subjects had a PFO and 2.5 % had an atrial septal aneurysm. At a mean follow-up of 6.6 years, 6.2 % of subjects had suffered a stroke. After adjustment of other risk factors, the presence of a PFO with or without an atrial septal aneurysm was not associated with increased stroke risk. In contrast, an isolated atrial septal aneurysm increased the stroke risk by nearly fourfold, yet the confidence interval for this association was quite broad. The SPARC study prospectively assessed 585 randomly sampled Olmsted County residents over age 45 years for the association of PFO, atrial septal aneurysm by transesophageal echocardiography, and the incidence of future stroke [47]. At baseline, 24.3 % of subjects were found to have a PFO and 1.9 % had an atrial septal aneurysm. During the 5.1 year median follow-up, the overall stroke rate was 7 %. After adjusting for age and other risk factors, PFO was not an independent predictor of stroke.

To further evaluate this issue, there have been three randomized controlled trials of PFO closure to determine whether this therapy reduces the incidence of recurrent stroke or embolization. The CLOSURE I investigators randomized 909 patients (ages 18–60 years) who presented with a cryptogenic stroke or transient ischemic attack (TIA) and a PFO to open-label percuta-

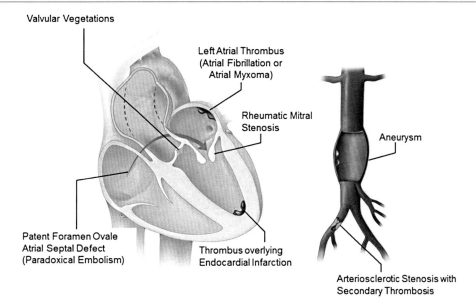

Fig. 25.1 Sources of arterial embolism. There are a number of potential sources of embolism resulting in acute arterial occlusion. These include cardiac sources, proximal aneurysms, or proximal ruptured atherosclerotic plaques with overlying thrombus. Cardiac sources include paradoxic emboli through patent foramen ovale and atrial or ventricular septal defects. Valvular diseases including bacterial or nonbacterial thrombotic endocarditis, fibroelastoma, or rheumatic valvular stenosis. Ventricular thrombi may form on the endocardial surface following large myocardial infarctions particularly if complicated by a ventricular aneurysm. Atrial fibrillation with atrial appendage thrombus formation is the most common source of cardiac embolism. Atrial myxoma or other intracardiac tumors may also first present with acute arterial occlusion following embolization underscoring the need for histopathologic assessment of all retrieved embolic material

neous closure (STARFlex closure device) or medical therapy [48]. Medical therapy included warfarin, aspirin, or both at the discretion of the local investigator. After a mean follow-up of 2 years, there was no difference in the primary end point of death within the first 30 days or death from neurologic causes from 31 days to 2 years. There were no differences in the rates of stroke or TIA. During the follow-up period, atrial fibrillation was significantly more common in the closure group compared to controls (5.7 vs. 0.7 %; $p<0.001$). The PC trial investigators randomized 414 patients (mean age 44 years) with cryptic embolism to undergo PFO closure with the Amplatzer PFO occluder or medical therapy [49]. Patients undergoing closure were treated with aspirin (at least 5 months) plus either ticlopidine or clopidogrel (1–6 months). Antithrombotic therapy for control subjects was left to the local investigators' discretion. After 4.1 years of follow-up, there was no difference in the composite primary efficacy outcome of death, stroke, TIA, or peripheral embolism between groups (3.4 vs. 5.2 %). Individual outcomes also did not differ between groups. Similarly, the RESPECT investigators found no benefit in PFO closure after randomizing 980 subjects with cryptogenic stroke [50].

In summary, the contribution of paradoxic embolism to patient suffering cryptogenic acute arterial occlusion remains unclear. While a devastating stroke may result from emboli as small as 1 mm in diameter, symptomatic peripheral arterial emboli require thrombus diameters of 10 mm or greater. Therefore, one would anticipate that a clinically relevant PFO participating in a peripheral paradoxic embolism must be of sufficient size to allow passage of a thrombus of such size. Moreover, it remains unclear whether the stroke data applies to such patients. Whether to offer percutaneous or surgical PFO closure to patients with cryptogenic stroke, TIA or peripheral embolism remains a complicated decision-making process. Our approach has been to involve a multidisciplinary team including cardiologists, stroke neurologists, and coagulation experts in the evaluation [51]. Each patient undergoes comprehensive transesophageal echocardiography, complete thrombophilia testing, thorough cross-sectional vascular imaging, and venous ultrasonography. For patients who would not otherwise require indefinite anticoagulation therapy and whose clinical picture strongly suggests a paradoxic event, elective PFO closure is offered after complete counseling regarding the risks and benefits of the procedure.

Atrial Fibrillation

Atrial fibrillation is an important cause of stroke, TIA, and peripheral embolization (Fig. 25.2) [52]. For patients with non-valvular atrial fibrillation, stroke accounts for 95 % of the thromboembolic complications with only 5 % affecting other arterial beds [53, 54]. Of these 5 %, atrial fibrillation-related thromboembolism accounts for considerable morbidity and mortality. For example, atrial fibrillation accounts for up to 95 % of acute arterial occlusion of the extremities, more than

Fig. 25.2 Sites of embolic acute arterial occlusion. The potential sites of acute arterial occlusion and their relative frequency of involvement are provided. Emboli tend to occlude arterial segments at bifurcation points where the arterial diameter abruptly narrows. Lower-extremity sites of involvement are nearly twice as common as upper extremity sites. Visceral vessels are much less frequently involved. (Adapted from Thromb Haemost. 2008;99:951–955)

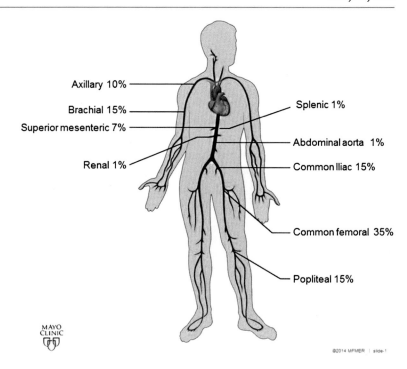

30 % of splenic infarction, more than half of renal infarctions, and nearly half of acute mesenteric ischemic events [55, 56]. For patients suffering a non-cerebral embolism, 85 % involved acute limb ischemia with the majority involving the lower compared to the upper extremities (2:1 ratio) [52]. Fifteen percent is involved in abdominal arteries, most frequently the mesenteric arteries (45 % of abdominal emboli). Moreover, the mortality rates for patients with atrial fibrillation associated acute arterial occlusion of the limb are significantly greater compared to those suffering an embolism in the setting of an acute coronary syndromes or local plaque rupture with secondary thrombotic arterial occlusion [56].

Compared to non-valvular atrial fibrillation, patients with valvular atrial fibrillation have a greater propensity for thromboembolism and particularly acute limb ischemia [57]. Valvular atrial fibrillation is defined as "AF in the association with rheumatic mitral stenosis, a mechanical or bioprosthetic heart valve, or mitral valve repair" [58]. Compared to non-valvular atrial fibrillation, patients with valvular atrial fibrillation carry a significantly greater risk of peripheral embolization compared to stroke [59]. For valvular atrial fibrillation, nearly half of thromboembolic events are to peripheral arteries compared to only 5 % for non-valvular atrial fibrillation [60]. For these reasons, even if atrial fibrillation is identified on the admission electrocardiogram, it is still important to perform an echocardiogram to distinguish "valvular" from "non-valvular" atrial fibrillation in these patients. While warfarin is an established effective therapy for atrial fibrillation regardless of underlying valvular status, the newer oral-specific factor inhibitors have not been adequately studied in "valvular atrial fibrillation" to recommend their use for this entity.

It is well established that atrial fibrillation represents a major cause of stroke and peripheral embolization. It is becoming more evident that an important percentage of patients with incident stroke or peripheral embolization will be found to have previously undiagnosed atrial fibrillation if appropriately screened. Identifying these patients requires careful and thorough monitoring. In a randomized, controlled study design, 441 patients over age 40 years with ischemic stroke and no prior history of atrial fibrillation or evidence of atrial fibrillation after 24 h of cardiac monitoring were randomized to either long-term cardiac monitoring using an implantable cardiac monitor or conventional follow-up [61]. By 6 months, atrial fibrillation was found in nearly 9 % of patients with extended monitoring. At 12 months, 12.4 % of patients were noted to have cryptic atrial fibrillation. Similarly, the Embrace investigators randomized 572 patients over age 55 years with cryptogenic stroke and no known atrial fibrillation to wearing a cardiac monitoring belt with a 30-day event-triggered loop recorder or additional 24 h Holter monitoring [62]. To get into the study, all patients underwent an initial 24 h Holter monitor. Thirty-day monitoring was superior to 24 h monitoring for the detection of atrial fibrillation. In the intervention group, atrial fibrillation was detected in 16.1 % compared to only 3.2 % in the control group.

For patients with acute arterial occlusion without an identifiable mechanism, prolonged cardiac monitoring for 30 days with either an implantable or wearable device appears to improve identification of atrial fibrillation. This identification has important therapeutic implications, whereas these patients would be treated with indefinite anticoagulant therapy as opposed to antiplatelet therapy.

Miscellaneous Causes

Hyperhomocysteinemia

Hyperhomocysteinemia is a risk factor for arterial occlusive disease and venous thromboembolism due to severely elevated plasma homocysteine concentrations [63–66]. Causes may be congenital (cystathionine β-synthase deficiency, methylene tetrahydrofolate reductase variant) or acquired (deficiencies in vitamin B6, vitamin B12, and folic acid). Proposed mechanisms by which hyperhomocysteinemia impacts arterial and venous thrombosis include direct toxic effects on the endothelium, enhanced platelet activation, oxidation of low-density lipoprotein cholesterol, an inflammatory reduction in endothelial thrombomodulin, and an increase in circulating von Willebrand factor and factor VIII [67]. To be a relevant pathogen for arterial occlusive disease and thrombosis, values must be more than modestly elevated. Hyperhomocysteinemia has been classified as either "moderate" (15–30 μM/L), "intermediate" (30–100 μM/L), or "severe" (>100 μM/L) [68]. There is a direct relationship between risk of vascular disease and concentration of homocysteine. Genetic testing for inherited causes of hyperhomocysteinemia should not be performed unless homocysteine levels are first found to be high, no other apparent acquired mechanisms are identified, and the results of such testing are anticipated to impact therapy for the patient or family members. While various therapeutic options effectively reduce homocysteine levels, the efficacy of these therapies to impact hard cardiovascular outcomes have been disappointing [69].

Paroxysmal Nocturnal Thrombophilia

Paroxysmal nocturnal thrombophilia (PNH) is a rare cause of thromboembolism. Thrombophilia of paroxysmal nocturnal hemoglobinuria is related to complement-mediated platelet activation, venous endothelial damage, and defects in fibrinolysis.

Thrombotic complications are the most common cause of mortality in PNH. Forty percent of patients will develop thrombotic complications, 85 % of which are venous and 15 % of which are arterial [70, 71]. Venous thrombosis in PNH has a predilection for the hepatic veins, portal and mesenteric venous systems, and the deep veins of the pelvis and lower extremities. Arterial thromboses have been described in cerebral, coronary, and pulmonary arteries [72, 73]. Diagnosis of PNH is made by the absence or near absence of two glycosyl-phosphatidyl-inositol (GPI)-linked antigens (e.g., CD55, CD59) in at least two cell lines (e.g., red cells, granulocytes) or the absence of the GPI anchor by fluorescent label. Treatment is in the form of anticoagulation therapy with warfarin or enoxaparin, which has shown definitive reduction in thromboses. Eculizumab is the first targeted therapy for a complement-mediated disease and has been used in the treatment of PNH. The drug is recombinant monoclonal antibody that selectively binds complement protein 5 (C5), preventing cleavage of C5 to C5a, a potent proinflammatory and prothrombotic mediator that activates the formation of the C5b-9 membrane attack complex [72, 74].

Summary

In summary, the congenital and acquired "thrombophilias" are infrequently the direct cause of acute arterial ischemic events. Most events arise from either thromboembolism from a cardiac source, proximal aneurysm, or proximal diseased artery. Thrombosis in situ at the site of a ruptured atherosclerotic plaque is also a common mechanism for such events. Less frequent mechanisms include arterial dissection, transection, arteritis, tumor or foreign body embolization, and vasospasm. In those patients for whom these mechanisms don't fit clinically, the vascular provider should consider diseases such as antiphospholipid antibody syndrome, heparin-induced thrombocytopenia, or myeloproliferative neoplasms. An evaluation for venous "thrombophilias" may be relevant if a paradoxic mechanism is implicated. For these patients, septal defect closure may be entertained after thorough multidisciplinary evaluation and testing. Lastly, previously undiagnosed atrial fibrillation is an important consideration particularly if significant valve disease can be identified by echocardiography. Identifying these patients will impact long-term therapy whereby indefinite anticoagulation is indicated.

References

1. Favaloro EJ, Wong RC. Antiphospholipid antibody testing for the antiphospholipid syndrome: a comprehensive practical review including a synopsis of challenges and recent guidelines. Pathology. 2014;46(6):481–95.
2. Lakos G, Favaloro EJ, Harris EN, Meroni PL, Tincani A, Wong RC, Pierangeli SS. International consensus guidelines on anticardiolipin and anti-β2-glycoprotein I testing: report from the 13th International Congress on Antiphospholipid Antibodies. Arthritis Rheum. 2012;64(1):1–10.
3. Giannakopoulos B, Krilis SA. The pathogenesis of the antiphospholipid syndrome. N Engl J Med. 2013;368(11):1033–44.
4. Giannakopoulos B, Passam F, Rahgozar S, Krilis SA. Current concepts on the pathogenesis of the antiphospholipid syndrome. Blood. 2007;109:422–30.
5. Pierangeli SS, Girardi G, Vega-Ostertag M, Liu X, Espinola RG, Salmon J. Requirement of activation of complement C3 and C5 for antiphospholipid antibody–mediated thrombophilia. Arthritis Rheum. 2005;52:2120–4.
6. Hojnik M, George J, Ziporen L, Shoenfeld Y. Heart valve involvement (Libman–Sacks endocarditis) in the antiphospholipid syndrome. Circulation. 1996;93:1579–87.

7. Kearon C, Gent M, Hirsh J, Weitz J, Kovacs MJ, Anderson DR, Turpie AG, Green D, Ginsberg JS, Wells P, MacKinnon B, Julian JA. A comparison of three months of anticoagulation with extended anticoagulation for the first episode of idiopathic venous thromboembolism. N Engl J Med. 1999;340(12):901–7.

8. Schulman S, Svenungsson E, Granqvist S, Duration of Anticoagulation Study Group. Anticardiolipin antibodies predict early recurrence of thromboembolism and death among patients with venous thromboembolism following anticoagulant therapy. Am J Med. 1998;104(4):332–8.

9. Galli M, Luciani D, Bertolini G, Barbui T. Lupus anticoagulants are stronger risk factors for thrombosis than anticardiolipin antibodies in the antiphospholipid antibody syndrome: a systematic review of the literature. Blood. 2003;101(5):1827–32.

10. De Groot PG, Lutters B, Derksen RH, Lisman T, Meijers JC, Rosendaal FR. Lupus anticoagulants and the risk of a first episode of deep venous thrombosis. J Thromb Haemost. 2005;3(9):1993–7.

11. Miyakis S, Lockshin MD, Atsumi T, Branch DW, Brey RL, Cervera R, Derksen RH, DE Groot PG, Koike T, Meroni PL, Reber G, Shoenfeld Y, Tincani A, Vlachoyiannopoulos PG, Krilis SA. International consensus statement on an update of the classification criteria for definite antiphospholipid syndrome (APS). J Thromb Haemost. 2006;4(2):295–306.

12. Crowther MA, Ginsberg JS, Julian J, Denburg J, Hirsh J, Douketis J, Laskin C, Fortin P, Anderson D, Kearon C, Clarke A, Geerts W, Forgie M, Green D, Costantini L, Yacura W, Wilson S, Gent M, Kovacs MJ. A comparison of two intensities of warfarin for the prevention of recurrent thrombosis in patients with the antiphospholipid antibody syndrome. N Engl J Med. 2003;349(12):1133–8.

13. Finazzi G, Marchioli R, Brancaccio V, Schinco P, Wisloff F, Musial J, Baudo F, Berrettini M, Testa S, D'Angelo A, Tognoni G, Barbui T. A randomized clinical trial of high-intensity warfarin vs. conventional antithrombotic therapy for the prevention of recurrent thrombosis in patients with the antiphospholipid syndrome (WAPS). J Thromb Haemost. 2005;3(5):848–53.

14. Schaefer JK, McBane RD, Black DF, Williams LN, Moder KG, Wysokinski WE. Failure of dabigatran and rivaroxaban to prevent thromboembolism in antiphospholipid syndrome: a case series of three patients. Thromb Haemost. 2014;112(5):947–50.

15. Linkins LA, Dans AL, Moores LK, Bona R, Davidson BL, Schulman S, Crowther M, American College of Chest Physicians. Treatment and prevention of heparin-induced thrombocytopenia: antithrombotic therapy and prevention of thrombosis, 9th ed: American College of Chest Physicians evidence-based clinical practice guidelines. Chest. 2012;141(2 Suppl):e495S–530S.

16. Warkentin TE. HIT paradigms and paradoxes. J Thromb Haemost. 2011;9 Suppl 1:105–17.

17. Lobo B, Finch C, Howard A, Minhas S. Fondaparinux for the treatment of patients with acute heparin-induced thrombocytopenia. Thromb Haemost. 2008;99(1):208–14.

18. Warkentin TE, Levine MN, Hirsh J, Horsewood P, Roberts RS, Gent M, Kelton JG. Heparin-induced thrombocytopenia in patients treated with low-molecular-weight heparin or unfractionated heparin. N Engl J Med. 1995;332(20):1330–5.

19. Pouplard C, Iochmann S, Renard B, Herault O, Colombat P, Amiral J, Gruel Y. Induction of monocytes tissue factor expression by antibodies to heparin-platelet factor 4 complexes developed in heparin-induced thrombocytopenia. Blood. 2001;97(10):3300–2.

20. Warkentin TE, Cook RJ, Marder VJ, Sheppard JA, Moore JC, Eriksson BI, Greinacher A, Kelton JG. Anti-platelet factor 4/heparin antibodies in orthopedic surgery patients receiving antithrombotic prophylaxis with fondaparinux or enoxaparin. Blood. 2005;106(12):3791–6.

21. Calaitges JG, Liem TK, Spadone D, Nichols WK, Silver D. The role of heparin-associated antiplatelet antibodies in the outcome of arterial reconstruction. J Vasc Surg. 1999;29(5):779–85.

22. Keeling D, Davidson S, Watson H, Haemostasis and Thrombosis Task Force of the British Committee for Standards in Haematology. The management of heparin-induced thrombocytopenia. Br J Haematol. 2006;133(3):259–69.

23. Warkentin TE, Greinacher A. Heparin-induced thrombocytopenia: recognition, treatment, and prevention: the seventh ACCP conference on antithrombotic and thrombolytic therapy. Chest. 2004;126(3 Suppl):311S–37.

24. Warkentin TE. Clinical presentation of heparin-induced thrombocytopenia. Semin Hematol. 1998;35(4 Suppl 5):9–16.

25. Ketha S, Smithedajkul P, Vella A, Pruthi R, Wysokinski W, McBane R. Adrenal haemorrhage due to heparin-induced thrombocytopenia. Thromb Haemost. 2013;109(4):669–75.

26. Tafur AJ, McBane 2nd RD, Wysokinski WE, Gregg MS, Daniels PR, Mohr DN. Natural language processor as a tool to assess heparin induced thrombocytopenia awareness. J Thromb Thrombolysis. 2012;33(1):95–100.

27. Warkentin TE, Kelton JG. A 14 year study of heparin-induced thrombocytopenia. Am J Med. 1996;101(5):502–7.

28. Warkentin TE, Elavathil LJ, Hayward CP, Johnston MA, Russett JI, Kelton JG. The pathogenesis of venous limb gangrene associated with heparin-induced thrombocytopenia. Ann Intern Med. 1997;127(9):804–12.

29. Nuttall GA, Oliver Jr WC, Santrach PJ, McBane RD, Erpelding DB, Marver CL, Zehr KJ. Patients with a history of type II heparin-induced thrombocytopenia with thrombosis requiring cardiac surgery with cardiopulmonary bypass: a prospective observational case series. Anesth Analg. 2003;96(2):344–50.

30. James C, Ugo V, Le Couédic JP, Staerk J, Delhommeau F, Lacout C, Garçon L, Raslova H, Berger R, Bennaceur-Griscelli A, Villeval JL, Constantinescu SN, Casadevall N, Vainchenker W. A unique clonal JAK2 mutation leading to constitutive signaling causes polycythemia vera. Nature. 2005;434(7037):1144–8.

31. Elliott MA, Tefferi A. Thrombosis and haemorrhage in polycythaemia vera and essential thrombocythaemia. Br J Haematol. 2005;128(3):275–90.

32. Finazzi G, Barbui T. How I, treat patients with polycythemia vera. Blood. 2007;109(12):5104–11.

33. Tefferi A, Barbui T. bcr/abl negative, classic myeloproliferative disorders: diagnosis and treatment. Mayo Clin Proc. 2005;80(9):1220–32.

34. Barbui T, Finazzi G, Carobbio A, Thiele J, Passamonti F, Rumi E, Ruggeri M, Rodeghiero F, Randi ML, Bertozzi I, Gisslinger H, Buxhofer-Ausch V, De Stefano V, Betti S, Rambaldi A, Vannucchi AM, Tefferi A. Development and validation of an International Prognostic Score of thrombosis in World Health Organization-essential thrombocythemia (IPSET-thrombosis). Blood. 2012;120(26):5128–33.

35. Gisslinger H, Gotic M, Holowiecki J, Penka M, Thiele J, Kvasnicka HM, Kralovics R, Petrides PE, ANAHYDRET Study Group. Anagrelide compared with hydroxyurea in WHO-classified essential thrombocythemia: the ANAHYDRET study, a randomized controlled trial. Blood. 2013;121:1720–8.

36. Barrio S, Gallardo M, Arenas A, Ayala R, Rapado I, Rueda D, Jimenez A, Albizua E, Burgaleta C, Gilsanz F, Martinez-Lopez J. Inhibition of related JAK/STAT pathways with molecular targeted drugs shows strong synergy with ruxolitinib in chronic myeloproliferative neoplasm. Br J Haematol. 2013;161:667–76.

37. Anía BJ, Suman VJ, Sobell JL, Codd MB, Silverstein MN, Melton 3rd LJ. Trends in the incidence of polycythemia vera among Olmsted County, Minnesota residents, 1935–1989. Am J Hematol. 1994;47(2):89–93.

38. Spivak JL, Silver RT. The revised World Health Organization diagnostic criteria for polycythemia vera, essential thrombocytosis, and primary myelofibrosis: an alternative proposal. Blood. 2008;112:231–9.

39. Berk PD, Goldberg JD, Donovan PB, Fruchtman SM, Berlin NI, Wasserman LR. Therapeutic recommendations in polycythemia vera based on Polycythemia Vera Study Group protocols. Semin Hematol. 1986;23(2):132–43.

40. Tefferi A, Rumi E, Finazzi G, Gisslinger H, Vannucchi AM, Rodeghiero F, Randi ML, Vaidya R, Cazzola M, Rambaldi A, Gisslinger B, Pieri L, Ruggeri M, Bertozzi I, Sulai NH, Casetti I, Carobbio A, Jeryczynski G, Larson DR, Müllauer L, Pardanani A, Thiele J, Passamonti F, Barbui T. Survival and prognosis among 1545 patients with contemporary polycythemia vera: an international study. Leukemia. 2013;27:1874–81.

41. Patrono C, Rocca B, De Stefano V. Platelet activation and inhibition in polycythemia vera and essential thrombocythemia. Blood. 2013;121:1701–11.

42. Hagen PT, Scholz DG, Edwards WD. Incidence and size of patent foramen ovale during the first ten decades of life: an autopsy study of 965 normal hearts. Mayo Clin Proc. 1984;59:17–20.

43. Schuchlenz HW, Weihs W, Horner S, Quehenberger F. The association between the diameter of a patent foramen ovale and the risk of embolic cerebrovascular events. Am J Med. 2000;109:456–62.

44. Homma S, Di Tullio MR, Sacco RL, Mihalatos D, Li Mandri G, Mohr JP. Characteristics of patent foramen ovale associated with cryptogenic stroke. A biplane transesophageal echocardiographic study. Stroke. 1994;25:582–6.

45. Overell JR, Bone I, Lees KR. Interatrial septal abnormalities and stroke: a meta-analysis of case-control studies. Neurology. 2000; 55:1172–9.

46. Di Tullio MR, Sacco RL, Sciacca RR, Jin Z, Homma S. Patent foramen ovale and the risk of ischemic stroke in a multiethnic population. J Am Coll Cardiol. 2007;49:797–802.

47. Meissner I, Khandheria BK, Heit JA, Petty GW, Sheps SG, Schwartz GL, Whisnant JP, Wiebers DO, Covalt JL, Petterson TM, Christianson TJ, Agmon Y. Patent foramen ovale: innocent or guilty? Evidence from a prospective population-based study. J Am Coll Cardiol. 2006;47:440–5.

48. Furlan AJ, Reisman M, Massaro J, Mauri L, Adams H, Albers GW, Felberg R, Herrmann H, Kar S, Landzberg M, Raizner A, Wechsler L, CLOSURE I Investigators. Closure or medical therapy for cryptogenic stroke with patent foramen ovale. N Engl J Med. 2012;366:991–9.

49. Meier B, Kalesan B, Mattle HP, Khattab AA, Hildick-Smith D, Dudek D, Andersen G, Ibrahim R, Schuler G, Walton AS, Wahl A, Windecker S, Jüni P, PC Trial Investigators. Percutaneous closure of patent foramen ovale in cryptogenic embolism. N Engl J Med. 2013;368:1083–91.

50. Carroll JD, Saver JL, Thaler DE, Smalling RW, Berry S, MacDonald LA, Marks DS, Tirschwell DL, RESPECT Investigators. Closure of patent foramen ovale versus medical therapy after cryptogenic stroke. N Engl J Med. 2013;368:1092–100.

51. Ford MA, Reeder GS, Lennon RJ, Brown RD, Petty GW, Cabalka AK, Cetta F, Hagler DJ. Percutaneous device closure of patent foramen ovale in patients with presumed cryptogenic stroke or transient ischemic attack: the Mayo Clinic experience. JACC Cardiovasc Interv. 2009;2(5):404–11.

52. McBane RD, Hodge DO, Wysokinski WE. Clinical and echocardiographic measures governing thromboembolism destination in atrial fibrillation. Thromb Haemost. 2008;99:951–5.

53. Hart R, Pearce LA, McBride R, Rothbart RM, Asinger RW, The Stroke Prevention in Atrial Fibrillation (SPAF) Investigators. Factors associated with ischemic stroke during aspirin therapy in atrial fibrillation: analysis of 2012 participants in the SPAF I-III clinical trials. Stroke. 1999;30(6):1223–9.

54. Fang MC, Singer DE, Chang Y, Hylek EM, Henault LE, Jensvold NG, Go AS. Gender differences in the risk of ischemic stroke and peripheral embolism in atrial fibrillation: the AnTicoagulation and Risk factors In Atrial fibrillation (ATRIA) study. Circulation. 2005;112(12):1687–91.

55. Frost L, Engholm G, Johnsen S, Møller H, Henneberg EW, Husted S. Incident thromboembolism in the aorta and the renal, mesenteric, pelvic, and extremity arteries after discharge from the hospital with a diagnosis of atrial fibrillation. Arch Intern Med. 2001;161(2):272–6.

56. Cambria RP, Abbott WM. Acute arterial thrombosis of the lower extremity. Its natural history contrasted with arterial embolism. Arch Surg. 1984;119(7):784–7.

57. Coulshed N, Epstein EJ, McKendrick CS, Galloway RW, Walker E. Systemic embolism in mitral valve disease. Br Heart J. 1970;32(1):26–34.

58. January CT, Wann LS, Alpert JS, Calkins H, Cleveland Jr JC, Cigarroa JE, Conti JB, Ellinor PT, Ezekowitz MD, Field ME, Murray KT, Sacco RL, Stevenson WG, Tchou PJ, Tracy CM, Yancy CW. 2014 AHA/ACC/HRS guideline for the management of patients with atrial fibrillation: a report of the American College of Cardiology/American Heart Association Task Force on practice guidelines and the Heart Rhythm Society. J Am Coll Cardiol. 2014;64:e1–76.

59. Blustin JM, McBane RD, Ketha SS, Wysokinski WE. Distribution of thromboembolism in valvular versus non-valvular atrial fibrillation. Expert Rev Cardiovasc Ther. 2014;12:1129–32.

60. Roy D, Marchand E, Gagne P, Cabot M, Cartier R. Usefulness of anticoagulant therapy in the prevention of embolic complications of atrial fibrillation. Am Heart J. 1986;112:1039–43.

61. Sanna T, Diener HC, Passman RS, Di Lazzaro V, Bernstein RA, Morillo CA, Rymer MM, Thijs V, Rogers T, Beckers F, Lindborg K, Brachmann J, CRYSTAL AF Investigators. Cryptogenic stroke and underlying atrial fibrillation. N Engl J Med. 2014;370:2478–86.

62. Gladstone DJ, Spring M, Dorian P, Panzov V, Thorpe KE, Hall J, Vaid H, O'Donnell M, Laupacis A, Côté R, Sharma M, Blakely JA, Shuaib A, Hachinski V, Coutts SB, Sahlas DJ, Teal P, Yip S, Spence JD, Buck B, Verreault S, Casaubon LK, Penn A, Selchen D, Jin A, Howse D, Mehdiratta M, Boyle K, Aviv R, Kapral MK, Mamdani M, EMBRACE Investigators. Atrial fibrillation in patients with cryptogenic stroke. N Engl J Med. 2014;370:2467–77.

63. Humphrey LL, Fu R, Rogers K, Freeman M, Helfand M. Homocysteine level and coronary heart disease incidence: a systematic review and meta-analysis. Mayo Clin Proc. 2008;83:1203–12.

64. Selhub J, Jacques PF, Bostom AG, D'Agostino RB, Wilson PW, Belanger AJ, O'Leary DH, Wolf PA, Schaefer EJ, Rosenberg IH. Association between plasma homocysteine concentrations and extracranial carotid-artery stenosis. N Engl J Med. 1995;332:286–91.

65. Bertoia ML, Pai JK, Cooke JP, Joosten MM, Mittleman MA, Rimm EB, Mukamal KJ. Plasma homocysteine, dietary B vitamins, betaine, and choline and risk of peripheral artery disease. Atherosclerosis. 2014;235:94–101.

66. Den Heijer M, Koster T, Blom HJ, Bos GM, Briet E, Reitsma PH, Vandenbroucke JP, Rosendaal FR. Hyperhomocysteinemia as a risk factor for deep-vein thrombosis. N Engl J Med. 1996;334:759–62.

67. D'Angelo A, Selhub J. Homocysteine and thrombotic disease. Blood. 1997;90:1–11.

68. Kang SS, Wong PW, Malinow MR. Hyperhomocysteinemia as a risk factor for occlusive vascular disease. Annu Rev Nutr. 1992;12:279–98.

69. Lonn E, Yusuf S, Arnold MJ, Sheridan P, Pogue J, Micks M, McQueen MJ, Probstfield J, Fodor G, Held C, Genest Jr J, Heart Outcomes Prevention Evaluation (HOPE) 2 Investigators. Homocysteine lowering with folic acid and B vitamins in vascular disease. N Engl J Med. 2006;354:1567–77.

70. Hillmen P, Lewis SM, Bessler M, Luzzatto L, Dacie JV. Natural history of paroxysmal nocturnal hemoglobinuria. N Engl J Med. 1995;333:1253–8.

71. Hall C, Richards S, Hillmen P. Primary prophylaxis with warfarin prevents thrombosis in paroxysmal nocturnal hemoglobinuria. Blood. 2003;102:3587–91.

72. Hillmen P, Muus P, Dührsen U, Risitano AM, Schubert J, Luzzatto L, Schrezenmeier H, Szer J, Brodsky RA, Hill A, Socié G, Bessler M, Rollins SA, Bell L, Rother RP, Young NS. Effect of complement inhibitor eculizumab on thromboembolism in patients with paroxysmal nocturnal hemoglobinuria. Blood. 2007;110:4123–8.

73. Heller PG, Grinberg AR, Lencioni M, Molina MM, Roncoroni AJ. Pulmonary artery hypertension in paroxysmal nocturnal hemoglobinuria. Chest. 1992;102:642–3.

74. Hillmen P, Young NS, Schubert J, Brodsky RA, Socié G, Muus P, Röth A, Szer J, Elebute MO, Nakamura R, Browne P, Risitano AM, Hill A, Schrezenmeier H, Fu CL, Maciejewski J, Rollins SA, Mojcik CF, Rother RP, Luzzatto L. The complement inhibitor eculizumab in paroxysmal nocturnal hemoglobinuria. N Engl J Med. 2006;355:1233–43.

Vasculitis

26

Michael Czihal and Ulrich Hoffmann

Introduction

The systemic vasculitides constitute a heterogeneous group of disorders characterized by inflammation of the blood vessels. Within the wide-ranging clinical spectrum of vasculitides, critical limb ischemia (CLI) represents a rather rare disease manifestation. However, some forms of vasculitis predominantly involve the large- and medium-sized arteries. Because noninflammatory arterial diseases also typically involve these arteries and specialists in Vascular Medicine are regularly confronted with the clinical picture, this chapter focuses primarily on vasculitides of medium- and large-sized vessels. Among the variety of other vasculitides, those carrying the potential to cause CLI are discussed comprehensively. As CLI caused by vasculitis usually requires a distinct treatment approach, particular emphasis is placed on how to differentiate inflammatory from noninflammatory arterial disease.

Classification of Vasculitis

Infectious vasculitis is extremely rare and characterized by direct invasion of microbial pathogens into the vessel wall. Noninfectious vasculitides are much more likely to be encountered in Vascular Medicine practice. Due to inconsistencies in the nomenclature, e.g., the use of eponyms or historic disease terms not reflecting the current state of knowledge, classification of the noninfectious vasculitides has been unnecessarily confusing in the past.

In 1990, the American College of Rheumatology proposed classification criteria, aimed to enable clinical researchers to differentiate one vasculitis form from another in order to unify inclusion criteria for clinical trials [1]. In 1994, the Chapel Hill Consensus Conference reached a consensus on names and specific definitions for the most common forms of noninfectious vasculitis. This consensus was revised in 2012 and provides the basis for today's nosology of vasculitis [2] (Table 26.1). The Chapel Hill nomenclature categorizes noninfectious vasculitides primarily according to type of vessels predominantly involved, but also integrates knowledge on etiology, pathophysiology, and clinical and pathological characteristics. However, one must be aware that, as a matter of principle, every type of vasculitis may affect vessels of any size [2].

Of note, some obviously inflammatory vasculopathies are not included in the Chapel Hill nomenclature, with Buerger's disease (see Chap. 21) being the most important of these from the vascular specialist's point of view.

Large Vessel Vasculitis (LVV)

According to the Chapel Hill nomenclature, the primary vasculitides predominantly involving the large- and medium-sized vessels are giant cell arteritis (GCA) and Takayasu arteritis (TA) [2].

M. Czihal, MD (✉) • U. Hoffmann, MD
Division of Vascular Medicine, Medical Clinic and Policlinic IV,
Hospital of the Ludwig Maximilians-University Hospital,
Pettenkoferstrasse 8a, Munich 80336, Germany

© Springer International Publishing Switzerland 2017
R.S. Dieter et al. (eds.), *Critical Limb Ischemia*, DOI 10.1007/978-3-319-31991-9_26

Table 26.1 Chapel Hill nomenclature of the primary systemic vasculitides [2]

Large vessel vasculitis (LVV)
Takayasu arteritis (TAK)
Giant cell arteritis (GCA)
Medium vessel vasculitis (MVV)
Polyarteritis nodosa (PAN)
Kawasaki disease (KD)
Small vessel vasculitis (SVV)
Antineutrophil cytoplasmic antibody (ANCA)-associated vasculitis (AAV)
Microscopic polyangiitis (MPA)
Granulomatosis with polyangiitis (Wegener's) (GPA)
Eosinophilic granulomatosis with polyangiitis (Churg-Strauss) (EGPA)
Immune complex SVV
Anti-glomerular basement membrane (anti-GBM) disease
Cryoglobulinemic vasculitis (CV)
IgA vasculitis (Henoch-Schönlein) (IgAV)
Hypocomplementemic urticarial vasculitis (HUV) (anti-C1q vasculitis)
Variable vessel vasculitis (VVV)
Behçet's disease (BD)
Cogan's syndrome (CS)
Single-organ vasculitis (SOV)
Cutaneous leukocytoclastic angiitis
Cutaneous arteritis
Primary central nervous system vasculitis
Isolated aortitis
Others
Vasculitis associated with systemic disease
Lupus vasculitis
Rheumatoid vasculitis
Sarcoid vasculitis
Others
Vasculitis associated with probable etiology
Hepatitis C virus-associated cryoglobulinemic vasculitis
Hepatitis B virus-associated vasculitis
Syphilis-associated aortitis
Drug-associated immune complex vasculitis
Drug-associated ANCA-associated vasculitis
Cancer-associated vasculitis
Others

Epidemiology

Being the most common form of vasculitis in Europe and North American countries, GCA can be considered also the most common inflammatory arteriopathy resulting in ischemia of the upper or lower limbs. GCA almost exclusively affects individuals aged 50 years and older, with women 2–3 times more frequently affected than men. In populations of Caucasian descent, annual incidence rates of up to 20/100,000

people have been reported, peaking in the 70–79 years age group [3]. There is a strong association with polymyalgia rheumatica (PMR).

TA is a rare disease, with annual incidence rates of less than 1 per million population in the USA and Europe. Higher incidence rates are found in Asian countries. The age of onset is typically before 40 years, and women are affected in up to 90 % of cases [4].

Pathophysiology

Both GCA and TA are characterized by a granulomatous panarteritis of the aorta and its major branches, going along with a variable systemic inflammatory response. The histological pattern is indistinguishable between both disorders and characterized by a segmental cell infiltrate composed of T lymphocytes, macrophages, and multinucleated giant cells, fragmentation of the internal elastic lamina, and myointimal hyperplasia [5].

A definite trigger eliciting the deregulated interaction between the arterial wall and the immune system has not been established yet. The typical vessel tropism observed in LVV could be the result of stimulation of distinct profiles of toll-like receptors mediating activation of vascular dendritic cells in different arterial territories [6]. Activated vascular dendritic cells attract CD4 T lymphocytes and macrophages by secretion of certain chemokines. In early and untreated vasculitis, interferon-γ-producing T_H1 T lymphocytes and interleukin-17-producing T_H17 T lymphocytes are abundant, surrounded by activated macrophages and multinucleated giant cells in granulomas [7].

Interferon-γ mediates macrophage activation as well as proliferation and migration of vascular smooth muscle cells [5]. Macrophages have various effector functions which differ according to their localization within the inflamed vessel wall. Macrophages recruited to the expanding intimal layer further stimulate migration and proliferation of medial smooth muscle cells by producing growth factors such as platelet-derived growth factor. Vascular remodeling by means of myointimal hyperplasia results in luminal stenosis or occlusion and is the fundament of tissue ischemia in LVV.

Differentiation of interleukin-17-producing T_H17 T lymphocytes is promoted by interleukin-6, a pleiotropic cytokine secreted by immune and vascular cells. The T_H17 subpopulation can be effectively suppressed by corticosteroid treatment, whereas the T_H1 subpopulation seems to persist in the arterial wall even under long-term corticosteroid treatment [7]. These findings have important clinical implications as they indicate that LVV is not a self-limiting disease and that structural vascular damage due to sustained arterial inflammation may occur in the long term despite immunosuppressive treatment.

Clinical Spectrum of GCA

Nowadays, GCA is recognized as a systemic vascular disease, with a variable disease pattern typically affecting the aorta and its major branches but also smaller-sized arteries such as the branches of the external carotid arteries (e.g., temporal and maxillary arteries) and ophthalmic arteries (e.g., posterior ciliary arteries) [8]. With increasing age, a continuous shift from extracranial large artery involvement to isolated cranial artery involvement can be seen, with a considerable overlap of both disease patterns in about 50 % of patients [9].

Best known are the cranial symptoms of the disease, comprising new-onset headache, jaw claudication due to ischemia of the mastication muscles, and tender and swollen superficial temporal arteries [3, 8]. Cranial GCA is frequently (in up to 20 % of cases) complicated by ischemic ocular complications, mainly AION, carrying a significant risk of uni- or bilateral persistent visual loss. Much less frequent is cerebral ischemia, mainly in the posterior circulation due to vertebral artery involvement. Forty to sixty percent of patients complain of symptoms of polymyalgia rheumatica, and about 40 % of patients suffer from systemic symptoms such as low-grade fever, fatigue, and weight loss [3].

Limb ischemia mainly occurs in early untreated disease but also has been reported to develop in known GCA during corticosteroid tapering [10, 11]. Applying modern noninvasive vascular imaging methods, involvement of the subclavian and axillary arteries has been observed in 25–75 % of patients (Fig. 26.1) [9, 12–14]. Obstructive lesions are typically localized in the axillary arteries, whereas the proximal subclavian arteries remain patent. Therefore, subclavian steal phenomenon is not a feature of extracranial GCA. Abundant collateralization via the subscapular and circumflex humeral arteries provides sufficient blood supply to the arms even in case of complete axillary occlusion (Fig. 26.2). The brachial arteries are rarely affected, but brachial artery involvement may increase the risk of hemodynamic decompensation due to impairment of the collateral inflow [10]. Bilateral involvement is a hallmark of upper extremity vasculitis in GCA [9, 12–14].

As a rule of thumb, vasculitis of the subclavian/arteries leads to luminal stenosis or occlusion in two thirds of cases and to symptomatic arm ischemia in only one third of cases [9]. In our cohort followed at a University Vascular Medicine Center, symptomatic upper limb ischemia was documented in every fifth patient suffering from GCA. The typical symp-

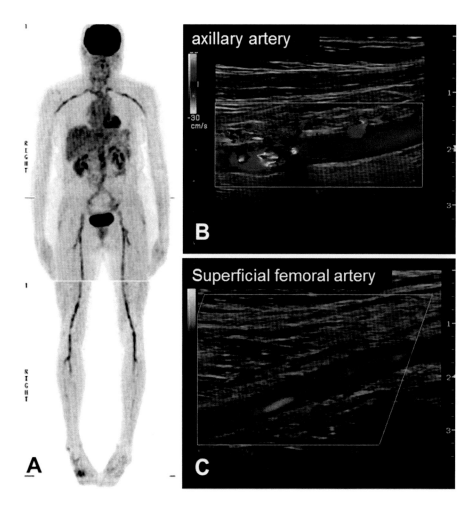

Fig. 26.1 Distribution of upper and lower extremity vasculitis in GCA, as visualized by PET (**a**) and CDS (**b**, **c**). *PET* ^{18}F-fluorodeoxyglucose-positron emission tomography, *CDS* color duplex sonography

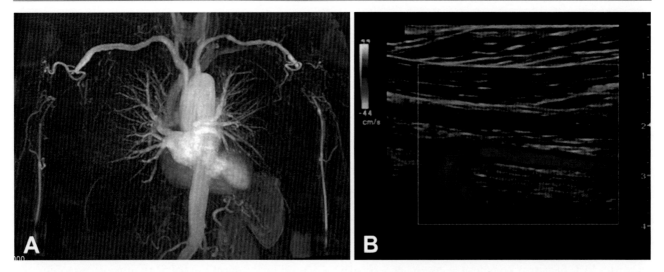

Fig. 26.2 Collateralization of axillary artery obstructions in GCA. MRA depicting bilateral axillary artery occlusions with abundant collateralization in a female patient with GCA (**a**). CDS revealing retro-grade flow in the left subscapular artery, filling the distal left axillary artery behind left axillary artery occlusion secondary to GCA (**b**). *MRA* magnetic resonance angiography, *CDS* color duplex sonography

toms of upper limb ischemia are intermittent claudication and Raynaud's phenomenon, with bilateral symptoms reported in 15–50 % of cases [9, 19]. Of note, classical cranial symptoms are absent in the majority of patients presenting with upper extremity ischemia as the leading disease manifestation [9]. Conversely, recognition of arm claudication in GCA may be impaired due to concomitant symptoms of polymyalgia rheumatica or ischemia of the brachial plexus.

Critical ischemia of the upper limbs with rest pain and/or digital necrosis seems to be essentially rare in GCA [9, 15]. Exceptional cases of digital necrosis due to upper limb ischemia in GCA requiring revascularization have been described in the literature [15]. We observed critical upper limb ischemia in a patient with bilateral occlusion of the axillary arteries expanding to the brachial arteries. Other, sporadic causes of upper limb ischemia in GCA include stent graft covering of the left subclavian artery's origin during thoracic endovascular aneurysm repair and small vessel vasculitis of the digital arteries.

It is very likely that lower extremity vasculitis in GCA has been misinterpreted as arteriosclerotic disease in many cases before noninvasive vessel wall imaging was introduced [8]. Applying these noninvasive vascular imaging modalities such as color duplex sonography (CDS) and ^{18}F-fluorodeoxyglucose-positron emission tomography (PET), rates of lower extremity arterial involvement between 25 and 50 % have been detected [12, 13, 16]. The disease process is bilateral in almost all cases, and the arterial segments predominantly affected are the femorocrural arteries (Fig. 26.3) [11, 12, 16]. The most important difference between upper and lower extremity vasculitis in GCA is that lower extremity vasculitis frequently results in extensive wall thickening of long arterial

segments. Multisegmental disease involving also the deep femoral arteries significantly impairs the capability of the femorocrural axis to collateralize arterial obstructions. Preexisting arteriosclerosis is common in the lower limbs in the age group affected by GCA and may further contribute to hemodynamic impairment.

The rate of symptomatic lower extremity vasculitis in our cohort of patients with GCA was 15 % [16]. The more than twofold increased risk of peripheral arterial disease observed in patients with polymyalgia rheumatica also might be attributable to occult lower extremity vasculitis [17]. The typical clinical presentation is bilateral and rapidly progressive calf claudication, frequently but not necessarily accompanied by arm claudication, cranial symptoms, and/or systemic manifestations [16]. Lower extremity vasculitis may be the only disease manifestation in rare cases and has been shown to result in CLI with tissue loss in a significant proportion of patients with GCA (15–30 % in published case series) [11, 16]. In some of the reported cases, spontaneous superficial femoral artery dissection contributed to hemodynamic deterioration (Fig. 26.3) [8, 16].

Clinical Spectrum of TA

Early TA is characterized by systemic symptoms, including fatigue, weight loss, night sweats, myalgia, carotidodynia, and low-grade fever, and therefore is referred to as "prepulseless phase" of TA. With advancing disease obstructions of the aortic branches occur, and progressing vascular symptoms dominate the clinical presentation ("pulseless phase") [4].

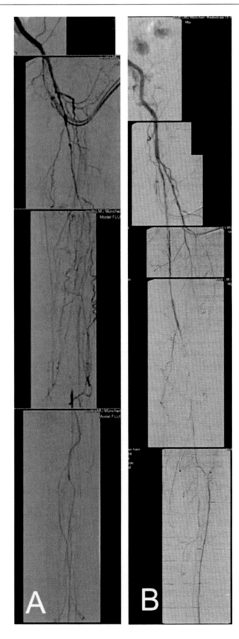

Fig. 26.3 Digital subtraction angiography showing the widespread character of lower extremity vasculitis in GCA with diffuse obstructions of the femorocrural arteries and impaired collateralization due to diffuse deep femoral artery involvement (**a**, **b**). Dissection of the proximal superficial femoral artery (**b**)

The supraaortic branches are almost always affected, and arm claudication, pulse loss, or subclavian bruits are prominent features of advanced TA. Contrasting to GCA, stenoses and occlusions typically involve the proximal subclavian arteries. Therefore, the subclavian steal phenomenon is not uncommon. As carotid involvement also frequently leads to significant stenoses, some patients will experience symp-tomatic cerebral ischemia. Arterial hypertension reflects renal ischemia secondary to (bilateral) renal artery stenosis, and symptomatic coronary involvement occurs occasionally. Symptomatic lower extremity ischemia is a rather infrequent manifestation of the disease, in most cases resulting from aortoiliac obstruction (Fig. 26.4).

Although many patients experience a significant time delay between symptom onset and diagnosis, CLI is quite uncommon due to excellent collateralization. By contrast, critical organ ischemia due to renal or coronary artery obstructions may occur.

Diagnosis of LVV

Assessment of arterial hemodynamics in limb ischemia with suspected underlying LVV follows the general principles of noninvasive vascular laboratory testing. Validated diagnostic criteria for the LVV are not existent. Moreover, it must be stressed that patients with extracranial GCA frequently do not meet the ACR classification criteria for cranial GCA [9]. Advanced noninvasive vascular imaging has dramatically improved the diagnosis of the LVV.

CDS can be considered the first-line imaging technique in suspected LVV [18]. CDS enables the investigator to accurately assess the arterial wall of the aortic branches for the presence of a hypoechogenic, circumferential, homogenous wall thickening as an almost pathognomonic sonographic sign of LVV (Fig. 26.1). Limited data available suggest that the circumferential, hypoechogenic wall thickening is highly specific for LVV, with a diagnostic accuracy comparable to that of PET imaging [12, 19]. However, this imaging modality is observer dependent, and the diagnostic accuracy may be hampered in the lower extremity arteries because of concomitant arteriosclerotic changes [16]. In every patient suspected to suffer from LVV, it is mandatory to screen the subclavian/axillary and common carotid arteries for the presence of vasculitis. In our experience, 75 % of patients with symptomatic lower extremity vasculitis also exhibited vasculitic wall thickening of the subclavian/axillary arteries [9]. The superficial temporal arteries should regularly be visualized in patients above the age of 50 suspected of suffering from GCA.

Cross-sectional imaging, i.e., PET combined with computed tomography (PET-CT) or magnetic resonance imaging (MRI), should be reserved for ambiguous cases and revascularization planning. Features of LVV include increased contrast enhancement (MRI, CT) and increased tracer uptake (PET-CT) of the thickened vessel wall. It is of outmost importance to realize that a pathological tracer uptake of the upper extremity arteries in PET/PET-CT is highly specific

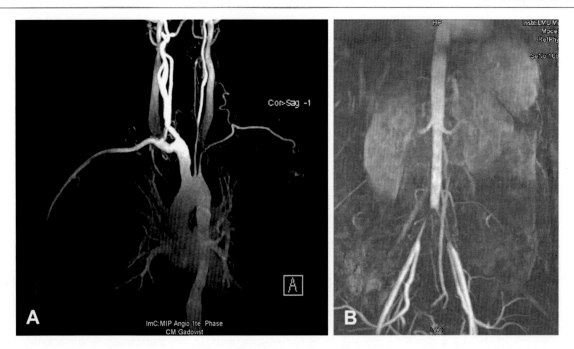

Fig. 26.4 MRA depicting long-segment tight stenosis of the left subclavian and carotid artery, occlusion of the left axillary artery, (**a**) and bilateral common iliac arteries (**b**) in patients with TA suffering from upper and lower extremity ischemia, respectively. *MRA* magnetic resonance angiography

for upper extremity vasculitis, whereas in the lower extremities, the specificity is reduced due to the increased tracer uptake seen with coexistent arteriosclerosis [18].

Digital subtraction angiography provides no information on the vessel wall morphology and thus is only indicated prior to revascularization (Fig. 26.3).

Medical Treatment of LVV

Systemic corticosteroids with an initial dose of 1 mg prednisone equivalent/kg/day (maximum 60 mg/day) remain the cornerstone of treatment in both GCA and TA [3, 4, 8]. In analogy to the treatment of GCA complicated by ocular ischemia, high-dose intravenous pulse treatment (1000 mg methylprednisolone) seems to be justified also in patients presenting with CLI on the basis of LVV. However, the benefit of this aggressive treatment approach is not proven and must be balanced against the potential risk of infection (particularly in those patients with ischemic ulcers). Corticosteroid tapering needs to be done very carefully and is allowed only in the absence of clinical and laboratory disease activity. After 3 months of treatment, one should aim at a dose of 10–15 mg prednisone equivalent/day. A minimum treatment duration of up to 2 years is recommended [3, 8]. However, relapses are common, and patients with GCA and widespread extracranial involvement and patients with TA appear to be particularly prone for a steroid-dependent or steroid-refractory disease course. As a result, more than 80 % of patients experience corticosteroid side effects. Unfortunately, only modest treatment effects have been documented for the conventional steroid sparing agents in the treatment of GCA and TA. A meta-analysis of three small randomized trials investigating adjunctive methotrexate treatment in GCA revealed a small benefit in terms of reduction of the cumulative corticosteroid dose and the recurrence rate [20]. Limited evidence for a potential benefit of other immunosuppressants such as azathioprine, cyclophosphamide, and leflunomide comes from case series. Randomized controlled studies failed to document a significant effect of the TNFα blockers infliximab and adalimumab as first-line treatment of GCA [21, 22]. However, these studies are in contrast to the results of open-label studies, documenting substantial treatment effects of TNFα blockers in refractory disease courses of TA [23]. Recently, promising results have been reported with the interleukin-6 receptor antagonist tocilizumab for achieving disease remission [23]. Currently, a randomized study investigating the effects of tocilizumab as adjunctive treatment in GCA is underway.

Although convincing data are lacking, antiplatelet treatment (aspirin) is recommended in addition to immunosuppressive medication in both types of LVV [3, 4, 8]. Because of the combination of aspirin with corticosteroids, proton pump inhibitors should be added to the medication. A benefit of adjunctive statin treatment is not evident. Under corticosteroid treatment, medical prevention of osteoporosis according to current guidelines is mandatory.

Treatment of Limb Ischemia in LVV

The current knowledge on surgical and endovascular treatment of LVV mainly comes from cohort studies having retrospectively evaluated patients with TA. Data on revascularization attempts in GCA are even less convincing, and randomized controlled trials are not available.

Two principal rules must be followed when considering invasive treatment of limb and organ ischemia in LVV. First, whenever possible, endovascular interventions and vascular surgery should be delayed until reaching complete clinical and laboratory remission of inflammatory disease activity [4, 8]. Second, revascularization procedures should be reserved for limb- or organ-threatening ischemia and for patients with ongoing severe symptoms despite optimal medical treatment. In this context, one should bear in mind the excellent collateralization of upper extremity arterial obstructions. We observed that every third patient with upper extremity claudication secondary to GCA became asymptomatic with medical treatment alone [24]. Patients with leg claudication secondary to GCA appear to have a similarly benign clinical course under conservative treatment, whereas in patients already suffering from CLI at the time of diagnosis, revascularization may be required [16].

Whether to prefer angioplasty with or without stent placement or bypass surgery depends on the localization of the lesion and the morphology of the obstruction (diffuse narrowing or long-segment occlusion vs. focal stenosis). As diffuse fibrotic changes of the vessel wall commonly are the morphologic basis of arterial obstruction and inflammation of the vessel wall may be still present to some extent, arterial lesions secondary to LVV exhibit a clear tendency for an increased rate of restenosis after endovascular treatment as compared to atherosclerotic obstructions. In a series of ten patients with GCA who underwent percutaneous transluminal angioplasty of the subclavian/axillary arteries for treatment of arm claudication, symptoms recurred in 50 % of patients after a mean follow-up of 24 months [25]. Limited data suggest that patency of bypass grafts is superior to an endovascular approach in arterial obstruction secondary to LVV. In a retrospective multicenter study including 79 patients with TA, the restenosis rate after a mean follow-up of 6.5 years was 64.5 % for endovascular procedures vs. 46.1 % after surgery in various arterial territories [26]. The most important predictor of restenosis was biological disease activity at the time of the procedure [26, 27]. It has been suggested that stent grafts may be superior to bare stents and plain old balloon angioplasty by disturbing nutrition of the intimal layer derived from the blood flow, but there are no firm data to support this hypothesis [28]. As of today, the theoretically promising use of drug-eluting stents and balloons cannot be judged due to a lack of data.

In our experience, bypass surgery in lower extremity vasculitis secondary to GCA is challenging due to diffuse arterial wall thickening involving also long segments of the crural arteries. The distal anastomosis typically is below the knee and the runoff thus may be poor. Both factors negatively influence the patency rates. As patients are usually under immunosuppressive treatment and frequently obese due to long-term corticosteroid use, surgery carries additional risks including infections and delayed wound healing. After bypass surgery, lifelong surveillance is required, with particular attention on development of anastomotic aneurysms which may occur at any time after surgery [29]. Postinterventional anticoagulation follows the general principles established in the treatment of arteriosclerotic disease.

To our knowledge, there are no systematic data available regarding the use of prostanoids or the selective phosphodiesterase-3 inhibitor cilostazol for treatment of limb ischemia secondary to LVV. We have limited experience with the use of intravenous prostanoids in addition to standard immunosuppressive treatment in two patients with critical lower limb ischemia secondary to GCA. Both patients experienced relief of rest pain and ulcer healing under prostanoid infusion and corticosteroid therapy [16].

Medium and Small Vessel Vasculitis

Necrotizing Vasculitides

Among the necrotizing vasculitides, Kawasaki disease (KD) and panarteritis nodosa (PAN) predominantly affect medium-sized arteries. Antineutrophil cytoplasmic antibody (ANCA)-associated vasculitides, i.e., microscopic polyangiitis (MPA), polyangiitis with granulomatosis (Wegener's; GPA), and eosinophilic polyangiitis with granulomatosis (Churg-Strauss; EGPA), primarily involve small arteries [2].

KD, a vasculitis of infants and young children, manifests as an acute febrile illness accompanied by erythematous oropharyngeal lesions, a morbilliform rash followed by skin desquamation of the palms and the soles of the feet, bilateral conjunctivitis, and lymphadenopathy. Myocarditis is a frequent finding, and coronary artery aneurysms represent the most severe complication. Less than 20 cases of severe peripheral ischemia with gangrene have been reported in the literature, almost exclusively in infants. The mechanisms of upper and lower limb ischemia in KD are poorly understood. Aneurysms of the subclavian/axillary or iliac arteries, as observed in some cases, could be potential sources of peripheral arterial embolism [30]. A variety of medical treatment approaches have been tried in addition to standard medical care with intravenous immunoglobulins with or without additional corticosteroids and high-dose aspirin. Favorable outcomes were anecdotally documented with anticoagulation alone or in combination with prostanoids [30, 31]. However, in the majority of cases, minor or major amputations had to be performed. Early diagnosis and treatment initiation appears to be crucial for avoiding severe complications including limb loss.

Limb ischemia is not a common complication of PAN and ANCA-associated vasculitides. In a retrospective cohort study of the French Vasculitis Study Group including 1304 patients, only 3.9 % and 3.1 % had Raynaud's phenomenon and digital necrosis, respectively, and less than 1 % underwent finger amputation [32]. CLI due to large artery obstructions is even more uncommon and has been reported only anecdotally. Single cases of GPA complicated by major amputations secondary to acute thrombotic lower limb arterial occlusions with repeated recurrent occlusions after local thrombolysis and surgical revascularization have been reported [33, 34].

PAN is characterized by its broad spectrum of clinical symptoms, arising from the systemic inflammatory process and from tissue ischemia. Any organ system can be affected, with ischemic infarctions of the skin, kidneys, and bowel commonly seen [35]. By contrast to MPA, pulmonary capillaritis and glomerulonephritis are no features of PAN. In a subset of patients, PAN develops secondary to hepatitis B infection. Diagnosis is based on histology or on the angiographic appearance, the latter characterized by multiple small aneurysms forming a "string of beds" (Fig. 26.5) [36]. For remission induction in cases of PAN with critical tissue ischemia, high-dose corticosteroids and cyclophosphamide pulse therapy are applied. When associated to hepatitis B, PAN can be treated with a combination of short-term corticosteroid treatment, plasma exchanges, and antiviral therapy. Noteworthy, angiographic abnormalities may regress under immunosuppressive treatment [35]. While there is an excessive mortality rate when left untreated, the disease relapse rate under adequate treatment seems to be lower than in other vasculitides.

The clinical features of the ANCA-associated vasculitides overlap considerably. In addition to pure vasculitic manifestations (particularly pulmonary capillaritis and glomerulonephritis), nonvasculitic manifestations are seen in granulomatosis with polyangiitis (granulomatous upper airway lesions) and eosinophilic granulomatosis with polyangiitis (asthma, hypereosinophilia). Most patients with MPA and GPA and some cases of EGPA are positive for ANCAs. The diagnosis is based on the combination of clinical and serological findings as well as tissue histology. Treatment is tailored according to the disease stage and severity. Remission induction still relies on corticosteroids and cyclophosphamide in severe cases. The monoclonal anti-CD20 antibody rituximab was shown to be equally effective as cyclophosphamide for remission induction and superior to azathioprine for maintenance therapy in ANCA-associated vasculitides [37].

Immune Complex Vasculitides

Cryoglobulinemic vasculitis (CV) is the prototype of immune complex-mediated vascular inflammation of small blood vessels. Cryoglobulins are immunoglobulins that precipitate

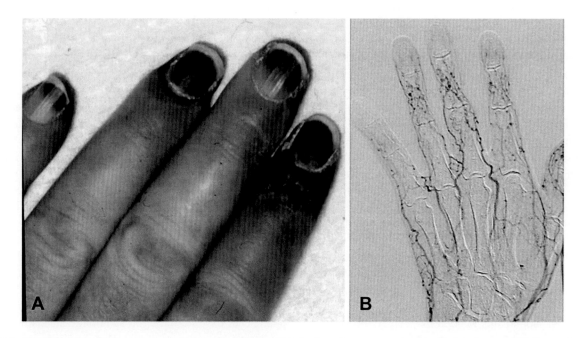

Fig. 26.5 Digital necroses due to severe finger ischemia in PAN (**a**). Digital subtraction angiography reveals digital artery occlusions and multiple microaneurysms (**b**). *PAN* panarteritis nodosa

at variable temperatures <37 °C in serum. Monoclonal cryo-globulins (type I cryoglobulinemia) are associated with hematological neoplasia, whereas mixed cryoglobulins (type II and III cryoglobulinemia) occur in infections, autoimmune disorders, and malignancies. The most important infectious cause of cryoglobulinemia is hepatitis C infection.

The major clinical manifestations of CV include purpura, arthralgia, fever, peripheral neuropathy, and glomerulone-phritis. The frequency of Raynaud's phenomenon is around 5 % [38]. Severe digital ischemia with necrosis is even more rare, but may complicate the disease course due to a signifi-cant risk of secondary infection [39].

Demonstration of cryoglobulins in the serum is required for diagnosis of the disease, with appropriate sample collec-tion and handling being indispensable. Treatment is contro-versial and should be modulated according to the underlying disease. The main columns of treatment are conventional immunosuppression, biologic treatment, and antiviral treat-ment of hepatitis C [39]. No specific data for treatment of distal ischemia in CV are available.

Variable Vessel Vasculitis

Behçet's Disease (BD)

BD is a rare inflammatory disorder of unknown origin with a strong association to HLA-B*51. Cases of BD cluster along the ancient Silk Road, extending from Eastern Asia to the Mediterranean region, but the disease is found world-wide. Males are more frequently and more severely affected, and the usual age of onset is between 20 and 40 years [40].

A distinctive vasculitis is thought to underlie many of the clinical manifestations of BD. Vasculitis in BD is unique in that it involves both arteries and veins of variable size and shows a tendency to formation of aneurysms and thrombus adherent to the vessel wall [41].

Recurrent oral apthoid ulcers are the pivotal symptoms, occurring in 98 % of cases. Other mucocutaneous lesions include genital ulcers and erythema nodosum-like lesions. Nearly 50 % of patients complain of arthritis/arthralgia, oftentimes as the initial symptom. Eye involvement is poten-tially sight threatening. Severe complications can also arise from central nervous system and cardiac involvement.

The reported rates of vascular complications ("vasculo-Behçet") vary between studies from 2 to 50 % [42]. Aneurysms of the pulmonary arteries are the most dangerous lesions, car-rying a significant risk of fatal hemoptysis [41]. The most com-mon vascular manifestations are superficial and deep venous thrombosis, frequently occurring early in the disease process. Deep venous thrombosis typically involves large proximal veins (e.g., inferior vena cava) and unusual sites (e.g., dural

sinus thrombosis) but carries a low risk of pulmonary embo-lism due to the adhesive nature of the thrombus [41].

Peripheral arterial lesions become clinically manifest in 1–7 % of cases, sometimes as the initial disease feature but more commonly several years (median 4–9 years) after dis-ease onset [42–45]. Arterial manifestations are significantly more common in males and in those patients suffering from deep venous thrombosis and pulmonary artery aneurysms [41–43, 45]. Arterial involvement in BD has been shown to negatively impact the response to immunosuppressive treat-ment as well as long-term survival [45].

The morphology of peripheral arterial lesions in BD is diverse, and any visceral or extremity artery may be involved. Multiple lesions can occur simultaneously at different sites [42, 45]. True and false aneurysms are the dominant lesion types, most commonly localized in the abdominal aorta and the lower extremity arteries [42–46]. Occlusions or stenoses are less common but are also mainly found in the lower extremity arteries [42–46]. CLI due to occlusion of native extremity arteries in BD is a rare clinical event [45]. However, CLI is not uncommon as a complication of graft occlusion after bypass surgery of arterial aneurysm (Fig. 26.6) [44, 47].

As specific histologic, laboratory, or imaging features are lacking, the diagnosis of BD is a clinical one. Widely used criteria used for the diagnosis of BD are as follows:

International study group for Behçet's disease diagnostic criteria [48]

Recurrent oral ulceration (at least three times within the previous year)
plus 2 of the following:
Recurrent genital ulceration
Eye lesions (retinitis or uveitis)
Skin lesions (erythema nodosum and/or papulopustular lesions)
Positive pathergy reaction

It is noteworthy that vascular involvement in BD frequently goes along with elevated humoral inflammatory markers [42, 45]. Vascular imaging should be noninvasive, because in BD every arterial puncture carries a risk of aneurysm forma-tion [41]. PET imaging may be of value in detecting arterial inflammation in BD [49].

Surgical revascularization has a high complication rate, mainly anastomotic false aneurysms and graft occlusions. Therefore, surgical repair should be reserved for treatment of large or progressive arterial aneurysms and for treatment of arterial occlusions with limb-threatening ischemia. Determining the appropriate sites of graft anastomoses in an unaffected arterial segment is challenging. Whether syn-thetic graft material may be chosen over autologous vein grafting remains a matter of debate. Some authors prefer synthetic grafts because of the possible vasculitic involve-ment of the superficial venous system [43, 44]. In recent

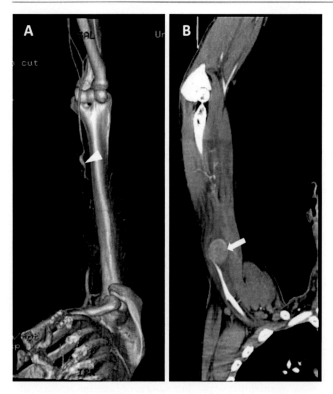

Fig. 26.6 Critical upper limb ischemia in BD related to bypass graft occlusion after revascularization of a large brachial artery aneurysm. Note the thrombosed anastomotic aneurysms at the proximal anastomosis (**b**, *arrow*) and arterial ectasia at the distal anastomosis (**a**, *arrowhead*). *BD* Behçet's disease

years, endovascular stent grafting has been attracting more and more interest. Although technical success was achieved in most cases, aneurysms at the femoral access sites and the proximal and distal stent margins evolved as relevant complications [46].

Rates of recurrent arterial lesions approach 40 % after 5 years, and retrospective data suggest that immunosuppressive treatment may reduce the risk of recurrent arterial disease in BD [45]. Immunosuppressive treatment thus is deemed mandatory in the management of BD with peripheral arterial involvement, with current guidelines recommending the use of corticosteroids and cyclophosphamide [50]. Azathioprine may be appropriate for maintenance therapy. As there is no firm evidence for a beneficial effect in BD with either venous or arterial involvement, anticoagulation is not recommended by the current guidelines [50]. However, the graft occlusion rate has been shown to be lower with anticoagulation or antiplatelet treatment, without an increased bleeding rate in a large retrospective study [45]. Therefore, we recommend anticoagulation after revascularization procedures according to current standards of practice. Smoking cessation is emphasized by data from retrospective studies indicating a possible relationship between cigarette smoking and the development of arterial complications [41].

Cogan's Syndrome (CS)

CS is a rare disorder typically affecting young adults and clinically characterized by inflammatory eye disease, sensorineural hearing loss, and vestibular dysfunction. Aortitis occurs in about 10 % of patients and goes along with a significant risk of developing severe aortic insufficiency. Coronary artery involvement may also occur, and rare cases exhibiting a disease pattern similarly to that of TA with inflammatory proximal stenoses of the supraaortic arteries have been described [51]. Vasculitis usually responds well to corticosteroids, and adjunctive treatment options include conventional immunosuppressants such as cyclophosphamide and biologicals including the TNFα blocker infliximab.

Other Vasculitides

Chronic Periaortitis (CP)

CP is a fibroinflammatory disorder originating from the adventitia of the abdominal aorta and the common iliac arteries. There is a significant overlap with retroperitoneal fibrosis, and up to 50 % of cases may be associated to IgG4-related systemic disease [52]. Destruction of the aortic wall can result in the development of inflammatory abdominal aortic aneurysm. Important symptoms include constitutional complaints, lower back pain, and lower extremity edema due to venous congestion. According to a large retrospective cohort study, 2 % of patients present with leg claudication [53]. However, CLI is not a disease feature of CP. Diagnosis necessitates confirmation of a periaortic pannus by vascular imaging and, whenever possible, histological analysis. The treatment is essentially the same than that of other LVV.

Systemic Sclerosis (SSc)

SSc is a systemic disease of unknown etiology characterized by vascular abnormalities (Raynaud's phenomenon, digital ischemia, and ulcers); activation of the immune system (indicated by the presence of several types of autoantibodies, particularly those directed against topoisomerase III and centromere proteins); and skin and organ fibrosis. According to the "vascular hypothesis" proposed by Campbell and Leroy in 1975, tissue fibrosis in SSc is the result of a complex pathophysiological cascade starting with vascular injury [54]. Vascular inflammation could contribute to this process finally resulting in intimal proliferation, fibrosis, and luminal thrombosis [55]. Of note, inflammatory vessel wall infiltrates were verified in the majority of SSc patients with severe digital ischemia requiring finger amputation [56].

Secondary Raynaud's phenomenon is the heralding symptom in more than 90 % of patients, and the majority of patients will develop ischemic digital ulcers during the disease course. Besides local infection, macrovascular disease is a major determinant of digital amputations. In addition to arterial obstructions of the digital arteries, occlusive involvement of the palmar and plantar arch and the distal arm and leg arteries is not uncommon [57]. Particularly, occlusive disease of the ulnar arteries has been shown to be highly prevalent in SSc and to be associated with the development of digital ischemia [58]. While the patient's prognosis is primarily affected by cardiopulmonary involvement, digital ischemia leads to severe impairment of quality of life.

Raynaud's phenomenon, abnormalities of nailfold capillaroscopy, and autoantibodies constitute major criteria of the preliminary conceptual framework for the very early diagnosis of SSc [59]. Besides clinical examination including Allen's test, noninvasive vascular laboratory investigations (digital photoplethysmography, digital pressure measurement) are of outmost importance in the evaluation of acral ischemia in SSc.

In addition to general management principles of Raynaud's phenomenon, as outlined in Chap. 23, the occurrence of digital ulcers requires treatment intensification [60]. Intravenous prostanoids (Iloprost) constitute the mainstay of ulcer treatment. The dual endothelin-1 receptor antagonist bosentan currently has its role in prevention of digital ulcers in patients who already experienced recurrent ulcers. The role of phosphodiesterase inhibitors, topical nitrates, statins, and antiplatelets is currently unclear. Results of small case series suggested a potential benefit of digital sympathectomy and ulnar artery revascularization by means of bypass surgery. Analgesics, antibiotics, and specialist wound care are important supportive measures.

HIV Arteriopathy

There is increasing evidence that infection with the human immunodeficiency virus (HIV) is a risk factor for peripheral arterial occlusive disease. A number of potential mechanisms are under discussion, with premature arteriosclerosis in association to aggravation of the cardiovascular risk profile by highly active antiretroviral treatment (protease inhibitors) considered to be among the most important factors. Recently, a case-control study provided evidence that leukocytoclastic vasculitis of the vasa vasorum and adventitial inflammation of the lower limb arteries could be a unique feature of CLI associated to HIV-associated arteriopathy [61]. However, the causality and the clinical implications of this association remain to be elucidated.

Approach to the Patient with Limb Ischemia and Suspected Vasculitis

First and foremost, the clinician should take some sort of vasculitis as a possible differential diagnosis of limb ischemia into account. Some red flags should raise suspicion of vasculitis as possible underlying etiology, as listed below:

- Rapidly progressive bilateral calf and/or foot claudication, particularly in the absence of traditional cardiovascular risk factors and in the presence of systemic symptoms or elevated inflammatory markers
- Symptomatic arm ischemia, particularly when occurring bilaterally or together with leg claudication
- Bilateral digital ischemia, particularly when occurring together with symptoms in other organ systems

As no single diagnostic test is fully diagnostic of vasculitis, a detailed medical history and thorough physical examination are essential for planning the further diagnostic workup. Imaging and laboratory tests contribute in assessing the vessel size(s) affected and the disease extent. Although not specific, normochrome anemia and thrombocytosis together with elevated humoral inflammatory parameters (ESR, CRP) are frequently found in patients with systemic vasculitides. Further serological testing should be considered when a small vessel vasculitis is considered as a differential diagnosis. Histology remains the diagnostic gold standard but is not feasible in most cases presenting with limb ischemia. The diagnostic workup is not only essential for establishing the diagnosis but also for assessment of disease severity, as current treatment approaches are tailored according to disease severity.

Summary

CLI secondary to a vasculitic process is uncommon. The most important step in identifying systemic vasculitis is to consider the possibility of its existence. This is of major clinical importance, as the diagnostic workup usually needs to be extended and the therapeutic approach differs substantially from that usually applied in arteriosclerotic disease. Among the vasculitides, those affecting the medium- and large-sized arteries (GCA, TA) are most important in Vascular Medicine practice. Immunosuppressive treatment, still primarily based on corticosteroids, is the pivotal treatment element. Indication for invasive treatment should be reserved for CLI and severely symptomatic patients, and invasive procedures should be postponed until disease remission is reached whenever possible.

References

1. Hunder GG, Bloch DA, Michel BA, Stevens MB, Arend WP, Calabrese LH, Edworthy SM, Fauci AS, Leavitt RY, Lie JT, et al. The American College of Rheumatology 1990 criteria for the classification of giant cell arteritis. Arthritis Rheum. 1990;33(8):1122–8.

2. Jennette JC, Falk RJ, Bacon PA, Basu N, Cid MC, Ferrario F, Flores-Suarez LF, Gross WL, Guillevin L, Hagen EC, Hoffman GS, Jayne DR, Kallenberg CG, Lamprecht P, Langford CA, Luqmani RA, Mahr AD, Matteson EL, Merkel PA, Ozen S, Pusey CD, Rasmussen N, Rees AJ, Scott DG, Specks U, Stone JH, Takahashi K, Watts RA. 2012 revised international Chapel Hill consensus conference nomenclature of vasculitides. Arthritis Rheum. 2013;65(1):1–11.

3. Salvarani C, Cantini F, Hunder GG. Polymyalgia rheumatica and giant-cell arteritis. Lancet. 2008;372(9634):234–45.

4. Mason JC. Takayasu arteritis-advances in diagnosis and management. Nat Rev Rheumatol. 2010;6(7):406–15.

5. Samson M, Audia S, Martin L, Janikashvili N, Bonnotte B. Pathogenesis of giant cell arteritis: new insight into the implication of CD161+ T cells. Clin Exp Rheumatol. 2013;31(1 Suppl 75):S65–73.

6. Pryshchep O, Ma-Krupa W, Younge BR, Goronzy JJ, Weyand CM. Vessel-specific toll-like receptor profiles in human medium and large arteries. Circulation. 2008;118(12):1276–84.

7. Deng J, Younge BR, Olshen RA, Goronzy JJ, Weyand CM. Th17 and Th1 T-cell responses in giant cell arteritis. Circulation. 2010;121(7):906–15.

8. Tatò F, Hoffmann U. Giant cell arteritis: a systemic vascular disease. Vasc Med. 2008;13(2):127–40.

9. Czihal M, Zanker S, Rademacher A, Tatò F, Kuhlencordt PJ, Schulze-Koops H, Hoffmann U. Sonographic and clinical pattern of extracranial and cranial giant cell arteritis. Scand J Rheumatol. 2012;41(3):231–6.

10. Assie C, Janvresse A, Plissonnier D, Levesque H, Marie I. Long-term follow-up of upper and lower extremity vasculitis related to giant cell arteritis: a series of 36 patients. Medicine (Baltimore). 2011;90(1):40–51.

11. Kermani TA, Matteson EL, Hunder GG, Warrington KJ. Symptomatic lower extremity vasculitis in giant cell arteritis: a case series. J Rheumatol. 2009;36(10):2277–83.

12. Aschwanden M, Kesten F, Stern M, Thalhammer C, Walker UA, Tyndall A, Jaeger KA, Hess C, Daikeler T. Vascular involvement in patients with giant cell arteritis determined by duplex sonography of 2×11 arterial regions. Ann Rheum Dis. 2010;69(7):1356–9.

13. Blockmans D, de Ceuninck L, Vanderschueren S, Knockaert D, Mortelmans L, Bobbaers H. Repetitive 18F-fluorodeoxyglucose positron emission tomography in giant cell arteritis: a prospective study of 35 patients. Arthritis Rheum. 2006;55(1):131–7.

14. Prieto-González S, Arguis P, García-Martínez A, Espígol-Frigolé G, Tavera-Bahillo I, Butjosa M, Sánchez M, Hernández-Rodríguez J, Grau JM, Cid MC. Large vessel involvement in biopsy-proven giant cell arteritis: prospective study in 40 newly diagnosed patients using CT angiography. Ann Rheum Dis. 2012;71(7):1170–6.

15. Schmidt WA, Moll A, Seifert A, Schicke B, Gromnica-Ihle E, Krause A. Prognosis of large-vessel giant cell arteritis. Rheumatology (Oxford). 2008;47(9):1406–8.

16. Czihal M, Tatò F, Rademacher A, Kuhlencordt P, Schulze-Koops H, Hoffmann U. Involvement of the femoropopliteal arteries in giant cell arteritis: clinical and color duplex sonography. J Rheumatol. 2012;39(2):314–21.

17. Warrington KJ, Jarpa EP, Crowson CS, Cooper LT, Hunder GG, Matteson EL, Gabriel SE. Increased risk of peripheral arterial disease in polymyalgia rheumatica: a population-based cohort study. Arthritis Res Ther. 2009;11(2):R50.

18. Schmidt WA. Ultrasound in vasculitis. Clin Exp Rheumatol. 2014;32(1 Suppl 80):S71–7.

19. Förster S, Tato F, Weiss M, Czihal M, Rominger A, Bartenstein P, Hacker M, Hoffmann U. Patterns of extracranial involvement in newly diagnosed giant cell arteritis assessed by physical examination, colour coded duplex sonography and FDG-PET. Vasa. 2011;40(3):219–27.

20. Mahr AD, Jover JA, Spiera RF, Hernández-García C, Fernández-Gutiérrez B, Lavalley MP, Merkel PA. Adjunctive methotrexate for treatment of giant cell arteritis: an individual patient data meta-analysis. Arthritis Rheum. 2007;56(8):2789–97.

21. Salvarani C, Macchioni P, Manzini C, Paolazzi G, Trotta A, Manganelli P, Cimmino M, Gerli R, Catanoso MG, Boiardi L, Cantini F, Klersy C, Hunder GG. Infliximab plus prednisone or placebo plus prednisone for the initial treatment of polymyalgia rheumatica: a randomized trial. Ann Intern Med. 2007;146(9):631–9.

22. Seror R, Baron G, Hachulla E, Debandt M, Larroche C, Puéchal X, Maurier F, de Wazieres B, Quéméneur T, Ravaud P, Mariette X. Adalimumab for steroid sparing in patients with giant-cell arteritis: results of a multicentre randomised controlled trial. Ann Rheum Dis. 2014;73(12):2074–81.

23. Tombetti E, Di Chio MC, Sartorelli S, Bozzolo E, Sabbadini MG, Manfredi AA, Baldissera E. Anti-cytokine treatment for Takayasu arteritis: state of the art. Intractable Rare Dis Res. 2014;3(1):29–33.

24. Czihal M, Piller A, Schroettle A, Kuhlencordt PJ, Schulze-Koops H, Hoffmann U. Outcome of giant cell arteritis of the arm arteries managed with medical treatment alone: cross-sectional follow-up study. Rheumatology (Oxford). 2013;52(2):282–6.

25. Both M, Aries PM, Müller-Hülsbeck S, Jahnke T, Schäfer PJ, Gross WL, Heller M, Reuter M. Balloon angioplasty of arteries of the upper extremities in patients with extracranial giant-cell arteritis. Ann Rheum Dis. 2006;65(9):1124–30.

26. Saadoun D, Lambert M, Mirault T, Resche-Rigon M, Koskas F, Cluzel P, Mignot C, Schoindre Y, Chiche L, Hatron PY, Emmerich J, Cacoub P. Retrospective analysis of surgery versus endovascular intervention in Takayasu arteritis: a multicenter experience. Circulation. 2012;125(6):813–9.

27. Park MC, Lee SW, Park YB, Lee SK, Choi D, Shim WH. Post-interventional immunosuppressive treatment and vascular restenosis in Takayasu's arteritis. Rheumatology (Oxford). 2006;45(5):600–5.

28. Qureshi MA, Martin Z, Greenberg RK. Endovascular management of patients with Takayasu arteritis: stents versus stent grafts. Semin Vasc Surg. 2011;24(1):44–52.

29. Miyata T, Sato O, Koyama H, Shigematsu H, Tada Y. Long-term survival after surgical treatment of patients with Takayasu's arteritis. Circulation. 2003;108(12):1474–80.

30. Kim NY, Choi DY, Jung MJ, Jeon IS. A case of refractory Kawasaki disease complicated by peripheral ischemia. Pediatr Cardiol. 2008;29(6):1110–4.

31. Chang JS, Lin JS, Peng CT, Tsai CH. Kawasaki disease complicated by peripheral gangrene. Pediatr Cardiol. 1999;20(2):139–42.

32. Lega JC, Seror R, Fassier T, Aumaître O, Quere I, Pourrat J, Gilson B, Sparsa A, Wahl D, Le Jeunne C, Decaux O, Mouthon L, Mahr A, Cohen P, Guillevin L, Pagnoux C, French Vasculitis Study Group (FVSG). Characteristics, prognosis, and outcomes of cutaneous ischemia and gangrene in systemic necrotizing vasculitides: a retrospective multicenter study. Semin Arthritis Rheum. 2014;43(5):681–8.

33. Bessias N, Moulakakis KG, Lioupis C, Bakogiannis K, Sfyroeras G, Kakaletri K, Andrikopoulos V. Wegener's granulomatosis presenting during pregnancy with acute limb ischemia. J Vasc Surg. 2005;42(4):800–4.

34. Lahmer T, Pongratz J, Härtl F, Heemann U, Schmid RM, Eckstein HH. Acute ischemia of the lower leg caused by granulomatosis with polyangiitis. Vasa. 2014;43(2):145–8.

35. Hernández-Rodríguez J, Alba MA, Prieto-González S, Cid MC. Diagnosis and classification of polyarteritis nodosa. J Autoimmun. 2014;48–49:84–9.

36. Stanson AW, Friese JL, Johnson CM, McKusick MA, Breen JF, Sabater EA, Andrews JC. Polyarteritis nodosa: spectrum of angiographic findings. Radiographics. 2001;21(1):151–9.

37. Kallenberg CG. Key advances in the clinical approach to ANCA-associated vasculitis. Nat Rev Rheumatol. 2014;10(8):484–93.

38. Trejo O, Ramos-Casals M, García-Carrasco M, Yagüe J, Jiménez S, de la Red G, Cervera R, Font J, Ingelmo M. Cryoglobulinemia: study of etiologic factors and clinical and immunologic features in 443 patients from a single center. Medicine (Baltimore). 2001;80(4):252–62.

39. Ramos-Casals M, Stone JH, Cid MC, Bosch X. The cryoglobulinaemias. Lancet. 2012;379(9813):348–60.

40. Saleh Z, Arayssi T. Update on the therapy of Behçet disease. Ther Adv Chronic Dis. 2014;5(3):112–34.

41. Calamia KT, Schirmer M, Melikoglu M. Major vessel involvement in Behçet's disease: an update. Curr Opin Rheumatol. 2011;23(1):24–31.

42. Fei Y, Li X, Lin S, Song X, Wu Q, Zhu Y, Gao X, Zhang W, Zhao Y, Zeng X, Zhang F. Major vascular involvement in Behçet's disease: a retrospective study of 796 patients. Clin Rheumatol. 2013;32(6):845–52.

43. Tuzun H, Seyahi E, Arslan C, Hamuryudan V, Besirli K, Yazici H. Management and prognosis of nonpulmonary large arterial disease in patients with Behçet disease. J Vasc Surg. 2012;55(1):157–63.

44. Koksoy C, Gyedu A, Alacayir I, Bengisun U, Uncu H, Anadol E. Surgical treatment of peripheral aneurysms in patients with Behcet's disease. Eur J Vasc Endovasc Surg. 2011;42(4):525–30.

45. Saadoun D, Asli B, Wechsler B, Houman H, Geri G, Desseaux K, Piette JC, du Huong LT, Amoura Z, Salem TB, Cluzel P, Koskas F, Resche-Rigon M, Cacoub P. Long-term outcome of arterial lesions in Behçet disease: a series of 101 patients. Medicine (Baltimore). 2012;91(1):18–24.

46. Yang SS, Park KM, Park YJ, Kim YW, Do YS, Park HS, Park KB, Kim DI. Peripheral arterial involvement in Behcet's disease: an analysis of the results from a Korean referral center. Rheumatol Int. 2013;33(8):2101–8.

47. Iscan ZH, Vural KM, Bayazit M. Compelling nature of arterial manifestations in Behcet disease. J Vasc Surg. 2005;41(1):53–8.

48. International Study Group for Behçet's Disease. Criteria for diagnosis of Behçet's disease. Lancet. 1990;335(8697):1078–80.

49. Cho SB, Yun M, Lee JH, Kim J, Shim WH, Bang D. Detection of cardiovascular system involvement in Behçet's disease using fluorodeoxyglucose positron emission tomography. Semin Arthritis Rheum. 2011;40(5):461–6.

50. Hatemi G, Silman A, Bang D, Bodaghi B, Chamberlain AM, Gul A, Houman MH, Kötter I, Olivieri I, Salvarani C, Sfikakis PP, Siva A, Stanford MR, Stübiger N, Yurdakul S, Yazici H, EULAR Expert Committee. EULAR recommendations for the management of Behçet disease. Ann Rheum Dis. 2008;67(12):1656–62.

51. Grasland A, Pouchot J, Hachulla E, Blétry O, Papo T, Vinceneux P, Study Group for Cogan's Syndrome. Typical and atypical Cogan's syndrome: 32 cases and review of the literature. Rheumatology (Oxford). 2004;43(8):1007–15.

52. Vaglio A, Pipitone N, Salvarani C. Chronic periaortitis: a large-vessel vasculitis? Curr Opin Rheumatol. 2011;23(1):1–6.

53. Kermani TA, Crowson CS, Achenbach SJ, Luthra HS. Idiopathic retroperitoneal fibrosis: a retrospective review of clinical presentation, treatment, and outcomes. Mayo Clin Proc. 2011;86(4):297–303.

54. Campbell PM, LeRoy EC. Pathogenesis of systemic sclerosis: a vascular hypothesis. Semin Arthritis Rheum. 1975;4:351–68.

55. Sunderkötter C, Riemekasten G. Pathophysiology and clinical consequences of Raynaud's phenomenon related to systemic sclerosis. Rheumatology (Oxford). 2006;45 Suppl 3:iii33-5.

56. Herrick AL, Oogarah PK, Freemont AJ, Marcuson R, Haeney M, Jayson MI. Vasculitis in patients with systemic sclerosis and severe digital ischaemia requiring amputation. Ann Rheum Dis. 1994;53(5):323–6.

57. Matucci-Cerinic M, Kahaleh B, Wigley FM. Review: evidence that systemic sclerosis is a vascular disease. Arthritis Rheum. 2013;65(8):1953–62.

58. Frerix M, Stegbauer J, Dragun D, Kreuter A, Weiner SM. Ulnar artery occlusion is predictive of digital ulcers in SSc: a duplex sonography study. Rheumatology (Oxford). 2012;51(4):735–42.

59. Hudson M, Fritzler MJ. Diagnostic criteria of systemic sclerosis. J Autoimmun. 2014;48–49:38–41.

60. Herrick AL. Contemporary management of Raynaud's phenomenon and digital ischaemic complications. Curr Opin Rheumatol. 2011;23(6):555–61.

61. Brand M, Woodiwiss AJ, Michel F, Nayler S, Veller MG, Norton GR. Large vessel adventitial vasculitis characterizes patients with critical lower limb ischemia with as compared to without human immunodeficiency virus infection. PLoS One. 2014;9(8), e106205.

Cholesterol Emboli

Muhamed Saric and Rose Tompkins

Introduction

Cholesterol embolization syndrome (CES) refers to the arterio-arterial embolization of plaque debris (predominantly cholesterol crystals) from an atheroma within proximal large caliber arteries, typically in the aorto-iliac-femoral system, to small, distal arteries and arterioles. This results in nonspecific constitutional symptoms and end-organ damage secondary to mechanical obstruction and a provoked inflammatory reaction [1]. Within the medical literature, several terms are synonymous with cholesterol embolization syndrome including atheroembolism, atheromatous embolization, cholesterol embolization, and cholesterol crystal embolization.

Cholesterol embolization is a rare disease that often presents insidiously secondary to the showering of microemboli into smaller distal arteries. This must be distinguished from the related but more common arterio-arterial thromboembolism that results from the acute embolization of larger fragments originating from thrombus overlying a complex atheromatous plaque, which can result in the sudden occlusion of larger downstream arteries with development of severe, acute ischemia [2].

The pathophysiology of CES consists of six key elements: presence of complex atherosclerotic plaque, plaque rupture, distal embolization of plaque debris, lodging of microemboli within distal arteries, foreign body reaction, and end-organ damage. CES can potentially affect any organ system resulting in a wide array of clinical manifestations. The clinical presentation, diagnosis, and management of CES will be reviewed.

M. Saric, MD, PhD (✉)
Echocardiography Lab, Leon H. Charney
Division of Cardiology, Department of Medicine,
New York University Langone Medical Center,
560 First Avenue, Tisch 11 East, New York, NY 10016, USA

R. Tompkins
Department of Cardiology, New York University
Langone Medical Center, New York, NY, USA

History

The first report of CES is believed to have occurred in 1844 by Fenger and colleagues in the Danish medical brochure Ugeskrift for Læger (Doctors' Weekly) with the autopsy description of Bertel Thorvaldsen, a Danish/Icelandic sculptor [3]. In 1862, this description was translated into German and made available to a wider medical audience [4]. The first autopsy series to provide a detailed description of the diffuse nature and multi-organ involvement of CES was published in 1945 from New York Hospital [5]. Then in the 1950s, the first observation of cholesterol crystals within the arteries of affected organs from frozen pathological specimens was described using polarized light microscopy [6]. To this day, biopsy remains the gold standard for definitive diagnosis of CES.

In 1957, Thurlbeck and Castleman were the first to report CES as a complication of vascular surgery [7]. This was followed by the classic description of pathognomonic retinal plaques in 1961 by Hollenhorst, an ophthalmologist from Mayo Clinic [8]. The blue toe syndrome was first described in 1973 by Karmody and later became synonymous with cholesterol embolization [9]. It was not until 1990 that the association was established between atheromatous aortic plaque visualized on transesophageal echocardiography (TEE) and clinical manifestations of CES; this significantly evolved our understanding of the underlying pathophysiology of CES [10].

Pathophysiology

The pathophysiology of CES consists of six key elements [1]:

1. The presence of atherosclerotic plaque in a proximal, large caliber artery (this can include the aorta, carotid arteries, iliac arteries, or femoral arteries)
2. Plaque rupture

3. Distal embolization of plaque debris including cholesterol crystals
4. Lodging of emboli into smaller caliber vessels leading to partial or complete occlusion
5. Foreign body inflammatory response to the cholesterol crystals
6. End-organ damage secondary to the combination of mechanical occlusion and the local inflammatory response

Atherosclerotic Plaque in a Proximal Artery

The development of generalized atherosclerosis is a lifelong process that begins in childhood and progresses to more advanced stages later in life. Histologically, atherosclerosis is localized to the arterial intima. In childhood to early adulthood, precursor lesions begin to form in the intimal layer that are characterized by fatty streaks containing layers of macrophage foam cells in combination with intracellular and extracellular lipid droplets. These clinically silent lesions then progress to more advanced stages overtime becoming more prevalent in the middle-aged and elderly. Once a lipid core develops, the lesion progresses through various histological stages of increasing complexity from an atheroma to fibroatheroma to a complex plaque associated with plaque hemorrhage, fissure, and ulceration, as well as development of overlying thrombus. These more advanced plaques can also develop calcifications. It is these advanced lesions that provide the source of cholesterol crystals for embolization in CES [11]. The histopathologic stages of atherosclerotic plaque are summarized in Table 27.1.

An advanced atheromatous plaque is composed of a necrotic core with an overlying fibrous cap (Fig. 27.1). The necrotic core contains cellular debris, macrophage foam cells, and various lipids. The foam cells contain oxidized low-density lipoprotein that is released into the extracellular space upon cell death. This cholesterol-rich material provides the primary source for cholesterol emboli. Cholesterol within a plaque can exist either in a soluble form or a crystalline form. Cholesterol crystals are typically found deep within the necrotic core of the plaque and represent more advanced atherosclerosis. Crystalline cholesterol can account for more

than 40 % of the total cholesterol contained within a plaque [12]. The fibrous cap of a plaque is composed of endothelial cells, smooth muscle cells, and connective tissue.

In the context of echocardiographic and radiologic imaging, atheromatous plaque is often classified as simple or complex. Simple plaques appear as smooth border lesions within the arterial luminal wall that have a wall thickness < 4 mm with absence of any mobile components. Complex plaques have a wall thickness ≥ 4 mm often with irregular, ulcerated luminal borders and evidence of mobile components consistent with overlying thrombus.

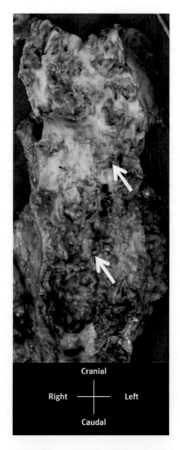

Fig. 27.1 Gross pathologic specimen of aortic atherosclerosis. The abdominal aorta is cut lengthwise to reveal severe advanced atherosclerosis (*arrow*)

Table 27.1 Stages of atherosclerotic plaque

Stage	Lesion classification	Histology	Age at onset	Clinical manifestation
I	Initial	Isolated macrophages, foam cells	Childhood and adolescence	Clinically silent
II	Fatty streak	Intimal fatty streak, intracellular lipid accumulation		
III	Intermediate	Stage II lesion with developing extracellular lipid pools		
IV	Atheroma	Developing extracellular lipid core	Fourth decade into advanced age	Clinically silent or overt
V	Fibroatheroma	Stage IV lesion with overlying fibrotic cap		
VI	Complicated plaque	Stage V lesion with evidence of fibrotic cap defect, hematoma/hemorrhage within lipid core, thrombus		

Based on data from Stary et al. [11]

Simple plaques have an intact fibrous cap that prevents communication between the cholesterol-rich necrotic core and the arterial lumen. Complex plaques often have disruption of the fibrous cap either by fissuring, ulceration, or rupture that exposes the plaque contents to the arterial lumen, thereby creating a potential source for cholesterol emboli. The aorto-iliac-femoral arterial system is the primary location of atheromatous plaques, and thus CES typically localizes to arterial beds of the abdomen and the lower extremities. Therefore, atheroembolism in the upper extremities is uncommon [13].

The risk of embolization is directly related to the presence, severity, and extent of atherosclerosis. This association was first shown in the previously mentioned autopsy series from the late 1940s. Among patients without significant atherosclerotic disease, no CES was observed. However, in patients with aortic plaques, the risk of atheroembolism increased linearly with increasing severity of atherosclerotic

disease; moderately eroded plaques were associated with a 1.3 % incidence of atheroembolism and severely eroded plaques with an increased incidence of 12.3 % [5].

Imaging of the Aorta

Aortic plaques can be visualized, characterized, and quantified by a variety of imaging modalities including transesophageal echocardiography (TEE), computed tomography (CT), and magnetic resonance imaging (MRI) [14]. TEE, predominantly two dimensional (2D), is typically the first-line imaging technique for the detection and measurement of aortic plaque (Fig. 27.2) [1]. The association between clinical embolization and advanced aortic atherosclerotic plaque visualized on TEE was first reported in 1990 [10]. Further studies later confirmed that aortic plaque detected by TEE represents a potential source for systemic emboli [15–17]. Noncalcified complex atheromas in the ascending aorta and aortic arch correlated with a higher risk where a plaque

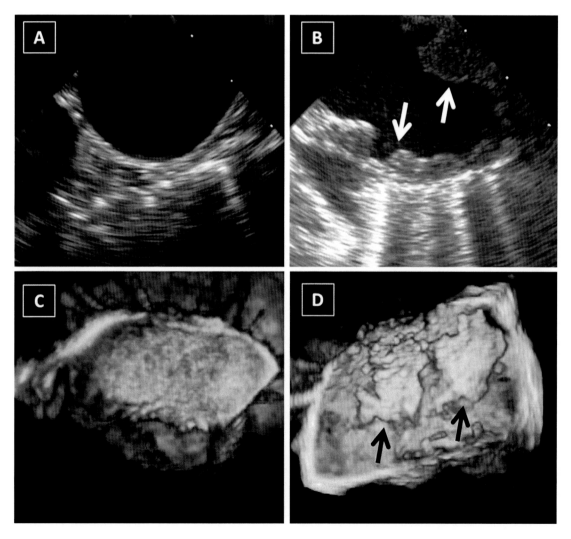

Fig. 27.2 2D and 3D TEE imaging of aortic plaque. (**a, b**) 2D TEE comparison of normal aortic arch (**a**) and severe ulcerated plaque (*arrows*) in the aortic arch. (**c, d**) 3D TEE demonstrates absence (**c**) and presence (**d**) of severe atherosclerotic plaque (*arrows*) in the aortic arch

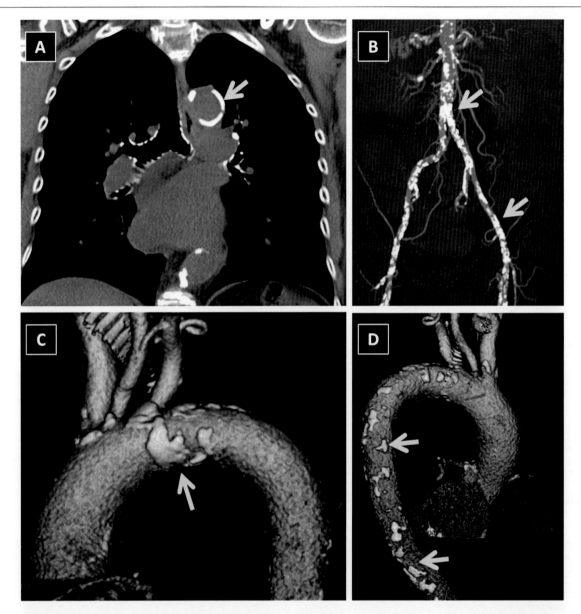

Fig. 27.3 CT imaging of aortic plaque. 2D CT (**a**, **b**) and 3D CT (**c**, **d**) imaging of atherosclerotic plaque in the aorta. (**a**) Coronal cut demonstrates severe calcified atherosclerotic plaque in the aortic arch (*arrow*). (**b**) Severe calcified plaque is seen in the entire abdominal aorta and its iliofemoral branches (*arrows*). (**c**, **d**) 3D-reconstructed CT images show diffuse focal plaque in the thoracic and abdominal aorta (*arrows*) (Courtesy of Dr. Robert Donnino, Veterans Affairs New York Harbor Healthcare System, New York, NY, and Departments of Medicine and Radiology, New York University School of Medicine, New York, NY)

thickness ≥4 mm measured on TEE emerged as a clinically important predictor of increased vascular embolic events [17–19]. These embolic events could have represented both arterial thromboembolism and atheroembolism. However, additional case reports with biopsy-proven CES found an association with complex aortic atheromas visualized on TEE, thereby strengthening not only the role of the aortic plaque in CES but also the role of TEE in detecting these plaques [20]. Real-time three-dimensional (3D) TEE is a newer imaging technique that may provide additional morphological detail of the plaque and could have an increasing clinical role in the future [21].

CT and MRI are additional imaging techniques that can be considered for detection and characterization of aortic plaque that may provide a less invasive and more comprehensive evaluation of aortic atherosclerosis relative to 2D and 3D TEE (Figs. 27.3 and 27.4) [22–24]. For imaging of the major branches of the thoracic aorta, CT and MRI are superior to TEE as TEE has a blind spot around the origin of the brachiocephalic artery due to interposition of the air-filled bronchi between the esophagus and the artery. In addition, the abdominal aorta is incompletely visualized on TEE as it is limited to the proximal abdominal aorta between the diaphragm and origin of the superior mesenteric artery.

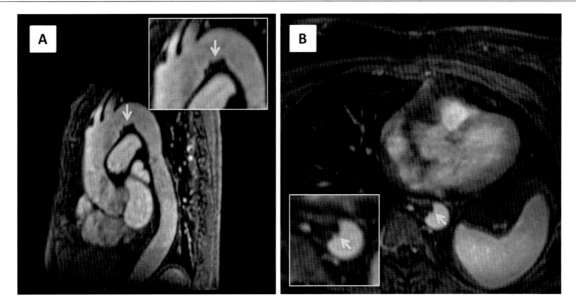

Fig. 27.4 MRI imaging of aortic plaque. (**a**) Magnetic resonance angiography (MRA) demonstrates a prominent ulcerated plaque (*arrow*) in the inferior aspect of the aortic arch in a near-sagittal cut. (**b**) MRA shows a protruding ulcerated plaque in the descending aorta (*arrow*) in an axial cut (Courtesy of Robert Donnino, Veterans Affairs New York Harbor Healthcare System, New York, NY, and Departments of Medicine and Radiology, New York University School of Medicine, New York, NY)

Therefore, for complete visualization of the aorta-iliac-femoral arterial system, CT or MRI is preferred.

Conventional arteriography has a low sensitivity for aortic plaque detection and often fails to detect plaques that are identified on other imaging modalities. In addition, arteriography is invasive and could lead to mechanical disruption of an aortic plaque and subsequent arterial cholesterol embolization or thromboembolism and, therefore, should generally be avoided [25].

Plaque Rupture

Rupture of the fibrous cap is a necessary event in the development of CES. This exposes the cholesterol-rich core of the atherosclerotic plaque to the arterial lumen. Plaque rupture can either be spontaneous or traumatic. Traumatic plaque rupture can be secondary to mechanical disruption from intra-arterial manipulation during catheter or surgical procedures. It remains controversial whether or not thrombolytic or anticoagulant therapy is an independent risk factor for plaque rupture and cholesterol embolization.

Spontaneous Atheroembolism

Spontaneous rupture of an aortic plaque shares similar mechanistic features to plaque rupture in other arterial beds. Plaque composition rather than plaque size is thought to play the principal role in plaque vulnerability. More vulnerable plaques often have larger lipid cores and thinning of fibrotic caps mediated by a complex interaction between inflammatory and extracellular matrix cells. Therefore, inflammation may play a critical role in altering plaque composition and thus increasing a plaque's vulnerability to spontaneous rupture [26].

The rate of spontaneous aortic plaque rupture in the general population has been extrapolated from older pathoanatomic series that were published in the era before the widespread use of intra-arterial cannulation for diagnostic and therapeutic purposes; this estimated rate ranged from <1 to 3.4 % [5, 27, 28]. However, the incidence of spontaneous plaque rupture leading to CES remains low even among higher-risk populations. One antemortem retrospective study of 519 patients with complex aortic plaque diagnosed by TEE found CES to occur at a rate of 1 % over a 3-year follow-up. For comparison, this CES rate is significantly lower than the 20 % rate of arterial thromboembolism observed in the same cohort [29].

Traumatic Plaque Rupture

Traumatic aortic plaque rupture can occur following intra-arterial manipulation during catheterization or cardiovascular surgery. Although cholesterol embolization has been reported in association with cardiac catheterization, it is considered a rare complication. The reported incidence of clinically apparent CES after cardiac catheterization is <2 % [30–32]. The data remains inconclusive regarding whether or not radial access versus femoral access results in a lower incidence of this complication [30, 33]. CES, particularly cerebral atheroembolism, has been a major concern following transcatheter aortic valve replacement (TAVR) with early registries reporting an incidence of 2.4–4 %. However, the incidence seems to be declining with the use of smaller catheters and more stringent patient selection criteria. The routine use of intra-arterial embolic protection devices may lead to an even further decline in embolization events [34].

CES in association with cardiovascular surgery is also rare. Risk is directly correlated with extent and severity of atherosclerosis in the ascending aorta. CES has been reported more frequently in association with coronary revascularization than valvular operations [35]. Off-pump cardiovascular surgeries may lead to less embolic events compared to the use of cardiopulmonary bypass techniques [36]. CES has also been a rare complication associated with carotid endarterectomy, carotid stenting, and abdominal aorta procedures including endovascular aneurysm repair (EVAR) [37–39].

Thrombolytic and Anticoagulation Therapy

The incidence of intra-plaque hemorrhage and an associated increase in plaque rupture leading to CES as a consequence of thrombolytic or anticoagulation therapy remains controversial. Case reports have suggested that CES can develop subsequent to thrombolytic therapy given for the acute management of various conditions including myocardial infarction and deep venous thrombosis. Although a small prospective trial of post-myocardial infarction patients treated with or without thrombolytic therapy failed to demonstrate a relationship [40], there still exists a controversy [41]. Similarly, case reports have suggested that anticoagulation is also associated with an increase in CES and that discontinuation of therapy can lead to clinical improvement [42, 43].

In addition to warfarin, the novel anticoagulants have also been suggested to play a role in development of CES [44]. However, it is difficult to determine if this is a causal relationship or merely an association. At this time, no randomized trials have specifically evaluated anticoagulation as an independent risk factor for development of CES. There is limited literature to support that the use of anticoagulation in patients with concurrent CES is safe and feasible among patients with a separate indication for anticoagulation [45]. Therefore, per current evidence, the causal relationship between cholesterol embolization and the use of anticoagulation and/or thrombolytic therapy can neither be proven nor refuted. Based on this unresolved controversy, routine use of anticoagulation among patients with CES is not generally recommended. However, use of anticoagulation in CES appears reasonable in patients with a separate indication for anticoagulation including atrial fibrillation, left ventricular thrombus, or mechanical prosthetic valve [1].

Embolization of Plaque Debris

Plaque rupture is thought to lead to a showering of plaque debris including cholesterol crystals to a variety of distal tissue and organs. Showering of microemboli typically occurs slowly

overtime and may not become clinically apparent until significant end-organ damage has occurred. This is in contrast to arterial thromboembolism where a large thrombus embolizes all at once. Currently, there are no diagnostic tests to definitively detect cholesterol microembolization in the absence of clinical findings; therefore, it is possible that there are many cases of silent cholesterol plaque embolization that have gone undiagnosed.

Lodging of Emboli into Smaller Caliber Vessels

Once released from a plaque, cholesterol crystals travel through the arterial circulation until they reach smaller caliber arteries or arterioles where they become lodged within their lumens. In routine biopsy specimens, cholesterol crystals are not visualized directly because they are washed away during standard specimen processing. However, characteristic ovoid or crescentic clefts within the lumens of the affected vessels can be seen; they represent voids in which the crystals had previously been located (Fig. 27.5) [46]. Direct visualization of cholesterol crystals is also possible if the biopsy specimen is preserved with liquid nitrogen then viewed with polarized microscopy; the crystals will demonstrate birefringence (double refraction of polarized light) [6].

Inflammatory Response

In addition to mechanical obstruction, cholesterol emboli incite an inflammatory reaction. This response has been well documented in an animal model and consists of three phases:

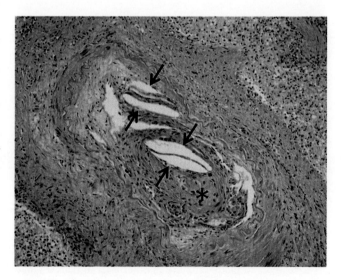

Fig. 27.5 Cholesterol clefts on histopathology. A hematoxylin-eosin-stained section of a small renal artery demonstrates several pathognomonic empty spaces referred to as cholesterol clefts (*arrows*) within the partly fibrosed (*asterisk*) lumen. Magnification 200× (Courtesy of Dr Amy Rapkiewicz, Department of Pathology, New York University Medical Center, New York, NY)

acute inflammation, foreign body reaction with intravascular thrombus formation, and endothelial proliferation and fibrosis. The acute inflammatory stage is marked histologically by local infiltration of polymorphonuclear cells and eosinophils. Over the following 24–48 h, the cholesterol crystals elicit a foreign body response leading to infiltration of mononuclear cells and their transformation into giant cells that phagocytizes the cholesterol crystals. Simultaneously, thrombus develops in the arterial lumen. In the final stages, there is a proliferation of endothelial cells within the wall of the affected vessel with an eventual progression to intravascular fibrosis that leads to long-term stenosis or complete obliteration of the artery. This results in tissue ischemia and necrosis manifested as end-organ damage [47].

End-Organ Damage

The mechanical obstruction and inflammatory response provoked by cholesterol emboli can affect virtually any organ. However, clinically CES is most apparent when the brain, kidney, gastrointestinal tract, and skin are affected. The end-organ manifestations seen within these tissues are further described.

Central Nervous System

Cholesterol emboli released from advanced atherosclerotic plaques within the ascending aorta, aortic arch, carotid arteries, and vertebral arteries can enter the central nervous system circulation. These atheroemboli can either result from spontaneous plaque rupture or from mechanical manipulation during intra-arterial catheter-based procedures or cardiovascular surgeries, as previously described. Showering of atheroemboli into the cerebral circulation can result in diffuse brain injury that is often characterized by global symptoms of confusion and memory loss rather than focal neurological deficits that are more typically seen with arterial thromboembolism [48]. Brain imaging can demonstrate multiple small areas of infarction in different vascular territories and/or border zone infarctions [49].

Transcranial Doppler (TCD) ultrasonography can be used to detect microemboli in the cerebral circulation. Microemboli appear as high-intensity transient signals superimposed on the background of standard spectral Doppler flow velocity tracings of red blood cells within the cerebral circulation. TCD has been employed intraoperatively to reveal a large number of microemboli showered into the cerebral circulation during both carotid and coronary artery manipulation. A limitation of this modality is its inability to distinguish atheroemboli from other microemboli including gas, fat, or calcium [50, 51].

The clinical consequence of these microemboli are negligible as a vast majority of patients will demonstrate some evidence of intraoperative cerebral microemboli on TCD, but only a very few patients will manifest postoperative neurological

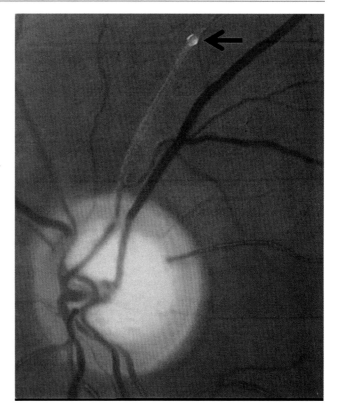

Fig. 27.6 Hollenhorst retinal plaque. Fundoscopic exam reveals characteristic Hollenhorst plaque (*arrow*) in a retinal artery branch (Courtesy of Dr Irene Cherfas Tsyvine, Department of Ophthalmology, New Jersey Medical School, Newark, NJ)

symptoms [52]. Even when new brain lesions suggestive of microembolization are visualized on MRI postoperatively, only a small percentage of patients have clinical findings of transient ischemic attack (TIA) or stroke [53].

Cholesterol emboli originating from atherosclerotic plaque in the ascending aorta, aortic arch, and carotid arteries can cause retinal artery occlusion. Amaurosis fugax is the typical clinical manifestation when there is retinal artery involvement. Retinal exam will often reveal pathognomonic Hollenhorst plaques, which are described as bright, orange-colored plaques seen at the bifurcation of the retinal arterioles (Fig. 27.6) [8].

Kidney

Atheroembolic renal disease should be considered in the differential diagnosis of unexplained acute renal insufficiency (ARI) among older adults. Histologically, atheroembolic renal disease affects predominantly the arcuate and interlobar renal arteries. Rarely, there can be involvement of the afferent arterioles and glomeruli. Renal biopsy is the gold standard for diagnosis but may not always be diagnostic given the patchy nature of disease [54]. Incidence of renal CES can be as high as 7 % among patients aged 60 years or older undergoing renal biopsy for ARI of unknown etiology [55].

In patients with histologically confirmed CES from any other tissue, renal involvement is frequent and can be found in up to 50 % of cases. Proteinuria and elevations in serum creatinine and blood urea nitrogen are the predominant manifestations, occurring in 54 %, 83 %, and 91 %, respectively [56]. Accelerated and difficult to control hypertension has also been described in renal CES and is thought to be secondary to the acute inflammatory response within the renal circulation [57].

Atheroembolic renal disease can result in acute, subacute, or chronic renal insufficiency. Subacute renal insufficiency can be precipitated by manipulation of the aorta during a vascular procedure. In contrast, chronic renal insufficiency is thought to develop from a spontaneous slow release of cholesterol emboli from advanced atherosclerotic plaque in the aorta over an extended period of time [1].

Renal impairment secondary to cholesterol embolization can resolve spontaneously or progress to end-stage disease often requiring renal replacement therapy. Progression to end-stage renal disease is frequent; in an observational study of 354 patients with renal atheroembolism inferred from either renal biopsy or concomitant retinal Hollenhorst plaques, more than 30 % of patients required hemodialysis by the end of a 2-year follow-up. In addition to poor renal recovery, atheroembolic renal disease has also been associated with decreased survival. The 1-year and 2-year survival rates have been reported as 83 % and 75 % respectively, which are lower than those than in other forms of renal disease requiring maintenance hemodialysis [58].

Gastrointestinal Tract

The gastrointestinal (GI) tract is another organ system that is commonly affected by cholesterol embolization. The prevalence of gastrointestinal involvement has been reported anywhere from 18.6 to 48 % of confirmed CES cases [59]. GI atheroembolism often results in abdominal pain and chronic intestinal bleeding secondary to mucosal ulceration and necrosis from bowel wall ischemia. Abdominal CT imaging is nonspecific and may show bowel edema or perforation. Endoscopy has a poor sensitivity, and many of these lesions tend to be microscopic. If endoscopic pathology is visualized, the findings are relatively nonspecific and may demonstrate congested mucosa, mucosal ulcerations or erosions, or focal areas of bluish or necrotic mucosa [60]. In more severe cases, massive bleeding can develop from pseudopolyp formation or frank bowel infarction with subsequent perforation [61].

In addition to bowel, atheroembolism has also been reported to affect other GI organs including the pancreas and gallbladder. Pancreatic involvement can be an uncommon cause of acute pancreatitis in elderly patients [62]. Cholesterol embolization can also be a rare etiology of acal-culous cholecystitis, especially following a recent vascular procedure [60].

Skin

The incidence of cutaneous manifestations in cholesterol embolization syndrome ranges from 35 to 96 % [63]. In one of the more comprehensive dermatologic case series of patients with confirmed CES, cutaneous findings were seen in 35 % of cases (78 of 223 patients). The most common skin manifestations are livedo reticularis (49 %), gangrene (35 %), cyanosis (28 %), ulceration (17 %), nodules (10 %), and purpura (9 %). Skin findings are located predominantly on the lower extremities; they are much less common on the trunk or upper extremities [64]. Cutaneous biopsies are reasonably sensitive for the diagnosis of CES and are positive in approximately 92 % of patients with skin manifestations [63].

Livedo reticularis appears as a rash of reddish blue spots distributed in a fishnet or lacy pattern. This finding represents a cyanotic response caused by restriction of blood flow due to narrowed arterioles within the skin. Although a common clinical finding that should raise suspicion for CES, especially in an elderly patient, livedo reticularis is not pathognomonic for atheroemboli and can be seen in other disorders that are associated with skin ischemia including polyarteritis nodosa, systemic lupus erythematous, cryoglobulinemia, and treatment with vasoconstrictive agents [63].

In the lower extremities, cholesterol crystal emboli can lead to the sudden development of blue or purple toes (Fig. 27.7) [13]. This finding was first described in 1976 by Karmody as a manifestation of CES [9]. Because the sudden

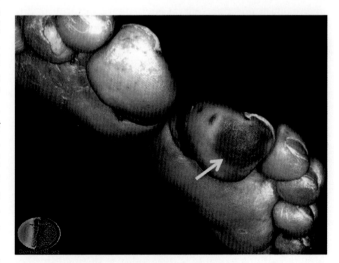

Fig. 27.7 Blue toes. An *arrow* points to bluish discoloration of the left big toe, a manifestation of microvascular ischemia in a patient with cholesterol embolization syndrome (Courtesy of Dr. Amanda Oakley, New Zealand Dermatological Society Incorporated; image reprinted with permission from DermNetNZ.org)

development of blue toes has a significant association with atheroembolism, the term blue toe syndrome is sometimes used clinically as a synonym for CES.

Development of blue toes represents microvascular ischemia, and although frequently seen in atheroembolic disease, it is a nonspecific finding than can also be seen in other conditions including vasculitis (polyarteritis nodosa), hypercoagulable states (antiphospholipid syndrome), hyperviscosity states (polycythemia vera), and endocarditis [65]. Toe and foot cyanosis in blue toe syndrome is more prevalent in dependent areas, typically blanches with moderate pressure, and is often asymmetric when both lower extremities are involved. If microvascular ischemia is severe, a spectrum of tissue necrosis can be seen ranging from superficial ulceration to gangrene (decay of dead tissue due to lack of a blood supply) [1].

Generally, when cutaneous manifestations are seen, they often occur in the context of palpable distal pulses because cholesterol crystal emboli are more likely to affect the smaller arteries and arterioles than the larger palpable arteries. Therefore, palpable distal pulses in the lower extremities may favor the diagnosis of CES over other forms of peripheral vascular disease. However, patients with atheroembolism often have other manifestations of advanced atherosclerotic disease including peripheral arterial disease that can independently cause diminished palpable pulses. Thus, absence of palpable pulses does not exclude CES [1]. Patients with blue toe syndrome secondary to CES are more likely to have other cutaneous manifestations including livedo reticularis.

Diagnosis of Cholesterol Emboli Syndrome

Diagnosis of CES is a challenge given that there is no definitive laboratory test or pathognomonic clinical presentation. The syndrome can affect any organ system and can present as a slow insidious process with nonspecific signs and symptoms mimicking a vast array of systemic illnesses. The cornerstone of diagnosis is predominantly clinical and based on the combination of signs and symptoms of end-organ damage in a patient with a recent history of an intra-arterial procedure and/or risk factors for advanced atherosclerosis (male, advanced age, hypertension, diabetes mellitus, hypercholesterolemia, and a history of tobacco use) [1].

Secondary to the provoked inflammatory response described above, patients can exhibit constitutional symptoms such as fever, weight loss, anorexia, fatigue, and generalized myalgia. There can also be an array of laboratory abnormalities; however, they are typically suggestive of rather than diagnostic of CES. Elevation of inflammatory markers such as erythrocyte sedimentation rate (ESR) and

C-reactive protein (CRP) is common and can be associated with a reactive leukocytosis. Hypocomplementemia has also been reported. Patients can have evidence of a normocytic anemia and thrombocytopenia. When there is renal involvement, the serum creatinine and blood urea nitrogen are often elevated, and proteinuria may be present.

Hypereosinophilia may also be a marker of CES. It has been reported in up to 80 % of CES cases, although the duration and degree of hypereosinophilia can be variable. One study found that the prevalence of eosinophilia ranged from 6 to 18 % of the total leukocyte count and persisted only for the first several days of the initial event [66]. The mechanism for hypereosinophilia in atheroembolism remains unknown. It is hypothesized to be cytokine mediated and may be related to release of interleukin-5 derived from vascular endothelium [67]. Similar to other laboratory findings, hypereosinophilia is not pathognomonic for CES. When associated with acute or progressive renal insufficiency, the differential diagnosis of hypereosinophilia includes systemic vasculitis, acute interstitial nephritis (AIN), and radiographic contrast-induced nephropathy (CIN) [66].

Given that the clinical and laboratory findings described thus far are not specific for the diagnosis of CES, it must be emphasized that a high degree of clinical suspicion is required in order to establish the diagnosis. If patient characteristics, clinical history, and laboratory findings are suggestive of atheroembolism, then an ophthalmologic exam demonstrating Hollenhorst plaques and/or aortic imaging revealing complex atherosclerotic plaques may further support the diagnosis, especially in the absence of a recent vascular procedure when spontaneous plaque rupture may be the underlying etiology.

Ultimately, pathological confirmation from a biopsy specimen remains the only definitive test for CES [68]. Technically any affected tissue can be targeted for biopsy, but the skin and skeletal muscle are the preferred sites secondary to the ease of the procedure and reduced patient discomfort. Cutaneous biopsies have a sensitivity of 92 % per one review [63]. Despite the utility of a biopsy in confirming the diagnosis of cholesterol embolization, biopsy is performed infrequently due to the concern that the biopsy sites may heal poorly given that these tissues are located in regions of restricted blood flow.

Treatment of Cholesterol Emboli Syndrome

At this time, no specific therapy is available for CES [69]. Management of atheroembolic disease focuses on supportive care for end-organ damage sustained and prevention of future cholesterol embolic events. In addition, measures should be taken to aggressively manage atherosclerotic disease risk factors including blood pressure control, lipid management, adequate glucose control, and smoking cessation.

Although no randomized trial data is available, there is some data to support the use of statin therapy. One retrospective study that included 519 patients with severe atherosclerosis visualized on TEE found that statin use was independently associated with a reduced incidence of future embolic events [29]. Another study that included 354 patients diagnosed with atherosclerotic renal disease reported a 50 % reduction in the need for renal replacement therapy or mortality among patients on statin therapy [58]. Future randomized trials may provide more evidence base for statin use in atheroembolic disease [70].

Antiplatelet therapy has been considered for the management of cholesterol embolization. However, there is no direct evidence that their use reduces recurrence of embolic events. Regardless, antiplatelet therapy is reasonable in CES considering that there is strong evidence to support that they reduce adverse cardiovascular events including myocardial infarction which is the leading cause of death among patients with atherosclerotic disease [71]. Angiotensin-converting enzyme inhibitors and/or angiotensin receptor blockers (ARB) are also reasonable to consider especially in patients with hypertension, diabetes, and/or renal involvement [72, 73]. There is limited data on the use of corticosteroids which may mitigate the inflammatory response in atheroembolic renal disease with a suggestion of favorable short-term outcomes. However, loss of benefit was seen in more long-term follow-up [74, 75].

As previously noted, the routine use of thrombolytic or anticoagulation therapy is not recommended given the uncertainty of their involvement in precipitating plaque rupture. Specifically, anticoagulation therapy should not be initiated in CES unless there are other established indications such as atrial fibrillation, left ventricular thrombus, deep venous thrombosis, or a mechanical prosthetic valve [1].

In patients with prior episode of CES, when considering future intra-arterial diagnostic or therapeutic interventions that involve the aorto-iliac-femoral system including angiography, percutaneous coronary revascularization, and cardiovascular surgery, risk of recurrent CES should be weighted carefully against benefits. Generally, elective intra-arterial procedures should be avoided.

Surgical or endovascular procedures may be a treatment option in patients with CES. They may be considered when a clear source of cholesterol emboli can be identified, the site is surgically or endovascularly accessible, and the patient is an appropriate surgical candidate. Such management is aimed at the surgical removal or endovascular exclusion of advanced atherosclerotic plaque felt to be the culprit. The data has shown this strategy to be effective in reducing the rate of future embolic events in appropriately selected patients [76, 77].

Conclusion

CES is a rare disease process with a high incidence of morbidity and mortality. The syndrome results from microembolization of plaque debris, including cholesterol crystals, from rupture of complicated atherosclerotic plaques found within large, proximal arteries usually in the aorta-iliac-femoral system. Plaque rupture can be spontaneous or as a result of aorta-iliac-femoral manipulation during intravascular catheter-based procedures or cardiovascular surgery. These microemboli become lodged within small caliber distal arteries and arterioles leading to mechanical obstruction and inflammation resulting in end-organ damage. Potentially, any organ can be affected resulting in variable clinical manifestations ranging from encephalopathy, gastrointestinal bleeding, renal insufficiency, livedo reticularis, and "blue toes." Constitutional symptoms such as fever, weight loss, and fatigue can also occur as a result of the acute inflammatory response. Nonspecific laboratory findings arising from this inflammatory response may include an elevated ESR, leukocytosis, and hypereosinophilia. Pathological diagnosis, obtained from biopsy of affected tissue, continues to be the gold standard for diagnosis. Treatment remains largely supportive.

References

1. Kronzon I, Saric M. Cholesterol embolization syndrome. Circulation. 2010;122(6):631–41.
2. Tunick PA, Kronzon I. Atheromas of the thoracic aorta: clinical and therapeutic update. J Am Coll Cardiol. 2000;35:545–54.
3. Fenger CE, Jacobsen JP, Dahlerup EA, Hornemann E, Collin T. Beretning af Obduktionen over Albert Thorvaldsen (autopsy report of Albert Thorvaldsen). Ugeskr Laeger. 1844;10(14–15):215–8. In literature, this article is often referenced from Panum's German translation as Obduktiosbericht (autopsy report).
4. Panum PL. Experimentelle Beiträge zur Lehre von der Embolie. Virchows Arch Pathol Anat Physiol. 1862;25:308–10.
5. Flory CM. Arterial occlusions produced by emboli from eroded aortic atheromatous plaques. Am J Pathol. 1945;21(3):549–65.
6. Octavio Rios C. Applications of polarized light in the clinical laboratory; research on cholesterol crystals in bile & biliary calculi. Rev Sanid Mil Peru. 1956;29(85):71–7.
7. Thurlbeck WM, Castleman B. Atheromatous emboli to the kidneys after aortic surgery. N Engl J Med. 1957;257(10):442–7.
8. Hollenhorst RW. Significance of bright plaques in the retinal arterioles. JAMA. 1961;178:23–9.
9. Karmody AM, et al. "Blue toe" syndrome. An indication for limb salvage surgery. Arch Surg. 1976;111(11):1263–8.
10. Tunick PA, Kronzon I. Protruding atherosclerotic plaque in the aortic arch of patients with systemic embolization: a new finding seen by transesophageal echocardiography. Am Heart J. 1990;120(3): 658–60.

11. Stary HC, et al. A definition of advanced types of atherosclerotic lesions and a histological classification of atherosclerosis. A report from the Committee on Vascular Lesions of the Council on Arteriosclerosis, American Heart Association. Circulation. 1995;92(5):1355–74.

12. Katz SS, et al. Cholesterol turnover in lipid phases of human atherosclerotic plaque. J Lipid Res. 1982;23(5):733–7.

13. Applebaum RM, Kronzon I. Evaluation and management of cholesterol embolization and the blue toe syndrome. Curr Opin Cardiol. 1996;11(5):533–42.

14. Tunick PA, et al. Diagnostic imaging of thoracic aortic atherosclerosis. AJR Am J Roentgenol. 2000;174(4):1119–25.

15. Tunick PA, Perez JL, Kronzon I. Protruding atheromas in the thoracic aorta and systemic embolization. Ann Intern Med. 1991;115(6):423–7.

16. Jones EF, et al. Proximal aortic atheroma. An independent risk factor for cerebral ischemia. Stroke. 1995;26(2):218–24.

17. Amarenco P, et al. Atherosclerotic disease of the aortic arch and the risk of ischemic stroke. N Engl J Med. 1994;331(22):1474–9.

18. Atherosclerotic disease of the aortic arch as a risk factor for recurrent ischemic stroke. The French Study of Aortic Plaques in Stroke Group. N Engl J Med. 1996;334(19):1216–21.

19. Cohen A, et al. Aortic plaque morphology and vascular events: a follow-up study in patients with ischemic stroke. FAPS Investigators. French Study of Aortic Plaques in Stroke. Circulation. 1997;96(11):3838–41.

20. Coy KM, et al. Transesophageal echocardiographic detection of aortic atheromatosis may provide clues to occult renal dysfunction in the elderly. Am Heart J. 1992;123(6):1684–6.

21. Piazzese C, Tsang W, Sotaquira M, Kronzon I, Lang RM, Caiani EG. Semiautomated detection and quantification of aortic plaques from three-dimensional transesophageal echocardiography. J Am Soc Echocardiogr. 2014;27(7):758–66.

22. Ko Y, et al. Significance of aortic atherosclerotic disease in possibly embolic stroke: 64-multidetector row computed tomography study. J Neurol. 2010;257(5):699–705.

23. Fayad ZA, et al. In vivo magnetic resonance evaluation of atherosclerotic plaques in the human thoracic aorta: a comparison with transesophageal echocardiography. Circulation. 2000;101(21):2503–9.

24. Harloff A, et al. 3D MRI provides improved visualization and detection of aortic arch plaques compared to transesophageal echocardiography. J Magn Reson Imaging. 2012;36(3):604–11.

25. Khatri IA, et al. Catheter-based aortography fails to identify aortic atherosclerotic lesions detected on transesophageal echocardiography. J Neuroimaging. 2005;15(3):261–5.

26. Shah PK. Molecular mechanisms of plaque instability. Curr Opin Lipidol. 2007;18(5):492–9.

27. Kealy WF. Atheroembolism. J Clin Pathol. 1978;31(10):984–9.

28. Cross SS. How common is cholesterol embolism? J Clin Pathol. 1991;44(10):859–61.

29. Tunick PA, et al. Effect of treatment on the incidence of stroke and other emboli in 519 patients with severe thoracic aortic plaque. Am J Cardiol. 2002;90(12):1320–5.

30. Fukumoto Y, et al. The incidence and risk factors of cholesterol embolization syndrome, a complication of cardiac catheterization: a prospective study. J Am Coll Cardiol. 2003;42(2):211–6.

31. Johnson LW, et al. Peripheral vascular complications of coronary angioplasty by the femoral and brachial techniques. Cathet Cardiovasc Diagn. 1994;31(3):165–72.

32. Saklayen MG, et al. Incidence of atheroembolic renal failure after coronary angiography. A prospective study. Angiology. 1997;48(7):609–13.

33. Kooiman J, et al. Risk of acute kidney injury after percutaneous coronary interventions using radial versus femoral vascular access: insights from the Blue Cross Blue Shield of Michigan Cardiovascular Consortium. Circ Cardiovasc Interv. 2014;7(2):190–8.

34. Webb JG, Wood DA. Current status of transcatheter aortic valve replacement. J Am Coll Cardiol. 2012;60(6):483–92.

35. Blauth CI, et al. Atheroembolism from the ascending aorta. An emerging problem in cardiac surgery. J Thorac Cardiovasc Surg. 1992;103(6):1104–11. discussion 1111–2.

36. Ascione R, et al. Retinal and cerebral microembolization during coronary artery bypass surgery: a randomized, controlled trial. Circulation. 2005;112(25):3833–8.

37. Sila CA. Neurologic complications of vascular surgery. Neurol Clin. 1998;16(1):9–20.

38. Rapp JH, et al. Cerebral ischemia and infarction from atheroemboli <100 micron in Size. Stroke. 2003;34(8):1976–80.

39. Toya N, et al. Embolic complications after endovascular repair of abdominal aortic aneurysms. Surg Today. 2014;44(10):1893–9.

40. Blankenship JC, Butler M, Garbes A. Prospective assessment of cholesterol embolization in patients with acute myocardial infarction treated with thrombolytic vs conservative therapy. Chest. 1995;107(3):662–8.

41. Konstantinou DM, et al. Cholesterol embolization syndrome following thrombolysis during acute myocardial infarction. Herz. 2012;37(2):231–3.

42. Hyman BT, et al. Warfarin-related purple toes syndrome and cholesterol microembolization. Am J Med. 1987;82(6):1233–7.

43. Bruns FJ, Segel DP, Adler S. Control of cholesterol embolization by discontinuation of anticoagulant therapy. Am J Med Sci. 1978;275(1):105–8.

44. Shafi ST, et al. A case of dabigatran-associated acute renal failure. WMJ. 2013;112(4):173–5. quiz 176.

45. Kim H, Zhen D, Lieske J, McBane R, Grande J, Sandhu G, Melduni R. Treatment of cholesterol embolization syndrome in the setting of an acute indication for anticoagulation therapy. J Med Case Rep. 2014;5:376–79.

46. Eliot RS, Kanjuh VI, Edwards JE. Atheromatous embolism. Circulation. 1964;30:611–8.

47. Gore I, McCombs HL, Lindquist RL. Observations on the fate of cholesterol emboli. J Atheroscler Res. 1964;4:527–35.

48. Soloway HB, Aronson SM. Atheromatous emboli to central nervous system. Report of 16 cases. Arch Neurol. 1964;11:657–67.

49. Ezzeddine MA, et al. Clinical characteristics of pathologically proved cholesterol emboli to the brain. Neurology. 2000;54(8):1681–3.

50. Spencer MP, et al. Detection of middle cerebral artery emboli during carotid endarterectomy using transcranial Doppler ultrasonography. Stroke. 1990;21(3):415–23.

51. Baker AJ, et al. Cerebral microemboli during coronary artery bypass using different cardioplegia techniques. Ann Thorac Surg. 1995;59(5):1187–91.

52. Ackerstaff RG, et al. The significance of microemboli detection by means of transcranial Doppler ultrasonography monitoring in carotid endarterectomy. J Vasc Surg. 1995;21(6):963–9.

53. Enevoldsen EM, et al. Cerebral infarct following carotid endarterectomy. Frequency, clinical and hemodynamic significance evaluated by MRI and TCD. Acta Neurol Scand. 1999;100(2):106–10.

54. Scolari F, et al. Cholesterol crystal embolism: a recognizable cause of renal disease. Am J Kidney Dis. 2000;36(6):1089–109.

55. Haas M, et al. Etiologies and outcome of acute renal insufficiency in older adults: a renal biopsy study of 259 cases. Am J Kidney Dis. 2000;35(3):433–47.

56. Fine MJ, Kapoor W, Falanga V. Cholesterol crystal embolization: a review of 221 cases in the English literature. Angiology. 1987;38(10):769–84.

57. Lye WC, Cheah JS, Sinniah R. Renal cholesterol embolic disease. Case report and review of the literature. Am J Nephrol. 1993;13(6):489–93.

58. Scolari F, et al. The challenge of diagnosing atheroembolic renal disease: clinical features and prognostic factors. Circulation. 2007;116(3):298–304.

59. Rushovich AM. Perforation of the jejunum: a complication of atheromatous embolization. Am J Gastroenterol. 1983;78(2):77–82.

60. Moolenaar W, Lamers CB. Cholesterol crystal embolization and the digestive system. Scand J Gastroenterol Suppl. 1991; 188:69–72.

61. Francis J, Kapoor WN. Intestinal pseudopolyps and gastrointestinal hemorrhage due to cholesterol crystal embolization. Am J Med. 1988;85(2):269–71.

62. Probstein JG, Joshi RA, Blumenthal HT. Atheromatous embolization; an etiology of acute pancreatitis. AMA Arch Surg. 1957;75(4):566–71. discussion 571–2.

63. Donohue KG, Saap L, Falanga V. Cholesterol crystal embolization: an atherosclerotic disease with frequent and varied cutaneous manifestations. J Eur Acad Dermatol Venereol. 2003;17(5):504–11.

64. Falanga V, Fine MJ, Kapoor WN. The cutaneous manifestations of cholesterol crystal embolization. Arch Dermatol. 1986;122(10): 1194–8.

65. O'Keeffe ST, et al. Blue toe syndrome. Causes and management. Arch Intern Med. 1992;152(11):2197–202.

66. Kasinath BS, Lewis EJ. Eosinophilia as a clue to the diagnosis of atheroembolic renal disease. Arch Intern Med. 1987;147(8): 1384–5.

67. Cecioni I, et al. Eosinophilia in cholesterol atheroembolic disease. J Allergy Clin Immunol. 2007;120(6):1470–1. author reply 1471.

68. Jucgla A, et al. Cholesterol embolism: still an unrecognized entity with a high mortality rate. J Am Acad Dermatol. 2006;55(5): 786–93.

69. Tunick PA, Kronzon I. Embolism from the aorta: atheroemboli and thromboemboli. Curr Treat Options Cardiovasc Med. 2001; 3(3):181–6.

70. Ueno Y, et al. Rationale and design of the EPISTEME trial: efficacy of post-stroke intensive rosuvastatin treatment for aortogenic embolic stroke. Cardiovasc Drugs Ther. 2014;28(1):79–85.

71. Smith Jr SC, et al. AHA/ACC guidelines for secondary prevention for patients with coronary and other atherosclerotic vascular disease: 2006 update: endorsed by the National Heart, Lung, and Blood Institute. Circulation. 2006;113(19):2363–72.

72. Yusuf S, et al. Effects of an angiotensin-converting-enzyme inhibitor, ramipril, on cardiovascular events in high-risk patients. The Heart Outcomes Prevention Evaluation Study Investigators. N Engl J Med. 2000;342(3):145–53.

73. Belenfant X, Meyrier A, Jacquot C. Supportive treatment improves survival in multivisceral cholesterol crystal embolism. Am J Kidney Dis. 1999;33(5):840–50.

74. Masuda J, et al. Use of corticosteroids in the treatment of cholesterol crystal embolism after cardiac catheterization: a report of four Japanese cases. Intern Med. 2013;52(9):993–8.

75. Nakayama M, et al. The effect of low-dose corticosteroids on short- and long-term renal outcome in patients with cholesterol crystal embolism. Ren Fail. 2011;33(3):298–306.

76. Keen RR, et al. Surgical management of atheroembolization. J Vasc Surg. 1995;21(5):773–80. discussion 780–1.

77. Shames ML, et al. Treatment of embolizing arterial lesions with endoluminally placed stent grafts. Ann Vasc Surg. 2002;16(5):608–12.

Venous Etiologies of Acute Limb Ischemia

John R. Hoch

Introduction

Acute limb ischemia is a rare complication of deep venous thrombosis (DVT). Phlegmasia cerulea dolens (PCD) and the subsequent development of venous gangrene are rare ischemic events that result from acute massive venous thrombosis of the total or near-total venous outflow of an extremity. Although the incidence of PCD and venous gangrene is unknown, the incidence of all forms of venous thromboembolism (VTE) has been estimated to be as high as one million cases per year in the United States [1]. Upper extremity PCD is rare, compared to lower extremity PCD, occurring in 2–5 % of all reported cases of PCD [2, 3].

PCD patients present with ischemic pain, cyanotic skin discoloration, and massive extremity swelling. Venous outflow obstruction causes massive fluid sequestration in the extremity, leading to shock with resulting mortality rates of 25–40 % [4]. The ischemia with PCD is secondary to venous hypertension and is reversible if treated early and aggressively. However, PCD may progress to irreversible venous gangrene in 40–60 % of patients, resulting in amputation rates of 12–50 % [4–7]. Patients with PCD also have a higher incidence of pulmonary emboli (12–40 %) than patients with submassive deep venous thrombosis, while 30 % of deaths reported from PCD are due to pulmonary embolism [3, 6, 8]. Successful management of both lower and upper extremity PCD is dependent upon early diagnosis, anticoagulation, aggressive fluid resuscitation, and relief of venous hypertension.

J.R. Hoch, MD (✉)
University of Wisconsin School of Medicine and Public Health,
600 Highland Ave., Madison, WI 53592, USA

Pathophysiology

The recognition and understanding of PCD as a clinical entity stretches back to the sixteenth century when, according to Haimovici, Fabricius Hildanus first proposed in 1593 that extremity gangrene could be secondary to venous thrombosis [9]. Hueter, in 1859, was the first to clearly outline the pathologic and clinical criteria for the diagnosis of "gangrene of venous origin" [5]. In 1862, Cruveilhier described accurately that venous thrombosis in these patients involved simultaneous thrombosis of the deep and superficial veins of an extremity [7]. Sixty-two years later, in 1924, Buerger described that gangrene can occur with venous thrombosis without larger artery thrombosis [5]. Fontaine and deSouza-Pereira demonstrated in 1937 that total venous occlusion of the lower extremity in a canine model resulted in gangrene [7]. The next year, Gregoire published a detailed description of ischemic venous thrombosis and used the term phlegmasia cerulea dolens (painful, blue, inflammation) to differentiate the condition from the more common nonischemic presentation of iliovenous thrombosis, termed phlegmasia alba dolens (painful, white, inflammation) [5]. Gregoire hypothesized that arterial spasm was responsible for the development of ischemia; however, his own use of acetylcholine and periarterial sympathectomy failed to achieve limb salvage. Amputation prevented mortality. Other authors in the 1930s, including Leriche, attributed the development of edema and ischemia to peripheral vasospasm [7]. DeBakey and Ochsner, in 1939, found the presence of "arterial spasm" after chemical phlebitis or iliofemoral vein ligation which was relieved by sympathectomy [7]. However by 1949, when they reported the largest series ($n = 56$) of PCD patients published in an American journal to that time, DeBakey and Ochsner attributed the development of ischemia to venous obstruction, stating that vasospasm was a less plausible explanation [10]. Brockman and Vasco created a canine hind limb model of ischemic venous thrombosis consisting of ligation of the entire iliofemoral venous system with the

R.S. Dieter et al. (eds.), *Critical Limb Ischemia*, DOI 10.1007/978-3-319-31991-9_28

filling of the distal veins with inert barium sulfate [8]. The dogs exhibited massive extremity swelling, cyanotic mottling of the skin, loss of distal pulses, tachycardia, and shock, with death ensuing in less than 24 h. No change in anterior tibial arterial pressures or flow amplitudes occurred after venous ligation, indicating no primary role for vasospasm in the development of PCD. The authors concluded that the cause of ischemia with venous occlusion is the collapse of arterioles and small arteries due to the combination of marked increases in tissue pressure, secondary to edema, and a drop in hydrostatic pressure due to shock. While the exact mechanism of ischemia remains unclear, Brockman and Vasco's conclusions are shared by most practitioners today.

Venous obstruction causes changes in the normal homeostasis between the influx and outflow of fluid occurring at the venous and arterial capillary beds. These changes lead to massive sequestration of fluid in the interstitial space, shock, collapse of arterioles and small arteries, and eventually ischemia and gangrene. Normal arterial capillary pressure exceeds the colloid osmotic pressure by 6–7 mmHg, leading to the passage of fluid into the interstitial space. The tissue pressure outside the capillaries is normally near zero. The colloid osmotic pressure at the venous end of the capillary normally exceeds the venous hydrostatic pressure by 11–15 mmHg which forces fluid back into the venous end of the capillary [8]. Massive venous occlusion causes the venous hydrostatic pressure to exceed the osmotic pressure, preventing absorption of fluid at the venous end of the capillary resulting in accumulation of interstitial edema. Venous pressure may increase 16–17-fold within 6 h of occlusion [11]. As the edema progresses, failure of extremity lymphatic outflow compounds the problem. Fluid continues to accumulate until a drop in hydrostatic pressure occurs due to arterial collapse. Interstitial pressures can reach 21–48 mmHg within 48 h after occlusion [8, 11]. Abnormal resting intramuscular compartment pressures in patients with PCD have been measured in the range of 37–70 mmHg [12–14]. The development of acute compartment syndrome with its coincident decrease in arterial perfusion acts as a second cause of ischemia in the extremity. Fasciotomy may improve limb salvage rates in patients with PCD and venous gangrene who develop acute compartment syndrome when combined with anticoagulation; however, fasciotomy is likely most effective if combined with attempts to relieve the venous obstruction [13–15].

Clinical deterioration to a state of shock occurs in patients with PCD due to massive sequestration of fluid in the extremity with venous obstruction. In a canine model of PCD, Brockman and Vasco reported loss of half of the blood volume into the extremity over 8 h. Intravenous volume replacement led to further third spacing of fluid and increased extremity edema. Haller estimated that 6–10 L of edema fluid builds up in a patient's extremity after 3–5 days of venous occlusion [16]. Therefore, rapid, aggressive fluid resuscitation is a critical element of the treatment of PCD.

All the factors contributing to the development of ischemia in patients with PCD are not known with clarity. The generally accepted theory of why ischemia develops in PCD involves a "critical closing pressure" for arteries that once exceeded leads to arterial collapse and subsequent arterial insufficiency and gangrene. Burton proposed that there are two forces at play in the arterial wall, transmural pressure and tension, that when in equilibrium, keep the vessel open [17, 18]. Hydrostatic pressure acts to distend the vessel, while wall tension acts to decrease the vessel's radius. Interstitial pressure normally approaches zero. The transmural pressure is the difference in venous hydrostatic and interstitial pressures. As interstitial pressure rises or hydrostatic pressure drops, the transmural pressure decreases. With venous obstruction, the interstitial and venous hydrostatic pressures initially markedly increase. With the onset of shock, the hydrostatic pressure drops while the interstitial pressure continues to rise. Eventually the transmural pressure will drop to a "critical closing pressure" that is exceeded by the wall tension, leading to vessel collapse [8, 18]. Brockman observed this phenomena in his canine model of PCD and demonstrated that vasospasm did not contribute to ischemia as the hemodynamics were the same after sympathectomy [8].

Etiology

All known risk factors for the development of venous thromboembolism are also associated with phlegmasia cerulean dolens and venous gangrene [18]. Reviews published in the 1960s by Brockman and Vasco and Haimovici found the most common risk factors associated with PCD to be: postoperative state (14–22 %), malignancy (12–18 %), postpartum condition (8–15 %), trauma (6–8 %), history of venous thromboembolism (3–11 %), inflammatory bowel disease (4–5 %), heart failure (5 %), and unknown (9–18 %) [3, 5]. Haimovici noted that patients with venous gangrene had a higher association with malignancy than patients with PCD but without gangrene (25 % vs. 12 %, respectively) [3]. A modern review of 62 patients with PCD identified between 1980 and 2008 found that malignancy is the strongest risk factor (33.9 %) today associated with the development of PCD and venous gangrene (Table 28.1) [4].

Trousseau in 1865 observed the association between malignancy and venous thrombosis when he described recurrent migratory thrombophlebitis in patients with cancer [19]. Patients with cancer have been estimated to have a 4–20 % chance of experiencing venous thrombosis [20]. Abnormalities of blood coagulation have been reported in up to 92 % of cancer patients [19]. Patients have presented with

Table 28.1 Risk factors of phlegmasia cerulea dolens (PCD)

Risk factors	Frequency	Percentage
Malignancy	21	33.9
Hypercoagulable state	9	14.5
Venous stasis	4	6.5
Contraceptive agent	3	4.8
IVC filter	2	3.2
May–Thurner syndrome	2	3.2
Aneurysm	2	3.2
Previous DVT	2	3.2
Trauma	2	3.2
Others	5	8.1
Nonspecified	10	6.1
Total	62	100

Source: From Chinsakchai K, Ten Duis K, Moll FL, et al. Trends in management of phlegmasia cerulea dolens. Vasc Endovasc Surg 2011; 45:5–14. Reprinted by permission of SAGE Publications
IVC inferior vena cava

PCD suffering from numerous types of cancer including pancreatic carcinoma, bronchoadenocarcinoma, testicular cancer, thyroid cancer, renal cell carcinoma, cholangiocarcinoma, and ovarian adenocarcinoma [21]. Between 10 and 16 % of patients with PCD will present without a discernable etiology, but 10 % of them will be diagnosed with a malignancy within 1 year [4, 22, 23]. While the exact pathogenic mechanism for the development of venous thrombosis in cancer patients remains elusive, we know it involves complex interactions between the tumor cell, host cells, and the coagulation system [23]. Tumors activate blood coagulation in part by abnormal expression of high levels of tissue factor (TF). Tissue factor is a constitutively expressed procoagulant, which causes the activation of the patients' extrinsic clotting pathway [24]. In addition to TF, plasma levels of factor VIIa, factor XIIa, and the thrombin–antithrombin complex are elevated in patients with malignancy [25]. Patients with PCD are more likely to progress to venous gangrene if they have cancer [3].

Patients with a hereditary hypercoagulable state (14.5 %; Table 28.1) constitute the second largest group of patients at risk for developing PCD and venous gangrene [4]. Patients with PCD have been diagnosed with factor V Leiden and prothrombin 20210A gene mutations and deficiencies in plasminogen, proteins C and S, and antithrombin [22]. Antiphospholipid syndrome (APS), an acquired thrombophilia, is also associated with the development of PCD. Diagnosis is confirmed after a thrombotic event with the finding of lupus anticoagulant or either anticardiolipin or beta-2-glycoprotein I antibodies [21]. Heparin-induced thrombocytopenia (HIT) may lead to PCD and venous gangrene [26]. Venous thrombosis as a complication of HIT occurs four times more frequently than arterial thrombosis [27]. Warfarin treatment of HIT-associated deep venous thrombosis will lead to progression to venous gangrene in

approximately 10 % of patients [27]. The development of venous gangrene in HIT patients with DVT is thought to be secondary to the warfarin-induced failure of the protein C anticoagulant pathway to downregulate the increased thrombin generation that occurs with HIT.

PCD is known to develop in patients with left common iliac vein compression by the right common iliac artery (May–Thurner syndrome) and in patients with inferior vena cava (IVC) filters [28, 29]. PCD has also been reported to occur in patients who develop DVT around an indwelling femoral venous catheter [30]. In Chinsakchai et al.'s recent review, the combined frequency of venous compression or venous indwelling foreign bodies was 6.4 % in patients with PCD [4]. Other causes of PCD and venous gangrene include immobilization, recent trauma, age, ulcerative colitis, mitral valve stenosis, intravenous drug use, venous stasis, the use of pharmacologic contraception, and pregnancy [4, 15, 18, 21, 22, 26, 28, 31].

PCD is estimated to occur in 2–5 % of patients with upper extremity deep vein thrombosis (UEDVT), while UEDVT accounts for up to 4 % of documented cases of DVT [2, 3, 32]. The etiology of UEDVT can be divided into primary and secondary causes. Primary UEDVT includes cases of effort-induced thrombosis (Paget–Schroetter syndrome) as well as unprovoked UEDVT. Secondary UEDVT accounts for 80 % of all cases [14]. Predisposing secondary factors include central and peripherally inserted central venous catheters (48 %), malignancy (38 %), immobility (14 %), prior DVT (7 %), implanted pacemakers, oral contraceptives, and left ventricular heart failure [14, 33]. Patients with UEDVT with an associated malignancy, hypercoagulable condition, or low cardiac output states are most likely to progress to PCD and/or venous gangrene [14].

Clinical Presentation

Venous thrombosis can be viewed as a disorder with a spectrum of clinical presentations. At its most benign, venous thrombosis presents with painless calf swelling due to calf vein thrombosis. As the thrombus burden extends into the proximal outflow veins of an extremity, the edema becomes more pronounced, the skin is pale, and the limb may be painful. The skin is pale and blanches without cyanosis due to subcutaneous edema without venous congestion. This stage of deep venous thrombosis has been termed phlegmasia alba dolens and is a common clinical presentation of ilio-femoral venous thrombosis [22]. Presentation with phlegmasia alba dolens was termed "milk leg" in the past due the preponderance of pregnant and postpartum woman with the condition presenting with iliac vein thrombosis secondary to uterine compression of the left common iliac vein against the pelvic rim. Patients presenting with phlegmasia alba dolens have significant swelling secondary to outflow obstruction, but they do not suffer from cyanosis and limb ischemia as they have patent venous collaterals. Without adequate therapy, patients with phlegmasia alba dolens will progress to phlegmasia cerulea dolens following the thrombosis of their venous collateral pathways. PCD is preceded by phlegmasia alba dolens in 50–60 % of patients [3, 15, 22].

The clinical presentation of patients with phlegmasia cerulea dolens is the triad of massive extremity swelling, cyanotic to purple skin discoloration, and severe ischemic extremity pain (Fig. 28.1). Although the onset of symptoms may be gradual, the majority of patients present acutely with progressive extremity swelling that takes on a tense and firm quality that is often described as "woody" in character but may be pitting. Ongoing fluid sequestration leads to the development of cutaneous blebs and bullae. Skin cyanosis progresses to mottling and progressive blue/purple skin discoloration. The changes start distally and

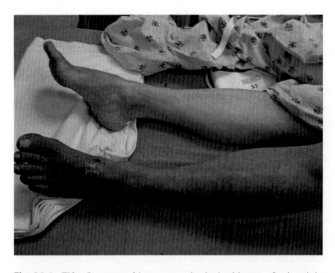

Fig. 28.1 Fifty-five-year-old woman, who had a history of prior right lower extremity deep vein thrombosis, presented to the emergency room complaining of a painful and swollen left lower extremity with bluish discoloration. The patient was found by duplex to have massive deep vein thromboses and no palpable left pedal pulses, consistent with phlegmasia cerulea dolens. From Khandker SR A case of a painful swollen leg. Ann Emerg Med 2012; 59:176,208. Reprinted by permission of Elsevier

progress proximally at varying rates. Bullae and cyanotic changes are most intense in the feet. Pain, due to ischemia, is a constant feature and is often agonizing and difficult to manage successfully. Ischemia is due to the venous obstruction coupled with the massive swelling and in some cases the development of acute compartment syndrome. Pain begins in the calf or femoral triangle but soon affects the entire extremity. Arterial insufficiency is progressive in untreated PCD. Palpable pedal pulses are present only in 17 % of patients with PCD, likely due in part to massive pedal edema [5]. Arterial continuous-wave Doppler signals are usually intact in uncomplicated PCD; however, loss of signals heralds venous gangrene (Table 28.2). The development of sensory and motor impairment occurs as the severity of PCD progresses from uncomplicated to impending gangrene [4]. Chinsakchai et al. graded severity of PCD as noncomplicated, impending venous gangrene and venous gangrene (Table 28.2) [4]. Patients with impending gangrene had changes in motor/sensory function with diminished pulses and skin blistering. Impending gangrene patients had a 22 % mortality and 7 % amputation rate compared to 0 % mortality and 20 % amputation rate in patients with uncomplicated PCD. Venous gangrene patients in their analysis had a 57 % mortality and 43 % amputation rate. The authors concluded that successful treatment outcome correlated with the initial graded severity of PCD and the surgeon's experience, not the type of therapy.

The massive sequestration of fluid in the extremity with PCD can lead to shock as well as to the development of acute compartment syndrome. Patients present with mild to severe shock states with signs of pronounced volume depletion including hypotension, tachycardia, and low urine output that require aggressive fluid resuscitation. Investigators in the 1960s estimated that up to 6–10 L of interstitial fluid loss occurs within 5–10 days of onset of PCD [16]. Fluid sequestration in calf and thigh muscular compartments leads to elevation in resting compartment pressures, with pressures in PCD patients recorded as high as 70 mmHg [12, 13]. Elevated compartment pressures compound the ischemia present secondary to venous obstruction and are the rational for the selective use of fasciotomy in managing patients with PCD [12, 13, 15].

Table 28.2 Grading severity of phlegmasia cerulea dolens

Severity	Cyanosis	Blistering skin	Gangrene	Sensory–motor function	Palpable distal pulses
1. Noncomplicated PCD	Y	N	N	++	++
2. Impending venous gangrene	Y	Y	N	+	+
3. Venous gangrene					
A. Toes or forefoot	Y	Y/N	Y	++/+/−	++/+/−
B. Above ankle	Y	Y/N	Y	−	−

Source: From Chinsakchai K, Ten Duis K, Moll FL, et al. Trends in management of phlegmasia cerulea dolens. Vasc Endovasc Surg 2011; 45:5–14. Reprinted by permission of SAGE Publications
PCD phlegmasia cerulea dolens

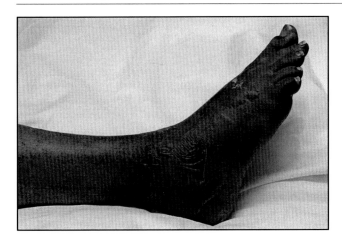

Fig. 28.2 Venous gangrene of the right lower extremity presenting 10 days after the onset of leg swelling. From Rosenbaum AN, ML, Yu RC, Rooke TW, et al. Venous gangrene and intravascular coagulation and fibrinolysis in a patient treated with rivaroxaban. Am J Med 2014; 127:e7-e8. Reprinted by permission of Elsevier

Venous gangrene develops in 40–60 % of patients with PCD with the time of onset usually between 2 and 8 days after developing PCD [3–6]. Gangrenous changes start distally with the majority of patients' gangrene limited to the toes and foot (Fig. 28.2). Gangrenous changes can occur with intact Doppler signals due to thrombosis at the microcirculation level. This has been termed superficial gangrene and occurs in 10–20 % of cases [8]. Gangrene can extend more proximal to the foot involving the musculature of the calf and thigh. The development of venous gangrene has a grim prognosis. Interventions to treat patients presenting with venous gangrene cannot reverse the gangrenous process so they are designed to reverse the ischemia in the extremity and resuscitate the patient. Despite the growing use of less invasive catheter-driven techniques, outcomes of patients with venous gangrene have not improved as evidenced by the recent systematic analysis illustrating 57 % mortality and 43 % amputation rates [4].

Patients with PCD have a higher incidence of pulmonary emboli (12–40 %) than patients with submassive deep venous thrombosis [3, 6, 8]. Patients with venous gangrene have a higher incidence of fatal pulmonary embolism (21 %) than patients with PCD (3.4 %) [3, 22]. Pulmonary embolism is fatal in 50 % of patients with ischemia venous thrombosis and responsible for 30 % of deaths reported from PCD [4, 6]. A recent literature review found that thrombus in patients with PCD localized to the IVC in 35 % of patients and the iliac veins in 50 % [4]. It makes empiric sense that patients with large proximal thrombus burdens would be more likely to develop pulmonary embolism.

Post-thrombotic syndrome (PTS), characterized by the development of pain, edema, venous ectasia, and skin induration of the affected limb, develops within 2 years after an extremity DVT in 23–60 % of patients who have experienced extremity deep vein thrombosis [34]. Some authors have reported that proximal deep vein thrombosis and persistent venous obstruction are risk factors for the development of PTS [35, 36]. Information on developing PTS in patients with PCD or venous gangrene is limited; however, the incidence of PTS has been reported to range between 46 and 94 % [6, 31].

The highest incidence of ischemic venous thrombosis occurs in the fifth and sixth decades, but PCD has been reported in patients from age 6 months to 87 years [3, 37]. Early reports of series of patients with PCD found a higher incidence of PCD in women than men (4:3 ratio) [5]. More recent series of patients reflect an older demographic and reveal a move toward an incidence ratio of PCD in men versus women of 1.5–1 [4, 38]. The left lower extremity is affected more often than the right in patients with PCD [3, 38]. This is felt due to the development of elevated venous pressure secondary to compression of the left common iliac vein as it passes posterior to the right common iliac artery. May and Thurner first described the anatomic variant that bares their name in 1957 [39]. Approximately 22–24 % of the population is felt to have this compressive physiology [15]. The majority of patients with iliac vein compression however are asymptomatic but can have elevated venous pressures placing them at an increased risk for subsequent development of DVT.

Upper extremity ischemic venous thrombosis is rare compared to lower extremity accounting for 2–5 % of all reported cases of PCD/venous gangrene [2, 3]. Haimovici's series of patients presenting with venous gangrene reported a 19 % incidence of upper extremity venous gangrene [3]. Clinical presentation mirrors the signs and symptoms of lower extremity ischemic venous thrombosis (Fig. 28.3). Patients with UEDVT who progress to ischemic venous thrombosis are more likely to have an underlying malignancy, hypercoagulable state, or low cardiac output condition [14, 40, 41]. Smith et al.'s retrospective review of the literature reported that the development of upper extremity venous gangrene was associated in 16 patients with either malignancy (31 %), hematologic abnormality (38 %), HIT (19 %), or IV infusions (44 %) and that 62 % of patients suffered from a severe systemic illness. Patients present with pain and cyanosis that begins in the fingers and progresses proximally. As PCD progresses to venous gangrene, arterial Doppler signals are lost and neurologic deficits ensue [2, 14, 40]. The majority of patients who present with venous gangrene have the combination of central and peripheral venous occlusion [40]. Patients who have central venous occlusion and low cardiac output states account for 12 % of patients. Unlike lower extremity PCD, a small number of patients with upper extremity PCD/venous gangrene do not have central vein (6 %) thrombosis but rather have a history of IV infusion in the affected extremity, peripheral vein thrombosis, and systemic illness causing a low cardiac output state [40]. The most central extent of gangrene

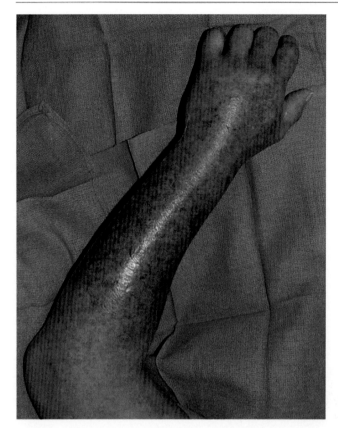

Fig. 28.3 Patient with stage IV non-small cell lung cancer presented to an emergency room with a 48-h history of *left upper extremity* swelling which had progressed over the previous 24 h to become painful, with tense edema and purpuric discoloration consistent with phlegmasia cerulean dolens. From Bedri ML, Khosravi AH, Lifchez SD Upper Extremity Compartment Syndrome in the Setting of Deep Venous Thrombosis and Phlegmasia Cerulea Dolens: Case Report. J Hand Surg 2009; 34:1859–1863. Reprinted by permission of Elsevier

has been reported to be the arm in 12 %, the forearm in 43 %, the hand in 19 %, and the fingers in 25 % [40]. Pulmonary embolisms have been reported in 19 % of upper extremity venous gangrene patients compared to only 1 % of patients with uncomplicated UEDVT [40].

The diagnosis of PCD and venous gangrene can usually be made based on the clinical findings of toxic-appearing patients with massive extremity edema, cyanotic to purple skin discoloration, and extreme pain in the extremity. However, further testing is necessary to confirm the diagnosis as well as to evaluate the extent of thrombus burden, assess for arterial insufficiency, and rule out compartment syndrome. A recent review of imaging modalities in a series of patients with ischemic venous thrombosis found that 37 % of patients underwent duplex ultrasound imaging (DUS), 34 % contrast venography, 15 % computed tomography angiography (CTA), 2 % magnetic resonance venography (MRV), and 26 % a combination of studies [4].

Duplex ultrasound imaging is a rapid, inexpensive, reliable noninvasive way to confirm your clinical diagnosis. White et al. compared DUS against contrast venography for the

diagnosis of proximal deep vein thrombosis and reported a sensitivity of 93 % and a specificity of 98 % for DUS [42]. Disadvantages of DUS include its operator dependence, decreased accuracy in obese patients, and decreased specificity in visualizing the extent of thrombus involving the IVC and iliac veins. Continuous-wave Doppler ultrasound is used for the calculation of ankle/brachial indices to quantify the presence of arterial insufficiency, while DUS color arterial imaging can be used in the PCD patient to noninvasively ascertain arterial anatomy and patency.

Contrast venography historically has been viewed as the "gold standard" to assess venous patency, but today it has been largely replaced by less invasive imaging. In cases of PCD, venography can be nondiagnostic in up to 20–25 % of cases [22]. Venography is expensive and can precipitate venous thrombosis in 2–3 % of cases [22]. Today, venous contrast venography is reserved for use in patients undergoing immediate catheter-directed thrombolysis (CDT), venous thrombectomy, or IVC filter insertion [4]. Contrast venography and CTA both utilize potentially nephrotoxic iodinated contrast whose potential harm is amplified by these patients' severe volume-depleted state.

CTA and MRV are important adjunctive techniques that allow for the characterization of thrombus extension into the IVC, iliac, subclavian, and/or axillary veins while also potentially identifying the precipitating cause for venous thrombosis such as May–Thurner syndrome, Paget–Schroetter syndrome, pelvic mass, or other malignancy. CTA and magnetic resonance imaging have the advantage of also evaluating the arterial vasculature at the same time the venous anatomy is examined (Fig. 28.4).

Recognizing the development of acute compartment syndrome in patients with PCD is critical to their successful management. Leg compartment pressure measurements can be obtained using the wick catheter technique or more simply with the Stryker Intra-Compartmental Pressure Monitor System (Stryker Instruments, Kalamazoo, Michigan). This is a bedside procedure that should be performed early in patient management. Markedly elevated compartment pressures in patients with PCD have been reported to average 50 mmHg in the anterior and 48 mmHg in the deep posterior compartments of the affected leg compared to 6 mmHg in the anterior and 3 mmHg in the deep posterior compartments of the patient's unaffected limb [13].

Treatment

Phlegmasia cerulea dolens and venous gangrene are rare clinical conditions that affect a heterogeneous population of patients making it unlikely that large randomized trials will be performed to establish optimal treatment recommendations to decrease the high mortality and amputation rates associated with these conditions. Evidenced-based treatment

Fig. 28.4 Patients with inferior vena cava thrombosis diagnosed with (**a**) MRV and (**b**) CTA; *arrow* indicates occluded IVC filter

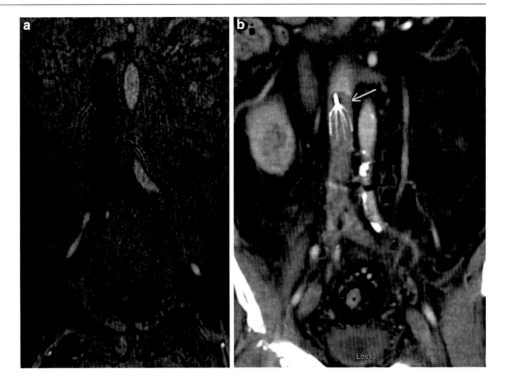

guidelines such as the American College of Chest Physicians (ACCP) Antithrombotic Therapy and Prevention of Thrombosis Guidelines recommend parental anticoagulation with unfractionated heparin for the treatment of uncomplicated iliofemoral deep vein thrombosis in order to decrease the propagation of thrombus and prevent pulmonary embolism (*Grade 1B, Strong Recommendation, Moderate Evidence*) [43]. Patients with PCD and venous gangrene similarly require anticoagulation to arrest thrombus progression and to preserve any patent venous collateral, but heparin has no effect on the venous outflow obstruction that leads to ischemia in the limb. Heparin alone has been shown to be ineffective in the treatment of venous gangrene [38]. PCD is a limb and life-threatening condition that requires aggressive efforts to reduce the thrombus burden in order to relieve the venous outflow obstruction, thus decreasing venous hypertension and limb edema, resulting in relief of ischemia and limb preservation. The authors of the ACCP Guidelines believe that thrombus removal strategies are indicated only in patients with impending venous gangrene despite optimal anticoagulant therapy [43]. Based on a systematic review and meta-analysis comparing the efficacy of systemic anticoagulation, surgical thrombectomy, and catheter-directed thrombolysis (CDT) for the treatment of iliofemoral deep vein thrombosis, the Joint Venous Committee of the Society for Vascular Surgery (SVS) and the American Venous Forum (AVF) published Clinical Practice Guidelines for the use of early thrombus removal strategies for acute deep vein thrombosis [44]. The authors recommend early thrombus removal strategies as the treatment of choice in patients with limb-threatening venous ischemia due to iliofemoral deep venous

thrombosis with or without associated femoropopliteal venous thrombosis (PCD; *Grade 1A, Strong Recommendation, High Level of Evidence*). Thrombus removal strategies include venous surgical or catheter-based thrombectomy, catheter-directed pharmacologic thrombolysis, and pharmacomechanical thrombolysis. An important benefit of iliofemoral thrombus removal compared to conventional anticoagulation alone is the reduction in the incidence of post-thrombotic syndrome [45].

Initial Management

The initial management of PCD includes anticoagulation, aggressive fluid resuscitation, pain management, bed rest, and severe elevation of the affected limb. Anticoagulation is by parental unfractionated heparin unless the PCD is HIT associated. In the setting of DVT and HIT, the ACCP makes weak recommendations for the use of argatroban, lepirudin, or danaparoid over other nonheparin anticoagulants in patients with normal renal function and for argatroban over other nonheparin anticoagulants in patients with impaired renal function (*Grade 2C, Weak Recommendation, Low Level of Evidence*) [46]. While low-molecular-weight heparin (LMWH) is effective in the treatment of proximal deep vein thrombosis and PE, there is no published evidence supporting the use of LMWH in PCD [4]. Limiting activity and severe limb elevation encourages venous drainage through patent collateral veins, if present. We attempt to elevate our patients' limbs at greater than a 45° angle. Severe elevation and anticoagulation may prevent noncomplicated PCD from progressing to impending limb loss [4]. Historically, these measures would be employed for 6–12 h in patients with noncomplicated PCD, reserving thrombus removal strategies for progression of symptoms [38]. Today, the trend is to initiate thrombus removal strategies earlier in the management course. Certainly there is agreement that patients presenting with venous gangrene and patients presenting with or progressing to impending venous gangrene should undergo thrombus removal as soon as they are resuscitated, as restoration of venous outflow is their best strategy to limit their mortality risk and avoid progression to limb loss [44].

Thrombus Removal Strategies

Thrombectomy

The SVS/AVF Guidelines suggest open surgical thrombectomy in selected patients who are candidates for anticoagulation but in who thrombolytic therapy is contraindicated (*Grade 2C, Weak Recommendation, Low Level of Evidence*) [44]. The primary advantage of thrombectomy is the rapid relief of venous and compartmental hypertension, which may prevent venous gangrene [13, 22, 47]. A randomized trial of venous thrombectomy coupled with creation of an arteriovenous fistula reported improved patency, lower venous pressures, less edema, and fewer post-thrombotic symptoms compared to anticoagulation after 10 years of follow-up [48]. Systematic review and meta-analysis by Casey et al. established that compared to anticoagulation, there are significant reductions in the development of post-thrombotic syndrome and venous reflux with surgical thrombectomy and a trend toward reduction in venous obstruction [49]. Disadvantages of open thrombectomy include high rates of rethrombosis, the use of general anesthesia, the more invasive nature of the procedure compared to CDT, the greater risk of complications, and the failure of thrombectomy to restore patency to distal thrombosed venous channels [22, 38]. Meta-analysis yielded no significant effect on mortality compared to anticoagulation [49]. A contemporary review of the use of surgical thrombectomy recorded from the American College of Surgeons National Surgical Quality Improvement Project (ACS NSQIP) database found that the 30-day mortality was 8.8 % and the composite morbidity was 25.3 % [1]. The procedure was combined with fasciotomy in 8.8 % and IVC filter placement in 2.2 %.

The technique of open surgical venous thrombectomy has been standardized over the past 20 years. It is best performed within 48 h of onset of thrombus formation, but the procedure can be successful at up to 7 days. Axial imaging is needed to define the extent of thrombus. Blood loss can be significant so we utilize a cell saver. PE accounts for up to two-thirds of deaths after thrombectomy so the intraoperative use of positive end-expiratory pressure ventilation with general anesthesia and postoperative anticoagulation is recommended [22]. Although controversial, we will place a retrieval IVC filter, via a jugular approach, when thrombus extends into the IVC. After femoral vein exposure, balloon embolectomy catheters are used to treat IVC and iliofemoral thrombus while a 6-in. Esmarch compression wrap is used to squeeze out thrombus from the infrainguinal veins. Plate et al. have demonstrated that the temporary use of a femoral arteriovenous fistula reduces early rethrombosis [48]. We recommend a combination of completion venography and intravascular ultrasound to confirm proximal thrombus removal. Left common iliac compression by the right common iliac artery discovered by completion venography (May–Thurner syndrome) should be treated by placement of a large-diameter self-expanding stent.

Percutaneous thrombectomy is an option for patients who have contraindications to thrombolytic therapy and who are too ill to undergo the general anesthesia required for open venous thrombectomy. Oguzkurt et al. reported a series of seven PCD patients who underwent manual percutaneous aspiration thrombectomy [50]. Patients were anticoagulated with systemic heparin and access obtained in the popliteal vein with a 10-Fr sheath, which was then used for aspiration. Retrievable IVC filters were placed when thrombus extended into the IVC. Manual aspiration successfully cleared the thrombus burden from the popliteal vein to the IVC in all patients. In this series, thrombolysis was used as an adjunct to manual aspiration if some residual nonocclusive thrombus was identified on completion venography.

Percutaneous vacuum-assisted thrombectomy (AngioVac; AngioDynamics, Latham, New York) is an evolving option for the treatment of PCD secondary to IVC thrombosis [51]. The AngioVac cannula is intended for use as a venous drainage cannula during extracorporeal bypass and is also approved for the removal of soft, fresh thrombi or emboli during extracorporeal bypass for up to 6 h (Fig. 28.5). The AngioVac cannula has been used off-label for treatment of IVC thrombosis in the setting of prior IVC filter insertion [51]. The AngioVac cannula is a 22-Fr device that can be inserted percutaneously through a 26-Fr sheath into the common femoral or jugular veins and advanced over a wire, using an internal dilator, into the IVC. Once in place, the tip can be expanded to 48 Fr where it serves as the suction end of a venovenous nonoxygenating bypass circuit that filters removed blood of any aspirated thrombus before returning the blood to the patient via a separate venous cannula. In a series of three patients, all patients had successful aspiration of thrombus and demonstrated clinical improvement (Fig. 28.6) [51]. The AngioVac is too large for treatment of infrainguinal deep vein thrombosis. It is a first-generation device, and users have complained that the rigidity of the cannula makes it difficult to manipulate. It is a labor-intensive procedure requiring time to set up and a pump technician to

Fig. 28.5 The AngioVac
venous drainage system. (**a**)
Schematic of the off-the-shelf
pump, filter, and reperfusion
cannula which allows
aspiration of venous thrombi;
(**b**) aspiration cannula.
AngioDynamics and
AngioVac are trademarks and/
or registered trademarks of
AngioDynamics, Inc. All
photographs are © 2015
AngioDynamics, Inc.

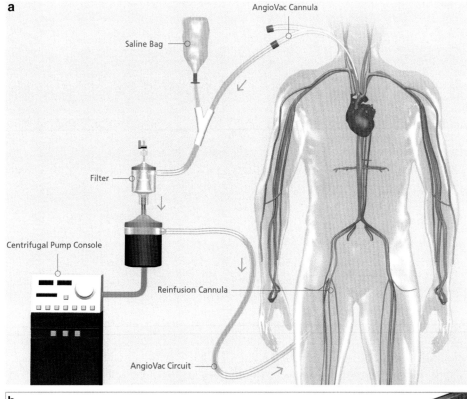

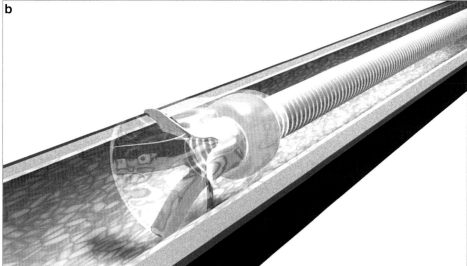

oversee the venovenous circuit. Both the AngioVac procedure and manual aspiration techniques can be used in patients
with contraindications to thrombolysis or used as adjunctive
procedures when thrombolysis has failed.

Catheter-Directed Thrombolysis

The SVS/AVF Guidelines suggest percutaneous catheter-
based technology (pharmacologic or pharmacomechanical)
as first-line therapy for early thrombus removal in patients with
iliofemoral deep vein thrombosis with or without extension
into the IVC (*Grade 2C, Weak Recommendation, Low Level*

of Evidence) [44]. Thrombolytic agents can be infused
directly into thrombus allowing lysis of both major veins and
small veins that would not be reachable by thrombectomy.
Comparing anticoagulation to CDT in patients with iliofemoral deep vein thrombosis, meta-analysis has shown that
CDT results in significant reductions in the risks of post-
thrombotic syndrome, venous reflux, and venous obstruction
[49]. Catheter-directed thrombolysis is associated with complete thrombus resolution in up to 90 % of patients with
PCD [15]. While safer and more efficient than systemic
thrombolysis, CDT is limited by prolonged infusions

Fig. 28.6 (**a**) Image of AngioVac aspiration cannula within the IVC, accessed via right jugular vein, prior to aspiration of venous thrombus from an IVC filter; (**b**) aspirated venous thrombus removed from an occluded IVC via the AngioVac system. AngioDynamics and AngioVac are trademarks and/or registered trademarks of AngioDynamics, Inc. All photographs are © 2015 AngioDynamics, Inc.

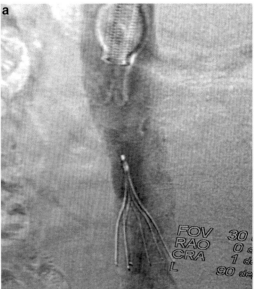 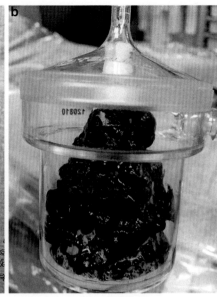

(averaging over 50 h), the necessity for ICU stays, and significant risk of major bleeding complications (8.3 %), including intracranial hemorrhage (0.2 %) [44, 52, 53]. The majority of bleeding complications however occur at the puncture site. Other complications of CDT include pulmonary embolism and recurrent thrombosis. Thery et al. reported that the incidence of PE was increased by CDT secondary to thrombus fragmentation or catheter manipulation [54]. These findings support the use of retrievable IVC filters in select patients undergoing CDT as the risk of PE is high in PCD and thrombolytic therapy acts to increase that risk. The volume of residual thrombus after completion of CDT correlates with the risk of recurrent DVT [55]. Only 5 % of patients with less than 50 % residual thrombus at completion of CDT experienced recurrent DVT compared to a 50 % risk of recurrent DVT in patients found to have >50 % residual thrombus present after CDT [55].

The transpopliteal vein approach is the commonest manner to access the iliofemoral veins and IVC. Alternatively the small saphenous vein, jugular vein, and tibial veins have been used for access. Catheters designed with variable lengths of multi-side-holed segments (Uni-Fuse Infusion Catheter, AngioDynamics, Latham, New York) are positioned within the thrombus. Patients are usually anticoagulated systemically with heparin, but the dose is adjusted to keep the activated partial thromboplastin (aPTT) time between 1.5 and 1.7 times higher than the upper limit of normal [45]. Recombinant tissue plasminogen activator (rt-PA) is then passively infused through the catheter at a dose of 0.5–1.0 mg/h. While the dose range is generally accepted, the total volume administered per hour in the literature ranges from 10 to 100 cc of saline. When treating large-diameter veins, we recommend an initial "pulse-spray" bolus of 2–5 mg rt-PA through the side-holed catheter prior to initiating the infusion. Thrombolytic

infusion times should be minimized by monitoring the thrombolytic process by follow-up venography at 8- to 24-h intervals and stopping therapy once no further lysis is achieved. We follow serum fibrinogen levels, hemoglobin, and aPTT every 6 h during rt-PA infusion.

Pharmacomechanical Thrombolysis

Pharmacomechanical catheter-directed thrombolysis (PCDT) combines CDT with a mechanical device designed to work in conjunction with the thrombolytic agent to achieve shorter thrombolytic infusion times and improve efficacy while decreasing lytic dosage and bleeding complications (Fig. 28.7). The SVS/AVF Guidelines suggest that a strategy of PCDT should be considered over CDT for the management of iliofemoral or IVC thrombosis if expertise and resources are available at your center (*Grade 2C, Weak Recommendation, Low Level of Evidence*) [44]. Pharmacomechanical devices can be categorized as ultrasound enhanced, rotational, or rheolytic. Although rotational and rheolytic devices have been used without thrombolysis, their success at achieving significant (>50 %) thrombus resolution is limited to approximately one-third of patients, leading the SVS/AVF to recommend against using these devices alone [44].

A review of 16 retrospective case series which reported the use of PCDT (rotational, rheolytic, or ultrasound-enhanced devices) in 481 patients found that PCDT resulted in clearing of >50 % of thrombus burden in 83–100 % of patients (Fig. 28.7) [56]. The majority of these studies reported no major bleeding complications and there were no deaths or strokes. Kim et al. retrospectively reported that PCDT achieved complete clot lysis in 84 % of iliofemoral

Fig. 28.7 Patient treated for left lower extremity phlegmasia cerulea dolens by pharmacomechanical catheter-directed thrombolysis (PCDT). (**a**) Patient's left lower extremity upon presentation; (**b**) venogram diagnosed left iliofemoral to popliteal occlusive venous thrombosis; (**c**) digital subtraction arteriogram (DSA) demonstrates resolution of iliofemoral thrombus after PCDT; (**d**) appearance of the left lower extremity 36 h after presentation. From Kalagher SD, Kane DD Phlegmasia cerulean dolens: before and after lysis. Intern Emerg Med 2015; 10:103–104. Reprinted by permission of Springer

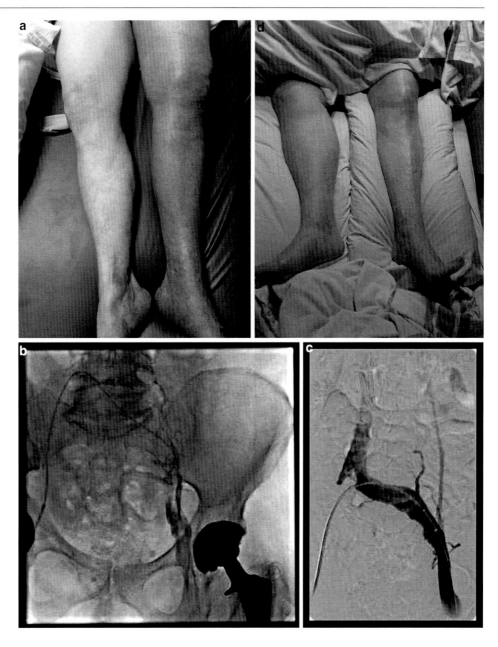

DVT patients compared to 81 % with CDT while doing so with a lower dose of thrombolytic agent and a shorter infusion time (PCDT 30 h vs. CDT 57 h) [57]. After retrospective review of their patients treated by CDT or PCDT, Lin et al. found similar rates of complete venous thrombus removal after CDT (70 %) and PCDT (75 %) [58]. However, significant reductions in intensive care unit and hospital length of stays were noted in the PCDT group, resulting in significant cost reductions [58]. The NIH-funded Acute Venous Thrombosis: Thrombus Removal with Adjunctive Catheter-Directed Thrombolysis (ATTRACT) Trial has recently completed enrollment of 692 patients with proximal DVT of less than 2 weeks duration [59]. Patients were randomized to receive PCDT with anticoagulation or anticoagulation alone.

PCDT consisted of delivery of rt-PA via "isolated thrombolysis" using the Trellis-8 Peripheral Infusion System (Medtronic, Minneapolis, Minnesota) or by "power-pulse thrombolysis" using the AngioJet Rheolytic Thrombectomy System (MEDRAD Interventional-Bayer, Minneapolis, MN) if the popliteal vein was patent [59]. An "infusion-first thrombolysis" strategy that amounted to CDT without an adjunctive device was employed if the popliteal vein was thrombosed. After the initial device and rt-PA treatment, investigators were allowed to continue with CDT for up to 30 h with a maximum dose of 35 mg rt-PA. Investigators were allowed to re-bolus rt-PA and use balloon maceration and aspiration or mechanical thrombectomy to eliminate residual thrombus. Iliac vein stenosis was treated with balloon angioplasty and/or stent placement. Once study follow-up is complete, the ATTRACT Trial will yield important information regarding the safety and efficacy of PCDT, its effects on the development of PTS, quality of life, and recurrent DVT. ATTRACT will have an impact on the management of PCD as speed of thrombus resolution is a critical factor in preventing the development of venous gangrene. Although a description of all available PCDT devices is outside the goals of this chapter, the most commonly used PCDT devices will be described.

Early rotational devices employed a high-velocity helix or nitinol cage to macerate thrombus; however, these types of rotational devices are less commonly used today than a newer version of rotational device, the Trellis-8. The Trellis device is a hybrid infusion catheter that isolates the thrombosed vein between two occluding balloons. Thrombolytic agent is infused into the thrombus between the balloons. A nitinol dispersion wire is inserted into the catheter that causes the catheter to take on a sinusoidal shape, which, when activated, rotates inside the vein at 500–3000 rpm for 5–15 min. This "isolated thrombolysis" technique results in pharmacomechanical lysis of the thrombus which, once liquefied, is aspirated from between the balloons. The advantage of the system is rapid mechanical breakdown of thrombus, while the balloons protect against PE and systemic dissemination of rt-PA. A recent retrospective series established the safety and utility of the Trellis system, reporting complete thrombus resolution in up to 86 % of limbs with a mean treatment time of 25 ± 11.5 min, mean tPA dose of 20.7 ± 12 mg, and no bleeding complications [60]. In another series the Trellis system was effective in 75 % of patients with IVC filter-related acute IVC occlusion, although adjunctive procedures including mechanical thrombectomy and balloon angioplasty were required [61]. Rotational devices have the disadvantage of potentially greater endothelial damage than rheolytic devices due to their mechanism of action. The Trellis device recently underwent factory recall and is currently not available for clinical use in the United States (December 2014).

The AngioJet Rheolytic Thrombectomy System is a catheter system that uses a high-pressure saline jet at the tip of the catheter to create a negative pressure gradient (Bernoulli principle) that acts to fracture thrombus and draw it back into the catheter to be aspirated [58, 62]. Less than one-quarter of patients treated with the AngioJet device alone, without the concomitant use of a thrombolytic agent, achieved >90 % of thrombus clearance [63]. Subsequent modifications of the device created a PCDT system termed the "power-pulse thrombolysis" technique. The catheter is positioned within the venous thrombus after which the aspiration outflow channel is temporarily closed. The device effectively becomes a thrombolytic infusion catheter which then uses its fluid jets at the catheter tip to power-pulse the lytic agent into the

thrombus while the catheter is advanced through the thrombus under fluoroscopic guidance. Once the thrombolytic agent has been power-pulsed into the thrombus, it is allowed to dwell for a minimum of 15 min after which the lytic agent is switched to saline and the outflow channel reopened allowing for thrombus and residual lytic agent aspiration by the device's rheolytic thrombectomy effect. Theoretically the advantage of the AngioJet over rotational devices is that there is less risk of endothelial injury due to minimal direct contact with the vessel wall. Hemolysis and hemoglobinuria are known complications of rheolytic thrombectomy which is magnified by prolonged AngioJet run times, especially in the IVC or iliac veins. It is recommended that the catheter should be run in 5-s intervals to minimize the risk of hemolysis [56]. Consequences of hemolysis after AngioJet therapy include renal insufficiency, pancreatitis, bradyarrhythmias, and hypotension [62, 64, 65]. Bradyarrhythmias, including bradycardia and asystole, have been reported in up to 12 % of patients with proximal DVT treated with the AngioVac device [64]. The mechanism is likely secondary to adenosine and potassium release due to hemolysis, although right heart stretch receptor activation due to cyclical high-pressure gradients is an alternative hypothesis.

In a retrospective series of patients with DVT, Lin et al. compared outcomes after CDT versus PCDT with the AngioJet device [58]. Complete thrombus resolution occurred in 75 % patients with PCDT and 70 % with CDT (NS). However, AngioJet PCDT patients had a significantly shorter ICU and hospital stays. Importantly, the mean thrombolytic infusion time for the AngioJet group was 76 ± 34 min versus 18 ± 8 h in the CDT group. There was no difference in long-term patency between groups. The Peripheral Use of AngioJet Rheolytic Thrombectomy with a Variety of Catheter Lengths (PEARL) registry was subsequently established to document procedural and patient outcomes with PCDT and the AngioJet device [62]. The PEARL registry reported that 95 % of patients initially treated by AngioJet PCDT achieved >50 % thrombus resolution and 58 % obtained 100 % of thrombus removal, with a median procedure time of 2 h. After the initial power-pulse technique, the addition of CDT was required in 61 % of patients. Overall 73 % of patients had their clot removal procedure completed within 24 h, and one-third required less than 6 h. The current retrospective and registry data suggest more rapid thrombus resolution occurs with PCDT compared to CDT, and it is this thrombus removal strategy that is recommended for patients with phlegmasia cerulean dolens and venous gangrene, where time is of the essence.

High-frequency, low-power ultrasound energy has been shown to disrupt the structure of venous thrombus, rendering it more susceptible to thrombolytic agents without fragmenting the clot [66]. Low-energy ultrasound disassociates fibrin strands to allow more effective thrombolysis with shorter and lower-dose administration [66–68]. The EkoSonic Endovascular System (EKOS; EKOS Corp, Bothell, WA) combines a multi-holed infusion catheter, through which tPA is infused, combined with a filament placed in the catheter's lumen, which contains multiple miniature ultrasound transducers placed along its treatment length. In addition to disassociating fibrin strands, the ultrasound waves drive the tPA away from the catheter and into the thrombus. EKOS has proven successful in treating both lower and upper extremity deep vein thromboses with complete clot lysis achieved in 54–85 % of patients (Fig. 28.8) [67, 68]. Successful thrombolysis rates of 92 % (50 % complete lysis) were seen with EKOS treatment of patients with chronic DVT (mean of 92d) [67]. A retrospective review comparing EKOS to standard CDT for treatment of iliofemoral deep vein thrombosis found similar resolution of thrombus load between treatment groups [69]. Although EKOS' mechanism of action would suggest that the EKOS treated patients would require lower doses of thrombolytic agent and shorter treatment times compared to CDT, there were no differences between groups. Therefore, we await a randomized trial comparing EKOS to CDT for the treatment of iliofemoral and/or IVC thrombus before its use is widely adapted.

Fig. 28.8 Treatment of IVC and iliofemoral thrombosis by PCDT using the EkoSonic Endovascular System (EKOS). (**a**) MRV demonstrating IVC and bilateral iliac vein thrombosis with an occluded IVC filter; (**b**) DSA of occluded left iliac and IVC, accessed from femoral vein; (**c**) EKOS catheter in position across occlusion; (**d**) DSA of patent IVC and left iliac system after PCDT. The left iliac stenosis was treated with a self-expanding stent (image not shown) (EKOS; EKOS Corp, Bothell, WA)

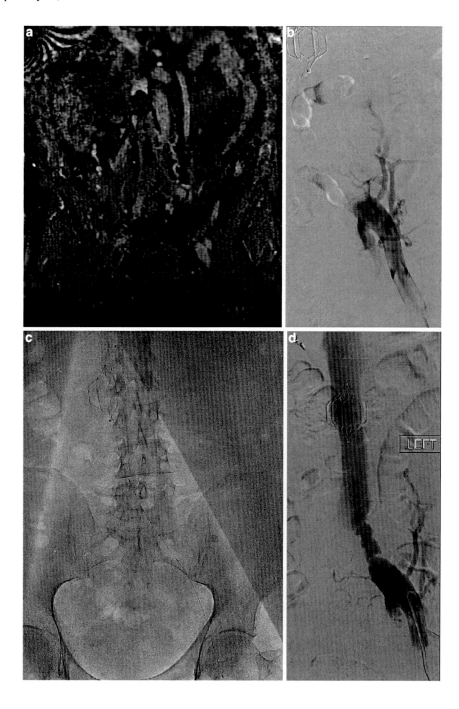

Thrombus removal strategies are as equally important in cases of upper extremity venous ischemia as they are for managing lower extremity PCD/venous gangrene. After systemic anticoagulation, venous thrombectomy, CDT, and PCDT have all been employed as attempts to remove the central venous obstruction, which is usually present, in an attempt to achieve limb preservation by relieving venous hypertension [2, 3, 14, 32, 40, 70]. In modern series, PCDT and CDT have become the favored treatment options over open thrombectomy [2, 14, 32, 40, 70]. In patients with both central and peripheral thromboses, it is recommended that thrombolysis be initiated to treat both the central and also the peripheral venous thrombi [32, 40, 70]. In the uncommon event of upper extremity PCD developing without central venous obstruction, the use of intra-arterial thrombolytic therapy has been proposed as a therapeutic option [40, 71].

Adjunctive Management Strategies

Periprocedural IVC Filters

The SVS/AVF Guidelines recommend against routine use of IVC filters in conjunction with CDT of iliofemoral venous thrombosis for the prevention of pulmonary embolism (Grade 1C) [44]. However, they also recommended that the risks vs. benefits of periprocedural retrievable IVC filters be considered in patients undergoing PCDT or who have IVC thrombus or markedly limited cardiac reserve (*Grade 2C, Weak Recommendation, Low Level of Evidence*) [44]. A prospective, randomized trial has shown that for the treatment of proximal DVT in patients considered to be at high risk, the combination of anticoagulation plus a permanent IVC filter was associated with a significantly lower risk of PE (1.1%) at 12 days compared to the anticoagulation alone group (4.8%) [72]. However, the filter group had a significantly higher risk of recurrent thrombosis at 2 years (20.8%) than the anticoagulation alone group (11.6%). The National Venous Registry reported only a 1% risk of PE in patients undergoing CDT, of which 71% had iliofemoral thrombus [73]. These findings suggest against the routine use of IVC filters if treating uncomplicated iliofemoral DVT with CDT. There is a lack of data to inform us of the risk of PE associated with the newer PCDT techniques. Case series suggest a low incidence of PE associated with PCDT; however, symptomatic PE has been reported [44, 74]. Patients presenting with PCD are considered a high-risk group as 12–40% of patients with venous ischemia develop symptomatic PE compared to approximately 7% of patients with uncomplicated iliofemoral venous thrombosis treated with anticoagulation [3, 6, 8, 75]. We recommend consideration of the use of periprocedural retrievable IVC filters in patients with venous ischemia undergoing PCDT because the morbidity of the filter is low and the baseline risk of PE in patients with venous ischemia is high.

Venous Stents

The SVS/AVF Guidelines recommend the use of self-expanding metallic stents for the treatment of iliocaval compressive or obstructive lesions identified after successful venous thrombus removal (*Grade 1C, Strong Recommendation, Low Level of Evidence*) [44]. Following thrombus removal by PCDT, CDT, or thrombectomy, venography is performed to identify any residual iliac vein stenosis or compression [44]. Lin et al. reported residual venous stenosis treated by balloon angioplasty and/or stenting in 82% and 78% of patients treated by PCDT and CDT, respectively [58]. The National Venous Registry reported that 33% of limbs treated by CDT required stent placement [73]. Stent placement in the iliac vein resulted in a 1-year patency rate of 74% compared with 53% for limbs without stents. Pull-back iliac venous pressures can be used to confirm the diagnosis of venous obstruction and assess the adequacy of therapy. Xue et al. demonstrated a significant drop in iliac vein pressures from 7.2 ± 4.6 cm H_2O prior to stenting down to 1.8 ± 2.8 cm H_2O after stenting [76]. Large diameter, flexible self-expanding stents should be used to treat regions of iliocaval narrowing. Intravascular ultrasound can aid in precise stent placement as it is more sensitive than venography [44]. The National Venous Registry reported that femoropopliteal venous stenting resulted in an 80% occlusion rate at 70 days; the SVS/AVF Guidelines recommend against stenting the femoral and popliteal veins (Grade 2C).

Fasciotomy in PCD

Lower extremity fasciotomy was commonly performed as an initial treatment strategy after anticoagulation in early series of patients with PCD and venous gangrene as it achieved significant decreases in interstitial pressures and improvement in venous outflow [3, 5, 7]. At the time, fasciotomy for PCD and venous gangrene patients was felt to be critical to avoid limb loss as it could be performed quickly before resorting to venous thrombectomy. Today thrombus removal strategies have replaced fasciotomy as the accepted management for venous ischemia. The trend toward faster relief of venous obstruction has continued as CDT and PCDT procedure times have dropped from a mean of over 50 h to where now 58% of limbs can obtain 100% of thrombus removal with a median procedure time of 2 h [44, 52, 53, 62]. Usually successful thrombus removal leads to decreases in compartment pressures. The SVS/AVF guidelines recommend fasciotomy if compartment pressures remain elevated (>30 mmHg) despite the attempt to relieve venous outflow obstruction (*Grade 2C, Weak Recommendation, Low Level of Evidence*) [44]. Although bleeding complications are common if CDT is continued after fasciotomy, the risk of bleeding should not deter the use of fasciotomy if the limb continues to be at risk after thrombus removal strategies have been attempted.

Although reports of the management of upper extremity PCD are rare, there does appear to be a consensus to consider fasciotomy treatment for acute compartment syndrome early in the course of the disease as elevated compartment pressures and neurologic deficits often develop prior to loss of arterial Doppler signals. Fasciotomy is not a substitute for thrombus removal, but it may be especially useful in patients with upper extremity PCD who do not have central venous thrombosis.

Role of Amputation

Extremity ischemia and gangrene of venous etiology differ from arterial ischemia and gangrene by the nature of the mechanism of ischemia as well as the clinical presentation and clinical course. Arterial ischemia occurs due to arterial blockage resulting in direct decrease in tissue perfusion resulting in deep tissue necrosis. Venous ischemia occurs due to venous obstruction with loss of collateral and the development of venous hypertension and fluid sequestration, which leads to small vessel collapse and eventual thrombosis starting at the microcirculatory level. Patients with arterial ischemia present with cool limbs, absence of swelling, skin pallor, and delayed capillary refill, while patients with venous ischemia have normal skin temperature, massive swelling, blue to purple skin color, and fast capillary refill. Patients with longer than 6 h of arterial ischemia will begin to have irreversible damage to nerves and muscle, which results in the need for amputation if arterial flow is not restored in short order. The onset of venous gangrene can be more insidious than arterial gangrene, and no evidence-based guidelines exist to guide the surgeon in the timing of interventions designed to relieve extremity venous hypertension. The gangrene that develops due to venous etiology is often more superficial than the deep tissue necrosis of arterial ischemia. Haimovici reported that 60 % of survivors of venous gangrene required only minor amputation or debridement and skin grafting [3]. Delay in arterial reconstruction or amputation in arterial ischemia can lead to myonecrosis and systemic consequences. In contrast, because of the common superficial nature of venous gangrene, amputation is delayed as long as possible while interventions are performed to restore venous outflow, allowing swelling to decrease and letting demarcation to occur.

Long-Term Management

The SVS/AVF Guidelines recommend that patients managed by early thrombus removal should be anticoagulated, according to the ACCP anticoagulation guidelines, with an initial course of unfractionated or low-molecular-weight heparin followed by oral anticoagulation (*Grade 1A, Strong*

Recommendation, High Level of Evidence) [43, 44]. The duration of anticoagulation should be a minimum of 90 days but is ultimately dependent upon the patient's risk factors. Every attempt should be made to identify the underlying medical condition that led to the onset of PCD. Anticoagulation should be extended for 6–12 months or until the identified risk factor is resolved. If the venous thrombosis was unprovoked or if risk factors are nonreversible, anticoagulation should be continued lifelong.

Patients with venous ischemia successfully treated with anticoagulation and thrombus removal are at high risk of developing post-thrombotic syndrome. The use of knee-length, 30–40 mmHg graduated compression stockings has been shown to reduce by 50 % he 2-year incidence of post-thrombotic syndrome [77]. Thus, the SVS/AVF Guidelines support the use of graduated elastic compression stockings for a minimum of 2 years after proximal venous thrombosis (*Grade 1A, Strong Recommendation, High Level of Evidence*) [44].

Conclusion

Phlegmasia cerulea dolens is a rare fulminant form of acute massive extremity venous thrombosis that progresses to venous gangrene unless it is recognized and treated early in its course. Venous ischemia historically carries a mortality risk of 25–40 % with an amputation rate of 12–50 % [4–7]. Modern management incorporates early diagnosis, aggressive volume resuscitation, anticoagulation, and the use of endovascular or open thrombus removal strategies that are capable of rapid resolution of obstructing thrombus. The ACCP and the Joint Guideline Committee of the SVS and AVF have published evidence-based treatment guidelines for the management of venous ischemia. Adoption of their recommendations may lead to improved clinical outcomes for patients presenting with PCD and venous gangrene.

References

1. Davenport DL, Xenos ES. Early outcomes and risk factors in venous thrombectomy: an analysis of the American College of Surgeons NSQIP dataset. Vasc Endovascular Surg. 2001;45(4):325–8.
2. Kammen BF, Soulen MC. Phlegmasia cerulea dolens of the upper extremity. J Vasc Interv Radiol. 1995;6(2):283–6.
3. Haimovici H. The ischemic forms of venous thrombosis. 1. Phlegmasia cerulea dolens. 2. Venous gangrene. J Cardiovasc Surg (Torino). 1965; 5(6):Suppl: 164–73.
4. Chinsakchai K, Ten Duis K, Moll FL, de Borst GJ. Trends in management of phlegmasia cerulea dolens. Vasc Endovascular Surg. 2011;45(1):5–14.
5. Brockman SK, Vasko JS. Phlegmasia cerulea dolens. Surg Gynecol Obstet. 1965;121(6):1347–56.
6. Veltchev LM, Kalniev MA, Todorov TA. Phlegmasia cerulea dolence- risk factors and prevention. Case report. J IMAB. 2009; 15(1):89–91.

7. Stallworth JM, Bradham GB, Kletke RR, Price Jr RG. Phlegmasia cerulea dolens: a 10-year review. Ann Surg. 1965;161:802–11.

8. Brockman SK, Vasko JS. The pathologic physiology of phlegmasia cerulea dolens. Surgery. 1966;59(6):997–1007.

9. Haimovici H. Gangrene of the extremities of venous origin; review of the literature with case reports. Circulation. 1950;1(2): 225–40.

10. DeBakey M, Ochsner A. Phlegmasia cerulean dolens and gangrene associated with thrombophlebitis. Surgery. 1949;26:16.

11. Snyder MA, Adams JT, Schwartz SI. Hemodynamics of phlegmasia cerulea dolens. Surg Gynecol Obstet. 1967;125:342–6.

12. Mesfin A, Lum YW, Nayfeh T, Mears SC. Compartment syndrome in patients with massive venous thrombosis after inferior vena cava filter placement. Orthopedics. 2011;34(3):229.

13. Qvarfordt P, Eklöf B, Ohlin P. Intramuscular pressure in the lower leg in deep vein thrombosis and phlegmasia cerulae dolens. Ann Surg. 1983;197(4):450–3.

14. Bedri MI, Khosravi AH, Lifchez SD. Upper extremity compartment syndrome in the setting of deep venous thrombosis and phlegmasia cerulea dolens: case report. J Hand Surg Am. 2009;34(10):1859–63.

15. Suwanabol PA, Tefera G, Schwarze ML. Syndromes associated with the deep veins: phlegmasia cerulea dolens, May-Thurner syndrome, and nutcracker syndrome. Perspect Vasc Surg Endovasc Ther. 2010;22(4):223–30.

16. Haller JA. Effects of deep femoral thrombophlebitis on the circulation of the lower extremities. Circulation. 1963;27:693–8.

17. Burton AC. On the physical equilibrium of small blood vessels. Am J Physiol. 1951;164(2):319–29.

18. Anderson Jr FA, Spencer FA. Risk factors for venous thromboembolism. Circulation. 2003;107(23 Suppl 1):I9–16.

19. Rickles FR, Edwards RL. Activation of blood coagulation in cancer: Trousseau's syndrome revisited. Blood. 1983;62(1):14–31.

20. Khorana AA, Francis CW, Culakova E, Kuderer NM, Lyman GH. Thromboembolism is a leading cause of death in cancer patients receiving outpatient chemotherapy. J Thromb Haemost. 2007;5(3):632–4.

21. Change G, Yeh JJ. Fulminant phlegmasia cerulea dolens with concurrent cholangiocarcinoma and a lupus anticoagulant: a case report and review of the literature. Blood Coagul Fibrinolysis. 2014;25(5):507–11.

22. Perkins JM, Magee TR, Galland RB. Phlegmasia cerulea dolens and venous gangrene. Br J Surg. 1996;83(1):19–23.

23. Elyamany G, Alzahrani AM, Bukhary E. Cancer-associated thrombosis: an overview. Clin Med Insights Oncol. 2014;8:129–37.

24. Mackman N. Role of tissue factor in hemostasis, thrombosis, and vascular development. Arterioscler Thromb Vasc Biol. 2004;24(6):1015–22.

25. Kakkar AK, DeRuvo N, Chinswangwatanakul V, Tebbutt S, Williamson RC. Extrinsic-pathway activation in cancer with high factor VIIa and tissue factor. Lancet. 1995;343(8981):1004–5.

26. Warkentin TE, Elavathil LJ, Hayward CP, Johnston MA, Russett JI, Kelton JG. The pathogenesis of venous limb gangrene associated with heparin induced thrombocytopenia. Ann Intern Med. 1997;127(9):804–12.

27. Warkentin TE. Venous thromboembolism in heparin-induced thrombocytopenia. Curr Opin Pulm Med. 2000;6(4):343–51.

28. Shem K. Phlegmasia cerulea dolens: rare complication of vena cava filter placement in man with paraplegia. J Spinal Cord Med. 2008;31(4):398–402.

29. Bazan HA, Reiner E, Sumpio B. Management of bilateral phlegmasia cerulea dolens in patient with subacute splenic laceration. Ann Vasc Dis. 2008;1(1):45–8.

30. Wood KE, Reedy JS, Pozniak MA, Coursin DB. Phlegmasia cerulea dolens with compartment syndrome: a complication of femoral vein catheterization. Crit Care Med. 2000;28(5):1626–30.

31. Cohen DJ, Briggs R, Head HD, Acher CW. Phlegmasia cerulea dolens and its association with hypercoagulable states: case reports. Angiology. 1989;40(5):498–508.

32. Muñoz FJ, Mismetti P, Poggio R, Valle R, Barrón M, Guli M, et al. Clinical outcome of patients with upper-extremity deep vein thrombosis: results from the RIETE Registry. Chest. 2008;133(1): 143–8.

33. Sullivan VV, Wolk SW, Lampman RM, Prager RL, Hankin FM, Whitehouse Jr WM. Upper extremity venous gangrene following coronary artery bypass. A case report and review of literature. J Cardiovasc Surg (Torino). 2001;42(4):551–4.

34. Ashrani AA, Heit JA. Incidence and cost burden of post-thrombotic syndrome. J Thromb Thrombolysis. 2009;28(4):465–76.

35. Prandoni P, Frulla M, Sartor D, Concolato A, Girolami A. Vein abnormalities and the post-thrombotic syndrome. J Thromb Haemost. 2005;3(2):401–2.

36. Stain M, Schönaueer V, Minar E, Bialonczyk C, Hirschl M, Weltermann A, et al. The post-thrombotic syndrome: risk factors and impact on the course of thrombotic disease. J Thromb Haemost. 2005;3(12):2671–6.

37. Hirschmann JV. Ischemic forms of acute venous thrombosis. Arch Dermatol. 1987;123(7):933–6.

38. Weaver FA, Meacham PW, Adkins RB, Dean RH. Phlegmasia cerulea dolens: therapeutic considerations. South Med J. 1988;81(3):306–12.

39. May R, Thurner J. The cause of the predominantly sinistral occurrence of thrombosis of the pelvic veins. Angiology. 1957;8(5): 419–27.

40. Levy MM, Bach C, Fisher-Snowden R, Pfeifer JD. Upper extremity deep venous thrombosis: reassessing the risk for subsequent pulmonary embolism. Ann Vasc Surg. 2011;25(4):442–7.

41. Smith BM, Shield GW, Riddell DH, Snell JD. Venous gangrene of the upper extremity. Ann Surg. 1985;201(4):511–9.

42. White RH, McGahan JP, Daschbach MM, Hartling RP. Diagnosis of deep-vein thrombosis using duplex ultrasound. Ann Intern Med. 1989;111(4):297–304.

43. Kearon C, Akl EA, Comerota AJ, Prandoni P, Bounameaux H, Goldhaber SZ, et al. Antithrombotic therapy for VTE disease: antithrombotic therapy and prevention of thrombosis, 9th ed: American College of Chest Physicians evidence-based clinical practice guidelines. Chest. 2012;141(2 Suppl):e419s–94.

44. Meissner MH, Gloviczki P, Comerota AJ, Dalsing MC, Eklöf BG, Gillespie DL, et al. Early thrombus removal strategies for acute deep venous thrombosis: clinical practice guidelines of the Society for Vascular Surgery and the American Venous Forum. J Vasc Surg. 2012;55(5):1449–62.

45. Enden T, Haig Y, Kløw NE, Slagsvold CE, Sandvik L, Ghanima W, et al. Long-term outcome additional catheter-directed thrombolysis versus standard treatment for acute iliofemoral deep vein thrombosis (the CaVenT study): a randomised controlled trial. Lancet. 2012;379(9810):31–8.

46. Linkins LA, Dans AL, Moores LK, Bona R, Davidson BL, Schulman S, et al. Treatment and prevention of heparin-induced thrombocytopenia: antithrombotic therapy and prevention of thrombosis, 9th ed: American College of Chest Physicians evidence-based clinical practice guidelines. Chest. 2012;141(2 Suppl):3e495S–530.

47. Comerota AJ, Paolini D. Treatment of acute iliofemoral deep venous thrombosis: a strategy of thrombosis removal. Eur J Vasc Endovasc Surg. 2007;33(3):351–60.

48. Plate G, Eklöf BG, Norgren L, Ohlin P, Dahlström JA. Venous thrombectomy for iliofemoral vein thrombosis—10-year results of a prospective randomized study. Eur J Vasc Endovasc Surg. 1997;14(5):367–74.

49. Casey ET, Murad MH, Zumaeta-Garcia M, Elamin MB, Shi Q, Edwin PJ, et al. Treatment of acute iliofemoral deep vein thrombosis. J Vasc Surg. 2012;55(5):1463–73.

50. Oguzkurt L, Ozkan U, Demirturk OS, Gur S. Endovascular treatment of phlegmasia cerulea dolens with impending venous gangrene: manual aspiration thrombectomy as the first-line thrombus removal method. Cardiovasc Intervent Radiol. 2011;34(6): 1214–21.

51. Smith SJ, Behrens G, Sewall LE, Sichlau MJ. Vacuum-assisted thrombectomy device (AngioVac) in the management of symptomatic iliocaval thrombosis. J Vasc Interv Radiol. 2014; 25(3):425–30.

52. Baldwin ZK, Comerota AJ, Schwartz LB. Catheter-directed thrombolysis for deep venous thrombosis. Vasc Endovascular Surg. 2004;38(1):1–9.

53. Vedantham S, Sista AK, Klein SJ, Nayak L, Razavi MK, Kalva SP, et al. Quality improvement guidelines for the treatment of lower-extremity deep vein thrombosis with use of endovascular thrombus removal. J Vasc Interv Radiol. 2014;25(9):1317–25.

54. Thery C, Asseman P, Amrouni N, Becquart J, Pruvost P, Lesenne M, et al. Use of a new removable vena cava filter in order to prevent pulmonary embolism in patients submitted to thrombolysis. Eur Heart J. 1990;11(4):334–41.

55. Aziz F, Comerota AJ. Quantity of residual thrombus after successful catheter-directed thrombolysis for iliofemoral deep venous thrombosis correlates with recurrence. Eur J Vasc Endovasc Surg. 2012;44(2):210–3.

56. Karthikesalingam A, Young EL, Hinchilffe RJ, Loftus IM, Thompson MM, Holt PJ, et al. A systematic review of percutaneous mechanical thrombectomy in the treatment of deep venous thrombosis. Eur J Vasc Endovasc Surg. 2011;41(4):554–65.

57. Kim HS, Patra A, Paxton BE, Khan J, Streiff MB. Adjunctive percutaneous mechanical thrombectomy for lower-extremity deep vein thrombosis: clinical and economic outcomes. J Vasc Interv Radiol. 2006;17(7):1099–104.

58. Lin P, Zhou W, Dardik A, Mussa F, Kougias P, Hedayati N, et al. Catheter-direct thrombolysis versus pharmacomechanical thrombectomy for treatment of symptomatic lower extremity deep venous thrombosis. Am J Surg. 2006;192(6):782–8.

59. Vedantham S, Goldhaber SZ, Kahn SR, Julian J, Magnuson E, Jaff MR, et al. Rationale and design of the ATTRACT study: a multicenter randomized trial to evaluate pharmacomechanical catheter-directed thrombolysis for the prevention of postthrombotic syndrome in patients with proximal deep vein thrombosis. Am Heart J. 2013;165(4):523–30.

60. Chaudhry MA, Pappy R, Hennebry TA. Use of the trellis device in the management of deep vein thrombosis: a retrospective single-center experience. J Invasive Cardiol. 2013;25(6):296–9.

61. Branco BC, Montero-Baker MF, Espinoza E, Gamero M, Zea R, Labropoulos N, et al. Pharmacomechanical thrombolysis in the management of acute inferior vena cava filter occlusion using the trellis-8 device. J Endovasc Ther. 2015;22(1):99–104.

62. Garcia MJ, Lookstein R, Malhotra R, Amin A, Blitz LR, Leung DA, et al. Endovascular management of deep vein thrombosis with rheolytic thrombectomy: final report of the prospective multicenter PEARL registry. J Vasc Interv Radiol. 2015;26:777–85. S1051-0443(15)00164-5.

63. Kasirajan K, Gray B, Ouriel K. Percutaneous AngioJet thrombectomy in the management of extensive deep venous thrombosis. J Vasc Interv Radiol. 2001;12(2):179–85.

64. Jeyabalan G, Saba S, Baril DT, Makaroun MS, Chaer RA. Bradyarrhythmias during rheolytic pharmacomechanical thrombectomy for deep vein thrombosis. J Endovasc Ther. 2010;17(3): 416–22.

65. Lebow M, Cassada D, Grandas O, Stevens S, Goldman M, Freeman M. Acute pancreatitis as a complication of percutaneous mechanical thrombectomy. J Vasc Surg. 2007;46(2):366–8.

66. Braaten JV, Goss RA, Francis CW. Ultrasound reversibly disaggregates fibrin fibers. Thromb Haemost. 1997;78(3):1063–8.

67. Dumantepe M, Tarhan A, Yurdakul I, Özler A. US-accelerated catheter-directed thrombolysis for the treatment of deep venous thrombosis. Diagn Interv Radiol. 2013;19(3):251–8.

68. Grommes J, Strijkers R, Greiner A, Mahnken AH, Wittens CH. Safety and feasibility of ultrasound-accelerated catheter-directed thrombolysis in deep vein thrombosis. Eur J Vasc Endovasc Surg. 2011;41(4):526–32.

69. Baker R, Samuels S, Benenati JF, Powell A, Uthoff H. Ultrasound-accelerated vs standard catheter-directed thrombolysis—a comparative study in patients with iliofemoral deep vein thrombosis. J Vasc Interv Radiol. 2012;23(11):1460–6.

70. Lessne ML, Bajwa J, Hong K. Fatal reperfusion injury after thrombolysis for phlegmasia cerulea dolens. J Vasc Interv Radiol. 2012;23(5):681–6.

71. Wlodarczyk ZK, Gibson M, Dick R, Hamilton G. Low-dose intra-arterial thrombolysis in treatment of phlegmasia cerulea dolens. Br J Surg. 1994;81(3):370–2.

72. Decousus H, Leizorovicz A, Parent F, Page Y, Tardy B, Girard P, et al. A clinical trial of vena caval filters in the prevention of pulmonary embolism in patients with proximal deep-vein thrombosis. Prévention du Risque d'Embolie Pulmonaire par Interrupption Cave Study Group. N Engl J Med. 1998;338(7):409–15.

73. Mewissen MW, Seabrook GR, Meissner MH, Cynamon J, Labropoulos N, Haughton SH. Catheter-directed thrombolysis for lower extremity deep venous thrombosis: report of a national multicenter registry. Radiology. 1999;211(1):39–49.

74. Protack CD, Bakken AM, Patel N, Saad WE, Waldman DL, Davies MG. Long-term outcomes of catheter directed thrombolysis for lower extremity deep venous thrombosis without prophylactic inferior vena cava filter placement. J Vasc Surg. 2007;45(5):992–7.

75. Partsch H. Therapy of deep vein thrombosis with low molecular weight heparin, leg compression and immediate ambulation. Vasa. 2001;30(3):195–204.

76. Xue GH, Huang XZ, Ye M, Liang W, Zhang H, Zhang JW, et al. Catheter-directed thrombolysis and stenting in the treatment of iliac vein compression syndrome with acute iliofemoral deep vein thrombosis: outcome and follow-up. Ann Vasc Surg. 2014;28(4): 957–63.

77. Padoni P, Lensing AW, Prins MH, Frulla M, Marchiori A, Bernardi E, et al. Below-knee elastic compression stockings to prevent the post-thrombotic syndrome: a randomized, controlled trial. Ann Intern Med. 2004;141:249–56.

Malignant and Benign Tumor-Induced Critical Limb Ischemia

29

Raymond A. Dieter, Jr., George B. Kuzycz,
Marcelo C. DaSilva, Raymond A. Dieter, III,
Anthony M. Joudi, and Morgan M. Meyer

Extremity ischemia represents one of the most devastating disabilities an individual may develop. The usual cause for critical circulatory ischemia is related to disease developing in an elderly individual. These diseases include the arteriosclerotic and diabetic conditions in a large proportion of the older patients. However, other causes of circulatory concerns may also develop on occasion. The less commonly occurring etiologies for critical limb ischemia involve both large and small vessel maladies. These include such lesions as the non-atherosclerotic arteriopathies, including Buerger's disease, vasculitis (large, medium, and small vessel), congenital abnormalities, and peripheral aneurysms [1].

The diagnoses of malignancy may also be a harbinger of serious and life-threatening events to come. Seldom does one consider malignancy as the cause of or to be associated with critical ischemia, gangrene, or loss of an extremity due to circulatory concerns. However, this situation does occur on occasion and may lead to loss of digits, an extremity, or even vascular-associated death. When one combines the two—ischemia of the extremity and a life-threatening malignancy—this may be an overwhelming situation for the individual both mentally and physically.

Case Reports

Patient #1

A middle-aged university professor was seen complaining of multiple physical changes during the previous 6 months. Initially, his dark brown to black hair had turned totally white during a 4-month period of time. He also noted a lack of energy and saw several physicians while developing gangrenous ulceration of his fingertips on both hands. Multiple laboratory tests and X-rays were not diagnostic. After several months of symptomatology progression and lack of diagnosis, he sought vascular consultation from us. On physical examination, he had pure white hair, ischemic changes and necrotic ulceration of his digits, and a suspicious mass or adenopathy deep in the right scalene area. Chest X-ray and CT (computerized tomography) examination failed to demonstrate any mass in the chest. During surgery, a right scalene "egg-sized" 4×6 cm mass was removed. Pathologic diagnosis was that of amelanotic melanoma. Extensive examination of his body surfaces failed to demonstrate any other lesion. Oncologic consultation, extensive ear, nose and throat examination, and radiologic gastrointestinal exam did not delineate a primary tumor. The entire visible mass had been removed. Additional oncologic consultation failed to demonstrate a beneficial course—including an antigen-antibody-induced program. A few months later, he developed a recurrence of the mass in the right scalene area. On resection the same pathologic diagnosis of amelanotic melanoma was established. Again no beneficial treatment program was found for this individual. His findings and photographs were presented at a world congress exempli-

R.A. Dieter, Jr., MD, MS (✉)
Northwestern Medicine, At Central DuPage Hospital,
Winfield, IL 60190, USA

International College of Surgeons, Cardiothoracic
and Vascular Surgery, Glen Ellyn, IL, USA

G.B. Kuzycz, MD
Thoracic and Cardiovascular Surgery, Cadence Hospital of
Northwestern System, Winfield, IL 60190, USA

M.C. DaSilva, MD
Thoracic Surgery, Harvard Medical School, Brigham and Women's
Hospital, Boston, MA 02115, USA

R.A. Dieter, III, MD
Division of Cardiothoracic Surgery, The University of Tennessee
Medical Center, Knoxville, TN 37920, USA

A.M. Joudi, MD
Loyola University Medical Center, Stritch School of Medicine,
Maywood, IL 60153, USA

M.M. Meyer, MD
Internal Medicine, Past President of the Illinois State Medical
Society, Lombard, IL 60148, USA

fying an ischemic paraneoplastic syndrome due to melanoma with secondary gangrene of the fingers [2].

Patient #2

An elderly male with a long history of smoking developed a cough and weight loss. On X-ray evaluation, he was found to have a carcinoma of the lung. At surgery, the tumor was found to be more central and required extensive dissection and lobectomy. Upon completion of surgery and closure of the chest, the patient was placed in the supine position and extubated. At this time, he was noted to have a morbid left lower extremity. No pulses were palpable in the left foot or in the left groin. Immediate exploration of the left common femoral artery with balloon catheter thromboendarterectomy was performed. Pathologic examination of the specimen was compatible with a squamous cell carcinoma tumor embolism. Postembolectomy, the patient's leg developed a pink color with palpable pulsations. The tumor embolus was felt to have originated in the left atrium and to have dislodged during surgical manipulation.

Patient #3

A previously healthy 26-year-old male with a 20-pack-year smoking history presented with acute left lower extremity ischemia, which began as he was exercising. He suddenly felt a "pop" in his left hip, followed by numbness, coldness, and pain from the calf to the left foot. On physical exam, the patient was in sinus rhythm, had no murmurs and no pulses in the left foot. An emergency CT angiogram revealed occlusion of the distal left common femoral artery, profunda femoral artery, superficial femoral artery, and distal vessels. A hypercoagulable lab work-up was negative. In surgery, he had a left femoral thromboembolectomy and four compartment fasciotomies. The transverse arteriotomy on the distal common femoral artery revealed a yellow, firm mass within the artery. A Fogarty embolectomy catheter was passed to the popliteal level and an additional embolus was retrieved (Fig. 29.1). An operative arteriogram demonstrated a patent femoral tibial system. The patient had an uneventful recovery.

Pathology examination of the specimens described a large clot with a thin rim of viable tumor cells at the periphery. The remainder of the clot appeared amorphous and eosinophilic with focal areas of calcification. The tumor cells were small and contained a small amount of ill-defined cytoplasm, ovoid nuclei, and formed focal rosette-like structures. The specimens stained positively for CD56, CK8/18, AE1/AE3, CD117, vimentin, synaptophysin (focally), and CD34 (focally). Initially, the tumor diagnosis was a small cell carcinoma. After the review, it was felt to be an undifferentiated cancer with spindle cell and neuroendocrine features. Three-

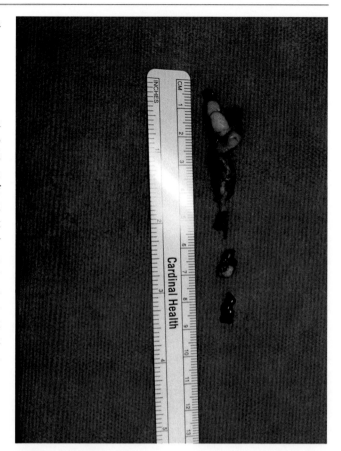

Fig. 29.1 Embolic angiosarcoma to the femoral artery causing acute ischemic symptoms

month follow-up CT scan of the chest demonstrated an increased cavitary ground-glass opacity in the right lower lobe and continued left pulmonary vein thrombosis. Repeat PET scan demonstrated interval development of the ground-glass opacity with mild FDG uptake (maximum SUV of 1.8) in the right lower lobe. A core needle biopsy demonstrated poorly differentiated carcinoma with neuroendocrine differentiation and appeared morphologically similar to the embolic lesion.

The patient underwent video-assisted thoracoscopic (VAT) right lower lobectomy. The surgical specimens stained positive for CD56 and CD117, as well as focally positive for MCK and CK7. Stains for CK20, p63, TTF-1, MOC-31, AFP, synaptophysin, and chromogranin were negative. Up to 30 % of the tumor cells showed reactivity for Ki67. Morphologically, the specimen demonstrated formation of primitive vascular channels with protrusion of neoplastic cells into the vascular spaces and abundant basement membrane production. The final pathologic diagnosis was angiosarcoma showing aberrant neuroendocrine differentiation. Lymph node biopsies and CT of the abdomen were negative for metastatic disease. The postoperative course was uneventful and he was discharged on postoperative day 3.

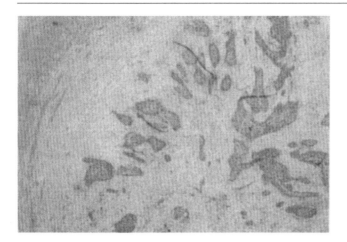

Fig. 29.2 Squamous cell carcinoma of the atrium showing tumor cells with normal muscle beyond

Patient #4

A 70-year-old Caucasian male was admitted to a small downstate community hospital in a wheelchair because of low back pain. He was short of breath and on evaluation was felt to have a carcinoma of the right lower lobe of the lung with probable bone metastases—including the spine. He came to see ourselves for a second opinion. Magnetic resonance (MR) study of the lumbar spine demonstrated a ruptured lumbar disc. Following lumbar discectomy, he was discharged home on continuous oxygen with the plan for future evaluation of his lung. Following repeat back surgery for another acutely ruptured disc, he had bronchoscopy and a right thoracotomy. A radical pneumonectomy with partial resection of the left atrium demonstrated the squamous cell tumor invasion of the cardiac muscle with a negative atrial myocardial resection margin for any remaining tumor, and he had no evidence of a dislodged embolic phenomenon (Fig. 29.2). Following the preoperatively anticipated prolonged postoperative period, the patient recovered and enjoyed a 6.5 year oxygen-free survival until developing high altitude pneumonia.

Patient #5

This middle-aged individual was admitted to the hospital with acute lower extremity ischemia. Open surgical balloon embolectomy of tumor bearing clot from the lower extremities relieved his symptoms. CT examination of the chest and cardiac catheterization demonstrated that this individual had a primary endocardial tumor (Fig. 29.3). Utilizing cardiopulmonary bypass and open cardiac surgery, the primary benign myxomatous endocardial tumor was resected. The patient made a full recovery without residual sequela.

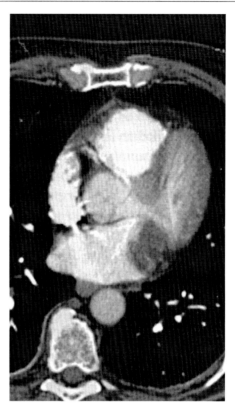

Fig. 29.3 Benign endocardial tumor demonstrated on CT scan

Patient #6

A middle-aged female with multiple complaints was admitted to the hospital. A previous gynecologic malignancy of the pelvis had been treated with extensive pelvic radiation and apparent control of the malignancy. Several years later, we were asked to see the patient with complaints of gastrointestinal and peripheral limb ischemic symptoms. Eventually, she required a colostomy and vascular surgical intervention. However, a few years later, she had progressive lower extremity difficulty with severe ischemic changes, marked lower abdominal and pelvic fibrosis, and extensive radiation-induced skin and soft tissue findings. Following repeated attempts to salvage her extremities, amputation and probable hemicorporectomy were offered—which she declined.

Patient #7

This patient had a long history of chronic lymphatic leukemia. However, chronic changes had developed in her right leg over time. Despite a mild anemia, the patient was able to live a moderately healthy life until she injured her foot. With the injury, a splinter was embedded in the right foot producing gangrenous changes, as a result of her leukemia and diminished circulation (Fig. 29.4).

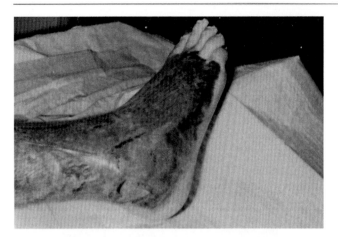

Fig. 29.4 Gangrene of the foot due to splinter in patient with chronic lymphatic leukemia

Table 29.1 Some examples of tumor-related extremity ischemia

Patient	Disease	Type of ischemia
1	Amelanotic melanoma	Paraneoplastic
2	Carcinoma lung	Embolic
3	Angiosarcoma	Embolic
4	Carcinoma lung	Embolic
5	Cardiac myxoma	Embolic
6	Gynecologic carcinoma	Radiation-induced fibrosis
7	Chronic leukemia	Foreign body gangrene

Discussion

As one begins to see from these case illustrations, the complexity of the situation for the dually afflicted individual is great—malignancy and ischemia. Two patients (#1, 2) of the above seven illustrative patients had markedly shortened survival after diagnosis of their tumor and associated ischemic process (1 year or less). Three patients (#4, 5, 7) were prolonged survivors of their malignant processes. Patient 1 had rapid progression of his primary malignant disease but eventual healing of his digits. Patient 6 had severe therapeutic complications of her malignancy. Patient 3 is a more recently treated and confusing patient. We await the longer-term progress of his primary malignant lung disease and treatment. Four patients are examples of a potential cardiovascular source for an embolus as demonstrated by the microscopic examinations of the pulmonary and cardiac tissues after resection. Patient 5 had a benign cardiac myxoma which embolized and did well postoperatively. The above cases demonstrate a diversity of etiologies as well as the complexity of therapy. As demonstrated, the diagnostic and therapeutic concerns for these patients present major challenges for both the patient and their treating physicians, as illustrated in Table 29.1. Further, these patients demonstrate the need for thromboembolectomy specimens to be examined microscopically in order to avoid missing the diagnosis of a tumor embolus.

Critical ischemia of the upper and lower extremities is not a rare occurrence. A number of these critical limb situations may end in amputation of a portion or all of an extremity. The pathophysiology of these lesions has been discussed extensively by Varu et al. They have classified the ischemic disease processes according to the patient's symptoms beginning with the asymptomatic individual and progressing to those with severe pain and loss of tissue or gangrene [3]. They further mention that individuals with critical limb ischemia have poor survival statistics and thus discussed the appropriateness of therapy, including gene, cell, and emergency therapy for individuals with tumors and critical limb ischemia. However, a number of their patients did show improvement in walking distance and the ankle—brachial index. Because of the high risk of leg amputation in the United Kingdom area (12,000 lower limb amputations in England during 2012 and 2013), a major review of the treatment of these individuals included the proposal of additional recommendations including a multidisciplinary team and rapid treatment initiation within the first 24 h of patient presentation [4]. In these critical acute, subacute, and chronic limb ischemia situations, a review of the management and options for these individual patients is well presented in an online outline of the nonoperative and operative interventions available, as well as various research-oriented studies [5]. Cell therapy, omental transplants, and wound V. A. C. are all discussed for the patient's benefit [6]. Despite the limitations of these concepts and therapeutic programs, treatments may be successful in a significant percentage of these patients.

Few authors discuss the occurrence of critical limb ischemia due to malignancy and its therapy except as case reports. We have illustrated a number of patients who had critical limb ischemia or the potential to develop critical ischemic changes of either the upper or lower extremity as a result of a malignant neoplasm or its therapy. In our experience, the incidence of such a relationship is very low, but the morbidity and potential effects are devastating. We have seen additional patients with other concerns related to tumors and have noted many of the signs or findings that may alert a physician to potential upcoming disasters. The multiple and various etiologies delineated above demonstrate the potential for tumor-induced peripheral ischemia and further demonstrate the need for critical examination of the diagnostic X-rays (especially thoracic CTs) and the patient's history and physical.

Various etiologies of tumor-induced peripheral ischemia are presented below (Table 29.2). The most common cause for such an acute tumor-induced ischemic calamity revolves around embolic phenomena from more central structures to the periphery. In our experience, most of these central lesions are located in the heart as a result of primary malignant or benign cardiac lesions or direct extension from pulmonary or mediastinal malignancies. Certainly, when one is considering major pulmonary surgery for a malignancy that is central in origin, one should closely review the CT (computerized

Table 29.2 Tumor-induced causes of extremity ischemia

Embolic sources
Benign tumors
Cardiac myxoma
Malignant tumors
Heart
Aorta
Lung
Mediastinum
Nuclear protein in testis (NUT) in childhood
Paraneoplastic syndromes
Pulmonary tumors
Gastric tumors
Melanomas
Ovarian tumors
Lymphoma/leukemias
Sarcoma
Vascular
Aortic intima
Aortic media
Soft tissue in unused arteriovenous fistulae
Cardiac
Chemotherapeutic agent therapy
Oncologic associated coagulation defects

Table 29.3 Possible tumor-induced symptomatology

Maybe confusing
Tumor manifestations
Paraneoplastic
Systemic tumor symptoms
Pain
Weight loss
Compression
Hemorrhage
Specific to tumor
Neurologic
Ischemic manifestations
Embolic
Paraneoplastic
Discoloration
Pain
Loss of function
Pulseless
Morbid
Clotting concerns

tomography studies) of the chest to be certain that there is no intracardiac or major pulmonary vessel involvement by the tumor that might embolize. A non-cardiopulmonary origin of an embolic tumor may also include the aorta [7].

Vascular sarcomas are rare but highly aggressive cancers, which affect less than 600 people in the United States each year, with angiosarcoma representing less than 1–3 % of all sarcoma diagnoses [8]. Peak incidence is reported in the seventh decade with men more affected than women. They are typically highly aggressive with a propensity for distant metastasis and a poor survival rate. A 2005 retrospective study of 125 angiosarcoma patients reported a median overall survival of 2.6 years and a 5-year survival rate of 31 % with 16 % of these patients presenting with metastatic disease at the time of diagnosis [9]. Angiosarcoma can arise in any part of the body, but is more common in soft tissue than in the bone, and the head and neck area appear to be the most common soft tissue site formation. The incidence of angiosarcoma of the breast has increased with the increased incidence of breast cancer, owing to the well-established risk factor of radiation. Other established risk factors include thorotrast exposure, chronic lymphedema, and vinyl chloride. In terms of visceral organ presentation, the heart (right atrium), liver, and spleen appear to be the most common sites of origin [8].

We have presented a case of a primary pulmonary angiosarcoma presenting in a 26-year-old male with none of these identifiable risk factors and a left common femoral metastatic thromboembolism and left leg ischemia. Other sources of a primary lesion were considered, given that the most common

site of angiosarcoma metastasis is widely recognized as the lung; however, an exhaustive work-up revealed no other identifiable lesions. As of 2012, it has been reported that there have only been about 20 cases of primary pulmonary angiosarcoma documented in the English literature [10]. They have been characterized as having insidious growth with extensive local invasion by the time of diagnosis. While this was not the case with our patient, it is unclear how long his primary lung lesion was present before his distant embolus had occurred. The PET scan had begun to show interval change in activity over a 7-month period. Radiologically, the common radiographic presentations of a primary pulmonary angiosarcoma may be multiple peripheral pulmonary nodules, a solitary mass with adjacent alveolar pattern and/or a variable degree of consolidation, and a ground-glass opacity which is thought to be related to intra-alveolar hemorrhage [10].

Multiple clinical problems may occur as a result of tumor-induced extremity ischemia including the possible need for amputation if lesser treatments are not successful. When one considers these various potential initiating processes, the manifestation may be confusing and difficult to diagnose and treat.

The Table 29.3 above outlines various manifestations resulting from an embolic, systemic, or compressive tumor creating ischemic considerations. Results of extrinsic vessel compression are less common than embolic or lumen filling tumor. Paraneoplastic manifestations such as those noted in our patient #1 with the amelanotic melanoma or in a patient with lung cancer are very unusual but more commonly are noted in patients with pulmonary crippling adenocarcinomas [11]. Other paraneoplastic symptoms such as ataxia or arthritic pains have been relieved with surgical resection of the pulmonary malignancy in several of our patients. When

Table 29.4 Tumors which may cause paraneoplastic ischemic manifestations

Lung
Adenocarcinoma
Squamous cell
Ovarian
Melanoma
Leukemia
Acute myelogenous
Lymphoma
Neuroendocrine carcinoma
Pheochromocytoma

Table 29.5 Types of tumor-induced extremity ischemia

Paraneoplastic syndromes
Circulating chemical agents
Coagulation disorders
Embolic
Direct vascular compression
Chemotherapeutic agents
Gemcitabine and carboplatin in ovarian chemotherapy

the etiology is not readily apparent for the patient's difficulty, a search for malignancy may be appropriate and necessary (Table 29.4). Pheochromocytoma, lymphomas, squamous cell carcinoma of the lung, and well-differentiated pulmonary neuroendocrine carcinoma have all been noted to present with a paraneoplastic syndrome [12–15]. Each of these patients presents a very difficult situation both in establishing the diagnosis and in the treatment of their lesion. Most importantly, one needs to be alert to the possibility of malignant or benign, such as a benign atrial myxoma, tumor etiology for these unusual peripheral hand and foot manifestations [16].

Lymphomas and leukemias may also be the etiologic source for the ischemic problem (Fig. 29.4). These malignancies may create the ischemic process in a number of manners. Upper arm ischemia due to compression of the great vessels or a dominant vessel such as the subclavian artery in association with venous thrombosis was noted by Daruwalla et al. [15]. New multiple embolic phenomena with organ infarction and extremity ischemia, as well as lymphoma-associated paraneoplastic ischemia of the digits, have been noted [17–19]. These lesions may involve the upper extremity, as well as the lower extremity, and create critical limb ischemia [20, 21].

Various carcinomas have been reported in association with acute or chronic limb ischemia. This list, as presented above (Table 29.3), would include carcinoma of the lung, esophagus, testicle, stomach, and ovary [22–26]. In addition, various sarcomas have been noted to initiate ischemic changes of the extremities, including the previous mentioned aortic intimal sarcoma [7]. Certainly, the unusual soft tissue sarcomas that may develop in arteriovenous fistula are a potential source for this problem, as well as the unusual nuclear protein in testis (NUT) midline carcinoma (NMC) [27, 28]. Sarcomas of the aorta may embolize either a proteinaceous material or actual portions of the tumor. On microscopic examination of the gelatinous embolic material, one may see spindle- and stellate-shaped cells with central necrosis. Of note, the mural sarcoma lesions of the aorta are usually less symptomatic and do not tend to embolize when compared to the intimal variety according to Raj [29].

Not only are embolic and direct tumor effects noted on occasion to cause limb ischemia, chemotherapeutic agents used for the treatment of malignancy may also initiate ischemic changes of the extremities (Table 29.5). There are a number of chemotherapeutic agents which may induce arterial ischemic events. Such ischemic events may include digital ischemia, myocardial infarction, cerebrovascular "accidents," and arterial thrombosis. Acute digital ischemia has been noted in patients receiving gemcitabine and carboplatin combination chemotherapy for ovarian carcinoma [30]. Such digital ischemia has also been noted in patients on gemcitabine and S-1 for systemic sclerosis [31]. Holstein et al. discussed their therapy for an ischemic patient under treatment with gemcitabine and carboplatin for urothelial carcinoma [32]. They utilized bilateral brachial plexus blockade, fractionated subcutaneous heparin, oral corticosteroids, aspirin, and iloprost to avoid digital amputation. The latter therapy has also been reported on a rare occasion to cause arterial thrombosis.

Treatment Modalities

Multiple approaches (Table 29.6) have been utilized for the treatment of limb ischemia in cancer patients [33]. The obvious question in many patients revolves around the potential benefit to the patient who may be in a severely deteriorated state and have a shortened survival expectation. The question as to the value of performing extensive complicated and expensive therapy for many of these individuals requires consideration by the physician, the patient, and the family members when there has been severe deterioration. This initial symptom once corrected may then lead to acute and long-term postoperative treatment of their primary malignant process. When the malignant process expectancy offers little hope, comfort care may be the best consideration. However, many of these individuals may be experiencing their first symptom due to the malignancy and thus may have a significant long-term survival potential when the acute limb ischemia process is corrected or alleviated [34]. Thus, evaluation of the risk and the options requires careful consideration. In a select group of these patients, resection of the primary cardiac tumor from the explanted heart followed by cardiac reconstruction and cardiac autotransplantation has

Table 29.6 Treatment options for tumor-induced extremity ischemia

Expectant or interventional decision
Observation
Spontaneous improvement
Urgent intervention
Emergency intervention
Drug therapy
Anticoagulation
Chemotherapy
Enzymatic—usually avoid
Surgical intervention
Embolectomy
Thrombectomy
Resection tumor
Cardiac autotransplantation
Bypass grafting
Amputation
Radiation
Long-term considerations
Patient care
Associated diseases
Cardiac
Diabetes
Blood pressure

been utilized with some long-term success [35–37]. More recently, more aggressive surgery has been utilized to resect the primary tumor, including aortic endografting and left atrial resection for more aggressive malignancies.

The treatment process one might utilize for the correction of the ischemic extremity may require both emergent and urgent intervention. A complete history and physical examination will aid in the determination of the best approach to the therapeutic decision and whether surgical or medical intervention is the most appropriate. If time permits, appropriate diagnostic laboratory and X-ray testing will aid in this decision analysis. Angiography and Doppler measurements may be diagnostic. Intervention, including balloon thromboembolic and bypass procedures, may be utilized as necessary. If the disease process is far advanced or no longer controllable, then more palliative measures may be utilized. Amputation will be required in a number of these individuals as both a short-term and long-term goal of increased survival. One should recognize, however, that operative therapy may be fraught with an increased mortality.

Other supportive therapy or possible curative therapy, including chemotherapy, radiation therapy, blood transfusions, and daily assistive care, must all be considered. Depending on the surgical approach, whether through the femoral or brachial arteries, the additional and appropriate tumor care may all be beneficial. In some cases, urokinase or other such agents have been utilized. Anticoagulation utilizing unfractionated heparin or low molecular weight heparin, followed by warfarin, will be utilized in many patients. Once

the acute phase is stable, then a determination as to the type and source of malignancy will follow. A number of authors have discussed the therapy and potential outcomes in patients with ischemia and malignancy [32–35]. Depending on the ischemia classification and the risk to the patients, Mouhayar et al. concluded that an invasive approach for the treatment of acute limb ischemia in cancer patients did not appear to have a prohibitively high mortality rate [38]. The 1-year survival rate is low and most likely is related to the prognosis of the malignancy and not to the ischemia itself. They further recommended that the patients with malignancy be managed utilizing established standards of care for such lesions. This is further emphasized by Singh et al. in the necessity for microscopic evaluation of embolic specimens in their patient with embolic germ cell tumor [39].

Malignancy-Associated Extremity Lymphedema

Edema of the upper and lower extremity may result from many causes and usually does not precipitate amputation. However, we have seen a number of patients with massive edema of the extremity consequent to their development of or treatment for a malignancy. The majority of these patients may be treated with conservative nonoperative modalities. But with the development of massive or elephantiasis type of lesions with loss of extremity function, ulceration, and weight concerns of the affected arm or leg, patients have been seen for surgical treatment consideration, including possible amputation with the provisional diagnoses of malignancy-related ischemia.

These patients may have had a radical inguinal lymph node dissection, pelvic carcinomatosis as a result of gynecologic or colonic neoplasms, or radical axillary lymph node dissection for carcinoma of the breast. Although most of these patients did not have ischemia in association with the massive function limiting edema of the extremity, they were seen with the concept of "need." Usually the patient was treated with a conservative nonoperative therapeutic program with reasonable patient acceptance along with treatment of the primary neoplastic process to include compression stockings, physiotherapy, intermittent compression, and elevation.

Some authors have utilized long saphenous vein sparing, fascia preserving dissection, sartorius transposition, microsurgery, and omental pedicle flap [40–42]. All of these procedures are designed to reduce the swelling and improve functionality of the extremity. Concomitant treatment of the underlying malignancy is a must in these patients. Usually, the patients do not have an ischemia component to their malady, although misinterpreted, but they certainly have a disabling/limiting affliction associated with their primary disease requiring intensive therapy and possibly using an ischemia therapy—omental grafting.

Summary

Malignancy-induced ischemia of the extremities may vary from the digits, to the hand, to the foot, or to a major amputation of an extremity. Treating these individuals presents many challenges both practically and ethically. We have seen a number of patients with these conditions and concerns. Many of the patients, when in the final stages of their life, have elected palliative or comfort care and avoidance of further aggressive treatment. Others in the initial phase of their diagnosis may elect to be progressive in their diagnostic evaluation and aggressive in their treatment program. We have only mentioned peripheral extremity (upper and lower) ischemia in this discussion, but have seen patients with tumor concerns and emboli to the brain (stroke) or to the intestinal tract vascularity. With the increasing population age and the increasing incidence of tumor diagnosis, you can expect to see more individuals with this combination of malignancy and extremity ischemia. Diagnostic and therapeutic programs will require a great deal of consideration. Usually the patient with the acute process will not be treated in the same manner as the patients with long-term atherosclerotic disease. However, maintenance medication, anticoagulation, and antitumor drugs, as well as interventional and open surgical procedures, may all be required in the treatment of these complex patients.

Acknowledgment Many thanks to Julie Stielstra, MLS, Manager, Libraries of Northwestern Cadence Health, Central DuPage Hospital, Winfield, Illinois, for her assistance in obtaining the appropriate reference materials. Also, thanks to Lynn Marie Murawski for her preparation assistance of this manuscript.

References

1. Silva MB, Choi L, Cheng CC. Chapter 63: peripheral arterial occlusive disease. In: , editor. Sabiston textbook of surgery. Philadelphia: Elsevier Saunders; 2012. pp. 1751–7.
2. Dieter RA Jr. Carcinoma and paraneoplastic syndromes XXXIII Biennial meeting International College of Surgeons, Taipei, 27–29 October 2002.
3. Varu VN, Hogg ME, Kibbe MR. Critical limb ischemia. J Vasc Surg. 2010;51(1):230–41.
4. UK all party parliamentary group condemns figures on regional variation in amputation rates. Vasc News/updates. BIBA. June 2014;20.
5. DynaMed. Management of critical limb ischemia. DynaMed Editor@ebscohost.com. 2013; EBSCO Industries, Inc., pp. 1–36.
6. Sumpio BE, Attinger CE. A multidisciplinary approach to limb preservation: the role of V.A.C. therapy. Wounds (suppl) 2009;(Sept): 1–19.
7. Barry N, Tsui J, Dick J, Baker D, Selvakumar S. Aortic tumor presenting as acute lower limb ischemia. Circulation. 2011;123:1785–7.
8. Cioffi A, Reichert S, Antonescu CR, Maki RG. Angiosarcomas and other sarcomas of endothelial origin. Hematol Oncol Clin North Am. 2013;27(5):975–88.
9. Fury MG, Antonescu CR, Van Zeek J, Brennan MF, Maki RG. A 14 - year retrospective review of angiosarcoma: clinical characteristics, prognostic factors, and treatment outcomes with surgery and chemotherapy. Cancer J. 2005;11(3):241–7.
10. Yang C-F, Chen T-W, Tseng G-C, Chiang I-P. Primary pulmonary angiosarcoma presenting as a solitary pulmonary nodule on image. Pathol Int. 2012;62(6):424–8.
11. Moulakakis K, Bessias N, Maras D, Andrikopoulos V. "Digital ischemia as a paraneoplastic manifestation of lung cancer" clinical image. Intern Med. 2010;49:199–200.
12. Lutchman D, Buchholz S, Keightley C. Phaeochromocytoma-associated critical peripheral ischaemia. Intern Med J. 2010;40:150–9.
13. Onitilo AA, Demos-Bertrand J, Depke J, Resnick JM, Engel J. Digital ischemia as a paraneoplastic consequence of squamous cell lung carcinoma. WMJ. 2012;111(3):138–41.
14. Karadeniz C, Kose F, Abali H, Sumbul A, Oquzkurt L, Karabacak T, Oberg K. Severe systemic vasoconstriction starting with acute limb ischemia leading to death in a patient with a well-differentiated pulmonary neuroendocrine carcinoma: a new paraneoplastic syndrome? Acta Oncol. 2012;51(1):124–7.
15. Daruwalla ZJ, Razak ARA, Duke D, Grogan L. Acute upper arm ischemia: a rare presentation of non-Hodgkin's lymphoma. Ir J Med Sci. 2010;179:589–92.
16. Roscher AA, Kato NS, Quan H, Padmanabham M. Intra-arterial Myxomas, clinical pathologic correlation based on two case studies, including historical review. Presented at the 5th World Congress of the International Society of Cardiothoracic Surgeons (ISCTS) Dorado, Puerto Rico, 4–8 June 1995.
17. Overton J, Nicklin A, Eleftheriou P, Frith D, Gravante G, Sapsford W. Recurrent acute lower-limb ischemia with multiple organ infarctions secondary to acute myeloid leukemia M1. Ann Vasc Surg. 2012;26(8):1128.e1–5.
18. Woei-A-Jin FJ, Tamsma JT, Khoe LV, den Hartog WC, Gerritsen JJ, Brand A. Lymphoma-associated paraneoplastic digital ischemia. Ann Hematol. 2014;93(2):355–7.
19. Mar N, Gorgan MA, Dailey ME, Vredenburgh JJ. Blue toes and a new pair of shoes–challenges in diagnosis and treatment of acute myelogenous leukemia. Am J Hematol. 2013;88(12):1090–3.
20. Belizna C, Pistorius MA, Planchon B. Lethal limb ischaemia in leukaemia. Case report and review of the literature. J Thromb Thrombolysis. 2009;28(3):354–7.
21. Kafetzakis A, Foundoulakis A, Loannou CV, Stavroulaki E, Koutsopoulos A, Katsamouris AN. Acute lower limb ischemia as the initial symptom of acute myeloid leukemia. Vasc Med. 2007;12(3):199–202.
22. Yong TY, Klebe S, Li JY. Acute critical leg ischemia: an uncommon initial manifestation of esophageal adenocarcinoma. J Palliat Med. 2009;12(9):841–4.
23. Le Ho H, Vauleon E, Boucher E, Gedouin D, Kerbrat P, Raoul JL. Acute ischemia of the lower limb during chemotherapy for testicular cancer: a report of 2 cases. Acta Oncol. 2009;486:9400–2.
24. Gibson CJ, Britton KA, Miller AL, Loscalzo J. Out of the blue. N Engl J Med. 2014;370:1742–8.
25. Schreffler SM, Paolo WF, Kloss BT. Spontaneous showering of tumor emboli in a patient with advanced primary lung cancer: a case report. Int J Emerg Med. 2012;5(1):27.
26. Griffin KJ, Bailey MA, Greenwood JP, Barker L, Nicholson T, Scott DJ. Ovarian mass causing paradoxical MI and leg ischemia. Case Rep Vasc Med. 2012;2012:702509.

27. Herbert PE, Crane JS. Soft tissue sarcomas in disused arteriovenous fistulae. Exp Clin Transplant. 2013;1:79–80.
28. Stein JJ, Boyes C, Costanza MJ, Amankwah KS, Corpron CA, Gahtan V. Bilateral lower extremity acute thromboembolism as first presentation for cancer in a child: an interesting report. J Pediatr Surg. 2012;47:2123–5.
29. Raj V, Joshi S, Hawlisch K, Wage R, Prasad S. An unusual cause of acute limb ischemia: aortic intimal sarcoma. Ann Thorac Surg. 2011;91(3):e33–5.
30. Staff S, Lagerstedt E, Seppanen J, Maenpaa J. Acute digital ischemia complicating gemcitabine and carboplatin combination chemotherapy for ovarian cancer. Acta Obstet Gynecol Scand. 2011;90(11):1296–7.
31. Zaima C, Kanai M, Ishikawa S, Kawaguchi Y, Masui T, Mori Y, Nishimura T, Matsumato S, Yanagihara K, Chiba T, Mimori T. A case of progressive digital ischemia after early withdrawal of gemcitabine and S–1 in a patient with systemic sclerosis. Jpn J Clin Oncol. 2011;41(6):803–6.
32. Holstein A, Batge R, Egberts EH. Gemcitabine induced digital ischemia and necrosis. Eur J Cancer Care (Engl). 2010;19(3):408–9.
33. Sanon S, Lenihan DJ, Mouhayar E. Peripheral arterial ischemic events in cancer patients. Vasc Med. 2011;16(2):119–30.
34. Silverberg D, Yalon T, Reinitz ER, Yakubovitch D, Segev T, Halak M. Acute limb ischemia in cancer patients: aggressive treatment is justified. Vascular. 2014. doi:10.1177/1708538114537048.

35. Ramlawi B, Al-jabbari O, Blau LN, Davies MG, Bruckner BA, Blackman SH, Ravi V, Benjamin R, Rodriguez L, Sharpira GM, Reardon MJ. Autotransplantation for the resection of complex left heart tumors. Ann Thorac Surg. 2014;98:863–8.
36. Moon MR. Commentary on "thoracic aortic endografting facilitates the resection of tumors infiltrating the aorta". J Thorac Cardiovasc Surg. 2014;147(5):1454–5.
37. Galvaing G, Tardy MM, Cassagnes L, Da Costa V, Chadeyros JB, Naamee A, Bailly P, et al. Ann Thorac Surg. 2014;97:1708–14.
38. Mouhayar E, Tayar J, Fasulo M, Aoun R, Massey M, Abi-Aad S, Ilieseu C, Ahrar K, Huynh T. Outcome of acute limb ischemia in cancer patients. Vasc Med. 2014;19(2):112–7.
39. Singh A, Jenkins DP, Dahdel M, Dhar S, Ratnatunga CP. Recurrent arterial embolization from a germ cell tumor invading the left atrium. Ann Thorac Surg. 2000;70:2155–6.
40. Abbas S, Seitz M. Systematic review and meta-analysis of the used surgical techniques to reduce leg lymphedema following radical inguinal nodes dissection. Surg Oncol. 2011;20(2):88–96.
41. Benoit L, Boichot C, Cheynel N, Arnould L, Chauffert B, Cuisenier J, Fraisse J. Preventing lymphedema and morbidity with an omentum flap after ilioinguinal lymph node dissection. Ann Surg Oncol. 2005;12(10):793–9.
42. Nakajima F, Nakajima R, Tsukamoto S, Koide Y, Yarita T, Kato H. Omental transposition for lymphedema after a breast cancer resection: report of a case. Surg Today. 2006;36(2):175–9.

Frostbite

Stephen M. Milner, Julie A. Caffrey, and Syed F. Saquib

Introduction

Studies have revealed that freezing of tissues produces inflammatory processes, similar to those found in thermal injury, with cell membrane disruption and ischemia reperfusion injury. The medical management has changed little since the recommendations emanating from the First World War, with prevention, rewarming, and delayed amputation being paramount. Currently, other options including thrombolytic therapy, hyperbaric oxygen, and sympathectomy have not proven to be superior to conventional treatment.

History

Frostbite was reported as early as 5000 years ago in a Chilean mummy with the right foot exhibiting loss of digits ascribed to cold injury [1]. Current management of the disorder dates back to treatment of military casualties, witnessed during the invasion of Russia in 1812, as described by Baron Dominique Larrey, Napoleon's military surgeon. He recognized the importance of rewarming and the injurious effects of the freeze-thaw-freeze cycle [2, 3]. Prophylactic measures to prevent frostbite were introduced by Munroe during First World War. In 1915, R.H. Jocelyn Swan, writing in the British Medical Journal, used the term "frost-bite" in soldiers and described symptoms of paresthesias and pain. He advocated painting the wounds with 2 % iodine solution and delaying amputation to await a natural separation at the junc-

tion of necrotic and viable tissue [4]. These recommendations remain just as true today.

Pathophysiology

When the temperature is less than 15 °C, the body undergoes an auto-thermoregulatory response with cycles of vasoconstriction and vasodilation, known as "the hunting reaction of Lewis." This preferentially decreases blood flow intermittently to the extremities to maintain core body temperature. Prolonged hypothermia leads to persistent vasoconstriction with hypoxia, acidosis, stasis of blood flow, and thrombosis [2, 5].

As tissue freezes parallel mechanisms act synergistically resulting in injury. The formation of extracellular ice crystals damages cell membranes, causing a change in the osmotic gradient, intracellular dehydration, electrolyte shifts, and ultimately cell death. As the temperature of the tissue continues to fall, formation and expansion of intracellular ice crystals also mechanically disrupt cells [2, 5]. Additionally progressive dermal ischemia augments the injury by an ischemia reperfusion response [2, 3]. Endothelial injury, tissue hypoxia, and thrombosis of blood vessels lead to a massive inflammatory cascade (Fig. 30.1). This triggers the release of prostaglandins and thromboxanes that lead to further vasoconstriction, platelet aggregation, and thrombosis, which is amplified during rewarming and recurrent freezing [2, 5]. Effective treatment must be aimed at prevention, rewarming to halt freezing, increasing blood flow to decrease hypoxia, and blocking the release of inflammatory mediators.

Clinical Manifestations

Frostbite affects primarily peripheral parts of the body, namely, hands, feet, ears, nose, and cheeks [3]. Predisposing risk factors include alcoholism, age 30–49 years old, improper

S.M. Milner, MBBS, BDS (✉)
J.A. Caffrey, DO, MS • S.F. Saquib, MD
Department of Plastic and Reconstructive Surgery, Johns Hopkins University School of Medicine, Baltimore, MD, USA

© Springer International Publishing Switzerland 2017
R.S. Dieter et al. (eds.), *Critical Limb Ischemia*, DOI 10.1007/978-3-319-31991-9_30

Fig. 30.1 Pathophysiology of frostbite

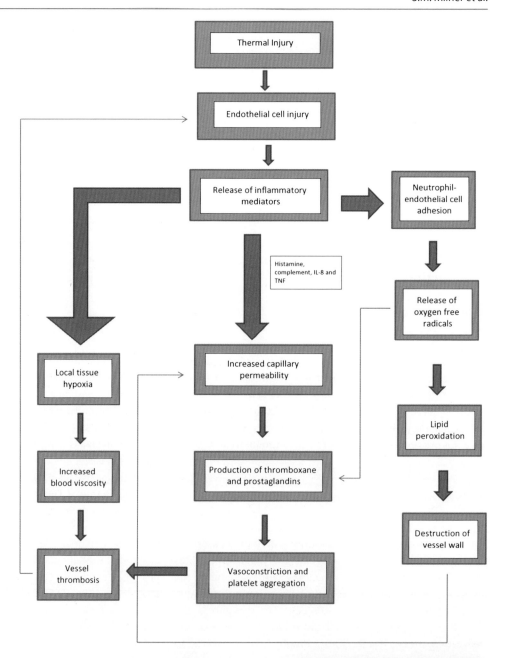

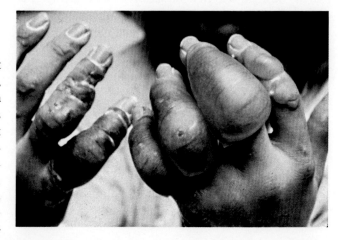

clothing, homelessness, infection, diabetes, and smoking. It can be classified practically as superficial, without tissue loss, or deep. Superficial frostbite often manifests as numbness, a central white plaque and surrounding erythema, or as blisters filled with a clear fluid and usually develops within the first 24 h (Fig. 30.2). The deeper variant characteristically presents with bluish-purple discoloration (Fig. 30.3) and hemorrhagic blisters that result in a hard black eschar and necrosis. Symptoms range from numbness that may progress to a feeling of clumsiness, throbbing pain and paresthesia to sensory loss, and increased cold sensitivity, which may persist for years after injury [5].

Fig. 30.2 Clear, fluid-filled blisters characteristic of superficial injury

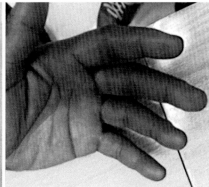

Fig. 30.3 Bluish-purple discoloration consistent with deeper injury

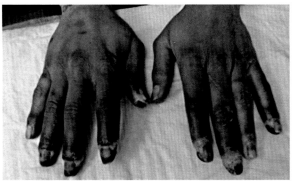
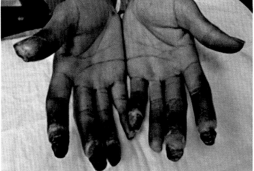

Fig. 30.4 Demarcation of viable and nonviable tissue 6 weeks after initial injury

Management

Hypothermia should be initially corrected to a core temperature above 35 °C before warming measures are implemented to the affected areas [6]. The frostbitten extremity should be placed in a water bath set at 38 °C containing an antiseptic solution such as chlorhexidine or povidone-iodine. Optimal thawing varies from 15 min to 1 h. Rewarming should stop once the affected tissue becomes pliable and appears a red/purple color. Adequate analgesia should be prescribed since rewarming can be extremely painful.

The debridement of blisters is controversial. There is no convincing literature or studies on the appropriate management of blisters with regard to drainage. Our protocol is to debride clear blisters and leave hemorrhagic ones intact.

A second strategy attempts to counter the inflammatory reaction with the use of NSAIDs and topical agents. Oral ibuprofen provides systemic antiprostaglandin activity. Topical aloe vera, a thromboxane synthetase inhibitor, can be applied to the wounds once they have been thawed and debrided. Injured extremities should be splinted and elevated to minimize swell-

ing. Prophylactic antibiotics are not indicated and tetanus toxoid should be administered according to standard guidelines.

Immediate amputation should be avoided. It is usual to wait a period of more than 6–12 weeks for demarcation to be established unless the patient has wet gangrene, liquefaction, or sepsis (Fig. 30.4).

With the advent of angiography, thrombolytic therapy has become another treatment option. There have been multiple studies published on the effectiveness of tissue plasminogen activator (rTPA). Bruen et al. showed a reduction of digital amputation rates from 41 to 10 % in those patients getting rTPA within 24 h of injury [2, 6].

Adjunctive therapies include hyperbaric oxygen therapy and sympathectomy. At this time, there is no level 1 data recommending the use of either therapy in the management of frostbite.

Summary

Frostbite, featuring heavily during wartime, is also commonly seen in the civilian population. The pathogenesis involves several mechanisms to include intra- and extracellular ice crystal formation, cell membrane rupture, and an ischemia reperfusion injury. Classifications follow the lines of those described in burn injury, namely, superficial and deep. Management must be aimed at prevention, rewarming, augmenting blood flow to decrease hypoxia, and inhibition of inflammatory mediators. Definitive treatment should be delayed until demarcation is seen between necrotic and viable tissue in order to maximally preserve tissue. Other modalities such as thrombolytic therapy, hyperbaric oxygen treatment, and sympathectomy are controversial.

References

1. Post PW, Donner DD. Frostbite in a pre-Columbian mummy. Am J Phys Anthropol. 1972;37(2):187–91.
2. Murphy JV, Barnwell PE, Roberts AHN, McGrouther DA. Frostbite: pathogenesis and treatment. J Trauma. 2000;48(1):171–8.
3. Zafren K. Frostbite: prevention and initial management. High Alt Med Biol. 2013;14(1):9–12.
4. Swan RHJ. The so-called "frost-bite". Proc.Roy.Soc.Med, 1914-1915, viii, Clin. Sect. 41-16.
5. Reamy BV. Frostbite: review and current concepts. J Am Board Fam Pract. 1998;11(1):34–40.
6. Handford C, Buxton P, Russell K, Imray C, McIntosh S, Freer L, Cochran A, Imray C. Frostbite: a practical approach to hospital management. Extreme Physiol Med. 2014;3:7.

Michael J. Feldman and Michael Fiore Amendola

Pathophysiology

Introduction

The pathophysiology of burn injury is well described [1] and is based on the depth of thermal injury and classically deemed as first, second, or third degree. Current nomenclature allows for a more detailed description of burn depth by stating how much of the dermis is injured. Previously classified second-degree burns are now categorized as superficial partial-thickness, mid-partial-thickness, and deep partial-thickness burns. Full-thickness injuries are analogous to previous described third-degree burns. Further classification of thermal injury now included fourth degree which involves the tendon, bone, or muscle. It is important to note that even a partial-thickness burn may require surgical intervention, can get infected, and/or cause a compartment syndrome if it is circumferential. The later of these presentations are the most worrisome due to the potential for conversion to a deeper tissue injury without the appropriate care.

Vascular bed responses to thermal injury have been examined and characterized in animal and human models. To date, these studies have been in prototypes with no known vascular disease or with unknown vascular perfusion. Many studies have well established that total circulating volume increases in a proportional response to percent body surface thermally injured [2, 3]. Elevated skin arterial flow has been described in the setting of thermal injury with concomitant increase in temperature [4]. This blood flow relationship is curvilinear in nature and is focused in the isolated burnt lower extremity with unchanged hemodynamics in the uninjured limb in the same patient [5]. Deep third-degree burn wounds, or full-thickness burns, have been found to be associated with a superficial vascular thrombosis [6] resulting in delayed increased blood flow to the skin which peaks at 1 week [3]. In contrast, superficial partial-thickness wound injuries do not impair the superficial vascular network, resulting in an immediate increase in superficial blood flow once circulatory blood volume is restored [3]. Muscle blood flow in the affected burnt limb has also been discovered to have unchanged skin perfusion [7]. Again, the limitation of this conceptual understanding of arterial and venous responses to thermal injury is that there is minimal to no existing underlying vascular disease.

Associated Disease States

The incidence of diabetes mellitus (DM) in the United States is expected to increase to a projected 15 cases per 1000 by 2050 [8]. One of the leading associated pathology states of diabetes is its known relation to arterial insufficiency in particular of the lower extremity small vessels. Additionally, peripheral neuropathy is a known complication. This latter manifestation is estimated to affect just over a quarter of all patients who suffer from diabetes [9]. As described by Kimball et al., the presence of lower extremity burns is expected to almost double in the next 50 years [10]. Reduced sensation to the foot is a large factor in foot burns as described in several case studies by Balakrishnan et al. in 1995 [11]. The University of Davis detailed their 10-year experience of 68 admissions of diabetic patients with foot burns half of which had neuropathy on admission [12]. Of these patients, roughly 16 % required either minor or major amputation secondary to their burn wound.

We reviewed 27 patients with diabetes and foot burns in our institute on an IRB-approved protocol to examine outcomes of patients admitted to our burn center from January

M.J. Feldman, MD (✉)
Division of Plastic and Reconstructive Surgery, Critical Care
Hospital, Virginia Commonwealth University,
8th Floor, 1213 East Clay St., Richmond, VA 23298, USA

M.F. Amendola, MA, MD
Division of Vascular Surgery, Department of Surgery, VCU
Medical Center, McGuire VA Medical Center,
Richmond, VA, USA

R.S. Dieter et al. (eds.), *Critical Limb Ischemia*, DOI 10.1007/978-3-319-31991-9_31

2008 to August 2011. These patients were compared to a control group matched by age, total body surface area of burn, complication, and length of hospitalization. Patients with underlying diabetes and thermal injury were found to have a higher rate of nosocomial infections as well as readmissions. These patients also tended to have longer hospital stays and presented at a later stage of their thermal injury. We also discovered that diabetic patients with foot burns respond appropriately to surgical intervention although they need more interventions comparatively [13].

It is well known that successful management of the underlying diabetes disease state is essential for wound healing and can be followed with serial hemoglobin A1C measurements. Elevated hemoglobin A1C has a known association with wound healing failure rates in diabetic patients. Diabetes not only makes one more susceptible to the burn injury but also worsens the extent of the injury by compromising the underlying arterial perfusion. The initial measure of this factor at admission can give the provider an idea of the patient's underlying diabetic state and forecast the potential future healing of the thermally injured extremity as well as serve as a surrogate marker for distal limb arterial insufficiency.

Assessment of Thermal Injury and Vascular Disease

General Burn Approach

Any patient who presents with thermal injury must be evaluated for concomitant trauma. One must not overlook life-threatening traumatic injuries in the setting of the obvious superficial or deep burn. That being said, the burn examination begins with assessment of the size of the burn. This involves all areas that are at least second degree or partial thickness in depth. First-degree burns are excluded in the determination of the patient's total body surface area affected because of known false elevation of calculated fluid requirements. As stated by the Baux formula [14], mortality is directly related to the patient's age and the total body surface area of thermal injury. This formula was recently updated based on the burn trauma database, which shows a less than one to one relationship to the Baux formula and mortality than 50 years ago [15]. There are multiple ways to determine total body surface area (TBSA) including: the rule of palms, the Lund-Browder chart, the rule of nines, as well as more modern flash-based or IOs-based apps.

General Vascular Approach

Underlying vascular disease can usually be ascertained based on a careful history prior to the thermal injury. For example, if a patient has more proximal arterial insufficiency (i.e., aortoiliac stenosis or obstruction), symptom complex usually focuses around pain with exertion in dedicated muscle groups (known as vascular claudication or simply claudication) involving the buttock, hip, or thigh. The majority of arterial insufficiency focuses in the lower extremity usually sparing the upper extremity. The reason for this incongruity disease distribution is currently unknown and has been the subject of only minimal research efforts [16]. For the simplicity of this chapter, we will focus on the lower extremity as a focal point of our comments.

Arterial insufficiency can be described on the spectrum of symptoms from claudication to rest pain. Intermittent claudication is classically described as calf symptoms ranging from fatigue to aching with exertion. Ischemic neuropathy involving the small unmyelinated A delta and C sensory fibers as well as intramuscular acidosis is thought to contribute to the etiology of this pain [17]. Once the activity has abated, pain subsides.

On the other extreme of the arterial insufficiency spectrum are patients with ischemic rest pain or critical limb ischemia. This is commonly described as pain that can awaken the patient from sleep and necessitates hanging their foot off the bed or walking to alleviate pain (usually centered in the foot). These patients have high risk of foot amputation and/or limb loss, while patients with claudication rarely progress to amputation [17]. These patients may also present with an element of tissue loss indicating a significant risk to progression to amputation if not addressed.

Part of the patient's history at initial presentation should be an assessment of associated vascular disease and predisposing risk factors. Patients with known claudication may also have a history of coronary artery disease and/or stroke. Well-described predisposing risk factors for arterial disease include but are not limited to hyperlipidemia, hypertension, chronic renal insufficiency, diabetes, and history of smoking.

In terms of underlying venous disease, there are known associations with obesity, immobility, diagnosed and undiagnosed carcinoma states, trauma, inherited hypercoagulability, and a history of deep venous thrombosis. It should be mentioned that many patients suffer from mild forms of chronic venous disorders including simple telangiectasia (spider veins) and reticular veins, varicose veins, and leg edema. Severe forms of this chronic venous disease stem from venous hypertension as related to venous valve incompetence (venous insufficiency) and to a lesser extent abnormal calf muscle pump function. This extreme aspect of the spectrum manifests hyperpigmented skin changes, dermal sclerosis, and potential skin ulceration. Venous insufficiency commonly leads to chronic wound states and only rarely leads to limb loss.

A history of venous insufficiency is usually that of heaviness or fullness in the lower limb with or without pain that is usually increased as the duration of the day wears on.

Additionally, patients with venous insufficiency could have history of deep venous thrombosis or recurrent ulceration on the medial aspects of the lower limb (gaiter region). Recurrent ulceration is an advanced presentation of venous insufficiency.

Patients with burns serve as a unique diagnostic problem due to routine swelling (making palpation of a pulse difficult), erythema (making skin assessment difficult), tenderness (making examination of the limb difficult for physical exam and duplex imaging), as well as acute presentation (making history taking challenging to ascertain underlying vascular disease).

The one aspect of examination that might be preserved in this type of patient is the contralateral limb. The majority of time patients will present with similar levels of arterial and/or venous insufficiency in their lower extremity limbs bilaterally. Closely examining and/or testing the unaffected or unburned limb might lead practitioners to an idea of the underlying vascular disease in the thermally injured lower extremity. Such assessment would lead to earlier vascular specialist consultation and potential intervention that might help with future burn wound healing.

Physical Exam

As in all aspects of disease, the cornerstone of vascular assessment of any given patient is the physical exam. In the setting of an acute thermal injury, the utility of the physical exam maybe limited secondary to the acute wound created by a thermal injury.

First assessment of any patient with presumed vascular disease is direct palpation of the femoral, popliteal, posterior tibial, and dorsalis pedis artery. When palpation a concurrent palpation of the radial artery to confirm in the mind of the practitioners that what they believe they are palpating is truly a pulse in the lower extremity. In the setting of a thermal injury, with ongoing resuscitation, pulses might be diminished based on low total body volume secondary to ongoing losses due to thermal injuries. It is important to assess the pulse exam of the contralateral possibly unaffected limb to provide an assessment of what the patient's arterial insufficiency was prior to the thermal injury with the assumption that vascular disease occurs with some regularity in a symmetrical fashion.

A secondary assessment is the use of a handheld Doppler for audible cataloging of perfusion. Doppler signal assessments range from triphasic waveforms (normal arterial flow; three distinct tones) to biphasic waveforms (moderate arterial insufficiency; two distinct tones) to monophasic waveforms (severe arterial insufficiency; single tone).

Ankle Brachial Index

Ankle brachial index (ABI) is an easily preformed bedside measurement to assess arterial perfusion. ABI is calculated by measuring the higher brachial pressure with a blood pressure cuff and handheld Doppler and dividing that pressure by the higher ankle pressure (posterior tibial artery, anterior tibial artery, or dorsalis pedis artery). To measure brachial and ankle pressures, a Doppler probe is placed beyond an inflated pressure cuff in line with an axial artery to assess when arterial perfusion is extinguished. The pressure cuff is released slowly, and when return of arterial signal is heard, then the pressure measurement is measured. This procedure is depicted in Fig. 31.1. It should be noted that posterior tibial, anterior tibial, and dorsalis pedis artery pressures can be obtained. Calcified atherosclerotic vessels may be noncompressible and thereby falsely elevate ABI. ABI values greater than or equal to 1.3 are considered unreliable, and additional imaging should be sought to assess the patient's perfusion. ABI values ranging from 0.90 to 1.3 indicate normal arterial perfusion.

As arterial insufficiency increases in the lower extremity, ABI decreases. A single level of arterial stenosis or occlusion is usually associated with ABI between 0.5 and 1.0 with multilevel disease less than 0.5. The utility of ABI measurement for initial triage of vascular patients is well known. In his ground breaking study, Yao [18] observed patients with intermittent claudication usually demonstrate an ABI between 0.5 and 0.9, but it may be as high as 1.0 or as low as 0.2. Patients presenting with pain at rest were found to have ABIs below 0.4 and those with impending gangrene generally a measure less than 0.3.

Arterial Duplex

Despite its common use, ABI has well-known limitations among patients with medial arterial calcifications, a common finding in diabetic and renal failure patients. Such arterial wall changes often falsely elevate ankle pressure measurements, and subsequent ABI measurements may be rendered as falsely negative. Based on the works of others [19, 20], our practice has been to use with increasing frequency arterial duplex examination of the tibial vessels to classify patients into various levels of arterial insufficiency. We have adopted an arterial assessment of peak ankle velocity (PAV). PAV is defined as the highest arterial perfusion velocity at any tibial vessel in the limb of interest [21]. We have found in investigation of nondiabetic patients that a PAV ≤ 40 cm/s detects severe to critical arterial insufficiency. We have begun implementing this measure to assess our diabetic patient population that has known

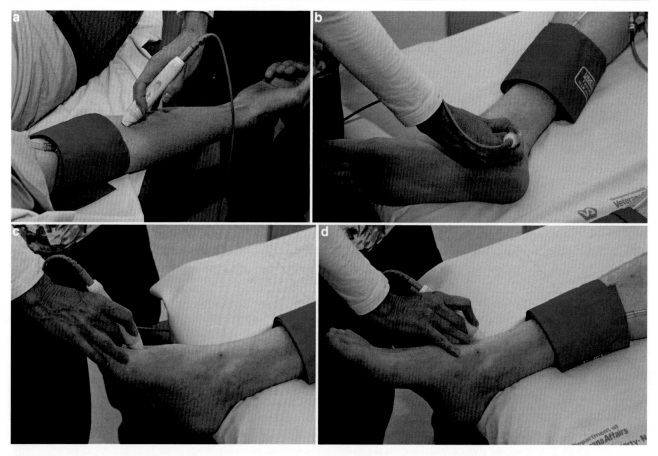

Fig. 31.1 Ankle brachial index measurements with Doppler probe and blood pressure cuff measurements. (**a**) Obtaining a brachial pressure measurement. (**b**) Obtaining a posterior tibial pressure measurement. (**c**) Obtaining a dorsalis pedis artery pressure measurement. (**d**) Obtaining an anterior tibial artery pressure measurement

limitations of ABI measurements. Arterial duplex examination of this sort is an easier assessment in a thermally injured lower extremity when application of blood pressure cuffs for ABI assessment might be problematic due to wound and/or patient tolerance.

Venous Duplex

Venous insufficiency can be measured with duplex interrogation and associated limb maneuvers to assess for physiological function of the venous system as well as occurrence of thrombus in the vein. Venous insufficiency leads to increased venous pressures in limbs (venous hypertension). Venous duplex with direct compression and flow assessments can be used to diagnose deep vein thrombosis. Venous valvular competency is essential to prevent regurgitation during relaxation of the lower limb muscles, protecting the superficial veins and capillaries from elevations in venous pressure [22]. Valvular incompetency causes an increase in superficial venous pressure (venous hypertension), resulting in the development of tissue trauma and eventual ulceration. This chronic ulcerative state usually does not result in limb loss;

however, in the setting of thermal injury, such claims might not hold true and have yet to be studied.

Other Imaging Modalities

Other modalities have been used in the measure of arterial insufficiency in the lower limb. These range from further noninvasive test such at segmental pressures, direct arterial duplex examination, and pulse volume recordings. Additionally, magnetic resonance imaging (MRI) and computer tomography angiography (CTA) technologies have utilized in the characterization arterial and venous insufficiency. The current gold standard for imaging of the arterial vasculature remains direct arterial puncture with subsequent angiogram. This later approach allows not only diagnosing arterial insufficiency but allows for possible endovascular intervention. This ability to intervene with minimal morbidly has resulted in a substantial increase in this treatment modality not only for severe presentation of arterial insufficiency but for venous disease as well. Endovascular interventions range in nature from balloon angioplasty to intra-arterial stent placement to percutaneous atherectomy, all of which has been addressed elsewhere in this volume.

Management of Vascular Disease

Arterial Disease Management

Once the need for vascular intervention is established, close collaboration with the burn surgery team should be maintained to optimize initial assessment, predict future treatment, and if need be intervene to aid in wound healing in the setting of thermal injury. Even patients with mild arterial insufficiency can potentially pose a challenge to the vascular specialist in that lower extremity wounds require increased perfusion for adequate healing [23]. Thus, the vascular consultant involvement early in the process is reasonable. Once level and severity of arterial disease has been confirmed, the vascular specialist will determine the risk-benefit ratio of an intervention versus conservative management for underlying arterial disease. This decision, in large part, should be based on the stability of the patient as well as the extent of the thermal injury. If initial injury to the extremity exists, intervention might not be warranted if wound burden of the thermal injury far exceeds the any functional outcome and amputation is contemplated. Again early consultation and active communication among all practitioners involved in the patient's care is needed to formulate a treatment plan that is tailored to the individual case.

With the advent of endovascular procedures, more and more morbid patients can be offered interventions to help restore some aspects of arterial perfusion. Additional open bypass of the lower extremity remains an option in select cases of thermal injury; however, due to the known wound complications of lower extremity bypass [24], this traditional restorative perfusion procedure has limited application in patients with extensive lower extremity burns.

Venous Disease Management

Interventions in patients with venous insufficiency are usually undertaken to prevent relapse of venous stasis disease. As found in the ESCHAR trial [25], a 12-month reduction in venous ulceration recurrences was found. This has led many practitioners to advocate for ablation of the superficial venous system and associated perforating veins in the treatment of advanced venous stasis disease.

Another aspect of the venous system that needs to be considered in the management of thermally injured patients is venous vascular access. The work of Gibron and coworkers recommend avoiding placement of central venous lines in limbs that will or have had fascial excision. This includes complete excision of the superficial venous system. Her article recognizes the difficulty in diagnosing venous congestion in these patients as typical findings are masked by the recent excision and resurfacing with split thickness skin grafts.

As such, she recommends maintaining a high index of suspicion as well as liberal use of lower extremity duplex scanning to assess for venous thrombosis. In the setting of acute or subacute venous thrombosis, treatment options include anticoagulation, bypass, and even lytic therapy, the last of which carries a high risk of complication in thermally injured patients who have recently been skin grafted [26].

Data regarding thromboembolic prophylaxis in burn patients remains sparse. One must always weigh the potential for increased bleeding while treating with anticoagulants with the devastating complication of deep vein thrombosis and/or pulmonary embolism. As is pointed out in the international consensus statement, recommendations for burn patients are generally based on extrapolation from other trauma patient populations. They recommend the use of low-molecular-weight heparin or unfractionated heparin in setting of underlying renal insufficiency, commonly found in the thermally injured. Another alternative is mechanical prophylaxis in the form of intermittent pneumatic compression stockings; however, this may not be an option with patients with lower extremity wounds [27]. That said, there is evidence that aside from improving venous hemodynamics, intermittent pneumatic compression stockings activated the fibrinolytic system by increasing levels of tissue plasminogen activator and prostacyclin [28] as well as tissue factor pathway inhibitor [29]. This has led us to use intermittent pneumatic compression stockings on the upper extremity when lower extremity wounds are present.

Compartment Syndrome

Circumferential burns can cause a compartment syndrome when the skin swells resulting in a reduction in blood flow to underlying compartments. This represents an acute threat to the limb with severely reduced arterial perfusion. This is addressed by releasing the injured skin through a procedure called escharotomies. Escharotomies typically involve the use of a cautery-type device to create a bivalve wound on the limb or trunk. Schematic representation of this procedure is shown in Fig. 31.2. Each incision site is placed along the midaxial plane. These incisions attempt to release burned skin from unburned skin. The incision is placed down to subcutaneous fat. Releases are performed until arterial flow is restored to the distal limb. This level of intervention is assessed by examining the limb involved, direct palpation compartments, evaluating peripheral pulses, and assessing capillary refill. Albeit the loss of distal arterial pulse is a late finding, practitioners should be vigilant to seek out changes in clinical examination, especially the occurrence of pain out of proportion to range of motion of the limb. If escharotomies are not undertaken, circumferential burns will require hourly neurovascular checks to monitor for perfusion.

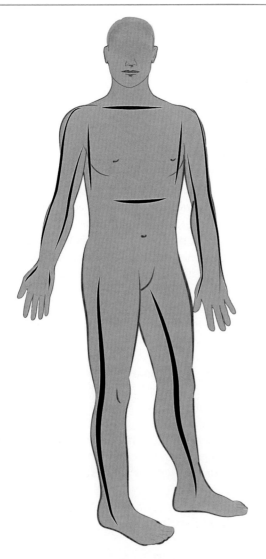

Fig. 31.2 Schematic representation of escharotomies of the trunk, lower limb, upper limb, and hand

Finger Escharotomies

Escharotomies are performed based on the location of the burn as well. In particular upper extremity locations with focus on the hand and digits are of great importance in the management of these patients. Releases are performed along the mid-axial plane of each digit as shown in Fig. 31.3. If one side is deemed enough to release pressure, then the surgeon would perform the incision on the non-pinch surface of the finger. One can determine the location of the incision by placing a mark at the junction between glabellar and dorsal skin. One may consider using traditional anatomic marking aids such as a line that connects the folds in the skin created by the interphalangeal joints depeding on obliteration of these landmarks by edema. The incision is carried, in general, from the tip of the finger to the base of the finger. This may be from burned to unburned skin. One should reassess the finger perfusion after creating

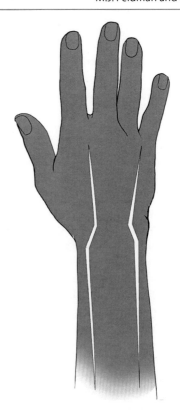

Fig. 31.3 Expanded schematic representation of escharotomies of the forearm and hand

the first incision. If perfusion is not restored, then completely bivalve the finger by creating an incision on the opposite side of the finger. One should avoid injuring the radial or ulnar neurovascular bundles.

Hand Escharotomies

The hand has nine known compartments in addition to the carpal tunnel. Each of these compartments needs to be taken into account when performing escharotomies. Again escharotomies have a different level of release with a similar incision versus fasciotomies undertaken for arterial reperfusion injury. One typically designs incisions along the dorsum of the hand in between the second and third and fourth and fifth metacarpal shafts. This is shown in Fig. 31.3. Additional incisions may be made along the edge of the glabellar skin over the thenar and hypothenar eminences if these areas are involved. For circumferential burns that cross the wrist, one would typically extend the dorsal incision across the wrist and combine them with forearm releases. All incisions are full thickness in nature, meaning the incision is extended through epidermis and dermis but not through the underlying fat. Incisions that involve fat tend to cause excessive bleeding as are thus avoided if at all possible. These incisions are typically created with electrocautery machine also known as the Bovie.

Following release, one would reassess compartment pressure, distal finger perfusion, and pulse examination. The goal is to reestablish a palpable pulse at the wrist and Doppler signals at the hand digital arch and fingers. The more distal vascular examination may be complicated by vasospasm which can make Doppler and physical examination findings difficult. If one has not established flow through the hand despite complete escharotomies, consider underlying compartment edema and the need for formal fasciotomies.

Forearm Escharotomies

Forearm escharotomies involve radial and ulnar mid-axial incisions to "bivalve" the forearm and release underlying pressure of the forearm compartments. This is indicated for deep partial-thickness or full-thickness, circumferential burns which are causing a compartment syndrome. Releases should improve blood flow to the flexor, extensor, and mobile wad compartments. The incisions are carried down to, but not through, the underlying fat. These incisions are typically created with Bovie cautery obtaining hemostasis simultaneously with the release. One would reassess perfusion after the release by feeling compartment pressure, assessing capillary refill of the fingers, palpating distal pulses, and a repeat Doppler examination. Consider a full fascial release should the escharotomy fail to provide reperfusion of the limb.

Upper Arm Escharotomies

Upper arm escharotomies involve both radial and ulnar mid-axial incisions to "bivalve" the upper arm and release underlying pressure to the upper arm. This is indicated for both deep partial-thickness and full-thickness circumferential burns which are causing a compartment syndrome. Release should aim to improve blood flow to both the flexor and extensor compartments of the upper arm. These incisions are carried down to, but not through, underlying fat. One would typically use a Bovie cautery to create the incisions and simultaneously obtain hemostasis as blood loss is to be minimized in large burns. Plan to reassess perfusion after the escharotomies have been completed as one must be prepared to perform fascial releases should perfusion not be restored to the underlying compartments.

Trunk Escharotomies

Escharotomies of the chest, abdomen, and back should be considered in patients with circumferential burns that appear to be constricting chest expansion and therefore limiting ventilation and/or oxygenation. The decision to release these compartments should be made in conjunction with the practitioners who are managing the patient's airway. While incisions are typically performed in deeper burn injuries, they are in our experience still painful and will require significant amounts of pain medication. In situations where the patient is having difficulty with oxygenation and/or ventilation, consider securing the airway before escharotomies are performed. All incisions are created with Bovie electrocautery down to, but not through, the underlying fat. The incisions on the chest are typically described as a "shield" pattern. These are carried out on both mid-axial locations of the axilla and connect via an inframammary incision below the breasts and may also have a separate incision to connect them at the level of the clavicles. This creates a pattern reminiscent of a knight's shield. The abdomen is typically release with bilateral mid-axial incisions.

Assessment of perfusion is via reevaluation of the patient's ventilatory status including pulse oximetry readings, peak airway pressures, changes in carbon dioxide levels, and tidal volumes. Abdominal pressure may be indirectly measured through the use of bladder pressures. Bladder pressures are obtained by clamping an indwelling Foley catheter distally, instilling approximately 30–50 mL of normal saline into the Foley, and then attaching the Foley to a pressure monitor after the patient and catheter are properly leveled. The Foley catheter must be clamped distally to ensure that the urine and saline form one contiguous unit. Normal bladder pressures are under 20 mmHg with abdominal hypertension considered greater than 20 mmHg, and possible intervention should be considered [30].

Neck Escharotomies

Neck escharotomies are typically performed with electrocautery Bovie down to the level of the fat on either side of the neck in a mid-axial plane. One should be careful to avoid injuring the external jugular venous system with these incisions. Always consider securing the airway with an endotracheal tube prior to performing a neck release.

Thigh Escharotomies

Escharotomies of the thighs are less common as these compartments have more space. The incisions are placed on either medial or lateral mid-axial lines of the thigh and extended from unburned skin to unburned skin if possible. One would aim to relieve pressure on both the flexor and extensor compartments.

Foot Escharotomies

Signs of compartment syndrome in the foot are difficult to assess especially in a patient with distracting injury and/or altered levels of consciousness. There are several methods for assessing compartment pressures in the foot including the Stryker needle puncture and measurement and/or arterial line measurement into the compartment of interest. Ultimately, one would not delay the release of a compartment based on these measurements alone, but would perform a release if there are clinical signs of compartment syndrome. Clinical signs include pain out of proportion to exam, sensory changes, pain on passive stretch, noncompressible compartments, tissue that is cooler to the touch versus contralateral limb, and a change in the pulse examination. Any change in the pulse examination would be later in the development of this process and may occur after tissue destruction has already begun. One should not delay releases until this occurs. Earlier, and more accurate, signs of compartment syndrome include pain out of proportion to examination and sensory changes [31].

Proposed Treatment Algorithm

Based on the principles of burn care in the acutely injured patient, we recommend the following algorithm (Fig. 31.4) for assessment and treatment of this special population of thermally injured patients. The first step of assessing patients with thermal injury is the initial trauma workup with appropriate volume resuscitation. The details of this particular initial step in assessment of this patient population is well known and followed under strict guidelines from the American College of Surgeons Advanced Trauma Life Support [32]. In the setting of thermal injury as stated above, it is of importance to assess patients for thermal injury of their torso or extremities for possible escharotomy. This portion of the algorithm represents an acute impending arterial insufficiency that is created by the initial thermal injury and mandates aggressive management by the burn surgeon in the care of these patients. It is of great importance to assess the patient early in his/her presentation for the indication for escharotomy. Also keep in mind that burn-related compartment syndromes may develop over time, and these patients require hourly neurovascular examinations for at least the first 24 h after the injury.

If initial assessment of the patient uncovers a potential arterial and/or venous insufficiency, appropriate vascular lab studies should be ordered to assess in particular arterial perfusion. The presence of diabetes should guide the clinician's choice of tests. The known limitations of diabetes in terms of compressibility of arteries and known inaccuracies of ABI measurements (i.e., ABI>1.3) dedicated arterial duplex examination and assessment of peak ankle velocities (PAV) should be undertaken. Consider enlisting the help of a vascular specialist if the patient has known arterial or venous insufficiency or studies suggest that these disease processes exist in a limb involved with a deep burn.

Key components in addition to a focused vascular history and physical exam is the assessment of patients with ankle brachial (ABI). If clinical grounds warrant arterial duplex examination should be obtained with peak ankle velocity (PAV) for characterization of possible underlying arterial disease.

Case Example

The patient is a 34-year-old male with a history of insulin-dependent diabetes, who accidentally burned himself using a heating pad to treat ankle pain. He presented a week later for treatment in our outpatient clinic. He was noted to have a full-thickness skin wound at that point with signs of local edema. This wound involved the left dorsal foot and medial malleolus as seen in Fig. 31.5.

Following admission, the patient underwent a preoperative workup including plain films that showed no fracture or dislocation. His admission laboratory work revealed a blood sugar of 156 mg/dL (normal value range 65–100 mg/dL) with a HgA1C of 9.3 % (normal value range 4.0–6.0 %) and a white cell count of 8.9×10^9/L (normal value range 3.7–9.7×10^9/L).

As is per our protocol, we began our assessment with a focused physical exam. On exam, the patient had non-palpable pulses in his dorsalis pedis artery, and due to the location of his thermal injury, we could not palpate his posterior tibial artery. We then proceeded to ABI measurements and obtained a left ABI of the posterior tibial vessel more proximal to the burned area of the lower extremity. The ABI calculated in this area was 1.34 and 1.38 for the dorsalis pedis and posterior tibial vessels, respectively. The contralateral ABI measures were 1.04 and 1.30 for the dorsalis pedis artery and posterior tibial arteries, respectively.

Secondary to the patient's falsely elevated ABI waveform analysis of these vessels were also undertaken. They demonstrated triphasic (normal) waveforms in all tibial vessels. This indicated that even in the setting of severe diabetes, this patient had preserved arterial perfusion to the affected limb, and thus no vascular consultation was warranted at the present time.

We then proceeded to surgical management of his wound. His initial excision was down to subcutaneous fat and deep reticular dermis. This tissue was protected with a vacuum-assisted closure device (VAC). Following several VAC changes, the wound was deemed ready for autografting (Fig. 31.6). A split thickness autograft was placed approximately a week after the initial excision (Fig. 31.7).

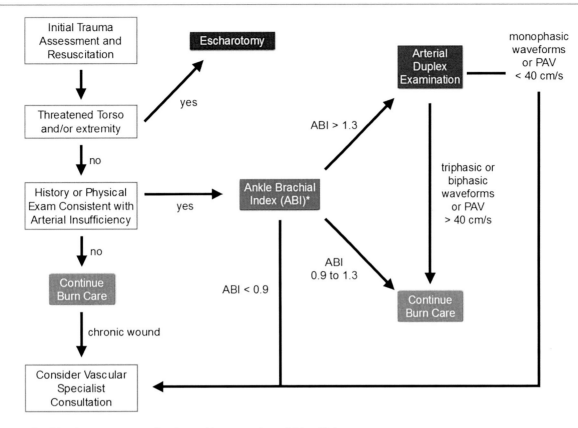

Fig. 31.4 Algorithm for management of patients with suspected arterial insufficiency

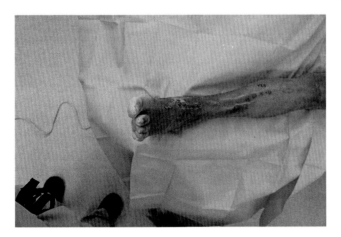

Fig. 31.5 Initial presentation to our clinic with left foot and lower extremity burn injury

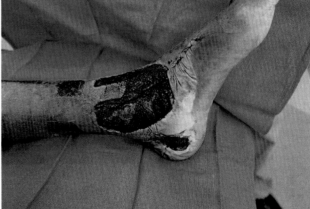

Fig. 31.6 Wound assessed post-excision day 4 showing result of vacuum-assisted wound care

Initial autograft take was noted to be complete; however, he went on to develop 50% loss of the autograft over the next 4 weeks. Local cultures were negative and laboratory work showed no elevation in white cell count. He underwent another local wound debridement and additional VAC therapy. Ultimately, he healed with meticulous wound care, antibiotic therapy, and strict blood sugar control (Figs. 31.8, 31.9, and 31.10).

This case highlights our experience with diabetic foot burns. While this patient achieved wound closure, it was at a significantly longer time period, required multiple surgeries,

and a higher complication rate possibly due to microvascular disease. If we had not achieved wound closure, then we would have reconsidered the involvement of a vascular specialist for further arterial assessment and possible endovascular treatment if needed. Ultimately, these patients do benefit from surgical intervention as demonstrated above; however, this must be coordinated with strict blood sugar control, wound management, and edema control. All of this should be discussed in detail with the diabetic burn patient in order to set expectations on admission.

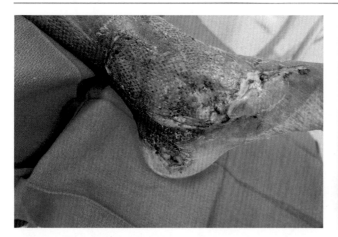

Fig. 31.7 Post-excision day 14 showing skin graft loss

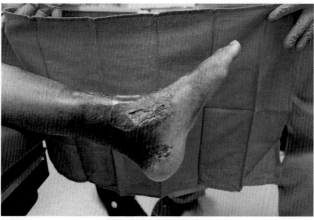

Fig. 31.9 Post-excision day 117 showing reepithelialization of wound bed

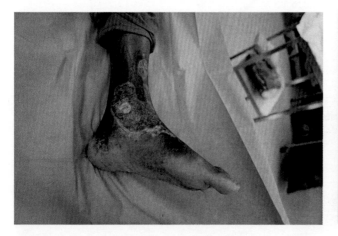

Fig. 31.8 Post-excision day 19 showing skin graft loss

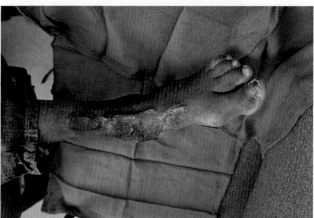

Fig. 31.10 Complete healing of the foot wound at 3 months and 25 days from initial hospitalization

Conclusions

This chapter reviews common vascular issues in thermal injuries with a focus on lower extremity wounds. The approach to all burn patients should focus on ruling out life-threatening injuries before focusing on the skin involvement itself. One should maintain a high index of suspicion for compartment syndrome in burn patients with circumferential wounds. Our aging population has higher rates of diabetes and comorbidities, which will exacerbate the effects of a burn injury. We have outlined an approach to these patients with a focus on their initial workup. Even under the best of circumstances, these patients should be counseled to expect higher rates of complications and longer hospital stays and require more surgeries to heal their wounds. Keep in mind, however, that surgical intervention can still be effective when paired with other methods to optimize blood flow and blood sugar control.

References

1. Kramer G. Pathophysiology of burn shock and burn edema. In: Herdon D, editor. Total burn. 4th ed. London: Saunders Publishers; 2012.
2. Baxter CR. Fluid volume and electrolyte changes of the early post-burn period. Clin Plast Surg. 1974;1(4):693–703.
3. Unger A, Haynes BW. Hemodynamic studies in severely burned patients. Surg Forum. 1960;10:356–61.
4. Wilmore D, Mason A, Johnson D, Pruitt B. Effect of ambient temperature on heat production and heat loss in burn patients. J Appl Physiol. 1975;38(4):593–7.
5. Aulick LH, Wilmore DW, Mason AD, Pruitt BA. Influence of the burn wound on peripheral circulation in thermally injured patients. Am J Physiol. 1977;233(4):H520–6.
6. Order SE, Moncrief JA. The burn wound. Springfield: Charles C Thomas; 1965.
7. Aulick HL, Wilmore DW, Mason AD, Pruitt BA. Muscle blood flow following thermal injury. Ann Surg. 1978;188(6):778–82.
8. Levin ME. Pathogenesis and management of diabetic foot lesions. In: Levin ME, O'Neal LW, editors. The diabetic foot. 5th ed. St Louis: C.V. Mosby Co.; 1988.

9. Gregg EW, Sorlie P, Paulose-Ram R, Gu Q, Eberhardt M, Wolz M. Prevalence of lower-extremity disease in the US adult population >=40 years of age with and without diabetes: 1999–2000 national health and nutrition examination survey. Diabetes Care. 2004; 27(7):1591–7.

10. Kimball Z, Patil S, Mansour H, Marano MA, Petrone SJ, Chamberlain RS. Clinical outcomes of isolated lower extremity or foot burns in diabetic versus non-diabetic patients: a 10-year retrospective analysis. Burns. 2013;39(2):279–84.

11. Balakrishnan C, Rak T, Meininger M. Burns of the neuropathic foot following use of therapeutic footbaths. Burns. 1995;21(8):622–3.

12. Barsun A, Sen S, Palmieri TL, Greenhalgh DG. A ten-year review of Lower extremity burns in diabetics: small burns that lead to major problems. J Burn Care Res. 2013;34(2):255–60.

13. Le B, Feldman M. Diabetic foot burns. Presented at the American College of Surgeons meeting in Chicago, IL, October 2, 2012.

14. Baux S. Contribution a l'Etude du traitement local des brulures thermigues etendues. Paris: These; 1961.

15. Osler T, Glance LG, Hosmer DW. Simplified estimates of the probability of death after burn injuries: extending and updating the baux score. J Trauma. 2010;68(3):690–7.

16. Edwards J. Upper extremity arterial disease: general considerations. In: Cronenwett J, Johnston K, editors. Rutherford's Vascular Surgery, 7th ed. Philadelphia. Saunders Elsevier; 2010.

17. White J. Lower extremity arterial disease: general considerations. In: Cronenwett J, Johnston K, editors. Rutherford's vascular surgery. 7th ed. Philadelphia: Saunders Elsevier; 2010.

18. Yao J. Hemodynamic studies in peripheral arterial disease. Br J Surg. 1970;57(10):761–6.

19. Bishara R, Taha W, Alfarouk M, Abdel Aal K, Wasfy S. Duplex detected ankle peak systolic velocity: a new parameter for the assessment of degree of peripheral ischemia. Int Angiol. 2004;23(4):368–72.

20. Bishara R, Taha W, Akladious I, Allam M. Ankle peak systolic velocity: new parameter to predict nonhealing in diabetic foot lesions. Vascular. 2009;17(5):264–8.

21. Taheri H, Amendola M, Pfeifer J, Albuquerque F, Levy M. Does peak ankle velocity (PAV) accurately reflect lower extremity arterial perfusion as assessed by ABI? J Vasc Surg. 2013;58(4):1154–5. Published abstract.

22. Lees T, Lambert D. Patterns of venous reflux in limbs with skin changes associated with chronic venous insufficiency. Br J Surg. 1993;80(6):725–8.

23. Marston W. Wound healing. In: Cronenwett J, Johnston K, editors. Rutherford's vascular surgery. 7th ed. Philadelphia: Saunders Elsevier; 2010.

24. Zhang J, Curran T, McCallum J, Wang L, Wyers M, Hamdan A. Risk factors for readmission after lower extremity bypass in the American College of Surgeons National Surgery Quality Improvement Program. J Vasc Surg. 2014;59(5):1331–9.

25. Barwell J, Davies C, Deacon J, Harvey K, Minor J, Sassano A. Comparison of surgery and compression with compression alone in chronic venous ulceration (ESCHAR study): randomised controlled trial. Lancet. 2004;363(9424):1854–9.

26. Gibran N, Heimbach H, Nicholis S. Iliofemoral venous thrombosis following fascial excision of a deep burn of the lower extremity: case report. J Trauma. 1992;33(6):912–3.

27. Nicolaides A, Hull R, Fareed J, Cardiovascular Disease Educational and Research Trust; European Venous Forum; North American Thrombosis Forum; International Union of Angiology and Union Internationale du Phlebologie. Burns. Clin Appl Thromb Hemost. 2013;19(2):161.

28. Summaria L, Caprini J, McMillan R, Sandesara J, Axelrod C, Mueller M. Relationship between postsurgical fibrinolytic parameters and deep vein thrombosis in surgical patients treated with compression devices. Am Surg. 1988;54(3):156–60.

29. Chouhan V, Comerota A, Sun L, Harada R, Gaughan J, Rao A. Inhibition of tissue factor pathway during intermittent pneumatic compression: a possible mechanism for antithrombotic effect. Arterioscler Thromb Vasc Biol. 1999;19(11):2812–7.

30. Hobson KG, Young KM, Ciraulo A, Palmieri TL, Greenhalgh DG. Release of abdominal compartment syndrome improves survival in patients with burn injury. J Trauma. 2002;53(6):1129–33.

31. Whitesides TE, Heckman MM. Acute compartment syndrome: update on diagnosis and treatment. J Am Acad Orthop Surg. 1996;4(4):209–18.

32. Chapleau W, Al-khatib J, Haskin D, LeBlanc P, Cardenas G, Borum S, Torres N, Abi Saad G, Al Ghanimi O, Al-Harthy A, Al Turki S, Ali J, Allerton D, Androulakis JA, Arca MJ, Armstrong JH, Atkinson JL, Ayyaz M, Baker A, Blake DP, Sallee R, Scruggs F, Bowyer MW, Brandt MM, Branicki FJ, Brasel K, Brighton G, Brown J, Bruna L, Burton RA, Bustraan J, Cabading V, Carvajal Hafemann C, Castagneto GH, Castro CL, Chaudhry Z, Chehardy P, Chennault RS, Chua WC, Chrysos E, Coimbra R, Collet e Silva F, Cooper A, Cortes Ojeda J, Cothren Burlew C, Chetty D, Davis KA, Domingues Cde A, di Silvio-lopez M, Doucet JJ, du Plessis HJ, Dunn JA, Dyson R, Dason M, Eastman AB, Elkholy AT, Falck larsen C, Fernandez FA, Foianini E, Foerster J, Frankel H, Gautam SC, Gomez GA, Gomez Fernandez AH, Guillamondegui OD, Guzman Cottallat EA, Hancock BJ, Henn R, Henny W, Henry SM, Herrera-Fernandez G, Hollands M, Horbowyj R, Hults CM, Jawa RS, Jover Navalon JM, Jurkovich GJ, Kaufmann CR, Knudson P, Kortbeek JB, Kosir R, Kuncir EJ, Ladner R, Lo CJ, Logsetty S, Lui KK, Lum SK, Lundy DW, Machado F, Mao P, Masood Gondal K, Maxson RT, Mcintyre C, Michael DB, Misra MC, Moore FO, Mori ND, Morrow CE Jr, Murphy SG, Nagy KK, Nicolau N, Oh HB, Omari OA, Ong HS, Olivero G, Pak-art R, Parry NG, Patel BR, Paul JS, Pereira PM, Poggetti RS, Poole A, Recalde Hidrobo M, Price RR, Primeau S, Quintana C, Razek TS, Roden R, Roed J, Romero M, Rotondo MF, Sabahi M, Schaapveld N, Schipper IB, Schoettker P, Schreiber MA, Serafico EC, Serrano JC, Siegel B, Siritongtaworn P, Skaff D, Smith RS, Sorvari A, Sutter PM, Sutyak J, Svendsen LB, Taha WS, Tchorz K, Lee Wt, Tisminetzky G, Trostchansky Jl, Truskett P, Upperman J, van den Ende Y, Vennike A, Vikström T, Voiglio E, Weireter LJ Jr, Wetjen NM, Wigle RL, Wilkinson S, Winchell RJ, Winter R, Yelon JA, Zarour AM. Thermal injuries. In: ATLS: advanced trauma life support for doctors (student course manual). 9th ed. Chicago: American College of Surgeons; 2012. Chapter 9.

Diabetic Foot

Joseph C. Babrowicz Jr., Richard F. Neville,
and Anton N. Sidawy

Introduction

While arterial occlusive disease causing limb ischemia is a
major factor in diabetic foot ulceration, it is only part of a
complex interaction of multiple factors leading to the serious
risks and complications of the diabetic foot.

Diabetes mellitus is among the leading causes of mortality and major morbidity in the United States. According to
the National Diabetes Statistics Report for 2014, approximately 1.7 million new cases of diabetes were diagnosed in
2012. In 2012, 29.1 million Americans, or 9.3 % of the population, had diabetes. Eighty-six million Americans age 20
and older had prediabetes and 25.9 % of seniors had diabetes
in 2012 [1]. Boulton reports that up to 50 % of older diabetics will be affected by a manifestation of diabetic foot such
as neuropathy. The lifetime risk for foot ulcer in diabetic
patients may be as high as 25 % and up to 80 % of amputations in diabetics are preceded by a diabetic foot ulcer [2]. In
2010 about 73,000 nontraumatic lower limb amputations
were performed in diabetics over the age of 20. About 60 %
of nontraumatic lower limb amputations in adults occur in
diabetics [1].

It is well accepted that peripheral artery disease (PAD) is
common in patients with diabetes. In the EURODIALE
Study, approximately 50 % of all patients with diabetic foot
ulcers had PAD [3]. The seriousness of social and economic
implications of diabetic foot disease on individual patient
cannot be overstated. Therefore, an understanding of the
pathophysiology, diagnosis, and treatment of the diabetic
foot is paramount for any physician involved in the care of
patients with diabetes and/or limb ischemia.

J.C. Babrowicz Jr., MD • R.F. Neville, MD
A.N. Sidawy, MD, MPH (✉)
Department of Surgery, George Washington University,
Washington, DC, USA

Pathophysiology

Neuropathy, PAD, and infection are generally considered a
triad of leading factors in the development of diabetic foot
ulceration. However, while neuropathy and PAD are clear
risk factors for diabetic foot ulceration, Boulton suggests
that infection is a result of, and not a risk factor for, ulceration [2]. Numerous other factors, such as age, prior foot
ulcer or amputation, and foot deformity, play a role in foot
ulcer formation as well. Understanding the multiple factors
leading to diabetic foot ulcer formation can be instrumental
in developing strategies to prevent these ulcers.

Diabetic Peripheral Neuropathy

Worldwide, diabetes is the most common cause of neuropathy, and diabetic neuropathies are among the most common
long-term complications of diabetes [2, 4, 5]. An international consensus group defined diabetic neuropathy (DN) as
the "presence of symptoms and/or signs of peripheral nerve
dysfunction in people with diabetes after the exclusion of
other causes" [6]. Of the several forms of DN (Table 32.1),
chronic sensorimotor diabetic peripheral neuropathy and
peripheral sympathetic autonomic neuropathy play the greatest role in diabetic foot ulceration [4, 6]. Neuropathy is a
major risk factor for developing foot ulceration, and according to Boulton, "in patients with significant neuropathy without a history of ulceration, the annual risk of developing an
ulcer is five to seven times higher than in those without neuropathy" [6].

The clinical features of DN may be best recognized by
understanding the "painful painless foot." This term is attributed to Dr. Paul Brand through his work with patients with
leprosy. He recognized that neuropathic patients often
experience severe painful neuropathic symptoms, but on
examination have complete sensory loss to all modalities
[6]. Smith describes the clinical features of DN as presenting

© Springer International Publishing Switzerland 2017
R.S. Dieter et al. (eds.), *Critical Limb Ischemia*, DOI 10.1007/978-3-319-31991-9_32

349

Table 32.1 Clinical classification of diabetic neuropathies

Polyneuropathy	Mononeuropathy
Sensory	Isolated peripheral
Acute sensory	Mononeuritis multiplex
Chronic sensorimotor	
Autonomic	Truncal
Cardiovascular	
Gastrointestinal	
Genitourinary	
Peripheral sympathetic	
Proximal motor (amyotrophy)	
Truncal	

Items in bold type are important in the etiopathogenesis of diabetic foot problems
From Boulton A. Diabetic Neuropathy: Is Pain God's Greatest Gift to Mankind? Semin Vasc Surg. 2012:25:61–65. Reprinted with permission from Elsevier

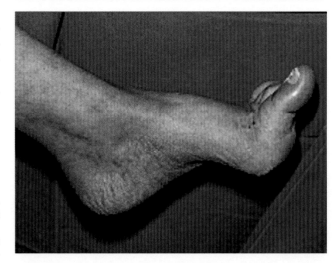

Fig. 32.1 At risk foot. Neuropathic diabetic foot with at risk "claw foot" deformity. From Boulton A. Diabetic Neuropathy: Is Pain God's Greatest Gift to Mankind? Semin Vasc Surg. 2012:25:61–65. Reprinted with permission from Elsevier

either "positive" or "negative" sensory symptoms or being asymptomatic. Positive symptoms are described as abnormal excessive sensations such as pricking, tingling, or burning. These sensations may be downright painful. Negative symptoms are characterized by numbness or sensory loss. Some patients are not aware of their sensory loss and may consider themselves as asymptomatic [5].

Typical sensorimotor neuropathy presents with a symmetric stocking distribution sensory loss described by the patients as a feeling of the limb being asleep or numb [4, 6]. Other patients will describe neuropathic painful symptoms such as burning discomfort, electrical sensations, or stabbing pain.

Motor neuropathy is also a component of overall diabetic neuropathy, thus the term sensorimotor neuropathy, and leads to small muscle wasting in the foot and absent ankle reflexes. The clinical presentation of motor nerve dysfunction is wasting of the small muscles in the feet and absent ankle reflexes. This chronic motor denervation results in malfunction of the intrinsic muscles of the foot that distorts foot architecture. Chronic metatarsal flexion, extensor subluxation of the toes, proximal migration of the metatarsal fat pad, and an imbalance in the action of the toe flexors and extensors lead to a "claw foot deformity." More importantly, with dislocation of the metatarsophalangeal joints, the heads of the metatarsals become more prominent, driven downward, and become the striking surface during ambulation. Other bony prominences become abnormal pressure points as well, and combined with a loss of pain sensation, the overlying skin is subject to repeated injury and ulceration. This so-called claw foot as depicted in Fig. 32.1 is characterized by clawing of the toes, prominent metatarsal heads, and a high arch. The "claw foot" deformity represents a high-risk diabetic neuropathic foot and is associated with increased risk of ulcer formation [7, 8].

Charcot foot (CF) is another form of foot deformity associated with diabetic neuropathy. CF can be acute or chronic.

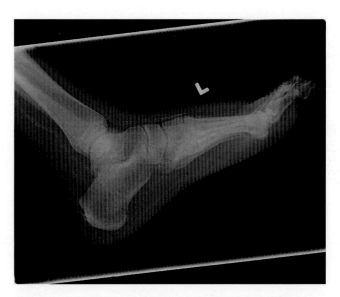

Fig. 32.2 Charcot foot. Radiographic example of a Charcot foot

Acute CF can mimic a foot infection where the foot is markedly red, warm, and swollen. Pain is often minimal or absent. The midfoot is usually most affected. Ongoing mechanical stresses lead to ligament strain, fracture-dislocations of the forefoot bones, midfoot collapse, and severe foot deformity and joint instability [9]. Figure 32.2 shows a radiograph of a Charcot foot.

Peripheral autonomic dysfunction affecting the sympathetic nervous system is also present in diabetic neuropathy. Autonomic dysfunction leads to loss of sweat and oil gland function resulting in dry skin prone to cracking and fissure formation. The cracked skin can breakdown and become a portal of entry for bacteria [2, 8].

Mechanisms of DSP

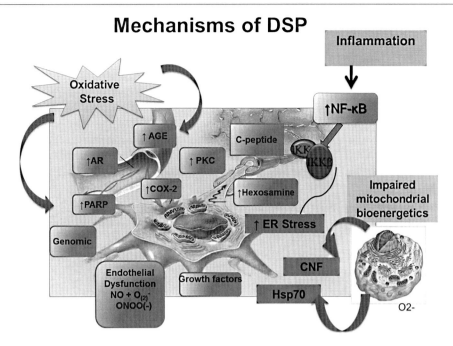

Fig. 32.3 Mechanisms of distal symmetric polyneuropathy (DSP). Proposed mechanisms of diabetic distal symmetric polyneuropathy (DSP). *AGE* advanced glycation end products, *AR* aldose reductase, *CNF* ciliary neurotrophic factor, *COX-2* cyclooxygenase 2, *ER* endoplasmic reticulum, *Hsp70* heat shock protein 70, *IKKβ* inhibitor of nuclear factor, *κB* kinase subunit β, *NF-kB* nuclear factor κB, *PARP* poly(ADP ribose) polymerase, *PKC* protein kinase C. The neuron displayed in the figure was drawn by the Juvenile Diabetes Research Foundation (JDRF) for the University of Michigan Center for Diabetes Complications, and it is reproduced here with permission from Helen Nickerson, PhD, Senior Scientific Program Manager JDRF. Reproduced from Albers JW, Rodica P-B. Diabetic Neuropathy: Mechanisms, Emerging Treatments, and Subtypes. Curr Neurol Neurosci Rep. 2014 Aug;14(8):473. Reprinted with permission from Springer

As one examines diabetic neuropathy, it becomes evident that there is a wide spectrum of presenting symptoms in these patients. Boulton emphasizes that, "neuropathic symptoms correlate poorly with sensory loss and their absence must never be equated with lack of foot ulcer risk." It has been observed that, "any patient that walks into clinic with a foot ulcer but without a limp must have neuropathy because those with normal pain sensation would not be able to put weight on the lesion" [7]. This observation lead Dr. Paul Brand to state that, "Pain is God's greatest gift to mankind" as it pertained to the protective nature of foot pain in the prevention of foot ulcers.

The pathogenesis of diabetic neuropathy is not completely understood and is likely multifactorial involving hyperglycemia, duration of diabetes, age-related neuronal degeneration, and other common factors such as hypertension, hyperlipidemia, and obesity [4]. According to Smith, "neuropathy likely results from a combination of direct axonal injury due to the metabolic consequences of hyperglycemia, insulin resistance, and toxic adiposity, and endothelial injury and microvascular dysfunction leading to nerve ischemia" [5]. The multiple biochemical pathways involved in the development of neuropathy may include increased mitochondrial production of free radicals, increased formation of glycation end products, downregulation of the soluble receptor for glycation end products, increased activity of the polyol or sorbitol pathway with accumulation of protein kinase C, activation of poly(ADP ribose) polymerase, cyclooxygenase 2 activation, endothelial dysfunction, peroxynitrite and protein nitration, and altered Na^+/K^+-ATPase pump function. These pathways alter neuronal activity, mitochondrial function, membrane permeability, and endothelial function. Ultimately these changes promote segmental demyelination, Wallerian degeneration, and microangiopathy and induce neuronal apoptosis leading to axonal and neuronal degeneration [4, 5]. In Fig. 32.3 Smith depicts this complex interaction of multiple pathways leading to neuropathy and the reader is referred to his thorough review of the mechanisms for further details [4].

Peripheral Artery Disease

Initial understanding of PSD in the diabetic population was mistakenly ascribed to the theory of small vessel disease or microvascular occlusion of the arterioles. This led to the assumption that diabetics with arterial insufficiency causing ulcers could not be revascularized and would need amputations. Subsequent decades of experience and research have shown that the predominant cause of ischemia in diabetic patients is macrovascular occlusion of the leg arteries, most commonly the tibial arteries, due to atherosclerosis [8].

PAD in diabetes alters vascular function at the macro-vascular and microvascular levels. On a macrovascular level, the formation of standard atheromatous plaques in diabetics is similar to nondiabetics. The pattern of involvement has some unique characteristics in diabetics with the larger iliac and femoral arteries commonly spared of hemodynamically significant disease. However, the popliteal and tibial arteries are more frequently involved compared to nondiabetics. While atherosclerosis affects the femoral and popliteal arteries in both diabetics and nondiabetics, the infragenicular occlusive disease in the anterior tibial, posterior tibial, and peroneal arteries is the classic distribution in diabetic patients (Fig. 32.4). It is not unusual to see diabetic patients with ischemic foot lesions having a palpable popliteal pulse with

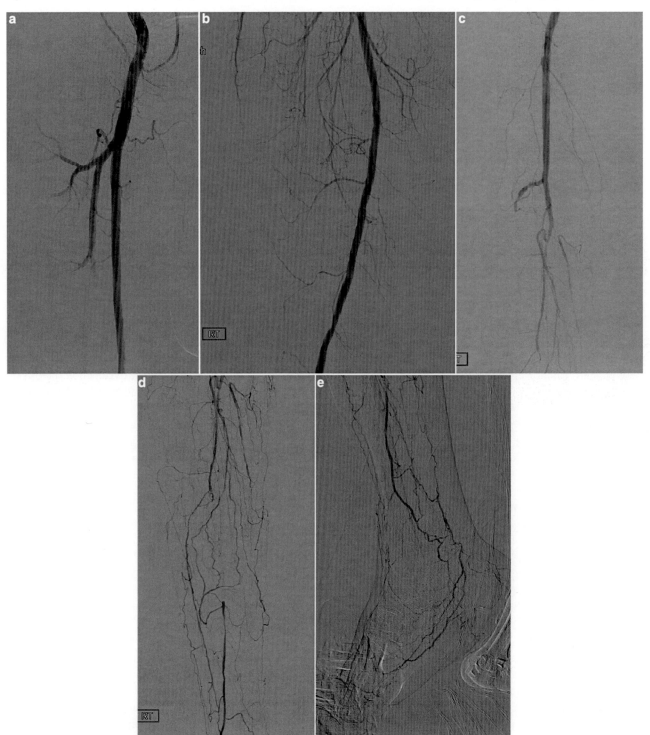

Fig. 32.4 Angiogram of diabetic foot patient. Serial angiograms of diabetic limb patient demonstrating relatively well-preserved femoral and popliteal arteries with severe tibial artery occlusive disease

occlusive disease isolated to the infragenicular arteries. Fortunately, the foot vessels are often spared in diabetics, even in the face of severe tibial level disease, which is important to the success of distal revascularization. A study based on arteriography showed no difference in occlusive disease in the arterial system of the foot when diabetics were compared to nondiabetics [10]. Diabetes can also lead to a hypercoagulable state through alterations in platelet function, coagulation, and blood rheology, thus potentially adding to arterial occlusive disease.

On a microvascular level, the arterial disease in diabetics is best described as nonocclusive microcirculatory impairment. This should not be confused with the term "small vessel disease" that refers to the common misconception of an untreatable occlusive lesion in the microcirculation. The concept of diabetic small vessel occlusive disease often leads to inappropriate management of diabetic patients with nonhealing foot lesions. The formation of these lesions in the presence of normal palpable foot pulses led to the misconception that diabetic patients have microvascular occlusive disease, which causes skin ischemia and formation of foot lesions. Dispelling the notion of "small vessel disease" has been fundamental to diabetic limb salvage, because arterial reconstruction is almost always possible and successful in these patients. In the presence of foot ischemia, the restoration of pulsatile blood flow using vein bypass may be necessary to heal the lesion. In this situation diabetic patients showed the same propensity to healing as nondiabetics. Infrainguinal vein bypasses in diabetics have comparable patency and limb salvage rates to those performed in nondiabetics [11].

Whereas there is no occlusive disease in the microcirculation, multiple structural and physiologic abnormalities result in functional microvascular impairment [12]. Endothelial cell dysfunction as a result of hyperglycemia and hyperinsulinemia plays a major role in this functional defect [13]. Nitric oxide (NO) is the main vasodilator released by the endothelium and causes vasodilation by diffusing into the vascular smooth muscle cells (VSMC) thereby stimulating cyclic guanosine 3′5′-monophosphate-mediated relaxation. NO is synthesized in the endothelial cell through the action of an endothelial-specific NO synthase (ecNOS). The expression of ecNOS is reduced in response to hyperglycemia and hyperinsulinemia [13]. Also, loss of NO homeostasis at the microcirculatory level creates a proinflammatory environment with damaging oxygen-free radical species released into the vasculature and surrounding tissues.

Another effect of hyperglycemia is the nonspecific glycosylation of proteins, so-called advanced glycosylation end products (AGEs). AGEs impair the actions of NO by stimulating the formation of free oxygen radicals that react with NO and convert it to a prooxidant. AGEs also displace disulfide cross-linkages in collagen proteins thereby diminishing the charge in the capillary basement membrane and altering its diffusion properties [14]. These basement membrane alterations contribute to increased vascular permeability and inflammation. AGEs activate and upregulate the expression of endothelial AGE receptors—these add to the local inflammatory state by increasing leukocyte chemotaxis and transformation into foam cells which contribute to increasing local oxidative stress [15]. One result of this increase in inflammation is an increase in C-reactive protein (CRP) which is strongly related to widespread acceleration of atherosclerosis and promotion of endothelial cell apoptosis [16]. These and other mechanisms result in the impaired microvasculature marked by a characteristic thickening of the capillary basement membrane which does not affect arteriolar luminal diameter or blood flow but does impair nutrient and substrate flow into the adjacent tissues. This, coupled with autonomic dysfunction at the capillary level described earlier, severely hinders the hyperemic response to injury, inflammation, and infection.

The macrovascular component of PAD in diabetics is due to atherosclerosis. The atheromatous changes occur in a similar fashion as in nondiabetics, but in an accelerated way. This acceleration could be due to the previously described diabetes-driven increases in inflammation that worsen the course of "normal" plaque pathophysiology, changes in platelet and coagulation system function, and the high coincidence of hypertension among diabetics due to diabetic nephropathy.

Another common finding among diabetics is extensive medial calcification of the arteries. This is a process that can occur either at or separate from sites of atheromatous plaque and in diabetics is characteristically found throughout the arteries of the legs. There are several different disease states and proposed pathways for this abnormal calcification of the media; in diabetics both hyperinsulinemia and hyperglycemia are implicated. Both have been shown to alter gene and protein expression in endothelial and vascular smooth muscle cell (VSMC) that directly result in "osteoblast-like" activity of the VSMC and pericyte cells of the artery [17]. An example is the abnormal expression of proteins like osteopontin by these cells. Osteopontin coupled with chronic inflammation and high presence of oxygen-free radicals and C-reactive protein within the vessel wall leads to the deposition of calcium-phosphate complexes that mineralize within the media. Although this is generally a nonobstructive lesion, it leads to noncompliant arteries unable to augment flow in response to increased demand and, depending on the luminal diameter of the vessel, long segmental stenoses that disturb normal blood flow.

As mentioned before, the formation of atheromatous plaques in diabetics is similar in most regards to nondiabetics, but the pattern of involvement has a unique characteristic in diabetics. Despite sometimes widespread calcinosis, the larger iliofemoral arteries are commonly spared of hemodynamically significant disease. However, in diabetics the popliteal and infra-popliteal vessels are more frequently involved than the larger arteries and more frequently diseased compared to nondiabetics [18]. The foot vessels are relatively spared in diabetics, even in the face of severe tibioperoneal level disease, which is important to the success of revascularization [19].

In addition to the effects on the endothelium and VSMC, diabetes also leads to a hypercoagulable state through alterations in platelet function, coagulation, and blood rheology. Platelet uptake of glucose is unregulated in hyperglycemia and results in increased oxidative stress which enhances platelet aggregation. These platelets also have increased expression of glycoprotein Ib and IIb/IIIa receptors which are important in thrombosis and platelet adhesion. The coagulation system is affected by diabetic-related increases in tissue factor expression by VSMC and endothelial cells and increases in plasma concentrations of factor VII. Hyperglycemia is also associated with a decreased concentration of antithrombin and protein C, impaired fibrinolytic function, and excess plasminogen activator inhibitor-1 [20]. Blood rheology is altered as a consequence of an increase in viscosity and fibrinogen content due to hyperglycemia.

In summary, the effects of PAD in diabetics confer alterations in the microvascular functioning and macrovascular supply that lead to ischemia. Because of the synergistic consequences of both processes, the actual degree of ischemia can be greater than suspected, and even relatively minor trauma or infection can be made worse due to vascular insufficiency. The contribution of neuropathy with even moderate levels of ischemia is particularly worrisome as these "neuroischemic" feet are more prone to ulceration and infection [21, 22].

Infection

As previously mentioned, infection is more a result of than a true cause of diabetic foot ulceration. The structural and functional alterations of the arteriole and capillary walls, most notably, membrane basement thickening, associated with diabetes add to the likelihood of an ulcer becoming infected. The thickened basement membrane blocks leukocyte migration and hinders hyperemic and vasodilatory response to injury. This may block the normal inflammatory signs associated with infection. Erythema, rubor, cellulitis, and tenderness may be absent. The normal systemic signs of infection like fever, tachycardia, and leukocytosis may be absent as well [8]. Failure by the diabetic patient to recognize the onset of infection in an ulcer can have dire consequences. The risk of amputation correlates directly with increasing severity of infection as confirmed by Lavery in 2007 [23]. This study of 1666 diabetic patients showed increased risk of amputation, higher level amputation, and lower extremity-related hospitalization in patients with increased severity of infection based on the Infectious Disease Society of America (IDSA) classification of wound infection.

Classification of the Diabetic Foot

Discussion of the pathophysiology of diabetic foot ulcers leads into a discussion about classification schemes for the threatened limb. The 2014 Society for Vascular Surgery document details the evolution of classification schemes for critical limb ischemia and the threatened limb. To date, any one of the existing systems failed to include all three major pathophysiologic components of the threatened diabetic foot. In fact, the original 1978 definition of critical limb ischemia actually excluded patients with diabetes altogether. These existing systems tended to concentrate on only one of the causative factors such as perfusion (Fontaine and Rutherford) or foot wound (Wagner and University of Texas) [24]. A complete summary of the previous systems is provided in Table 32.2.

The 2014 SVS document calls the new classification system "The Society for Vascular Surgery Lower Extremity Threatened Limb Classification System." Under this new system, risk stratification is based on wound, ischemia, and foot infection. Shorthand for the system is WIfI (**W**ound, **I**schemia, and **f**oot **I**nfection). It is the intention of this system to, "provide more precise description of the disease burden to allow accurate outcomes assessment and comparison between similar groups of patients and alternative therapies." The system takes into account that, "wound healing depends not only on the degree of ischemia, but also on the extent and depth of the wound and the presence and severity of infection." The entire WIfI system is outlined in Table 32.3.

Assessment of the Diabetic Foot

Screening

Screening patients at risk for diabetic foot ulceration should be based on those factors that may lead a diabetic down the final common pathway to foot ulceration. It is commonly believed that neuropathy, deformity, and trauma interact to ultimately cause ulceration. Therefore, the history and physical examination of the diabetic patient should concentrate on identifying signs and symptoms of these mechanisms.

In 2008, a task force of the American Diabetes Association was assembled to address and construct a comprehensive foot examination for diabetic patients [25]. According to the document, diabetic patients should be assessed for their risk of foot ulceration by exploring key features of their history and following a thorough physical

Table 32.2 Summary and comparison of existing diabetic foot ulcer, wound, and lower extremity ischemia classification systems

Classification system	Ischemic rest pain	Ulcer	Gangrene	Ischemia	Infection	Comments
Rutherford	Yes, category 4/6	Category 5, minor tissue loss, nonhealing ulcer, focal gangrene with diffuse pedal ischemia	Category 6, major tissue loss extending above TM level, functional foot no longer salvageable (although in practice often refers to extensive gangrene, potentially salvageable foot with significant efforts)	Yes, cutoffs for CLI, category 4: resting AP <40 mmHg, flat or barely pulsatile ankle or forefoot PVR; TP <30 mmHg category 5/6: AP <60 mmHg; flat or barely pulsatile ankle or forefoot PVR; TP <40 mmHg	No	Pure ischemia model PAD classification system includes milder forms of PAD (categories 1–3); categories 4–6 based on cutoff values for CLI; no spectrum of ischemia, does not acknowledge potential need for revascularization with <CLI cutoff depending on wound extent/infection; not intended for patients with diabetes; wound classes not sufficiently detailed; omits infection as a trigger
Fontaine	Yes, class III/IV	Class IV/IV, ulcer and gangrene grouped together	Class IV/IV, ulcer and gangrene grouped together	Cutoff values for CLI based on European consensus document: ischemic rest pain >2 weeks with AP <50 mmHg or TP <30 mmHg ulcer and gangrene; AP <50 mmHg, TP <30 mmHg, absent pedal pulses in patient with diabetes	No	Pure ischemia model; no clear definitions of spectrum of hemodynamics; minimal description of wounds; infection omitted
PEDIS	No	Yes, grades 1–3; grade 1: superficial full-thickness ulcer, not penetrating deeper than the dermis; grade 2: deep ulcer, penetrating below the dermis to subcutaneous structures involving fascia, muscle, or tendon; grade 3: all subsequent layers of the foot involved including bone and/or joint (exposed bone, probing to bone)	No	Yes, three grades; CLI cutoff grade 1: no PAD symptoms, ABI >0.9, TBI >0.6, TcPO$_2$ >60 mmHg; grade 2: PAD symptoms, ABI <0.9, AP >50 mmHg, TP >30 mmHg, TcPO$_2$ 30–60 mmHg; grade 3: AP <50 mmHg, TP <30 mmHg, TcPO$_2$ <30 mmHg	Yes, grades 1–4; see IDSA classification (Table 32.3)	Primarily intended for DFUs; ulcer grades validated; includes perfusion assessment, but with cutoff for CLI; gangrene not separately categorized; includes validated IDSA infection categories
UT	No	Yes, grades 0–3 ulcers; grade 0: pre- or postulcerative completely epithelialized lesion; grade 1: superficial, not involving tendon, capsule, or bone; grade 2: penetrating to tendon/capsule; grade 3: penetrating to bone or joint	No	Yes ± based on ABI <0.8	Yes, ± wounds with frank purulence or >2 of the following (warmth, erythema, lymphangitis, edema, lymphadenopathy, pain, loss of function) considered infected	Primarily intended for DFUs; includes validated ulcer categories; PAD and infection included, but only as ± with no grades/spectrum
Wagner	No	Grade 0: pre- or postulcerative lesion; grade 1: partial/full-thickness ulcer; grade 2: probing to tendon or capsule; grade 3: deep ulcer with osteitis; grade 4: partial foot gangrene; grade 5: whole foot gangrene	Ulcer and gangrene grouped together; gangrene due to infection not differentiated from gangrene due to ischemia; also includes osteomyelitis	No	No for soft tissue component; included only as osteomyelitis	Orthopedic classification intended for diabetic feet; no hemodynamics; gangrene from infection not differentiated from that due to ischemia; osteomyelitis included; soft tissue infection not separated from bone infection

(continued)

Table 32.2 (continued)

Classification system	Ischemic rest pain	Ulcer	Gangrene	Ischemia	Infection	Comments
S(AD) SAD system	No	Yes, grades 0–3 based on area and depth; grade 0: skin intact; grade 1: superficial, <1 cm²; grade 2: penetrates to tendon, periosteum, joint capsule, 1–3 cm²; grade 3: lesions in bone or joint space, >3 cm²	No	Pulse palpation only, no hemodynamics	Yes, 1 = no infection; 2 = cellulitis; 3 = osteomyelitis	Intended for DFUs; also includes neuropathy; does not mention gangrene; no hemodynamic information; perfusion assessment based on pulse palpation only
Saint Elian	No	Yes, grades 1–3 based on depth; grade 1: superficial wound disrupting entire skin; grade 2: moderate or partial depth, down to fascia, tendon, or muscle but not bone or joints; grade 3: severe or total, wounds with bone or joint involvement, multiple categories including area, ulcer number, location, and topography	No	Yes, grades 0–3; grade 0: AP >80 mmHg, ABI 0.9–1.2; grade 1: AP 70–80 mmHg, ABI 0.7–0.89, TP 55–80 mmHg; grade 2: AP 55–69 mmHg, ABI 0.5–0.69, TP 30–54 mmHg; grade 3: AP <55 mmHg, ABI <0.5, TP <30 mmHg	Yes, grades 0–3; grade 0: none; grade 1: mild; erythema 0.5–2 cm, induration, tenderness, warmth, and purulence; grade 2: moderate, erythema >2 cm, abscess, muscle tendon, joint, or bone infection; grade 3: severe, systemic response (similar to IDSA)	Detailed system intended only for DFUs; detailed comprehensive ulcer classification system and hemodynamic categories for gradation of ischemia; gangrene not considered separately infection system similar to IDSA
IDSA	No	No	No	No	Yes, uninfected, mild, moderate, and severe (Table 32.3)	Validated system for risk of amputation related to foot infection, but not designed to address wound depth/complexity or degree of ischemia
SVS lower extremity threatened limb classification	Yes, wound/clinical class 0–3	Yes, grades 0–3; grouped by depth, location and size, and magnitude of ablative/wound coverage procedure required to achieve healing	Yes, grades 0–3; grouped by extent, location and size, and magnitude of ablative or wound coverage procedure required to achieve healing	Yes, ischemia grades 0–3; hemodynamics with spectrum of perfusion abnormalities; no cutoff value for CLI; grade 0: unlikely to require revascularization	Yes, IDSA system (Table 32.3)	Includes PAD + diabetes with spectrum of wounds, ischemia, and infection, scaled from 0 to 3; no cutoff for CLI. Need for revascularization depends on degree of ischemia, wound, and/or infection severity; ulcers/gangrene categorized based on extent and complexity of anticipated ablative surgery/coverage

ABI ankle-brachial index, *AP* ankle pressure, *CLI* critical limb ischemia, *DFUs* diabetic foot ulcers, *IDSA* Infectious Disease Society of America, *PAD* peripheral artery disease, *PEDIS* perfusion, extent/size, depth/tissue loss, infection, sensation, *PVR* pulse volume recording, *SAD* sepsis, arteriopathy, denervation, *SVS* Society for Vascular Surgery, *TcPO2* transcutaneous oxygen pressure, *TP* toe pressure, *UT* University of Texas

From Mills JL Sr, et al. The Society for Vascular Surgery Lower Extremity Threatened Limb Classification System: Risk stratification based on wound, ischemia, and foot infection (WIfI). J Vasc surg. 2014 Jan;59(1):220–34.e1-2. Reprinted with permission from Elsevier Limited

Table 32.3 Society for Vascular Surgery Lower Extremity Threatened Limb (SVS WIfI) Classification System

I. **W**ound
II. **I**schemia
III. **f**oot **I**nfection
WIfI score

W: Wound/clinical category

SVS grades for rest pain and wounds/tissue loss (ulcers and gangrene):

0 (ischemic rest pain, ischemia grade 3, no ulcer), 1 (mild), 2 (moderate), and 3 (severe)

Grade	Ulcer	Gangrene	
0	No ulcer	No gangrene	
Clinical description: ischemic rest pain (requires typical symptoms + ischemia grade 3), no wound			
1	Small, shallow ulcer(s) on distal leg or foot; no exposed bone, unless limited to distal phalanx	No gangrene	
Clinical description: minor tissue loss. Salvageable with simple digital amputation (one or two digits) or skin coverage			
2	Deeper ulcer with exposed bone, joint, or tendon; generally not involving the heel; shallow heel ulcer, without calcaneal involvement	Gangrenous changes limited to digits	
Clinical description: major tissue loss salvageable with multiple (≥3) digital amputations or standard TMA ± skin coverage			
3	Extensive, deep ulcer involving forefoot and/or midfoot; deep, full-thickness heel ulcer ± calcaneal involvement	Extensive gangrene involving forefoot and/or midfoot; full-thickness heel necrosis ± calcaneal involvement	

Clinical description: extensive tissue loss salvageable only with a complex foot reconstruction or nontraditional TMA (Chopart or Lisfranc); flap coverage or complex wound management needed for large soft tissue defect

I: Ischemia

Hemodynamics/perfusion: measure TP or TcPO$_2$ if ABI incompressible (>1.3)

SVS grades 0 (none), 1 (mild), 2 (moderate), and 3 (severe)

Grade	ABI	Ankle systolic pressure (mmHg)	TP, TcPO2 (mmHg)
0	≥0.80	>100	≥60
1	0.6–0.79	70–100	40–59
2	0.4–0.59	50–70	30–39
3	≤0.39	<50	<30

fI: foot Infection:

SVS grades 0 (none), 1 (mild), 2 (moderate), and 3 (severe: limb and/or life threatening)

SVS adaptation of Infectious Diseases Society of America (*IDSA*) and International Working Group on the Diabetic Foot (IWGDF) perfusion, extent/size, depth/tissue loss, infection, sensation (*PEDIS*) classifications of diabetic foot infection

(continued)

Table 32.3 (continued)

Clinical manifestation of infection	SVS	IDSA/PEDIS infection severity	
No symptoms or signs of infection	0	Uninfected	
Infection present, as defined by the presence of at least two of the following items: • Local swelling or induration • Erythema >0.5 to ≤2 cm around the ulcer • Local tenderness or pain • Local warmth Purulent discharge (thick, opaque to white, or sanguineous secretion) Local infection involving only the skin and the subcutaneous tissue (without involvement of deeper tissues and without systemic signs as described below) Exclude other causes of an inflammatory response of the skin (e.g., trauma, gout, acute Charcot neuro-osteoarthropathy, fracture, thrombosis, venous stasis)	1	Mild	
Local infection (as described above) with erythema >2 cm or involving structures deeper than skin and subcutaneous tissues (e.g., abscess, osteomyelitis, septic arthritis, fasciitis) No systemic inflammatory response signs (as described below)	2	Moderate	
Local infection (as described above) with the signs of SIRS, as manifested by two or more of the following: • Temperature >38° or <36 °C • Heart rate >90 beats/min • Respiratory rate >20 breaths/min or $PaCO_2 < 32$ mmHg • White blood cell count >12,000 or <4000 cu/mm or 10 % immature (band) forms	3	Severe[a]	

(32.3 a) Key summary points for use of Society for Vascular Surgery Lower Extremity Threatened Limb (SVS WIfI) Classification System

1. Table 32.3, the full system, is to be used for initial, baseline classification of all patients with ischemic rest pain or wounds within the spectrum of chronic lower limb ischemia when reporting outcomes, regardless of form of therapy. The system is not to be employed for patients with vasospastic and collagen vascular disease, vasculitis, Buerger's disease, acute limb ischemia, or acute trauma (mangled extremity)

2. Patients with and without diabetes mellitus should be differentiated into separate categories for subsequent outcomes analysis

   a. Presence of neuropathy (±) should be noted when possible in patients with diabetes in long-term studies of wound healing, ulcer recurrence, and amputation, since the presence of neuropathy (loss of protective sensation and motor neuropathic deformity) influences recurrence rate

3. In the Wound (W) classification, depth takes priority over size. Although we recommend that a wound, if present, be measured, a shallow, 8-cm^2 ulcer with no exposed tendon or bone would be classified as grade 1

   a. If a study of wound healing vs. Wound (W) grade were performed, wounds would be classified by depth and could also be categorized by size: small (<5 cm^2), medium (5–10 cm^2), and large (>10 cm^2)

4. TPs are preferred for classification of ischemia (I) in patients with diabetes mellitus, since ABI is often falsely elevated. TcPO$_2$, SPP, and flat forefoot PVRs are also acceptable alternatives if TP is unavailable. All reports of outcomes with or without revascularization therapy require measurement and classification of baseline perfusion

5. In reporting the outcomes of revascularization procedures, patients should be restaged after control of infection, if present, and/or after any debridement, if performed, prior to revascularization

   a. Group a patients: no infection within 30 days or simple infection controlled with antibiotics alone

   b. Group b patients: had infection that required incision and drainage or debridement/partial amputation to control

From Mills JL Sr, et al. The Society for Vascular Surgery Lower Extremity Threatened Limb Classification System: Risk stratification based on wound, ischemia, and foot infection (WIfI). J Vasc surg. 2014 Jan;59(1):220–34.e1-2. Reprinted with permission from Elsevier Limited

Patients with diabetes should have TP measurements. If arterial calcification precludes reliable ABI or TP measurements, ischemia should be documented by TcPO$_2$, SPP, or PVR. If TP and ABI measurements result in different grades, TP will be the primary determinant of ischemia grade

Flat or minimally pulsatile forefoot PVR = grade 3

TMA transmetatarsal amputation, *ABI* ankle-brachial index, *PVR* pulse volume recording, *SPP* skin perfusion pressure, *TP* toe pressure, *TcPO2* transcutaneous oximetry, *PACO2* partial pressure of arterial carbon dioxide, *SIRS* systemic inflammatory response syndrome, *ABI* ankle-brachial index, *PVR* pulse volume recording, *SPP* skin perfusion pressure, *TcPO2* transcutaneous oximetry, *TP* toe pressure

[a]Ischemia may complicate and increase the severity of any infection. Systemic infection may sometimes manifest with other clinical findings, such as hypotension, confusion, vomiting, or evidence of metabolic disturbances, such as acidosis, severe hyperglycemia, new-onset azotemia

examination. The major risk factors for diabetic foot ulcer formation are outlined in [25].

The history must consider signs and symptoms consistent with the key issues of prior ulceration, foot deformity, neuropathy, and arterial occlusive disease. While the history is usually very revealing, it must be kept in mind that many patients will describe themselves as asymptomatic. Therefore, a detailed and methodical exam of the feet is paramount [25]. Once the history and physical has been obtained as outlined by the task force document, the risk of developing a foot ulcer can be determined. This risk classification may then be used to determine the timing and extent of referral to members of the treatment team. Details of the risk classification and referral scheme are outlined in [25].

Noninvasive Assessment for PAD

When the diabetic patient has history and physical findings worthy of further assessment for PAD, the noninvasive vascular laboratory offers studies that are well established and easily obtained in most circumstances.

An ankle-brachial index (ABI) is usually the initial step in the objective noninvasive assessment of the patient with suspected peripheral arterial occlusive disease. The study compares the higher of the systolic blood pressure at either the dorsalis pedis or posterior tibial arteries on each limb to the higher of the two brachial artery systolic pressures. A ratio is calculated by placing the ankle pressure value over the brachial pressure value. The generally accepted normal value range is from 1.0 to 1.2. An ABI less than 0.6 generally indicates that a foot ulcer is unlikely to heal without revascularization [26].

In diabetic patients with medial calcinosis, the tibial artery walls may not be compressible. Therefore, the ABI value may be unobtainable or misleading. The noncompressible tibial artery wall usual leads to a supranormal value for the ABI such as 1.3. In such circumstances the clinician must be suspicious that the ABI is not reliable for that patient especially in the absence of palpable pulses and alternative noninvasive measures for arterial occlusive disease should be considered.

The digital arteries usually remain compressible in diabetic patients. Therefore, the measurement of a toe-brachial index (TBI) may be useful when the ABI measurement is unreliable. A TBI greater than 0.75 is generally accepted as normal, while a value below 0.25 suggests critical limb ischemia. An absolute toe pressure greater than 55 mmHg suggests adequate perfusion to heal a foot ulcer [26]. An obvious limitation of the TBI occurs when the toes are absent such as following a transmetatarsal amputation.

If the TBI cannot be obtained due to missing digits, another useful noninvasive study is the pulse volume recording (PVR). In this study blood pressure cuffs are placed at multiple levels along each leg and segmental pressures and pulse waveforms are measured and recorded. As the degree of arterial occlusive disease increases, the waveforms will change from triphasic to biphasic and then monophasic. This study allows measurement and comparison of occlusive disease longitudinally from proximal to distal arterial segments, as well as laterally from one leg to the other leg. A gradient between any consecutive longitudinal segments or from side to side suggests significant arterial occlusive disease between the segments. The PVR is particularly useful in diabetic patients since the study is not affected by medial calcinosis [26].

Duplex ultrasound imaging can provide anatomic and physiologic information with regard to arterial stenosis and/or occlusion. This information may be used to guide selective angiographic imaging or even sometimes may be sufficient enough to guide endovascular intervention or operative therapy [26].

Contrast Imaging of PAD

Historically, most diabetic PAD has been imaged with contrast angiography when planning a revascularization procedure. While catheter-based contrast angiography remains the workhorse of vascular imaging, newer techniques of computerized tomographic angiography and magnetic resonance angiography are becoming more refined and useful for planning vascular reconstruction. Each modality must be examined with regard to its benefits and drawbacks when specifically applied to the diabetic patient.

Catheter-Based Contrast Angiography

Digital subtraction angiography remains the gold standard for lower extremity arterial imaging. The high-resolution images produced on current flat-panel image intensifiers allow for great detail of even the small tibial and pedal artery segments. The flat-panel systems have larger field of view than conventional image intensifiers and can produce the same image acquisition with less radiation and contrast volume. The computer processing techniques of masking and road mapping allow for easier endovascular interventions. One of the greatest benefits of contrast angiography is that it can quickly go from diagnostic to treatment modalities with ease.

The drawbacks of contrast angiography are related to the need to access the vascular system and the use of intravascular contrast agents. The latter issue is particularly problematic in diabetic patients as they often have renal insufficiency along with their vascular disease.

Arterial access can lead to well-known complications of arterial puncture such as hematoma or bleeding, dissection, pseudoaneurysm formation, and embolism. These mechanical complications can be minimized by the use of ultrasound guidance for arterial puncture and smallest diameter sheaths and catheters for interventions.

A more difficult set of problems comes from the need for iodinated contrast agents for contrast angiography. According to Pompeselli, the typical contrast agents are iodine-containing agents that are ionic or nonionic. The ionic compounds have a higher osmolality than the nonionic compounds. The common side effects of contrast agents like nausea, vomiting, and pain in the artery being studied are related to hyperosmolality. Thus, the use of nonionic agents has mostly supplanted that of ionic agents [27]. Allergic reaction is also more common with ionic agents and might be avoided by combining their use with the administration of steroids and antihistamines prior to angiography [27].

The incidence of contrast-induced nephrotoxicity (CIN) is higher in diabetic patients, particularly in type I diabetics. Preexisting renal dysfunction, which is more common in diabetics, is a significant risk factor for developing nephropathy. The risk of CIN can be reduced by prehydration with intravenous normal saline or sodium bicarbonate solution. The type of contrast agent and volume of contrast are not independent factors in the development of nephrotoxicity [27, 28].

Other strategies to reduce the risk of CIN include the use of half-strength contrast to reduce contrast volume and the use of CO_2 for more proximal larger vessels such as the aorta, iliac, and femoral arteries. The use of gadolinium as contrast for patients with renal insufficiency has mostly been stopped for reasons that will be discussed later. Finally, selective catheterization deep into the vascular tree, such as the distal superficial femoral artery, can be used to better image the popliteal and tibial arteries and reduce contrast volumes.

Computerized Tomographic Angiography

High-speed spiral CT scanners that acquire raw data over continuous volume rather than discontinuous slices allow for collection of major amounts of data that may be reformatted into three-dimensional reconstruction of the vascular system. The benefits of CT angiography (CTA) include rapid acquisition times with the contrast administered intravenously. CTA also provides good resolution of the tibial arteries. According to Schaper, two meta-analyses showed that sensitivity and specificity for detecting a stenosis of at least 50 % per segment were 92–95 % and 93–96 %, respectively. The disadvantages of CTA include the use of relatively high doses of ionizing radiation and ionic contrast agents. Most CTA angiogram protocols require more contrast volume than conventional angiogram and therefore carry risk of nephrotoxicity [27, 28]. Other disadvantages include potential artifacts caused by the artificial reconstruction of the images in postprocessing. The artifacts may include motion artifact, volume averaging, and stair-step artifact. Differentiating calcium in the vessel wall from intravascular contrast can also be difficult. Knowing how to alter the CT image "window" may be crucial to differentiating calcium from contrast, particularly in the small tibial vessels.

Magnetic Resonance Angiography

Magnetic resonance angiography (MRA) is a noninvasive imaging modality that can be helpful in PAD patients. MRA can be done with or without contrast. When done without contrast, the usual MR technique employs time-of-flight (TOF) angiography and rapid sequence T1-weighted images. This technique is designed to, "accentuate the signal from flowing blood and attenuate that from non-moving structures and tissues with signal characteristics different from blood" [27]. Thus the bloodstream appears white or brighter on the displayed images.

Contrast-enhanced MRA is a low invasive imaging method. The contrast agent gadolinium is administered after an unenhanced mask image of the body part under study is obtained. In this way contrast-enhanced MRA is similar to digital subtraction angiography. Contrast-enhanced MRA offers superior image resolution and has mostly replaced noncontrast MRA. However, contrast-enhanced MRA has some drawbacks such as long acquisition times that require proper timing of the image acquisition. The quality of images as a function of time is referred to as temporal resolution. Improper timing of image acquisition can lead to problems such as venous contamination of the arterial images [27].

Much more problematic and limiting to the use of gadolinium for contrast-enhanced MRA is the condition known as nephrogenic systemic fibrosis (NSF). In NSF the skin thickens and contracts on the extremities and trunks. Some cases have reported organ fibrosis as well. As a result of NSF, patients may suffer severe physical limitations and hardships, organ damage, or even death. NSF after gadolinium administration has occurred in patients with all levels of renal insufficiency or failure. NSF has not been reported in patients with normal renal function. It is currently recommended that gadolinium contrast agents not be administered in patients with glomerular filtration rates less than 30 mL/min or acute renal insufficiency [27].

Management of the Diabetic Foot

Treatment selection and timing of treatment for diabetic foot ulcers depend on factors such as the extent of the foot wound, infection, and ischemia. First one should determine if a foot is salvageable. A foot with extensive non-reconstructable tissue loss or advanced sepsis from the foot should be considered for primary amputation. Other individual patient circumstances such as severe medical comorbidities, lower extremity contractures, and nonfunctional bedridden status must be considered and should likely lead the surgeon to suggest primary amputation.

Medical Management

Medical management of the diabetic foot begins with preventive care. This includes strict glycemic control and modification of other cardiovascular risk factors like hypertension, hypercholesterolemia, and smoking. According to a review by Singh, patient education about proper foot care and hygiene improves short-term knowledge and may modestly reduce risk of foot ulceration and amputation in diabetics. The review also found that when physicians were educated with the LEAP (Lower Extremity Amputation Prevention) project, documented foot care education improved from 38 to 48 % over 9 months, appropriate foot care self-management increased from 32 to 48 %, and there was a trend toward reduced lower extremity amputations [29].

The first active step in treating any diabetic foot ulcer, particularly neuropathic ulcers, is off-loading and weight-bearing restriction. The ulcer must be protected from excessive pressure by special shoes or padding. Cavanaugh reviewed practices for off-loading the diabetic foot for ulcer prevention and healing. He found that standard therapeutic footwear is not effective in ulcer healing. He concludes that the total contact cast is the most effective modality to heal an uncomplicated plantar ulcer in a short time frame [30]. Clearly, input from a podiatrist is paramount at this stage.

When a limb-threatening diabetic foot infection is identified, the patient requires immediate hospitalization and intravenous antibiotics. Empiric broad-spectrum antibiotics should be started as most diabetic foot infections are polymicrobial. Deep wound cultures should be obtained, hopefully, prior to initiating the antibiotics. Table 32.4 summarizes several of the antibiotic trials for treatment of diabetic foot infections. The largest trial by Lipsky in 2005, like the remaining studies, did not show any difference in eradication rates, clinical outcomes, and adverse events between the

Table 32.4 Summary of antibiotic trials for diabetic foot infections

Author	Antibiotic regimens	Design	Patients (no.)	Treatment duration (days)	Reported results	95 % CI	P
Grayson 1994	Ampicillin/sulbactam	Randomized, double-blind, single-center	48	13±6.5	81 % cure; 67 % eradication		NS
	Imipenem/cilastatin		48	14.8±8.6	85 % cure; 75 % eradication		
Lipsky 2004	Linezolid IV or PO, ± aztreonam	Randomized, open-label, multicenter	241 (5 % aztreonam)	17.2±7.9	81 % overall cure	−0.1 to 20.1	NS
	Ampicillin/sulbactam, or amoxicillin/ clavulanate ± vancomycin or aztreonam		120 (9.6 % vancomycin, 2.5 % aztreonam)	16.5±7.9	71 % overall cure		
Clay 2004	Ceftriaxone + metronidazole	Randomized, open-label, single-center	36	44	72 % treatment success		NS
	Ticarcillin/clavulanate		34	4	76 % treatment success		
Harkless 2005	Piperacillin/ tazobactam ± vancomycin	Randomized, open-label, multicenter	155	9 median	81 % cure or improvement	12.9–9.1	0.124
	Ampicillin/ sulbactam ± vancomycin		159	10 median	83.1 % cure or improvement		
Lipsky 2005	Daptomycin ± aztreonam or metronidazole	Randomized, open-label, multicenter	47 (38 % aztreonam)	7–14	66 % cure	−14.4 to 21.8	NS
	Comparator (vancomycin or semisynthetic PCN) ± aztreonam or metronidazole		56	7–14	70 % cure		
			(29)				
			(27)				
			(41 % aztreonam)				
Lipsky 2005	Ertapenem ± vancomycin	Randomized, double-blind, multicenter	295 (2.3 % vancomycin)	11.1	87 % favorable clinical response	−6.3 to 9.1	NS
	Piperacillin/ tazobactam ± vancomycin		291 (1.7 % vancomycin)	11.3	83 % favorable clinical response		

CI confidence interval, IV intravenous, PCN penicillin, PO oral administration
From Kalish J, Hamdan A. Management of diabetic foot problems. J Vasc Surg. 2010;51:476–86. Reprinted with permission from Elsevier Limited

Table 32.5 Summary of randomized trials comparing hyperbaric oxygen therapy to standard wound care

Author	Patients	Treatment sessions	Reported results	P
Faglia 1996	Five HBOT + standard wound care	38.8 ± 8	8.6 % major amputation (RR, 0.26; 95 % CI, 0.08–0.84)	0.016
	33 standard wound care		33.3 % major amputation	
Abidia 2003	Eight HBOT	30	62.5 % ulcer healing	
			100 % median ↓ wound area 6 weeks	0.027
			100 % median ↓ wound area 6 months	NS
	Eight control (air)	30	12.5 % ulcer healing	
			52 % median ↓ wound area 6 weeks	
			95 % median ↓ wound area 6 months	
Kessler 2003	14 HBOT + standard wound care	20	Ulcer size decrease	
			42 % ± 25 % (day 15)	0.037
			48 % ± 30 % (day 30)	NS
	14 standard wound care		22 ± 17 % (day 15)	
			42 ± 27 % (day 30)	
Duzgun 2008	50 HBOT + standard wound care	60–90	66 % healing without surgery	<0.05
			8 % distal amputation	<0.05
			0 % major amputation	<0.05
	50 standard wound care		0 % healing with surgery	<0.05
			48 % distal amputation	<0.05
			34 % major amputation	<0.05

CI confidence interval, *HBOT* hyperbaric oxygen therapy, *RR* relative risk
From Kalish J, Hamdan A. Management of diabetic foot problems. J Vasc Surg. 2010;51:476–86. Reprinted with permission from Elsevier Limited

study drugs. One should notice the relatively high failure rates of 11–12 % for moderate infections and 19–30 % for severe infections. This highlights the limitation of treating diabetic foot ulcers with antibiotics alone [8].

Hyperbaric oxygen treatment may be an adjunct to facilitate wound healing in diabetic foot ulcers. The beneficial mechanisms of hyperbaric oxygen therapy are reported to include an antimicrobial effect and increased oxygenation at the ulcer tissue bed via stimulation of angiogenesis [8, 31]. Table 32.5 summarizes trials comparing hyperbaric oxygen therapy to standard wound care for healing diabetic foot ulcers. A 2010 study by Londahl compared patients with chronic diabetic foot ulcers receiving either hyperbaric oxygen therapy (*n* = 47) or hyperbaric air therapy (*n* = 41). At 1-year follow-up, 53 % of the HBO patients remained healed versus 28 % of the hyperbaric air patients. In an accompanying editorial, Boulton suggests that, "this study puts HBO on firmer ground for diabetic patients with chronic foot ulcers who do not respond to standard therapy and in whom vascular reconstruction is not possible" [31].

Surgical Management

One key to understanding the surgical management of diabetic foot ulcers and infections is that they often extend deeper into the foot than apparent from the skin surface. A deep space abscess is frequently present when the wound looks fairly innocuous externally. Figure 32.5 shows the

effects of a deep space infection. The goal of surgical intervention is to evacuate any abscess, remove necrotic tissue, and minimize the risk of further infection and tissue damage. Fisher has proposed a stepwise surgical approach to management of diabetic foot infections [32]. This strategy is depicted in Fig. 32.6. First, an initial skin incision must be made that will allow access to and drainage of all infected tissues while taking into account future surgical plans like eventual wound closure. These incisions are directed by an understanding of the three major plantar spaces: the medial, central, and lateral spaces. Next the wound is investigated in order to locate all possible abscess collections, foreign bodies, necrotic tissues, tracts, and fistulas. Debridement then removes all nonviable tissues. Wound lavage and copious irrigation help reduce the bacterial burden in the wound. The choice of irrigation fluid, normal saline versus antibiotic solution, is likely less important than the volume of irrigation and is left to operator's choice. Final closure of the wound may be attempted once infection is under control and adequate viable soft tissues are present. Closure most often occurs after serial debridement, local wound care, and negative pressure wound therapy to prepare the wound bed.

Revascularization

The indications for revascularization in diabetics are no different as compared to nondiabetic patient population. These indications include the usual incapacitating claudication, rest

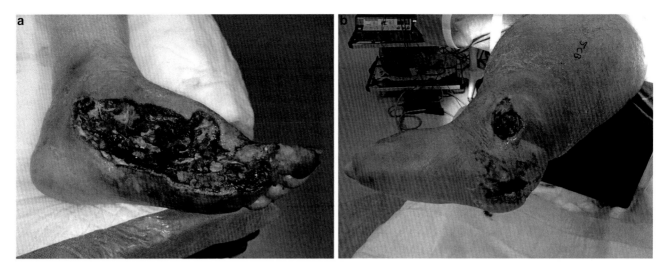

Fig. 32.5 Examples of diabetic foot infection. (**a**) Diabetic foot with extensive deep space infection after initial debridement. (**b**) Severe diabetic foot infection and ulceration in patient with Charcot foot

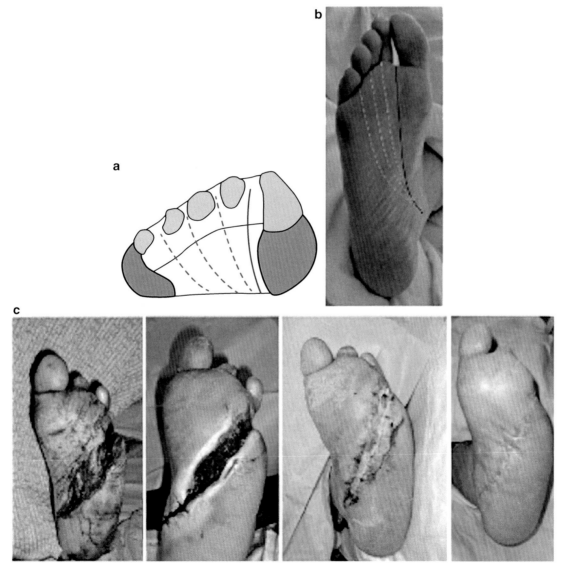

Fig. 32.6 Surgical incisions for diabetic foot infections. From Fisher TK, Scimea CL, Bharara M, Mills JL Sr, Armstrong DG. A step-wise approach for the surgical management of diabetic foot infections. J Vasc Surg. 2010 Sep;52(3 Suppl):72S–75S. Reprinted with permission from Elsevier

pain, and tissue loss such as ulcers or gangrene. After physical exam and noninvasive physiological testing, the severity of arterial ischemia should be determined. In some cases appropriately selected diabetic foot ulcers may heal without revascularization and this is guided by the physiologic testing. If the decision is made to revascularize the diabetic limb in order to heal an ischemic ulcer, the goal of therapy is to restore pulsatile blood flow to the foot.

The classic distribution of arterial occlusive disease in diabetics involves the tibial vessels. Therefore, diabetic limb salvage often involves infragenicular, or distal, revascularization. Ipsilateral greater saphenous vein is the conduit of choice for surgical distal revascularization. When vein is used for distal bypasses in diabetics, comparable patency and limb salvage rates can be obtained as for those performed in nondiabetics [11]. Of note, these results are comparable despite more bypasses performed for limb salvage in the diabetic group.

Diabetic patients often present with extensive tissue loss in the foot. The relative value of endovascular versus open surgical revascularization for diabetic limb salvage must be considered when choosing a revascularization strategy. Endovascular therapy for critical limb ischemia leads to high restenosis rates attributable to risk factors of age, diabetes, and chronic renal failure [34]. In 2010, Abularrage assessed the influence of diabetes on long-term outcomes of percutaneous transluminal angioplasty, with or without stenting in patients with peripheral vascular disease. He concluded that diabetes is an independent predictor of decreased long-term primary patency after PTA/stent [33].

We have presented data that indicate surgical bypass provides faster and more complete healing with wounds greater than 2-cm diameter when compared to endovascular revascularization [34]. Bypasses ($n=142$) and endovascular procedures ($n=148$) were performed for limb salvage in a cohort of patients that had 58 % diabetics. Of those presenting with larger wounds, 76 % healed completely after bypass compared with only 41 % after endovascular therapy. This difference only reached statistical significance in the group with initial wounds greater than 2-cm diameter. Median time to healing was also 34 days faster in the surgical group compared to the endovascular group. While the study has selection bias and a variety of endovascular techniques making firm conclusions difficult, we prefer bypass as the first choice for patients with tissue loss and long-segment tibial artery occlusive disease. Endovascular therapy is offered for limb salvage in critical limb ischemia patient that is deemed too high risk for surgery.

Surgical Bypass Options

Ipsilateral greater saphenous vein is the conduit of choice for distal bypass to tibial arteries. However, despite the use of duplex ultrasound vein mapping, 30 % of patients that need distal revascularization do not have adequate saphenous vein. That percentage increases to 50 for patients needing reoperation for limb salvage. Alternative conduits include arm vein, lesser saphenous vein, composite veins, and polytetrafluoroethylene (PTFE) with or without adjunctive techniques. The results of these alternative conduits are not equivalent to saphenous vein bypass [35–38].

Historically, tibial artery bypasses using PTFE anastomosed directly to the artery have dismal results. One-year patency rates between 20 and 50 % with 3-year patency rates of 12–40 % have been reported [39, 40]. Failure of the bypass is secondary to the technical difficulties of anastomosing the noncompliant prosthetic graft to a small diseased often calcified artery and aggressive myointimal hyperplasia that forms at the toe and heel of the graft [41].

Adjunctive procedures have been devised to increase patency of the prosthetic tibial bypasses. These maneuvers have included the Miller cuff and the Taylor "patch." The goal of these adjuncts was to optimize anastomotic surface area, provide a biological buffer, and possibly provide a mechanical buffer by increasing compliance at the anastomosis by placing a segment of vein between the prosthetic graft and the recipient tibial artery. These adjuncts improved prosthetic graft patency, but were technically challenging. Our group popularized the distal vein patch (DVP) technique [42, 43]. In this technique a segment of suitable vein is attached to the recipient artery as a simple Linton vein patch. The PTFE graft is then anastomosed to the vein patch to complete the bypass. In an early series, the DVP bypass resulted in 62 % primary patency rate and 79 % limb salvage at 4-year follow-up. The addition of a distal arteriovenous fistula to the DVP (the patchula) resulted in 62 % patency and 57 % limb salvage at 24 months in a patient cohort otherwise being considered for primary amputation [44].

The "angiosome" concept divides the body into three-dimensional vascular territories supplied by specific source arteries [45]. The foot has six angiosomes arising from the posterior tibial artery (three), anterior tibial artery (one), and peroneal arteries (two). A full description of the arteries and their related angiosomes is provided by Attinger [46]. Direct revascularization involves the artery supplying the angiosome in which the wound is located. Indirect revascularization involves an artery that does not directly perfuse the ischemic angiosome. A study by our group demonstrated a significant advantage in wound healing when direct revascularization was performed (91 %) compared to indirect revascularization (62 %). Similar conclusions were found when a study looked at direct versus indirect endovascular revascularization [47]. When there is a choice of target vessels for revascularization, one should consider the artery that will directly perfuse the angiosome feeding the wound in question.

The Limb Salvage Team

It is well established that limb salvage teams can reduce the rate of major amputations in diabetic foot ulcer patients. Kim et al. states that the major amputation rate is reduced by more than 50 % when diabetic foot patients are treated by a team approach [48]. Driver et al. cite several studies that show as much as a 78 % reduction in major amputations after implementing a multidisciplinary team for diabetic foot patients [49]. They site another study of a podiatry and vascular surgery team that produced 83 % limb salvage rates at 5 years. Through economic modeling and studies, Driver shows that multidisciplinary limb salvage care following established guidelines is cost effective and even cost saving compared to usual fragmented care. Sumpio et al. found that establishing an identifiable limb salvage "center" can increase patient referrals for participating physicians [50].

The multidisciplinary limb salvage team optimally includes vascular surgeons, podiatrists, interventionalists, infectious disease specialists, plastic and reconstructive surgeons, diabetologists, physical therapists, and orthotists. Kim et al. discuss the role of the podiatrist in prevention and treatment of diabetic foot ulcers [48]. Kim nicely describes the importance of podiatrists as "biomechanical surgeons" as they "rebalance and reconstruct the biomechanically unstable or mal-positioned foot." Rogers et al. detail the "irreducible minimum" of a diabetic podiatrist and vascular surgeon for a "toe and flow" program to prevent, diagnose, and treat diabetic foot patients and their complications [51].

References

1. Centers for Disease Control and Prevention. National diabetes statistics report: estimates of diabetes and its burden in the United States, 2014. Atlanta: U.S. Department of Health and Human Services; 2014.
2. Boulton AJ. The pathway to foot ulceration in diabetes. Med Clin North Am. 2013;97(5):775–90. doi:10.1016/j.mcna.2013.03.007.
3. Prompers L, Schaper N, Apelqvist J, Edmonds M, Jude E, Mauricio D, et al. Prediction of outcome in individuals with diabetic foot ulcers: focus on the differences between individuals with and without peripheral arterial disease. The EURODIALE Study. Diabetologia. 2008;51:747–55. doi:10.1007/s00125-008-0940-0.
4. Albers JW, Rodica P-B. Diabetic neuropathy: mechanisms, emerging treatments, and subtypes. Curr Neurol Neurosci Rep. 2014;14(8):473. doi:10.1007/s11910-014-0473-5.
5. Smith AG, Singleton JR. Continuum: lifelong learning in neurology. Peripher Neuropathy. 2012;18(1):60–84. doi:10.1212/01.CON.0000411568.34085.3e.
6. Boulton A. Diabetic neuropathy: is pain god's greatest gift to mankind? Semin Vasc Surg. 2012;25:61–5. doi:10.1053/j.semvascsurg.2012.04.009.
7. Boulton AJ. What you can't feel can hurt you. J Vasc Surg. 2010;52:28S–30S. doi:10.1016/j.jvs.2010.06.005. Review.
8. Kalish J, Hamdan A. Management of diabetic foot problems. J Vasc Surg. 2010;51:476–86. doi:10.1016/j.jvs.2009.08.043.
9. Blume PA, Sumpio B, Schmidt B, Donegan R. Charcot neuropathy of the foot and ankle: diagnosis and management strategies. Clin Podiatr Med Surg. 2014;31(1):151–72.
10. Menzoian JO, LaMorte WW, Panniszyn CC, Mcbride DJ, Sidawy AN, Logerfo FW, et al. Symptomatology and anatomic patterns of peripheral vascular disease: differing impact of smoking and diabetes. Ann Vasc Surg. 1989;3:224–8.
11. Rosenblatt MS, Quist WC, Sidawy AN, Paniszyn CC, Logerfo FW. Lower extremity vein graft reconstruction: results in diabetic and non-diabetic patients. Surg Gynecol Obstet. 1990;171:331–5.
12. LoGerfo FW. Vascular disease, matrix abnormalities, and neuropathy: implications for limb salvage in diabetes mellitus. J Vasc Surg. 1987;5(5):793–6.
13. Veves A, Akbari CM, Primavera J, Donaghue VM, Zacharoulis D, Chrzan JS, et al. Endothelial dysfunction and the expression of endothelial nitric oxide synthetase in diabetic neuropathy, vascular disease, and foot ulceration. Diabetes. 1998;47(3):457–63.
14. Brownlee M, Cerami A, Vlassara H. Advanced glycosylation end products in tissue and the biochemical basis of diabetic complications. N Engl J Med. 1998;318(20):1315–21.
15. Sheehan P. The consensus panel of the American Diabetes Association. Peripheral arterial disease in people with diabetes. Diabetes Care. 2003;26:3335.
16. Ridker PM, Cushman M, Stampfer MJ, Tracy RP, Hennekens CH. Plasma concentration of C-reactive protein and risk of developing peripheral vascular disease. Circulation. 1998;97(5):425–8.
17. Hayden MR, Tyaqi SC, Kolb L, Sowers JR, Khanna R. Vascular ossification-calcification in metabolic syndrome, type 2 diabetes mellitus, chronic kidney disease, and calciphylaxis-calcific uremic arteriopathy: the role of sodium thiosulfate. Cardiovasc Diabetol. 2005;4:4.
18. Menzoian JO, LaMorte WW, Paniszyn CC, McBride KJ, Sidawy AN, LoGerfo FW, et al. Symptomatology and anatomic patterns of peripheral vascular disease: Differing impact of smoking and diabetes. Ann Vasc Surg. 1989;3(3):224–8.
19. Akbari CM, Pompeselli Jr FB, Gibbons GW, Campbell DR, Pulling MC, Mydiarz D, et al. Lower extremity revascularization in diabetes: late observations. Arch Surg. 2000;135(4):452–6.
20. Schneider DL, Sobel BE. Diabetes and thrombosis. In: Johnstone MT, Veves A, editors. Diabetes and cardiovascular disease. Totowa: Humana Press; 2001. p. 149.
21. Boyko EJ, Ahroni JH, Cohen V, Nelson KM, Heagerty PJ. Prediction of diabetic foot ulcer occurrence using commonly available clinical information: the Seattle Diabetic Foot Study. Diabetes Care. 2006;29(6):1202–7.
22. Lavery LA, Armstrong DG, Wunderlich RP, Mohler MJ, Wendel CS, Lipsky BA. Risk factors for foot infections in individuals with diabetes. Diabetes Care. 2006;29(6):1288–93.
23. Avery LA, Armstrong DG, Murdoch DP, Peters EJG, Lipsky B. Validation of the Infectious Diseases Society of America's diabetic foot infection classification system. Clin Infect Dis. 2007;44(4):562–5. Epub 2007 Jan 17.
24. Mills JL Sr, Conte MS, Armstrong DG, Pompeselli FB, Schanzer A, Sidawy AN, Andros G; Symptomatology and anatomic patterns of peripheral vascular disease: Differing impact of smoking and diabetes. Society for Vascular Surgery Lower Extremity Guidelines Committee. J Vasc surg. 2014;59(1):220–34.e1-2. doi:10.1016/j.jvs.2013.08.003. Review.
25. Boulton A, Armstrong DG, Albert SF, Fryberg RG, Hellman R, Kirkman MS, et al. Comprehensive foot examination and risk assessment: a report of the task force of the foot care interest group of the American Diabetes Association, with endorsement by the American Association of Clinical Endocrinologists. Diabetes Care. 2008;31(8):1679–85. doi:10.2337/dc08-9021.

26. Anderson C. Noninvasive assessment of lower extremity hemodynamics in individuals with diabetes mellitus. J Vasc Surg. 2010;52 (3 Suppl):76S–80S. doi:10.1016/j.jvs.2010.06.013. Review. PMID; 20804937.

27. Pomposelli F. Arterial imaging in patients with lower extremity ischemia and diabetes mellitus. J Vasc Surg. 2010;52(3 Suppl):81S–91S. doi:10.1016/j.jvs.2010.06.013. Review.

28. Schaper NC, Andros G, Apelqvist J, Bakker K, Lammer J, Lepantalo M, et al. Diagnosis and treatment of peripheral arterial disease in diabetic patients with a foot ulcer. A progress report of the International Working Group on the Diabetic Foot. Diabetes Metab Res Rev. 2012;28 Suppl 1:218–24. doi:10.1002/dmrr.2255. Review.

29. Singh N, Armstrong DG, Lipsky BA. Preventing foot ulcers in patients with diabetes. JAMA. 2005;293(2):217–28. Review.

30. Cavanagh PR, Bus SA. Off-loading the diabetic foot for ulcer prevention and healing. Plast Reconstr Surg. 2011;127 Suppl 1:248S–56S. doi:10.1097/PRS.0b013e3182024864.

31. Boulton A. Hyperbaric oxygen in the management of chronic diabetic foot ulcers. Curr Diab Rep. 2010;10(4):355–6. doi:10.1007/s11892-010-0121-7.

32. Fisher TK, Scimea CL, Bharara M, Mills Sr JL, Armstrong DG. A step-wise approach for the surgical management of diabetic foot infections. J Vasc Surg. 2010;52(3 Suppl):72S–5S. doi:10.1016/j.jvs.2010.06.011. Review.

33. Abularrage CJ, Conrad MF, Hackney LA, Paruchuri V, Crawford RS, Kwolek CJ, et al. Long-term outcomes of diabetic patients undergoing endovascular infrainguinal interventions. J Vasc Surg. 2010;52:312–22.

34. Neville RF, Sidawy AN. Surgical bypass: when is it best and do angiosomes play a role? Semin Vasc Surg. 2012;25(2):102–7. doi:10.1053/j.semvascsurg.2012.04.001.

35. Bergan JJ, Veith FJ, Bernhard VM, Yao JS, Flinn WR, Gupta SK, et al. Randomization of autogenous vein and polytetrafluoroethylene grafts in femoral-distal reconstruction. Surgery. 1982;92(6):921–30.

36. Veith FJ, Gupta SK, Ascer E, White-Flores S, Samson RH, Scher LA, et al. Six-year prospective randomized comparison of autologous saphenous vein and expanded polytetrafluoroethylene grafts in infrainguinal arterial reconstruction. J Vasc Surg. 1986;3(1):104–14.

37. Calligaro KD, Sytrek JR, Dougherty MJ, Rua I, Raviola CA, DeLaurentis DA. Use of arm vein and lesser saphenous vein compared with prosthetic grafts for infrapopliteal arterial bypass: are they worth the effort? J Vasc Surg. 1997;26(6):919–24.

38. Holzenbien TJ, Pomposelli FB, Miller A, Contreras MA, Gibbons GW, Campbell DR, et al. Results of a policy with arm veins used as the first alternative to an unavailable ipsilateral greater saphenous vein for infrainguinal bypass. J Vasc Surg. 1996;23(1):130–40.

39. Hobson RW, Lynch TG, Jamil Z, Karanfilian RG, Lee BC, Padberg Jr FT, et al. Results of revascularization and amputation in severe lower extremity ischemia: a five-year clinical experience. J Vasc Surg. 1985;2(1):174–85.

40. Whittemore AD, Kent KC, Donaldson MC, Couch NP, Mannick JA. What is the proper role of polytetrafluoroethylene grafts in infrainguinal reconstruction? J Vasc Surg. 1989;10(3):299–305.

41. Bassiouny HS, White S, Glagov S, Choi E, Giddens DP, Zarins CK. Anastomotic intimal hyperplasia: mechanical injury or flow induced. J Vasc Surg. 1992;15(4):708–16.

42. Neville RF, Attinger C, Sidawy AN. Prosthetic bypass with a distal vein patch for limb salvage. Am J Surg. 1997;174(2):173–6.

43. Neville RF, Tempesta B, Sidawy AN. Tibial bypass for limb salvage using polytetrafluoroethylene and a distal vein patch. J Vasc Surg. 2001;33(2):266–71.

44. Neville RF, Dy B, Singh N, DeZee KJ. Distal vein patch with an arteriovenous fistula: a viable option for the patient without autogenous conduit and severe distal occlusive disease. J Vasc Surg. 2009;50(1):83–8. doi:10.1016/j.jvs.2008.12.052.

45. Taylor GI, Palmer JH. The vascular territories (angiosomes) of the body: experimental study and clinical applications. Br J Plast Surg. 1987;40(2):113–41.

46. Attinger C, Evans KK, Bulan E, Blume P, Cooper P. Angiosomes of the foot and ankle and clinical implications for limb salvage: reconstruction, incisions, and revascularization. Plast Reconstr Surg. 2006;117(7 Suppl):261S–93S.

47. Lida O, Soga Y, Hirano K, Kawasaki D, Suzuki K, Miyashita Y, et al. Long-term results of direct and indirect endovascular revascularization based on the angiosome concept in patients with critical limb ischemia presenting with isolated below-the-knee lesions. J Vasc Surg. 2012;55(2):363–70.e5. doi:10.1016/j.jvs.2001.08.014.

48. Kim PJ, Attinger C, Evans KK, Steinberg JS. Role of the podiatrist in diabetic limb salvage. J Vasc Surg. 2012;56(4):1168–72. doi:10.1016/j.jvs.2012.06.091.

49. Driver VR, Fabbi M, Lavery LA, Gibbons G. The cost of diabetic foot: the economic case for the limb salvage team. J Am Podiatr Med Assoc. 2010;100(5):335–41.

50. Sumpio BE, Armstrong DG, Lavery LA, Andros G, SVS/APMA Writing Group. The role of interdisciplinary team approach in the management of the diabetic foot: a joint statement from the Society for Vascular Surgery and the American Podiatric Medical Association. J Vasc Surg. 2010;51(6):1504–6. doi:10.1016/j.jvs.2010.04.010.

51. Rogers LC, Andros G, Caporusso J, Harkless LB, Mills JL Sr, Armstrong DG. Toe and flow: essential components and structure of the amputation prevention team. J Vasc Surg. 2010;52(3 Suppl):23S–7S. doi:10.1016/j.jvs.2010.06.004. Review

Critical Limb Ischemia and the Angiosome Model

Alexander Turin and Robert S. Dieter

Introduction

Peripheral artery disease (PAD), as its name might suggest, refers to atherosclerosis of the arteries of the peripheral vasculature defined as partial or complete obstruction of at least one of the peripheral arteries [1]. Prior terminology for PAD, including peripheral vascular disease, peripheral arterial occlusive disease, and arteriosclerosis obliterans, all describe a spectrum of disease related to the stenosis or occlusion of upper or lower extremity arteries. The prevalence of PAD is more than 200 million people globally and is associated with considerable morbidity and mortality [2]. Risk factors for the development of PAD include tobacco use, diabetes, and hypercholesterolemia, among others, and symptoms can include intermittent claudication, rest pain, and ulceration [3]. Progressive PAD can result in critical limb ischemia (CLI), which is defined as PAD with hemodynamic compromise often manifesting as "distal leg pain at rest with or without the presence of ulcers or gangrene" [1]. Treatments range from lifestyle modification to open surgical revascularization and endovascular therapy.

The principle of treatment with regard to revascularization, whether surgical or endovascular, begins with an understanding of the basic principles of anatomy. There are three major arteries below the knee that supply the foot and are the primary sites of intervention. The anterior tibial artery gives off the dorsalis pedis artery and supplies primarily the anterior compartment of the leg and dorsum of the foot. The posterior tibial artery gives off the medial and lateral plantar branches which supply the medial instep and lateral/plantar forefoot, respectively, as well as the calcaneal branch that supplies a portion of the medial ankle and plantar heel. Lastly, the peroneal artery gives off the lateral calcaneal branch supplying the lateral ankle and portion of the plantar heel as well as the anterior perforator which supplies the anterior ankle.

Angiosome Model of Revascularization

It follows that there may be a correlation between the tissue loss seen in CLI and the distribution of stenosis or occlusion of the supplying arteries. Interestingly, this research began in 1987 in the realm of plastic surgery. Taylor and Palmer [4] examined the blood supply of 2000 fresh cadavers and isolated limbs in order to determine a better method for planning incisions and skin flaps. They injected cadavers with ink to determine the subsequent vascular territories of major arteries and perforating blood vessels. Taylor and Palmer hence coined the term "angiosome," defined as an area of the foot that corresponds to areas supplied by the anterior tibial, posterior tibial, and peroneal arteries and their branches. As such, there is a total of six angiosomes in the foot as summarized in Table 33.1 and as outlined in Fig. 33.1. Though this is a relatively novel concept in the lower extremities, this model is already being used in other fields, most notably in percutaneous coronary intervention determining which vessel to target with myocardial reperfusion [5].

It was not until 2006 that Attinger et al. [6] proposed applying the concept of angiosomes beyond the realm of plastic and reconstruction and into interventions for CLI. Attinger postulated that revascularization of the major artery supplying the angiosome with present ischemia or ulceration should be more efficacious than revascularization of one of the other two major arteries. Hence, direct revascularization (DR) is intervention upon an artery which correlates with the affected angiosome; indirect revascularization (IR), then, is when the intervened-upon artery does not correlate with the affected angiosome.

A. Turin, MD (✉)
Internal Medicine, Loyola University Medical Center,
2160 S. 1st Ave., Room 769, Maywood, IL 60153, USA

R.S. Dieter, MD, RVT
Medicine, Cardiology, Vascular and Endovascular Medicine,
Loyola University Medical Center, Maywood, IL, USA

© Springer International Publishing Switzerland 2017
R.S. Dieter et al. (eds.), *Critical Limb Ischemia*, DOI 10.1007/978-3-319-31991-9_33

Table 33.1 Arteries and angiosomes of the foot

Artery	Origin	Distribution	Angiosome[a]
Anterior tibial artery	Popliteal artery	Anterior compartment of the leg	Dorsalis pedis: anterior compartment and dorsum of foot and toes (1)
Posterior tibial artery	Tibioperoneal trunk	Posterior compartment of the leg	Medial plantar: medial instep (2)
		Lateral compartment of the leg	Lateral plantar: lateral forefoot, plantar forefoot (3)
			Calcaneal branch: medial ankle, plantar heel (4)
Peroneal (fibular) artery	Tibioperoneal trunk	Posterior compartment of the leg	Lateral calcaneal: lateral ankle, plantar heel (5)
			Anterior perforator: anterior ankle (6)

[a]Branches of main artery and subsequent angiosomes numbered sequentially in parentheses

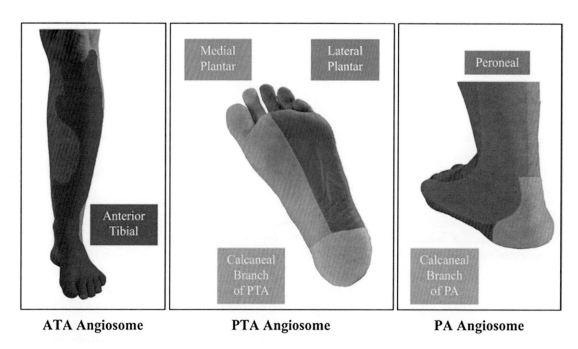

ATA Angiosome   **PTA Angiosome**   **PA Angiosome**

Fig. 33.1 Color-coded model of angiosomes stratified by primary supplying artery. *PTA* posterior tibial artery, *ATA* anterior tibial artery, *PA* peroneal artery. From Iida et al. Long-term results of direct and indirect endovascular revascularization based on the angiosome concept in patients with critical limb ischemia presenting with isolated below-the-knee lesions. J Vasc Surg 2012;55:363-370. Reprinted with permission from Elsevier Limited

Review of Current Data on the Angiosome Model

There has been a fair amount of research investigating the angiosome model as it applies to CLI and revascularization. Neville et al. [7] published one of the initial retrospective reports in 2009 in which 60 wounds with tissue loss due to ischemia underwent angiogram and intervention with surgical bypass. Preoperative angiograms were correlated with the lesion and, in blinded fashion, were compared to operative reports and subsequently classified as DR if the bypass was to the artery directly feeding the ischemic region, and IR if it was not. While approximately half of the patients underwent both DR and IR, there was no significant difference in mean time to healing, but there was a statistically significant difference in complete wound healing rate (91 % in the DR group compared with 62 % in the IR group). There was also a fourfold increase in amputation rate in the IR group (eight compared with two in the DR group) that was not powered enough for statistical significance. Iida et al. [8] conducted a retrospective review in 2010 of 203 limbs that underwent endovascular repair and found limb salvage to be significantly higher in patients who received DR as compared to IR (86 % vs 69 % at 1 year with a similar percentage extended through 4 years of follow-up). Another retrospective study [9] 2 years later of almost 400 limbs with CLI showed similar results. Amputation-free survival was much higher in the DR group (71 % vs 50 % at 1 year and 49 % vs 29 % at 4 years). Lastly, Soderstrom et al. [10] retrospectively reviewed 250 foot ulcers and found that patients who underwent DR had improved healing rates but not limb salvage or overall 1-year survival.

Similar studies, however, have been unable to find significant differences between DR and IR. Alexandrescu et al. [11], in a retrospective review of >200 wounds, found no difference in limb salvage rates at 12, 24, and 36 months and further showed no difference in overall mortality rates between DR and IR groups. Both Azuma et al. [12] and Fossaceca et al. [13] also reviewed >200 wounds and again showed no significant difference between DR and IR with respect to limb salvage at 1 and 2 years, respectively, and wound healing. Lastly, Berceli et al. [14], though not specifically investigating the angiosome hypothesis, noted that both forefoot and heel ulcers had equivalent rates of healing with bypass of the dorsalis pedis artery. As this is part of the anterior tibial angiosome, this effectively represents the DR and IR groups, respectively, and again illustrates the lack of significant findings between these interventions.

With data both in support of and against the angiosome model, two recent meta-analyses published in 2014 attempted to address the controversy [15, 16]. Biancari et al. [15] evaluated nine studies and found that DR may significantly improve wound healing and limb salvage rates compared to IR. Risk of unhealed wound was lower after DR with a hazard ratio of 0.64, and risk of major amputation was lower with a hazard ratio of 0.44. Huang et al. [16] similarly found that DR improves time to amputation (HR 0.61) and time to wound healing (HR 1.38). However, despite these findings, the above studies and meta-analyses are very limited in their methods and conclusions, and the meta-analysis was not able to account for the confounding differences between studies and groups. The majority of trials mentioned and included in the meta-analyses are retrospective reviews, and there are no randomized controlled trials evaluating the efficacy of DR as compared to IR. Moreover, there is a significant lack of consistency in study design, namely, the lack of consistent outcome measures. Several trials address time to wound healing or limb salvage, but few address all-cause mortality or even limited mortality in their outcomes data.

Though it seems somewhat unexpected to find a lack of overwhelming data in support of DR, there are some hypotheses and evidence to potentially explain the discrepancies. Varela et al. [17] retrospectively reviewed 76 total procedures of ischemic ulcers for patients revascularized by either endovascular or surgical means. Angiograms and operative reports were reviewed and patients were assigned into three separate groups, rather than two: DR and IR as usual, as well as a third group, designated "IR with collaterals" (IRc). While healing rate and limb salvage rates were statistically significant between DR and IR patients, there was no difference in the DR and IRc groups. This suggests that the presence of collaterals effectively transforms IR into a type of DR. These collaterals track through the vessels of the pedal or plantar arch and their presence or absence is referred to as pedal arch patency (Fig. 33.2). However, further studies have found variable results. Kret et al. [18] found improved wound healing in the DR group, but this was not influenced by the pedal arch patency. A study by Rashid et al. [19] investigated the patency of the pedal arch as a measure of collateral flow and found no statistically significant difference in amputation-free survival or time to wound healing in groups treated with DR or IR, regardless of the status of the pedal arch, except that no pedal arch flow did have an association with longer healing rates. An alternative explanation is the presence of inflammation; one multivariate analysis [9] showed that the presence of elevated levels of C-reactive protein (CRP) was an independent prognostic factor for major amputation in the IR but not the DR group, suggesting that worsening inflammation may favor a direct approach. This is similar to data seen in both endovascularly and surgically revascularized patients in whom elevated CRP was associated with an increased risk of amputation, regardless of surgical or endovascular, direct or indirect approach [20].

Surgical or Endovascular Approach: Is There a Difference?

Both surgical bypass and percutaneous transluminal angioplasty are potential approaches for revascularization of PAD. Both of these methods have been included in the aforementioned data with respect to the angiosome hypothesis in somewhat of an interchangeable light. However, these approaches are neither synonymous, nor do they engender the same results. Dick et al. [21] prospectively followed a cohort of approximately 400 patients with CLI for 1 year and stratified them into intervention groups including surgical, endovascular, and medically managed cohorts; surveillance and repeat revascularization were done, if deemed clinically necessary. In patients without diabetes, clinical improvement was seen regardless of intervention type. However, in diabetics, there appeared to be a benefit to repetition of revascularization that approached the clinical success seen in nondiabetics. Mode of revascularization, however, was not significant among the groups. Conversely, Spillerova et al. [20] retrospectively reviewed 744 patients who underwent endovascular or surgical repair and were further stratified into DR and IR groups. Surgical bypass with a DR strategy seemed to be most successful compared to the other permutations with respect to wound healing, but there were no

Fig. 33.2 Pre- and post-revascularization images of loop technique recanalization of deep plantar artery, with intact complete pedal arch seen post-revascularization. From Graziani L. The Loop Technique for the Plantar Arch Reconstruction. Endovascular Interventions. Page 675/676, Fig 59.5 (c) and (k). Reprinted with permission from Springer

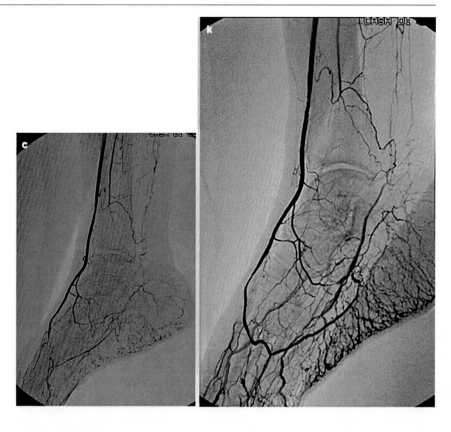

effects on overall survival. Lastly, in the BASIL trial [22], 450 patients with CLI were randomized to either surgical or endovascular repair and found no difference in mortality rates overall. However, those randomized to surgery did have a significant increase in overall survival by approximately 7 months *if they were still living at 2 years of follow-up*. This implies that healthier patients without comorbidities such as diabetes, coronary artery disease, stroke, smoking history, and age who would likely succeed postoperatively may have improved mortality with surgical bypass rather than endovascular repair.

Future Studies

Clearly, there is still work to be done to determine the most efficacious and appropriate methods and approach for revascularization in patients with PAD and CLI. Recent work by Kagaya et al. [23] describes the "real angiosome," addressing the problem of truly mapping anatomically accurate and patient-specific angiosomes rather than those defined by cadaveric studies from the 1980s. Near-infrared tissue oximetry was used to measure tissue oxygen saturation (StO_2) which, at a threshold of 50 %, was used to define areas of ischemia (Fig. 33.3). These correlated very well to areas of ulceration with 14 of 16 ulcers surrounded by low StO_2 tissue; 11/16 were matched accurately with the current principle of the angiosome model. Future studies investigating tissue oxygen saturation, transcutaneous oxygen tension, skin perfusion pressure, and dyes for subcutaneous or microvascular flow mapping may be on the horizon.

Conclusions

PAD and CLI are extremely prevalent conditions that are responsible for a large proportion of both morbidity and mortality in a vast quantity of patients. Treatment of these lesions involves revascularization, either with surgical bypass or endovascular therapy. The angiosome model, proposed by Taylor and Palmer [4] in 1987, is an anatomically accurate and medically sound theory for revascularization of arteries that supply the area of ischemia or ulceration. The data available, however, is limited due to methodology and results, and while there is some support for DR, trials are inconsistent. Part of the doubt may be explained by collaterals in circulation that make IR more effective or by elevated inflammation (as measured by inflammatory markers) that in turn make IR less effective. As for type of intervention, a surgical approach may be beneficial in healthier patients who are more likely to survive beyond 2 years, and multiple revascularizations may benefit patients with diabetes. Future work in angiosome mapping may help pave the way for randomized controlled trials and studies with more consistent outcomes to obtain accurate evidence to determine the most appropriate therapy in these patients.

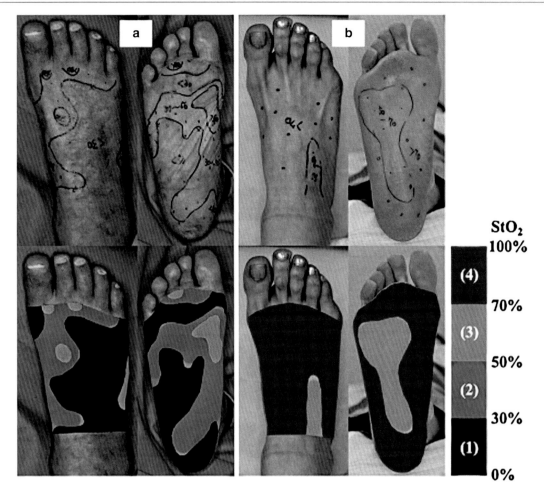

Fig. 33.3 Example of StO$_2$ foot mapping in a patient with CLI (**a**) and control (**b**). From Kagaya Y et al. "Real Angiosome" Assessment from Peripheral Tissue Perfusion Using Tissue Oxygen Saturation Foot-mapping in Patients with Critical Limb Ischemia. *Eur J Vasc Endovasc Surg* 2014;47:433–41. Reprinted with permission from Elsevier Limited

References

1. Hiatt WR, Goldstone J, Smith SC, McDermott M, Moneta G, Oka R, Newman AB, Pearce WH. Atherosclerotic peripheral vascular disease symposium II: nomenclature for vascular diseases. Circulation. 2008;118:2826–9.
2. Fowkes FGR, Rudan D, Rudan I, Aboyans V, Denenberg JO, McDermott MM, Norman PE, Sampson UKA, Williams LJ, Mensah GA, Criqui MH. Comparison of global estimates of prevalence and risk factors for peripheral artery disease in 2000 and 2010: a systematic review and analysis. Lancet. 2013;382:1329–40. doi:10.1016/S0140-6736(13)61249-0.
3. Criqui MH, Aboyans V. Epidemiology of peripheral artery disease. Circ Res. 2015;116:1509–26. Available from: http://www.sciencedirect.com/science/article/pii/B9781437729306000161.
4. Taylor GI, Palmer JH. The vascular territories (angiosomes) of the body: experimental study and clinical applications. Br J Plast Surg. 1987;40:113–41.
5. Antonopoulos AG, Thomopoulos M, Trikas A. The role of the angiosome model in percutaneous intravascular and surgical reperfusion treatment of peripheral artery disease of the lower limbs. Hell J Cardiol. 2014;55:52–7. Available from: http://www.ncbi.nlm.nih.gov/pubmed/24412085.
6. Attinger CE, Evans KK, Bulan E, Blume P, Cooper P. Angiosomes of the foot and ankle and clinical implications for limb salvage: reconstruction, incisions, and revascularization. Plast Reconstr Surg. 2006;117:261S–93S.
7. Neville RF, Attinger CE, Bulan EJ, Ducic I, Thomassen M, Sidawy AN. Revascularization of a specific angiosome for limb salvage: does the target artery matter? Ann Vasc Surg. 2009;23:367–73. doi:10.1016/j.avsg.2008.08.022.
8. Iida O, Nanto S, Uematsu M, Ikeoka K, Okamoto S, Dohi T, Fujita M, Terashi H, Nagata S. Importance of the angiosome concept for endovascular therapy in patients with critical limb ischemia. Catheter Cardiovasc Interv. 2010;75:830–6.
9. Iida O, Soga Y, Hirano K, Kawasaki D, Suzuki K, Miyashita Y, Terashi H, Uematsu M. Long-term results of direct and indirect endovascular revascularization based on the angiosome concept in patients with critical limb ischemia presenting with isolated below-the-knee lesions. J Vasc Surg. 2012;55:363–70. doi:10.1016/j.jvs.2011.08.014.
10. Söderström M, Albäck A, Biancari F, Lappalainen K, Lepäntalo M, Venermo M. Angiosome-targeted infrapopliteal endovascular revascularization for treatment of diabetic foot ulcers. J Vasc Surg. 2013;57:427–35. doi:10.1016/j.jvs.2012.07.057.
11. Alexandrescu V, Vincent G, Azdad K, Hubermont G, Ledent G, Ngongang C, Filimon A-M. A reliable approach to diabetic

neuroischemic foot wounds: below-the-knee angiosome-oriented angioplasty. J Endovasc Ther. 2011;18:376–87.

12. Azuma N, Uchida H, Kokubo T, Koya A, Akasaka N, Sasajima T. Factors influencing wound healing of critical ischaemic foot after bypass surgery: is the angiosome important in selecting bypass target artery? Eur J Vasc Endovasc Surg. 2012;43:322–28. doi:10.1016/j.ejvs.2011.12.001.

13. Fossaceca R, Guzzardi G, Cerini P, Cusaro C, Stecco A, Parziale G, Perchinunno M, De Bonis M, Carriero A. Endovascular treatment of diabetic foot in a selected population of patients with below-the-knee disease: is the angiosome model effective? Cardiovasc Intervent Radiol. 2013;36:637–44.

14. Berceli SA, Chan AK, Pomposelli J, Gibbons GW, Campbell DR, Akbari CM, Brophy DT, LoGerfo FW. Efficacy of dorsal pedal artery bypass in limb salvage for ischemic heel ulcers. J Vasc Surg. 1999;30:499–508.

15. Biancari F, Juvonen T. Angiosome-targeted lower limb revascularization for ischemic foot wounds: systematic review and meta-analysis. Eur J Vasc Endovasc Surg. 2014;47:517–22. doi:10.1016/j.ejvs.2013.12.010.

16. Huang T-Y, Huang T-S, Wang Y-C, Huang P-F, Yu H-C, Yeh C-H. Direct revascularization with the angiosome concept for lower limb ischemia. Medicine (Baltimore). 2015;94, e1427. Available from: http://content.wkhealth.com/linkback/openurl?sid=WKPTLP:landingpage&an=00005792-201508040-00033.

17. Varela C, Acín F, de Haro J, Bleda S, Esparza L, March JR. The role of foot collateral vessels on ulcer healing and limb salvage after successful endovascular and surgical distal procedures according to an angiosome model. Vasc Endovascular Surg. 2010;44:654–60.

18. Kret MR, Cheng D, Azarbal AF, Mitchell EL, Liem TK, Moneta GL, Landry GJ. Utility of direct angiosome revascularization and runoff scores in predicting outcomes in patients undergoing revascularization for critical limb ischemia. J Vasc Surg. 2014;59:121–8. doi:10.1016/j.jvs.2013.06.075.

19. Rashid H, Slim H, Zayed H, Huang DY, Wilkins CJ, Evans DR, Sidhu PS, Edmonds M. The impact of arterial pedal arch quality and angiosome revascularization on foot tissue loss healing and infrapopliteal bypass outcome. J Vasc Surg. 2013;57:1219–26. doi:10.1016/j.jvs.2012.10.129.

20. Spillerova K, Biancari F, Leppäniemi A, Albäck A, Söderström M, Venermo M. Differential impact of bypass surgery and angioplasty on angiosome-targeted infrapopliteal revascularization. Eur J Vasc Endovasc Surg. 2015;49:412–19. Available from: http://linkinghub.elsevier.com/retrieve/pii/S107858841400700X.

21. Dick F, Diehm N, Galimanis A, Husmann M, Schmidli J, Baumgartner I. Surgical or endovascular revascularization in patients with critical limb ischemia: influence of diabetes mellitus on clinical outcome. J Vasc Surg. 2007;45:751–61.

22. Bradbury AW. Bypass versus angioplasty in severe ischaemia of the leg (BASIL) trial: what are its implications? Semin Vasc Surg. 2009;22:267–74. doi:10.1016/j.jvs.2010.02.002.

23. Kagaya Y, Ohura N, Suga H, Eto H, Takushima A, Harii K. "Real angiosome" assessment from peripheral tissue perfusion using tissue oxygen saturation foot-mapping in patients with critical limb ischemia. Eur J Vasc Endovasc Surg. 2014;47: 433–41. Available from: http://www.ncbi.nlm.nih.gov/pubmed/24412085.

Principles of Endovascular Treatment of Critical Limb Ischemia

34

Robert S. Dieter

History of Endovascular Treatment for Critical Limb Ischemia

Dotter and Judkins, in 1964, described a series of 15 endovascular procedures in nine patients on 11 limbs [1]. Eight of their patients had gangrene, whereas the others had claudication or rest pain. In five of the eight patients, an amputation was averted; an additional amputation was delayed by 3 months. One patient functionally had a hybrid procedure. Their technique involved an "ordinary coil-spring catheter guide of about 0.05 in. OD is passed down the lumen until its tip has traversed the stenosis to reach the lumen beyond." Notably, some of these vessels were occluded, and some have suggested that this represents the first report of subintimal guidewire placement. Continuing with the procedure, "a tapered, radiopaque, Teflon dilating catheter of approximately 0.1 in. OD is then slipped over the guide and advanced until it, too, has traversed the block, thereby enlarging the preexisting or newly opened lumen." And, "where desirable and possible, a second dilating catheter of nearly 0.2 in. OD is passed over the first" [1]. Beyond opening the door to a paradigm shift in how these patients can be treated, Dotter and Judkins also were robust in following these patients longitudinally with objective studies—with plethysmography and segmental pressures.

Building upon this, Dorros, Jaff et al. published their series from 1983 to 1996 of 284 limbs in 235 patients with CLI [2]. They had a 92 % success rate in the ability to dilate the tibioperoneal lesions. At 5 years, there was a 91 % limb salvage rate, bypass surgery was performed in 8 %, and survival was only 56 % (lower with more advanced disease) [2]. Notably, the complication rate was low—one procedurally related death, emergency vascular surgery in three patients (arterial access repair, 2; no emergent bypasses, amputation, 1), one infection, one compartment syndrome, one patient required transfusion, and 20 patients (7 %) developed acute renal failure [2].

Natural History of Critical Limb Ischemia Without Revascularization ("Usual Care")

Natural history studies of critical limb ischemia are limited and have inherent methodological flaws, biased by patient selection. Nonetheless, there are some studies that provide insights into what can be expected from optimal medical therapy. In a series of patients by Marston et al. between 1999 and 2005, they followed 142 patients (169 limbs) with both PAD and a full-thickness ulceration that were not revascularized [3] (Table 34.1). These patients carried the traditional risk factors: mean age of 70 years, 70 % were diabetics, and chronic renal insufficiency (serum creatinine > 2.5 mg/dL) in 28 %. Within 6 months, 19 % required a major amputation and by 1 year 23 %. Foot-sparing amputations were performed in 28 % of limbs. Complete wound healing was seen in 25 % of patients at 6 months and 52 % by 1 year. Limb loss was associated with a lower ABI: with an ABI <0.5, major amputation rate is 28 % (6 months) and 34 % (12 months) compared with 10 % (6 months) and 15 % (12 months) with an ABI > 0.5. The only risk factor that was found to be associated with wound closure was the initial size of the wound [3].

Frequency of Vascular Studies Prior to Amputation

Endovascular treatment of critical limb ischemia assumes that the patient has undergone a vascular assessment. Surprisingly, though, vascular evaluation is not routine prior to amputations. In a study of 17,463 Medicare patients from 2000 to 2010 who underwent nontraumatic amputation, only 68.4 % had some type of arterial evaluation within 2 years of

R.S. Dieter, MD, RVT (✉)
Cardiology, Vascular and Endovascular Medicine,
Loyola University Medical Center, Maywood, IL, USA

© Springer International Publishing Switzerland 2017
R.S. Dieter et al. (eds.), *Critical Limb Ischemia*, DOI 10.1007/978-3-319-31991-9_34

the amputation. In decreasing frequency of testing were: ABI (47.5%), arterial duplex (38.7%), invasive angiography (31.1%), CT-angiography (6.7%), and MRA (5.6%) [4]. Frequency of arterial testing varied by the level of amputation: foot, 62.5%; below the knee, 76.7%; and above the knee, 62.5%. The rate of arterial testing increased, though minimally, over the study period: 65.7% (2002) to 69.2% (2010). The utilization of ABI, arterial duplex, and CT-A all increased over time, whereas invasive angiography remained the same and MRA use declined (Table 34.2). Attention should be made to reduce racial disparities in revascularization rates [5].

Noninvasive Evaluation to Predict Healing and Outcomes

Arterial insufficiency represents one component to the multiple etiologies contributing to lower extremity ulcerations [6]. Arterial insufficiency is the etiology of approximately 50% of foot ulcerations while <25% of above foot ulcerations [7]. The use of noninvasive studies can help determine the likelihood of ischemic rest pain as well as wound healing in order to guide endovascular therapies. Typically, without local trauma or infection, less flow is required for maintenance of intact integument than is required for wound healing. It is for this reason that it is important to distinguish these cutoffs. Ischemic rest pain may develop at an absolute ankle pressure of ≤50 mmHg and absolute toe pressure of ≤30 mmHg, whereas nonischemic etiologies should be sought in patients with rest pain and pressures above these cutoffs [7]. Review of the literature will reveal other cutoffs, and some have used a cutoff for absolute tissue ischemia with an ankle pressure of ≤35 mmHg in nondiabetic patients and ≤55 mmHg in diabetics [8]. Conversely, ankle pressures

≤70 mmHg or toe pressures ≤50 mmHg may be seen in patients with ischemic tissue loss (Fontaine IV or Rutherford category 5 or 6) [7]. Further confirmation of an ischemic component can be from a severely dampened or flat pulse volume recording ("PVR").

Despite efforts to predict which patients require aggressive intervention, it should be remembered that fewer than half of the patients with CLI, requiring a below the knee amputation, had symptoms up to 6 months prior [9]. Coupled with data that shows only about 75% of below the knee amputations heal by primary or secondary intention, 15% require an above the knee amputation, and 10% will die in the perioperative amputation period, highlighting the need for revascularization strategies which minimize physiological stress, patient morbidity, and mortality. Depending on the initial level and type of amputation, reamputation rates for the ipsilateral limb at 1 year in diabetic patients are approximately 25 and 60% by 5 years; contralateral amputations at 5 years are as high as 50% [10].

The decision to proceed with endovascular revascularization must be weighed against surgical revascularization, at times, even weighed against conservative and adjunctive therapies. There is a paucity of well-designed trials which compare endovascular to surgical revascularization, let alone various endovascular techniques/devices against each other [11].

Anatomic Levels of Arterial Disease Encountered in Critical Limb Ischemia

In an early series of tibioperoneal angioplasty in 284 limbs, 59% were found to have some form of inflow treatment prior to the infrapopliteal angioplasty [2]. In a study by Tartari et al., evaluating the efficacy of subintimal angioplasty as the first choice of revascularization in patients with critical limb ischemia, out of 109 limbs, 27 (25%) of the lesions were isolated to the femoropopliteal segment, 36 (33%) had combined femoropopliteal and tibial lesions, and 46 (42%) were isolated to the tibial vessels [12]. Since this was a study of infrainguinal occlusions, iliac lesions were not included in the analysis. Gray et al. demonstrated that in 446 patients with CLI undergoing revascularization, 36% had isolated

Table 34.1 Natural history of untreated critical limb ischemia

	Six months (%)	One year (%)
Wound healing	25	52
Major amputation (overall)	19	23
Limb loss ABI<0.5	28	34
Limb loss ABI>0.5	10	15

Table 34.2 Frequency of vascular testing prior to amputation

	ABI (%)	Arterial duplex (%)	Invasive angiography (%)	CT-angiography (%)	MRA (%)	Any testing (%)
Overall	47.5	38.7	31.1	6.7	5.6	
Foot amputation						62.5
Below the knee amputation						76.7
Above the knee amputation						62.5
2002						65.7
2010						69.2

tibial disease, 64% had multilevel disease, and 8% had both suprainguinal and infrainguinal diseases [13]. In a series of 229 limbs with critical limb ischemia, aortoiliac disease was found in 1.7%, iliofemoral in 5.2%, "iliodistal" 3.9%, femoropopliteal 22.7%, femorodistal 35.4%, and below the knee only 31% [14]. It is estimated that about 13–25% of patients with CLI will not be amenable to revascularization; ultimately, although lesions may be amenable to endovascular treatment, the clinician must keep in mind that the patient and limb may not ultimately be able to be healed due to comorbidities and other contributing factors [14, 15].

A consecutive series of diabetic patients with critical limb ischemia by Graziani et al. highlights the anatomic complexity which is encountered when an endovascular approach is taken. Of 417 patients, there were 2893 lesions identified. Over half (55%) of the lesions were occlusions. Only 1% of the stenosis were in the iliac arteries, whereas 74% of the below the knee vessels were identified involved. Of these below the knee lesions, 66% were occlusions (50% were >10 cm in length). In 55% there was at least one patent tibial artery and in 28% of the patients, all three of the tibial vessels were occluded. Not surprisingly, TcPO2 correlated to the extent of vascular involvement [16]. TASC II uses a TcPO2 threshold of ≤30 mmHg for diagnosis of CLI and if <20 mmHg revascularization is often necessary for wound healing; similarly, skin perfusion pressure (SPP) using laser Doppler of <30 mmHg is frequently seen in patients with CLI [17].

Faglia et al., in a series of nearly 1000 diabetic limbs, determined the level of disease contributing to CLI. Lesions of >50% were found in the iliac artery, femoral artery, or popliteal artery in 6.7%, entirely in the below the knee arteries (infrapopliteal) in 31.8%, and in both the fem-pop and infrapopliteal segments in 61.4% of patients [18].

Angiosomes

Angiosome-directed interventions will be reviewed in a separate chapter. However, the ability to achieve revascularization of the "appropriate" angiosome artery can be technically difficult, if not impossible, endovascularly. Outcomes, although seemingly should be improved with this approach, often times oversimplify the relationship between the tibial vessel above the ankle and the status of the plantar vessels and plantar arch. Acin et al. analyzed the outcomes of infrapopliteal artery interventions relative to the number of tibial vessels attempted, number of patent tibial vessels, and if direct revascularization (angiosome appropriate) or indirect revascularization (ulcer supplied by collaterals) [19]. They found that ulcer healing at 1 year was equivalent between the direct (66.0%) and indirect (68.0%) revascularization strategies as was limb salvage at 2 years (88.9% vs 84.8%, respectively) [19]. Indirect revascularization without collat-

erals resulted in a 7.1% 1 year ulcer healing rate, though limb salvage at 2 years in this group was 59.0%. Amputation-free survival at 24 months was statistically equivalent between the groups (direct revascularization, 67.5%; indirect revascularization through collaterals, 73.3%; and 61.9% indirect revascularization without collaterals) [19]. Amputation-free survival at 2 years was lower in the group in which there were no patent (<30% residual stenosis) tibial vessels (43.8%), but statistically equivalent between runoff "1" and runoff ">1" groups (64.3% vs 76.6%) [19]. Further contributing to the confusion surrounding whether angiosome-guided revascularization enhances outcomes is data from Kawarada et al. They evaluated the skin perfusion pressure after revascularization of either the anterior tibial or posterior tibial artery. They found that comparing the dorsal side to the plantar side, anterior tibial artery revascularization, 64 and 58%, demonstrated higher dorsal post-intervention skin perfusion pressure and change in skin perfusion pressure; posterior tibial artery revascularization resulted in higher plantar skin perfusion pressures in 47 and 40% had a higher post change in skin perfusion pressure. They concluded that "single tibial artery revascularization, whether of the ATA or PTA, yielded comparable improvements in microcirculation of the dorsal and plantar foot. Approximately half of the feet revascularized had a change in microcirculation that was not consistent with the 2D angiosome theory" [20].

TASC II

The TransAtlantic Inter-Society Consensus (TASC) II has developed a scheme by which lesions can by approached from an anatomic perspective. Lesions are classified A–D. Type A lesions are preferentially treated with an endovascular approach, whereas type D lesions are best suited for surgical revascularization [7]. These recommendations were published in 2007, however, and there have been significant advancements in endovascular techniques which have allowed for the greater utilization of endovascular procedures for lesions that otherwise would have been reserved for vascular surgery. The Society of Cardiac Angiography and Interventions has published expert consensus statements which address appropriate endovascular treatment of lesions based upon anatomy and symptom status [21, 22].

Technical Considerations

The goal of this chapter is not to discuss particular methodologies or techniques but rather to provide an overview of endovascular principles and particularly to discuss outcomes with an endovascular strategy. For an exhaustive review on endovascular techniques, please refer to our sepa-

Table 34.3 Clinical scenarios in which treatment of infrapopliteal artery disease may be considered

Appropriate care	• Moderate-severe claudication (RC 2–3) with two- or three-vessel IP disease (if the arterial target lesion is focal) • Ischemic rest pain (RC 4) with two- or three-vessel IP disease (to provide direct flow to the plantar arch and to maximize volume flow to the foot) • Minor tissue loss (RC 5) with two- or three-vessel IP disease (to provide direct flow to the plantar arch and to maximize volume flow to the foot) • Major tissue loss (RC 6) with two- or three-vessel IP disease (to prevent major amputation[a] and to facilitate healing a minor amputation[b])
May be appropriate care	• Moderate-severe claudication (RC 2–3) with two- or three-vessel IP disease (occlusion or diffuse disease) • Ischemic rest pain (RC 4) with one- or two-vessel IP disease (to provide direct flow to the plantar arch and in two vessel, to maximize volume flow to the foot) • Minor tissue loss (RC 5) with one-vessel IP disease (to provide direct flow to the plantar arch and to maximize volume flow to the foot)
Rarely appropriate care	• Mild claudication (RC 1) with one-, two-, or three-vessel IP disease • Moderate-severe (RC 2–3) claudication symptoms with one-vessel IP disease • Major tissue loss (RC 6) with one-vessel IP disease

From Gray BH, Diaz-Sandoval LJ, Dieter RS, Jaff MR, White CJ. SCAI Expert consensus statement for infrapopliteal arterial intervention appropriate use. Catheter Cardiovasc Intervent 2014;84(4):539–45. Reprinted with permission from John Wiley and Sons

RC = Rutherford classifications for chronic limb ischemia one-vessel infrapopliteal disease implies that two tibial arteries are without hemodynamically significant stenosis or occlusion; two-vessel infrapopliteal disease implies that one tibial artery is without hemodynamically significant stenosis or occlusion; three-vessel infrapopliteal disease implies that all three tibial arteries have hemodynamically significant stenosis and/or occlusion; no significant infrapopliteal disease implies that all three tibial are without hemodynamically significant stenosis or occlusion. Severe stenosis = luminal narrowing 70–99 %, moderate stenosis = luminal narrowing 50–69 %, mild stenosis = luminal narrowing <50 %, and occlusion = no flow through the arterial segment. Tibioperoneal trunk disease affects both the posterior tibial and peroneal arteries so would be consistent with two-vessel disease. Focal infrapopliteal lesion = discrete area of narrowing that can be treated with a single 15-mm-long balloon/stent; multiple lesions = more than one focal lesion in noncontiguous arterial segments; diffuse lesion = a continuous segment of disease treated with >15 mm long balloon/stent

[a]Major amputation = removal of the leg either above or below the knee, but above the ankle

[b]Minor amputation = removal of the foot or portions of it [i.e., isolated toe(s)]

rate textbook, *Endovascular Interventions: A Case Based Approach* [23].

The Society for Cardiovascular Angiography and Interventions (SCAI) published expert consensus statements on appropriate revascularization of lower extremity arterial disease [21, 22]. Table 34.3 details how to approach a patient with infrapopliteal disease. These recommendations follow a rational and logical approach to the clinical scenario based upon the patients symptoms classification paired to the artery anatomy.

Access

Arterial access is dictated by a number of factors, including lesion location, body habitus, and local tissue issues (such as hernias, scar tissue, infection, etc.). Furthermore, it is not uncommon for catheter or wire length to limit approaches. Although radial access can be used for some aortoiliac lesions, it is difficult for even a 90 cm sheath to engage the iliac arteries in some patients from a radial approach. Similarly, if a contralateral common femoral approach is used, equipment may not reach the contralateral dorsalis pedis artery. As such, the interventionalist must be cognizant of catheter limitations, access vessel diameters that may limit equipment being used, as well as hemostasis issues. A variety of techniques are available—even high anterior tibial access

[24]. Antegrade crossing for tibial intervention is unsuccessful in up to 20 % of patients. In a study of 51 failed antegrade crossing attempts, a transcollateral approach (11.8 %) or pedal access (88.2 %) was utilized resulting in an 86.3 % success rate [25]. Direct digital arterial access has also been utilized for revascularization.

Lesion Crossing

There are a number of techniques described for lesion crossing. For stenosis, true lumen crossing is relatively straightforward, particularly with road mapping techniques. Occlusions however can be crossed with an attempt to remain in the true lumen. The longer the occlusion or more calcified the lesion, remaining true lumen can be difficult.

Bolia et al. first introduced subintimal angioplasty (SIA or percutaneous intentional extraluminal recanalization—PIER) in 1989. Their report of the inadvertent creation of a subintimal channel in the popliteal artery and subsequent angioplasty introduced a new technique which allows an alternative than true lumen lesion crossing [26]. True lumen crossing in long-segment chronic total occlusions (CTOs) can be difficult and identification of the vessel course can be challenging. In a study by Hynes et al. comparing the "pre-SIA" period and the period after the introduction of SIA, "post-SIA" over 15 years, the limb salvage rate increased from 42 to 70 %, in the pre to post SIA period. The post revascularization limb salvage rate increased from 72 to 86 % and the 30-day morbidity, mortality, and length of stay were shorter [27]. Zhu et al. evaluated the efficacy of subintimal angioplasty in the dorsalis pedis or plantar arteries in diabetic patients with CLI [28]. They were successful in 83.3 % of cases with limb salvage rate of 94.6 % [28]. Many of the techniques used for tibial artery occlusions were originally developed for the treatment of coronary artery CTO. The controlled antegrade and retrograde tracking and dissection (CART)/reverse CART technique is one such method, originally described by Surmely in 2006 [29]. When balloons are simultaneously inflated/deflated, the technique is referred to as "confluent balloon technique" [30]. Similarly, the parallel wire technique in which after the first guidewire enters the false lumen, a second wire is used with the first wire as a guide, was first introduced by Japanese coronary CTO experts [31].

There are, however, no randomized controlled trials comparing SIA to other lesion crossing techniques and vascular endpoints are diverse across studies. In an analysis of 11 studies, involving approximately 1400 limbs, Brennan found that technical success in patients with CLI was 87.7 %. One-year primary patency was 55.8 % (four studies) and 1-year limb salvage rate was 91.1 % (six studies) [32]. This data again highlights the disparity between primary patency (relatively low) and the limb salvage rates (relatively high). Another systematic review of SIA demonstrated that technical success is higher in femoral or femoropopliteal arteries compared to crural vessels [33]. Complication rates were reported at about 15 % and ranged from puncture site hematoma, perforation, or distal embolization with a range of 2–20 % across studies. One-year primary and assisted primary patency rates are about 50 % with limb salvages rates about 80–90 % [33]. Vraux et al. demonstrated a 77 % success rate of SIA for tibial vessels with 1-year primary patency rates of 46 and 87 % 1-year limb salvage rates [34].

The utilization of a transcollateral approach has allowed increased success rates where antegrade crossing has failed. The ability to access the target vessel via collaterals and treat the occlusion has the advantage of one access point (as opposed to a separate pedal access). Current small profile balloons will generally track well and allow for dilation in this retrograde manner. After angioplasty, the vessel can either be rewired from an antegrade approach or the retrograde wire externalized, maintaining lumen access [25].

Complications of Endovascular Interventions

Complications of endovascular interventions, including contrast induced nephropathy, must be weighed against the potential benefit to the patient. Embolization from peripheral interventions can lead to additional procedures, prolonged

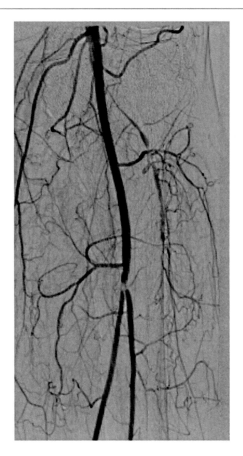

Fig. 34.1 Tibial embolization post intervention

hospital stays, convert a stable patient into acute limb ischemia, and in some cases loss of limb or death. Distal embolization is seen in 1–100 % of peripheral interventions. Rates are dependent upon how embolic debris is detected—"hits" by ultrasound, capture with filters, or clinically relevant embolization. When an embolic protection device is used for endovascular interventions, Mendes et al. found macroscopic debris in almost 70 % of cases [35]. Embolization leads to increased reintervention (20 % vs 3 %) and amputation rates (11 % vs 3 %) [35]. Embolization rates are likely related to lesion complexity (occlusions), and atherectomy devices appear to have a higher rate of embolization (Fig. 34.1).

All percutaneous vascular interventions carry the risk of the development of an access-related arteriovenous fistula (0.4 %) or pseudoaneurysm. Interventional procedures, presumably due to the use of anticoagulation, increase the risk from approximately 0.05–2.0 % for diagnostic cases to 2–6 % for interventional procedures [36]. Other risk factors include increasing sheath size, female gender, and inadequate compression post sheath removal [23]. Spontaneous resolution of small pseudoaneurysms <2–3 cm in patients not on anticoagulation can be expected in almost 90 % of patients. Pseudoaneurysm morphology guides treatment strategies. Generally, if the pseudoaneurysm is small, without an identifiable neck, has a concomitant arteriovenous fistula, or is in very close proximity to other vessels, then ultrasound-guided compression (or even non-ultrasound-guided compression) should be attempted first (approximately ≥75 % success rate); otherwise, the pseudoaneurysm is treated with ultrasound-guided thrombin injection (≥90–95 % success rate).

"Endo-First" Strategy for the Treatment of Critical Limb Ischemia

Dosluoglu et al. reported on limb salvage and survival after adoption of an endovascular first approach to critical limb ischemia [37]. The 30-day mortality trend was lower in the endovascular vs open group (2.8 % vs 6.0 %, $p = 0.079$). Five-year limb salvage rates were equivalent to 78 %, amputation-free survival in the endovascular group was 30 % vs 39 % in the surgical group, and overall survival was equivalent to 36 % vs 46 % [37]. Although primary patency rates were equivalent at 5 years (50 % vs 48 %), the assisted primary patency rates (70 % vs 59 %) and the secondary patency rates (73 % vs 64 %) favored the endovascular first approach [37].

A retrospective analysis of 1053 patients with critical limb ischemia by Soga et al. compared treatment with either bypass surgery or endovascular therapy first for limb revascularization [38]. At 3 years, the groups were equivalent in limb salvage (85.4 % vs 88.7 %), amputation-free survival (62.1 % vs 60.5 %), and overall survival rates (69.2 % vs 65.8 %). A matched pair analysis confirmed the equivalency between the two groups [38].

Jones et al. performed a meta-analysis of studies with patients with critical limb ischemia comparing the effectiveness of endovascular versus surgical revascularization [39]. Overall, 23 studies (only one randomized control trial) were used in the analysis. There was no difference in overall mortality between 1 and 2 years or after 3 years. The rates of lower extremity amputation were equivalent at <2 years, at 2–3 years, and at >5 years. Amputation-free survival was equivalent between the groups at these time points, as well. Endovascular treatment had higher primary patency and secondary patency at 1 year and at 2–3 years [39].

In an analysis of 202 patients involving 229 limbs with critical limb ischemia, May et al. evaluated the efficacy of an endovascular first approach [14]. Patients preferentially underwent an endovascular approach unless there were contraindications to angiography (11 patients), anatomy not amenable to percutaneous intervention (20 patients), or those that failed an endovascular approach (16 patients). Ultimately, 198 limbs underwent endovascular revascularization. One hundred and forty-four of these required no further intervention (72.7 % of those underwent endovascular intervention), 38 (19.2 %) required a secondary endovascular intervention, and 16 (8.1 %) required bypass surgery after an initial endo-vascular approach, but with continued impaired perfusion and wound nonhealing (mean 37±58 days after the initial endovascular intervention) [14]. The mortality rates at 30 days, 12 months, and 24 months were 5.2 %, 20 %, and 27 %, respectively. However, the cumulative limb salvage rates and amputation-free survival at 1 year were 78 and 75.5 % and, at 2 years, 74 and 57.6 % [14]. Interestingly, in this study, the investigators opted not to report the vessel patency, citing reluctance of asymptomatic patients to undergo further testing, but also "limb preservation is the ultimate condition that matters most to the patients."

Another study, by Garg et al., evaluated the difference between endovascular first approach and surgical bypass [40]. Their findings support an equivalent outcome between the two strategies in regard to 5-year survival and limb salvage, but more secondary procedures after an initial open strategy. Patients with end-stage renal disease, below the knee interventions, or gangrene had a lower amputation-free survival rate [40].

Endovascular Approach Does Not Compromise Surgical Targets

BASIL Trial

Despite being published in 2005, the Bypass versus Angioplasty in Severe Ischemia of the Leg (BASIL): multicenter, randomized controlled trial remains one of the landmark trials comparing surgical revascularization versus endovascular treatment for CLI [41]. This trial randomized 452 patients with CLI and infrainguinal PAD to either a surgery first or angioplasty; follow-up was for 5.5 years. The lesions were similar in distribution between the two arms. The majority of the patients in the angioplasty arm (80 %) had SFA lesions treated and 62 % also had more distal vessels treated. At 1 year, 56 % of patients treated with surgery and 50 % of patients treated with angioplasty were alive with their trial leg intact. Re-intervention rates were lower with a surgery-first approach—both by intention to treat (18 % vs. 26 %) and by actual treatment (17 % vs. 28 %). Amputation-free survival at 1 year and 3 years was similar (surgery, 68 and 57 %; angioplasty, 71 and 52 %), and there were no differences in survival between the arms. There was a trend toward a higher earlier mortality with surgery (at 6 months) which by 2 years, survival favored the surgical group. Health-related quality of life, short form 36 (SF36), and EuroQoL (EQ5D) were similar between groups [41]. Only about 20 % of the patients screened for the BASIL trial were actually enrolled, and there was a 20 % immediate technical failure rate in the angioplasty arm, higher than most studies. One of the most important findings in the BASIL trial was that angioplasty did not compromise future surgical bypass operations.

Santo et al. compared outcomes of lower extremity bypass for CLI in patients with and without prior endovascular interventions [42]. Of 314 patients who underwent autologous vein bypass, 19% had prior lower extremity endovascular interventions. There was no difference between the groups for patency rates, limb salvage rates, or amputation-free survival [42]. Additional data from Uhl et al. evaluated prior crural interventions on patency and limb salvage rates in patients who subsequently undergo bypass surgery [43]. They found no difference in limb salvage rates at 1 year in patients with prior endovascular interventions versus those without (82.3% vs 71.6%) nor graft occlusion rates at 30 days (19.4% vs 17.9%) [43].

Pedal Bypass After Crural Peripheral Vascular Intervention

Pedal access for an endovascular approach to the treatment of CLI results in an access site occlusion in approximately 2% of patients. Acutely, this can be recognized and treated in an antegrade fashion [25]. Pedal access likely does not limit future bypass in the majority of limbs.

These studies, coupled with the BASIL trial, confirm that an endovascular approach is reasonable for this patient population and generally offers competitive, if not equivalent, outcomes with surgical bypass. The treating physician should remember to individualize patient care based upon the patient and anatomy. Applying a similar treatment paradigm, as was developed by Dr. Raymond A Dieter Jr., for thoracic oncology, to peripheral revascularization can help the clinician determine the best initial and subsequent strategy for treatment. The "ORC" scheme is as follows: "O" is for operability, from a physiological stress standpoint (including renal function), which is best for the patient, open surgery, or endovascular therapy; "R" is for resectability, but here it would indicate the ability to either bypass (conduits, distal vasculature, infection, etc.) or perform endovascular therapy; and "C" is curability—if the patient has life-threatening gangrene or an ulceration that ultimately will never heal, then amputation rather than revascularization may be preferred [44] (Table 34.4).

Table 34.4 ORC classification modified for CLI treatment

"O"—operability	Is the patient an acceptable candidate for either endovascular or open surgical repair
"R"—resectability	Is there a distal target for bypass; is endovascular lesion crossing possible/trentable
"C"—curability	Will healing occur after revascularization, or are there significant comorbid conditions (e.g., infection, edema, immobility, etc.) that preclude healing

Outcomes After Endovascular Intervention

When treating the patient with critical limb ischemia, the clinician must have a clear understanding of the limb specific goals of therapy. Objective performance goals ("OPGs") have been developed by the Society for Vascular Surgery and endovascular infrapopliteal interventions have been found to meet the OPG endpoints for CLI [45]. When treating patients with rest pain, long-term patency is very important since restenosis will lead to recurrent rest pain; however, patients with ischemic ulceration require patency long enough for wound healing and the prevention of limb loss. The term "subcritical" ischemia (Fontaine III or Rutherford category 4) has been used to help differentiate patients as well as expectations of revascularization. A review of 20 publications, involving over 6000 patients, demonstrated differential outcomes for patients with subcritical ischemia and an ankle pressure above 40 mmHg compared to those with tissue loss and/or an ankle pressure less than 40 mmHg [46]. The natural history of non-revascularized limbs ("conservative" treatment) in patients with subcritical ischemia and an ankle pressure >40 mmHg was that at 1 year 27% were alive without an amputation. At 1 year, 95% of the patients with critical limb ischemia treated conservatively underwent an amputation. However, those with critical limb ischemia undergoing revascularization, only 25% required a major amputation. Not unexpected, the 1-year mortality in patients with critical limb ischemia was 26%, regardless of treatment modality (and, at 1 year, 69% of the critical limb ischemia patients who underwent revascularization were alive without an amputation) [46].

The patency of the plantar arch vessels can ultimately determine the success or failure of an endovascular intervention. The toe brachial index compared to the ankle brachial index can provide some noninvasive evidence of the status of the pedal arch vessels prior to an angiogram and intervention. Graziani has been able to demonstrate the ability to pass 0.014″ guidewires and angioplasty balloons into the plantar arteries and appropriately dilate in order to enhance foot/toe perfusion. It should be emphasized that both the AP and lateral angiographic views help delineate the arterial anatomy of the plantar arch vessels. Typically, diabetic patients have more extensive pedal arch vessel involvement relative to nondiabetics.

Patients with renal failure do particularly poor. CLI in this patient population is addressed in a separate chapter. Briefly, estimated freedom from amputation at 1 year ranges from 65 to 86% and at 5 years approximately 40% freedom from amputation [47]. From an anatomic and not patient perspective, it is thought that these patients have worse pedal arch circulation (Fig. 34.2).

Fig. 34.2 Demonstrating
significant pedal arch and
digital calcification (*arrows*)

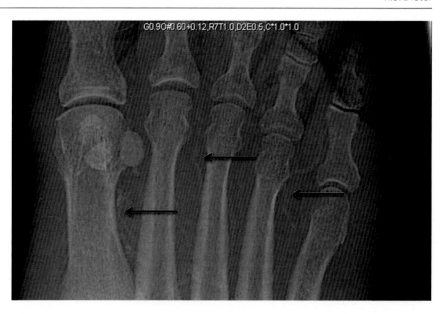

Timeline for Wound Healing After Endovascular Revascularization

It is difficult to compare the timeline for healing after endo-vascular interventions across studies, due to confounding variables and rates of re-intervention. Fernandez et al. com-pared the impact of multilevel intervention (fem-pop and tibial) versus isolated tibial interventions on wound healing [48]. Patients with multilevel disease had a lower initial ABI (0.53 vs 0.74) prior to the intervention, but after endo-vascular intervention, the ABI was similar (0.86 versus 0.88). Despite equivalent post-intervention ABIs, the limb salvage rate was higher in the multilevel disease group (87 % vs 69 %). The time to wound healing was shorter in the multilevel group (7.7 months vs 11.5 months) despite similar rates of re-intervention (18 % vs 13 %). It is postu-lated that the group with isolated tibial disease have poorer pedal runoff as well as more extensive distal disease which contribute to overall lower limb salvage rates [48]. In the XCELL trial which evaluated the use of stenting with the Xpert stent (Abbott Vascular, Illinois) for below the knee lesions in patient with CLI, the 6-month ulcer healing rate was 49 % and the 1-year complete healing rate was 54.4 % (with a 68.5 % binary restenosis rate) [49]. However, the 1-year amputation-free survival rates were 100 % (Rutherford 4), 77.3 % (Rutherford 5), and 55.2 % (Rutherford 6); the freedom from major amputation at 1 year was 100 % (Rutherford 4), 90.9 % (Rutherford 5), and 70.1 % (Rutherford 6). This highlights the discordance between limb salvage and ulcer healing.

Restenosis and Impact on Recurrent Ulcerations

Restenosis rates following tibial artery interventions vary by study and potentially by treatment modality. Restenosis rates differ by treatment modality, lesion length, and indication for treatment and patient comorbidities. A study by Saqib et al. demonstrated a restenosis rate of 41 % at 4 months with a 59 % 1-year primary patency rate [50]. Thirty-two percent of patients with restenosis had a persistent wound, 42 % of patients with restenosis had worsening of their wound, rest pain developed in 16 %, and 10 % were asymptomatic. This data suggests that most restenosis, at least early, are not asymptomatic and restenosis is suggested by failure of wound healing. In their study, limb loss was 27 % in patients with restenosis versus 4 % in those without restenosis. Interestingly, restenosis was seen more frequently in patients who presented with gangrene (63 % vs 38 %) suggesting the inflammatory milieu may contribute to restenosis. There was a trend toward higher restenosis in patients with renal insuf-ficiency, but not in patients with diabetes, statin use status, or smoking. Thirty-six percent of patients required an addi-tional intervention after the first re-intervention, yielding an overall 87 % limb salvage rate [50]. Patients with connective tissue disease after revascularization appear to be at higher risk of limb loss [51].

For patients with femoropopliteal lesions treated with self-expanding stents, in-stent complete occlusion was seen in 5.2 %, 11.2 %, and 16.4 % at 1, 3, and, 5 years in the mul-ticenter, retrospective analysis by Dohi et al. [52]. Predictors of stent occlusion included female gender, TASC C/D lesions, and those with critical limb ischemia. Patients with stent occlusion had a hazard ratio of 6.35 for major amputation and 21.1 for major adverse limb event.

In data which is concordant with podiatry literature suggesting that albumin, potentially as a marker of nutritional status and perhaps as an acute phase reactant, predicts outcomes, Chang et al. found that albumin <3.0 g/dL predicted poor outcomes (poorer sustained clinical success and increased amputation rates) in patients undergoing endovascular procedures for limb salvage [53]. The rate of sustained clinical success increased for every one mg/dL increase in albumin levels. Furthermore, multivariate analysis demonstrated that patients with coronary artery disease, low albumin, end-stage renal disease, and atrial fibrillation correlated with low sustained clinical success [53].

In an analysis of 246 patients undergoing endovascular treatment, Ryer et al. evaluated the outcomes of patients who failed after an initially successful procedure for chronic limb ischemia [54]. Due to duplex findings of restenosis, nonhealing of an ulceration, loss of a previously palpable pulse, or return of clinical symptoms, 18% were found to have restenosis after their initial intervention. The majority of these restenosis were found in the 1–18-month time frame (78%) with the mean time to detection, 8.7 months. The authors found that 82% of these patients were eligible for a secondary endovascular intervention, 11% only for bypass surgery, and 4% required an amputation. The overall limb salvage in those undergoing a secondary endovascular intervention was 86% at 1 year [54].

secondary patency for angioplasty at 1, 6, 12, 24 months: 83.3%, 73.8%, 68.2%, 63.5%; primary patency for surgery at 1, 6, 12, 24 months: 93.3%, 85.8%, 81.5%, 76.8%; secondary patency for surgery at 1, 6, 12, 24 months: 94.9%, 89.3%, 85.9%, 81.6%; limb salvage rates at 1, 6, 12, 24 months for angioplasty vs surgery: 93.4% vs 95.1%, 88.2% vs 90.9%, 86.0 vs 88.5%, 83.8 vs 85.2%). The authors concluded, "The technical success and subsequent durability of crural angioplasty are limited compared with bypass surgery, but the clinical benefit is acceptable because limb salvage rates are equivalent to bypass surgery" [56]. Criticisms of this meta-analysis include small sample size of the trials included, non-uniform evaluation of vessel patency, different clinical endpoints used, and inclusion in some studies of patients with intermittent claudication [55]. Duplex scanning, compared to angiography, after tibial interventions has been demonstrated to both over and underestimate rates of restenosis [57]. It has been shown that tibial restenosis can delay wound healing, but this does not mean that once healed, that restenosis will lead to recurrent ulcerations [58]. According to the data from drug-eluting stents versus bare metal stents, though generally demonstrating superior patency rates, these rates do not necessarily reflect improved limb salvage rates. Finally, limb salvage should be differentiated from wound healing. Lo et al., in a study evaluating infrapopliteal angioplasty, found a limb salvage rate of 84% at 1 year, but only 63% complete healing of the wound at 1 year; at 6 months, complete wound healing was seen in only 15% of patients [59]. Nonetheless, it is generally accepted that long-term patency after endovascular therapy for CLI is not necessary after initial healing.

Is Long-Term Patency Necessary for Wound Healing?

The general consensus is that only short-/midterm patency is required for wound healing and the adage "less blood flow is required to keep a wound healed than is required to heal a wound" has essentially become a dogma. As such, long-term patency of endovascular interventions for CLI may not be as necessary as patency "long enough to achieve healing" [55]. In a meta-analysis of 30 studies (1990–2006, most between 2000 and 2006) with 2404 patients receiving crural angioplasty and 242 undergoing popliteal to distal vein bypass surgery, Romiti et al. evaluated the clinical outcomes of patients with critical limb ischemia [56]. Although the primary and secondary patency rates were significantly less with angioplasty than bypass surgery at all time points measured (1 month, 6 months, 1 year, and 2 years), the limb salvage rate was equivalent at all time points (primary patency for angioplasty at 1, 6, 12, 24 months: 77.4%, 65.0%, 58.1%, 51.3%;

Impact of Runoff Vessels on Patency Rates for Lower Extremity Interventions

In patients requiring endovascular treatment of superficial femoral artery lesions, there has been concern regarding the number of the runoff vessels impacting long-term durability of patency. Lee and Katz evaluated the patency of stented femoropopliteal segments and determined that runoff was associated with TASC classification. Furthermore, the number of patent tibials at time of stenting did not affect limb salvage, either [60]. An alternative explanation is the evaluation of runoff in terms analogous to coronary artery, TIMI flow rates. Hiramori et al. found that femoropopliteal stent patency was dependent upon post-procedural runoff grade, but not on the number of runoff vessels [61]. Conceptually, the runoff grade accounts for the quality of the tibial vessels, more importantly than the number. This also may reflect the flow beyond what an ABI measures and accounts for why the post-procedural ABI did not predict stent patency [61].

Single-vessel runoff via the peroneal artery, significant plantar arch disease, and renal insufficiency or failure are predictive of poorer outcomes after endovascular therapy for CLI [62]. Lazaris et al. reported 1-year patency of 81% in patients with more than one vessel runoff compared to 25% in those with single-vessel runoff [63]. Furthermore, for every one centimeter in angioplasty length, the hazard for reocclusion was 1.02 [63].

Cost Analysis

In the BASIL trial, the costs of surgery versus angioplasty for limb salvage favored angioplasty, especially the inpatient and 1-year follow-up costs. Surgical costs at 1 year were about a third higher than those assigned to angioplasty [41]. The patients assigned to surgery also spent more time in the intensive care unit and hospital overall [41]. In this trial, reintervention rates are higher with angioplasty than surgery, but due to lower costs associated with the procedure and shorter hospital stays, costs remain lower with angioplasty at 1 year.

Risk Factors for Post-revascularization Health-Care-Associated Infections After Revascularization

Patients undergoing revascularization are at risk for health-care-related infections. Patients undergoing bypass surgery had a 3.41 higher OR of developing an infection than those undergoing endovascular revascularization [64]. Similarly, those with gangrene had a 1.39 OR higher rate of developing health-care-related infection after surgery. Results were consistent between bypass and thromboendarterectomy.

Upper Extremity Critical Limb Ischemia

Upper extremity critical limb ischemia is uncommon and will only be briefly discussed in this chapter. Thoracic outlet syndrome will be reviewed in a separate chapter.

Atherosclerosis leading to critical limb ischemia of the upper extremities is rare. More common etiologies include Buerger's disease (thromboangiitis obliterans), vasculitis, embolization, or steal syndromes from hemodialysis access. Occasionally, repetitive trauma such as the hypothenar hammer syndrome or the "crutch" syndrome can result in hand or upper extremity ischemia. Rarely, patients with severe atherosclerotic disease of the upper extremity, below the brachial artery, will present. Furthermore, palmar arch atherosclerotic occlusive disease can also contribute to steal symptoms. Given the small vessel size, an endovascular approach is often first line for these patients. Gandini et al. present a patient with long-standing diabetes and renal failure

who presented with rest pain and digital ulceration [65]. In their case, they were unable to cross the occluded ulnar artery in an antegrade fashion. However, by accessing the radial artery and using the superficial palmar arch to access the ulnar artery, they were successful in crossing the occlusion and performing angioplasty.

Patients that have previously undergone arteriovenous fistula or graft placement in the forearm are at risk for both steal and the development of CLI if the feeder artery (e.g., radial artery in a radiocephalic arteriovenous fistula) occludes. In a small series by Kawarada et al., five limbs in four patients, all of which had chronic kidney disease, three limbs with a previous arteriovenous fistula, were treated in a percutaneous fashion using either 3 or 4 Fr sheaths; balloon sizes ranged from 2.5 mm for the radial (one limb) or ulnar (four limbs) arteries and 2.0 mm for the palmar arch (two limbs) [66]. Their technical success was 100% with clinical success in 100% with a mean follow-up of 11 months [66]. High fistula flow rates can also result in hand ischemia, though procedures designed to limit fistula flow often result in thrombosis of the fistula.

Randomized controlled trial supporting lower extremity interventions for CLI is only recently emerging. The data supporting upper extremity interventions is generally limited even more to case reports and small series. A case series by Dieter et al. has demonstrated the clinical efficacy of stenting for subclavian artery stenosis (coronary subclavian steal) [67]. Case reports of brachial artery occlusions leading to hand CLI have been reported. The use of a self-expanding stent in this region helps prevent stent compression and allows for more durable results [68].

Follow-Up Post-Endovascular Intervention

Post-intervention Surveillance

After endovascular treatment for CLI, it is unclear what represents the best surveillance strategy for the patient and limb. The patient requires appropriate risk factor modification and caution regarding appropriate contralateral foot care. It is hypothesized that endovascular interventions maintain collateral patency better than does lower extremity bypass, and as such, restenosis or occlusion of a previously treated vessel may not lead to a clinical recurrence. Consequently, although many interventionalists will obtain a baseline, post intervention, ABI, or toe pressure, the best surveillance strategy remains debatable. Saarinen et al. systematically evaluated patients after endovascular treatment for CLI with baseline; 1-, 3-, and 6-month ABI, toe pressure, and duplex [69]. For most patients, clinical status or the toe pressure adequately predicted restenosis/occlusion. However, there was no correlation in 30% of the cases between duplex ultrasound and the clinical findings; in 29% of cases, the toe pressure and the duplex findings were discordant [69]. This highlights the importance of clinical judgment despite seemingly adequate noninvasive vascular studies.

In an interesting analysis of 39 patients (40 limbs), Wakassa et al. evaluated both the healing time as well as the gradient of peak systolic velocities both before and after endovascular intervention for CLI [70]. The investigators measured the mean of the peak systolic velocity of three tibial arteries, and a gradient was calculated subtracting the pretreatment mean from the post-endovascular procedure mean. They found that the limb salvage and wound healing rates were independent of this change in increase inflow. Furthermore, the median time for healing was 26.5 weeks (range: 4–130 weeks) [70]. This study underscores the complexity of wound healing in patients with CLI and perhaps the complexity of post intervention surveillance.

Post-Peripheral Vascular Intervention Antiplatelet/Anticoagulant Therapy

In 2012, the Cochrane Collaboration published a systematic review of data regarding the use of different anticoagulants/antiplatelets on restenosis or reocclusion following the endovascular treatment of peripheral arterial disease [71]. Although there is significant heterogeneity in the studies, anatomic distribution of the intervention (all aortoiliac or lower), Rutherford stage (II–VI), and methods of treatment (angioplasty, stent, etc.), the results do provide some insights into how to approach the long-term medical regimen post-peripheral vascular intervention for these patients. Below is a summary:

- Aspirin versus aspirin + dipyridamole:
  - Primary patency at 14 days: equivalent
- High-dose aspirin (900 or 1000 mg) versus low-dose (50–300 mg) aspirin:
  - <1-month occlusion: equivalent
  - Six-month patency: equivalent
  - One-year patency: two of four trials showed a slight advantage for high-dose aspirin (OR 0.78 and OR 0.90)
  - Two-year patency (one trial): equivalent
  - Gastrointestinal side effects were generally more frequent in the high-dose aspirin group
- Aspirin + dipyridamole versus vitamin K antagonist
  - No difference at 1-, 3-, 6-, and 12-month follow-up
- Clopidogrel + aspirin versus low molecular weight heparin followed by warfarin
  - No difference in restenosis at 24 h, 1 month, 6 months, 1 year, 18 months
  - Fewer bleeding events with clopidogrel + aspirin
- Cilostazol + aspirin versus ticlopidine + aspirin
  - Statistically significant reduction in restenosis with cilostazol + aspirin at 1, 2, and 3 years

- Abciximab versus control
  - Significant heterogeneity in studies
  - Pooled data demonstrated no benefit at 24 h nor 3 months
  - Pooled data suggested a reduction in primary occlusion at 6 months
  - Bleeding tended to be higher in the abciximab group
- Low molecular weight heparin versus unfractionated heparin
  - Significant reduction in restenosis at 3 weeks, 3 months, and 6 months
  - No significant differences in bleeding rates

Adjunct Therapies to Aid in Healing

Critical limb ischemia is complex in its etiology, and reestablishment of in-line, pulsatile flow to the extremity is not always sufficient to allow healing of the wound. As such, it may be necessary to employ adjunctive therapies to facilitate wound healing. Infections must be treated, edema resolved, nutritional status optimized, and wound off-loaded. Hyperbaric oxygen has a role for some patients. Intermittent pneumatic compression devices ("ArtAssist") as an adjunct to wound care have demonstrated increased wound healing and limb salvage rates, and sitting TcPO2 was high in the intermittent compression therapy group. The device delivers intermittent pressures of 85–95 mmHg, every 2 s with a rapid rise time (0.2 s), with three cycles per minute and three sessions of 2 h each per day [72].

Multidisciplinary Team

Patients with critical limb ischemia have significant comorbidities and an astounding mortality rate. Although it may be easy to view these patients as simply not getting enough blood supply to their extremity, this approach does the patient a disservice. Beyond revascularization, be it with an endovascular, surgical, or hybrid approach, these patients require aggressive risk factor modification and a multidisciplinary approach to their care. Collaboration with podiatry, surgical, and medical disciplines often leads to a more comprehensive patient and limb care [73].

References

1. Dotter CT, Judkins MP. Transluminal treatment of arteriosclerotic obstruction: description of a new technic and a preliminary report of its applications. Circulation. 1964;30:654–70.
2. Dorros G, Jaff MR, Dorros AM, Mathiak LM, He T. Tibioperoneal (outflow lesion) angioplasty can be used as primary treatment in

235 patients with critical limb ischemia: five-year follow-up. Circulation. 2001;104:2057–62.

3. Marston WA, Davies SW, Armstrong B, Farber MA, Mendes RC, Fulton JJ, Keagy BA. Natural history of limbs with arterial insufficiency and chronic ulceration treated without revascularization. J Vasc Surg. 2006;44:108–14.

4. Vemulapalli S, Greiner MA, Jones WS, Patel MR, Hernandez AF, Curtis LH. Peripheral arterial testing before lower extremity amputation among medicare beneficiaries, 2000 to 2010. Circ Cardiovasc Qual Outcomes. 2014;7:142–50.

5. Hughes K, Seetahal S, Oyetunji T, Rose D, Greene W, Chang D, Cornwell III E, Obisesan T. Racial/ethnic disparities in amputation and revascularization: a nationwide inpatient sample study. Vasc Endovascular Surg. 2014;48:34–7.

6. Dieter RS, Chu WW, Pacanowski Jr JP, McBride PE, Tanke TE. The significance of lower extremity peripheral arterial disease. Clin Cardiol. 2002;25(1):3–10.

7. TASC II inter-society consensus on peripheral arterial disease. Eur J Vasc Endovasc Surg. 2007;33 Suppl 1:S1-75.

8. Dieter RS, Dieter RA Jr, Dieter RA III, editors. Peripheral arterial disease. New York: McGraw-Hill; 2009.

9. Dormandy J, Belcher G, Broos P, Eikelboom B, Laszlo G, Konrad P, et al. Prospective study of 713 below-knee amputations for ischaemia and the effect of a prostacyclin analogue on healing. Hawaii Study Group. Br J Surg. 1994;81(1):33–7.

10. Izumi Y, Satterfield K, Lee S, Harkless LB. Risk of reamputation in diabetic patients stratified by limb and level of amputation. Diabetes Care. 2006;29:566–70.

11. Beard JD. Which is the best revascularization for critical limb ischemia: endovascular or open surgery? J Vasc Surg. 2008; 48:11S–6S.

12. Tartari S, Zattoni L, Rizzati R, Aliberti C, Capello K, Sacco A, Mollo F, Benea G. Subintimal angioplasty as the first-choice revascularization technique for infrainguinal arterial occlusions in patients with critical limb ischemia. Ann Vasc Surg. 2007;21:819–28.

13. Gray BH, Grant AA, Kalbaugh CA, Blackhurst DW, Langan 3rd EM, Taylor SA, Cull DA. The impact of isolated tibial disease on outcomes in the critical limb ischemic population. Ann Vasc Surg. 2010;24:349–59.

14. May KK, Robless PA, Sidhu HRS, Chua BSY, Ho P. Limb salvage in patients with peripheral arterial disease managed by endovascular first approach. Vasc Endovascular Surg. 2014;48:129–33.

15. Lumsden AB, Davies MG, Peden EK. Medical and endovascular management of critical limb ischemia. J Endvasc Ther. 2009;16 Suppl II:II31–62.

16. Graziani L, Silvestro A, Bertone V, Manara E, Andreini R, Sigala A, Mingardi R, DeGiglio R. Vascular involvement in diabetic subjects with ischemic foot ulcer: a new morphologic categorization of disease severity. Eur J Vasc Endovasc Surg. 2007;33:453–60.

17. Falluji N, Mukherjee D. Critical and acute limb ischemia: an overview. Angiology. 2014;65:137–46.

18. Faglia E, Paola LD, Clerici G, Clerissi J, Graziani L, Fusaro M, Gabrielli L, Losa S, Stella A, Gargiulo M, Mantero M, Caminiti M, Ninkovic S, Curci V, Morabito A. Peripheral angioplasty as the first-choice revascularization procedure in diabetic patients with critical limb ischemia: prospective study of 993 consecutive patients hospitalized and followed between 1999 and 2003. Eur J Vasc Endovasc Surg. 2005;29:620–7.

19. Acin F, Varela C, de Maturana IL, de Haro J, Bleda S, Rodriguez-Padilla J. Results of infrapopliteal endovascular procedures performed in diabetic patients with critical limb ischemia and tissue loss from the perspective of an angiosome oriented revascularization strategy. Int J Vasc Med. 2014;2014:270539. doi: 10.1155/2014/270539. Epub 2014 Jan 6.

20. Kawarada O, Yasuda S, Nishimura K, Sakamoto S, Noguchi M, Takahi Y, et al. Effect of single tibial artery revascularization on microcirculation in the setting of critical limb ischemia. Circ Cardiovasc Interv. 2014 Oct;7(5):684-91. doi: 10.1161/CIRCINTERVENTIONS.113.001311. Epub 2014 Aug 19.

21. Gray BH, Diaz-Sandoval LJ, Dieter RS, Jaff MR, White CJ. SCAI expert consensus statement for infrapopliteal arterial intervention appropriate use. Catheter Cardiovasc Interv. 2014;84(4): 539–45.

22. Klein AJ, Feldman DN, Aronow HD, Gray BH, Gupta K, Gigliotti OS, Jaff MR, Bersin RM, White CJ. Appropriate use criteria: a Society for Cardiovascular Angiography and Interventions (SCAI) consensus statement for aorto-iliac intervention. Catheter Cardiovasc Interv. 2014.

23. Dieter RS, Dieter RA, Dieter RA, editors. Endovascular interventions: a case based approach. New York: Springer; 2014.

24. Iida T, Iida O, Okamoto S, Dohi T, Nanto K, Uematsu M. Endovascular therapy with novel high anterior tibial artery puncture for limb salvage in a case of critical limb ischemia. Cardiovasc Interv Ther. 2014;29(4):363–7.

25. Montero-Baker M, Schmidt A, Bräunlich S, Ulrich M, Thieme M, Biamino G, Botsios S, Bausback Y, Scheinert D. Retrograde approach for complex popliteal and tibioperoneal occlusions. J Endovasc Ther. 2008;15:594–604.

26. Bolia A, Brennan J, Bell PR. Recanalisation of femoro-popliteal occlusions. Improving success rates by subintimal recanalization. Clin Radiol. 1989;40:325.

27. Hynes N, Mahendran B, Manning B, Andrews E, Courtney D, Sultan D. The influence of subintimal angioplasty on level of amputation and limb salvage rates in lower limb critical ischemia: a 15-year experience. Eur J Vasc Endovasc Surg. 2005;30:291–9.

28. Zhu YQ, Zhao JG, Liu F, Wang JB, Cheng YS, Li MH, Wang J, Li J. Subintimal angioplasty for below-the-knee arterial occlusions in diabetic patients with chronic critical limb ischemia. J Endovasc Ther. 2009;16:604–12.

29. Surmely JF, Tsuchikane E, Katoh O, Nishida Y, Nakayama M, Nakamura S, Oida A, Hattori E, Suzuki T. New concept for CTO recanalization using controlled antegrade and retrograde subintimal tracking: the CART technique. J Invasive Cardiol. 2006; 18:334–8.

30. Kawarada O, Sakamoto S, Harada K, Ishihara M, Yasuda S, Ogawa H. Contemporary crossing techniques for infrapopliteal chronic total occlusions. J Endovasc Ther. 2014;21:266–80.

31. Mitsudo K, Yamashita T, Asakura Y, Muramatsu T, Doi O, Shibata Y, Morino Y. Recanalization strategy for chronic total occlusions with tapered and stiff-tip guidewire. The results of CTO new techniQUE for STandard procedure (CONQUEST) trial. J Invasive Cardiol. 2008;20:571–7.

32. Brennan RP. Subintimal angioplasty in critical limb ischemia: a literature review. R Coll Surg Ireland Stud Med J. 2011;4:39–45.

33. Met R, van Lienden KP, Koelemay MJW, Bipat S, Legemate DA, Reekers JA. Subintimal angioplasty for peripheral arterial occlusive disease: a systematic review. Cardiovsac Intervent Radiol. 2008;31:687–97.

34. Vraux H, Bertoncello N. Subintimal angioplasty of tibial vessel occlusions in critical limb ischemia: a good opportunity? Eur J Vasc Endovasc Surg. 2006;32:663–7.

35. Mendes BC, Oderich GS, Fleming MD, Misra S, Duncan AA, Kalra M, Cha S, Gloviczki P. Clinical significance of embolic events in patients undergoing endovascular femoropopliteal interventions with or without embolic protection devices. J Vasc Surg. 2014;59:359–67.

36. Horn-Dzijan M, Langwieser N, Groha P, Bradaric C, Linhardt M, Bottiger C, Byrne RA, Kopara T, Godel J, Hadamitzky M, Ott I, von Beckerath N, Kastrati A, Laugwitz KL, Ibrahim T. Safety and efficacy of a potential treatment algorithm by using manual compression repair and ultrasound-guided thrombin injection for the management of iatrogenic femoral artery pseudoaneurysm in a large patient cohort. Circ Cardiovasc Interv. 2014;7:207–15.

37. Dosluoglu HH, Lall P, Harris LM, Dryjski ML. Long-term limb salvage and survival after endovascular and open revascularization for critical limb ischemia after adoption of endovascular-first approach by vascular surgeons. J Vasc Surg. 2012;56:361–71.

38. Soga Y, Mii S, Lida O, Okazaki J, Kuma S, Hirano K, Suzuki K, Kawasaki D, Yamaoka T, Kamoi D, Shintani Y. Propensity score analysis of clinical outcome after bypass surgery vs. endovascular therapy for infrainguinal artery disease in patients with critical limb ischemia. J Endovasc Ther. 2014;21:243–53.

39. Jones WS, Dolor RJ, Hasselblad V, Vemulapalli S, Subherwal S, Schmit K, Heidenfelder B, Patel MR. Comparative effectiveness of endovascular and surgical revascularization for patients with peripheral artery disease and critical limb ischemia: systematic review of revascularization in critical limb ischemia. Am Heart J. 2014;167:489–98.

40. Garg K, Kaszubski PA, Moridzadeh R, Rockman CB, Adelman MA, Maldonado TS, Veith FJ, Mussa FF. Endovascular-first approach is not associated with worse amputation-free survival in appropriately selected patients with critical limb ischemia. J Vasc Surg. 2014;59:392–9.

41. BASIL Trial Participants. Bypass versus angioplasty in severe ischaemia of the leg (BASIL): multicenter, randomized controlled trial. Lancet. 2005;366:1925–34.

42. Santo VJ, Dargo P, Azarbal AF, Liem TK, Mitchell EL, Landra GJ, Moneta GL. Lower extremity autologous vein bypass for critical limb ischemia is not adversely affected by prior endovascular procedure. J Vasc Surg. 2014;60:129–35.

43. Uhl C, Hock C, Betz T, Topel I, Steinbauer M. Pedal bypass surgery after crural endovascular intervention. J Vasc Surg. 2014;59:1583–7.

44. Dieter Jr RA, Kuzucz G, Dieter III RA, Dieter RS. The ORC patient/tumor classification- a new approach: a new challenge with special consideration for the lung. J Cancer Ther. 2011;2:172–5.

45. Varela C, Acin F, de Maturana IL, de Haro J, Bleda S, Paz B, Esparza L. Safety and efficacy outcomes of infrapopliteal endovascular procedures performed in patients with critical limb ischemia according to the Society for Vascular Surgery Objective Performance Goals. Ann Vasc Surg. 2014;28:284–94.

46. Wolfe JHN, Wyatt MG. Critical and subcritical ischemia. Eur J Vasc Endovsac Surg. 1997;13:578–82.

47. Silverberg D, Yalon T, Rimon U, Reinitz ER, Yakubovitch D, Schniderman J, Halak M. Endovascular treatment of lower extremity ischemia in chronic renal failure patients on dialysis: early and intermediate term results. IMAJ. 2013;15(12):734–8.

48. Fernandez N, McEnaney R, Marone LK, Rhee RY, Leers S, Makaroun M, Chaer RA. Multilevel versus isolated endovascular tibial interventions for critical limb ischema. J Vasc Surg. 2011;54:722–9.

49. Rocha-Singh KJ, Jaff M, Joye J, Laird J, Ansel G, Schneider P; on behalf of the VIVA Physicians. Major adverse limb events and wound healing following infrapopliteal artery stent implantation in patients with critical limb ischemia: the XCELL trial. Catheter Cardiovasc Interv. 2012;80:1042–51.

50. Saqib UN, Domenick N, Cho JS, Marone L, Leers S, Makaroun MS, Chaer RA. Predictors and outcomes of restenosis following tibial artery endovascular interventions for critical limb ischemia. J Vasc Surg. 2013;57:692–9.

51. Harries RL, Ahmed M, Whitaker C, Majeed MU, Williams DT. The influence of connective tissue disease in the management of lower extremity ischemia. Ann Vasc Surg. 2014;28:1139–42.

52. Dohi T, Iida O, Soga Y, Hirano K, Suzuki K, Takahara M, Uematsu M, Nanto S. Incidence, predictors, and prognosis of in-stent occlusion after endovascular treatment with nitinol stents for femoropopliteal lesions. J Vasc Surg. 2014;59:1009–15.

53. Chang S-H, Tsai Y-J, Chou H-H, Wu T-Y, Hsieh C-A, Cheng S-T, Huang H-L. Clinical predictors of long-term outcomes in patients with critical limb ischemia who have undergone endovascular therapy. Angiology. 2014;65:315–22.

54. Ryer EJ, Trocciola SM, DeRubertis B, Lam R, Hynecek RL, Karwowski J, Mureebe L, McKInsey JF, Morrissey NJ, Kent KC, Faries PL. Analysis of outcomes following failed endovascular treatment of chronic limb ischemia. Ann Vasc Surg. 2006;20:440–6.

55. Baumann F, Diehm N. Restenosis after infrapopliteal angioplasty-clinical importance, study update and further directions. Vasa. 2013;42:413–20.

56. Romiti M, Albers M, Brochado-Neto FC, Durazzo AE, Pereira CA, De Luccia N. Meta-analysis of infrapopliteal angioplasty for chronic critical limb ischemia. J Vasc Surg. 2008;47:975–81.

57. Bosiers M, Peeters P, D'Archambeau O, Hendriks J, Pilger E, Düber C, Zeller T, Gussmann A, Lohle PN, Minar E, Scheinert D, Hausegger K, Schulte KL, Verbist J, Deloose K, Lammer J. AMS INSIGHT investigators. Absorbable metal stent implantation for treatment of below-the-knee critical limb ischemia: 6-month analysis. Cardiovasc Intervent Radiol. 2009;32:424–35.

58. Iida O, Soga Y, Kawasaki D, Hirano K, Yamaoka T, Suzuki K, Miyashita Y, Yokoi H, Takahara M, Uematsu M. Angiographic restenosis and its clinical impact after infrapopliteal angioplasty. Eur J Vasc Endovasc Surg. 2012;44:425–31.

59. Lo RC, Darling J, Bensley RP, Giles KA, Dahlberg SE, Hamdan AD, Wyers M, Schermerhorn ML. Outcomes following infrapopliteal angioplasty for critical limb ischemia. J Vasc Surg. 2013;57:1455–63.

60. Lee JJ, Katz SG. The number of patent tibial vessels does not influence primary patency after nitinol stenting of the femoral and popliteal arteries. J Vasc Surg. 2012;55:994–1000.

61. Hiramori S, Soga Y, Tomoi Y, Tosaka A. Impact of runoff grade after endovascular therapy for femoropopliteal lesions. J Vasc Surg. 2014;59:720–7.

62. Georgakarakos E, Papanas N, Papadaki E, Georgiadis GS, Maltezos E, Lazarides MK. Endovascular treatment of critical ischemia in the diabetic foot: new thresholds, new anatomies. Angiology. 2012;64:583–91.

63. Lazaris AM, Salas C, Tsiamis AC, Vlachou PA, Bolia A, Fishwick G, Bell PR. Factors affecting patency of subintimal infrainguinal angioplasty in patients with critical limb ischemia. Eur J Vasc Endovasc Surg. 2006;32:668–74.

64. Daryapeyma A, Ostlund O, Wahlgren CM. Healthcare associated infections after lower extremity revasculzarization. Eur J Vasc Endovasc Surg. 2014;48:72–7.

65. Gandini R, Angelopoulos G, Da Ros V, Simonetti G. Percutaneous transluminal angioplasty for treatment of critical hand ischemia with a novel endovascular approach: "the radial to ulnar artery loop technique.". J Vasc Surg. 2010;51:760–2.

66. Kawarada O, Yokoi Y, Higashimori A. Angioplasty of ulnar or radial arteries to treat critical hand ischemia: use of 3- and 4-French systems. Catheter Cardiovasc Interv. 2010;76:345–50.

67. Fergus T, Pacanowski Jr JP, Dieter RS, et al. Subclavian-coronary steal: diagnosis and treatment. Angiology. 2007;58:372–5.

68. Nasser F, Cavalcante RN, Galastri FL, de Amorim EJ, Telles MAP, Travassos FB, De Fina B, Affonso BB. Endovascular stenting of brachial artery occlusion in critical hand ischemia. Ann Vasc Surg. 2014;28:1564e1-3.

69. Saarinen E, Laukontaus SJ, Alback A, Venermo M. Duplex surveillance after endovascular revascularization for critical limb ischemia. Eur J Vasc Endovasc Surg. 2014;47:418–21.

70. Wakassa TB, Benabou JE, Puech-Leao P. Clinical efficacy of successful angioplasty in critical ischemia—a cohort study. Ann Vasc Surg. 2014;28:143–1148.

71. Robertson L, Ghouri MA, Kovacs F. Antiplatelet and anticoagulant drugs for prevention of restenosis/reocclusion following peripheral endovascular treatment (review). Cochrane Database Syst Rev.

2012; issue 8. Art no.:CD002071. doi:10.1002/14651858. CD002071.pub3

72. Kavros SJ, Delis KT, Turner NS, Voll AE, Liedl DA, Gloviczki P, Rooke TW. Improving limb salvage in critical ischemia with intermittent pneumatic compression: a controlled study with 18 month follow up. J Vasc Surg. 2008;47:543–9.

73. Van Gils CC, Wheeler LA, Mellstrom M, Brinton EA, Mason S, Wheeler CG. Amputation prevention by vascular surgery and podiatry collaboration in high-risk diabetic and nondiabetic patients. Diabetes Care. 1999;22:678–83.

Endovascular Technologies for Chronic Critical Limb Ischemia

Ambrose F. Panico, Asif Jafferani, Paul A. Johnson, John J. Lopez, John R. Laird, and Robert S. Dieter

Peripheral artery disease (PAD) rates have risen globally over the past decade. PAD currently affects one in ten people over 70 years of age [1]. The prevalence of PAD in patients with risk factors such as diabetes, hypertension, and obesity may be as high as 26 % [2]. With the increasing rate of associated risk factors and the overall aging population, the incidence of PAD will likely continue to climb. When suitable, percutaneous intervention is frequently used as a treatment of lower extremity occlusive artery disease and, in many cases, has shown more satisfactory results than more invasive techniques [3–5]. One of the main challenges of using endovascular interventions continues to be preventing restenosis of the altered segment of vessel.

Mechanism of Balloon Angioplasty and Stenting

Use of percutaneous transluminal angioplasty (PTA) also referred to as balloon angioplasty in the treatment of occlusive arterial disease relies on several mechanisms of increasing the arterial lumen diameter. First, pressure from the balloon causes a controlled dissection of the intima and media, while

A.F. Panico, DO • A. Jafferani, MBBS
Cardiology, University of Wisconsin, Madison, WI, USA

P.A. Johnson, BS
Loyola University Chicago, Stritch School of Medicine, Loyola University, Maywood, IL, USA

J.J. Lopez, MD
Medicine, Cardiology, Loyola University Medical Center, Maywood, IL, USA

J.R. Laird, MD
Internal Medicine, Cardiovascular Medicine UC Davis Vascular Center, Sacramento, CA, USA

R.S. Dieter, MD, RVT (✉)
Medicine, Cardiology, Vascular and Endovascular Medicine, Loyola University Medical Center, Maywood, IL, USA

simultaneously compressing the atherosclerotic plaque. Contents of the plaque are pushed longitudinally and axially in the vessel wall as the balloon expands [6]. The acute benefit is limited by arterial response to this insult resulting in elastic recoil causing up to a 40 % reduction in the lumen diameter [6, 7]. Deploying a stent during this process assists in increasing lumen area by providing scaffolding for the artery wall that almost completely prevents the elastic recoil [6]. Additionally, dissection creates intimal flaps that increase the risk of acute or subacute vessel closure. Stenting helps reduce the risk of immediate closure by keeping the flaps pressed between the scaffolding and arterial wall [8].

Pathophysiology of Restenosis

Studies have shown that restenosis is dictated by elastic recoil, negative/constrictive remodeling, and neointimal hyperplasia [6, 9]. In stented segments, the structural support of struts effectively eliminates the effects of recoil and negative remodeling, making neointimal hyperplasia the limiting factor of long-term maintenance of arterial patency [10–12]. This process is incited by the increased inflammation from the chronic presence of the stent. Smooth muscle cells from the media are stimulated to migrate and proliferate, causing luminal narrowing.

Several mechanisms behind restenosis have been studied in animal models. There are three major aspects of the process: denudation of the endothelium, disruption of the intima, and penetration of the smooth muscles in the vascular media [7, 9, 12]. Each injury to the vessel contributes to late restenosis through the attempted repair mechanism. Denudation of the epithelial surface results in the release of pro-inflammatory and procoagulant factors, adhesion molecules, and growth stimulators. Rupturing the plaque and disruption of the endothelium expose subepithelial collagen to the lumen contents. Circulating and locally released vonWillebrand factor binds the collagen surface, allowing platelet adherence and activation. Injury results in the activation of platelets, plaque rupture, release of growth factors, inflam-

© Springer International Publishing Switzerland 2017
R.S. Dieter et al. (eds.), *Critical Limb Ischemia*, DOI 10.1007/978-3-319-31991-9_35

matory cytokines, reactive oxygen species combined, and macrophage chemotactic factors [7, 9, 13]. This environment along with fibrin deposition and thrombosis aids in cellular migration by providing a matrix [7]. Platelet degranulation releases mitogens that promote further cell activation and proliferation [12, 14, 15]. Smooth muscle cells and fibroblasts then migrate to the site of injury. Eventually, this process of repair results in smooth muscle migration from the media to the intima above the stent, followed by cellular proliferation. The end result is a neointimal scar consisting mainly of collagen, proteoglycans, and vascular smooth muscle cells [7, 9, 12, 13].

Animal models with verification through human studies have experimentally determined the time and order of the vascular proliferative response after stent implantation. Deployment of the stent initiates the process as described above. Acutely, there is an invasion of inflammatory cells around the struts with associated platelet adherence and deposition of fibrin. In the following few weeks, the struts are covered in immature neointima, consisting of macrophages and alpha-actin-negative spindle cells. Smooth muscle cells then differentiate and begin proliferating, while additional extracellular matrix is deposited by fibroblasts. Several weeks to months later, there is a re-endothelialization process that concludes the proliferative response.

Endovascular Interventions for Critical Limb Ischemia in the Lower Extremity

The management of lower extremity PAD can be quite complex and presents a number of very unique clinical and therapeutic challenges especially in the setting of critical limb ischemia (CLI). The underlying complex nature of PAD has limited the success of a number of endovascular therapeutic modalities in the treatment of CLI; these clinical challenges have been the driving force behind the development and advancement in endovascular therapies. This review will aim to highlight the historical challenges of endovascular intervention in the treatment of CLI as well as focus on the advancements which have been developed. While the primary focus of this chapter is treatment/management of CLI, included are several studies which evaluated CLI, symptomatic ischemia, and intermittent claudication as inclusion criteria. While some of the presented trials included both above- and below-the-knee lesions in the reported data (and are therefore presented as such), every effort was made to separate and present the available data by anatomic location, as the treatment and results for each of the reviewed therapeutic modalities may differ between above- and below-the-knee lesions. A summary of the important individual studies appears in Table 35.1.

Table 35.1 Summary of important studies evaluating endovascular technologies in lower extremity peripheral artery disease (including critical limb ischemia)

Trial name	Study population	Outcomes measured (major)	Results
Percutaneous transluminal angioplasty			
Dorros et al. [NR] [18]	235 patients (284 ischemic limbs)	Technical success [E]	95 %
		5-year limb salvage [E]	91 %
Söder et al. [NR] [19]	121 de novo lesions and 67 chronic total occlusions	Primary angiographic success [E]	84 % vs 61 %*
Trocciola et al. [NR] [21]	58 patients with claudication and 63 patients with CLI	Primary patency at 3, 6, and 9 months [E]	100, 98, and 85 % vs 89, 80, and 72 %
		Limb salvage at 12 months (CLI only) [E]	91 %
PTA vs bypass			
BASIL [R] [5]	224 in PTA arm and 228 in bypass arm	6-month amputation-free survival [E]	48 vs 60 (HR 1.07, CI 0.72; 1.6)
Bare-metal stents			
Vogel et al. [NR] [24]	41 patients (68 % for limb salvage)	Primary patency at 6, 12, and 24 months [E]	95, 84, and 84 %
		Limb salvage at 6, 12, and 24 months [E]	92, 89, and 89 %
RESILIENT [R] [25]	134 patients in the BMS arm and 72 patients in PTA arm	Primary patency at 12 months [E]	81.3 % vs 36.7 %*
		Freedom from TLR at 12 months [E]	87.3 % vs 45.1 %*
STROLL [NR] [26]	250 patients	Primary patency at 1 year [E]	81.70 %
		Freedom from 30 days' MAEs [S]	100 %
SUPERB [NR] [32]	264 patients (265 lesions)	Primary patency at 1 year [E]	78.90 %
Stent grafts			
Saxon et al. [R] [41]	97 in stent-graft arm and 100 patients in PTA arm	Technical success [E]	95 % vs 66 %*

(continued)

Table 35.1 (continued)

Trial name	Study population	Outcomes measured (major)	Results
		Primary patency at 1 year [E]	65 % vs 40 %*
Kedora et al. [R] [42–44]	40 patients (50 limbs) in stent-graft arm and	Primary patency at 1 year [E]	73.5 % vs 74.2 %
	40 patients (50 limbs) in bypass arm	Primary patency at 4 years [E]	59 % vs 58 %
VIBRANT [R] [45]	72 patients in stent-graft arm	Primary patency at 3 years [E]	24.2 % vs 25.9 %
	And 76 patients in BMS arm	Freedom from 30 days of MAEs [S]	98.6 % vs 100 %
VIPER [NR] [46]	113patients (119 limbs)	Primary patency at 1 year [E]	73 %
		30 days of procedure-related MAEs [S]	0.80 %
VIASTAR [R] [47]	72 patients in stent-graft arm	Primary patency at 1 year [E]	70.9 % vs 55.1 %
	And 69 patients in BMS arm	30 days of procedure-related MAEs [S]	15 % vs 13 %
Drug-eluting stents			
Femoropopliteal disease			
SIROCCO I [R] [55]	18 patients in DES arm and 18 patients in BMS arm	6-month in-stent mean percent diameter stenosis by	22.6 % vs 30.9 %
		quantitative angiography [E]	
SIROCCO II [R] [56, 57]	29 patients in DES arm and 28 patients in BMS arm	6-month in-stent mean luminal diameter [E]	4.94 mm ± 0.69 vs 4.76 mm ± 0.54
STRIDES [NR] [59]	104 patients	In-stent binary restenosis at 6 months [E]	14 % (CI 7.8;22.2)
Zilver PTX [R] [60, 61]	236 patients in DES arm vs 238 in primary PTA arm	Primary patency at 1 year in primary randomization [E]	83.1 % vs 32.8 %*
	120 patients with acute PTA failure randomized to	Event-free survival at 1 year in primary randomization [S]	90.4 % vs 82.6 %*
	provisional DES (61) or BMS arms (59)		
Infrapopliteal disease			
Falkowski et al. [R] [69]	25 patients in DES arm and 25 patients in BMS arm	Restenosis rate at 6 month [E]	16 % vs 76 %*
ACHILLES [R] [70]	99 patients in DES arm and 101 patients in PTA arm	In-stent binary restenosis at 12 months [E]	22.4 % vs 41.9 %*
YUKON-BTK [R] [71]	82 patients in DES arm and 79 patients in BMS arm	Primary patency at 1 year [E]	80.6 % vs 55.6 %*
DESTINY [R] [73]	74 patients in DES arm and 66 patients in BMS arm	Primary patency at 1 year [E]	85 % vs 54 %*
Cryoplasty			
Femoropopliteal disease			
Cold [R] [78]	46 patients in PTA arm and 40 patients in cryoplasty arm	Technical success [E]	54 % vs 35 %*
Infrapopliteal disease			
BTK Chill [NR] [80]	108 patients	Technical success [E]	97.30 %
		Absence of amputation at 6 and 12 months [E]	93.4 % and 85.2 %
		Cryoplasty-related complications [S]	One dissection, two residual stenoses, three required additional stenting
CLIMB [NR] [81]	100 patients	Primary patency at 12 months [E]	55.9 ± 7.4 %
Cutting balloon angioplasty			
Canuad et al. [NR] [84]	16 patients in the claudication arm	Primary patency at 12 and 24 months [E]	82.1 % and 82.1 %
	116 patients in the CLI arm	Primary patency at 12 and 24 months [E]	64.4 % and 51.9 %
Amighi et al. [R] [86]	21 patients in the CBA arm and 22 patients in the PTA arm	Restenosis rates at 6 months [E]	62 % vs 32 %*
Drug-eluting balloons			
Femoropopliteal disease			
THUNDER [R] [94, 95]	48 patients in DEB arm, 54 patients in PTA arm,	Late lumen loss at 6 months [E]	0.4 mm ± 1.2*, 1.7 mm ± 1.8, 2.2 mm ± 1.6
	52 patients in paclitaxel in contrast medium arm		

(continued)

Table 35.1 (continued)

Trial name	Study population	Outcomes measured (major)	Results
FEMPAC [R] [96]	45 patients in DEB Arm vs 42 patients in PTA arm	Late lumen loss at 6 months [E]	0.5 mm ± 1.1 vs 1.0 mm ± 1.1*
LEVANT I [R] [97]	49 patients in DEB arm vs 52 patients in PTA arm	Late lumen loss at 6 months [E]	0.46 mm ± 1.13 vs 1.09 mm ± 1.07*
LEVANT II [R] [98]	316 patients in DEB arm vs 160 patients in PTA arm	Primary patency at 1 year [E]	65.2 % vs 52.6 %*
		Freedom from MAEs [S]	83.9 % vs 79 %
PACIFIER [R] [99]	44 cases in DEB vs 47 cases in PTA arm	Late lumen loss at 6 months [E]	−0.01 mm [CI −0.29; 0.26] vs 0.65 mm [CI 0.37; 0.93]
DEBELLUM [R] [100, 101]	44 lesions in DEB vs 48 in PTA arm	Late lumen loss at 6 months [E]	
IN.PACT SFA [R] [102]	220 patients in DEB vs 111 in PTA arm	Primary patency at 1 year [E]	82.2 % vs 52.4 %*
Infrapopliteal disease			
DEBATE-BTK [R] [110]	65 patients in DEB arm vs 67 patients in PTA arm	Binary restenosis at 12 months [E]	27 % vs 74 %*
DEBELLUM [R] [100, 101]	13 lesions in DEB vs 17 in PTA arm	Late lumen loss at 6 months [E]	
IN.PACT DEEP [R] [111]	239 patients in DEB arm vs 119 patients in PTA arm	Clinically driven TLR (CD-TLR) at 12 months [E]	9.2 % vs 13.1 %
		Late lumen loss at 12 months [E]	0.61 mm ± 0.78 vs 0.62 mm ± 0.78
		Composite of death, amputation, and CD-TLR at 6 months [S]	17.7 % vs 15.8 %

BMS bare-metal stent, *CBA* cutting balloon angioplasty, *CI* 95 % confidence interval, *CLI* critical limb ischemia, *DEB* drug-eluting balloon, *DES* drug-eluting stent, *E* primary efficacy endpoint, *HR* hazards ratio, *NR* nonrandomized study, *PTA* percutaneous tissue angioplasty, *R* randomized controlled trial, *S* primary safety endpoint, *TLR* target lesion revascularization

*Significant difference ($p < 0.05$)

Percutaneous Transluminal Angioplasty

Some of the earliest angioplasty data were reported in the Trans-Atlantic Inter-Society Consensus document for the management of peripheral arterial disease (TASC I) which summarized the results of 19 different registries dating back to the early 1990s [16]. Primary technical success rates ranged between 80 and 100 % and limb salvage rates between 88 % and 54 % at 17 and 24 months, respectively, with low rates of complication between 2 and 6 %. Dormandy et al. published these results showing that the endovascular treatment of lower limb ischemia with unassisted balloon angioplasty has primary patency rates of 61 %, 51 %, and 48 % at 1, 3, and 5 years, respectively [16].

Subsequently, based on their results in a study of 53 patients with infrapopliteal disease, Bakal et al. proposed that the restoration of linear flow to the distal leg was the most important predictor of success [17]. They found the rate of limb salvage was 80 % when straight-line flow was restored and approached 0 % when distal flow remained obstructed. Dorros et al. published their results of a prospective, nonrandomized consecutive series of 235 CLI patients (284 ischemic limbs, 529 tibioperoneal lesions) treated between 1983 and 1996 [18]. Primary success was reported

in 95 % (270) of ischemic limbs. At 5-year follow-up, the rate of limb salvage was 91 % (5 above-the-knee (ATK) and 18 below-the-knee (BTK) amputations) with a cumulative survival of 56 %. Söder and associates subsequently published results of a prospective trial of 60 patients (72 limbs) in which primary angiographic success was 84 % in treatment of stenosis and 61 % in chronic total occlusions, with 10-month restenosis rates of 32 and 52 %, respectively [19]. Limb salvage at 18 months based on Kaplan–Meier analysis was found to be 80 %. These results in conjunction with the fact that PTA carries lower morbidity and mortality, shorter hospitalization, and does not preclude surgery are a very attractive option for the management of CLI [20].

While PTA alone as an intervention has showed promising results, it is imperative to understand how PTA compares to PTA with adjunctive therapies. In a retrospective review published by Trocciola et al., the clinical success, patency, and limb salvage rates after endovascular repair were evaluated in patients with PAD who presented with either claudication ($n = 58$) or critical ischemia ($n = 63$) [21]. In all, 199 lesions were treated with PTA + subintimal angioplasty (tibial lesions) or adjunctive stenting (self-expanding nitinol stents if femoropopliteal lesions and balloon-expandable stainless steel for tibial lesions). At 3, 6, and 9 months in the claudicant group, primary patency rates recorded were 100 %,

98 %, and 85 %, respectively, while in the critical ischemia group, the 3-, 6-, and 9-month primary patency rates were reported as 89 %, 80 %, and 72 % with limb salvage rate of 91 % at 12 months. Results cemented the role of PTA ± adjunctive therapies as an acceptable mode for intervention with acceptable patency at 12 months for both claudication and CLI.

PTA vs Surgical Bypass

As CLI patients often present with multiple medical comorbidities and are often considered high risk for high-risk vascular surgery, it is imperative to understand the comparison between PTA and bypass surgery. The Bypass versus Angioplasty in Severe Ischemia of the Leg (BASIL) trial was a randomized controlled multicenter trial comparing PTA ($n = 224$) versus surgery ($n = 228$) as first-line therapy in 452 patients with severe limb ischemia secondary to infrainguinal disease [5]. Both groups were followed for a primary endpoint of amputation-free survival. At 6 months, there was no significant difference in amputation-free survival (48 vs 60, HR 1.07, 95 CI 0.720–1.6) and no difference in health-adjusted quality of life; there was however a significant increase in hospital cost (roughly one third higher for surgery arm over the first year). The authors, however, did report a significant reduction in amputation-free survival and all-cause mortality in the surgical bypass arm beyond 2 years of follow-up from randomization. Thus, surgery may be a better choice for patients expected to survive beyond 2 years of the procedure; otherwise, PTA is a viable option for intervention in these patients.

Bare-Metal Stents vs Angioplasty

There have been many trials comparing balloon angioplasty to balloon angioplasty with bare-metal stent (BMS) for superficial femoral artery (SFA) stenosis in patients with critical limb ischemia or claudication. Cumulative results published in a Cochrane review compared the two treatments head-to-head in regard to the duplex patency, angiographic patency, ankle-brachial index, treadmill walking distance, and quality of life [22]. The completed review included 11 trials with a total of 1387 patients (average age of 69). Patients were followed for up to 2 years. The results of the review found a significant improvement in duplex patency at 6 (six studies, 578 patients) and 12 months (9 studies, 858 patients) in the group who received PTA + stent versus PTA alone; this early benefit however was lost when followed out to 24 months. In regard to angiographic patency, four studies (329 patients) confirmed the short-term patency benefit in the PTA + stent group at 6 months; this too however was lost

by 12 months (5 studies, 384 patients). ABI and treadmill walk test were found to have no statistically significant difference between groups. Perhaps the most interesting parameter followed in 3 of the 11 studies was assessment in quality of life (660 patients); there was unfortunately no significant difference between treatment groups. While the study showed that there was a statistically significant difference in short-term patency with PTA + stenting, there was no sustained benefit to the combination intervention over PTA alone.

A meta-analysis published by Mwipatayi et al. compared the short- and long-term results of primary PTA versus primary stenting in 1362 patients from seven RCTs (934 patients underwent angioplasty and 482 underwent stenting) [23]. Both groups were assessed in regard to primary patency at 12 months and post-intervention ABI. Primary patency at 12 months ranged from 45 to 84.2 % in the angioplasty arm and 63–90 % in the stenting arm; there was no statistically significant difference between groups (OR 0.989, 95 % CI 0.623–1.57, $p = 0.962$). Additionally, both groups exhibited similar occlusion rates at 12 months (19 and 22 %, respectively). Despite these results, there was however a nonstatistically significant trend toward improved ABI in the angioplasty group as compared to the primary stenting group (three studies with balloon-expandable stents, two studies with self-expandable stents).

Nitinol Self-Expanding Stents

The practice of stenting in peripheral arterial disease (predominantly using balloon-expandable and self-expanding stainless steel stents) was primarily in the setting of suboptimal results with PTA alone [16]. The advent of self-expanding nitinol stents, which allow for constant radial force to be exerted on the arterial wall and increased flexibility, made it possible to consider deployment as an option for primary therapy in femoropopliteal lesions. Individual trials and stents will be reviewed to highlight their utility.

Vogel et al. reported their results of a retrospective analysis of 41 patients who underwent placement of a nitinol stents either in the femoral ($n = 35$) or above-the-knee popliteal arteries ($n = 6$) [24]. They reported that 68 % of patients studied underwent intervention for the indication of limb salvage. They were followed from 1999 to 2002 for both primary patency and limb salvage. The 6-month, 1-year, and 2-year primary patency rates and limb salvage rates were 95 %, 84 %, and 84 % and 92 %, 89 %, and 89 %, respectively.

Laird et al. published their results from the prospective, Randomized Study Comparing the Edwards Self-Expanding Lifestent versus Angioplasty Alone in Lesions Involving the SFA and/or Proximal Popliteal Artery (RESILIENT) trial [25]. Two Hundred and six patients were enrolled and randomized to either intervention with a self-expanding nitinol stent ($n = 134$) or PTA ($n = 72$). Immediate technical success (<30% stenosis) was superior in the stent group compared to the angioplasty group (95.8% vs 83.9%, $p < 0.01$), with stents also having better primary patency (81.3% vs 36.7%, $p < 0.0001$) and freedom from TLR at 12 months (87.3% vs 45.1%, $p < 0.0001$), respectively. Stent fractures occurred in 3.1% of stents at 12 months with none resulting in loss of patency or TLR.

Gray et al. published the results of the S.M.A.R.T. Self-Expanding Nitinol Stent for the Treatment of Atherosclerotic Lesions in the Superficial Femoral Artery (STROLL) trial [26]. The trial was a single-arm, prospective, open-label multicenter trial (39 US centers) comprising of 250 patients to assess safety and efficacy of the S.M.A.R.T. Vascular Stent System stent (Cordis, Johnson & Johnson, Warren, NJ) in the treatment of SFA disease in patients with symptomatic limb ischemia. Primary patency rates at 1 year were reported as 81.7% by Kaplan–Meier estimate. There were no major adverse events reported in the first 30 days (death, index limb amputation, clinically driven TLR), and only four patients (2%) experienced single-stent strut fracture at 1 year without associated loss of stent patency.

Supera Stent

The Supera Peripheral Stent System (Abbott Vascular, Santa Clara, CA) is an interwoven nitinol stent constructed from six pairs of nitinol wires forming closed loops at both ends. The design of this stent aims to counteract concerns for stenting in femoral and popliteal vessels relating to rate of stent fractures and consequent restenosis. The biomechanics of this helical stent impart greater radial compression resistance and flexibility without unwanted chronic outward force or barotrauma against the artery, theoretically making it ideal for SFA and popliteal interventions. Clinical experience has been very encouraging. Registry data from Leipzig, Germany, have reported accumulated experience in SFA (137 stents) and popliteal (125 stents) lesions, with 12-month patency rates of 84.7% ± 3.6% and 87.7 ± 3.7%, respectively [27, 28]. In the second study with popliteal lesions, about 23% of the patients had CLI. In another registry from the United States with 39 stent cases, primary patency rate at 1 year remained at 79.2% [29]. Most patients (74%) in this study had CLI. Another Chinese registry also reported a patency rate of about 79% in 82 cases [30], with 42% of the study sample having CLI at baseline. Similarly, George et al. reported a primary patency of about 86% at 1 year in 98 limbs with Supera stents [31]. Thirty-one percent of the cases had CLI. None of these studies have reported any stent fractures.

In order to further evaluate this stent system, the Comparison of the SUpera PERipheral System to a Performance Goal Derived from Balloon Angioplasty Clinical Trials in the Superficial Femoral Artery (SUPERB) was designed as a single-arm study which evaluated a total of 265 lesions (264 patients) in the SFA or proximal popliteal artery with the use of the Supera stent [32]. Primary patency at 1 year was 78.9% which was statistically significant when compared with the performance goal of 66%. Primary safety endpoint at 1 year was freedom from death, target lesion revascularization (TLR), or amputation in the index limb and was reported at 99.2%, again comparing favorably with the performance goal (88%). At VIVA 2014, 3-year follow-up results were reported [33]. TLR rates were 89%, 84%, and 82% at 1, 2, and 3 years' follow-up. Post hoc analysis also revealed differences in primary patency varying with the deployed stent length. Nominally deployed stents (i.e., post-deployment stent being within ±10% of labeled length) had a higher patency than those deployed elongated (i.e., greater than their labeled length). Of note, during the 3-year follow-up, there was only one case of stent fracture.

Stent Grafts

The role of stent grafts in the treatment of peripheral vascular disease of the lower limb has been extensively evaluated, yet consensus about its role is difficult to achieve. The stent grafts (also known as covered stents, PTFE vascular prosthesis, etc.) were initially used for percutaneous interventions for aneurysms and pseudoaneurysms as well as to deal with complications relating to endovascular interventions [34], though later were also extensively evaluated for primary use in PAD especially femoropopliteal and aortoiliac disease. The main advantage of the covered stent is that the expanded polytetrafluoroethylene (ePTFE) graft material lining the stent serves to limit neointimal hyperplasia. The stent can also cover friable lesions potentially limiting distal embolization [34]. There are however a number of potential disadvantages which include problems with edge restenosis, higher rates of thromboses in the covered stents, and potential coverage of side branches or collaterals in the vascular bed, which can potentially worsen symptoms if the stent graft fails [35]. Almost all experience in the femoropopliteal vasculature comes with the Viabahn (formerly Hemobahn; W. L. Gore and Associates, Flagstaff, AZ) endoprosthesis [36–40] which is FDA approved for this indication. The Viabahn stent consists of a self-expanded nitinol stent encapsulated in ePTFE and more recently has undergone modifications to the device including heparin-bound luminal surface to reduce device thrombogenicity [34].

Saxon and colleagues reported on a randomized, premarket approval, multicenter trial of the Viabahn endoprosthesis compared to the PTA for treatment of symptomatic SFA PAD [41]. A hundred patients were assigned to the PTA and

97 to the stent-graft arm, with about 11% of total patients having CLI. Immediate technical success was substantially higher in the stent graft group as compared to the PTA (95% vs 66%) and the 1-year primary patency was also reported to be higher in the stent-graft group (65% vs 40%).

Subsequently, further research accumulated and stent grafts were also compared with bypass grafts. Kedora et al. reported a randomized controlled trial (RCT) in which stent grafts were used in 40 patients (50 limbs), with another 40 patients (50 limbs) having open surgical femoral above-knee popliteal bypass [42]. Proportion of the study sample with CLI was 26%. At median follow-up of 18 months, no significant difference was present between stent-graft and surgical bypass arms in terms of primary or secondary patency. Two-year and later 4-year follow-up on these patients still showed no difference between stent grafts and surgical bypass (59% vs 58% primary patency at 4 years) [43, 44]. This trial, thus, gave some evidence that stent grafts may be equal to surgical bypass for femoropopliteal disease.

In order to evaluate expanded indications for the use of stent grafts, particularly in TASC I C and D lesions, the GORE VIABAHN Endoprosthesis versus Bare Nitinol Stent in the Treatment of Long Lesion Superficial Femoral Artery Occlusive Disease (VIBRANT) trial was conducted to compare the Viabahn-covered stent with bare-nitinol stent in TASC I C and D lesions [45]. At 3-year follow-up, there was no difference in primary patency for the Viabahn stent as compared to the BMS (24.2%; 95% CI, 12.2–38.5% vs 25.9%; 95% CI, 10.3–45.0%). Even though higher-assisted primary and secondary patency rates were achieved in both arms, no additional benefit was demonstrated with the use of the stent graft in such cases (BMS had significantly higher-assisted primary patency, no difference in rates of secondary patency between the two arms).

Following this, the heparin-bonded Viabahn was studied in a single-arm multicenter registry, the Gore Viabahn Endoprosthesis with Heparin Bioactive Surface in the Treatment of Superficial Femoral Artery Obstructive Disease (VIPER) study [46]. One hundred and thirteen patients with 119 limbs were included in this trial, with about 61% TASC II C and D lesions and 12% with CLI. The mean lesion length was 19 cm. Primary patency rate at 12 months' follow-up was 73%, with secondary patency rate of 92%. A logistic regression analysis done to identify factors affecting loss of patency identified age and oversizing at the proximal end were independently associated with loss of patency.

The efficacy of the Viabahn stent graft in long femoropopliteal lesions was retested in the Viabahn Endoprosthesis with PROPATEN Bioactive Surface Versus Bare Nitinol Stent in the Treatment of Long Lesions in Superficial Femoral Artery Occlusive Disease (VIASTAR) trial [47]. A total of 141 patients with femoropopliteal lesions 10–35 cm in length were randomized 1:1 in the Viabahn and

BMS subgroups. About 16% of the patients presented as CLI. Primary patency rates at 1 year showed a trend toward benefit for the stent graft in the intention-to-treat (ITT) analysis (70.9%; 95% CI, 0.58–0.80 vs 55.1%; 95% CI, 0.41–0.67); this difference became significant when analyzed as treatment-per-protocol (TTP) (78.1%; 95% CI, 0.65–0.86 vs 53.5%; 95% CI. 0.39–0.65). No differences however were present in TLR rates. In lesions >20 cm, however, stent grafts were significantly superior in terms of primary patency to the BMS (71% vs 37%).

Drug-Eluting Stent

Drug-eluting stents (DES) have been the mainstay of percutaneous revascularization strategies for coronary arteries. With the incidence of restenosis seen in peripheral artery disease interventions, DES technologies have been specifically developed to respond to the specific needs of the femoropopliteal as well as below-the-knee arterial revascularization.

Review of the Basics

Ideal Drug to Inhibit Restenosis

Complex regulation and our incomplete understanding of the cell cycle justify some of the difficulties in developing appropriate drug therapy to inhibit neointimal hyperplasia and restenosis (Fig. 35.1). The presence of redundant systems of promoting neointimal growth makes it unlikely that drugs with a highly specific target and mechanism will be effective inhibitors or restenosis [6]. An ideal drug would act locally, without systemic effects, and selectively inhibit the activation of vascular smooth muscle cells while allowing normal progression of re-endothelialization [10]. The base metal of the stent and polymer aiding in drug adherence must both be inflammatorily unreactive. This was especially problematic with early stent materials and copolymers that stimulated restenosis due to their pro-inflammatory or prothrombotic properties [10, 12, 13, 48].

Overview of Candidate Drugs

Recovery from endovascular injury parallels early tumor development and the normal injury repair process [7, 13]. As such, immunosuppressant and antitumor drugs have been a major area of focus in trying searching for locally deliverable, effective agents in preventing neointimal hyperplasia [7, 13]. Paclitaxel and sirolimus are currently the drugs with the most encouraging results for usage in peripheral arteries.

Paclitaxel

In the late 1960s, paclitaxel was first isolated from the bark of the Pacific yew tree, *Taxus brevifolia*, and has since become an important chemotherapeutic agent. The mechanism of action for paclitaxel, and others in the taxane family of drugs, is to inhibit cellular division by preventing breakdown of tubulin. Taxanes accomplish this by binding with high affinity to the β subunit of assembled tubulin while poorly binding to the soluble tubulin components. Polymerized tubulin with bound paclitaxel is stabilized against degradation [49, 50]. By interfering with normal tubulin activity, multiple regulatory pathways in the cell cycle are disrupted creating a mitotic block at the transition between G2 and M (Fig. 35.1) along with disturbing signal transduction and migration of smooth muscle cells [6, 13, 50]. The lipophilic characteristics of paclitaxel make it ideally suited for absorption into damaged vascular tissue [6, 51].

Sirolimus (Rapamycin) and Rapamycin Analogs

In the 1970s, sirolimus was isolated from the fermentation products of the soil bacteria *Streptomyces hygroscopicus* on Easter Island. Sirolimus is a macrocyclic lactone with weak antibiotic and was initially being developed as an antifungal but was found to strongly suppress the immune system. Sirolimus and a structurally similar macrolide, tacrolimus (FK506), share an intracellular receptor; however, there functions differ. Both bind to FK-binding protein 12 (FKBP12), forming a tertiary complex, but the complexes then interact with different regulatory mechanisms. The tacrolimus–FKBP12 complex inhibits calcineurin halting the cell cycle at the G0/G1 transition, whereas sirolimus–FKBP12 prevents the cytokine-mediated G1/S transition (Fig. 35.1) [9].

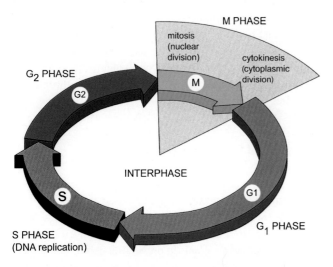

Fig. 35.1 Simplified diagrammatic representation of the cell cycle with stages affected by sirolimus and paclitaxel identified. *G* gap phase, *S* synthesis phase, *M* mitosis phase

Inside the cell, the mechanism of inhibition begins with the complexing of sirolimus to FKBP12 and their interaction with the mammalian target of rapamycin (mTOR). The kinase activity of mTOR is essential in proper regulation of the cell cycle. Some of its targets with regulatory roles are 70 kd S6 protein kinases (regulators of translation that are critical to the cell cycle), the eukaryotic initiation factor eIF4F, G1-controlling cyclin-dependent kinases, and p27 (reduces phosphorylation of Rb) [6, 9, 12, 13, 52]. The combined effect on inhibiting mTOR is to arrest the cell cycle in G1. Sirolimus has additional inhibition of cytokine signals that would activate stimulated T-cells and promote migration of smooth muscle cells. One suggested reason for how sirolimus halts the cell cycle is that it induces a cellular survival process reminiscent to nutrient deprivation resulting in autophagy where the G1/S transition is prevented by the release of intracellular amino acids [53].

Several stents using analogs and derivatives of sirolimus were developed, and two were approved for use in coronary artery disease. These second-generation drug-eluting coronary stents used everolimus (a sirolimus analog) and zotarolimus (a sirolimus derivative), both of which are more lipophilic than sirolimus, increasing their cellular uptake [54].

Femoropopliteal Disease

Initial enthusiasm for DES in femoropopliteal disease was marred with the less than ideal results for sirolimus and everolimus DES technologies. The Sirolimus-Coated Cordis Self-expandable Stent (SIROCCO) I trial was the first study, which utilized a sirolimus-eluting stent (SES) in above-the-knee lesions [55]. In this study, participants were randomized to the sirolimus-coated shape-memory alloy-recoverable technology (S.M.A.R.T.) stent (Cordis, Johnson & Johnson, Warren, NJ) or the same stent without the sirolimus coating. The study was designed as a multicenter, randomized controlled trial, in which 36 patients have obstructive, de novo, native, or restenotic lesions with a diameter stenosis of >70 % in the superficial femoral artery (SFA). The primary endpoint of the study, namely, the mean in-stent percent stenosis as detected by quantitative angiography at 6 months, was 22.6 % as compared to 31 % for the uncoated stent group. Though the difference was nonsignificant, there was a trend toward benefit for the SES group. The occlusion and in-stent restenosis rates (ISR) were also 0 % for the SES as compared to 5.9 and 23.5 %, respectively, in the uncoated stent group. Improvements in the Rutherford–Becker class (RBC) and ankle-brachial indices (ABIs) were uniformly seen in both groups at 6 months.

The findings of this study were expanded upon by the Sirolimus-Coated Cordis SMART Nitinol Self-expandable

Stent for the Treatment of Obstructive Superficial Femoral Artery Disease (SIROCCO) II trial which randomized 57 patients in the sirolimus-coated SMART stent and uncoated stent groups [56]. Inclusion criteria were similar, and the study demonstrated that there was no difference in the primary endpoint of in-stent mean luminal diameter between the sirolimus-coated and uncoated groups (4.94 mm±0.69 and 4.76 mm±0.54). There was a trend toward reduction in stent late lumen loss in DES as compared to the uncoated stent which was however nonsignificant. Follow-up at 24 months demonstrated that improvement in ABI and freedom from claudication were maintained in both groups with no difference seen in the restenosis rates (23% in the DES vs 21% in the uncoated group) [57]. It has been hypothesized that the failure of the sirolimus-coated SMART stent is due to the lower-dose concentration of sirolimus on the stent as compared to its coronary counterpart (90 mcg/cm^2 vs 140 mcg/cm^2 of stent area) or due to its rapid eluting kinetics (7 days vs 30 days) [58], though this potential problem has not been studied further.

It seems that mTOR inhibitors did not have much success overall in PAD of above-the-knee vessels. In another single-arm study, the first-in-human Superficial Femoral Artery Treatment with Drug-Eluting Stents (STRIDES) study, everolimus-eluting stents were evaluated for the treatment of de novo or restenosis lesions in the femoral and proximal popliteal arteries [59]. All patients had chronic PAD with RBC of 2–5 (17% of patients having CLI). A total of 104 patients with 106 lesions were enrolled in 11 European centers. Ninety-eight percent device success rate was immediately achieved and 6-month rates of ISR remained at 14%. Six-month primary patency rates were 94%±2.3 dropping to 68%±4.6 however at 12 months. These are very much comparable to historical rates observed for bare-nitinol stents; hence, this study failed to create a role for everolimus DES in the treatment of femoropopliteal PAD lesions.

A breakthrough, however, came in the form of the paclitaxel-eluting stent, the Zilver PTX (Cook Medical, Bloomington, IN). The Zilver PTX trial was a randomized controlled trial designed to compare percutaneous transluminal angioplasty (PTA) with the Zilver PTX DES in treatment of symptomatic de novo or restenotic lesions of above-the-knee femoropopliteal artery segment [60]. Since PTA often fails acutely, a secondary randomized assignment post-PTA failure compared assignment of the Zilver PTX with the Zilver bare-nitinol stent (Cook Medical, Bloomington, IN). Four hundred seventy-nine patients (238 in the PTA group and 241 in the DES group) were enrolled in this multicenter trial. Nine percent of the total patients were with CLI. Due to acute PTA failure, secondary randomization was done in 120 patients which were divided in the provisional BMS (59 patients) and provisional DES (61 patients) groups. The primary endpoints were 12-month event-free survival and primary patency rates. Paclitaxel DES showed significantly improved event-free survival (90.4% vs 82.6%, respectively) and primary patency (83.1% vs 32.8%). Of note, the patency rates with optimal PTA (defined as the group excluding acute PTA failure) and PTA with provisional stent (again not counting acute PTA failure as loss of patency) also remained at only 65.3 and 73.4%; thus, paclitaxel DES patency rates, regardless, remained significantly superior. Secondary outcomes showed that provisional DES was significantly superior to provisional BMS in the acute PTA failure group (90% vs 73%, respectively). These differences have remained at 2 years follow-up as well [61] suggesting that the Zilver PTX does not demonstrate the adverse late catch-up phenomenon seen in STRIDES and SIROCCO studies. The trial, however, was not designed to evaluate the stent's usefulness in the CLI subgroup.

The Zilver PTX stent was also examined in TASC II C/D lesions. The Zilver PTX single-arm study was a prospective, multicenter study involving 787 patients with de novo or restenotic femoropopliteal lesions >50% stenosis, with a total of 900 lesions treated with the Zilver PTX stent [62]. Among these, a subgroup analysis was performed on 135 lesions >15 cm corresponding to the TASC II C/D subgroup lesions, with 84% of these lesions having total occlusion. The primary patency rate for these lesions remained at 77.6% at 12 months with freedom from target lesion revascularization (TLR) at about 85%. Twenty-one major adverse events (MAEs) were observed in this population including two deaths, while the remaining being TLRs. Stent fracture rates remained at 2%. Compared with historical surgical bypass patency rates of 85% for venous bypass and 67% for prosthetic grafts, the authors concluded that the Zilver PTX offers a viable option for these complex lesions in patients with comorbidities or other factors precluding surgical bypass. This, however, remains to be explored in further randomized controlled studies.

Infrapopliteal Disease

In contrast with above-the-knee disease, drug-eluting stents found early application and use for below-the-knee disease. Coronary stents have been studied in the tibial vessels with significant success reported in smaller studies [63–65]. These have been subsequently replicated in RCTs as well. Among the nonrandomized studies, sirolimus for below-the-knee (SiroBTK) was a nonrandomized, single-arm study using the Cypher sirolimus-eluting stent (SES) (Cordis, Johnson & Johnson, Warren, NJ) for treatment of patients with severe intermittent claudication or critical limb ischemia (CLI) due to infrapopliteal PAD [66]. One hundred and six SES were implanted in 62 arteries in 30 patients. The overall primary patency rate at 1 year measured by TLR was 97%

with the event-free survival calculated at 92.5%. Eighty-seven percent of the patients were CLI prior to treatment, whereas at 12 months the number had decreased to 3.7%. Recurrence of CLI or failure to heal chronic ulcers was often due to new, de novo lesions. No adverse effects as a direct consequence of the stent were observed.

Similarly, the PReventing Amputations using Drug eluting StEnts (PaRADISE) trial was another single-arm, non-randomized trial designed to study the utility of DES in the treatment of BTK lesions in patients with CLI [67]. Interestingly, there were no exclusion criteria as everyone, even patients with concomitant above-the-knee lesions, was treated with DES. The CYPHER SELECT SES and the Taxus paclitaxel-eluting stents (PES) (Boston Scientific, Maple Grove, MN) were used in this study. One hundred and six patients (118 limbs) received a total of 228 stents. The 3-year cumulative risk of amputation was $6 \pm 2\%$ with survival rates of $71 \pm 5\%$ and amputation-free survival of $68 \pm 5\%$. Overall RC scores 4 and 5 did significantly better than score 6 (both improving to 97–98% vs 86% for score 6 on follow-up). These results compared favorably by the comparison with historical controls from the TASC II document and the BASIL study as reported by the authors [5, 68].

Among randomized controlled trials (RCT), earlier trials were rather limited in their scope for examining the effectiveness of DES for the treatment of below-the-knee lesions. Falkowski et al. presented the first trial which examined the role of Cypher stent compared with a BMS counterpart in reducing the restenosis rates in crural arteries at 6 months' follow-up. Fifty patients were randomized 1:1 in the two groups (32% with CLI), and at 6 months, restenosis rates were significantly lower in the SES group (16% vs 76%) [69].

The ACHILLES trial was a multicenter randomized controlled trial comparing the efficacy of SES with PTA in the treatment of de novo as well as restenotic infrapopliteal PAD lesions using angiographic 1-year binary restenosis rates as endpoint [70]. Two hundred patients were enrolled in the trial with 99 randomized to the CYPHER SELECT arm. The primary endpoint was reached by 22% of SES patients as compared to 42% in the PTA arm ($p = 0.019$). The difference was even more significant in diabetics (17% vs 53%). No difference was however there in rates of death, target lesion revascularization rates, or index limb amputation rates though there was a trend favoring the SES arm. This trial, like others, suggests that long-term patency is improved with DES, but may not be necessary for initial limb salvage.

Another SES, Yukon (Translumina, Hechingen, Germany), was compared with BMS in the YUKON Below-the-Knee (YUKON-BTK) randomized, double-blind trial [71]. A total of 161 patients (82 randomized to the SES arm) were enrolled with 47% having CLI. The primary endpoints of 1-year freedom from TLR significantly favoring the SES

arm (44% in the SES arm vs 19% in the BMS) with primary patency rates at 1 year significantly higher in the SES subgroup (81% vs 56%). The hazard ratio for restenosis calculated by the authors for the BMS was 3.2 (95% confidence interval 1.5–6.7), with significant improvements in the RBC and ABI observed. Subgroup analysis in the CLI patients showed benefit from SES for primary patency but did not reach statistical significance (75% vs 56.5%). Again, no significant differences were seen in median RBC score improvement, healing of chronic ulcers at baseline, or improvement in ABI among the two subgroups, though there was a trend favoring the SES. Long-term follow-up to about 3 years for this trial reported the SES showed significantly higher event-free survival than the BMS (66% vs 44%) with significantly improved RBC scores for the SES as compared to the BMS groups [72]. The long-term event-free survival benefit becomes even more significant in the CLI subgroup (58% vs 32%). These late findings becomes all the more important as 1-year results did not show statistical difference between SES and BMS arms in the CLI subgroup, thus indicating that in the long run, SES may be the better option for revascularization in CLI patients.

The Drug Eluting Stents in the Critically Ischemic Lower Leg (DESTINY) compared the everolimus-eluting XIENCE V (Abbott Vascular, Santa Clara, CA) with bare-metal stents for the treatment of de novo tibial arterial lesions in patients with chronic CLI [73]. A total of 140 patients were enrolled in this multicenter trial with 74 in the XIENCE V arm. Primary patency rates were significantly favorable for the XIENCE V arm (85% vs 54%) with significantly greater freedom from TLR also achieved (92% vs 65%); however, there was no difference obtained in survival rates or improvement in the Rutherford–Becker class between the two groups. This was attributed to the authors to the lack of power in the study design to test these hypotheses.

A meta-analysis of these trials by Fusaro et al. reported that drug-eluting stents reduce the rates of TLR (odds ratio (OR) 0.31; CI 0.18–0.54), restenosis (OR 0.25; CI 0.15–0.43), and amputation (OR 0.50; CI 0.26–0.97) significantly with no impact on the rates of death or improvement in the RBC score as compared to control therapy (balloon angioplasty or BMS implantation) [74]. It must be noted that PES were not used in any of the RCTs; thus, their role in below-the-knee arterial lesions remains undefined. An older meta-analysis of nonrandomized studies by Biondi-Zoccar and colleagues does suggest that for BTK lesions, SES performed significantly better than PES in terms of primary patency (93% vs 30%) and target vessel revascularization (TVR) (7% vs 31%) [75]. These results, however, must be used with caution as the studies included generally had low sample sizes and only one study which examined the role of PES was included in this analysis.

Beyond Stents: New Technologies for Endovascular Interventions

As techniques/technologies have continued to advance, the limitations of PTA continue to become more evident, mostly secondary to the inability to address the immediate technical complications leading to procedural failure. In addition to the advent of stents, a number of balloon angioplasty technologies have been developed to address these major technical complications. Such advances include cryoplasty, cutting balloons, brachytherapy (not included in this review), and drug-eluting balloons.

Cryoplasty

The lone cryoplasty system available today, PolarCath (Boston Scientific, Natick, MA) catheter, utilizes a low-pressure (~8 atm) double-balloon system, which in addition to applying compressive pressure causes a cold-induced injury to the lesion. The application of the 30-s cryotherapy cools the vessel wall to roughly -10°C; the physiologic effects of cooling are believed to create a uniform rigidity in the vessel wall altering both collagen fibrils and inducing smooth muscle apoptosis. The PolarCath system thus allows for a uniform mechanical load to be achieved between the vessel wall balloon interface, which is believed to decrease significant amounts of plaque dissection, vessel recoil, and intimal hyperplasia.

Femoropopliteal Disease

The published results of the cryoplasty safety registry of non-complex femoropopliteal lesions showed a 10-month patency rate of 82% in the 102 patients studied [76, 77]. The COLD study was a prospective single-center trail to evaluate the efficacy and safety of cryo- versus conventional angioplasty in focal popliteal artery lesions [78]. Eighty-six patients were enrolled and randomized into each arm (46 in conventional PTA arm and 40 in cryo arm); patients were equally matched with a mean age of 72 and were assessed for a primary endpoint of target lesion patency and secondary endpoint of treatment success (without need for subsequent stenting). Both arms were followed at 3, 6, 9, and 15 months with duplex ultrasound. Initial success rate was 35% in cryoplasty versus 54% in the conventional PTA, with no statistically significant difference in rate of dissection, need for stent placement secondary to dissection, or target lesion patency at 9 months' follow-up. Despite a lower primary anatomic success rate in the cryoplasty group, there was, however, a nonsignificant trend toward greater patency in the cryoplasty arm at 9 months' follow-up (79.3%±7.5 vs 66.7%±8.1 ($p=0.14$)).

Similar results were published by Spiliopoulos et al. in another prospective randomized controlled single-center trial comparing cryoplasty versus conventional PTA of femoropopliteal artery lesions in diabetic patients, with CLI being present in 41.4% of the cryoplasty arm and 38.7% of the conventional arm [79]. Initial technical success (<30% stenosis and no need for adjunctive stenting) was 58% in cryoplasty versus 64% in conventional arm ($p=0.29$), a nonsignificant trend toward increased binary restenosis (HR 1.3, 95% CI 0.6–2.6, $p=0.45$) and no statistically significant differences in patient survival or limb salvage at 3 years when compared to a Kaplan–Meier model. There were however significantly lower rates of primary patency (HR 2.2, 95% CI 1.1–4.3) and higher repeat intervention secondary to recurrent symptoms in the cryoplasty group (HR 2.5, 95% CI 1.2–5.3).

Infrapopliteal Disease

Das et al. published the 12-month follow-up results, from the 16-center prospective BTK Chill trial which included 108 patients to evaluate the efficacy of cryoplasty for below-the-knee (BTK) occlusive disease in patients with CLI [80]. Pts were followed at 1, 3, and 12 months for acute technical success (≤50% stenosis and continuous in-line flow to the foot) and absence of major amputation at 6 months as primary endpoints and secondary endpoints of cryoplasty-associated complications and absence of major amputations out to 12 months' follow-up. Immediate technical success was achieved for 97.3% of threatened limbs, with major amputation avoided in 93.4% and 85.2% of patients at 6 and 12 months, respectively. There was only one clinically significant dissection, two patients with residual stenosis >50%, three patients requiring adjunctive stenting, and only 21% of patients requiring subsequent intervention at 1 year. Cryoplasty appears to be a reasonable, safe, and effective method of treating infrapopliteal disease in patients with CLI.

Bosiers et al. published their data from the CLIMB registry of 100 patients with CLI who underwent intervention with cryoplasty for infrapopliteal lesions [81]. They were all followed out to 12 months with a primary endpoint of patency (based on duplex) and secondary endpoints of immediate success, limb salvage, and survival at 12 months. They reported 95% immediate technical success rates with 17% requiring adjunct stent placement and patency (55.9%±7.4%), limb salvage (93.8±2.5%), and survival (81.8±3.9%) at 12 months. Results of the CLIMB registry supported the use of cryoplasty as an effective treatment modality; however, it was speculated that the success rates of cryoplasty-based interventions in below-the-knee lesions was comparable to that of conventional angioplasty.

Cutting Balloon Angioplasty (CBA)

Cutting balloon (CB) catheters use a low-pressure balloon (~8 atm) mounted with either 3–4 longitudinal or helical/elliptical microsurgical blades, which cut directly into the vessel with inflation of the balloon. Cutting directly into the vessel wall causes controlled disruption of the internal elastic lamina, which reduces elastic recoil, vessel wall injury, and ideally restenosis [82].

The efficacy and safety of CBA in treating de novo infrainguinal arterial lesions have been studied in a number of small series and have shown promising results [83–85]. Rabbi et al. published the results of a small case series including 11 patients who underwent CBA, 82% of which underwent intervention for the indication of CLI [85]. They reported good initial technical success rates of 90.09%, with primary patency and limb salvage at 3 months of 88% and 100%, respectively. Canuad et al. published the results of a substantially larger series, which included 128 patients who underwent interventions in both femoropopliteal and infrapopliteal lesions for both claudication and CLI, with a combined initial success rate of 96.30% and complication rate of 8.90% [84]. Patients were followed up at 12- and 24-month intervals with primary patency rates of 82.1 and 82.1% (claudication group) and 64.40% and 51.90% (CLI group), respectively. Additional endpoints at 12- and 24-month limb salvage (84.2% and 76.9%) and survival (92.6% and 88.5%) were also reported in the cohort of CLI patients. Similar rates of limb salvage (89.5%) at 12 months' follow-up were reported by Ansel et al. in a series of 73 patients who underwent intervention for symptomatic CLI [83].

Amighi et al. published the results of their randomized controlled trial comparing CBA to conventional PTA at 6 months in pts with de novo superficial femoral artery (SFA) lesions manifesting as either claudication or CLI [86]. Forty-three patients were randomly assigned to either CBA or PTA and followed for 6 months with duplex ultrasound to assess for restenosis. At 6-month follow-up, restenosis rates were 32 and 62% ($p=0.048$) and freedom from symptoms 73% and 38% ($p=0.059$) in the PTA and CBA groups, respectively. There was no significant difference in ABI or pain-free walking distance.

Despite no major difference between modalities in treatment of de novo lesions, there does however appear to be some advantage favoring CB-PTA in restenotic lesions in bypass vein grafts. Initially reported by Engelke et al. in 2002, CBA was shown to be superior to PTA and comparable to open surgical revision in selected pts with infrainguinal graft stenosis [87]. In their series of 15 patients (16 lesions), CBA was technically successful in 15/16 lesions without any short-term clinical complications. While two lesions were complicated by local restenosis and one graft occlusion was observed, the cumulative primary and secondary patency rates at 6 months were 84 and 92%, with patency rates of 67 and 83% when followed out to 12 and 18 months, respectively. Subsequent results were not uniformly replicated. While the risk of early restenosis rates was still promising, the risk of long-term restenosis persisted.

In a single-center retrospective review evaluating endovascular therapies to treat failing infrapopliteal bypass vein grafts, 30 patients were identified by angiograms between 2006 and 2012 and followed with duplex US at 1, 3, and 6 months for surveillance [88]. Of the 30 patients included in the study, nine underwent intervention for symptoms of persistent or recurrent limb ischemia. Intervention techniques included cutting balloon angioplasty (83%, $n=25$), PTA (7%, $n=2$), and stent placement (10%, $n=3$). Procedural success was achieved in all 30 cases with no procedural complications, amputations, or death reported in 30 days follow-up and extended patency rates of 37% and 31% at 12 and 24 months, respectively.

Scoring Balloon Angioplasty (SBA)

The AngioSculpt (ASC) (AngioScore Inc., Fremont, CA) catheter is composed of a balloon that is encircled by three nitinol spiral struts which allow for targeted lesion scoring on inflation, designed to treat complex diffuse fibrocalcific lesions.

Scheinert et al. published the results of a multicenter study of 42 patients with 56 targeted lesions who underwent SBA for infrapopliteal disease, 38 of which (90.5%) presented with symptomatic CLI [89]. Lesion morphology varied in regard to complexity of calcification, length, and anatomic location (bifurcation and ostial lesions). The ASC was successfully deployed in 98.2% of lesions attempted with dissection and adjunctive stenting required in 10.7% (6/56), and no significant device slippage or perforations were observed. The device was used in a wide variety of lesion morphologies with a low complication rate

In a subsequent retrospective analysis covering 1 year of procedural data, Bosiers and his colleagues assessed the efficacy and safety of SBA in treating infrapopliteal lesions in patients with symptomatic CLI [90]. They were evaluated for the primary endpoints of 1-year survival ($83.0\pm6.6\%$), primary patency ($61.0\pm9.3\%$), limb salvage ($86.3\pm6.4\%$), and major safety endpoint of 1-month complication-free survival (96.8%).

Drug-Eluting Balloons

Drug-eluting balloons (DEBs), also known as drug-coated balloons, represent the next step in the evolution of effective treatment strategies for atherosclerotic vascular disease.

Stent technology, particularly the drug-eluting stents, solved much of the problems, and their use in coronary angioplasty has cemented over the years; however, development of late restenosis and neointimal hyperplasia coupled with the need for effective long-term antiplatelet therapy for preventing stent thrombosis meant that further evolution of technologies was needed to develop an effective therapy for extracardiac atherosclerotic vascular disease [91]. DEBs were found to be effective in preventing neointimal proliferation and therefore were accepted as alternatives to plain old balloon angioplasty and stenting-based interventions in the coronary circulation. This has recently been expanded to the peripheral arterial disease as well, as DEBs were well suited to adapt to the unique challenges encountered in the intervention for PAD lesions.

Femoropopliteal Lesions

The femoropopliteal artery interventions present certain unique challenges not encountered in the coronary circulation. This vessel encounters significant longitudinal stretching, external compression, and torsion and flexion forces, which pose a greater risk for stent fractures and eventual restenosis [92, 93]. Furthermore, prior to the Zilver PTX studies, DES was not found to have significant benefit over BMS for the treatment of femoropopliteal lesions. Hence, DEBs were also investigated during this time for their usefulness in prevention of restenosis in these lesions.

The Local Taxane with Short Exposure for Reduction of Restenosis in Distal Arteries (THUNDER) trial was the first to examine the utility of paclitaxel-eluting balloons in the treatment of femoropopliteal lesion [94]. A total of 154 patients with de novo or restenotic lesions in the femoropopliteal segment were distributed in three different treatment arms using uncoated balloons (UCB) as control, the prototype PACCOCATH DEB (now known as Cotavance, MEDRAD Interventional, Indianola, PA) paclitaxel-coated balloon (PCB), and paclitaxel dissolved in the contrast medium. 16.2 % of the entire study sample had CLI. Eighty-three percent of the patients underwent angiographic follow-up at 6 months. Mean late lumen loss (LLL) was significantly lower in PCB arm than the control arm (0.4 ± 1.2 mm vs 1.7 ± 1.8 mm) with no difference seen in the group with paclitaxel in the contrast medium as compared to the control arm. Restenosis rates were also thus significantly lower in the PCB group as compared to UCB (17 % vs 44 %). Rates of TLR were not significantly different in the three groups at 6 months; however, PCB showed a clear benefit at 12 (10 % vs 48 %) and 24 months' follow-up as compared to UCB (15 % vs 52 %). Five-year follow-up results of the follow-up of this trial were presented in the Transcatheter Cardiovascular Therapeutics (TCT) 2011 [95]. Freedom from TLR rates was still significantly higher in the PCB subgroup (70 % vs 30 %). These results are very encouraging for the success of PCBs in revascularization of PAD.

Another early study, the Femoral Paclitaxel (FEMPAC) study, compared the efficacy of again the prototype PACCOCATH PCB versus UCB in the treatment of femoropopliteal PAD [96]. Eighty-seven patients were randomized in the two groups. The primary endpoint of late lumen loss at 6 months was again significantly lower in the PCB arm (0.5 ± 1.1 mm vs 1.0 ± 1.1 mm) with significantly lower restenosis rates (19 % vs 47 %). Interestingly, as opposed to other studies, the RBC improved significantly in the PCB group at 6 months, though significant numbers of CLI patients were not involved in this study (5.7 % at baseline).

The Lutonix Paclitaxel-Coated Balloon for the Prevention of Femoropopliteal Restenosis (LEVANT I) was designed to examine the Lutonix PCB (also known as the Moxy, C.R. Bard, New Hope, MN) as compared to UCB in the treatment of femoropopliteal PAD in 101 patients [97]. Six-month LLL data showed significant lumen loss in the PCB subgroup (0.46 ± 1.13 mm vs 1.09 ± 1.07 mm). TLR and MAE rates up to 24 months follow-up showed no difference among the groups. As a follow-up, the LEVANT II study was designed to rigorously test this PCB against standard balloon angioplasty in a large, global, multicenter trial [98]. Four hundred and seventy-six patients were randomized 2:1 for treatment of native femoropopliteal disease, with primary efficacy endpoint being 12 months and rates of primary patency being defined as freedom from restenosis and TLR. Interestingly, in order to reduce bias, the authors excluded bailout stenting as a cause of TLR. Primary patency at 12 months was significantly superior for the PCB (65 % vs 53 %) though TLR at 12 months (per the above definition) did not show any significant difference between the two groups (88 % vs 83 %). However, a post hoc analysis which included bailout stenting as TLR showed a significant difference (85 % vs 76 %, respectively). The primary safety endpoint which was composite of periprocedure death, freedom from index limb amputation, re-intervention, or index limb-related death also showed that the PCB was significantly superior to the control (84 % vs 79 %). On the basis of these results, the Lutonix PCB was given FDA approval for femoropopliteal PAD interventions.

Another randomized trial, PACIFIER, compared the IN.PACT Pacific paclitaxel-eluting balloon (Medtronic, Santa Rosa, CA) and UCB in 85 patients undergoing femoropopliteal PTA [99]. Mean LLL at 6 months was significantly lower in the PCB group (-0.01 mm [CI -0.29; 0.26] vs 0.65 mm [0.37; 0.93]) with lower rates of restenosis (8.6 % vs 32.4 %). Furthermore, PCB-treated patients had significantly lower TLR at 12 months (7 % vs 28 %) and rates of MAE (7 % vs 35 %). However, the number of CLI patients was quite low in the study sample (~5 %). Another closely related DEB, the IN.PACT Admiral (Medtronic, Santa Rosa, CA), was used in the Drug-Eluting Balloon Evaluation for Lower Limb MUltilevel TreatMent (DEBELLUM) randomized trial [100, 101]. DEBELLUM was designed to cater both femoropopliteal and BTK lesions, and therefore among a total of 50 patients randomized 1:1 in the DEB (57 lesions) versus PTA (65 lesions) arms, 44 lesions were in the femoropopliteal segment in DEB arm, whereas 48 were in the PTA sub-arm. Thirty-eight of the patients had CLI. LLL showed benefit for DEB over PTA in femoropopliteal segment subgroup analysis (0.61±0.8 mm vs 1.84±0.3 mm).

Newer evidence has come in the form of the recently published results of the IN.PACT SFA trial [102]. This trial was designed as a multicenter, RC trial to assess the IN.PACT Admiral against PTA in two phases, IN.PACT SFA I in Europe and IN.PACT SFA II conducted in the United States, jointly referred to as the IN.PACT SFA. This trial enrolled 331 patients who were randomized 2:1 to the DEB versus PTA arms; however, the proportion of CLI patients was only 5.4%. The results from the two phases of the trial were pooled based upon nonsignificant treatment-by-trial phase interaction value using the Cox proportional hazards regression. The pooled results indicated that the DEB group had significantly higher primary patency at 12 months (82.2% vs 52.4%) with significantly lower TLR rates (2.4% vs 20.6%). No difference in functional measures of quality of life were detected, though the PTA group did require 8.6 times more repeat TLR to achieve the same functional outcome as the DEB group. Evidence from this trial further strengthens the role of DEB in the primary treatment of femoropopliteal symptomatic PAD, though further trials are needed for CLI patients.

Though head-to-head comparison of DEB with DES is limited, a retrospective study by Zeller et al. aimed to compare their performance in TASC II C/D femoropopliteal lesions [103]. Two hundred and twenty-eight patients (131 DCB and 97 DES) were analyzed in this study, with propensity score analysis used to minimize bias. Around 13% of the patients had CLI. The IN.PACT Admiral and the IN.PACT Pacific balloons were used in the DEB arm, whereas the Zilver PTX was used in the DES arm. There were no differences in rates of binary stenosis (24% vs 30%), TLR rates (16% vs 19%), and event-free survival rates, though there was a trend toward benefit of DEB with provisional BMS subgroup when analyzed against DEB only and DES subgroups in terms of TLR and event-free survival. This, however, did not reach statistical significance.

This analysis, however, still does not clarify the potential role of the DEBs in the modern revascularization era as compared to DES and other strategies already available for revascularization. The question of the place for DES is not addressed in the ACC/AHA guidelines for the management of patients with peripheral artery disease (last updated in 2011) [104]. In the interim, however, a Bayesian network meta-analysis was conducted by Katsanos et al. and published recently in the Journal of Vascular Surgery [105]. This meta-analysis aimed to compare the performance of bare-nitinol stents, covered stents, PES, SES, and PCB with PTA or with each other in the treatment of femoropopliteal disease. In all, 16 RCTs with 2532 patients were analyzed which dealt with the above question. While covered stents had reportedly the highest immediate technical success, followed by uncovered stents, vascular restenosis at different points in follow-up (median reported to be 22 months) was lowest with the PES (RR, 0.43; 95% credible interval (CrI), 0.16–1.18; probability best 45), closely followed by PCB (RR, 0.43; 95% CrI, 0.26–0.67; probability best 42%). TLR rates were, however, lowest in PCB (RR, 0.36; 95% CrI, 0.23–0.55; probability best 56%) followed by the PES (RR, 0.42; 95% CrI, 0.16–1.06; probability best 33%) (Figs. 35.2 and 35.3). It must be remembered that there was significant heterogeneity in the trials themselves, as the lesion lengths varied in different regions, with trials dealing with covered stents generally reporting on longer lesions, with BMS trials reporting on shorter lesions and others with intermediate lesion size. Data on the use of adjunctive therapies and durations such as dual antiplatelet therapy, statins, etc. was frequently underreported in the primary trials themselves. Finally, the design of the interventions themselves varied, for example, it is unclear at this time which PCB design is better in terms of performance in different arterial territories. Nevertheless, the evidence generated through this meta-analysis prominently points out that DES and DEB are complimentary and may find wide-scale acceptability for use in the PAD of the femoropopliteal vessels.

DEBs Combined with Other Therapies in Femoropopliteal Lesions

As DEBs are a variant of the PTA, combination of DEB with stenting or other potential therapies to reduce restenosis is an attractive concept. The Drug-Eluting Balloon in Peripheral Intervention for the Superficial Femoral Artery (DEBATE-SFA) aimed to compare the IN.PACT Admiral (Medtronic, Santa Rosa, CA) PEB with BMS with PTA + BMS for femoropopliteal artery stenosis or occlusion [106]. A total of 104 patients were randomized in the two groups, with 74% reported to have CLI. PEB + BMS was significantly more effective in preventing binary restenosis (17% vs 47%), with freedom from TLR showing benefit (without establishing significance) for the PCB + BMS group. Subgroup analysis also showed that in longer lesions as well (>100 mm), PEB + BMS was significantly more effective in reducing restenosis and LLL.

Similarly, in heavily calcified lesions, DEBs can be combined with often-used atherectomy to further improve upon lesion and vessel patency. Cioppa et al. reported their unique approach of combining directional atherectomy with DEB in

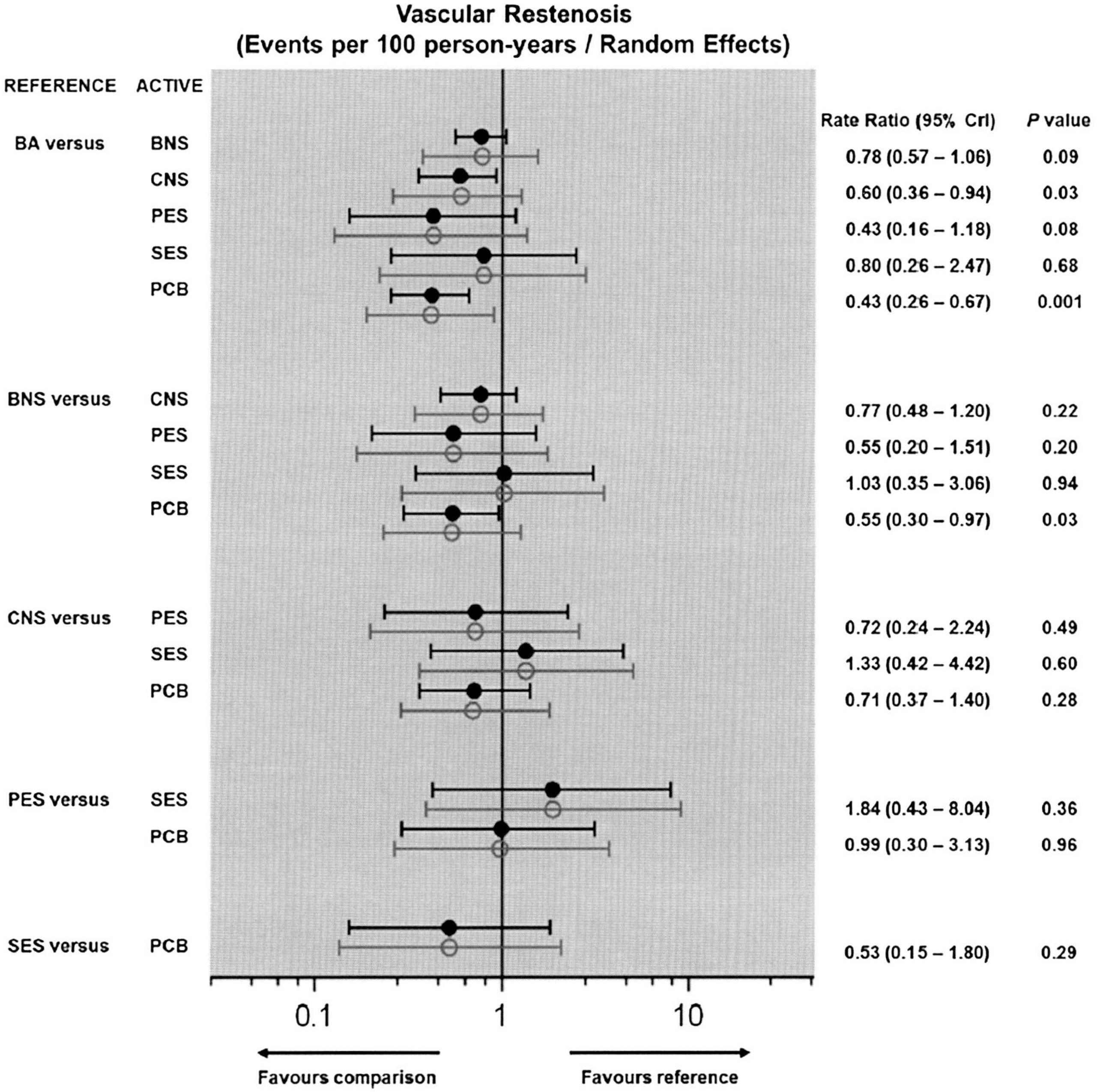

Vascular Restenosis
(Events per 100 person-years / Random Effects)

REFERENCE	ACTIVE		Rate Ratio (95% Crl)	P value
BA versus	BNS		0.78 (0.57 – 1.06)	0.09
	CNS		0.60 (0.36 – 0.94)	0.03
	PES		0.43 (0.16 – 1.18)	0.08
	SES		0.80 (0.26 – 2.47)	0.68
	PCB		0.43 (0.26 – 0.67)	0.001
BNS versus	CNS		0.77 (0.48 – 1.20)	0.22
	PES		0.55 (0.20 – 1.51)	0.20
	SES		1.03 (0.35 – 3.06)	0.94
	PCB		0.55 (0.30 – 0.97)	0.03
CNS versus	PES		0.72 (0.24 – 2.24)	0.49
	SES		1.33 (0.42 – 4.42)	0.60
	PCB		0.71 (0.37 – 1.40)	0.28
PES versus	SES		1.84 (0.43 – 8.04)	0.36
	PCB		0.99 (0.30 – 3.13)	0.96
SES versus	PCB		0.53 (0.15 – 1.80)	0.29

0.1   1   10

Favours comparison   Favours reference

Fig. 35.2 Random effects forest plot of pooled estimates of vascular restenosis. The *black lines* denote 95 % credible intervals (*CrIs*) and the *gray lines* denote 95 % prediction intervals. The numbers represent odds ratios (ORs) and 95 % CrIs. *BA* balloon angioplasty, *BNS* bare-nitinol stent, *CNS* covered nitinol stent, *PCB* paclitaxel-coated balloon, *PES* paclitaxel-eluting stent, *SES* sirolimus-eluting stent. From Katsanos K. et al. Bayesian network meta-analysis of nitinol stents, covered stents, drug-eluting stents, and drug-coated balloons in the femoropopliteal artery. J Vasc Surg. 2014;59(4):1123-33 E. Reprinted with permission from Elsevier Limited

heavily calcified femoropopliteal lesions [107]. In this single-center registry, 30 patients (40 % with CLI) underwent revascularization of heavily calcified (calcium score >3) femoropopliteal lesions, with the combined use of directional atherectomy using the TurboHawk system (Covidien, Plymouth, CO) followed by the IN.PACT Admiral DEB. Technical and procedural success was achieved in all cases, and primary patency at 1-year follow-up was 90 %.

Amputation-free survival and improvement in RBC scores were also achieved in all cases.

Following the above study, a randomized, pilot trial, Directional Atherectomy Followed by a Paclitaxel-Coated Balloon to Inhibit Restenosis and Maintain Vessel Patency (DEFINITIVE-AR) was designed to evaluate directional atherectomy and anti-restenosis therapy with DEBs (DAART) as compared to DEB alone in the femoropopliteal

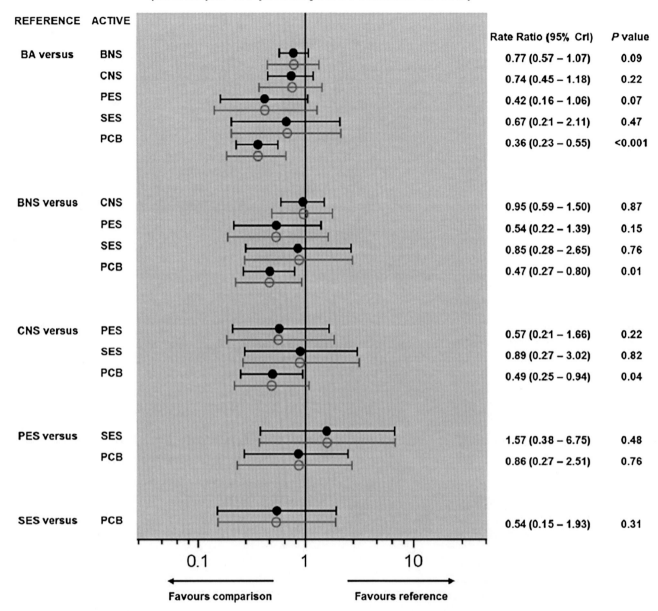

Fig. 35.3 Random effects forest plot of pooled estimates of target lesion revascularization (TLR). The *black lines* denote 95 % credible intervals (*CrIs*) and the *gray lines* denote 95 % prediction intervals. The numbers represent odds ratios (ORs) and 95 % CrIs. *BA* balloon angioplasty, *BNS* bare-nitinol stent, *CNS* covered nitinol stent, *PCB* paclitaxel-coated balloon, *PES* paclitaxel-eluting stent, *SES* sirolimus-eluting stent. From Katsanos K et al. Bayesian network meta-analysis of nitinol stents, covered stents, drug-eluting stents, and drug-coated balloons in the femoropopliteal artery. J Vasc Surg. 2014;59(4):1123-33 E. Reprinted with permission from Elsevier Limited

segment [108]. Patients with symptomatic PAD (RBC scores 2, 3, and 4) with ≥70 % stenosis, restenosis, or occlusion of the segment were included in this study. Of 121 patients enrolled in this multicenter study, 19 with severe calcification (defined as circumferential calcification extending >5 cm) were included in a nonrandomized DAART Severe Ca^{++} Arm, whereas the remaining were randomized to the DAART (48) versus DCB (54) arms. The SilverHawk and

TurboHawk atherectomy systems (Covidien, Plymouth, CO) were used in the DAART arm, while the Cotavance DEB was used in this study. Preliminary results at 12 months' follow-up indicate that DAART demonstrated significantly higher technical success rates (89.6 % vs 64.2 %) and lower rates of flow-limiting dissections (2 % vs 19 %), with a nonsignificant trend of lower bailout stenting in the DAART arm (0 % vs 3.7 %). These benefits were also retained in the DAART

Severe Ca++ Arm. At 12 months, there was a trend, albeit nonsignificant of improved patency in DAART arm versus DES in >10-cm lesions by ultrasound (96.8 % vs 85.9 %) and angiography (90.9 % vs 60.8 %). Furthermore, improved patency was also observed in patients with severely calcified lesions (70.4 % with ultrasound; 58.3 % with angiography). The study has a planned 24 months' follow-up as well, which is awaited, while at the same time it yields important information on the potential role of DAART in special lesion characteristics.

Below-the-Knee Lesions

The infrapopliteal arterial segment atherosclerotic disease is characterized by often diffuse, long, calcific lesions, making conventional stent implantation difficult [109]. Frequently, multiple stents are needed to be implanted, and the frequency of bifurcation lesions makes this all the more challenging. DEBs, therefore, offer an attractive alternative to this problem. Unfortunately, they have not found as wide of an appeal in infrapopliteal lesions as in the above-the-knee lesions as examined above.

The first experience for DEB use in BTK lesions was reported by Schmidt et al. in their single-armed registry using the IN.PACT Amphirion (Medtronic, Santa Rosa, CA) in 104 patients (109 limbs) with BTK lesions and CLI or severe claudication [110]. About 83 % of treated limbs were classified as having CLI and mean lesion length was reported as 176±88 mm. Three months' follow-up in 84 limbs angiographically showed a restenosis rate of 27 %. At mean follow-up of about a year in 86 patients with 91 limbs (17 deaths in this period, 1 lost to follow-up), clinical improvement occurred in 91 % limbs. TLR rates were 17 % and limb salvage rates in CLI patients were close to 96 %.

Following this study, two other RCTs examined the role of the IN.PACT Amphirion in the treatment of BTK lesions. The Drug-Eluting Balloon in Peripheral Intervention for Below the Knee Angioplasty Evaluation (DEBATE-BTK) was a randomized trial examining the use of DEB in diabetic patients with CLI undergoing revascularization for BTK lesions [109]. One hundred and thirty-two patients (158 lesions) were randomized in DEB (80 lesions) and PTA (78 lesions) arms. Binary restenosis rates at 12 months showed significant superiority for the DEB arm (27 % vs 75 %). Freedom from TLR was significantly higher in the DEB subgroup, with 12-month MAEs also significantly lower in this subgroup (31 % vs 51 %).

The DEBELLUM trial was aimed at comparing the performance of DEB versus PTA in all lower limb lesions (see above) [100, 101]. The IN.PACT Amphirion was used for BTK lesions in this trial as well. Thirteen lesions, in which post-dilation with DEB was carried out, were compared with 17 other lesions with conventional PTA. None of the BTK lesions had provisional stenting done. At 12 months' follow-up, DEB lesions had significantly lower LLL (0.66±0.9 mm vs 1.69±0.5 mm). Overall, the trial showed benefit for the use of DEB in lower extremities, with overall LLL (0.64±0.9 mm vs 1.81±0.1 mm) and TLR (12 % vs 35 %) significantly lower in the DEB subgroups.

However, recent results from the Study of IN.PACT Amphirion drug-eluting balloon versus Standard PTA for the Treatment of Below the Knee Critical Limb Ischemia (IN.PACT DEEP) trial have significantly challenged the role of the DEB in BTK lesions [111]. A total of 358 patients were randomized (2:1) in the IN.PACT Amphirion DEB versus PTA across 13 European centers. Predominantly, patients presented in Rutherford class 5. Primary endpoint of clinically driven TLR (CD-TLR; defined as TLR associated with worsening of Rutherford class and/or worsening of previous wounds or development of new wounds) at 12 months was comparable in the two arms (9.2 % in DEB category vs 13.1 % in PTA category). LLL was also nonsignificant in the comparison (0.61±0.78 mm vs 0.62±0.78 mm, respectively). The primary safety endpoint which was a composite of death, amputation, and CD-TLR was also comparable (17.7 % vs 15.8 %); however, there was a nonsignificant trend toward higher amputation rates in the DEB group at 12 months (8.8 % vs 3.6 %; p-value=0.08). The trial, however, was not powered enough to detect significant differences in amputation rates as an endpoint. Interestingly, the rates of amputation in the PTA arm of the IN.PACT DEEP have been lower than those observed historically in similar CLI patients [112, 113] in spite of the fact that the PTA group had longer lesions and deeper PAD associated wounds. According to Laird et al., the IN.PACT Amphirion's design is different from other DEBs studied in the SFA, which allows a lower amount of the drug to be released over time in the lesion wall [114]. This may have contributed to this device's failure to improve upon rates of TLR observed in the PTA arm. Following this trial, the IN.PACT Amphirion was withdrawn from the market by Medtronic; however, the role of DEBs in treating BTK lesion still needs to be further explored.

Adjunctive Devices Useful in Special Circumstances

Atherectomy

Excimer Laser

Laser-based endovascular therapies for plaque removal and debulking while initially met with challenges have advanced substantially. Initial laser-based technologies utilized heat-tipped, continuous-wave catheters and were quickly abandoned secondary to high complication/restenosis rates.

Advances such as the Excimer laser-assisted system (Spectranetics Corporation, Colorado Springs, Co) utilize flexible fiberoptic catheters to deliver 308-nm ultraviolet (UV) light waves directly to the plaque. The improved design along with a short penetration depth of only 50 µm allows for direct ablation of the plaque on contact alone, without causing thermal damage to the surrounding tissues. Scheinert et al. published early data, which showed promising primary technical success rates of 90.5 % with primary and secondary patency rates of 33 % and 75.9 %, respectively [115]. The Peripheral Excimer Laser Angioplasty (PELA) trial supported previous data showing comparable primary patency rates between laser and PTA as determined by ultrasound, 48 % and 58 %, respectively [116].

Subsequent advancements in laser technology came in the form of the Turbo-Booster catheter (Spectranetics Corporation, Colorado, Co) which aimed to improve technical success by offering a custom guided catheter that allowed for directional ablation of the vascular tissue, thereby allowing the ability to create a channel larger than the catheter itself and thus creating a larger lumen. In the CLiRpath Excimer Laser System to Enlarge Lumen Openings (CELLO) study, using this new directional technology, the catheters demonstrated patency rates (<50 % residual stenosis) of 59 % and 54 % at 6 and 12 months, respectively [117]. Target lesion revascularization was required in 23.1 % of the study participants.

Excisional and Orbital Atherectomy

Atherectomy devices are used to debulk and remove atherosclerotic plaques without causing stretch-related injury as is observed with primary balloon angioplasty (PBA). There have been few recent trials comparing atherectomy to balloon angioplasty. A two-center, prospective, randomized controlled trial compared atherectomy with adjunctive PBA versus PBA alone using the SilverHawk atherectomy catheter (Covidien, Plymouth, Co) in the treatment of infrainguinal disease [118]. Fifty-eight patients were randomized (36 vessels involved in the atherectomy arm and 48 vessels in PBA arm) and followed for the primary endpoint of TLR at 1 year, secondary outcome rate of "bailout" stent placement, and rate of TVR. Results of the study showed no statistically significant difference in TLR at 1 year (16.7 % vs 11.1 %) or TVR (21.4 % vs 11.1 %). There was however a significant difference in the need for bailout stent placement (27.6 % in atherectomy arm and 62.1 % in PTA arm; $p = 0.017$). Major adverse outcomes were similar between groups; however, there was a significant difference in distal microembolization (64.7 % ($n = 17$) vs 0 % ($n = 10$)) when an embolic filter was used [118].

The prospective, multicenter, single-arm DEFINITIVE Ca^{++} study was designed to evaluate the effectiveness and safety of the SilverHawk and TurboHawk (Covidien, Plymouth, CO) catheters when used with a distal embolic protection device [119]. The 30-day freedom from MAE was 93.1 %, primary effectiveness endpoint (≤50 % residual diameter stenosis) was 92 %, and technical success with a mean residual diameter stenosis of 33.3 % was also achieved (further reduced to 24.1 % with adjunctive therapy). The clinical improvement to asymptomatic status (RBC = 0) at 30 days increased from 0 to 52.3 %, with 88.5 % of patients experiencing a symptomatic improvement of one or more RBC categories.

Jetstream

Jetstream systems (Bayer Health System) offer both single (SC) and expandable-cutter (XC) options. The XC system achieves graded atherectomy using two sets of rotating stainless steel blades. The first set of blades lies within a fenestrated metal housing situated at the tip of the catheter; this set allows cutting in a diameter just over 3 mm when rotated clockwise. The secondary set of blades are hinged and mounted just proximal from the distal housing; these also allow for cutting to a diameter of 3 mm when rotated counterclockwise. The SC design has a longer working shaft, which allows for its use in the revascularization of more distal lesions and is available in sizes ranging from 1.6 to 1.85 mm. Both systems work by the principle of differential cutting, allowing for fibrous and calcified tissue/plaque to be preferentially cut sparing the normal compliant vascular tissue. Prior to approval, the Jetstream device was studied by Zeller et al. in the Pathway PVD trial [120]; lesion crossing and debulking success rate was 99 %, minor embolic events were observed in 10 % of cases, and perforations were seen in 2 % ($n = 4$). Patients were followed at 6 and 12 months for major adverse events which were reported as 19 % and 25 % DM and 31.5 % non-DM; most of these events were TLR 15 % and 26 % (20 % DM and 28 % in non-DM).

Devices for Interventions in Chronic Total Occlusions

Chronic CLI with Chronic Total Occlusions (CTOs) presents as a special challenging subpopulation of patients. Previously, endovascular therapeutic options used to be limited; however, a number of devices are available currently to allow cap penetration, lesion crossing, and entry into the true lumen. Furthermore, a special technique developed by Bolia et al. known as subintimal angioplasty (SIA) also allows significant improvement in lesion crossing for CTOs [121]. This technique is dependent upon gaining subintimal access at a suitable point, lesion crossing, and then reentry into the true lumen to establish vascular access. Reentry, thus, is a pivotal movement in this technique, and failure in this step leads to a majority of failures while using the SIA approach. For this reason, an entire generation of true-lumen reentry devices was also developed which significantly increase the effectiveness of this technique. A review on both classes of devices follows.

Lesion Crossing Devices

Frontrunner

The Frontrunner CTO Catheter (Cordis, Johnson & Johnson, Warren, NJ) was one of the earliest devices available for lesion crossing. This catheter uses blunt microdissection done by opening and closing of a hinged jaw at the blunt end of the catheter, allowing guidewire penetration for angioplasty. Several studies have reported its usefulness, with a small number of complications which include minor perforations and distal extension of dissections [122–124]. Shetty et al. reported a series of 26 TASC D femoral and popliteal CTOs, in which the use of this device was associated with about a 96 % success rate and no complications [125].

Crosser

The Crosser CTO Recanalization system (Bard Peripheral Vascular, Tempe, AZ) is another one of the earlier devices relying on high-frequency (20 kHz), low-amplitude vibrations to break the CTO cap. A number of studies have reported a success rate in the order of 70 % for this device [126–128]. However, one study by Khalid et al. with 27 CTO lesions reported a success rate of only 41 % for the catheter [129]. Further evidence has also accumulated over the years regarding the device's usefulness. Results from the Peripheral Approach To Recanalization In Occluded Totals (PATRIOT) study were reported [130]. PATRIOT was a single-arm, multicenter study held across the United States, in which 85 patients with a failed attempt at crossing a CTO were evaluated with the use of the Crosser catheter. Almost half of the patients present as CLI (49.5 %). Successful crossing and guidewire advancement to the distal lumen were reported in about 84 % cases with procedural success achieved in 81 % cases. The safety endpoint of the study was freedom from clinically significant perforation at 30 days which was achieved in 99 % of the cases. Thus, the Crosser system still remains useful in interventions for CTOs.

Vibrational Angioplasty

Another earlier technique, vibrational angioplasty involved connecting a guidewire to a device which imparts mechanical vibrations to it. This guidewire is used to break the CTO cap and allow lesion crossing. Small case series had reported a success rate of 92–100 % [131, 132]. In a review of 28 CTO

lesions in 27 patients, Kapralos et al. reported a technical success rate of 89 % [133]. Technical failures in these cases were due to severely calcified lesions causing inability to cross them intraluminally even after successful cap penetration.

Excimer Laser Angioplasty

The excimer laser angioplasty is very similar to its counterpart in atherectomy techniques, with the caveat that the laser here only allows a path to be ablated photochemically across the atherosclerotic plaque for a guidewire to be placed. The CVX-300 Excimer Laser System (Spectranetics, Colorado Springs, CO) with the Turbo Elite catheter (Spectranetics) has been widely studied, with technical success rates above 80 % [134–136]. Most frequently, this is done in a gradual step-by-step technique, with smaller attempts at ablation followed by attempts at guidewire advancement repeated in multiple steps. Usual adverse events reported include vascular perforation, reocclusion, or distal thromboembolism.

Wildcat and Kittycat

The Wildcat and Kittycat (Avinger, Redwood City, CA, USA) are devices with a distal tip having wedges which are able to rotate both in the clockwise and anticlockwise direction. The device can be engaged in two different configurations, passive and active, the latter of which allows exposure of the wedges out of the catheter. Kittycat is similar to the Wildcat, however with a smaller crossing profile. The Wildcat catheter was evaluated in the single-arm, multicenter CONNECT study, in which the Wildcat was used in 84 femoropopliteal lesions with previous conventional guidewire failure [137]. Technical success was reported in 89 % of cases. Around 11 % of these patients were defined as CLI (with ABI <0.4) and showed significant improvement in ABIs (only 1.3 % in this category at 30 days follow-up). There were about 5 % clinically significant perforation rates, which were sealed with balloon inflation.

Ocelot

One of the newer devices in this category, the Ocelot System (Avinger, Redwood City, CA, USA), is a device with a distal tip having spiral wedges allowing clockwise and counterclockwise rotation to allow penetration through the CTO. Additionally, it has a viewing system based on optical coherence tomography (OCT) allowing real-time visualization of the catheter, also enabling discrimination of the plaque from healthy tissue allowing appropriate manipulation of the catheter. Initial experience from a European single-arm study involving 33 CTOs was quite encouraging with technical success rate reported to be 94 % without any adverse events [138]. Interventionalists also rated the catheter and the OCT system across different performance studies as mostly excellent to good. The CONNECT II, a larger, nonrandomized, multicenter study, examined the utility of the Ocelot system in 100 patients and reported a 97% technical success rate [139].

TruePath

The TruePath CTO Device (Boston Scientific, Maple Grove, MN) is another new catheter which has a diamond-coated, radiopaque, distal tip, revolving at 13,000 rpm to access through the CTO. The catheter was reported in a study of 85 participants with lower extremity CTOs, in which the technical success rate was reported at 80% [140]. There was only one clinically significant perforation requiring intervention. In another smaller registry, the procedural success rate was 100%, though in three cases, the guidewire passed into the subintimal space requiring the use of a reentry device [141].

Reentry Devices

Outback

The Outback LTD Re-Entry Catheter (Cordis, Johnson & Johnson, Warren, NJ) is a device which employs a hollow needle which is used to gain entry from the subintimal plane into the true lumen. The catheter has two radiopaque markers which allow the correct positioning of the device under fluoroscopy. Smaller studies have noted considerable success with the use of this device. Among larger studies, Bausback et al. reported a 91.5% technical success rate with a procedural success rate of 90.7% in their retrospective review of 118 cases [142]. In 32% of the cases, CLI was the indication for the procedure. Gandini reported an RCT in which the Outback catheter was compared with manual reentry in a total of 52 patient cases [143]. While technical success was achieved in all cases, the Outback device was successful in reentry within 5 cm of the dissection while also significantly reducing mean procedural and fluoroscopy time (36.0 ± 9.4 min and 29.8 ± 8.9 min compared to 55.4 ± 14.2 min and 39.6 ± 13.9 min, respectively). No device-related complications were reported.

Pioneer

The Pioneer Plus Re-Entry Catheter (Volcano Corporation, San Diego, CA) is an intravascular ultrasound (IVUS)-guided catheter which allows it to gain reentry into the true lumen. The lumen of the vessel distal to the CTO can be visualized via the IVUS allowing a needle to be deployed from the device at an appropriate position which gains access from the subintimal space to the true lumen allowing guidewire passage. Smaller studies have reported good success rates in the order of 95–100% with the use of the catheter with no significant adverse effects [144, 145].

BridgePoint System: Viance and Enteer

The BridgePoint system (now simply known as the Chronic Total Occlusion System, Boston Scientific, Maple Grove, MN) is a novel device system consisting of CrossBoss Catheter, Stingray Balloon Catheter, and Stingray guidewire, which is primarily designed for coronary CTOs but has been used in peripheral interventions as well. The CrossBoss Catheter is designed for intraluminal cap penetration of a CTO. The CrossBoss has a rotating tip with a torque device, which allows rotation and penetration of the device into the CTO cap. In instances in which the device fails to enter the CTO intraluminally and SIA is attempted, the Stingray System helps as a reentry device system. The Stingray Catheter has a self-orienting flat-topped balloon, which allows the Stingray guidewire to gain access into the true lumen via a port adjacent to the lumen. The device is reported to have success in the coronary circulation; however, Banerjee et al. in his report of 17 cases described 100% success with the use of the CrossBoss Catheter in PAD CTOs [146]. Only two of the cases required a reentry device.

Another similar system consists of the Viance Crossing Catheter and the Enteer Re-entry System (Covidien, Mansfield, MA). This device system, which works similarly as the system above, has been specifically evaluated in PAD CTOs in the Peripheral Facilitated Antegrade Steering Technique in Chronic Total Occlusions (PFAST-CTO) trial [147]. In this study, 66 patients with lower extremity CTOs were attempted to be crossed with the Viance catheter. In those in which the catheter failed at crossing, SIA was attempted with the use of the Enteer Re-entry System. Technical success rate with the Viance catheter was 84%, while it was 86% in 21 cases requiring the use of the reentry device. Overall, technical success rate of the system was 85% with 3% MAE rate at 1 month.

Embolic Protection Devices

Distal embolization is well known as a complication following lower extremity peripheral endovascular interventions, especially in the setting of single-vessel runoff. While these complications are well appreciated in the literature, the role of embolic protection is not quite as well understood.

Karnabatidis et al. conducted a prospective study of 48 patients who underwent endovascular interventions of infra-aortic lesions (64.6% above knee and 35.4% below) to assess the burden of distal embolization [148]. The SpiderFX Embolic Protection Device (Covidien, Plymouth, MN), a heparin-coated nitinol filter basket, was used for distal protection. Procedural success was reached in 93.8% with three reported failures (one vasospasm, one distal embolus, one side branch occlusion). Debris was collected in 49/50 filters deployed and retrieved with a reported total average area collected of 2.76 ± 6.49 mm^2 and major particle diameter of >1 mm in 58.0 % and >3 mm in 12 % of all particles.

A number of small studies since have shown similar results and confirmed that distal embolization is considerable in peripheral interventions. Results of a single-center prospective registry published by Shammas et al. evaluated the rates of distal embolization as well as the safety and efficacy of distal protection devices [149]. Their DEEP EMBOLI registry looked at 20 patients with 28 vascular lesions who underwent treatment with the excimer laser ± adjunctive stenting ($n = 17$, 60.7 %). The SpiderFX filter was used in all cases and was deployed and retrieved successfully with no complications. The primary angiographic endpoint (<30 % residual stenosis or 30–50 % stenosis with <20 mmHg gradient across the lesion) was reached in 100 % of patients. Clinically significant embolic debris (≥2 mm) was collected in ~20 % of retrieved filters.

While a number of small single-center studies have confirmed the regular occurrence of distal embolization in peripheral endovascular intervention, it is not completely clear if the use of embolic protection devices (EPDs) is indicated in all cases. High-risk factors for distal embolism include major embolic debris, increased lesion length, increased reference vessel diameter, chronic total occlusions, thrombosed bypass grafts, stent thromboses, subacute symptoms (fresh clot), and CLI patients with single-vessel runoff [148, 150].

Shrikhande et al. reviewed available prospective registry data to examine incidence of distal embolization occurring during the treatment of 2137 lesions in 1029 patients undergoing atherectomy using four different atherectomy devices [151]. Significantly, they found an overall embolization rate of 1.6 % (based on pre- and post-runoff angiograms) with higher rates of embolization seen in both more complex lesions and chronic total occlusions when compared to de novo lesions (3.2 % vs 2.4 % vs 0.9 %, respectively, $p = 0.01$). There was also significant variance in rates of embolization observed between devices/techniques used. Jetstream and Diamondback 360 (Cardiovascular Systems Inc., St Paul, MN) had a combined embolization rate of 22 % that was significantly higher than with PTA alone (0.9 %), PTA plus stent (0.7 %), SilverHawk atherectomy (1.9 %), and laser atherectomy (3.6 %).

It is clear that the incidence of both macro- and microembolization is significant in lower extremity endovascular interventions and that the safety and efficacy of EPDs are clear. Large randomized controlled trials are needed to truly define the role of routine EPD use. Furthermore, better risk stratification and algorithms based upon patient, lesion, and treatment characteristics are needed.

Summary

While significant advances have been made in the endovascular treatment of PAD, more studies are needed to gauge the efficacy of this technology in patients with CLI. These patients have a complex clinical course, and even though a number of studies for newer device technologies do incorporate a subset of CLI patients, in the end, widespread acceptability of these device technologies will depend upon reasonable demonstration of safety and efficacy in such patients. Furthermore, all these treatment modalities, including surgical options, should not be treated as all or none options. Some guidance is offered in published guidelines regarding appropriate use of the intervention strategies [152, 153]; however, it is the individual patient and the nature of their disease process which should dictate appropriate selection of treatment options and a combination of therapy options can always be selected. Thus, it is up to the physician to be best aware of the evidence guiding the treatment therapies so that the best care plan can be offered to each individual patient.

References

1. Fowkes FG, Rudan D, Rudan I, Aboyans V, Denenberg JO, Mcdermott MM, et al. Comparison of global estimates of prevalence and risk factors for peripheral artery disease in 2000 and 2010: a systematic review and analysis. Lancet. 2013;382(9901):1329–40. doi:10.1016/S0140-6736(13)61249-0.

2. Beckman JA, Paneni F, Cosentino F, Creager MA. Diabetes and vascular disease: pathophysiology, clinical consequences, and medical therapy: part II. Eur Heart J. 2013;34(31):2444–52. doi:10.1093/eurheartj/eht142.

3. Gray BH, Laird JR, Ansel GM, Shuck JW. Complex endovascular treatment for critical limb ischemia in poor surgical candidates: a pilot study. J Endovasc Ther. 2002;9(5):599–604. doi:10.1583/1545-1550(2002)009<0599:Cetfcl>2.0.Co;2.

4. Malas MB, Enwerem N, Qazi U, Brown B, Schneider EB, Reifsnyder T, et al. Comparison of surgical bypass with angioplasty and stenting of superficial femoral artery disease. J Vasc Surg. 2014;59(1):129–35. doi:10.1016/J.Jvs.2013.05.100.

5. Adam DJ, Beard JD, Cleveland T, Bell J, Bradbury AW, Forbes JF, et al. Bypass versus angioplasty in severe ischaemia of the leg (BASIL): multicentre, randomised controlled trial. Lancet. 2005;366(9501):1925–34. doi:10.1016/S0140-6736(05)67704-5.

6. Bennett MR. In-stent stenosis: pathology and implications for the development of drug eluting stents. Heart. 2003;89(2):218–24.

7. Fattori R, Piva T. Drug-eluting stents in vascular intervention. Lancet. 2003;361(9353):247–9. doi:10.1016/S0140-6736(03)12275-1.

8. Ozaki Y, Violaris AG, Serruys PW. New stent technologies. Prog Cardiovasc Dis. 1996;39(2):129–40. doi:10.1016/S0033-0620(96)80022-3.

9. Regar E, Sianos G, Serruys PW. Stent development and local drug delivery. Br Med Bull. 2001;59:227–48.

10. Hehrlein C, Arab A, Bode C. Drug-eluting stent: the "magic bullet" for prevention of restenosis? Basic Res Cardiol. 2002;97(6):417–23. doi:10.1007/S00395-002-0379-2.

11. Inoue S, Koyama H, Miyata T, Shigematsu H. Pathogenetic heterogeneity of in-stent lesion formation in human peripheral arterial disease. J Vasc Surg. 2002;35(4):672–8.

12. Schwertz DW, Vaitkus P. Drug-eluting stents to prevent reblockage of coronary arteries. J Cardiovasc Nurs. 2003;18(1):11–6.

13. Lemos PA, Regar E, Serruys PW. Drug-eluting stents in the treatment of atherosclerotic coronary heart disease. Indian Heart J. 2002;54(2):212–6.

14. Heldman AW, Cheng L, Jenkins GM, Heller PF, Kim DW, Ware Jr M, et al. Paclitaxel stent coating inhibits neointimal hyperplasia at 4 weeks in a porcine model of coronary restenosis. Circulation. 2001;103(18):2289–95.

15. Neville RF, Sidawy AN. Myointimal hyperplasia: basic science and clinical considerations. Semin Vasc Surg. 1998;11(3):142–8.

16. Dormandy JA, Rutherford RB. Management of peripheral arterial disease (PAD). Tasc Working Group. Transatlantic Inter-Society Consensus (TASC). J Vasc Surg. 2000;31(1 Pt 2):S1–296.

17. Bakal CW, Sprayregen S, Scheinbaum K, Cynamon J, Veith FJ. Percutaneous transluminal angioplasty of the infrapopliteal arteries: results in 53 patients. AJR Am J Roentgenol. 1990;154(1):171–4. doi:10.2214/Ajr.154.1.2136784.

18. Dorros G, Jaff MR, Dorros AM, Mathiak LM, He T. Tibioperoneal (outflow lesion) angioplasty can be used as primary treatment in 235 patients with critical limb ischemia: five-year follow-up. Circulation. 2001;104(17):2057–62.

19. Soder HK, Manninen HI, Jaakkola P, Matsi PJ, Rasanen H, Kaukanen E, et al. Prospective trial of infrapopliteal artery balloon angioplasty for critical limb ischemia: angiographic and clinical results. J Vasc Interv Radiol. 2000;11(8):1021–31.

20. Tsetis D, Belli AM. The role of infrapopliteal angioplasty. Br J Radiol. 2004;77(924):1007–15.

21. Trocciola SM, Chaer R, Dayal R, Lin SC, Kumar N, Rhee J, et al. Comparison of results in endovascular interventions for infrainguinal lesions: claudication versus critical limb ischemia. Am Surg. 2005;71(6):474–9. Discussion 9-80.

22. Chowdhury MM, Mclain AD, Twine CP. Angioplasty versus bare metal stenting for superficial femoral artery lesions. Cochrane Database Syst Rev. 2014;6:CD006767. doi:10.1002/14651858. CD006767.pub3.

23. Mwipatayi BP, Hockings A, Hofmann M, Garbowski M, Sieunarine K. Balloon angioplasty compared with stenting for treatment of femoropopliteal occlusive disease: a meta-analysis. J Vasc Surg. 2008;47(2):461–9. doi:10.1016/j.jvs.2007.07.059.

24. Vogel TR, Shindelman LE, Nackman GB, Graham AM. Efficacious use of nitinol stents in the femoral and popliteal arteries. J Vasc Surg. 2003;38(6):1178–84. doi:10.1016/j.jvs.2003.09.011.

25. Laird JR, Katzen BT, Scheinert D, Lammer J, Carpenter J, Buchbinder M, et al. Nitinol stent implantation versus balloon angioplasty for lesions in the superficial femoral artery and proximal popliteal artery: twelve-month results from the resilient randomized trial. Circ Cardiovasc Interv. 2010;3(3):267–76. doi:10.1161/Circinterventions.109.903468.

26. Gray WA, Feiring A, Cioppi M, Hibbard R, Gray B, Khatib Y, et al. S.M.A.R.T. Self-expanding nitinol stent for the treatment of atherosclerotic lesions in the superficial femoral artery (STROLL): 1-year outcomes. J Vasc Interv Radiol. 2014. doi:10.1016/j. jvir.2014.09.018.

27. Scheinert D, Grummt L, Piorkowski M, Sax J, Scheinert S, Ulrich M, et al. A novel self-expanding interwoven nitinol stent for complex femoropopliteal lesions: 24-month results of the SUPERA SFA registry. J Endovasc Ther. 2011;18(6):745–52. doi:10.1583/11-3500.1.

28. Scheinert D, Werner M, Scheinert S, Paetzold A, Banning-Eichenseer U, Piorkowski M, et al. Treatment of complex atherosclerotic popliteal artery disease with a new self-expanding interwoven nitinol stent: 12-month results of the Leipzig SUPERA

29. Leon Jr LR, Dieter RS, Gadd CL, Ranellone E, Mills Sr JL, Montero-Baker MF, et al. Preliminary results of the initial United States experience with the Supera woven nitinol stent in the popliteal artery. J Vasc Surg. 2013;57(4):1014–22. doi:10.1016/J. Jvs.2012.10.093.

30. Chan YC, Cheng SW, Ting AC, Cheung GC. Primary stenting of femoropopliteal atherosclerotic lesions using new helical interwoven nitinol stents. J Vasc Surg. 2014;59(2):384–91. doi:10.1016/J. Jvs.2013.08.037.

31. George JC, Rosen ES, Nachtigall J, Vanhise A, Kovach R. SUPERA interwoven nitinol Stent Outcomes in Above-Knee IntErventions (SAKE) study. J Vasc Interv Radiol. 2014;25(6):954–61. doi:10.1016/j.jvir.2014.03.004.

32. Rosenfield K, Editor. Comparison of the Supera peripheral system to a performance goal derived from balloon angioplasty clinical trials in the superficial femoral artery. Vascular Interventional Advances (Viva), Las Vegas. 2012.

33. Garcia L. Comparison of the Supera peripheral system to a performance goal derived from balloon angioplasty clinical trials in the superficial femoral artery (SUPERB): 3 year results. Vascular Interventional Advances (Viva); 2014 Nov; Las Vegas. 2014.

34. Laird JR, Armstrong EJ. Stents for femoropopliteal disease: are some things better covered up? J Am Coll Cardiol. 2013;62(15):1328–9. doi:10.1016/J.Jacc.2013.06.031.

35. Saxon RR, Coffman JM, Gooding JM, Ponec DJ. Long-term patency and clinical outcome of the Viabahn stent-graft for femoropopliteal artery obstructions. J Vasc Interv Radiol. 2007;18(11):1341–9. doi:10.1016/J.Jvir.2007.07.011. Quiz 50.

36. Bauermeister G. Endovascular stent-grafting in the treatment of superficial femoral artery occlusive disease. J Endovasc Ther. 2001;8(3):315–20. doi:10.1583/1545-1550(2001)008<0315:Esgit t>2.0.Co;2.

37. Hartung O, Otero A, Dubuc M, Boufi M, Barthelemy P, Aissi K, et al. Efficacy of Hemobahn in the treatment of superficial femoral artery lesions in patients with acute or critical ischemia: a comparative study with claudicants. Eur J Vasc Endovasc Surg. 2005;30(3):300–6. doi:10.1016/J.Ejvs.2005.04.027.

38. Jahnke T, Andresen R, Muller-Hulsbeck S, Schafer FK, Voshage G, Heller M, et al. Hemobahn stent-grafts for treatment of femoropopliteal arterial obstructions: midterm results of a prospective trial. J Vasc Interv Radiol. 2003;14(1):41–51.

39. Lammer J, Dake MD, Bleyn J, Katzen BT, Cejna M, Piquet P, et al. Peripheral arterial obstruction: prospective study of treatment with a transluminally placed self-expanding stent-graft. International Trial Study Group. Radiology. 2000;217(1):95–104. doi:10.1148/Radiology.217.1.R00se0595.

40. Saxon RR, Coffman JM, Gooding JM, Natuzzi E, Ponec DJ. Long-term results of ePTFE stent-graft versus angioplasty in the femoropopliteal artery: single center experience from a prospective, randomized trial. J Vasc Interv Radiol. 2003;14(3):303–11.

41. Saxon RR, Dake MD, Volgelzang RL, Katzen BT, Becker GJ. Randomized, multicenter study comparing expanded polytetrafluoroethylene-covered endoprosthesis placement with percutaneous transluminal angioplasty in the treatment of superficial femoral artery occlusive disease. J Vasc Interv Radiol. 2008;19(6):823–32. doi:10.1016/J.Jvir.2008.02.008.

42. Kedora J, Hohmann S, Garrett W, Munschaur C, Theune B, Gable D. Randomized comparison of percutaneous Viabahn stent grafts vs prosthetic femoral-popliteal bypass in the treatment of superficial femoral arterial occlusive disease. J Vasc Surg. 2007;45(1):10–6. doi:10.1016/j.jvs.2006.08.074. Discussion 6.

43. Mcquade K, Gable D, Hohman S, Pearl G, Theune B. Randomized comparison of ePTFE/nitinol self-expanding stent graft vs prosthetic femoral-popliteal bypass in the treatment of superficial

femoral artery occlusive disease. J Vasc Surg. 2009;49(1):109–15. doi:10.1016/j.jvs.2008.08.041. 116.e1–9; discussion 116.

44. Mcquade K, Gable D, Pearl G, Theune B, Black S. Four-year randomized prospective comparison of percutaneous ePTFE/nitinol self-expanding stent graft versus prosthetic femoral-popliteal bypass in the treatment of superficial femoral artery occlusive disease. J Vasc Surg. 2010;52(3):584–90. doi:10.1016/j.jvs.2010.03.071. discussion 590-1, 591.e1–591.e7.

45. Geraghty PJ, Mewissen MW, Jaff MR, Ansel GM. Three-year results of the VIBRANT trial of VIABAHN endoprosthesis versus bare nitinol stent implantation for complex superficial femoral artery occlusive disease. J Vasc Surg. 2013;58(2):386–95.e4. doi:10.1016/j.jvs.2013.01.050.

46. Saxon RR, Chervu A, Jones PA, Bajwa TK, Gable DR, Soukas PA, et al. Heparin-bonded, expanded polytetrafluoroethylene-lined stent graft in the treatment of femoropopliteal artery disease: 1-year results of the VIPER (Viabahn Endoprosthesis with Heparin Bioactive Surface in the Treatment of Superficial Femoral Artery Obstructive Disease) trial. J Vasc Interv Radiol. 2013;24(2):165–73. doi:10.1016/j.jvir.2012.10.004. quiz 174.

47. Lammer J, Zeller T, Hausegger KA, Schaefer PJ, Gschwendtner M, Mueller-Huelsbeck S, et al. Heparin-bonded covered stents versus bare-metal stents for complex femoropopliteal artery lesions: the randomized VIASTAR trial (Viabahn endoprosthesis with PROPATEN bioactive surface [VIA] versus bare nitinol stent in the treatment of long lesions in superficial femoral artery occlusive disease). J Am Coll Cardiol. 2013;62(15):1320–7. doi:10.1016/J.Jacc.2013.05.079.

48. Thierry B, Merhi Y, Bilodeau L, Trepanier C, Tabrizian M. Nitinol versus stainless steel stents: acute thrombogenicity study in an ex vivo porcine model. Biomaterials. 2002;23(14):2997–3005.

49. Jordan MA, Wilson L. Microtubules as a target for anticancer drugs. Nat Rev Cancer. 2004;4(4):253–65. doi:10.1038/Nrc1317.

50. Kataoka T, Grube E, Honda Y, Morino Y, Hur SH, Bonneau HN, et al. 7-Hexanoyltaxol-eluting stent for prevention of neointimal growth: an intravascular ultrasound analysis from the Study to COmpare REstenosis rate between QueST and QuaDS-QP2 (SCORE). Circulation. 2002;106(14):1788–93.

51. Virmani R, Liistro F, Stankovic G, Di Mario C, Montorfano M, Farb A, et al. Mechanism of late in-stent restenosis after implantation of a paclitaxel derivate-eluting polymer stent system in humans. Circulation. 2002;106(21):2649–51.

52. Stepkowski SM. Molecular targets for existing and novel immunosuppressive drugs. Expert Rev Mol Med. 2000;2(4):1–23. doi:10.1017/S1462399400001769.

53. Kamada Y, Funakoshi T, Shintani T, Nagano K, Ohsumi M, Ohsumi Y. Tor-mediated induction of autophagy via an Apg1 protein kinase complex. J Cell Biol. 2000;150(6):1507–13.

54. Claessen BE, Henriques JP, Dangas GD. Clinical studies with sirolimus, zotarolimus, everolimus, and biolimus A9 drug-eluting stent systems. Curr Pharm Des. 2010;16(36):4012–24.

55. Duda SH, Pusich B, Richter G, Landwehr P, Oliva VL, Tielbeek A, et al. Sirolimus-eluting stents for the treatment of obstructive superficial femoral artery disease: six-month results. Circulation. 2002;106(12):1505–9.

56. Duda SH, Bosiers M, Lammer J, Scheinert D, Zeller T, Tielbeek A, et al. Sirolimus-eluting versus bare nitinol stent for obstructive superficial femoral artery disease: the SIROCCO II trial. J Vasc Interv Radiol. 2005;16(3):331–8. doi:10.1097/01.Rvi.0000151260.74519.Ca.

57. Duda SH, Bosiers M, Lammer J, Scheinert D, Zeller T, Oliva V, et al. Drug-eluting and bare nitinol stents for the treatment of atherosclerotic lesions in the superficial femoral artery: long-term results from the SIROCCO trial. J Endovasc Ther. 2006;13(6):701–10. doi:10.1583/05-1704.1.

58. Singh KP, Sharma AM. Critical limb ischemia: current approach and future directions. J Cardiovasc Transl Res. 2014;7(4):437–45. doi:10.1007/S12265-014-9562-8.

59. Lammer J, Bosiers M, Zeller T, Schillinger M, Boone E, Zaugg MJ, et al. First clinical trial of nitinol self-expanding everolimus-eluting stent implantation for peripheral arterial occlusive disease. J Vasc Surg. 2011;54(2):394–401. doi:10.1016/J.Jvs.2011.01.047.

60. Dake MD, Ansel GM, Jaff MR, Ohki T, Saxon RR, Smouse HB, et al. Paclitaxel-eluting stents show superiority to balloon angioplasty and bare metal stents in femoropopliteal disease: twelve-month Zilver PTX randomized study results. Circ Cardiovasc Interv. 2011;4(5):495–504. doi:10.1161/Circinterventions.111.962324.

61. Dake MD, Ansel GM, Jaff MR, Ohki T, Saxon RR, Smouse HB, et al. Sustained safety and effectiveness of paclitaxel-eluting stents for femoropopliteal lesions: 2-year follow-up from the Zilver PTX randomized and single-arm clinical studies. J Am Coll Cardiol. 2013;61(24):2417–27. doi:10.1016/J.Jacc.2013.03.034.

62. Bosiers M, Peeters P, Tessarek J, Deloose K, Strickler S. The Zilver® PTX® Single Arm Study: 12-month results from the TASC C/D lesion subgroup. J Cardiovasc Surg (Torino). 2013;54(1):115–22.

63. Bosiers M, Deloose K, Verbist J, Peeters P. Percutaneous transluminal angioplasty for treatment of "below-the-knee" critical limb ischemia: early outcomes following the use of sirolimus-eluting stents. J Cardiovasc Surg (Torino). 2006;47(2):171–6.

64. Siablis D, Karnabatidis D, Katsanos K, Kagadis GC, Kraniotis P, Diamantopoulos A, et al. Sirolimus-eluting versus bare stents after suboptimal infrapopliteal angioplasty for critical limb ischemia: enduring 1-year angiographic and clinical benefit. J Endovasc Ther. 2007;14(2):241–50. doi:10.1583/1545-1550(2007)14[241:Svbsas]2.0.Co;2.

65. Siablis D, Kraniotis P, Karnabatidis D, Kagadis GC, Katsanos K, Tsolakis J. Sirolimus-eluting versus bare stents for bailout after suboptimal infrapopliteal angioplasty for critical limb ischemia: 6-month angiographic results from a nonrandomized prospective single-center study. J Endovasc Ther. 2005;12(6):685–95. doi:10.1583/05-1620mr.1.

66. Commeau P, Barragan P, Roquebert PO. Sirolimus for below the knee lesions: mid-term results of SiroBTK study. Catheter Cardiovasc Interv. 2006;68(5):793–8. doi:10.1002/Ccd.20893.

67. Feiring AJ, Krahn M, Nelson L, Wesolowski A, Eastwood D, Szabo A. Preventing leg amputations in critical limb ischemia with below-the-knee drug-eluting stents: the PaRADISE (PReventing Amputations using Drug eluting StEnts) trial. J Am Coll Cardiol. 2010;55(15):1580–9. doi:10.1016/J.Jacc.2009.11.072.

68. Norgren L, Hiatt WR, Dormandy JA, Nehler MR, Harris KA, Fowkes FG. Inter-Society Consensus for the Management of Peripheral Arterial Disease (TASC II). J Vasc Surg. 2007;45(Suppl S):S5–67. doi:10.1016/J.Jvs.2006.12.037.

69. Falkowski A, Poncyljusz W, Wilk G, Szczerbo-Trojanowska M. The evaluation of primary stenting of sirolimus-eluting versus bare-metal stents in the treatment of atherosclerotic lesions of crural arteries. Eur Radiol. 2009;19(4):966–74. doi:10.1007/S00330-008-1225-1.

70. Scheinert D, Katsanos K, Zeller T, Koppensteiner R, Commeau P, Bosiers M, et al. A prospective randomized multicenter comparison of balloon angioplasty and infrapopliteal stenting with the sirolimus-eluting stent in patients with ischemic peripheral arterial disease: 1-year results from the ACHILLES trial. J Am Coll Cardiol. 2012;60(22):2290–5. doi:10.1016/J.Jacc.2012.08.989.

71. Rastan A, Tepe G, Krankenberg H, Zahorsky R, Beschorner U, Noory E, et al. Sirolimus-eluting stents vs. bare-metal stents for treatment of focal lesions in infrapopliteal arteries: a double-blind, multi-centre, randomized clinical trial. Eur Heart J. 2011;32(18):2274–81. doi:10.1093/eurheartj/ehr144.

72. Rastan A, Brechtel K, Krankenberg H, Zahorsky R, Tepe G, Noory E, et al. Sirolimus-eluting stents for treatment of infrapopliteal arteries reduce clinical event rate compared to bare-metal stents: long-term results from a randomized trial. J Am Coll Cardiol. 2012;60(7):587–91. doi:10.1016/J.Jacc.2012.04.035.

73. Bosiers M, Scheinert D, Peeters P, Torsello G, Zeller T, Deloose K, et al. Randomized comparison of everolimus-eluting versus bare-metal stents in patients with critical limb ischemia and infrapopliteal arterial occlusive disease. J Vasc Surg. 2012;55(2):390–8. doi:10.1016/j.jvs.2011.07.099.

74. Fusaro M, Cassese S, Ndrepepa G, Tepe G, King L, Ott I, et al. Drug-eluting stents for revascularization of infrapopliteal arteries: updated meta-analysis of randomized trials. JACC Cardiovasc Interv. 2013;6(12):1284–93. doi:10.1016/J.Jcin.2013.08.007.

75. Biondi-Zoccai GG, Sangiorgi G, Lotrionte M, Feiring A, Commeau P, Fusaro M, et al. Infragenicular stent implantation for below-the-knee atherosclerotic disease: clinical evidence from an international collaborative meta-analysis on 640 patients. J Endovasc Ther. 2009;16(3):251–60. doi:10.1583/09-2691.1.

76. Laird J, Jaff MR, Biamino G, Mcnamara T, Scheinert D, Zetterlund P, et al. Cryoplasty for the treatment of femoropopliteal arterial disease: results of a prospective, multicenter registry. J Vasc Interv Radiol. 2005;16(8):1067–73. doi:10.1097/01.Rvi.0000167866.86201.4e.

77. Laird JR, Biamino G, Mcnamara T, Scheinert D, Zetterlund P, Moen E, et al. Cryoplasty for the treatment of femoropopliteal arterial disease: extended follow-up results. J Endovasc Ther. 2006;13 Suppl 2:II52–9.

78. Jahnke T, Mueller-Huelsbeck S, Charalambous N, Trentmann J, Jamili A, Huemme TH, et al. Prospective, randomized single-center trial to compare cryoplasty versus conventional angioplasty in the popliteal artery: midterm results of the cold study. J Vasc Interv Radiol. 2010;21(2):186–94. doi:10.1016/J.Jvir.2009.10.021.

79. Spiliopoulos S, Katsanos K, Karnabatidis D, Diamantopoulos A, Kagadis GC, Christeas N, et al. Cryoplasty versus conventional balloon angioplasty of the femoropopliteal artery in diabetic patients: long-term results from a prospective randomized single-center controlled trial. Cardiovasc Intervent Radiol. 2010;33(5):929–38. doi:10.1007/S00270-010-9915-X.

80. Das TS, Mcnamara T, Gray B, Sedillo GJ, Turley BR, Kollmeyer K, et al. Primary cryoplasty therapy provides durable support for limb salvage in critical limb ischemia patients with infrapopliteal lesions: 12-month follow-up results from the BTK Chill Trial. J Endovasc Ther. 2009;16(2 Suppl 2):II19–30. doi:10.1583/08-2652.1.

81. Bosiers M, Deloose K, Vermassen F, Schroe H, Lauwers G, Lansinck W, et al. The use of the cryoplasty technique in the treatment of infrapopliteal lesions for critical limb ischemia patients in a routine hospital setting: one-year outcome of the Cryoplasty CLIMB Registry. J Cardiovasc Surg (Torino). 2010;51(2):193–202.

82. Cejna M. Cutting balloon: review on principles and background of use in peripheral arteries. Cardiovasc Intervent Radiol. 2005;28(4):400–8. doi:10.1007/S00270-004-0115-4.

83. Ansel GM, Sample NS, Botti Jr IC, Tracy AJ, Silver MJ, Marshall BJ, et al. Cutting balloon angioplasty of the popliteal and infrapopliteal vessels for symptomatic limb ischemia. Catheter Cardiovasc Interv. 2004;61(1):1–4. doi:10.1002/Ccd.10731.

84. Canaud L, Alric P, Berthet JP, Marty-Ane C, Mercier G, Branchereau P. Infrainguinal cutting balloon angioplasty in de novo arterial lesions. J Vasc Surg. 2008;48(5):1182–8. doi:10.1016/J.Jvs.2008.06.053.

85. Rabbi JF, Kiran RP, Gersten G, Dudrick SJ, Dardik A. Early results with infrainguinal cutting balloon angioplasty limits distal dissection. Ann Vasc Surg. 2004;18(6):640–3. doi:10.1007/S10016-004-0103-9.

86. Amighi J, Schillinger M, Dick P, Schlager O, Sabeti S, Mlekusch W, et al. De novo superficial femoropopliteal artery lesions: peripheral cutting balloon angioplasty and restenosis rates--randomized controlled trial. Radiology. 2008;247(1):267–72. doi:10.1148/Radiol.2471070749.

87. Engelke C, Morgan RA, Belli AM. Cutting balloon percutaneous transluminal angioplasty for salvage of lower limb arterial bypass grafts: feasibility. Radiology. 2002;223(1):106–14. doi:10.1148/Radiol.2231010793.

88. Westin GG, Armstrong EJ, Javed U, Balwanz CR, Saeed H, Pevec WC, et al. Endovascular therapy is effective treatment for focal stenoses in failing infrapopliteal vein grafts. Ann Vasc Surg. 2014;28(8):1823–31. doi:10.1016/J.Avsg.2014.07.015.

89. Scheinert D, Peeters P, Bosiers M, O'sullivan G, Sultan S, Gershony G. Results of the multicenter first-in-man study of a novel scoring balloon catheter for the treatment of infra-popliteal peripheral arterial disease. Catheter Cardiovasc Interv. 2007;70(7):1034–9. doi:10.1002/Ccd.21341.

90. Bosiers M, Deloose K, Cagiannos C, Verbist J, Peeters P. Use of the AngioSculpt scoring balloon for infrapopliteal lesions in patients with critical limb ischemia: 1-year outcome. Vascular. 2009;17(1):29–35.

91. Schnorr B, Albrecht T. Drug-coated balloons and their place in treating peripheral arterial disease. Expert Rev Med Devices. 2013;10(1):105–14. doi:10.1586/Erd.12.67.

92. Kasapis C, Gurm HS. Current approach to the diagnosis and treatment of femoral-popliteal arterial disease. A systematic review. Curr Cardiol Rev. 2009;5(4):296–311. doi:10.2174/157340309789317823.

93. Scheinert D, Scheinert S, Sax J, Piorkowski C, Braunlich S, Ulrich M, et al. Prevalence and clinical impact of stent fractures after femoropopliteal stenting. J Am Coll Cardiol. 2005;45(2):312–5. doi:10.1016/J.Jacc.2004.11.026.

94. Tepe G, Zeller T, Albrecht T, Heller S, Schwarzwalder U, Beregi JP, et al. Local delivery of paclitaxel to inhibit restenosis during angioplasty of the leg. N Engl J Med. 2008;358(7):689–99. doi:10.1056/Nejmoa0706356.

95. Tepe G, editor. 5-Year thunder follow-up: patients with pad treated with uncoated versus paccocath paclitaxel coated balloons. J Am Coll Cardiol. 2011; 58(20s1):B151-B151. doi:10.1016/j.jacc.2011.10.572.

96. Werk M, Langner S, Reinkensmeier B, Boettcher HF, Tepe G, Dietz U, et al. Inhibition of restenosis in femoropopliteal arteries: paclitaxel-coated versus uncoated balloon: femoral paclitaxel randomized pilot trial. Circulation. 2008;118(13):1358–65. doi:10.1161/Circulationaha.107.735985.

97. Scheinert D, Duda S, Zeller T, Krankenberg H, Ricke J, Bosiers M, et al. The LEVANT I (Lutonix paclitaxel-coated balloon for the prevention of femoropopliteal restenosis) trial for femoropopliteal revascularization: first-in-human randomized trial of low-dose drug-coated balloon versus uncoated balloon angioplasty. JACC Cardiovasc Interv. 2014;7(1):10–9. doi:10.1016/J.Jcin.2013.05.022.

98. FDA. FDA executive summary prepared for the June 12, 2014 meeting of the Circulatory System Devices Advisory Panel Bard Lutonix® 035 Drug Coated Balloon PTA Catheter. 2014.

99. Werk M, Albrecht T, Meyer DR, Ahmed MN, Behne A, Dietz U, et al. Paclitaxel-coated balloons reduce restenosis after femoro-popliteal angioplasty: evidence from the randomized PACIFIER trial. Circ Cardiovasc Interv. 2012;5(6):831–40. doi:10.1161/Circinterventions.112.971630.

100. Fanelli F, Cannavale A, Boatta E, Corona M, Lucatelli P, Wlderk A, et al. Lower limb multilevel treatment with drug-eluting balloons: 6-month results from the DEBELLUM randomized trial. J Endovasc Ther. 2012;19(5):571–80. doi:10.1583/Jevt-12-3926mr.1.

101. Fanelli F, Cannavale A, Corona M, Lucatelli P, Wlderk A, Salvatori FM. The "DEBELLUM"--lower limb multilevel treatment with drug eluting balloon--randomized trial: 1-year results. J Cardiovasc Surg (Torino). 2014;55(2):207–16.

102. Tepe G, Laird J, Schneider P, Brodmann M, Krishnan P, Micari A, et al. Drug-coated balloon versus standard percutaneous transluminal angioplasty for the treatment of superficial femoral and/or popliteal peripheral artery disease: 12-month results from the IN.PACT SFA randomized trial. Circulation. 2014. doi:10.1161/Circulationaha.114.011004.

103. Zeller T, Rastan A, Macharzina R, Tepe G, Kaspar M, Chavarria J, et al. Drug-coated balloons vs. drug-eluting stents for treatment of long femoropopliteal lesions. J Endovasc Ther. 2014;21(3):359–68. doi:10.1583/13-4630mr.1.

104. Rooke TW, Hirsch AT, Misra S, Sidawy AN, Beckman JA, Findeiss L, et al. Management of patients with peripheral artery disease (compilation of 2005 and 2011 ACCF/AHA Guideline Recommendations): a report of the American College of Cardiology Foundation/American Heart Association Task Force on Practice Guidelines. J Am Coll Cardiol. 2013;61(14):1555–70. doi:10.1016/J.Jacc.2013.01.004.

105. Katsanos K, Spiliopoulos S, Karunanithy N, Krokidis M, Sabharwal T, Taylor P. Bayesian network meta-analysis of nitinol stents, covered stents, drug-eluting stents, and drug-coated balloons in the femoropopliteal artery. J Vasc Surg. 2014;59(4):1123–33.e8. doi:10.1016/j.jvs.2014.01.041.

106. Liistro F, Grotti S, Porto I, Angioli P, Ricci L, Ducci K, et al. Drug-eluting balloon in peripheral intervention for the superficial femoral artery: the DEBATE-SFA randomized trial (drug eluting balloon in peripheral intervention for the superficial femoral artery). JACC Cardiovasc Interv. 2013;6(12):1295–302. doi:10.1016/j.jcin.2013.07.010.

107. Cioppa A, Stabile E, Popusoi G, Salemme L, Cota L, Pucciarelli A, et al. Combined treatment of heavy calcified femoro-popliteal lesions using directional atherectomy and a paclitaxel coated balloon: one-year single centre clinical results. Cardiovasc Revasc Med. 2012;13(4):219–23. doi:10.1016/J.Carrev.2012.04.007.

108. Zeller T. 12-month results: directional atherectomy followed by a paclitaxel-coated balloon to inhibit restenosis and maintain vessel patency (DEFINITIVE-AR). Vascular Interventional Advances (Viva); 2014 Nov; Las Vegas. 2014.

109. Liistro F, Porto I, Angioli P, Grotti S, Ricci L, Ducci K, et al. Drug-eluting balloon in peripheral intervention for below the knee angioplasty evaluation (DEBATE-BTK): a randomized trial in diabetic patients with critical limb ischemia. Circulation. 2013;128(6):615–21. doi:10.1161/Circulationaha.113.001811.

110. Schmidt A, Piorkowski M, Werner M, Ulrich M, Bausback Y, Braunlich S, et al. First experience with drug-eluting balloons in infrapopliteal arteries: restenosis rate and clinical outcome. J Am Coll Cardiol. 2011;58(11):1105–9. doi:10.1016/J.Jacc.2011.05.034.

111. Zeller T, Baumgartner I, Scheinert D, Brodmann M, Bosiers M, Micari A, et al. Drug-eluting balloon versus standard balloon angioplasty for infrapopliteal arterial revascularization in critical limb ischemia: 12-month results from the IN.PACT DEEP randomized trial. J Am Coll Cardiol. 2014;64(15):1568–76. doi:10.1016/J.Jacc.2014.06.1198.

112. Laird JR, Zeller T, Gray BH, Scheinert D, Vranic M, Reiser C, et al. Limb salvage following laser-assisted angioplasty for critical limb ischemia: results of the LACI multicenter trial. J Endovasc Ther. 2006;13(1):1–11. doi:10.1583/05-1674.1.

113. Romiti M, Albers M, Brochado-Neto FC, Durazzo AE, Pereira CA, De Luccia N. Meta-analysis of infrapopliteal angioplasty for chronic critical limb ischemia. J Vasc Surg. 2008;47(5):975–81. doi:10.1016/J.Jvs.2008.01.005.

114. Laird JR, Armstrong EJ. Drug-coated balloons for infrapopliteal disease: digging deep to understand the impact of a negative trial.

115. Scheinert D, Laird Jr JR, Schroder M, Steinkamp H, Balzer JO, Biamino G. Excimer laser-assisted recanalization of long, chronic superficial femoral artery occlusions. J Endovasc Ther. 2001;8(2):156–66. doi:10.1583/1545-1550(2001)008<0156:Elarol>2.0.Co;2.

116. Laird J, editor. Peripheral excimer laser angioplasty (PELA) Trial results. 14th Annual Scientific Symposium Transcatheter Cardiovascular Therapeutics; 2002; Washington, DC.

117. Dave RM, Patlola R, Kollmeyer K, Bunch F, Weinstock BS, Dippel E, et al. Excimer laser recanalization of femoropopliteal lesions and 1-year patency: results of the CELLO registry. J Endovasc Ther. 2009;16(6):665–75. doi:10.1583/09-2781.109-2781.

118. Shammas NW, Coiner D, Shammas GA, Dippel EJ, Christensen L, Jerin M. Percutaneous lower-extremity arterial interventions with primary balloon angioplasty versus Silverhawk atherectomy and adjunctive balloon angioplasty: randomized trial. J Vasc Interv Radiol. 2011;22(9):1223–8. doi:10.1016/J.Jvir.2011.05.013.

119. Roberts D, Niazi K, Miller W, Krishnan P, Gammon R, Schreiber T, et al. Effective endovascular treatment of calcified femoropopliteal disease with directional atherectomy and distal embolic protection: final results of the DEFINITIVE Ca(+)(+) trial. Catheter Cardiovasc Interv. 2014;84(2):236–44. doi:10.1002/Ccd.25384.

120. Zeller T, Krankenberg H, Steinkamp H, Rastan A, Sixt S, Schmidt A, et al. One-year outcome of percutaneous rotational atherectomy with aspiration in infrainguinal peripheral arterial occlusive disease: the multicenter pathway PVD trial. J Endovasc Ther. 2009;16(6):653–62. doi:10.1583/09-2826.1.

121. Bolia A, Miles KA, Brennan J, Bell PR. Percutaneous transluminal angioplasty of occlusions of the femoral and popliteal arteries by subintimal dissection. Cardiovasc Intervent Radiol. 1990;13(6):357–63.

122. Charalambous N, Schafer PJ, Trentmann J, Humme TH, Stohring C, Muller-Hulsbeck S, et al. Percutaneous intraluminal recanalization of long, chronic superficial femoral and popliteal occlusions using the Frontrunner XP CTO device: a single-center experience. Cardiovasc Intervent Radiol. 2010;33(1):25–33. doi:10.1007/S00270-009-9700-X.

123. Mossop P, Cincotta M, Whitbourn R. First case reports of controlled blunt microdissection for percutaneous transluminal angioplasty of chronic total occlusions in peripheral arteries. Catheter Cardiovasc Interv. 2003;59(2):255–8. doi:10.1002/Ccd.10529.

124. Mossop PJ, Amukotuwa SA, Whitbourn RJ. Controlled blunt microdissection for percutaneous recanalization of lower limb arterial chronic total occlusions: a single center experience. Catheter Cardiovasc Interv. 2006;68(2):304–10. doi:10.1002/Ccd.20703.

125. Shetty R, Vivek G, Thakkar A, Prasad R, Pai U, Nayak K. Safety and efficacy of the frontrunner XP catheter for recanalization of chronic total occlusion of the femoropopliteal arteries. J Invasive Cardiol. 2013;25(7):344–7.

126. Al-Ameri H, Mayeda GS, Shavelle DM. Use of high-frequency vibrational energy in the treatment of peripheral chronic total occlusions. Catheter Cardiovasc Interv. 2009;74(7):1110–5. doi:10.1002/Ccd.22163.

127. Gandini R, Volpi T, Pipitone V, Simonetti G. Intraluminal recanalization of long infrainguinal chronic total occlusions using the Crosser system. J Endovasc Ther. 2009;16(1):23–7. doi:10.1583/08-2520.1.

128. Staniloae CS, Mody KP, Yadav SS, Han SY, Korabathina R. Endoluminal treatment of peripheral chronic total occlusions using the Crosser(R) recanalization catheter. J Invasive Cardiol. 2011;23(9):359–62.

129. Khalid MR, Khalid FR, Farooqui FA, Devireddy CM, Robertson GC, Niazi K. A novel catheter in patients with peripheral chronic

total occlusions: a single center experience. Catheter Cardiovasc Interv. 2010;76(5):735–9. doi:10.1002/Ccd.22607.

130. Laird J, Joye J, Sachdev N, Huang P, Caputo R, Mohiuddin I, et al. Recanalization of infrainguinal chronic total occlusions with the crosser system: results of the PATRIOT trial. J Invasive Cardiol. 2014;26(10):497–504.

131. Michalis LK, Tsetis DK, Katsamouris AN, Rees MR, Sideris DA, Gourtsoyiannis NC. Vibrational angioplasty in the treatment of chronic femoropopliteal arterial occlusions: preliminary experience. J Endovasc Ther. 2001;8(6):615–21. doi:10.1583/1545-1550(2001)008<0615:Vaitto>2.0.Co;2.

132. Tsetis DK, Michalis LK, Rees MR, Katsamouris AN, Matsagas MI, Katsouras CS, et al. Vibrational angioplasty in the treatment of chronic infrapopliteal arterial occlusions: preliminary experience. J Endovasc Ther. 2002;9(6):889–95. doi:10.1583/1545-1550(2002)009<0889:Vaitto>2.0.Co;2.

133. Kapralos I, Kehagias E, Ioannou C, Bouloukaki I, Kostas T, Katsamouris A, et al. Vibrational angioplasty in recanalization of chronic femoropopliteal arterial occlusions: single center experience. Eur J Radiol. 2014;83(1):155–62. doi:10.1016/J.Ejrad.2013.09.026.

134. Boccalandro F, Muench A, Sdringola S, Rosales OR. Wireless laser-assisted angioplasty of the superficial femoral artery in patients with critical limb ischemia who have failed conventional percutaneous revascularization. Catheter Cardiovasc Interv. 2004;63(1):7–12. doi:10.1002/Ccd.20084.

135. Steinkamp HJ, Rademaker J, Wissgott C, Scheinert D, Werk M, Settmacher U, et al. Percutaneous transluminal laser angioplasty versus balloon dilation for treatment of popliteal artery occlusions. J Endovasc Ther. 2002;9(6):882–8. doi:10.1583/1545-1550(2002)009<0882:Ptlavb>2.0.Co;2.

136. Steinkamp HJ, Werk M, Haufe M, Felix R. Laser angioplasty of peripheral arteries after unsuccessful recanalization of the superficial femoral artery. Int J Cardiovasc Intervent. 2000;3(3):153–60. doi:10.1080/14628840050516064.

137. Pigott JP, Raja MI, Davis T. A multicenter experience evaluating chronic total occlusion crossing with the Wildcat catheter (the CONNECT study). J Vasc Surg. 2012;56(6):1615–21. doi:10.1016/J.Jvs.2012.06.071.

138. Schwindt A, Reimers B, Scheinert D, Selmon M, Pigott JP, George JC, et al. Crossing chronic total occlusions with the Ocelot system: the initial European experience. EuroIntervention. 2013;9(7):854–62. doi:10.4244/Eijv9i7a139.

139. Selmon MR, Schwindt AG, Cawich IM, Chamberlin JR, Das TS, Davis TP, et al. Final results of the chronic total occlusion crossing with the ocelot system II (CONNECT II) study. J Endovasc Ther. 2013;20(6):770–81. doi:10.1583/13-4380mr.1.

140. Bosiers M, Diaz-Cartelle J, Scheinert D, Peeters P, Dawkins KD. Revascularization of lower extremity chronic total occlusions with a novel intraluminal recanalization device: results of the ReOpen study. J Endovasc Ther. 2014;21(1):61–70. doi:10.1583/12-4083r.1.

141. Banerjee S, Sarode K, Das T, Hadidi O, Thomas R, Vinas A, et al. Endovascular treatment of infrainguinal chronic total occlusions

using the TruePath device: features, handling, and 6-month outcomes. J Endovasc Ther. 2014;21(2):281–8. doi:10.1583/13-4527r.1.

142. Bausback Y, Botsios S, Flux J, Werner M, Schuster J, Aithal J, et al. Outback catheter for femoropopliteal occlusions: immediate and long-term results. J Endovasc Ther. 2011;18(1):13–21. doi:10.1583/10-3248.1.

143. Gandini R, Fabiano S, Spano S, Volpi T, Morosetti D, Chiaravalloti A, et al. Randomized control study of the outback LTD reentry catheter versus manual reentry for the treatment of chronic total occlusions in the superficial femoral artery. Catheter Cardiovasc Interv. 2013;82(3):485–92. doi:10.1002/Ccd.24742.

144. Al-Ameri H, Shin V, Mayeda GS, Burstein S, Matthews RV, Kloner RA, et al. Peripheral chronic total occlusions treated with subintimal angioplasty and a true lumen re-entry device. J Invasive Cardiol. 2009;21(9):468–72.

145. Smith M, Pappy R, Hennebry TA. Re-entry devices in the treatment of peripheral chronic occlusions. Tex Heart Inst J. 2011;38(4):392–7.

146. Banerjee S, Hadidi O, Mohammad A, Alsamarah A, Thomas R, Sarode K, et al. Blunt microdissection for endovascular treatment of infrainguinal chronic total occlusions. J Endovasc Ther. 2014;21(1):71–8. doi:10.1583/12-4009mr.1.

147. Gray WA, editor. Peripheral facilitated antegrade steering technique in chronic total occlusions. Vascular Interventional Advances (Viva), Las Vegas. 2012.

148. Karnabatidis D, Katsanos K, Kagadis GC, Ravazoula P, Diamantopoulos A, Nikiforidis GC, et al. Distal embolism during percutaneous revascularization of infra-aortic arterial occlusive disease: an underestimated phenomenon. J Endovasc Ther. 2006;13(3):269–80. doi:10.1583/05-1771.1.

149. Shammas NW, Coiner D, Shammas GA, Christensen L, Dippel EJ, Jerin M. Distal embolic event protection using excimer laser ablation in peripheral vascular interventions: results of the DEEP EMBOLI registry. J Endovasc Ther. 2009;16(2):197–202. doi:10.1583/08-2642.1.

150. Allie DE. To PROTECT or not to PROTECT? In lower extremity angioplasty procedures, "Why Not?" is the question! J Endovasc Ther. 2008;15(3):277–82. doi:10.1583/08-2397c.1.

151. Shrikhande GV, Khan SZ, Hussain HG, Dayal R, Mckinsey JF, Morrissey N. Lesion types and device characteristics that predict distal embolization during percutaneous lower extremity interventions. J Vasc Surg. 2011;53(2):347–52. doi:10.1016/J.Jvs.2010.09.008.

152. Gray BH, Diaz-Sandoval LJ, Dieter RS, Jaff MR, White CJ. SCAI expert consensus statement for infrapopliteal arterial intervention appropriate use. Catheter Cardiovasc Interv. 2014;84(4):539–45. doi:10.1002/Ccd.25395.

153. Klein AJ, Pinto DS, Gray BH, Jaff MR, White CJ, Drachman DE. SCAI expert consensus statement for femoral-popliteal arterial intervention appropriate use. Catheter Cardiovasc Interv. 2014;84(4):529–38. doi:10.1002/Ccd.25504.

Surgical Revascularization of Chronic Limb Ischemia

Sarah P. Pradka, Vahram Ornekian,
and Cameron M. Akbari

General Considerations

The approach to the patient with CLI, including the choice of revascularization technique, depends on the patient's presentation and the CLI classification. For example, the patient with extensive foot ulceration and/or gangrene (Fontaine stage IV CLI) will require normal perfusion to the foot for limb salvage, with the goal of restoration of a normal foot pulse. In order to maximize the chances of successful limb salvage, targeted revascularization to the specific angiosome should always be the first choice [1].

As the majority of CLI patients have diabetes, and because diabetic vascular disease tends to be most pronounced in the tibial vessels, this will almost always require infrainguinal surgical bypass to the target vessel. Proximal bypass to the popliteal or tibio-peroneal arteries may restore foot pulses, but the characteristic pattern of occlusive disease in the diabetic patient usually requires more distal bypass grafting, often to the dorsalis pedis, distal posterior tibial, or plantar artery.

In contrast, the patient presenting with ischemic rest pain (Fontaine stage III CLI) without tissue loss may be significantly ameliorated with more proximal revascularization. This may include femoral endarterectomy with profundaplasty alone in the patient with concomitant superficial femoral artery occlusion or bypass to an isolated popliteal segment.

Active infection in the foot is commonly encountered in the complicated ischemic diabetic foot. However, it is not a contraindication to lower extremity revascularization, as long as the infectious process is controlled and located remotely from the proposed incisions. Adequate control implies absence of sepsis and resolution of cellulitis, lymphangitis, and edema, especially in areas of proposed incisions required to expose the distal artery or saphenous vein.

Preoperative Surgical Considerations

Essential to the success of surgical revascularization is appropriate and accurate preoperative planning. High-quality arteriography should include visualization of planned target vessels, localization and extent of disease in the proximal vessels (including aorta and iliac arteries), and, if needed, pressure measurements across suspected inflow lesions. Based on the pattern of vascular disease in the diabetic patient, with sparing of the pedal vessels, the arteriogram must include the foot vessels in both the lateral and anterior views for a complete assessment (Fig. 36.1). Although others have performed distal revascularization based on duplex ultrasound or CT angiography alone, the author's preference is to always have a high-quality arteriography prior to any infrainguinal bypass.

Autogenous ipsilateral saphenous vein is the preferred conduit for all infrainguinal bypass grafts. High-quality conduit is central to successful bypass and has direct implications for both short-term and long-term patency results. Preoperative bilateral saphenous vein mapping with duplex ultrasound should always be performed, assessing for caliber and size, phlebitic changes, wall thickening, and accessory branching (Fig. 36.2). Saphenous vein grafts should have a minimum diameter of 2 mm, ideally 3 mm or more, as smaller veins have been shown to yield inferior short- and long-term patency [2]. If the great saphenous vein is inadequate, consideration may be given to either arm vein or prosthetic graft; if the former is chosen, duplex scanning should be performed of the upper extremities as well.

As with any major operation, appropriate medical stabilization and optimization of the patient should be performed prior to proceeding with surgical revascularization. This may

S.P. Pradka, MD (✉) • V. Ornekian, MD, MS
Vascular Surgery, Washington Hospital Center,
Washington, DC, USA

C.M. Akbari, MD
Vascular Surgery, Georgetown University Hospital,
Washington, DC, USA

© Springer International Publishing Switzerland 2017
R.S. Dieter et al. (eds.), *Critical Limb Ischemia*, DOI 10.1007/978-3-319-31991-9_36

Fig. 36.1 Lateral and AP arteriogram of the foot. Note that on the lateral projection, a vessel which resembles the dorsalis pedis artery is seen (*red arrow*). However, the AP projection confirms only lateral tarsal runoff (*yellow arrow*), and no true dorsalis pedis artery is present

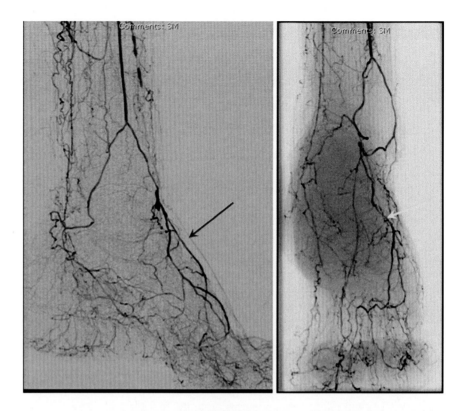

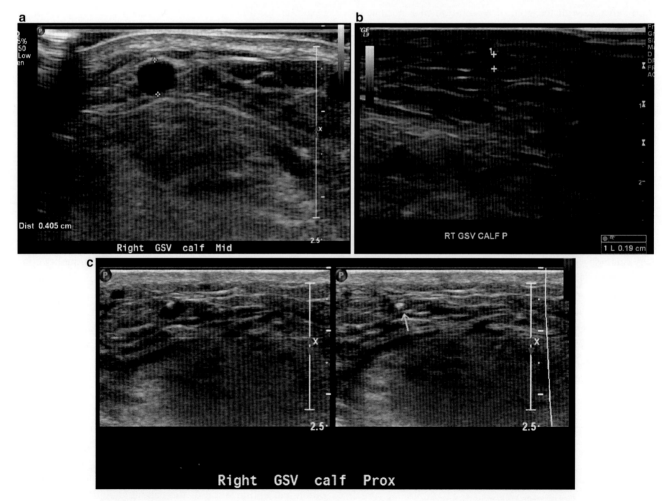

Fig. 36.2 Adequate-sized great saphenous vein by duplex (**a**) in contrast to a non-usable small-sized vein (**b**). Duplex can also demonstrate previous phlebitic changes or thrombus within the saphenous vein (**c**)

involve cardiac stress testing, coronary angiography, and echocardiography. Many patients with long-standing foot ulceration may be nutritionally depleted, and preoperative assessment and intervention may prevent postoperative wound and systemic complications.

Diabetic patients also present unique challenges to the surgeon as hyperglycemia has been linked to poor perioperative outcomes. Good glycemic control around the time of surgery, employing a multidisciplinary team of endocrine and nutrition specialists, can improve chances of success and reduce infection rates. Diabetics have lower rates of limb salvage and reduced long-term survival overall; however, several institutional series and randomized trials have demonstrated that diabetes per se is not a risk factor for graft failure. Vein grafts in diabetics in fact have superior patency, which is explained by the preponderance of shorter distal-origin grafts in those patients [2].

As noted previously, many patients with CLI will present with foot ulceration or gangrene, with concomitant foot infection. Control of infection is mandatory prior to surgical revascularization, to prevent the risk of systemic sepsis, wound, and graft infection. In the patient with diabetes, classical signs of infection may not always be present in the infected foot due to the consequences of neuropathy, alterations in the foot microcirculation, and leukocyte abnormalities. Fever, chills, and leukocytosis may be absent in the majority of diabetic patients with extensive foot infections, and hyperglycemia is often the sole presenting sign [3]. Infections should be adequately drained, as diabetic patients simply cannot tolerate undrained pus or infection. Because most infections are polymicrobial, cultures should be obtained from the base or depths of the wound after debridement so that appropriate antibiotic treatment may ensue. If adequately controlled with antibiotics and surgical drainage (if necessary), the infectious process can be controlled within 5–7 days, even in patients with systemic sepsis, and the patient may subsequently be revacularized.

Surgical Considerations: Inflow Operations

The term "inflow operation" refers to any procedure performed on a vessel at or proximal to the inguinal ligament, which restores normal flow into the femoral segment. These include aortobifemoral bypass, iliac-femoral bypass, common femoral endarterectomy, and profundaplasty, as well as extra-anatomic bypasses such as axillo-femoral and femoral-femoral bypass. Because they are performed on larger vessels with expected higher patency rates, prosthetic grafts are utilized for almost all inflow bypasses. With greater success and application of endovascular procedures, especially in the aortoiliac segment, these procedures are being performed with less frequency. Nevertheless, they continue

to be an important component of the treatment plan for revascularization, especially after endovascular failure or infection.

Aortobifemoral bypass represents the "gold standard" of patency and durability for inflow operations, with 5-year primary patency of approximately 85 % [4]. The aorta is exposed via a midline or retroperitoneal incision, and the proximal anastomosis may be performed to the infrarenal aorta in almost all cases. Even if there is occlusive disease present, endarterectomy of the infrarenal aorta may be performed, followed by the proximal anastomosis to the endarterectomized aorta (Fig. 36.3). Each limb of the graft is tunneled anatomically to the respective groin and the distal anastomoses are performed to the common femoral arteries. The author's preference is to extend the anastomosis onto the profunda, so as to prevent late thrombosis of the limb secondary to unrecognized stenoses at the profunda or superficial femoral artery origins. In instances of redo operations or groin infection, the anastomosis may be performed onto the profunda directly, with a lateral approach to the profunda, which avoids the femoral region altogether (Fig. 36.4).

A hybrid approach to the aortoiliac segment involving aortouniiliac angioplasty with concomitant femoral-femoral bypass is another option for patients who are poor candidates

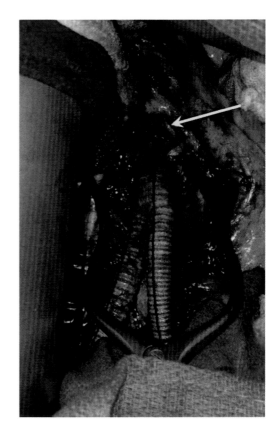

Fig. 36.3 Proximal anastomosis of an aortobifemoral graft sewn to endarterectomized infrarenal aorta. The *yellow arrow* points to the left renal vein

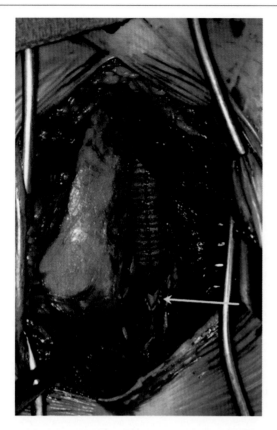

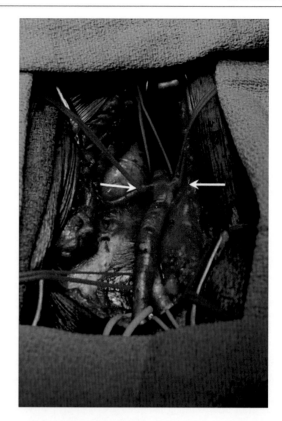

Fig. 36.4 Distal anastomosis of an aortobifemoral graft sewn to the second profunda segment, approached laterally, in a patient with an infected heavily scarred groin from a previous femoral-femoral graft. Note the vein patch onto the profunda (*yellow arrow*), with the Dacron graft sewn onto the patch

Fig. 36.5 The femoral vessels as well as the distal external iliac artery proximal to the circumflex branches (*white arrows*) are dissected free prior to femoral endarterectomy

for open aortic surgery. This approach is associated with similar patency to open aortafemoral bypass in patients with focal iliac occlusive disease (<5 cm) [5].

Because of the challenges associated with percutaneous endovascular treatment of common femoral artery disease, common femoral endarterectomy and profundaplasty is utilized commonly and may be combined with concomitant iliac or superficial femoral-popliteal-tibial angioplasty. The femoral vessels are exposed, and as the occlusive process often extends proximally to the external iliac artery, the distal external iliac artery above the circumflex branches is also exposed (Fig. 36.5). Arteriotomy is made extending onto the profunda and all plaque is removed (Figs. 36.6 and 36.7), followed by patch closure with vein, prosthetic patch, or bovine pericardium (Fig. 36.8). If concomitant iliac or distal endovascular intervention is planned, a sheath may be placed directly through the patch after restoration of flow (Fig. 36.9), and a simple suture used to close the hole after the sheath is removed. In some cases, the occlusive process within the profunda may be too bulky for endarterectomy or may result in extensive thinning of the artery. In these instances, a short

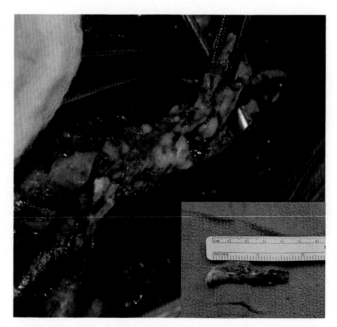

Fig. 36.6 Standard endarterectomy of the common femoral, proximal superficial femoral, and profunda femoris arteries, with inset showing plaque removed

Fig. 36.7 Following complete thrombo-endarterectomy. Note the widely patent orifices of both the superficial femoral and profunda arteries

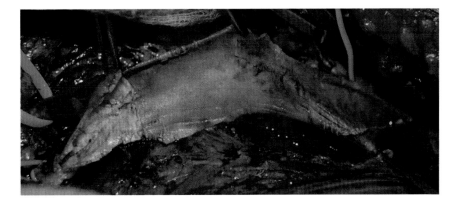

Fig. 36.8 The arteriotomy is closed with a bovine pericardial patch

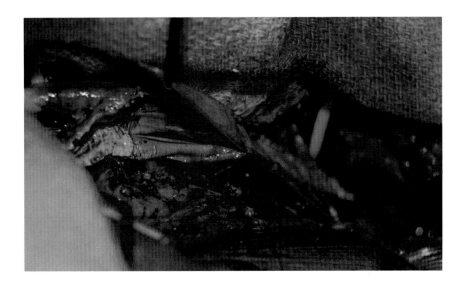

bypass from the common femoral to the profunda may be performed, with excellent results (Fig. 36.10).

Although axillo-femoral and femoral-femoral bypasses are associated with lower patency rates as compared to the aortobifemoral bypass, their principal advantages lie in the fact that they are markedly less invasive. By avoiding an abdominal incision and aortic cross clamping, these operations may be performed in high-risk patients with poor cardiopulmonary reserve; in some cases, the operation may be performed under local anesthesia in those patients in whom general anesthetic is contraindicated. In addition, by virtue of their extra-anatomic location, they may be utilized in instances of groin sepsis when placement of a prosthetic graft is undesirable.

Surgical Considerations: Infrainguinal Bypass

Infrainguinal bypass is the most commonly performed surgical revascularization among patients with CLI. Several principles are noteworthy. Autogenous saphenous vein is the preferred conduit for all infrainguinal bypass operations, even to the above-knee popliteal artery. In addition to its superior primary patency compared to prosthetic, autogenous vein also carries less risk of graft infection, which can be devastating.

The saphenous vein graft can be prepared in several ways. The simplest is a reversed configuration, in which the vein is harvested off its bed, reversed, and then placed either subcutaneously or deep to the muscle and fascia after the proximal anastomosis is performed. Because of the inherent disadvantage of the size discrepancy between the smaller distal portion of the vein and the larger proximal artery, the non-reversed and in situ techniques may be employed, in which the valves are rendered incompetent by cutting them with an atraumatic valvulotome. The non-reversed translocated technique is identical to the reversed technique except that the valves are cut, whereas the in situ technique leaves the vein in the bed, with mobilization only of the proximal and distal portions and tributary ligation without harvesting the vein. In both of these, the larger proximal vein is utilized for the proximal anastomosis, allowing for an easier anastomosis both proximally and distally.

Fig. 36.9 After completion of the patch closure (*top panel*), a sheath may be inserted for iliac or more distal intervention

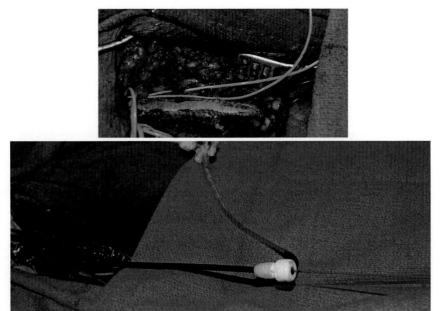

Fig. 36.10 Vein bypass from the common femoral to the profunda (*white arrow*)

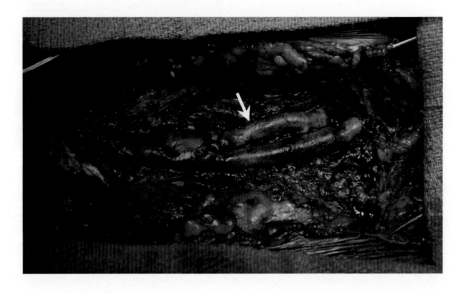

The type of configuration utilized—reversed, non-reversed translocated, or in situ—has no effect on patency, and multiple series have confirmed that all yield virtually identical results when performed correctly [6]. Ultimately the decision as to the type of configuration should depend on the surgeon's experience with each technique and vein graft size. My preference is either a reversed graft when the vein is of a uniformly large caliber and for shorter bypasses or non-reversed translocated for smaller veins and for long bypasses (such as femoral-tibial). If a non-reversed configuration is used, I prefer to inspect the vein with an angioscope and cut all the valves under direct angioscopic guidance, which allows for precise valve lysis without any risk of intimal injury or retained valve, both of which can have an adverse effect on patency and outcome (Fig. 36.11) [7].

The vein may be harvested through a continuous incision, small "skip" incisions, or endoscopically. There has been increasing enthusiasm for endoscopic vein harvest, as it may decrease postoperative recovery time, edema, and wound complications. However, this should be tempered against the risk of occult vein injury during harvest, including vein spasm, which can have implications for patency [8]. My preference continues to be harvesting vein through a contin-

Fig. 36.11 Angioscopic evaluation and angioscopy-guided valve lysis (*labeled*)

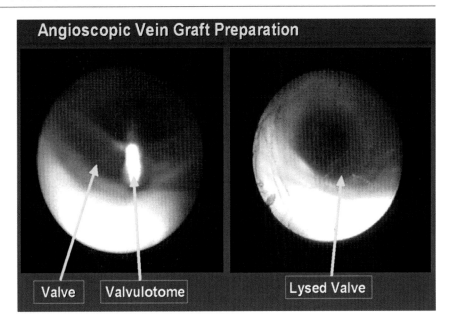

Fig. 36.12 Exposure and harvest of the saphenous vein through a continuous incision without flaps. Note the vein is fully exposed, allowing for meticulous harvest and prevention of spasm. The incision is created directly overlying the vein, and no thin flaps are created, which maximizes the chance for successful wound healing

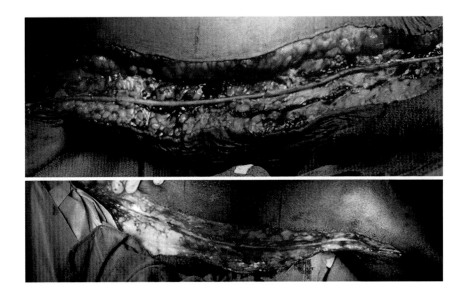

uous incision which is meticulously created to avoid any skin flaps (Fig. 36.12). Periadventitial papaverine or nitroglycerin injection overcomes vein spasm, and the vein is gently distended with solution and then harvested off its bed. With careful incision placement, avoiding skin flaps, and with layered accurate closure, I have found the risk of significant wound complications to be minimal. Additionally, I prefer to place all grafts deep to surgical incisions, such that grafts originating from the femoral artery are tunneled deep to the muscle and fascia down to the below-knee popliteal space. This obviates the risk of graft infection or exposure should a wound complication occur, which is discussed in more detail later in this chapter.

The proximal and distal anastomoses are almost always performed end to side. All adventitia should be removed from the vein at the site of proposed anastomosis to avoid kinking at the "heel" of the graft, which can be a cause of subsequent graft stenosis or failure. Redundancy at the proximal and distal anastomoses should also be avoided. The graft should have a natural curve with the native artery, with the anastomosis on the anterior aspect, so as to minimize twisting of the graft (Fig. 36.13). A hand-held continuous wave Doppler is used to insonate the distal anastomosis and distal artery. Completion imaging with angiography or duplex ultrasound was at one time considered standard at the end of a bypass, but these rarely detect correctable technical problems that would otherwise be missed with careful physical exam. Completion imaging should be done if there is a weak pulse or Doppler signal distal to the graft.

Recognizing the pattern of vascular disease in diabetes, in which the femoropopliteal segment is often spared of the atherosclerotic occlusive process, shorter bypass grafts to the tibial vessels with origin from the popliteal or distal superficial femoral artery may be performed. Extensive experience has shown that, in the absence of more proximal occlusive disease, such grafts yield the same patency results as grafts taken from the common femoral artery [9]. This allows for reconstruction in those patients with limited saphenous vein, shortened operative time, and incision length and avoids potentially troublesome groin wound complications.

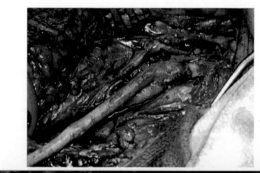

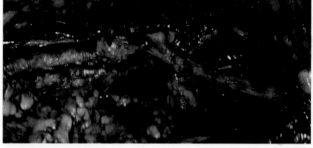

Fig. 36.13 Proximal (*top panel*) and distal (*bottom panel*) anastomoses of a femoral-tibial graft. Note absence of kinking or "pull" on the anastomosis, with no redundancy

As an example of a short bypass graft from the popliteal artery, a typical popliteal to dorsalis pedis bypass graft is illustrated in Figs. 36.14, 36.15, and 36.16. The saphenous vein is harvested from the upper leg and will be translocated subcutaneously in the lower leg, where no incision has been made, which minimizes the risk of graft infection with any wound complication (Fig. 36.14). After preparation of the vein graft with angioscopy, the proximal anastomosis is performed in an end-vein to side-artery fashion to the popliteal artery (Fig. 36.15). After completion of the anastomosis, the graft is placed in the previously created tunnel to the dorsalis pedis incision under arterial pressure (to avoid kinking or twisting of the graft), and the distal anastomosis is then performed (Fig. 36.16). Estimated blood loss is usually 150 ml or less.

In many patients with CLI, the only suitable target for revascularization is a distal inframalleolar vessel, such as the plantar or tarsal artery. Bypass to these vessels, though technically challenging, can be performed successfully through accurate angiographic visualization preoperatively, anatomic knowledge of the plantar and tarsal vessels, and incorporating meticulous surgical and vein harvest techniques (Figs. 36.17, 36.18, and 36.19). Increasing experience has shown excellent short-term and long-term patency and limb salvage rates, which is highly encouraging in this particular subset of patients who are often advised to undergo limb amputation [10].

Unfortunately, good quality ipsilateral greater saphenous vein is not available in 20–40 % of patients, due to prior use of vein for coronary or lower extremity bypass, vein ablation, or other anatomic factors [11]. The decision for an alternative source of conduit should be made with consideration of the patient's comorbidities. Contralateral saphenous vein offers the best outcomes of all the alternative sources of autogenous vein, but I prefer to use it only for those patients who have a palpable foot pulse or near-normal noninvasive arterial studies. An estimated 20 % of patients will require bypass for that contralateral leg within 5 years, although harvest of the contralateral vein does not

Fig. 36.14 Popliteal to dorsalis pedis bypass, with translocated vein harvested from the upper thigh (*solid dark arrow*). Note the vein graft is translocated to a subcutaneous position where no incision has been made in the calf and lower leg (*dashed dark arrow*)

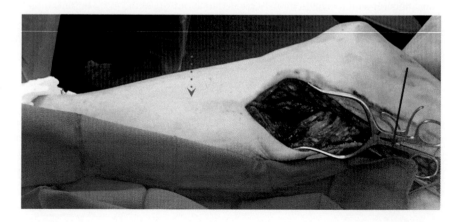

Fig. 36.15 Same patient as in Fig. 36.14, demonstrating the proximal anastomosis to the below-knee popliteal artery

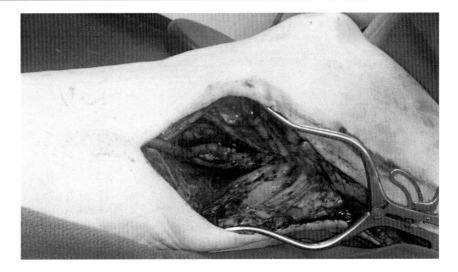

Fig. 36.16 Same patient as in Fig. 36.14. The graft has been tunneled subcutaneously to the dorsalis pedis artery and the distal anastomosis has been performed

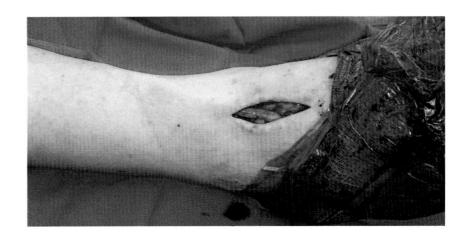

seem to affect the approximately 10 % rate of contralateral limb loss [11]. Upper extremity veins can also be used, particularly for shorter bypasses. Upper extremity vein can be spliced to produce a longer bypass, with patency only slightly inferior to greater saphenous vein [12]. However, arm vein should not be sacrificed for patients with advanced chronic kidney disease who may rely on autogenous dialysis access for survival.

Due to limitations in available autogenous conduit, about 25 % of infrainguinal bypasses for CLI are performed with prosthetic graft, usually polytetrafluoroethylene (PTFE) [13]. Although only one half of below-knee bypasses with PTFE remain patent after 2 years, this may be adequate to heal a wound for a patient who otherwise faces imminent limb loss [14]. Vein cuffs or patches at the distal anastomoses of prosthetic tibial bypasses have resulted in improved patency rates in some series [15]. My preference is to perform a vein patch at *both* the proximal and distal anastomoses. The patch is sewn widely onto the recipient vessel, with a generous PTFE anastomosis on the top of the patch

(Fig. 36.20). The vein patch protects the lumen of the recipient artery, to allow it to remain patent even if the prosthetic graft develops a flush occlusion. I have yet to encounter a patient who presents with severe limb ischemia secondary to proximal propagation of thrombus in the native artery if the bypass is done in that fashion.

The relatively poor long-term patency of below-knee prosthetic bypass has led to development of several modified grafts. Some grafts feature structural elements such as removable rings for external support or a hood for the distal anastomosis. Heparin-bonded PTFE has also been developed, which has a bioactive surface that is intended to reduce thrombus formation and myointimal hyperplasia.

Cryopreserved cadaveric vein has been promoted as an alternative to prosthetic bypass, particularly for patients with elevated risk of graft infection. However, these advantages are mostly theoretical, as cadaveric vein has never demonstrated superiority over prosthetic conduit in terms of patency or limb salvage [16]. The use of cadaveric vein is also limited by its cost, which is several-fold higher than PTFE.

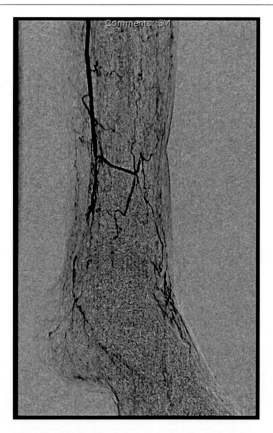

Fig. 36.17 Arteriogram of the foot in a 60-year-old patient with a gangrenous hallux, demonstrating only a plantar vessel in the foot

Complications

Both systemic and local complications are increased in patients who undergo bypass for critical limb ischemia, with an estimated 30 % patients experiencing a major systemic and/or local perioperative complication [17]. Perioperative cardiac complications are the most common systemic complication, occurring in 4–10 % of CLI patients, and include arrhythmias, congestive heart failure, and myocardial infarction [18]. Perioperative use of beta-blockers may reduce this risk. Judicious use of fluids, intraoperative monitoring with liberal use of nitrates, and a high index of suspicion for myocardial ischemia remain important tenets of postoperative care.

Wound infections complicate at least 10 % of lower extremity bypasses, but are often under-reported [17, 18]. The spectrum ranges from simple cellulitis which may be treated with antibiotics alone, to extensive soft tissue infection with graft involvement. Most often, the sequence is that of an indolent infection which results in a small area of wound dehiscence and fibrinous exudate. Unfortunately, this can mask deeper involvement, which can result in a catastrophic outcome if the graft is involved (Fig. 36.21). The most important treatment is prevention. Accurate and precise

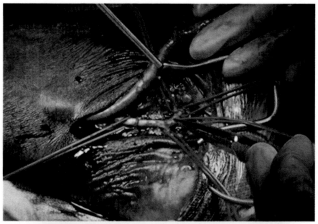

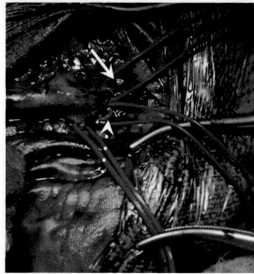

Fig. 36.18 Same patient as in Fig. 36.17. The plantar vessels have been exposed and the vein graft is prepared for distal anastomosis (*top panel*). Distal anastomosis performed to the junction of the medial and lateral plantar arteries (*solid* and *dashed arrows*) (*bottom panel*)

tissue approximation and closure, avoidance of flaps, judicious use of antibiotics, prevention of lymph leaks, and clean dressings all can help prevent wound complications. Additionally, as stated previously, I avoid placing grafts in the subcutaneous space of a surgically created incision. In the femoral location, use of a rotational sartorius muscle flap is quite helpful to cover the graft prophylactically [19].

Results

Patency rates and limb salvage after surgical revascularization vary widely, principally according to the anatomic location, though other factors (such as redo procedures, type of conduit, and indication) also are important determinants. The highest patency rates are seen with in-line (anatomic) inflow operations, with 5-year aortobifemoral bypass averaging 85 % [20]. Similar rates are seen following isolated

Fig. 36.19 Angiogram 1 year postoperatively and duplex 2 years postoperatively of the patient from Fig. 36.17, demonstrating a widely patent graft

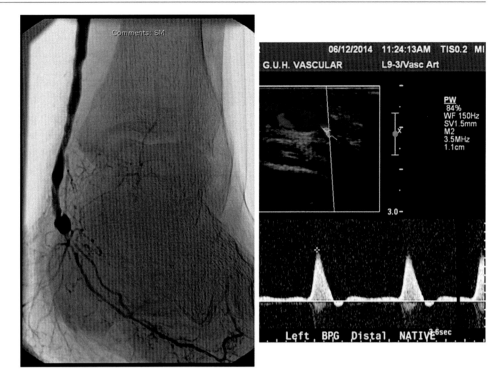

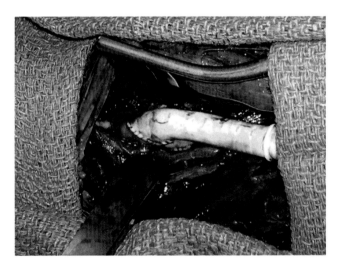

Fig. 36.20 Distal anastomosis of a PTFE graft with distal vein patch to the peroneal artery. Note the wide vein patch on the native artery with the PTFE graft anastomosed to the patch

profundaplasty or femoral endarterectomy. For extra-anatomic bypass, the results are obviously lower, with 5-year patency for femoral-femoral bypass averaging 65 % [21]. Among axillo-bifemoral grafts, the patency rates are even lower, averaging between 40 and 60 % at 3 years.

The incidence of early (<30 days) postoperative graft occlusion varies according to graft location, conduit, indication for bypass, and surgeon. Approximately 4–7 % of infrainguinal bypasses fail within 30 days, but the incidence is significantly higher for tibial bypasses, prosthetic grafts, emergency or limb salvage procedures, and patients who are female, African-American, or continue to smoke [22]. Early graft occlusion should raise suspicion for a technical problem: inadequate inflow or outflow, poor-quality vein, trauma to the vein during harvesting, or an error in creation of an anastomosis. Unless otherwise dictated at the time of the original operation, or otherwise mitigating circumstances, early graft occlusion is an indication for immediate re-exploration and graft thrombectomy. Most importantly, an underlying cause (such as an anastomotic flap or clamp injury) should be sought and addressed, as the outcome is more favorable when the cause is corrected. If there is no identifiable technical cause, less common factors such as thrombophilia should be considered.

Bypass grafts with saphenous vein provide the highest patency rates among infrainguinal revascularization. In situ and reversed vein graft primary patency at 1 year and 4 years averages approximately 85 % and 65 %, respectively, again with no difference based on vein configuration. For perimalleolar bypass grafts, secondary patency is approximately 60 % at 5 years, with limb salvage rates in excess of 80 % at 5 years. For reasons that are not totally clear, African-American women experience significantly worse long-term graft patency and limb salvage. Interestingly, diabetes and ESRD are major risk factors for death and limb loss, but are not independently associated with graft occlusion [2].

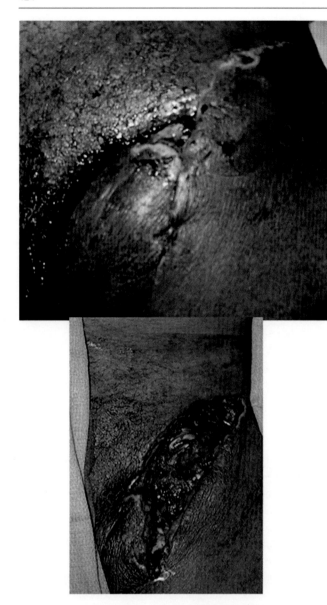

Fig. 36.21 Four weeks following left femoral to tibial bypass, complicated by a superficial wound dehiscence, this patient presented with bleeding in the groin incision (*top panel*) with a large infected pseudoaneurysm by CT scan. This necessitated emergent groin exploration with debridement and graft removal (*bottom panel*)

Approximately 35 % of infrainguinal vein bypasses will develop a hemodynamically significant stenosis, most commonly in the first postoperative year [23]. Intermediate vein graft failure (30 days to 2 years postoperatively) is more likely related to intimal hyperplasia. Surveillance of grafts with duplex ultrasound allows detection of stenoses prior to failure of the bypass, as interventions for stenoses are more successful than those for occlusion. A duplex ultrasound is typically obtained at 1, 3, 6, and 12 months postoperatively, every 6 months for another 2 years, then yearly. Patients with an abnormal first duplex scan or multiple risk factors

for vein graft failure may benefit from more frequent surveillance [23].

The reported patency data for prosthetic grafts vary widely, with expected 1-year patency between 35 and 75 %. Multiple factors may explain this wide variation. At least some of the reports are 20 years or older; additionally, variables such as use of a distal vein cuff, anticoagulation, and outflow are widely discrepant or not even reported. More recent data certainly support the use of prosthetic grafts to the popliteal or tibial location when good-quality autogenous vein is not available.

The relatively poor long-term patency of prosthetic grafts in the below-knee position has led to development of heparin-bonded PTFE. Intermediate results are encouraging, with primary patency of 61 % for below-knee popliteal and 52 % for tibial bypasses [24]. Although these bypasses have primary patency that is inferior to vein, rates of limb salvage and amputation-free survival are similar [25].

In addition to patency, quality of life scores must be considered when recommending infrainguinal bypass to a patient with CLI, as these surgeries require considerable recovery time and only a small minority of patients will have an "optimal" outcome of uncomplicated surgery, successful wound healing, maintenance of functional status, and freedom from reoperation [26]. In the CLI population, the surgical wounds will typically take 6–8 weeks to heal and ischemic ulcers may take several months or even years. In fact, a quarter of patients will still have an open wound 6 months after surgery and a quarter will die before the wound is healed [26]. Furthermore, among patients who are independent and ambulatory preoperatively, only about 55 % maintain that status on discharge, and only 68 % are independent and ambulatory at 3 years.

Choice of Surgical Revascularization or Endovascular Procedure

Several professional societies have published recommendations with regard to surgical versus endovascular intervention, but these are only guidelines, not clinical practice standards. For example, TASC A lesions are generally treated endovascularly and TASC D lesions with surgery, with a flexible approach to TASC B and C disease. The ultimate decision as to whether to pursue surgical revascularization depends on patient variables and comfort level of the surgeon. Notwithstanding the debates on which should be performed first, it is axiomatic that the patient with CLI is best served by an aggressive approach to limb salvage, which, by definition, incorporates both endovascular and surgical approaches.

The results of the Bypass Versus Angioplasty for Severe Limb Ischemia (BASIL) and other smaller nonrandomized series suggest that an endovascular-first approach is warranted in almost all patients, provided that it may be performed without "burning a bridge" for future surgical revascularization. The BASIL trial was the first and only intention-to-treat randomized controlled trial comparing endovascular intervention to primary surgical bypass for severe limb ischemia. Over half of the patients died by the end of the study, emphasizing their precarious medical condition. At 2 years, there was no difference in amputation-free survival or overall survival for patients who received primary bypass, although there was a slight increase in overall survival and amputation-free survival for those patients who lived past 2 years [27]. Costs were equal at 3 years. Based on these results, an endovascular option is preferred for patients with an expected survival of fewer than 2 years. Finally, in the analysis of quality of life, the worst outcome was seen among patients undergoing major limb amputation. Conclusively, it can be stated that limb amputation should be avoided, and surgical revascularization plays an integral part of that goal.

References

1. Alexandrescu V, Soderstrom M, Venermo M. Angiosome theory: fact or fiction? Scand J Surg. 2012;101(2):125–31.
2. Schanzer A, Hevelone N, Owens CD, Belkin M, Bandyk DF, Clowes AW, et al. Technical factors affecting autogenous vein graft failure: observations from a large multicenter trial. J Vasc Surg. 2007;46(6):1180–90.
3. Akbari CM, Macsata R, Smith BM, Sidawy AN. Overview of the diabetic foot. Semin Vasc Surg. 2003;16(1):3–11.
4. Hertzer NR, Bena JF, Karafa MT. A personal experience with direct reconstruction and extra-anatomic bypass for aortoiliofemoral occlusive disease. J Vasc Surg. 2007;45(3):527–35.
5. Aburahma AF, Robinson PA, Cook CC, Hopkins ES. Selecting patients for combined femorofemoral bypass grafting and iliac balloon angioplasty and stenting for bilateral iliac disease. J Vasc Surg. 2001;33 Suppl 2:S93–9.
6. Gupta AK, Bandyk DF, Cheanvechai D, Johnson BL. Natural history of infrainguinal vein graft stenosis relative to bypass grafting technique. J Vasc Surg. 1997;25(2):220–5.
7. Miller A, Stonebridge PA, Tsoukas AI, Kwolek CJ, Gibbons GW, et al. Angioscopically directed valvulotomy: a new valvulotome and technique. J Vasc Surg. 1991;13(6):813–20.
8. Santo VJ, Dargon PT, Azarbal AF, Liem TK, Mitchell EL, Moneta GL, et al. Open versus endoscopic great saphenous vein harvest for lower extremity revascularization of critical limb ischemia. J Vasc Surg. 2014;59(2):427–34.
9. Reed AB, Conte MS, Belkin M, Mannick JA, Whittemore AD, Donaldson MC. Usefulness of autogenous bypass grafts originating distal to the groin. J Vasc Surg. 2002;35(1):54–5.
10. Hughes K, Domeniq CM, Hamdan AD, Schermerhorn M, Aulivola B, Blattman S, et al. Bypass to plantar and tarsal arteries: an acceptable approach to limb salvage. J Vasc Surg. 2004;40(6):1149–57.
11. Chew DK, Owens CD, Belkin M, Donaldson MC, Whittemore AD, Mannick JA, et al. Bypass in the absence of ipsilateral greater saphenous vein: safety and superiority of the contralateral greater saphenous vein. J Vasc Surg. 2002;35(6):1085–92.
12. Faries PL, Arora S, Pomposelli Jr FB, Pulling MC, Smakowski P, Rohan DI, et al. The use of arm vein in lower-extremity revascularization: results of 520 procedures performed in eight years. J Vasc Surg. 2000;31(1 Pt 1):50–9.
13. Simons JP, Schanzer A, Nolan BW, Stone DH, Kalish JA, Cronenwett JL, et al. Outcomes and practice patterns in patients undergoing lower extremity bypass. J Vasc Surg. 2012;55(6):1629–36.
14. Albers M, Battistella VM, Romiti M, Rodriques AA, Pereira CA. Meta-analysis of polytetrafluoroethylene bypass grafts to infrapopliteal arteries. J Vasc Surg. 2003;37(6):1263–9.
15. Griffiths GD, Nagy J, Black D, Stonebridge PA. Randomized clinical trial of distal anastomotic interposition vein cuff in infrainguinal polytetrafluoroethylene bypass grafting. Br J Surg. 2004;91(5):560–2.
16. Chang CK, Scali ST, Feezor RJ, Beck AW, Waterman AL, Huber TS, et al. Defining utility and predicting outcome of cadaveric lower extremity bypass grafts in patients with critical limb ischemia. J Vasc Surg. 2014;14(1):1120–3.
17. LaMuraglia GM, Conrad MF, Chung T, Hutter M, Watkins MT, Cambria RP. Significant perioperative morbidity accompanies contemporary infrainguinal bypass surgery: an NSQIP report. J Vasc Surg. 2009;50(2):299–304.
18. Goshima KR, Mills Sr JL, Hughes JD. A new look at outcomes after infrainguinal bypass surgery: traditional reporting standards systematically underestimate the expenditure of effort required to attain limb salvage. J Vasc Surg. 2004;39(2):330–5.
19. Fischer JP, Nelson JA, Rohrbach JI, Wu LC, Woo EY, Kovach SJ, et al. Prophylactic muscle flaps in vascular surgery: the Penn Groin Assessment Scale. Plast Reconstr Surg. 2012;129(6):940e–49e.
20. Chiu KW, Davies RS, NIghtingale PG, Bradbury AW, Adam DJ. Review of direct anatomical open surgical management of atherosclerotic aorto-iliac occlusive disease. Eur J Vasc Endovasc Surg. 2010;39(4):460–71.
21. Kim YW, Lee JH, Kim HG, Huh S. Factors affecting the long-term patency of crossover femorofemoral bypass graft. Eur J Vasc Endovasc Surg. 2005;30(4):376–80.
22. Soma G, Greenblatt DY, Nelson MT, Rajamanickam V, Havlena J, Fernandes-Taylor S. Early graft failure after infrainguinal arterial bypass. Surgery. 2014;155(2):300–10.
23. Tinder CN, Chavanpun JP, Bandyk DF, Armstrong PA, Back MR, Johnson BL, et al. Efficacy of duplex ultrasound surveillance after infrainguinal vein bypass may be enhanced by identification of characteristics predictive of graft stenosis development. J Vasc Surg. 2008;48(2):613–8.
24. Pulli R, Dorigo W, Castelli P, Dorucci V, Ferilli F, De Blasis G, et al. Midterm results from a multicenter registry on the treatment of infrainguinal critical limb ischemia using a heparin-bonded ePTFE graft. J Vasc Surg. 2010;51(5):1164–77.e1.
25. Dorigo W, Pulli R, Castelli P, Dorrucci V, Ferilli F, De Blasis G, et al. A multicenter comparison between autologous saphenous vein and heparin-bonded expanded polytetrafluoroethylene (ePTFE) graft in the treatment of critical limb ischemia in diabetics. J Vasc Surg. 2011;54(5):1332–8.
26. Nicoloff AD, Taylor Jr LM, McLafferty RB, Moneta GL, Porter JM. Patient recovery after infrainguinal bypass grafting for limb salvage. J Vasc Surg. 1998;27(2):256–63.
27. Bradbury AW, Adam DJ, Bell J, Forbes JF, Fowkes FG, Gillespie I. Bypass versus Angioplasty in Severe Ischaemia of the Leg (BASIL) trial: an intention-to-treat analysis of amputation-free and overall survival in patients randomized to a bypass surgery-first or a balloon angioplasty-first revascularization strategy. J Vasc Surg. 2010;51 Suppl 5:5S–17S.

Hani Slim, Elias Khalil, Hiren Mistry,
Raghvinder Singh Gambhir, Domenico Valenti,
and Hisham Rashid

Introduction

The revascularization of patients with critical leg ischaemia (CLI) is essential for limb salvage and healing tissue loss. Both infrainguinal bypass surgery and angioplasty are established techniques in the treatment of these patients. The healing of tissue loss is dependent on several factors, but re-establishing direct blood flow is mandatory to achieve this process. The role of the pedal arch in the treatment of patients with CLI has not been fully studied. The quality of the pedal arch could impact on the ability of a successful revascularization in healing tissue loss, as well as the long-term durability of both surgical and radiological treatment of patients with CLI.

In this chapter the authors will address the importance of the pedal arch in the healing process of tissue loss in patients undergoing infrapopliteal bypass surgery and its impact on patency and major amputation rates in relation to the quality of the pedal arch. This will also be linked with the angiosome concept for revascularization which is also dependent on the quality of the pedal arch in achieving tissue loss healing.

Anatomy of the Pedal Arch

The blood supply to the foot and ankle is mainly supplied by the anterior tibial and dorsalis pedis arteries and its anastomosis with the posterior tibial artery and terminal branches, the medial and lateral plantar arteries, forming together the pedal arch. Both the anterior and posterior tibial arteries also receive communicating branches from the peroneal artery and supply the heel with the lateral calcaneal artery (Fig. 37.1).

H. Slim, MD • E. Khalil, MD, MSc
H. Mistry, MBBS • R.S. Gambhir, MD
D. Valenti, DM, PhD • H. Rashid, MSc (✉)
Department of Vascular Surgery, King's College Hospital,
Denmark Hill, London SE5 9RS, UK

The dorsalis pedis and the plantar arteries arise as the terminal branches of the anterior and posterior tibial arteries. The anterior tibial artery continues as the dorsalis pedis when it crosses the ankle joint and is often the main blood supplier to the forefoot. After passing to the first interosseous space, the dorsalis pedis artery splits into the first metatarsal artery and the perforating deep plantar artery. By passing deeply between the heads of the first interosseous muscle, the deep plantar artery enters the sole of the foot where it unites with the lateral plantar artery to give rise to the deep plantar arch. Proximally, the lateral tarsal artery branches off the dorsalis pedis artery and runs beneath the extensor digitorum brevis muscle to join the arcuate artery, forming a dorsal arterial loop. The arcuate artery splits from the dorsalis pedis artery and runs to the lateral aspect of the forefoot under the extensor tendons. By running across the bases of the lateral four metatarsals, the arcuate artery supplies the second, third and fourth dorsal metatarsal arteries. Perforating branches connect these vessels that run distally to the toes, to the plantar metatarsal arteries and to the plantar arch. Each dorsal metatarsal artery supplies the dorsal aspect of two adjoining toes by dividing into two dorsal digital arteries. The dorsal arteries generally do not reach the end of the digits and this area is supplied by dorsal branches of the plantar digital arteries.

The posterior circulation of the foot derives its blood supply from the posterior tibial artery. At its terminal division under the flexor retinaculum, the tibial artery continues as the medial and lateral plantar arteries. The medial plantar artery gives rise to deep and superficial branches. As the smaller branch of the posterior tibial artery, the deep branches of the medial plantar artery supply the first toe, whereas its superficial branch supplies the skin of the sole on the medial side and has digital branches. Anatomic variations exist whereby the superficial branch anastomoses with the deep plantar arch or lateral plantar artery forming a superficial plantar arch. The lateral plantar artery, being the largest branch of the posterior tibial artery, runs laterally and anteriorly. The deep plantar arch is formed by the lateral plantar artery crossing

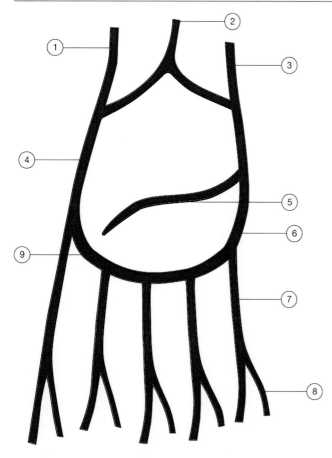

Fig. 37.1 Schematic diagram demonstrating the pedal arch and its components. (1) Anterior tibial artery, (2) peroneal artery, (3) posterior tibial artery, (4) dorsalis pedis artery, (5) medial plantar artery, (6) lateral plantar artery, (7) tarsal arteries, (8) digital arteries and (9) deep plantar artery. Graphic designer: Mariam Rashid

the foot and arching medially and connecting with the deep plantar artery. Along its course, it branches into four plantar metatarsal arteries, three perforating branches and several branches supplying the muscles, fascia and skin of the sole. Near the base of the proximal phalanges, the plantar metatarsal arteries divide to form the plantar digital arteries that supply adjacent toes. The plantar digital arteries are the main blood supply to the distal toes and the nail bed which they reach via perforating and dorsal branches.

Venous System of the Foot

Similar to the anatomical division in the lower limb, the venous system of the foot can be separated into superficial and deep veins. As paired veins, the deep veins accompany all arteries internal to the deep fascia. Superficial veins are not accompanied by arteries and are found subcutaneously. Contrary to the venous drainage in the leg, the deep and superficial veins of the foot mainly drain into the superficial system.

The distal dorsal digital and plantar digital veins continue proximally as the dorsal metatarsal veins. Subsequently, these drain to the dorsal venous arch of the foot. The remainder of the dorsum of the foot is drained by the proximal dorsal venous network, which together with the dorsal venous arch lies subcutaneously. The plantar venous system can be divided into veins draining either the median border or the lateral border of the sole. The medial system joins the dorsal venous network to form the medial marginal vein which continues more proximally as the great saphenous vein. Lateral veins of the plantar venous network join the lateral part of the dorsal venous arch to form the lateral marginal vein. The lateral marginal vein proximally continues as the small saphenous vein. Throughout the entire lower limb, perforating veins begin the one way shunting of blood, an intrinsic pattern essential to the function of the musculo-venous pump [1].

Anomalies of the Pedal Arch

The pedal arch, as an essential anastomosis between the anterior and posterior tibial arteries in the foot, occurs in several anatomical variations and has been the subject of study in several pioneering studies [2, 3]. The circulation in the foot has been divided into superficial and deep plantar arches. The plantar arch is formed when the deep plantar artery joins the deep branch of the lateral plantar artery. The contribution of each artery differs among individuals. Based on a study by Ozer et al., the pedal arch has been divided into three anatomical categories [4]:

Type I: the dorsalis pedis artery is predominant with a large terminal portion anastomosing with a slender terminal portion of the lateral plantar artery. This configuration was present in 48 % of the cases. More specifically, the first metatarsal plantar artery branched off the widest part of the deep plantar arch and had the largest diameter of the plantar metatarsal arteries.

Type II: the lateral plantar artery is predominant in which its terminal portion is larger than that of the dorsalis pedis artery. This configuration was present in 38 % of the specimens. Here it was the fourth plantar metatarsal artery that originated from the thickest part of the deep plantar arch, making the fourth plantar artery the widest plantar metatarsal artery.

Type III: a balanced type in which both arteries contributed equally to the pedal arch. This configuration was seen in 14 % of the dissections. Interestingly, the thinnest part of the plantar arch was located between the second and third plantar metatarsal artery.

Several other studies have investigated the different anatomical variations of the arterial supply to the foot. Also, these studies have shown that the dorsalis pedis is most often the predominant artery in 40–82% of cases [3, 5]. In most cases, the dorsalis pedis artery is a continuation of the anterior tibial artery. Less often, the dorsalis pedis can also arise from the anterior communicating branch of the peroneal artery (6.7%). However, the dorsalis pedis is not always present and several studies have reported on a small or even absent dorsalis pedis in 1.9–14.2% of the cases [2, 5–8]. Papon et al., in a dissection of 20 specimens, found the deep plantar artery present in only 16 cases. This artery was found to be easily accessible via the dorsal route, making it a possible anatomic site for the performance of a distal bypass [9].

Likewise, anatomical variations exist with an absent arcuate artery. When the arcuate artery is present, it most often branches from the dorsalis pedis directly (90%) and less often from the lateral tarsal artery (10%) [5]. The posterior tibial artery is more consistent in terms of location and presence and found to be absent in 0.18–2% of cases only [2, 6].

The deep plantar arch gives off four plantar metatarsal arteries, four perforating branches and numerous branches to joints, muscles, etc. By penetrating through the first, second, third and fourth interosseous space, the perforating branches anastomose with the dorsal metatarsal arteries. A superficial plantar arch is formed when superficial branches from the lateral plantar artery and the medial plantar artery form and give off the first to the fifth common plantar digital arteries. This configuration, however, is only found in 2–8% of the studies and was more often absent [3, 4].

The Angiosome Concept

In 1987, Taylor and Palmer published an elaborated study covering the anatomy of the whole human body describing their angiosome theory [10]. They defined the angiosome as a 'three-dimensional jigsaw made up of composite blocks of tissue supplied by named source arteries. The arteries supplying these blocks of tissue are responsible for the supply of the skin and the underlying structures'. They identified five distinctive angiosomes in the leg and foot territory which are supplied by the anterior tibial (and dorsalis pedis), peroneal and posterior tibial arteries (with its terminal branches, the medial and lateral plantar arteries). However, Taylor and Palmer also described well-established anastomoses that exist between the angiosomes territorial distribution of different arteries. They also described finer arterial connections existing between the different angiosomes describing them as 'choke vessels'. These 'choke vessels' link neighbouring angiosomes but also demarcate the border of each angiosome.

This angiosome concept has generated great interest in peripheral vascular disease, with several studies extrapolating this model on the treatment of patients with CLI and tissue loss.

In 2006, Attinger et al. published their first study looking into the angiosomal distribution in the ankle and foot region in cadavers concluding the presence of six angiosomes supplied by the anterior tibial/dorsalis pedis (one angiosome), the posterior tibial (three angiosomes) and the peroneal (two angiosomes) arteries [11].

However, Attinger et al. also stated that the blood flow to the foot and ankle is redundant because the three major arteries feeding the foot have multiple arterial–arterial connections. The 'choke vessels' described by Taylor and Palmer illustrate a type of connection between different angiosomes, as well as the true anastomoses where no change in arterial calibre occurs. The anastomosis between the dorsalis pedis and the posterior tibial arteries perfectly demonstrate this type of connection.

Neville et al. published their study about the clinical implications of foot and ankle angiosomes on revascularization and limb salvage in CLI patients undergoing distal bypass surgery [12]. In the direct revascularization group, there was 91% complete healing with only 9% major amputation rate. While in the indirect revascularization group, only 62% healed with a 38% major amputation rate ($p=0.03$). However, the total time to healing was not significantly faster in patients undergoing direct revascularization. The authors concluded that direct revascularization of the angiosome specific to the anatomy of the wound leads to a higher rate of healing and limb salvage, recommending that consideration should be given to revascularization of the artery directly feeding the ischemic angiosome. This is in line with a recent meta-analysis of 1290 limb revascularizations showing that direct revascularization leads to improved wound healing and limb salvage when compared to indirect revascularization [13].

Similar studies exploring this same angiosome concept in revascularization in CLI patients undergoing both infrapopliteal bypass surgery and angioplasty were published. These studies, however, reached different conclusions about the importance of this concept in healing tissue loss and limb salvage in patients with CLI. Most of these studies did not include data regarding the pedal arch quality in relation to the angiosome revascularized. The authors believe that there is a strong correlation between the angiosome concept and the quality of the foot arch in influencing the healing process of tissue loss in patients with CLI following revascularization. This could explain the contradicting results previously published using the concept of angiosomes in CLI.

In clinical practice, healing of tissue loss can be achieved significantly fast in spite of the severe disease of the angiosome artery supplying the area of tissue loss. This is well demonstrated by this diabetic patient presenting with severe plantar foot sepsis requiring emergency debridement of the medial aspect of the foot sole, heal and hallux (Fig. 37.2).

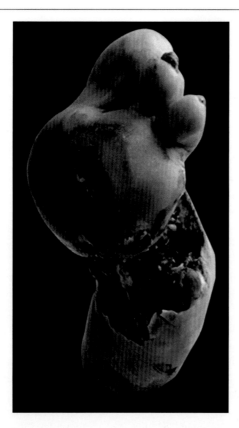

Fig. 37.2 Extensive necrosis and tissue loss following debridement of severe sepsis in the plantar surface of the foot

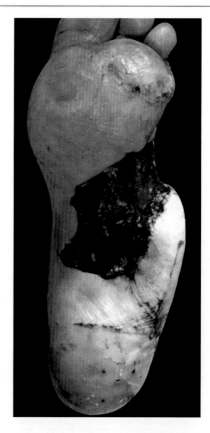

Fig. 37.3 Excellent granulation tissue following repeat bedside debridement and negative pressure wound therapy few weeks later without any attempt of revascularization

The patient was noted to have very good perfusion at the time of surgery. A duplex scan performed post-operatively demonstrated complete occlusion of the posterior tibial artery and severe stenosis of the peroneal artery with triphasic flow in the dorsalis pedis artery. The patient was managed with intravenous antibiotics, regular bedside debridement and negative pressure wound therapy. Within 2 weeks, the patient developed healthy granulation tissue (Fig. 37.3) that was easily covered by a split-thickness skin graft (Fig. 37.4).

Based on the angiosome concept, this patient with extensive tissue loss in the angiosomal territory of the posterior tibial artery (demonstrated to be occluded on duplex scan) would not have been expected to heal so rapidly. This patient through a complete pedal arch has perfused the plantar region of the foot through retrograde flow from the dorsalis pedis artery, through its deep plantar artery, to the lateral plantar artery, hence achieving complete healing.

This and similar cases have prompted the authors to study the healing process of patients with CLI undergoing infrapopliteal bypass surgery and correlate the outcome to the quality of the pedal arch and direct angiosome revascularization.

The angiosome concept is an anatomic rather than a physiologic study, as stated by Taylor and Palmer in a letter published in 1992 [14]. Taylor and Palmer even stated that they were careful not to make this extrapolation. Thus, applying this concept wholly to patients with CLI may not be as rewarding as hoped because these patients do have generalized peripheral arterial disease spreading down to the pedal arch. The other limiting factor for the application of this concept on patients with CLI is the severely diseased foot run-off and the poor quality of the pedal arch allowing only half of the patients to be selected for the appropriate angiosome revascularization [15, 16]. The authors however believe that the angiosome principle should still be applied to all patients with suitable foot run-off. However, when reporting outcomes of this revascularization policy, the quality of the pedal arch should always be included in the data analysis to be able to accurately assess the success of this treatment from an angiosome point of view.

Surgical Bypass

Using distal (crural) and ultra-distal (pedal) bypasses in the treatment of patients with CLI is a well-established treatment modality with proven good outcomes. The outcomes of these two complex procedures have been previously shown to have very comparable results regardless of the comorbidities of patients undergoing these complex procedures. However, it

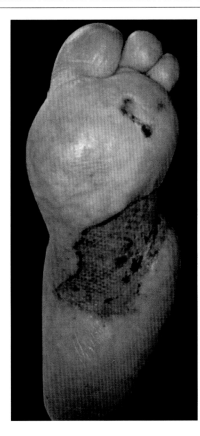

Fig. 37.4 Complete healing after split-thickness skin graft 5 weeks after initial emergency debridement

was shown that the distal bypass group had a higher number of threatened grafts identified during the surveillance programme when compared to the ultra-distal group (40.6% and 26.9%, respectively), although the need for secondary intervention was not statistically significant between the two groups ($p=0.6349$) [17].

The outcome of bypasses is influenced by several factors including the quality of the conduit used and more importantly the quality of the run-off arteries. Rutherford et al. have proposed in their detailed publication a scoring system for scoring all factors that could influence the outcome in infrainguinal bypasses including diabetes, smoking and hyperlipaemia, as well as a run-off scoring system [18]. The wall quality and the internal diameter of the autologous vein used have also influenced the patency rates of these grafts. However, veins with an internal diameter as small as 2 mm have been successfully used with good patency rates [19].

The authors have used a simple classification in reporting the outcome of distal and ultra-distal bypasses passed on the quality of the pedal arch. Three categories were identified: complete (CPA), incomplete (IPC) or no pedal arch (NPA) with either anterior or posterior tibial component, based on angiographic findings prior to bypass surgery [15].

Atherosclerotic Classification of the Pedal Arch

Several classifications for run-off scoring are available in the literature. However, the most used classification is that of Rutherford et al. described in their detailed article about the recommended standards for reporting lower extremity ischaemia. This classification based on the extent of the occlusive disease in the pedal arch was divided into five categories; (1) no primary pedal artery patent, (2) partially patent or fully patent beyond critical in-line occlusive lesion, (3) in-line continuity with patent outflow vessels but incomplete arch, (4) one or more subcritical stenoses distally but no in-line and (5) fully patent pedal run-off (<20% stenosis) [18]. These categories were scored from 3 to 0 where 3 had the worst extent of disease.

However, for a simple preoperative assessment and a classification that offers an angiosomal analysis of the revascularization, the authors have classified the pedal arch based on the digital subtraction angiography (DSA) studies into three categories; complete pedal arch (CPA), incomplete pedal arch (IPA) and no pedal arch (NPA), depending on the extent and the distribution of atherosclerotic occlusive plaque across the pedal arch and its dorsalis pedis and posterior tibial arterial components.

An arch is considered *complete* if the dorsalis pedis component is in direct continuation, through its perforating branch (deep plantar artery), with the posterior tibial artery and its lateral plantar branch without any significant interruption. This could occur with either an occluded or patent anterior tibial and posterior tibial arteries at the level of the ankle (Fig. 37.5).

An *anterior incomplete* pedal arch (Fig. 37.6) is an arch that only includes the dorsalis pedis artery component without any direct connection to the posterior tibial artery or its lateral plantar branch. Whereas, a *posterior incomplete* pedal arch (Fig. 37.7) is an arch that only includes the posterior tibial artery component and its lateral plantar branch without a direct connection to the dorsalis pedis artery.

An *anterior* and *posterior no pedal arch* (Figs. 37.8 and 37.9) is when no pedal arch could be demonstrated; however, the tarsal and digital arteries were filled through collaterals from the anterior and posterior tibial arteries, respectively.

In a study of 167 infrapopliteal bypasses for CLI, preoperative digital subtraction angiography (DSA) showed that only 31 (19%) had CPA, while 104 (62%) had IPA and 32 (19%) had NPA, demonstrating the rarity of the complete pedal arch in these patients with CLI [15]. These findings were also confirmed in a recent study by Kret et al., which showed only 33% of patients undergoing distal bypass surgery for CLI had a complete CPA, whereas 67% had an IPA [16].

Fig. 37.5 (**a**) Completely patent pedal arch with both components; anterior and posterior tibial arteries occluded at ankle level. (**b**) Completely patent pedal arch with both components; anterior and posterior tibial arteries patent. Graphic designer: Mariam Rashid

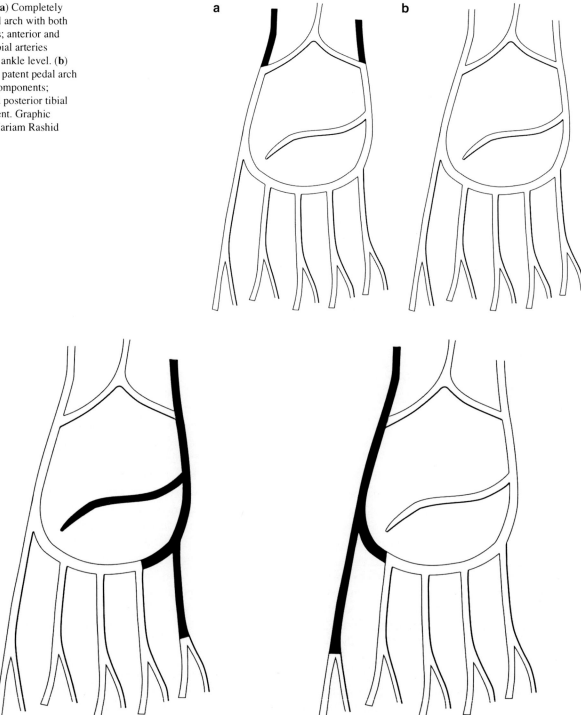

Fig. 37.6 An incomplete pedal arch with an anterior tibial and dorsalis pedis arteries component. Graphic designer: Mariam Rashid

Fig. 37.7 An incomplete pedal arch with a posterior tibial and lateral plantar arteries component. Graphic designer: Mariam Rashid

Assessing the Pedal Arch

Assessing the quality of the pedal arch prior to surgery could be very challenging. This could be due to the advanced occlusive disease of the crural vessels and the pedal arch with severe low flow state in patients with severe chronic CLI. The usage of digital subtraction angiography (DSA) with targeted crural and pedal arch biplane images could still fail to demonstrate the presence of available outflow arteries suitable for successful pedal bypasses. Denying these patients the surgical revascularization option could result in

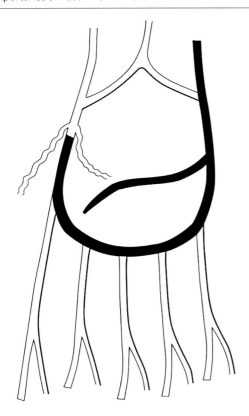

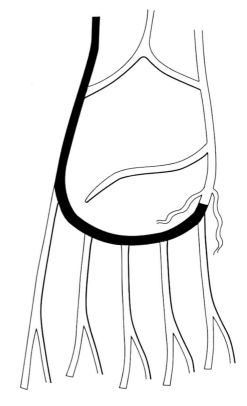

Fig. 37.8 No pedal arch with collateral filling of the tarsal arteries from the dorsalis pedis artery. *Graphic designer*: Mariam Rashid

Fig. 37.9 No pedal arch with collateral filling of the tarsal arteries from the lateral plantar artery. *Graphic designer*: Mariam Rashid

non-healing of tissue loss with a high risk of major amputation. Hence, all effort should be made to identify pedal arteries using more than one imaging modality if necessary.

In a study comparing gadobenate dimeglumine (Gd-BOPTA)-enhanced magnetic resonance angiography (MRA) of the pedal vasculature with selective digital subtraction angiography in patients with peripheral arterial occlusive disease, Gd-BOPTA-enhanced MRA was able to delineate significantly more patent vessels without segmental occlusions and more metatarsal arteries than selective DSA [20]. These results were also confirmed in a later study using contrast-enhanced MRA with a three-dimensional capability that has been proven to be superior to DSA and ultrasound scan in pedal vasculature imaging in CLI detecting potential pedal bypass target arteries [21].

McCarthy et al., comparing preoperative colour-coded duplex imaging and dependent Doppler ultrasonography with intraoperative DSA, showed there was a very good agreement between these two modalities in predicting pedal arch patency and the predominant feeding vessel in patients undergoing crural and pedal bypasses for CLI [22]. The authors rely heavily on the preoperative assessment of the pedal arteries using colour-coded duplex (Figs. 37.10, 37.11, and 37.12) with accurate measurement of the pedal arteries diameters and collateral flow in all patients undergoing pedal bypass surgery. This modality has been very beneficial in patients with no demonstrable pedal arteries on conventional DSA with successful revascularization using ultra-distal bypasses.

In extreme cases, where only pedal arteries could be detected with hand-held Doppler, the authors have performed on-table exploration of the pedal artery and proceeded with successful ultra-distal bypass. This technique has also been successfully reported by Pomposelli et al. in a series of dorsalis pedis bypasses in diabetic patients where in 16 of 28 (57%) cases, no artery was seen but an audible Doppler signal was present and successful bypass was still feasible [23].

Pedal Bypass Patency in Relation to the Quality of Pedal Arch

Few articles have reported patency rates outcome for distal or ultra-distal bypasses in relation to the quality of the pedal arch. Panayiotopoulos et al. showed that the patency rates of femorotibial and peroneal bypasses depend on the number of calf vessels, the presence of straight flow to the foot and the presence of patent pedal vessels [24]. In this study, the authors classified the outflow circulation into categories based on the number of crural vessels available, as well as the number of the vessels crossing the ankle joint. The number of vessels crossing the ankle was shown to be extremely significant ($P < 0.0001$) in graft patency, irrespective of the state of the pedal vessels. If no artery crossed the ankle, the patency rate was only 7% at 6 months. Whereas, if one artery crossed the ankle, the patency improved to 37%, but if two arteries were

Fig. 37.10 Colour-coded duplex demonstrating a patent medial plantar artery with severely damped wave form

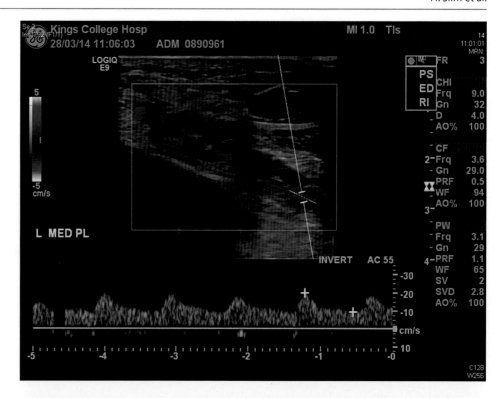

Fig. 37.11 Colour-coded duplex demonstrating a patent but diseased dorsalis pedis artery

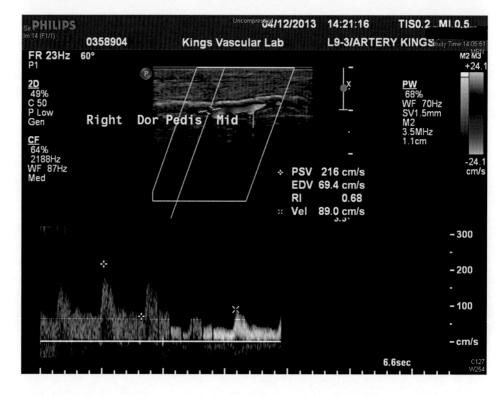

present the outcome was 70 % at 2 years. The 2-year patency associated with two vessels was better than that associated with no patent pedal vessels (58 % vs 6 % at 2 years).

Davies et al., in a study of 90 patients, have also demonstrated similar outcomes with a cumulative patency for grafts with a complete, incomplete and occluded pedal arch as defined by pulse-generated run-off. The 12-month cumulative patency rates were 78 %, 90 % and 38 %, respectively (P < 0.0001) [25].

The authors have studied the patency rates in 167 infrapopliteal bypasses in patients with CLI in relation to the quality of the pedal arch as classified earlier (Figs. 37.13 and 37.14). This showed a 1-year primary patency rates in the

Fig. 37.12 Colour-coded
duplex demonstrating a
severely disease dorsalis pedis
artery with a patent lumen of
0.24 cm

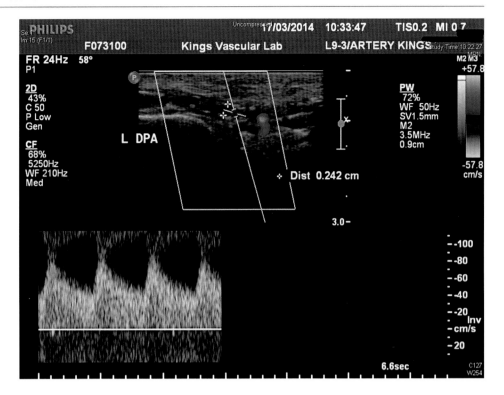

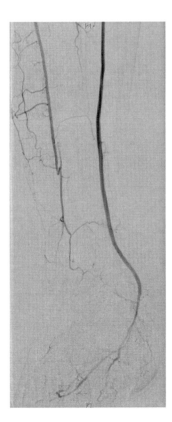

Fig. 37.13 DSA demonstrating a posterior tibial bypass at the malleolar level running into diseased medial and lateral plantar arteries

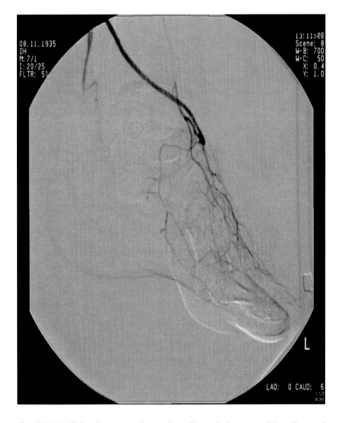

Fig. 37.14 DSA demonstrating a dorsalis pedis bypass with a diseased
incomplete pedal arch

CPA, IPA and NPA groups of 58.4%, 54.6% and 63.8%, respectively ($P=0.5168$), and secondary patency rates of 86.0%, 84.7% and 88.8%, respectively ($P=0.8940$). These results did not achieve statistical difference between the three groups, hence concluding that the quality of the pedal arch did not impact on the patency rates in these patients.

Major Amputation Rate in Relation to the Quality of the Pedal Arch

The authors have studied the major amputation rate and the amputation-free survival in patients with CLI undergoing distal and ultra-distal bypass surgery. This was analysed based on the quality of the pedal arch divided in the three groups complete, incomplete and no pedal arch based on the preoperative angiographic findings. Although there was a trend to have better outcome in the CPA, there was no statistically significant difference between the three groups for the major amputation rate and the amputation-free survival at 48 months (CPA, 67.2%; IPA, 69.7%; and NPA, 45.9%; $P=0.3883$) [15].

Kret et al. have reported similar outcomes with major amputation rates compared between the CPA and IPA groups [16]. However, Biancari et al., using the Rutherford classification of pedal arch disease, showed that in patients with completely open or mildly diseased run-off, the graft patency, leg salvage and survival rates were significantly better than if outflow run-off was compromised [26].

Azuma et al. also showed that the limb salvage rates in patients with CLI undergoing distal bypass surgery, on the direct revascularization and indirect revascularization groups in matched pairs, were statistically insignificant at 97.8% and 92.3% at 2 years, respectively ($p=0.855$) [27].

Pedal Bypass Tissue Loss Healing Outcome in Relation to the Quality of the Pedal Arch

Wound healing in patients with CLI is influenced by several factors including diabetes, end-stage renal disease (ESRD), successful angiosome revascularization, control of ongoing sepsis and nutritional status of the patient.

Azuma et al. demonstrated in a study of 249 CLI undergoing distal bypass surgery that the angiosome concept seems unimportant, at least in non-ESRD patients. However, the location and extent of ischaemic wounds, as well as the comorbidities, could be more relevant than the angiosome in terms of wound healing. The wound healing rate in the indirect revascularization group after matching using a propensity score method was slightly slower than that of the direct revascularization group, but this observation did not reach statistical significance [27].

The authors have studied the healing of 141 CLI with ischaemic feet tissue loss undergoing distal and ultra-distal bypasses. The results were correlated to the quality of the pedal arch and the direct angiosome revascularization [15].

The majority of tissue loss in the foot was in the posterior tibial artery angiosome (86%) compared to 10% in the anterior tibial artery angiosome and 4% in the peroneal artery angiosome. Based on preoperative diagnostic DSA, a CPA was only present in 31 of 141 patients (22%) compared to 88 (62%) with IPA and 22 (16%) with NPA. Although as a unit policy the authors have always attempted to target the angiosome artery, however, direct revascularization of the specific angiosome was only feasible in 66 patients (47%) compared with the nonspecific angiosome in 75 (53%). By following the angiosome vascularization principle, this did not achieve any statistical significant difference between direct angiosome revascularization (DAR) and non-DAR (Fig. 37.15). However, the healing and time-to-healing rates were directly influenced by the quality of the pedal arch. In patients with NPA, wound healing was significantly reduced compared to CPA or IPA ($p=0.0264$). The study also demonstrated that wound healing was significantly compromised in patient with NPA undergoing non-DAR.

Kret et al. studied the outcome in 109 cases of CLI undergoing distal bypass surgery. Direct revascularization, according to pedal angiosomes, provided more efficient wound healing. Unfortunately, this was only possible in one-half of the patients and did not affect amputation-free or overall survival. However, in this series, the direct revascularization group was associated with improved run-off scores. They also showed that comparing patients with and without a CPA revealed similar wound healing between groups (IPA, 63%, $n=36$ vs CPA, 68%, $n=19$; $P=0.67$), as well as median time to complete wound healing as determined by Kaplan–Meier

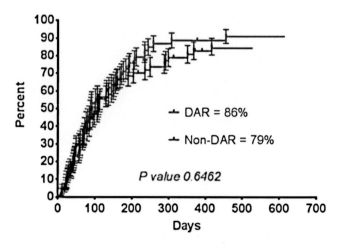

Fig. 37.15 Kaplan–Meier survival curves showing a log-rank P value of 0.6462 in patients healing following direct angiosome revascularization (DAR) and non-DAR

analysis (IPA, 124 days vs CPA, 116 days; log-rank, $P=0.64$) [16]. These results are very similar to the authors' personal series. However, Kret et al. did not include the NPA patients in their series, a group we have found to be significantly difficult to heal. These two studies clearly demonstrate that an IPA will still allow the healing of tissue loss regardless of its site.

In patients with CLI with NPA but still underwent a successful pedal bypass, where healing has been demonstrated to be significantly slower in this group, we believe that the endovascular reconstruction of the pedal arch either on-table or as a staged procedure can achieve rapid healing.

The authors believe that studies with large series examining this healing process in patients with diseased pedal arch and applying the angiosome concept is still needed to be able to reach a final conclusion on the importance this treatment policy in patients with severe CLI.

Loop Angioplasty of the Pedal Arch

The importance of a patent pedal arch for the healing of foot tissue loss has led to attempts to recanalize the whole pedal arch using complex endovascular techniques. The 'pedal-plantar loop' technique was developed by Fusaro et al. [28] which allows the recanalization of both pedal and plantar arteries and their anatomical anastomosis in order to restore direct arterial in-flow from both anterior and posterior tibial vessels. This complex technique, using sub-intimal angioplasty and retrograde pedal cannulation, could achieve full recanalization of the pedal arch with establishing reperfusion to the foot and heel allowing rapid healing of the tissue loss (Figs. 37.16, 37.17, 37.18, and 37.19).

Manzi et al. [29] reported a large series of 135 patients with CLI undergoing this technique with technical success in 85 % of the cases. They also reported clinical improvement in functional status which was obtained and maintained after an average of 12 months, with a significant improvement of transcutaneous oxygen tension after 15 days. This technique is however difficult to reproduce in a standard unit, requiring advanced endovascular skills and techniques. Also, in the unfortunate situations when acute thrombosis of the pedal arch occurs following recanalization, this could end up in major amputation.

The authors have used this pedal-plantar loop technique on-table and in the immediate postoperative period as a planned hybrid procedure, in patients undergoing ultra-distal bypass, with success but in a small number of selected patients. We however believe that these hybrid techniques of extreme open and endovascular procedures will be particularly useful in the so labelled 'no-option' CLI, hence reducing the risk of major amputation in these patients.

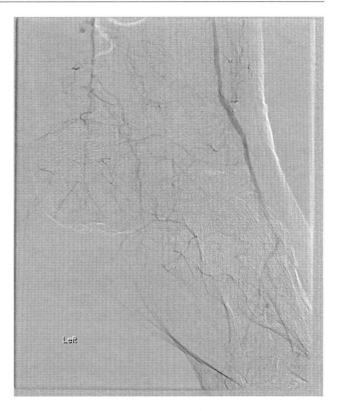

Fig. 37.16 DSA showing a dorsalis pedis artery running into a severely disease pedal arch in a diabetic patient with a non-healing amputation site of her lateral four toes

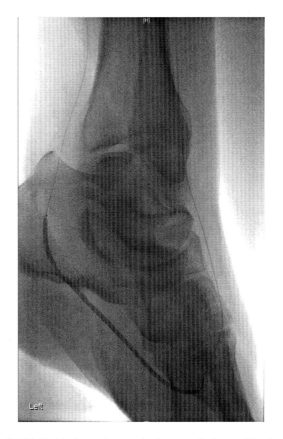

Fig. 37.17 Pedal-plantar loop angioplasty; angioplasty of the lateral plantar artery

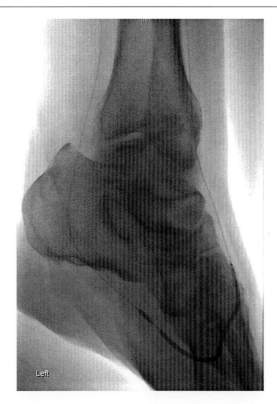

Fig. 37.18 Pedal-plantar loop angioplasty; angioplasty of the plantar arch

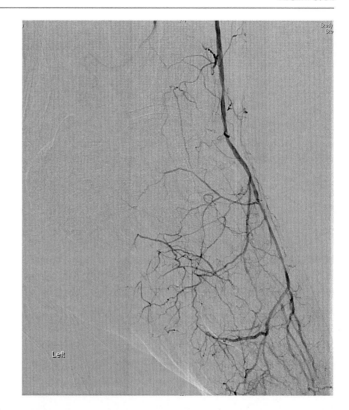

Fig. 37.19 Successful partial canalization of the pedal arch with better filling of the tarsal arteries

References

1. Moore KL, Agur AMR, Dalley AF. Clinically oriented anatomy. 7th, North American Edition. 2013. 978-1451119459.
2. Adachi B. Das Arteriensystem der Japaner. Kyoto: Maruzen; 1928, p. 242–51.
3. Dubreuil-Chambardel L. Variations des arteres du pelvis et du membre inferieur. Paris: Mason; 1925. p. 271.
4. Ozer MA, Govsa F, Bilge O. Anatomic study of the deep plantar arch. Clin Anat. 2005;18(6):434–42.
5. Yamada T, Gloviczki P, Bower TC, Naessens JM, Carmichael SW. Variations of the arterial anatomy of the foot. Am J Surg. 1993;166(2):130–5; discussion 135.
6. Robertson GS, Ristic CD, Bullen BR. The incidence of congenitally absent foot pulses. Ann R Coll Surg Engl. 1990;72(2):99–100.
7. Chavatzas D. Revision of the incidence of congenital absence of dorsalis pedis artery by an ultrasonic technique. Anat Rec. 1974; 178(2):289–90.
8. Reich RS. The pulses of the foot: their value in the diagnosis of peripheral circulatory disease. Ann Surg. 1934;99(4):613–22.
9. Papon X, Brillu C, Fournier HD, Hentati N, Mercier P. Anatomic study of the deep plantar artery: potential by-pass receptor site. Surg Radiol Anat. 1998;20(4):263–6.
10. Taylor GI, Palmer JH. The vascular territories (angiosomes) of the body: experimental study and clinical applications. Br J Plast Surg. 1987;40(2):113–41.
11. Attinger CE, Evans KK, Bulan E, Blume P, Cooper P. Angiosomes of the foot and ankle and clinical implications for limb salvage: reconstruction, incisions, and revascularization. Plast Reconstr Surg. 2006;117 Suppl 7:261S–93S.
12. Neville RF, Attinger CE, Bulan EJ, Ducic I, Thomassen M, Sidawy AN. Revascularization of a specific angiosome for limb salvage: does the target artery matter? Ann Vasc Surg. 2009;23(3):367–73.
13. Biancari F, Juvonen T. Angiosome-targeted lower limb revascularization for ischemic foot wounds: systematic review and meta-analysis. Eur J Vasc Endovasc Surg. 2014;47(5):517–22.
14. Taylor GI, Palmer JH. Angiosome theory. Br J Plast Surg. 1992;45(4):327–8.
15. Rashid H, Slim H, Zayed H, Huang DY, Wilkins CJ, Evans DR, et al. The impact of arterial pedal arch quality and angiosome revascularization on foot tissue loss healing and infrapopliteal bypass outcome. J Vasc Surg. 2013;57(5):1219–26.
16. Kret MR, Cheng D, Azarbal AF, Mitchell EL, Liem TK, Moneta GL, et al. Utility of direct angiosome revascularization and runoff scores in predicting outcomes in patients undergoing revascularization for critical limb ischemia. J Vasc Surg. 2014;59(1):121–8.
17. Slim H, Tiwari A, Ahmed A, Ritter JC, Zayed H, Rashid H. Distal versus ultradistal bypass grafts: amputation-free survival and patency rates in patients with critical leg ischaemia. Eur J Vasc Endovasc Surg. 2011;42(1):83–8.
18. Rutherford RB, Baker JD, Ernst C, Johnston KW, Porter JM, Ahn S, et al. Recommended standards for reports dealing with lower extremity ischemia: revised version. J Vasc Surg. 1997;26(3):517–38.
19. Slim H, Tiwari A, Ritter JC, Rashid H. Outcome of infra-inguinal bypass grafts using vein conduit with less than 3 millimeters diameter in critical leg ischemia. J Vasc Surg. 2011;53(2):421–5.
20. Kreitner KF, Kunz RP, Herber S, Martenstein S, Dorweiler B, Dueber C. MR angiography of the pedal arteries with gadobenate dimeglumine, a contrast agent with increased relaxivity, and comparison with selective intraarterial DSA. J Magn Reson Imaging. 2008;27(1):78–85.
21. Langer S, Kramer N, Mommertz G, Koeppel TA, Jacobs MJ, Wazirie NA, et al. Unmasking pedal arteries in patients with critical ischemia using time-resolved contrast-enhanced 3D MRA. J Vasc Surg. 2009;49(5):1196–202.
22. McCarthy MJ, Nydahl S, Hartshorne T, Naylor AR, Bell PR, London NJ. Colour-coded duplex imaging and dependent Doppler

ultrasonography in the assessment of cruropedal vessels. Br J Surg. 1999;86(1):33–7.

23. Pomposelli Jr FB, Marcaccio EJ, Gibbons GW, Campbell DR, Freeman DV, Burgess AM, et al. Dorsalis pedis arterial bypass: durable limb salvage for foot ischemia in patients with diabetes mellitus. J Vasc Surg. 1995;21(3):375–84.

24. Panayiotopoulos YP, Tyrrell MR, Owen SE, Reidy JF, Taylor PR. Outcome and cost analysis after femorocrural and femoropedal grafting for critical limb ischaemia. Br J Surg. 1997;84(2):207–12.

25. Davies AH, Magee TR, Parry R, Horrocks M, Baird RN. Evaluation of distal run-off before femorodistal bypass. Cardiovasc Surg. 1996;4(2):161–4.

26. Biancari F, Alback A, Ihlberg L, Kantonen I, Luther M, Lepantalo M. Angiographic runoff score as a predictor of outcome following

femorocrural bypass surgery. Eur J Vasc Endovasc Surg. 1999; 17(6):480–5.

27. Azuma N, Uchida H, Kokubo T, Koya A, Akasaka N, Sasajima T. Factors influencing wound healing of critical ischaemic foot after bypass surgery: is the angiosome important in selecting bypass target artery? Eur J Vasc Endovasc Surg. 2012;43(3):322–8.

28. Fusaro M, Dalla Paola L, Biondi-Zoccai G. Pedal-plantar loop technique for a challenging below-the-knee chronic total occlusion: a novel approach to percutaneous revascularization in critical lower limb ischemia. J Invasive Cardiol. 2007;19(2):E34–7.

29. Manzi M, Fusaro M, Ceccacci T, Erente G, Dalla Paola L, Brocco E. Clinical results of below-the knee intervention using pedal-plantar loop technique for the revascularization of foot arteries. J Cardiovasc Surg (Torino). 2009;50(3):331–7.

Endovascular and Thrombolytic Therapy for Upper and Lower Extremity Acute Limb Ischemia

38

Sarah S. Elsayed and Leonardo C. Clavijo

Introduction

Definition

This chapter focuses on the endovascular treatment options for acute limb ischemia (ALI) of the upper and lower extremities, namely, endovascular and thrombolytic therapies. ALI is associated with a high risk of loss of limb and life and thus requires prompt diagnosis, which can be challenging [1]. ALI is defined as a vascular emergency characterized by an abrupt loss of limb perfusion that threatens tissue viability presenting within 14 days of symptom onset [2].

Prevalence

More than 200,000 patients suffered from lower extremity ALI in the USA in 2000. Estimated hospital mortality was 10 % and >1 in eight underwent in-hospital amputation [2]. Using Medicare claim data from 1998 to 2009, Baril et al. showed that there has been a decrease in the incidence of hospitalization for lower extremity ALI from 45.7 to 26 per 100,000. The percentage of patients undergoing surgical intervention decreased from 57.1 to 51.5 %, and those undergoing endovascular intervention increased from 15 to 33.1 % [3]. ALI of the upper extremities is rare and has been reported as 1:4–5 ratio of upper to lower extremity ALI [4].

Clinical Classification of ALI

There are four clinical categories of ALI. Table 38.1 reveals the differences between various clinical limb scenarios and their prognoses, which serves as a helpful guide to type of intervention [5]. Rutherford proposed an algorithm for ALI; after history and physical and Doppler exam confirm an ALI diagnosis and heparin is initiated, patients in categories I (if early intervention is appropriate) and IIA should undergo diagnostic angiography. These patients may undergo catheter-directed thrombolysis (CDT) with or without mechanical thrombectomy or surgical thrombo-embolectomy. For category IIB and III (if early) patients, one must consider emergent surgery and late category III, delayed amputation [5].

Clinical Presentation

A meticulous history should be taken to identify the onset of symptoms (14 days or more), which may dictate indication for intervention and screening for possible embolic source. This may include a cardiac source, such as arrhythmia, recent percutaneous intervention, trauma, connective tissue disease, and cancer [4–7]. A complete physical exam should be done with focus on the symptomatic extremity (pallor, pulses, sensory, motor) as mentioned in Table 38.1.

Investigations

According to the American College of Cardiology Foundation/American Heart Association (ACCF/AHA) 2013 Guidelines for Management of Patients with Peripheral Arterial Disease (PAD), the recommendations are as follows (Table 38.2) [8]:

Electronic supplementary material: The online version of this chapter (doi:10.1007/978-3-319-31991-9_38) contains supplementary material, which is available to authorized users. Videos can also be accessed at http://link.springer.com/chapter/10.1007/978-3-319-31991-9_38.

S.S. Elsayed, MD • L.C. Clavijo, MD, PhD (✉)
Interventional Cardiology, Division of Cardiovascular Medicine, University of Southern California, Los Angeles, CA, USA

Table 38.1 Clinical categories of acute limb ischemia

Category	Prognosis	Sensory loss	Motor deficit	Arterial Doppler	Venous Doppler
I: Viable	No immediate threat	None	None	Audible	Audible
IIA: Marginally threatened	Salvageable if promptly treated	Minimal (toes) or none	None	Inaudible	Audible
IIB: Immediately threatened	Salvageable if immediately revascularized	More than toes, rest pain	Mild/moderate	Inaudible	Audible
III: Irreversible	Major tissue loss, permanent nerve damage inevitable	Profound, anesthetic	Profound, paralysis (rigor)	Inaudible	Inaudible

Data from: Rutherford RB. Clinical Staging of Acute Limb Ischemia as the Basis for Choice of Revascularization Method: When and How to Intervene. Semin Vasc Surg 2009;22:5–9

Table 38.2 ACCF/AHA 2013 guidelines for management of patients with PAD

Level of recommendation	
Class I (Level of Evidence: B)	Patients with ALI and a salvageable extremity should undergo an emergent evaluation that defines the anatomic level of occlusion and leads to prompt endovascular or surgical revascularization
Class III (Level of Evidence: B)	Patients with ALI and a nonviable extremity should not undergo an evaluation to define vascular anatomy or efforts to attempt revascularization

Data from: Anderson JL et al. Management of Patients with Peripheral Artery Disease (Compilation of 2005 and 2011 ACCF/AHA Guideline Recommendations). Circulation 2013;127:1425–43

Etiology

There are numerous etiologies for ALI in the lower extremity (LE) and upper extremity (UE) [4, 5]:

- Thrombosis (in situ)
- Embolic
  - Cardiac: atrial fibrillation, left atrial appendage thrombus, left ventricular thrombus, myocardial infarction
  - Paradoxical: patent foramen ovale and deep venous thrombosis
  - Atherosclerotic: aortic atheroma, thrombosed popliteal aneurysm (LE)
- Vasculitis
- Trauma
- Iatrogenic
- Malignancy
- Thoracic outlet syndrome (UE)
- Subclavian aneurysm (UE)

Treatment

There are three treatment options for ALI, which depend on multiple factors, including duration of symptoms, ALI clinical category, patient comorbidities/functional status, and availability of treatment options per institution [5].

- Catheter-directed thrombolysis (CDT)
- CDT with percutaneous mechanical thrombectomy (PMT)
- Surgical thrombo-embolectomy (Table 38.3)
- Ouriel et al. (Rochester trial) randomized patients to surgery (revascularization or amputation as required, $n=57$) versus thrombolysis (with urokinase 4000 IU/min, $n=57$) [9, 14].
  - There was a survival benefit in the thrombolysis group (84%) compared to surgical group (58%), $p=0.01$.
  - In-hospital complications were 16% and 41% in the thrombolysis and surgical groups, respectively, $p=0.001$.
  - There was no difference in limb salvage.
  - At 30 days, stroke rates were 1.8% and 0%, and hemorrhage rates were 10.5% and 1.8% in the thrombolysis and surgical groups, respectively.
- The STILE trial included 393 patients from 31 centers and randomized them to surgery versus thrombolysis as the initial treatment for ALI [9]. Two different thrombolytic regimens were used (rt-PA 0.05 mg/kg/h or urokinase 250,000 IU bolus followed by 4000 IU/min, in addition to heparin 5000 IU bolus intravenously then infusion 1000 unit/h+ASA 325 mg).
  - The trial was stopped early due to adverse events in the thrombolysis group at 1 month (in both bypass and native artery subgroups).
  - At 6-month follow up:

Table 38.3 Treatment strategy according to ALI clinical categories by Rutherford

Category	
I: Viable	Endovascular (CDT ± PMT) or surgical
IIA: Marginally threatened	Endovascular (CDT ± PMT) or surgical
IIB: Immediately threatened	Surgical (but operating room availability may be delayed) so consider endovascular
III: Irreversible	Amputation

Data from: Rutherford RB. Clinical Staging of Acute Limb Ischemia as the Basis for Choice of Revascularization Method: When and How to Intervene. Semin Vasc Surg 2009;22:5–9

Three large randomized trials have evaluated thrombolysis versus surgery for acute limb ischemia of the lower extremity [1, 9]:

- Rochester trial [14]
- Surgery versus Thrombolysis for Ischemia of the Lower Extremity (STILE) (1994)
  - ALI <14 days
  - Ischemia >14 days
- STILE subanalysis (1996)
  - Occluded bypass
  - Native artery occlusion
- Thrombolysis or Peripheral Arterial Surgery (TOPAS) (1998)

  Patients with <14 days' duration of symptoms:
  Thrombolysis group had significantly reduced rate of death and amputation (15.3 % versus 37.5 %, $p=0.01$).
  Patients with >14 days' duration of symptoms:
  Thrombolysis group had reversed (increased) trend of death and amputation (17.8 % versus 9.9 %, $p=0.08$) that did not reach significance.
- Hemorrhage occurred in 5.6 % and 0.7 % in the thrombolysis and surgery groups, respectively.
- Catheter placement failed in 28 % of patients in the thrombolysis group.
- Patients divided into <14 days' duration and >14 days' duration was a post hoc division not stratified in the original protocol.
- Over 80 % of patients had symptoms >14 days.

- The STILE subgroup analyses at 12 months (low number of patients):
  - Comerota (bypass grafts):
    Reduced amputation rate (<14 days' duration group).
    Overall, the thrombolysis group had higher rate of continued ischemia, claudication, or critical limb ischemia (73 % versus 50 %, $p=0.01$).
    Increased morbidity in prosthetic grafts compared to autogenous grafts ($p=0.038$).
  - Weaver (native artery):
    Recurrent ischemia (64 % versus 35 %, $p=0.0001$) and major amputation (10 % versus 0 %, $p=0.0024$) were higher in the thrombolysis group.
    Very few patients were included in subgroup analysis.
    Some patients failed to receive a catheter, but were included in the thrombolysis group.
- The TOPAS trial included 213 patients from 79 centers. All patients had class II ischemia for <14 days. Three different urokinase thrombolysis regimens were used (2000 IU/min versus 4000 IU/min versus 6000 IU/min for first 2 h). All regimens were followed by 2000 IU/min.
  - Comparison between thrombolysis (optimal dose 4000 IU/min) and surgery was done.
  - No significant difference was seen in 1-year mortality or amputation-free survival between groups.
- Meta-analysis of the previously mentioned trials showed the following:
  - No significant difference in limb salvage or death at 30 days, 6 months, or 1 year between initial treatment with surgery and thrombolysis.
  - Stroke was more likely to occur at 30 days in the thrombolysis group.
  - Major hemorrhage was more likely to occur at 30 days in the thrombolysis group.
  - Failure to place catheter was a major problem in STILE (Tables 38.4, 38.5, 38.6, and 38.7).

Therapeutic Infusion Systems Commercially Available in the USA

- AngioDynamics (Queensbury, NY): Pulse Spray, Unifuse Infusion Catheter, SpeedLyser Infusion System.
- Covidien (Mansfield, MA): Cragg-McNamara Valved Infusion Catheter, MicroMewi Infusion Catheter with Multiple Sideholes, ProStream Infusion Wire.
- Merit Medical Systems, Inc. (South Jordan, UT): Fountain Infusion Catheter with Squirt Fluid Dispensing System, Mistique Infusion Catheter, Fountain Occluding Wire.

Table 38.4 Summary of major outcome in three large randomized trials

Trial	Limb salvage at 6 months (%)			Limb salvage at 12 months (%)			Survival at 6 months (%)			Survival at 12 months (%)		
	Surg	Endo	P value	Surg	Endo	P value	Surg	Endo	P value	Surg	Endo	P value
Rochester	–	–	–	82	82	–	–	–	–	58	84	0.01
STILE												
<14 days	70	88.9	0.02	–	–	–	25.7	54	0.011	–	–	–
>14 days	97	87	0.01	–	–	–	–	–	–	–	–	–
STILE subanalysis												
Bypass	–	–	–	70	82	0.011	–	–	–	100	94	0.290
Native	100	93.3	<0.05	100	90	0.0024	87.4	92.7	NS	85.1	89.3	NS
TOPAS	74.8	71.8	0.43	69.9	65	0.23	–	–	–	83	80	NS

Data from: van den Berg JC. Thrombolysis for acute arterial occlusion. J Vasc Surg 2010;52:512–5
– not available, *NS* not significant. In STILE results: survival column corresponds to composite endpoint (trial stopped). In TOPAS results: limb salvage column corresponds to amputation-free survival

Table 38.5 ACCF/AHA 2013 guidelines for the management of patients with PAD

Level of recommendation	
Class I (Level of Evidence: A)	CDT is an effective and beneficial therapy in patients with ALI (Rutherford category I, IIa) with symptoms <14 days' duration
Class IIa (Level of Evidence: B)	Mechanical thrombectomy devices may be used as adjunctive therapy in patients with ALI due to peripheral arterial occlusion
Class IIb (Level of Evidence: B)	CDT or thrombectomy may be considered in patients with ALI (Rutherford category IIb) of >14 days' duration

Data from: Anderson JL et al. Management of Patients with Peripheral Artery Disease (Compilation of 2005 and 2011 ACCF/AHA Guideline Recommendations). Circulation 2013;127:1425–43

Table 38.6 Thrombolytic drugs, mechanisms of action, half-life, and protocols in CDT for ALI [10, 11]

Drug	Mechanism of action	Half-life (min)	Protocol
Urokinase	Cleavage of the arginine–valine bond in plasminogen leading to active plasmin	7–20	*No longer used in the USA* Multiple protocols in the UK: 240,000 IU/h in the first 4 h followed by 120,000 IU/h for up 48 h (with or without 250,000 IU bolus)
Streptokinase	Irreversible binding and activation of SK to plasminogen. Indirect activation. Vaguely fibrin specific	12–18	*No longer used*
Alteplase (rt-PA, t-PA)	Tissue plasminogen activator produced by recombinant DNA technology. Fibrin-enhanced conversion of plasminogen to plasmin. It produces limited conversion of plasminogen in the absence of fibrin	3–6	Weight-based scheme: 0.001–0.02 mg/Kg/h Non-weight-based scheme: 0.12–2.0 mg/h. Maximum dose: 40 mg
Reteplase (r-PA)	Similar to alteplase. Lower fibrin binding and superior penetration ability	14–18	From 0.25 to 1.0 mg/h. Maximum: 20 IU in 24 h
Tenecteplase (t-NK)	Similar to alteplase. Greater binding affinity for fibrin	20–24	Bolus infusion of 1–5 mg, followed by infusions ranging from 0.125 to 0.5 mg/h

Data from: Karnabatidis D et al. Quality Improvement Guidelines for Percutaneous Catheter-Directed Intra-Arterial Thrombolysis and Mechanical Thrombectomy for Acute Lower-Limb Ischemia. Cardiovasc Intervent Radiol 2011;34:1123–1136

Table 38.7 Percutaneous mechanical thrombectomy/thrombolysis/embolectomy device examples commercially available in USA

Company name	Product name	Mode of operation
Argon Medical Devices, Inc. (designed by Rex Medical) (Athens, TX)	Cleaner	Battery-operated, handheld drive unit initiates the mechanical rotation of an atraumatic, wall-contact, 9-mm sinusoidal vortex wire for effective thrombus maceration
Bayer (Minneapolis, MN)	AngioJet	High-velocity water jets enclosed in catheter utilize the Bernoulli principle for capture, micro-fragmentation, and removal
Covidien (Mansfield, MA)	Trellis	Mechanical oscillation of sinusoidal wave catheter with two compliant balloons surrounding the treatment zone; this allows for isolation of thrombus and targeted, thrombolytic infusion
EKOS Corporation (Bothell, WA)	EkoSonic Endovascular System with Rapid Pulse Modulation	Ultrasound-accelerated thrombolysis simultaneously delivers ultrasound and thrombolytics to target clot; high-frequency, low-power ultrasonic energy loosens and thins the clot's fibrin structure, allowing thrombolytic agents to access more receptor sites. At the same time, ultrasonic pressure forces the drug deep into the clot and keeps it there so it does not escape downstream
Medtronic (Minneapolis, MN)	Export	Aspiration catheter
Vascular Solutions (Minneapolis, MN)	Pronto	Aspiration catheter
Arrow International, a division of Teleflex (Asheboro, NC)	Single Lumen Double Lumen	Embolectomy balloon catheter
Edwards Lifesciences (Irvine, CA)	Fogarty	Embolectomy balloon catheter

Table 38.8 Complications related to thrombolytic therapy

Complication	Incidence (%)		
	Overall	Urokinase	rt-PA
Hemorrhagic stroke	1–2.3	0.6	2.8
Major hemorrhage	<5.1	6.2	8.4
Minor hemorrhage	14.8	21.9	43.8
Mortality	<1	3	5.6
Peri-catheter thrombosis	3–16.7	–	–
Catheter-related trauma	1.2–1.4	–	–
Compartment syndrome	2	–	–
Distal embolization	<1	–	–

Data from: van den Berg JC. Thrombolysis for acute arterial occlusion. J Vasc Surg 2010;52:512–5
rt-PA recombinant tissue plasminogen activator – not available

- Spectranetics Corporation (Colorado Springs, CO): Tapas Targeted Drug Delivery System.

Procedural Complications

Complications related to surgery include stroke, hemorrhage, reoperation, and cardiopulmonary complications (Table 38.8) [12].

Long-Term Outcomes

Long-term data are lacking in patients with ALI. At 1 year, survival was 80 % in most trials, and amputation-free survival was 65–70 % in TOPAS [1]. Byrne et al. showed that endovascular therapy with CDT or PMT in patients with ALI is beneficial, with a major amputation rate of 15 % at 15 months [6]. Predictors of limb loss in this study were end-stage renal disease and poor pedal outflow.

Example Case 1

- **History**: A 59-year-old woman with history of 30-pack year tobacco use and recent axillary bifemoral bypass surgery at another hospital presented to the emergency room with excruciating right lower extremity rest pain that started at 4 a.m.
- Physical exam:
  - Cold mottled right leg with decreased sensation and intact motor strength.
  - No palpable pulses except for femoral 1+. Doppler signal was found at the popliteal level but not distal.
- **Plan**: Urgently, patient was taken to the cardiac catheterization laboratory, and an angiogram was performed of the native bilateral lower extremity arteries and of the axillary bifemoral bypass graft (Image 1).

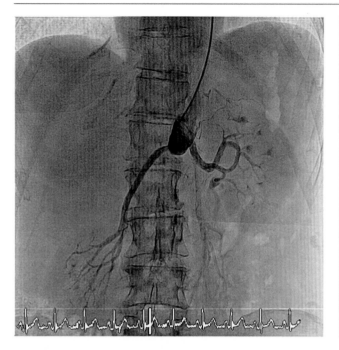

Fig. 38.1 Aortogram showing occlusion of the aorta just distal to the renal arteries

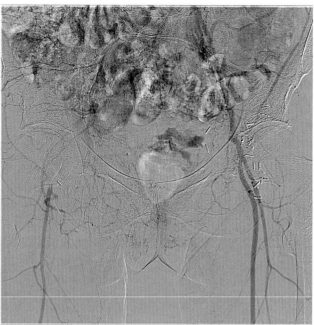

Fig. 38.2 Angiogram showing occluded axillary bifemoral bypass graft, reconstitution of the common femoral arteries. The right SFA is occluded

- **Aortogram with bilateral lower extremity and bypass graft angiogram**:
  - Occlusion of the aorta just distal to the renal arteries and occluded right axillary femoral bypass with reconstitution of the common femoral arteries bilaterally.
  - The right superficial femoral artery (SFA) was occluded, and the profunda artery was patent providing collaterals to the above-knee popliteal artery.
  - The left SFA and profunda arteries are patent.
  - There was a severe proximal stenosis of the axillary bifemoral bypass graft.
  - **Intervention**: AngioJet thrombectomy, catheter-directed thrombolysis of the axillary right femoral bypass graft, and angioplasty of the severe proximal stenosis with excellent result. Occluded SFA prior to intervention was completely patent after CDT and mechanical thrombectomy (Figs. 38.1 and 38.2).
  - Axillary bifemoral bypass graft angiogram before and after intervention (Videos 38.1 and 38.2) (Figs. 38.3 and 38.4).

- **Physical Exam**:
  - Left leg was cool, decreased sensation on sole of foot, intact motor strength.
  - Right leg with normal pulses. Left leg with 2+ femoral, non-palpable popliteal, posterior tibial, and dorsalis pedis pulses but with Doppler signal present.
- **Plan**: Patient was taken urgently to the cardiac catheterization laboratory for aortogram and left lower extremity angiogram.
- **Angiogram**:
  - Aorta, iliacs, common femoral, SFA, and profunda arteries were normal.
  - The popliteal artery was occluded at mid-portion.
  - Faint reconstitution of anterior tibial and posterior tibial arteries was visualized.
- **Intervention**: CDT of the popliteal artery was performed. Twenty-four hours later, repeat angiogram showed residual thrombus; thus, AngioJet thrombectomy was done with excellent results. Three-vessel runoff was visualized after intervention (Fig. 38.5).

Example Case 2

- **History**: A 33-year-old woman with history of multiple miscarriages and cocaine use presented with left lower extremity claudication pain for 1 week and rest pain for 2 days. She complained of left leg coolness and sensitivity to touch.

Summary

- ALI is associated with a high risk for morbidity and mortality, especially if left untreated or not treated promptly.
- Survival and limb salvage are the ultimate goals.
- Rutherford categories should be used to classify patients with ALI.

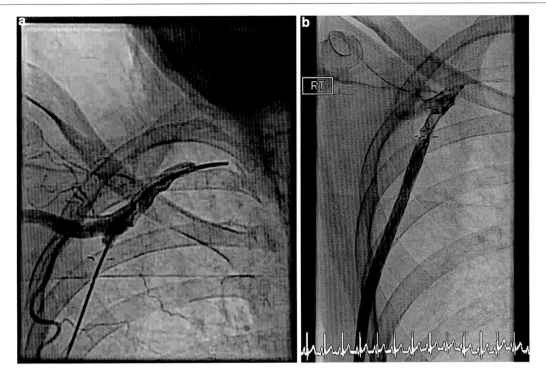

Fig. 38.3 (a) and (b) showing axillary bypass graft before and after intervention

Fig. 38.4 (a) and (b)
showing SFA before
(occluded) and after (patent)
intervention

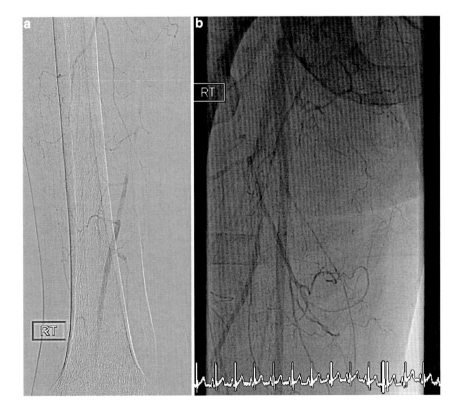

Fig. 38.5 (**a**) and (**b**) showing popliteal artery before and after intervention

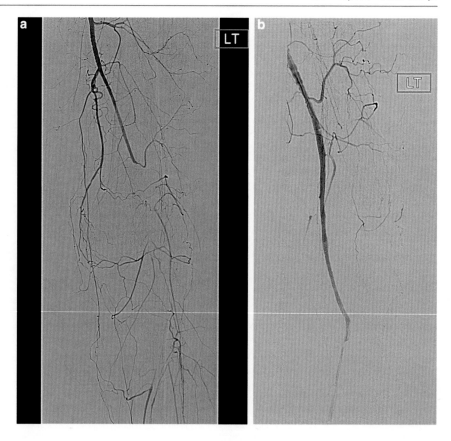

- Patients with Rutherford categories I and IIA can be treated via endovascular or surgical approaches. CDT with or without mechanical thrombectomy is effective and beneficial for these categories.
- On the other hand, patients with Rutherford category IIB can undergo emergent surgery or endovascular therapy (if resources are not available for surgery).
- Rutherford category III is irreversible and patients should undergo amputation.
- Three large randomized trials have evaluated thrombolysis versus surgery for ALI; however, there are no contemporary trials using the newer, current thrombolytic agents.
- After reviewing the available randomized data, survival and limb salvage are similar in thrombolysis and surgery groups.
- CDT has similar major amputation outcomes compared to PMT in patients with mild to moderate ALI [6, 13].

References

1. van den Berg JC. Thrombolysis for acute arterial occlusion. J Vasc Surg. 2010;52:512–5.

2. Vemulapalli S, Curtis LH. Putting the vascular back into cardiovascular research ST-segment-elevation myocardial infarction as a blueprint for improving care in patients with acute limb ischemia. Circulation. 2013;128:89–91.

3. Baril DT, Ghosh K, Rosen AB. Trends in the incidence, treatment, and outcomes of acute lower extremity ischemia in the United States Medicare population. J Vasc Surg. 2014;60(3):669–77.e2.

4. Hernandez-Richter T, Angele MK, Helmberger T, et al. Acute ischemia of the upper extremity: long-term results following thrombo-embolectomy with the Fogarty catheter. Langenbecks Arch Surg. 2001;386:261–6.

5. Rutherford RB. Clinical staging of acute limb ischemia as the basis for choice of revascularization method: when and how to intervene. Semin Vasc Surg. 2009;22:5–9.

6. Byrne RM, Taha AG, Avgerinos E, et al. Contemporary outcomes of endovascular interventions for acute limb ischemia. J Vasc Surg. 2014;59:988–95.

7. Sultan S, Evoy D, Saad Eldin A, et al. Atraumatic acute upper limb ischemia: a series of 64 patients in a Middle East tertiary vascular center and literature review. Vasc Endovascular Surg. 2001;35:181–97.

8. Anderson JL, Halperin JL, Albert NM, et al. Management of patients with peripheral artery disease (compilation of 2005 and 2011 ACCF/AHA guideline recommendations): a report of the American College of Cardiology Foundation/American Heart Association Task Force on Practice Guidelines. Circulation. 2013;127:1425–43.

9. Berridge DC, Kessel DO, Robertson I. Surgery versus thrombolysis for initial management of acute limb ischemia. Cochrane Database Syst Rev. 2013;6:CD002784.

10. Karnabatidis D, Spiliopoulos S, Tsetis D, et al. Quality improvement guidelines for percutaneous catheter-directed intra-arterial thrombolysis and mechanical thrombectomy for acute lower-limb ischemia. Cardiovasc Intervent Radiol. 2011;34:1123–36.

11. Rajan DK, Patel NH, Valji K, et al. Quality improvement guidelines for percutaneous management of acute limb ischemia. J Vasc Interv Radiol. 2009;20:S208–18.

12. Kempe K, Starr B, Stafford JM, et al. Results of surgical management of acute thromboembolic lower extremity ischemia. J Vasc Surg. 2014;60(3):702–7.

13. Comerota AJ, Gravett MH. Do randomized trials of thrombolysis versus open revascularization still apply to current management: what has changed? Semin Vasc Surg. 2009;22:41–6.

14. Ouriel K, Shortell CK, DeWeese JA, et al. A comparison of thrombolytic therapy with operative revascularization in the initial treatment of acute peripheral arterial ischemia. J Vasc Surg. 1994;19(6):1021–30.

Surgical Treatment for Acute Limb Ischemia

Pegge M. Halandras

Introduction

Patients suffering from acute limb ischemia (ALI) are at risk for significant morbidity and mortality. Successful surgical revascularization in this high-risk group is dependent on maintaining a systematic treatment approach. First, this chapter will review those clinical findings important for recognizing ALI. The classification of an affected limb according to its predicted viability will be discussed. Ultimately this categorization will help determine the urgency or futility of restoring blood flow to an ischemic leg. Finally, characteristics of the two major causes of ALI, embolus and thrombosis, will be explored to illustrate various treatment approaches for revascularization.

Diagnosis

Timely diagnosis and accurate recognition of the etiology of decreased limb perfusion is essential for successful treatment of ALI. History should be focused on determining the onset of symptoms and symptoms are most commonly due to pain. Duration, location, and severity can provide important clues about the source of the ischemia and institution of an appropriate treatment plan. In addition, past and recent medical history is important to establish as this may suggest an etiology and the urgency of intervention. If a patient has a history of claudication or previous vascular surgery, collaterals may have developed and result in less severe presenting symptoms or even a delay in presentation. In contrast, if a patient has a history of atrial fibrillation or aneurysmal disease, an embolic source may be responsible.

P.M. Halandras, MD (✉)
Division of Vascular Surgery and Endovascular Therapy,
Department of Surgery, Loyola University Chicago,
2160 S. First Ave., Building 110, Maywood, IL 60153, USA

This patient will present with sudden and severe onset of ischemic symptoms that may be urgently and effectively treated with embolectomy.

Physical exam findings of ALI have traditionally correlated with six signs and symptoms referred to as the "six Ps." These include pain, pallor, poikilothermia, pulselessness, paresthesia, and paralysis (Fig. 39.1). Careful physical exam allows identification of the level of occlusion, the viability of the limb, the urgency of revascularization efforts, and the decision to proceed with endovascular versus surgical modalities. For instance, a patient with complaints of bilateral lower-extremity pain, lack of femoral pulses, mottling to the proximal lower extremities, and complete lack of lower-extremity motor or sensory function is most likely suffering from an aortoiliac occlusion. This patient's ischemic event should be urgently addressed and carries a high risk of morbidity and mortality. This presentation is contrast with a patient presenting with a palpable femoral pulse and a painful, pale foot that is numb but without motor dysfunction. In contrast to the first scenario, the less severe presentation may allow more detailed evaluation of the cause for acute limb ischemia. Additional diagnostic studies may be obtained prior to revascularization. The two previous clinical scenarios also highlight the importance of comparing both lower extremities during the physical exam. This comparison will help establish a baseline of the degree of peripheral vascular disease and assist with identifying if the acute ischemic event is secondary to an embolus or thrombosis.

Proper identification of the degree of acute ischemia is the cornerstone of management for this entity. Reporting standards approved by the Joint Council of the Society for Vascular Surgery and the North American Chapter of the International Society for Cardiovascular Surgery for acute limb ischemia were first proposed in 1986 and revised in 1997 [1]. Acute limb ischemia should be categorized according to the criteria illustrated in Table 39.1. These criteria are frequently referred to as the Rutherford classification. Categories are based on the presenting viability of a threatened limb, prognosis of intervention, and physical exam findings. These exam findings include evaluation of sensory function, motor function, and Doppler exam. This categorization tool will assist with developing a treatment algorithm. Category I refers to a viable limb that can be investigated with further diagnostic studies and does not require prompt revascularization. Category III refers to acutely ischemic limbs with loss of motor and sensory function along with tissue loss. Category III limbs are frequently managed with primary amputation as revascularization efforts may result in a painful, nonfunctional limb. Finally, category II can be subdivided into two levels of severity. Category IIa refers to a marginally threatened limb with retained motor function and minimal numbness restricted to the toes. Category IIb refers to an immediately threatened limb with more severe pain such as rest pain and most importantly, mild or moderate motor dysfunction. Patients in category IIa require prompt revascularization and those patients in category IIb require immediate revascularization. Therefore, patients categorized in either category I or III do not represent the management dilemma involved with correctly identifying and managing those patients in the subcategories of category II. Historically, patients categorized as IIb were not candidates for endovascular treatment due to the need for immediate revascularization. Due to advances in therapy, endovascular revascularization can now be performed concurrently with diagnostic studies. For instance, an arteriogram can be performed in the same setting as restoration of flow in an expedient manner with pharmacomechanical thrombolytic therapy. Therefore, revascularization efforts for category II patients should proceed regardless of endovascular versus surgical techniques according to the urgency dictated by the subcategorization into a marginally threatened IIa versus immediately threatened IIb limb.

After determining if a patient is a revascularization candidate, proper management is also dependent on identifying the underlying cause of the acute limb ischemia. Acute limb ischemia occurs typically in the setting of either an embolic or a thrombotic event. Thrombotic events are estimated to be responsible for 85 % of cases of ALI. Embolic events occur less commonly and make up roughly 15 % of events [2]. Proper identification of the responsible etiology will assist with the type of intervention performed and the durability of this intervention.

An embolic event involves lodging of material in a vessel with obstruction of distal limb perfusion. The majority of emboli are secondary to thrombus with a cardiac origin [3]. Cardiac emboli frequently result from arrhythmias, thrombus formation after myocardial infarction, valvular destruction, cardiac tumors, or paradoxical emboli. Thrombus from proximal aneurysmal disease and embolization of proximal atherosclerotic plaque may also be responsible. Finally, emboli secondary to an endovascular intervention may be due to dislodgement of thrombus by catheters and wires or thrombus formation with prolonged sheath placement.

The second type of event, thrombosis, should be suspected in patients with a history of peripheral vascular disease. Atherosclerotic plaque rupture may cause thrombosis of the vessel at this site and result in occlusion of the vessel with limited collateral flow. Other sources of thrombosis include arterial dissection causing distal occlusion of distal outflow, hypercoagulable states, trauma resulting in intimal damage or flap creation, low-flow states created by hypotension or vasoactive drugs, and compartment syndrome.

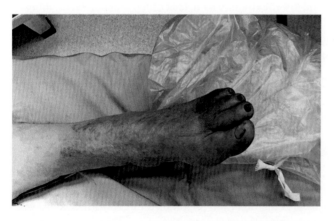

Fig. 39.1 Typical findings with acute limb ischemia including pain, pulselessness, coolness, neurogenic dysfunction, and skin demarcation

Table 39.1 Clinical categories or Rutherford classification for acute limb ischemia

Category	Description/prognosis	Sensory loss	Motor loss	Arterial Doppler signal	Venous Doppler signal
I. Viable	Not immediately threatened	None	None	Audible	Audible
II. Threatened					
a. Marginally	Salvageable with *prompt* treatment	Minimal	None	Inaudible	Audible
b. Immediately	Salvageable with *immediate* revascularization	Moderate, rest pain	Mild to moderate	Inaudible	Audible
III. Irreversible	Major tissue loss, permanent nerve damage	Profound, complete	Profound, paralysis	Inaudible	Inaudible

Management

Once the diagnosis of acute limb ischemia is made and the viability of the affected limb has been categorized, patients should undergo systemic heparinization. The main goal of heparin administration is to prevent propagation of thrombus and thereby, prevent worsening of ischemia. Most often, intravenous, unfractionated heparin is utilized.

Electrocardiogram is routinely obtained and will help establish if a patient has a possible arrhythmia responsible for the ALI. In addition, a metabolic panel should be obtained and can help guide diagnostic studies and interventional methods based on a patient's renal function. Finally a complete blood count, prothrombin time, and partial thromboplastin time should also be obtained. Other studies should be collected, such as a baseline fibrinogen level if thrombolytic therapy is being considered and a baseline creatine phosphokinase level if compartment syndrome following revascularization is a concern. The next step in management involves the decision to obtain imaging studies. The classification of ALI guides the need for emergent intervention versus the luxury of imaging to more specifically delineate the etiology and treatment for ALI. Imaging modalities include formal ultrasound studies, arteriography, computed tomographic angiography (CTA), and magnetic resonance angiography (MRA). Ultrasound can help identify the level of occlusion and status of distal outflow but is operator dependent. In addition, ultrasound does not routinely identify proximal sources accurately and may not be easily obtained during off-hours. Arteriography accurately diagnoses the level of obstruction and status of distal runoff. Also, patients that will be more effectively treated with percutaneous interventions versus surgery (embolectomy or bypass) can be identified. As previously stated, patients categorized as category IIb and requiring immediate revascularization were not traditionally candidates for formal arteriography performed in an interventional suite. The recent institution of hybrid operating room suites now makes postponing intervention for an arteriogram less of an issue as the study can be performed prior to surgical interventions with little delay. CTA may be performed relatively expediently but should not delay intervention in patients with category IIb ALI. In addition, those patients with renal insufficiency or those expected to need significant contrast administration for revascularization efforts may not be candidates for CTA. Finally, MRA is traditionally an imaging modality that is time consuming, may be contraindicated in those with metal implants or renal insufficiency, and is typically reserved for those patients not needing immediate revascularization.

Imaging can demonstrate clear differences between emboli and thrombotic events. Emboli frequently lodge at arterial bifurcations such as the femoral bifurcation and remaining vessels may be normal appearing. Occlusions can be sharply demarcated with a crescent shape and without associated collateral vessels. These findings are in contrast to thrombotic events that typically affect areas prone to atherosclerotic disease. An example is the superficial femoral artery at the adductor canal. Patients suffering from thrombosis may have more evidence of significant atherosclerotic disease including robust collateral vessel development and peripheral vascular disease bilaterally [4].

To summarize, a patient is diagnosed with ALI and categorized according to the Rutherford classification system. Affected patients are then promptly heparinized and additional diagnostic tests such as labs and ECGs are obtained. Obtaining additional imaging prior to revascularization is dependent on the categorization of limb viability. Patients requiring immediate revascularization (class IIb), patients without a percutaneous solution (i.e., thrombosed bypass graft without an option for percutaneous revascularization), or those who felt to be more expediently managed with open embolectomy are typically managed with an open surgical intervention.

Strategies for Surgical Revascularization

Surgical revascularization techniques for ALI consist of thromboembolectomy, endarterectomy, patch angioplasty, and bypass. Thromboembolectomy involves passing a Fogarty balloon catheter past an embolus or through a thrombosed bypass graft or artery. The balloon is inflated while removing the catheter in an attempt to clear the responsible occlusion (Fig. 39.2). Those patients presenting with an absent femoral pulse and presumed suprainguinal occlusion affecting the distal aorta, iliac system, or occluded suprainguinal bypass may undergo femoral artery exposure with subsequent thromboembolectomy (Fig. 39.3). Those patients with a focal embolus in the common femoral artery or superficial femoral artery due to an arrhythmia may also be treated with embolectomy. Finally, an occluded infrainguinal bypass that cannot be safely or effectively managed with thrombolysis or pharmacomechanical thrombectomy can be managed with thromboembolectomy. This intervention may require both a femoral and popliteal exposure and requires thoughtful evaluation of the bypass graft. The decision to salvage a bypass graft is directly dependent on the type of bypass conduit (venous or prosthetic), availability of additional native conduit, and timing of thrombosis (acute or chronic). If the bypass is prosthetic, there is less incentive to salvage the bypass if thrombus is not easily removed or anastomotic problems cannot be improved. If the bypass graft is acutely thrombosed, this is likely due to a technical problem that may be repaired with restoration of flow through the bypass graft. This scenario is in contrast to midterm and late thrombosis of a bypass. Midterm failure is defined as 3–24

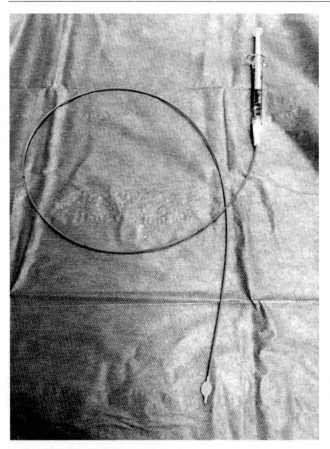

Fig. 39.2 Fogarty catheter used for thromboembolectomy

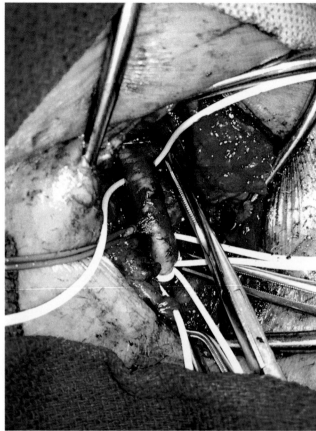

Fig. 39.3 Exposure of the femoral artery to be used for thromboembolectomy, endarterectomy, or bypass target

months after initial bypass and attributed to hyperplasia. Late graft thrombosis is defined as greater than 2 years after bypass and many times is directly attributed to distal progression of atherosclerotic disease [5]. Consequently, scenarios involving midterm or late graft occlusion may require more extensive revascularization techniques to be detailed below.

Following thromboembolectomy, adequacy of intervention should be determined to guide further management. Frequently, the limb will be evaluated to determine if the appearance has improved. Palpable pulses may have returned or Doppler signals may now be detected. Apart from these physical exam findings, passage of a Fogarty catheter allows tactile sensation of potential areas of stenosis. In addition, the character of inflow and back bleeding from an affected artery or discontinuation of thrombotic retrieval may offer clues about the adequacy of an intervention. Although frequently used, the true accuracy of these measures has been debated in the literature [6, 7]. Completion arteriogram offers a more definitive method to investigate for completeness of thrombus or embolus removal. Likewise, the extent of native artery disease or anastomotic stenosis that may be responsible for reocclusion can be identified and corrected. Retrospective analysis of patients treated with routine versus selective completion angiogram confirmed lower reocclusion rates at 24 months in patients with both thrombosis and

embolic etiologies of ALI [8]. Despite these findings, consensus regarding the mandatory performance of a completion arteriogram does not exist in the literature [6, 8].

The discovery of a flow-limiting stenosis or anastomotic stenosis on arteriogram can frequently be treated with endarterectomy or endarterectomy with patch angioplasty of an offending lesion (Figs. 39.4 and 39.5).

Infrainguinal bypass is commonly reserved for patients with long-segment occlusion or diffuse disease. Infrainguinal bypass is also performed when a Fogarty catheter will not pass due to vessel occlusion and intraoperative arteriogram confirms a distal arterial target for bypass [9]. In addition, some surgeons do not advocate performing thrombectomy for a thrombosed infrainguinal bypass but instead proceeding with a new bypass primarily [10]. Finally, a thrombosed aneurysm or aneurysm embolizing mural thrombus may require ligation and exclusion of the aneurysm with a bypass or interposition graft (Fig. 39.6). A successful bypass involves confirming both adequate inflow and outflow to support this revascularization. Securing adequate conduit for the bypass is important as well. Native venous conduit (i.e., greater saphenous vein, small saphenous vein, cephalic vein, or basilic vein) is the most preferred conduit. Although observed to have inferior patency rates as compared to native

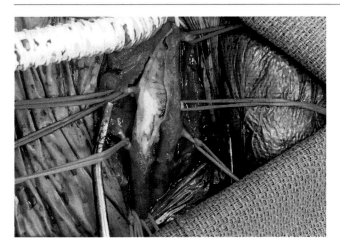

Fig. 39.4 Femoral endarterectomy with removal of plaque extending into the profunda and superficial femoral artery

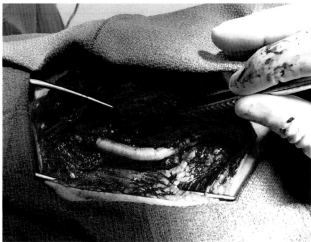

Fig. 39.6 Interposition bypass of a superficial femoral artery aneurysm. Aneurysm was excised secondary to an embolization event resulting in acute limb ischemia

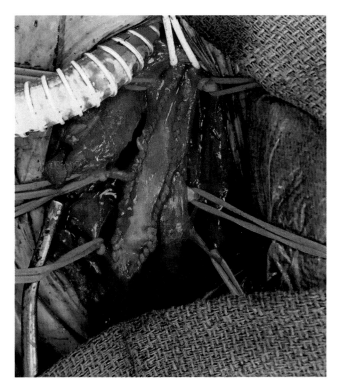

Fig. 39.5 Patch angioplasty of femoral artery after endarterectomy

conduit, prosthetic bypass (i.e., PTFE or Dacron) may also be utilized in surgical fields free from infection.

In some instances, inflow cannot be reestablished. This may occur with native aortoiliac thrombosis, thrombosis of a suprainguinal bypass graft, or malperfusion from a dissection. In these emergent situations, extra-anatomic bypass may provide the most expedient method of revascularization. Examples of extra-anatomic bypass include axillary–femoral bypass, axillary–bifemoral bypass, femoral–femoral bypass, and axillary–popliteal bypass (Fig. 39.7).

Currently, revascularization is frequently a combination of both percutaneous and open surgical techniques [7]. This

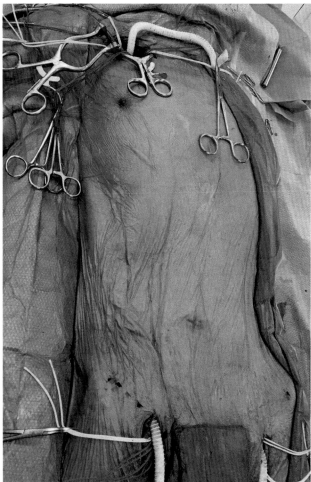

Fig. 39.7 Axillary–bifemoral bypass utilizing right axillary artery for inflow

hybrid approach routinely involves exposure of the femoral artery or, less frequently, exposure of the below-knee trifurcation. This allows access for thromboembolectomy.

If the thrombectomy is felt to be inadequate or suspicious for completeness, intraoperative arteriogram may be performed. If residual thrombus is noted, intra-arterial infusion of a thrombolytic agent may be performed. Likewise, mechanical thrombectomy or suction aspiration techniques may also be used to address this residual thrombus. In addition, intraoperative arteriogram may document a persistent stenosis or an iatrogenic dissection from thromboembolectomy that can be treated with angioplasty and/or stenting [7, 9, 10].

Following revascularization, anticoagulation in the immediate postoperative period is recommended. The duration of anticoagulation is debatable and influenced by the origin of the inciting event. Cardiac emboli may require further imaging with echocardiogram to look for a source. If an aortoiliac source is suspected, imaging with CT or MR may help identify arterial thrombus or aneurysmal disease conducive to endovascular or open repair. If anticoagulation is contraindicated, antiplatelet therapy should be taken at the very least.

Unfortunately, in some instances, a patient may present with a non-salvageable limb. A surgeon must have the ability to objectively evaluate the patient with acute limb ischemia. If a patient presents with a category III limb that has no sensation, no motor function, tissue loss, and absent Doppler signals, revascularization should not be attempted (Fig. 39.8).

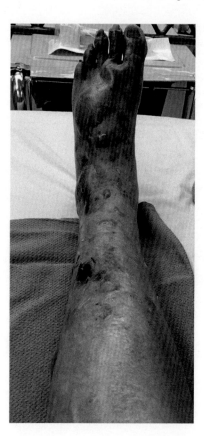

Fig. 39.8 Nonviable category III limb with tissue loss and no detectable motor or sensory function

Instead, primary amputation is the recommended treatment plan. A reported 10 % of patients presenting with ALI are not salvageable and a higher level of amputation is often required due to compromised calf muscle [6].

Compartment Syndrome

Successful revascularization of an acutely ischemic limb can be complicated by the development of compartment syndrome. Compartment syndrome after reperfusion is defined as muscle compartment hypertension that develops in a fixed space. Ischemia results in the depletion of cellular energy stores and cellular dysfunction. Once reperfused, reactive oxygen radicals are generated and result in a cascade of events culminating in cellular swelling and increased interstitial edema. This edema ultimately results in venous outflow obstruction causing increased venule and subsequent capillary pressure. Increased capillary pressure results in additional fluid transudation and cellular swelling that creates higher intracompartmental pressure. As the pressure increases, arterial inflow is blocked and therefore, delivery of nutrients to tissue ceases. This ultimately leads to irreversible tissue infarction [11].

Compartment syndrome should be suspected in limbs with pain that is more severe than expected or if a patient experiences pain in an affected compartment with passive movement. As the syndrome progresses, muscle paralysis, paresis, and paresthesia may develop. Affected limbs may become indurated with absent or diminished distal pulses [11]. Many other factors must also be considered when contemplating to perform fasciotomies to prevent or treat compartment syndrome after revascularization. The severity of ischemia, duration of ischemia, and presence of peripheral artery disease with associated collaterals should all be considered when assessing the risk of developing compartment syndrome. A more definitive measurement is the detection of elevated intracompartmental pressure with an intracompartmental pressure monitoring system. Compartment pressures greater than 20 mmHg are an indication for fasciotomies and the anterior lower leg compartment is the most commonly involved with ALI [6].

Fasciotomy is the treatment of choice for compartment syndrome. It is frequently performed at the conclusion of a revascularization procedure if there is a high suspicion a patient develops the signs and symptoms detailed above postoperatively. The main goal of this intervention is to prevent neuromuscular ischemia and necrosis. A four-compartment (deep and superficial posterior, anterior, and lateral) fasciotomy is recommended and can be achieved through lateral and medial lower-leg incisions (Fig. 39.9). Alternatively, all four compartments may be released via a single anterolateral incision. Technical success is rooted in both timely intervention and the quality of the procedure. To

Fig. 39.9 Four-compartment fasciotomy through two lower-leg incisions. (**a**) Lateral incision allows access for release of the anterior and lateral compartments. (**b**) Medial incision allows access for release of the superficial posterior and deep posterior compartments

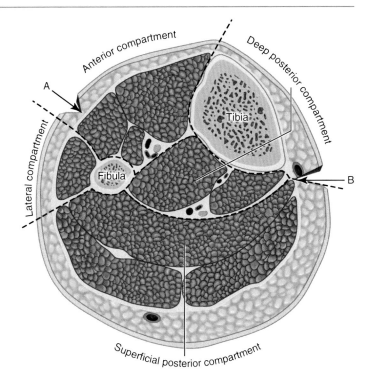

be effective, an adequate skin incision with complete longitudinal fascial decompression of compartments must be performed.

Conclusion

Overall, patients presenting with ALI are at high risk for significant morbidity and mortality. Despite aggressive intervention for limb salvage, studies have reported 30-day amputation rates up to 16 %. In addition, multiple studies indicate a 1-month mortality rate of 9–16 % [12–14].

Initial assessment involves categorizing an ischemic limb according to its viability. Threatened limbs or category II limbs should be expediently revascularized. Careful history and physical exam can assist with distinguishing between acute embolic and acute thrombotic events. In the past, this would primarily guide the open surgical approach used for revascularization. More recently, treatment strategies employ a combination of both surgical and percutaneous techniques. Despite these advances, morbidity and mortality rates remain high in this high-risk patient population.

References

1. Rutherford RB, Baker JD, Ernst C, et al. Recommended standards for reports dealing with lower extremity ischemia: revised version. J Vasc Surg. 1997;26:517–38.

2. Dormandy J, Heeck L, Vig S. Acute limb ischemia. Semin Vasc Surg. 1999;12:148–53.
3. Abbott WM, Maloney RD, McCabe CC, et al. Arterial embolism: A 44-year perspective. Am J Surg. 1982;143:460–4.
4. O'Connell JB, Quinones-Baldrich WJ. Proper evaluation and management of acute embolic versus thrombotic limb ischemia. Semin Vasc Surg. 2009;22:10–6.
5. Owens CD, Ho KJ, Conte MS. Lower extremity vein graft failure: a translational approach. Vasc Med. 2008;13:63–74.
6. Norgren L, Hiatt WR, Dormandy JA, et al. Inter-Society Consensus for the Management of Peripheral Arterial Disease (TASC II). J Vasc Surg. 2007;45 Suppl S:S5.
7. de Donato G, Setacci F, Sirignano P, et al. The combination of surgical embolectomy and endovascular techniques ma improve outcomes of patients with acute lower limb ischemia. J Vasc Surg. 2014;59:729–36.
8. Zaraca F, Stringari C, Ebner JA, Ebner H. Routine versus selective use of intraoperative angiography during thromboembolectomy for acute lower limb ischemia: analysis of outcomes. Ann Vasc Surg. 2010;24:621–7.
9. Pemberton M, Varty K, Nydahl S, Bell PRF. The surgical management of acute limb ischaemia due to native vessel occlusion. Eur J Vasc Endovasc Surg. 1999;17:72–6.
10. Yeager RA, Moneta GL, Taylor LM, et al. Surgical management of severe acute lower extremity ischemia. J Vasc Surg. 1992;15:385–93.
11. Arato E, Kurthy M, Sinay L, et al. Pathology and diagnostic options of lower limb compartment syndrome. Clin Hemorheol Microcirc. 2009;41:1–8.
12. Campbell WB, Ridler BM, Szymanska TH. Two-year follow-up after acute thromboembolic limb ischaemia: the importance of anticoagulation. Eur J Vasc Endovasc Surg. 2000;19:168–73.
13. Eliason JL, Wainess RM, Proctor MC, et al. A national and single institutional experience in the contemporary treatment of acute lower extremity ischemia. Ann Surg. 2003;238:382–9.
14. Tawes RL, Harris EJ, Brown WH, et al. Arterial thromboembolism. A 20-year perspective. Arch Surg. 1985;120:595–9.

Sympathectomy Revisited: Current Status in the Management of Critical Limb Ischemia

Pawan Agarwal and Dhananjaya Sharma

Introduction

Lumbar sympathectomy (LS) has been used in the treatment of various vascular and neurological disorders of lower extremities for close to 80 years [1].

The concept of sympathetic denervation as a mode of therapy for arterial occlusive disease was first described by Jaboulay in 1889 in the form of periarterial sympathectomy on femoral artery. Leriche [2] states that results are disappointing due to reinnervation and vasospasm within weeks of operation. Lumbar sympathectomy (LS) or section of the lumbar sympathetic chain and excision of one or more ganglia was introduced by Royle in 1923 in the treatment of spastic paralysis of the lower extremity, and he observed after lumbar sympathectomy that the skin and toes of ipsilateral foot became warm and dry due to increased circulation. By the 1940s, lumbar sympathectomy became the primary surgical treatment of atherosclerotic occlusive disease and its sequelae in the lower extremity because it was often the only alternative to amputation. However, the development of direct arterial reconstructive procedures in the 1950 diminished the importance of LS as a primary operation.

LS is acknowledged to have a role in the treatment of patients with reflex symptomatic dystrophy (causalgia), vasospastic disorders like acrocyanosis and Raynaud's syndrome, hyperhidrosis of the hand and feet, symptomatic vasospasm, and non-reconstructable arterial occlusive disease. A literature survey finds its miscellaneous uses for frostbites, desiccation of chronically moist ulcerations between the toes, chronic renal pain, rectal tenesmus, and sympathetically maintained intractable pain due to malignant reasons. Although it is the most commonly performed operation in the developing countries for critical limb ischemia (CLI), there is considerable controversy about its usefulness.

Anatomy

In the lower extremity, the lumbar sympathetic system exerts anatomic control over the vasoconstriction and sweating. Preganglionic neurons in the lateral gray substances of the spinal cord from the level of T10 to L2 or L3 send axons along the ventral nerve roots to the lumbar sympathetic ganglia via white rami communicantes. Preganglionic fibers then synapse within the ganglion or ascend or descend as the interganglionic part of the sympathetic chain to synapse with postganglionic neurons in the ganglion of the chain. The postganglionic fibers exit through gray rami communicantes to accompany the peripheral nerves.

Postganglionic fibers may arise from the first to the fourth or even fifth lumbar ganglion to travel with the lumbar and sacral nerves to the lower extremities. The foot and leg below the knee are primarily supplied by postganglionic fibers from the L3 level and below [3].

The lumbar sympathetic trunk contains 4–5 ganglia. They lay retroperitoneally in front of the vertebral column along the medial borders of the psoas major muscles. Four ganglia are usually found in the lumbar chain, but the number may vary between two and eight, and rarely one continuous ganglion is found [4].

Although the variations in position of the ganglia are common, the second and the fourth lumbar ganglia are the more constant ones.

The number of rami of any ganglion and their position between the spinal nerves and lumbar sympathetic trunk

Disease is very old and not much about it has changed. It is we who change as we learn to recognize what was formerly imperceptible.—Charcot

P. Agarwal, MS, MCh, DNB, MNAMS, PhD (✉)
Department of Surgery, NSCB Government Medical College, Nagpur Road, Garha, Jabalpur 482003, MP, India

D. Sharma, MS, PhD, DSc
Department of Surgery, Government NSCB Medical College, Nagpur Road, Garha, Jabalpur 482003, MP, India

© Springer International Publishing Switzerland 2017
R.S. Dieter et al. (eds.), *Critical Limb Ischemia*, DOI 10.1007/978-3-319-31991-9_40

show considerable variation. Cross communication between the right and left sympathetic trunk are also variable [5]. Knowledge of these variations in the anatomic structure may be helpful in performing correctly a lumbar sympathectomy. It is to be mentioned here that because most vascular problems that may require sympathectomy are confined to the foot, resection of 2nd–4th lumbar ganglia is necessary.

The Procedure

There are three approaches for lumbar sympathectomy anterior, anterolateral, and posterior. The anterolateral approach is most popular because the incision is well tolerated, dissection remains retroperitoneal, exposure is adequate, and both sides can be done in one sitting. Anterior approach is selected when any associated intra-abdominal or intraperitoneal procedures like repair of aortic aneurysm are undertaken or other intraperitoneal procedure. Posterior approach is not favored because it is associated with severe postoperative paraspinal muscle spasm.

In anterolateral approach patient lies supine with 30° tilt to opposite side. A transverse incision is placed in the loin extending from anterior axillary line to lateral border of rectus (Fig. 40.1). Muscles are split, and peritoneum is displaced medially and forward off the posterior abdominal wall (Figs. 40.2 and 40.3), the genital vessels and ureter being raised along with it. After proper dissection the lumbar sympathetic chain is located medial to the psoas muscle and lies over the transverse process of lumbar spine. The left lumbar ganglia lie adjacent and lateral to the abdominal aorta and on the right, just beneath the edge of the inferior vena cava.

Tactile identification of the lumbar chain by plucking discloses a characteristic "snap" as a result of tethering of the nodular chain by rami communicantes. Other vertical band-like structures in this region like genitofemoral nerve, paravertebral lymph nodes, or ureter do not recoil as briskly. Once identified the midportion of the sympathetic chain is dissected free of surrounding tissues and retracted with a right-angled clamp or a nerve hook to draw it up (Fig. 40.4). The first lumbar ganglion is sought high up in under the crus of the

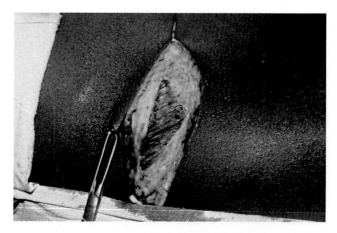

Fig. 40.2 Muscles are split in full length of skin incision

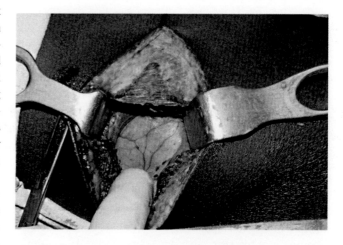

Fig. 40.3 Peritoneum is displaced medially and forward off the posterior abdominal wall

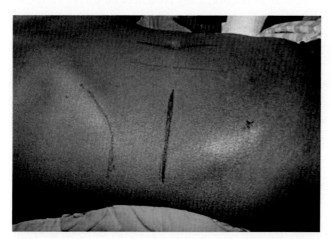

Fig. 40.1 Transverse incision is placed in the loin extending from anterior axillary line to lateral border of rectus

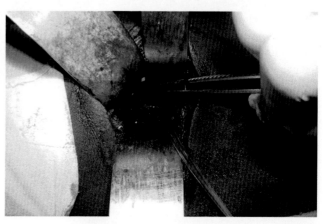

Fig. 40.4 Sympathetic chain is dissected free of surrounding tissues and retracted with a right-angled clamp or a nerve hook

diaphragm, and fourth ganglion is obscured by common iliac vessels. The surgeon facilitates orientation and ganglion numbering by identifying the sacral promontory and an adjacent lumbar vein that usually crosses the sympathetic chain in front of or behind the third lumbar ganglion. The chain and at least two lumbar ganglia are removed and hemostasis done [6].

The technique of laparoscopic LS has gained popularity in recent times. The time-tested instruments, dissection maneuvers along with videoscopic magnification, that have proved so effective in thoracoscopic dorsal sympathectomy are employed in LS [7].

Complications of Lumbar Sympathectomy

Major complications result from failure to appreciate normal anatomic relationships with resultant injury to the genitofemoral nerve, ureter, lumbar veins, aorta, and inferior vena cava. The most common complications following LS are post-sympathectomy neuralgia, sexual dysfunction, and failure to achieve the desired objectives of pain relief or tissue healing.

Post-sympathectomy Neuralgia

It usually begins 1–2 weeks after LS and appears in up to 50 % of patients. It is localized to the thigh (anterolateral), worse at night, and rarely responds to medications. It usually remits spontaneously within 8–12 weeks.

Sexual Dysfunction

It consists of retrograde ejaculation, and occurs in 25–50 % patients undergoing bilateral LS including the L1 sympathetic ganglia.

Failed Lumbar Sympathectomy

Failure to achieve the desired objective of pain relief or tissue healing is blamed on several factors. These include an incomplete sympathectomy as a result of a technically incomplete operation or as a result of cross innervation that makes a complete sympathectomy impossible. The latter recurrence may be caused by regenerating nerves or increased function of previously inconsequential crossed fibers.

Surgical vs. Chemical Sympathectomy

Surgical sympathectomy is defined as the surgical ablation of the cervicothoracic or lumbar sympathetic chain by means of open or laparoscopic procedure. Chemical sympathectomy

is the percutaneous ablation of the cervicothoracic or lumbar sympathetic chain by the injection of phenol or alcohol solution. This procedure promotes a prolonged but not permanent sympathetic denervation.

Review

On the one hand, the advent of laparoscopic lumbar sympathectomy and reports of LS in conjunction with omental transposition have maintained interest in this procedure. On the other hand, rapid development of various arterial reconstructive procedures, description of distraction osteosynthesis, and availability of gene transfer technology has added to the confusion concerning the proper place of this procedure in the management of thromboangiitis obliterans (Buerger's disease) and other CLIs. Being aware of these inconsistent opinions, we decided to try and define the place of LS for the management of thromboangiitis obliterans by evaluating the currently available evidence and to answer the following questions:

What are the physiological reasons for outcome after LS? What are the controversies for the use of LS for CLI? Is it possible to predict the therapeutic response to LS? What are the indications of LS today?

What Are the Physiological Reasons for Outcome After LS?

Clinical response after lumbar sympathectomy is variable and transitory. This can be partially explained by physiological changes in the skin and muscle blood flow after sympathectomy. The resting blood flow in human skeletal muscle is 2–5 ml/100 g/min; elimination of all sympathetic vasoconstrictive activity only increases this flow to 6–9 ml/100 g/min in contrast with exercising muscle which will have the flow rate of 50–75 ml/100 g/min. [8]. Ischemia and exercise both produce metabolic substances locally, which cause maximal vasodilatation, despite sympathetic discharge; therefore, there is no physiological basis to use lumbar sympathectomy for patients with intermittent claudication since they already have maximal arteriolar vasodilatation [9, 10]. While sympathectomy cannot increase exercise hyperemia, it increases the collateral blood flow provided there are enough collateral vessels and vascular pliability. Sympathectomy increases the transient blood flow through the collaterals in an ischemic extremity as a result of the decrease in peripheral resistance due to opening of arteriovenous anastomoses with marked reduction in peripheral resistance, thereby increasing blood flow. These arteriovenous anastomoses have little or no intrinsic myogenic tone but are dependent upon sympathetic vasoactivity to control their diameter [11–13]. All these mechanisms increase the skin blood flow and result in increased skin temperature, rather than true nutritional capillary blood flow [14]. Therefore, its use in rest pain and ischemic ulceration is well accepted. The vasomotor tone is usually normalized in 2 weeks to 6 months after operation; this transient effect of LS can be explained by Cannon's law of supersensitivity of denervated sympathetic endings to circulating catecholamines and return of vasomotor tone by alternate pathways [15, 16]. The division of afferent pain fibers traveling in the sympathetic chain may be an alternative basis for the success of lumbar sympathectomy, especially in rest pain [17].

What Are the Controversies for the Use of LS for CLI?

The place of LS in the treatment of CLI of the lower limbs remains controversial; inconsistent opinions on its value can be divided into those who are against and those who are not.

Against

Assessment of cutaneous blood flow in the foot in patients with critical limb ischemia failed to detect improvement in nutritional blood flow after LS [18]. Investigators assessing microcirculation (with intra-arterial injection of radioisotopes) in the feet of patients with TAO found that LS does not improve microcirculation and concluded that there is breakdown of the microvascular defense system from the beginning of the disease [19]. In fact, even the presumed increased sympathetic nerve activity which may respond to LS has not been demonstrated which points to a local vascular abnormality in TAO [20]. LS, like any other surgical procedure, is not without its share of complications which include failure of adequate denervation, brief paralytic ileus, hyperhidrosis in parts of the body which remain normally innervated, sexual dysfunction, and post-sympathectomy neuralgia. The detractors and skeptics conclude that a weak case can be made for sympathectomy for ischemic rest pain when arterial surgery is impractical, but there is no reliable evidence to support its use in intermittent claudication [21]. An additional limitation is that assessment of response to lumbar sympathectomy is difficult because selection of cases is usually empirical as ischemia is difficult to quantitate objectively. Different expectations in different patient groups and continuation of precipitating factors like smoking further compound the issue, thereby illustrating the pitfalls of applying physiological data to such a variability of pathological processes. This makes comparison between different reported series very difficult.

For

Empirically derived evidence in favor of LS for management of CLI comes from innumerable clinical studies, which support the continued use of the procedure, coupled with local tissue management in the treatment of selected patients with localized pre-gangrenous lesions or superficial ischemic ulcerations in whom arterial reconstructive operation is not feasible or who refuse major vascular surgery [22–27]. Studies on long-term outcome of TAO after LS are not completely discouraging [28]. Even if LS provides only short-term pain relief and ulcer healing without long-term benefit in majority of patients, it remains a useful tool [29]. Research workers from Russia have shown that LS reduces pathogenetically reliable orthostatic and post-orthostatic spasm of the diseased arteries. Specific complications after LS are remarkably low and almost always transient, and these cannot be arguments against the use of LS; in fact, LS has been safely done under local anesthesia also. LS have been justifiably called a "goal line last ditch stand" and should be considered before a major amputation [30, 31].

Is it Possible to Predict the Therapeutic Response to LS?

Although lumbar sympathectomy can benefit patients with critical limb ischemia, many derive no benefit from the procedure. This has prompted research workers to study various predictive tests, which might allow LS to be done only in those patients who are likely to benefit by this procedure. These tests can be classified into:

Clinical assessment of degree of ischemia: Good response is expected if there is no evidence of a somatic neuropathy and if the tissue damage is not too extensive, i.e., only rest pain, night pain, or digital gangrene is present [32, 33]. Deep infection or gangrene is a bad prognostic sign and its presence predicts failure of LS [30, 34].

Tests of vasomotor tone: These include an increase of 2 degrees or more in skin temperature of the ipsilateral great toe after lumbar sympathetic block, preoperative assessment of sympathetic nerve function by means of acetylcholine sweat-spot test, foot vascular resistance index, the use of Hillestad's reactive hyperemia test, segmental impedance plethysmography (irrigraphy), skin thermometry, measurement of arterial blood flow and resistance in the foot and in the leg, reactive hyperemia under photoplethysmographic control, and thermographic test using reserpine injected in the femoral artery [35–38].

Assessment of Collateral Circulation

1. Angiography has been used, but quantification of data is difficult and so is the prediction of response to LS.
2. Doppler ultrasound can determine the pressure in the thigh and ankle and has been used as a predictive test. Good response is expected if ankle systolic pressure is above 60 mmHg, preoperative ankle-brachial index (ABI) is >0.3, or if the distal thigh/arm index is >0.6 [24, 28, 31, 32]. Another important predictive parameter is patency of superficial femoral artery which has been found to be related to successful outcome of the patients [27].

    Tests for verification of completeness of sympathetic denervation, although available, are difficult to perform and interpret [38–43]. The poor prediction of outcome may be related to preexisting damage to the sympathetic fibers [39].
3. Transcutaneous oximetry (TCPO2) has also been found useful, as there is high correlation between ABI and TCPO2. If transmetatarsal TCPO2 is <30 mmHg, an amputation is likely to be needed [41, 42].

What Are the Indications of LS Today?

The majority of the reports show benefits in terms of relief of rest pain after lumbar sympathectomy in the range of 60–75 %, which is better than the percentage assumed in natural history. This suggests that lumbar sympathectomy has a definite role in CLI. Short-term efficacy of LS in terms of relief of symptoms is 60 %, while in long run the effectiveness of treatment lasted in only 50 % of patients. Its results in terms of limb conservation and relapses are disappointing due to extensive breakdown of regional microcirculation by disease process and normalization of vasomotor tone within 2 weeks to 6 months after operation. Sympathectomy gives best results in younger cooperative patients with short history who have stopped smoking, in nondiabetics (because microvascular lesions reduce peripheral vasodilatation), and in patients with rest pain and ischemic ulcers, healing of amputation stump, and distal involvement of vessels. Ankle-brachial pressure index (ABPI) >0.3 and a patent femoral artery are prerequisites for the success of lumbar sympathectomy.

Summary

Despite the lack of objective evidence-based support, LS continues to hold a place in the treatment of refractory ischemic ulceration or persistent rest pain, especially when there is a distal ischemia, which is not suitable for direct arterial surgery. There is no physiological basis to use lumbar sympathectomy for patients with intermittent claudication. The nonspecificity

of the indications and lack of simple methods to predict success of this procedure have led to many conflicting reports; however, the toe-temperature response following peripheral nerve block, transcutaneous oximetry (TCPO$_2$), or ankle-brachial pressure index (ABPI) correlates best with the effect of LS. Among the patients with rest pain and no distal ulcerations, pain relief is obtained in 76 % at 3 months after LS in those who did not require amputation [17, 25, 44]. LS does not exempt the patient from a subsequent amputation as the vasomotor tone is usually normalized in 2 weeks to 6 months after operation. Therefore the healing effect of LS on an ulcer may become negligible after this "grace period" [29]. The relapsing and remitting nature of intermittent claudication makes the study of natural history of claudication difficult; hence, the patient selection and results vary considerably, and this is the reason for conflicting reports in different studies. No controlled trial has been done till now to compare the natural history of PIDs with the results of LS. LS may not produce the dramatic improvements seen after reconstructive surgery but should be considered as first-line management in selected patients. For many avoidance of further surgery will be achieved after LS, but should the procedure fail to secure appropriate relief of symptoms, reconstructive surgery can still be offered without disadvantage [45]. The magnitude of changes in blood flow and sympathetic activity is similar for LS and chemical sympathectomy.

The combination of noninvasive vascular assessment and good clinical judgment may well lead to selective use of lumbar sympathectomy in the management of symptomatic atherosclerotic occlusive disease when it is of the severity to require surgical procedure and where arterial reconstruction is not feasible because of diffuse distribution of disease and poor distal runoff.

In summing up, it is difficult to improve upon Smithwick's observation on LS made in 1957: The effect of sympathectomy upon the peripheral circulation is physiological in nature. In order to predict the outcome, appropriate studies are needed before and after operation, which will demonstrate the physiological effect. In addition to this, certain physiological information regarding the state of peripheral circulation is essential. Failure to obtain the necessary data before and after operation is the basic reason why the selection of cases for sympathectomy is unsatisfactory today and the outcome unpredictable or speculative for the most part [46].

References

1. Ewing M. The history of lumbar sympathectomy. Surgery. 1971;70:790–6.
2. Leriche R. Some researches on the peri-arterial sympathetics Ann Surg. 1921 Oct; 74(4):385–393.
3. Littooy FN, Baker WH. Use of lumber sympathectomy in lower extremity vascular disease. In: Harrett F, Hirsch SA, editors.

Vascular surgery of the lower extremity. USA: CV Mosby; 1985. p. 184–91.

4. Haimovici H. lumbar sympathectomy. In: Haimovici H, editor. Vascular surgery. Principles and Techniques. USA: ACC USA; 1984. p. 925–39.

5. Webber RH. An analysis of Sympathetic trunk, communicating rami, sympathetic roots and visceral rami in the lumber region in man. Ann Surg. 1955;118:420.

6. Rutherford RB. lumbar sympathectomy indications and technique. In: Rutherford RB, editor. Vascular surgery. 5th ed., vol. V. W.B. Philadelphia: Saunders; 2000. p. 1069–78.

7. Kathouda N, Wattanasirichaigoon S, Tang E, et al. Laparoscopic lumbar sympathectomy. Surg Endosc. 1997;11:257.

8. Folkow B, Neil E. Circulation. New York: Oxford University Press; 1971.

9. Myers KA, Irwin WT. An objective study of lumbar sympathectomy I: intermittent claudication. Br Med J. 1966;I:879–83.

10. Fyfe T, Quin RO. Phenol sympathectomy in the treatment of intermittent claudication: a controlled clinical trial. Br J Surg. 1975;62:68–71.

11. Scarpino JH, Delaney JP. Lumbar sympathectomy and arteriovenous shunting. Surg Forum. 1971;22:176–8.

12. Cronenwett JL, Lindenauer SM. Direct measurement of arteriovenous anastomotic blood flow after sympathectomy. Surgery. 1977;82:82–9.

13. Moore WS, Hall AD. Effects of lumbar sympathectomy on skin capillary blood flow in arterial occlusive disease. J Surg Res. 1973;14:151–7.

14. Lindenauer SM, Cronenwett JL. What is the place of lumbar sympathectomy? Br J Surg. 1982;69(Suppl):S32–3.

15. Cannon WB, Rosenbluth A. The supersensitivity of denervated structures. New York: McMillan; 1949.

16. Monro PAG. Sympathectomy: an anatomical and physiological study with clinical applications. London: Oxford University Press; 1959.

17. Cotton LT, Cross FW. Lumbar sympathectomy for arterial disease. Br J Surg. 1985;72:678–83.

18. Welch GH, Leiberman DP. Cutaneous blood flow in the foot following lumbar sympathectomy. Scand J Clin Lab Invest. 1985;45:621–6.

19. Nishikimi N, Sakurai T, Shionoya S, Oshima M. Microcirculatory characteristics in patients with Buerger's disease. Angiology. 1992;43:312–9.

20. Iwase S, Okamoto T, Mano T, Kamiya A, Niimi Y, Qi F, et al. Skin sympathetic outflow in Buerger's disease. Auton Neurosci. 2001;87:286–92.

21. Gordon A, Zechmeister K, Collin J. The role of sympathectomy in current surgical practice. Eur J Vasc Surg. 1994;8(2):129–37.

22. Allen TR. Current status of lumbar sympathectomy. Am Surg. 1976;42:89–91.

23. Kim GE, Ibrahim IM, Imparato AM. Lumbar sympathectomy in end stage arterial occlusive disease. Ann Surg. 1976;183:157–60.

24. Janoff KA, Phinney ES, Porter JM. Lumbar sympathectomy for lower extremity vasospasm. Am J Surg. 1985;150:147–52.

25. Baker DM, Lamerton AJ. Operative lumbar sympathectomy for severe lower limb ischaemia: still a valuable treatment option. Ann R Coll Surg Engl. 1994;76:50–3.

26. Holiday FA, Barendregt WB, Slappendel R, Crul BJ, Buskens FG, van der Vliet JA. Lumbar sympathectomy in critical limb ischaemia: surgical, chemical or not at all? Cardiovasc Surg. 1999;7:200–2.

27. Perez-Burkhardt JL, Gonzalez-Fajardo JA, Martin JF, Carpintero Mediavilla LA, Mateo Gutierrez AM. Lumbar sympathectomy as isolated technique for the treatment of lower limbs chronic ischemia. J Cardiovasc Surg (Torino). 1999;40:7–13.

28. Shigematsu H, Shigematsu K. Factors affecting the long-term outcome of Buerger's disease (thromboangiitis obliterans). Int Angiol. 1999;18:58–64.

29. Lau H, Cheng SW. Buerger's disease in Hong Kong: a review of 89 cases. Aust N Z J Surg. 1997 May;67:264–9.

30. Blumenberg RM, Gelfand ML. Lumbar sympathectomy for limb salvage: a goal line stand. Am J Surg. 1979;133:241–5.

31. Lantsberg L, Goldman M, Khoda J. Should chemical sympathectomy precede below-knee amputation? Int Surg. 1996;81:85–7.

32. Walker PM, Key JA, MacKay IM, Johnston KW. Phenol sympathectomy for vascular occlusive disease. Surg Gynecol Obstet. 1978;146:741–4.

33. Walker PM, Johnston KW. Predicting the success of a sympathectomy: a prospective study using discriminant function and multiple regression analysis. Surgery. 1980;87:216–21.

34. Persson AV, Anderson LA, Padberg Jr FT. Selection of patients for lumbar sympathectomy. Surg Clin North Am. 1985;65:393–403.

35. Shanik G, Hayes A, Barnes RW. Foot vascular resistance index: a noninvasive method to assess foot vasomotor tone. Surgery. 1975;78:446–52.

36. Pistolese GR, Speziale F, Taurino M, Spartera C, Faraglia V. Criteria for prognostic evaluation of the results of lumbar sympathectomy: clinical, haemodynamic and angiographic findings. J Cardiovasc Surg (Torino). 1982;23:411–4.

37. Kruse CA. Thirty year experience with predictive lumbar sympathectomy. Method for selection of patients. Am J Surg. 1985;150:232–6.

38. Altomare DF, Regina G, Lovreglio R, Memeo V. Acetylcholine sweat test: an effective way to select patients for lumbar sympathectomy. Lancet. 1994;344:976–8.

39. Collins Jr GJ, Rich NM, Clagett GP, Salander JM, Spebar MJ. Clinical results of lumbar sympathectomy. Am Surg. 1981;47:31–5.

40. Lee BY, Ostrander LE, Aquino-Chu G, Madden RE. Distal thigh/arm index as a predictor of success for lumbar sympathectomy. J Rehabil Res Dev. 1993;30:383–7.

41. Ballard JE, Eke CC, Bunt TJ, Killen JD. A preoperative evaluation of transcutaneous oxygen measurements in the management of diabetic foot problems. J Vasc Surg. 1995;22:185–92.

42. de Goote P, Millaire A, Deklunder G, Marache P, Decoulx E, Ducloux G. Comparative diagnostic value of ankle-to-brachial index and transcutaneous oxygen tension at rest and after exercise with intermittent claudication. Angiology. 1995;46:115–22.

43. Bohler U, Wienert V. Dermofluorography as a possibility for therapeutic control following sympathectomy. Int J Microcirc Clin Exp. 1996;16:195–7.

44. Bloor K. Natural history of arteriosclerosis of the lower extremities. Ann R Coll Surg. 1961;28:36–52.

45. Norman PE, House AK. The early use of lumbar sympathectomy in peripheral vascular disease. J Cardiovasc Surg. 1988;29:717–22.

46. Smithwick RH. Lumbar sympathectomy in the treatment of obliterative vascular diseases of the lower extremities. Surgery. 1957;42:567–78.

Spinal Cord Stimulation

41

Pawan Agarwal and Dhananjaya Sharma

Peripheral vascular disease (PVD) and critical limb ischemia (CLI) should be treated with surgical or endovascular technique to restore a pulsatile blood flow as distally as possible, particularly in patients with ischemic ulcers or gangrene. However, some patients cannot be revascularized or they do not reach a complete resolution of rest pain, so they need other treatment to improve their quality of life. Spinal cord stimulation (SCS), also known as neuromodulation, delivers small electrical fields to the spinal cord. These electrical fields mask areas of pain by changing the pain messages to the brain. Spinal cord stimulation is reserved for patients who have severe debilitating chronic pain that is limiting their daily life and who have already tried all reasonable, more conservative therapies, such as analgesics and physiotherapy.

SCS was first described by Melzack and Wall in 1965 and used in spine-related disorders to relieve neurogenic pain [1]. Spinal cord stimulation has been first proposed in the clinical practice for treatment of intractable pain by Shealy in 1967 [2]. In 1976 Cook first reported its efficacy in control of ischemic pain associated with peripheral disease and diabetic vasculopathy [3]. It is aimed to reduce the unpleasant sensory experience of pain and the consequent functional and behavioral effects that pain may have.

The selection of candidates for spinal cord stimulation is a critical factor for producing acceptable outcomes. For SCS implantation patients should be 18 years of age or older, have moderate to severe chronic pain measuring greater than five out of ten on a pain rating scale, have tried and not responded to conservative treatments, be willing to stop or reduce excessive medication, and use pain management strategies and be able to manage the technical demands of the equip-

ment. The primary purpose of SCS is to improve quality of life (QOL) and physical function by reducing the severity of pain and its associated characteristics.

Indications of SCS

- High probability of successful pain reduction:
  1. Chronic radicular pain (cervical and lumbar)/failed back surgery syndrome
  2. Complex regional pain syndrome (CRPS), types I and II
  3. Painful peripheral neuropathies and mononeuropathies
  4. Angina pectoris refractory to conventional drug therapy and not amenable to surgical bypass
  5. Painful ischemic peripheral vascular disease not amenable to conventional drug therapy or surgical bypass
- Low probability of successful pain reduction:
  1. Neuropathic pain following spinal cord injury
  2. Central pain (e.g., poststroke pain)
  3. Nerve root avulsion (e.g., brachial plexus avulsion)
- Unknown probability of pain reduction (case reports of successful treatment):
  1. Postherpetic neuralgia
  2. Axial low back pain (improving with new lead arrays and programming)
  3. Phantom limb pain

Contraindications

1. Pain due to arthritis or spinal instability
2. Widespread pain syndromes
3. Anatomical problems when it is not possible to implant a spinal cord stimulation system safely like major spinal deformity, extensive spinal metalwork, or extensive spinal scar tissue in the epidural space
4. Active infective illness or local site infection
5. Psychiatric illnesses/untreated drug addiction/metal allergy

P. Agarwal, MS, MCh, DNB, MNAMS, PhD (✉)
Department of Surgery, NSCB Government Medical College, Garha, Nagpur Road, Jabalpur 482003, MP, India

D. Sharma, MS, PhD, DSc
Department of Surgery, Government NSCB Medical College, Nagpur Road, Garha, Jabalpur 482003, MP, India

© Springer International Publishing Switzerland 2017
R.S. Dieter et al. (eds.), *Critical Limb Ischemia*, DOI 10.1007/978-3-319-31991-9_41

Complications of a Spinal Cord Stimulator

1. Painful battery/connection site
2. Infection (less than 5%)
3. Bleeding
4. Severe headache
5. Mechanical failure of device
6. Unpleasant stimulation/failure to capture the area of pain
7. Allergic reaction
8. Decrease in pain relief with time
9. Nerve damage leading to nerve pain, numbness, and weakness
10. Paralysis (rare two patients in one million)

Mechanism of SCS

Although the clinical benefits of SCS are clear and its success rate remains high, the mechanisms have not been completely understood. Melzack and Wall in 1965 suggested gate-control theory that SCS stimulates the afferent fibers of the dorsal column by closing the gate of pain transmission to reduce pain [1]. But there is little evidence that SCS influences nociceptive pain.

The mechanisms of action may differ depending on the type of pain targeted for treatment. For example, its effect on neuropathic pain may be secondary to stimulation-induced suppression of central excitability, whereas the beneficial effect of SCS on ischemic pain may be related to stimulation-induced inhibition of sympathetic nervous system influences and antidromic vasodilation, which increases blood flow and reduces oxygen demand [4]. Until now, two theories can explain the effects of SCS. One is the antidromic mechanism which states that, at the spinal L2-5 segments, SCS activates interneurons containing extracellular signal-regulated kinase (ERK), protein kinase B (AKT), and possibly other intracellular signaling molecules, and subsequently stimulates the spinal terminals of transient receptor potential vanilloid receptor-1 (TRPV1) containing sensory fibers. The neural information is transmitted from the site of stimulation in the spinal segments to the nerve endings in the peripheral tissues and results in the production and release of vasodilators, including calcitonin gene-related peptide (CGRP). CGRP, as the most powerful vasodilator, leads to SCS-induced vasodilation directly. And the subsequent release of nitric oxide may be associated with vascular smooth muscle relaxation and peripheral blood flow increase in response to SCS. Another theory is that SCS induces decreased sympathetic efferent activity and subsequently reduces vasoconstriction and enhances blood flow in the lower limbs and feet. This is called the sympathetic mechanism. The two mechanisms are complementary, and the balance between them is affected by tonic sympathetic activity, SCS intensity, and individual patients or animal strains [5–8].

Techniques of Stimulation

Stimulation of the spinal cord is done by an implanted electrode powered by an implanted pulse generator (IPG). Electrodes may be inserted percutaneously via an epidural needle or surgically implanted via laminotomy. Electrodes may be bipolar or multipolar, and multiple electrodes may be used. Pulse generation is achieved by a fully implantable battery-powered device. Rechargeable battery systems may be preferred for some patients such as those with high current use, including those with multiple electrodes. Following IPG insertion, the patient may switch the device on and off with a hand-held programmer and may vary voltage and frequency within physician-determined limits. IPG battery life is variable but is usually between 2 and 8 years depending on the pattern of use and the output required. The commonest organism to infect SCS systems is *Staphylococcus aureus*. Patients scheduled for SCS should be screened for methicillin-resistant *Staphylococcus aureus* less than 4 weeks before the procedure to allow rational choice of antibiotic prophylaxis at the time of surgery. Compatibility of SCS with magnetic resonance imaging (MRI) is problematic. Therefore, if MRI is needed, it may be necessary to remove the SCS system.

Discussion

Around the world, some 14,000 patients undergo spinal cord stimulator implants each year [4]. Spinal cord stimulation (SCS) delivers mild electrical stimulation to nerves along the spinal column, modifying nerve activity to minimize the sensation of pain reaching the brain. Since the therapy first entered routine use in the 1980s, improvement since battery and microprocessor power and the ability to integrate position sensors are contributing to have a longer life-span, lower maintenance, and more precise control of the system. Spinal cord stimulation was approved by the FDA in 1989 to relieve pain from nerve damage and now accounts for about 70% of all neuromodulation treatments. Despite technical progress, the treatment of patients with inoperable chronic CLI is still challenging; 33% patients at 6 months and 51% at 2 years have to undergo amputation [9].

Augustinsson et al. used spinal cord stimulation in 34 patients with severe limb ischemia; all had resting pain and most had ischemic ulcers. Arterial surgery was technically impossible in all cases. 94% of the patients experienced pain relief. SCS healed ulcers in 50% of patients and 70% of the patients showed improved skin temperature. Only 38% of the stimulated arteriosclerotic patients underwent amputations during a mean follow-up period of 16 months, as compared to 90% of a comparable group of unstimulated patients [10]. Studies on the effect of SCS for inoperable CLI caused by diabetes mellitus have also shown promising pain-relief effect after spinal cord stimulation [11].

Almost all of the studies show better pain relief after SCS treatment as compared with best medical treatment. However, pain reduction is not the only objective. Limb salvage and other clinical improvements are more important. A meta-analysis of six controlled trials including 444 patients in 2006 showed a lower amputation rate of 11% after 12 months of SCS compared with optimum medical treatment. In addition, SCS patients required fewer analgesics and showed significant improvement [12, 13].

Many authors have used transcutaneous oxygen pressure as predictive parameter for ulcer healing in end-stage vascular patients treated with spinal cord stimulation. Spinal cord stimulation appears to provide a major benefit for lesion in stage IV patients with non-reconstructable PVD. Patients with an initial TcPO2 > 10 mmHg will respond better to the stimulation therapy. Gersbach reported that a (*transcutaneous partial pressure of oxygen*) AtcpO2 > 20 Torr may be an indication for permanent DCS without trial stimulation and that conversely an AtcpO2 < 15 Torr would contraindicate DCS treatment. With AtcpO2 values in the 15–20 Torr range, a trial stimulation period may still be warranted. In stage III or IV ischaemic limb disease refractory to other modes of revascularization, DCS is an effective therapeutic option providing substantial symptomatic relief and a 1-year limb salvage rate of over 60%. Functional improvement, as measured by walking perimeter increase, is also significant. These results are superior to those obtained with sympathectomy or prostaglandin infusion and are comparable to those of femoro-infrapopliteal bypass grafting. SCS treatment of non-reconstructable critical leg ischemia provides a significantly better limb survival rate compared with conservative treatment. Patient selection based on TcpO2 and the results of trial screening further increase the probability of limb survival after SCS therapy [14–18].

There is no controversy regarding pain relief, ulcer healing, and improved quality of life with the use of SCS, but many authors question the effects on limb salvage but extent of amputation level was less in patients with severe inoperable leg ischemia [19–21].

Klomp et al. reported that although SCS is thought to be promising in the treatment of CLI, its true effect and cost-effectiveness have not been proved. Large randomized clinical trials are needed before SCS can be integrated in the standardized treatment algorithm. A systematic meta-analysis published in 2009 also showed insufficient evidence for higher efficacy of SCS compared with optimum medical treatment [22]. Some prognostic factors of amputation in patients with CLI have been found, but there is no evidence for a better treatment in any group [22, 23].

Truin et al. suggested that the success of SCS may be related to its timing in the development of chronic neuropathic pain. Early SCS 24 h after appearance of neuropathic pain may result in an increased number of responders to SCS and an increased duration of the effect as compared to late SCS after 16 days [24].

Pain relief caused by SCS is apparent; however, objective studies focused on assessment of microcirculatory blood flow of skin, including TcpO2 and video capillary results; before and after SCS are needed to prove its efficacy in improving circulation. Undoubtedly, SCS is still considered as an option for reducing the chance of amputation, when all conventional treatments fail to be effective, especially in patients who suffer from chronic ischemic pain. The patient must know and accept the risk of SCS, its complications, and high cost.

Conclusion

Persistent pain is common and interferes with person's life, both physically and psychologically. There is clinical evidence from randomized controlled trials to support use of SCS in pain from failed back surgical syndrome (FBSS), complex regional pain syndrome (CRPS), neuropathic pain, and ischemic pain. Pain relief from SCS has been confirmed in a majority of the studies, while limb salvage has not been proved. Not all patients are suitable for SCS; therefore a multidisciplinary pain management team is the most appropriate environment in which SCS should be offered. SCS may be delivered in parallel with other therapies and should be used as part of an overall rehabilitation strategy.

References

1. Melzack R, Wall PD. Pain mechanisms: a new theory. Science. 1965;150:971–9.
2. Shealy CN, Mortimer JT, Reswick JB. Electrical inhibition of pain by stimulation of the dorsal columns: preliminary clinical report. Anesth Analg. Jul–Aug 1967;46(4):489–91
3. Cook AW, Oygar A, Baggenstos P, Pacheco S, Kleriga E. Vascular disease of extremities: electrical stimulation of spinal cord and posterior roots. N Y State J Med. 1976;76:366–8.
4. Linderoth B, Foreman RD. Mechanisms of spinal cord stimulation in painful syndromes: role of animal models. Pain Med. 2006;7 Suppl 1:s14–26.
5. Wu M, Komori N, Qin C, Farber JP, Linderoth B, Foreman RD. Extracellular signal-regulated kinase (ERK) and protein kinase B (AKT) pathways involved in spinal cord stimulation (SCS)-induced vasodilation. Brain Res. 2008;1207:73–83.
6. Tanaka S, Komori N, Barron KW, Chandler MJ, Linderoth B, Foreman RD. Mechanisms of sustained cutaneous vasodilation induced by spinal cord stimulation. Auton Neurosci. 2004;114:55–60.
7. Wu M, Thorkilsen M, Qin C, Farber JP, Linderoth B, Foreman RD. Effects of spinal cord stimulation on peripheral circulation in stretozotocin-induced diabetic rats. Neuromodulation. 2007;10:217–23.
8. Wu M, Komori N, Qin C, Farber JP, Linderoth B, Foreman RD. Roles of peripheral terminals of transient receptor potential vanilloid-1 containing sensory fibers in spinal cord stimulation induced peripheral vasodilation. Brain Res. 2007;1156:80–92.

9. Transatlantic Inter-Society Consensus (TASC). Section D: chronic critical limb ischaemia. Management of peripheral arterial disease. Eur J Vasc Endovasc Surg. 2000;19 Suppl A:S144–243.

10. Augustinson LE, Carlson CA, Holm J, Jivergard L. Epidural electric stimulation in severe limb ischemia. Pain relief, increased blood flow and possible limb-saving effect. Ann Surg. 1985;202:104–10.

11. Pluijms W, Huygen F, Cheng J, Mekhail N, van Kleef M, Van Zundert J, et al. Evidence-based interventional pain medicine according to clinical diagnoses. 18. Painful diabetic polyneuropathy. Pain Pract. 2011;11:191–8.

12. Ubbink DT, Vermeulen H. Spinal cord stimulation for critical leg ischemia: a review of effectiveness and optimal patient selection. J Pain Symptom Manage. 2006;31 Suppl 4:S30–5.

13. Ubbink DT, Vermeulen H. Spinal cord stimulation for non-reconstructable chronic critical leg ischaemia. Cochrane Database Syst Rev. 2005;3:CD004001.

14. Claeys LG, Horsch S. Transcutaneous oxygen pressure as predictive parameter for ulcer healing in end-stage vascular patients treated with spinal cord stimulation. Int Angiol. 1996;15:344–9.

15. Gersbach P, Hasdemir MG, Stevens RD, Nachbur B, Mahler F. Discriminative microcirculatory screening of patients with refractory limb ischaemia for dorsal column stimulation. Eur J Vasc Endovasc Surg. 1997;13:464–71.

16. Gersbach PA, Argitis V, Gardaz JP, von Segesser LK, Haesler E. Late outcome of spinal cord stimulation for unreconstructable and limb-threatening lower limb ischemia. Eur J Vasc Endovasc Surg. 2007;33(6):717–24.

17. Galley D, Rettori R, Boccalon H, Medvedowsky A, Lefebvre JM, Sellier F, et al. La stimulation électrique médullaire dans les arteriopathies des membres inférieurs. Une étude multicentrique chez 244 patients. J Mal Vasc. 1992;17:208–13.

18. Amann W, Berg P, Gersbach P, Gamain J, Raphael JH, Ubbink DT. Spinal cord stimulation in the treatment of non-reconstructable stable critical leg ischaemia: results of the European Peripheral Vascular Disease Outcome Study (SCS-EPOS). Eur J Vasc Endovasc Surg. 2003;26:280–6.

19. Jivegard LE, Augustinsson LE, Holm J, Risberg B, Ortenwall P. Effects of spinal cord stimulation (SCS) in patients with inoperable severe lower limb ischaemia: a prospective randomized controlled study. Eur J Vasc Endovasc Surg. 1995;9:421–5.

20. Jivegard LE, Augustinsson LA, Carlsson CA, Holm J. Long-term results by epidural spinal electrical stimulation (ESES in patients with inoperable severe lower limb ischaemia. Eur J Vasc Surg. 1987;1:345–9.

21. Klomp HM, Spincemaille GH, Steyerberg EW, Habbema JD, van Urk H. Spinal-cord stimulation in critical limb ischaemia: a randomized trial. ESES study group. Lancet. 1999 Mar 27;353:1040–4.

22. Klomp HM, Steyerberg EW, Habbema JD, van Urk H, ESES study group. What is the evidence on efficacy of spinal cord stimulation in (subgroups of) patients with critical limb ischemia? Ann Vasc Surg. 2009;23:355–63. Epub 2009 Jan 6. Review.

23. Klomp HM, Steyerberg EW, van Urk H, Habbema JD, ESES Study Group. Spinal cord stimulation is not cost-effective for non-surgical management of critical limb ischaemia. Eur J Vasc Endovasc Surg. 2006;31:500–8.

24. Truin M, van Kleef M, Linderoth B, Smits H, Janssen SP, Joosten EA. Increased efficacy of early spinal cord stimulation in an animal model of neuropathic pain. Eur J Pain. 2011;15:111–7.

Omental Transplant for Revascularization in Critical Ischemic Limbs and Tissues

42

V.K. Agarwal, Jyoti Bindal, and Swati Bhargava

Ancient Egyptians coined the word "omentum" while embalming human bodies by looking at the omentum to assess their "omens." Hippocrates thought that the omentum in some way was connected with the regulation of the amount of fluid in the peritoneal cavity. Aristotle looked upon the omentum as a fatty apron, designed to protect the viscera from cold. From time immemorial, various purposeful functions were attributed to the greater omentum.

In the past, the omentum was considered to be an inert tissue without much biological significance. But since the beginning of the last century, innumerable studies and trials have been conducted by surgeons and scientists all over the world, which have proven that the omentum is a unique, physiologically dynamic tissue with immense therapeutic potential.

Now it has been well accepted throughout the years that the omentum is indeed an organ of exceptional versatility. The greater omentum in its natural state with its own blood supply has the ability to seal, to wall off, and to carry away through its many phagocyte cells foreign bacteria, foreign bodies, and dead tissue. Morrison [1] called the omentum "a special protective agency the abdominal policeman. It travels around the abdomen with considerable activity, and is attracted by some sort of inflammation in neighborhoods in which mischief is brewing," because it was shown to plug hernia orifices, to seal off infections and perforation, and to impart new blood supply to a detached uterine fibroid. It has been found wrapped around acute appendices, gall bladders,

and gangrenous intestines. There are indications that it could revascularize the intestine and other organs which had lost their blood supply.

Based on the arterialization properties of the omentum, Shaughnessy [2] attempted to provide the heart an alternative blood supply by taking the omentum to the myocardium with its vascular pedicle. Later the omentum was utilized in the repair of recurrent vesicovaginal fistulae, the technique subsequently popularized by Turner-Warwick [3]. The value of the omentum in relief of lymphedema was experimentally proven by Goldsmith and De los Santos [4]; Casten and Alday [5] used it for revascularization of the lower limb.

Anatomy of the Greater Omentum

The size of the omentum varies from 300 to 2000 g with a surface area of 300–1500 cm^2. The greater omentum is a large apron-like fold of visceral peritoneum that hangs down from the stomach. It extends from the greater curvature of the stomach, passing in front of the small intestines, and reflects on itself to ascend to the transverse colon before reaching to the posterior abdominal wall. Since the greater omentum appears to float on the surface of the intestines, it is the first structure observed when the abdominal cavity is opened. The omentum has a rich vascular supply with numerous characteristic capillary convolutions which are termed omental glomeruli due to their similarity to renal glomeruli. These capillary beds lie directly under the mesothelium (Fig. 42.1).

Structure

The greater omentum is the largest peritoneal fold. It consists of a double sheet of peritoneum, folded on itself so that it is made up of four layers. The two layers which descend from the greater curvature of the stomach and commencement of the duodenum pass in front of the small intestines, sometimes as low down as the pelvis; they then turn upon themselves

V.K. Agarwal, MBBS, MS (✉)
Surgery, M.G.M. Medical College, Sanjivini Nursing Home, 1-A, Phadnis Colony, A.B. Road, Indore, MP 452009, India

J. Bindal, MBBS, MS, LLB. PGDHM
Obstetrics and Gynecology, G.R. Medical College, Bungalow No. 11, J.A. Hospital Campus, Gwalior, MP, India

S. Bhargava, MBBS, MS (OBGY)
Obstetrics and Gynaecology, M.G.M. Medical College, 63, 64 Sampat Farms, Bicholi Mardana, Indore, MP 452016, India

© Springer International Publishing Switzerland 2017
R.S. Dieter et al. (eds.), *Critical Limb Ischemia*, DOI 10.1007/978-3-319-31991-9_42

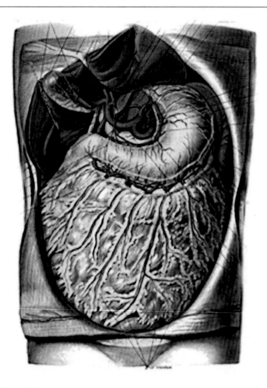

Fig. 42.1 Greater omentum

and ascend again as far as the transverse colon, where they separate and enclose that part of the intestine.

These individual layers may be easily demonstrated in the young subject, but in the adult, they are more or less inseparably blended.

The left border of the greater omentum is continuous with the gastrolienal ligament; its right border extends as far as the commencement of the duodenum.

The greater omentum is usually thin, presents a variegated appearance, and always contains some adipose tissue, which in obese people accumulates in considerable quantity.

Blood Supply

The greater omentum comprises of loaded arterial arcade constituting three influential vessels that descend from gastroepiploic artery along the stomach's greater curvature. The right, middle, and left omental branches that possess tiny intervening branches along with draining veins lying adjacently arise from the gastroepiploic system. The vascular supply to the omentum is mostly provided by anastomosis from the right direction and gastroepiploic arteries from the left direction.

The right and left gastroepiploic vessels provide the sole blood supply to the greater omentum. Both are branches of the celiac trunk. The right gastroepiploic is a branch of the

gastroduodenal artery, which is a branch of the common hepatic artery, which is a branch of the celiac trunk. The left gastroepiploic artery is the largest branch of the splenic artery, which is a branch of the celiac trunk. The right and left gastroepiploic vessels anastomose within the two layers of the anterior greater omentum along the greater curvature of the stomach. And form the gastroepiploic arch from which arise the right, middle, and left omental arteries. The middle vessel joining the right and the left forms the distal arcade on the free border of the omentum, the Barlow's arcade. There may be some variation in the pattern, and care should be observed during mobilization of these vessels (Fig. 42.2).

Biological Properties of the Greater Omentum

The greater omentum is a primitive part of the gastrointestinal system containing a vast network of blood vessels and lymphatics. The omentum performs a number of functions during episodes of peritonitis. The first of these is the rapid absorption and clearance of bacteria and foreign material from the peritoneal cavity. The omentum is the only site, other than the diaphragmatic stomata, that has a documented ability to absorb particles from the peritoneal cavity.

The second function of the omentum is to supply leukocytes to the peritoneal cavity. In experimental animals with peritonitis, the omentum appears to be the principal site by which firstly macrophages and then neutrophils migrate into the peritoneal cavity.

The third function of the omentum is to adhere and seal off areas of contamination. The omentum can rapidly produce a layer of fibrin by which it adheres to the contaminated area at the point of contact.

Neovascularization

The human omental microvascular endothelial cells (HOME cells) express the angiogenic peptide basic fibroblast growth factor. This process of neovascularization allows the omentum to provide vascular support to adjacent tissues such as the gut and promote function and healing in ischemic or inflamed tissue. Even if deprived of its own blood supply, it might survive by attacking arteries in the tissue in its vicinity, and Vineberg and Lwin [6] demonstrated in dogs that the free omental strips, within 3–8 days, had obtained a new blood supply from its vicinity. Free omental grafts, however, have a variable fate, they may gain a viable blood supply from the vicinity as stated earlier, or they may undergo complete infraction and necrosis. Infection greatly reduces the chance of the successful take of the free omental graft.

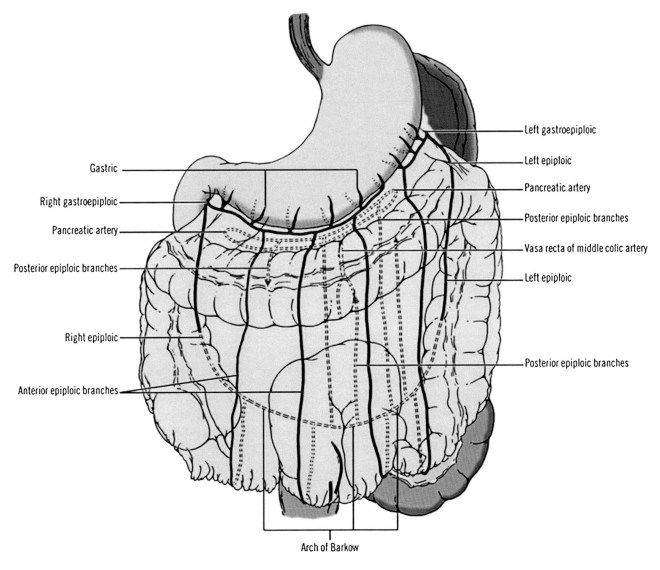

Gastric

Right gastroepiploic

Pancreatic artery

Posterior epiploic branches

Right epiploic

Anterior epiploic branches

Left gastroepiploic

Left epiploic

Pancreatic artery

Posterior epiploic branches

Vasa recta of middle colic artery

Left epiploic

Posterior epiploic branches

Arch of Barkow

Fig. 42.2 Blood supply — omentum

In the immediate operative period, a free omental graft behaves to some extent as an inert membrane, in that the biological defenses contained in the peritoneal adhesions may be denied adequate early access to the immediate area of operation, e.g., a suture line.

The result of the experimental work by Carter et al. [7] has shown that though a free omental graft may be used successfully, the pedicle omentum gives superior results, and its biological role is more reliable.

In a similar study, experimental and clinical results reported by Agarwal and Agarwal [8] were encouraging. In this clinical study, in 50 cases of critical ischemic limbs due to Buerger's disease, allografts were taken from patients undergoing laparotomy for any other diseases. Simultaneously experimental study was done in 20 dogs in two groups: Group I was without ligation of femoral artery in ten dogs, and Group II was studied with ligation of femoral artery in another ten dogs.

Results of clinical and experimental studies showed that even mismatched graft is taken up and revascularizes the ischemic limbs.

Special Properties of the Omentum

Recent studies have revealed that the omentum, apart from being a great source of various growth factors, neurotransmitters, neurotrophic factors, and inflammatory mediators, also contains omnipotent stem cells that can differentiate into a variety of cell types, this omnipotent stem cell having the power to migrate (Solvason and Kearney [9]). In a study, it was found that the human fetal omentum, liver, and spleen are sites of B cell generation, but it was also demonstrated that the pro/pre-B cell compartment (CD24+, sIgM−) is detected in the omentum and liver but not in the spleen as early as 8 weeks of gestation. From 8 to 12 weeks of gestation, the proportions of IgM+ cells that were pre-B cells (cIgM+/sIgM−) in the omentum and liver were $53 \pm 15\%$ and $45 \pm 13\%$, respectively, and IgM+ cells were not detectable in the spleen. After 12 weeks, the percentage of pre-B cells was unchanged in the fetal liver ($41 \pm 10\%$) but decreased significantly in the omentum ($25 \pm 14\%$); Pre-B cells were now detected in the spleen but at much lower percentages ($2 \pm 3\%$) than either the omentum or liver. The nuclear enzyme, Tdt, was detected in approximately 25% of the CD24+ cells in the omentum and liver during the 8–12-week time period; however, Tdt+ cells were not detected in the spleen. Approximately 40% of the mature B cells found in the omentum and spleen were CD5+ compared with only 20% in the liver. These results demonstrate that the fetal omentum, like the fetal liver and bone marrow, is a primary site of B cell development.

Solvason and Kearney [10] further studied the relationship between the omentum and liver during the development of Ly-1 B cells. The most obvious relationship between these two sites is that cells simply migrate from one location to the other, that is, precursor cells may migrate from the fetal liver into the fetal omentum and in this milieu give rise to exclusively Ly-1+ B cells or the sister population

García-Gómez et al. [11] studied angiogenic capacity of human omental stem cells. Human omental CD34+ cells were obtained from samples of human omentum by density gradient centrifugation in Ficoll. Proliferative pattern, marker expression (by flow cytometry), and angiogenic growth factor synthesis by omental cell cultures were determined.

In vivo angiogenic capacity of the cells was evaluated in rats. Omental stem cells showed a high rate of proliferation (Ki67 staining), expressed CD34 marker, and synthesized bFGF and VEGF. When implanted in rats, omental cells promoted neovascularization. Human omental cells were localized in rat tissue, mainly forming the endothelium of neo-vessels. Implantation of omental cells also facilitated angiogenesis of rat origin.

It was concluded that CD34+ cell population of human omentum could be responsible for the clinical benefit of omental transplantation by promoting angiogenesis and synthesizing angiogenic growth factors to facilitate revascularization of injured tissue.

Use of Inherent Properties of Omental in Limb Salvage

These revascularizing properties of the omentum learned over the years were based on clinical and experimental studies. The exact mechanism of action has eluded the surgeons for many years. It appears to be answered by these recent studies, which showed that the omentum is full of omnipotent stem cells having power to migrate.

With the development and refinement of microvascular surgery, most of the ischemic tissue and organs are salvaged by direct reconstructive surgery. But many times, we are faced with situation where, either due to technical difficulty or complications like graft failure, these ischemic tissues and organs is lost.

In such situations, we have used the properties of the omentum by developing a simple technique to lengthen it and mobilizing it extra-abdominally. This technique can be used in all parts of the body from the scalp to the toe, to revascularize in end-stage ischemic limbs in Burger's disease, where direct revascularization surgery is not feasible and amputation has to be done eventually [12]. We have been able to salvage limbs in 85% cases in 15 years of follow-up [13].

Preparation of an Omental Pedicle

Hoshino et al. [14] described the mobilization of the omentum from greater curvature of the stomach, and later Talwar et al. [15] described the technique of its elongation. Several techniques are available to mobilize and lengthen the omentum to reach inguinal region or mid-thigh. We have simplified the technique (Agarwal technique) to lengthen the omentum up to 1 m long with upper end attached to stomach.

Operative Technique

The blood supply to the omentum comes mainly from the right and left gastroepiploic arteries which join along the greater curvature of the stomach to form the gastroepiploic arterial arch. The three major omental arterial trunks—the right, middle, and left—arising from this gastroepiploic arch form vascular arcade in the free border of omentum Barlow's arcade which is not constant, and there are several variations. In some cases, it is not found on the free border of omentum but much higher which makes mobilization of omentum difficult. All the arteries are accompanied by veins (Fig. 42.2).

The abdomen is opened by left paramedian or median incision. The omentum is made free from its attachment to the colon and the stomach preserving the gastroepiploic arch. Attachment to the colon is avascular and easy to separate. To separate from the stomach, the ascending branches from the gastroepiploic arch to the stomach need to be divided. Depending upon the caliber, right or left gastroepiploic artery is divided. The omentum is then completely freed except for one pedicle attached to the stomach (Fig. 42.3). The omental graft is further designed using a cotton tape to get enough length to reach the ankle or wrist (Fig. 42.4).

In end-stage ischemic extremities, the lengthened omentum is brought out of the abdomen by an incision, lateral to deep inguinal region for lower extremity (Fig. 42.5) and near xiphisternum for the upper extremity, eye, and scalp (Fig. 42.6), and the abdomen is closed.

Further skin incisions are made at 4–5 sites, depending on the requirement; on the inner part of the thigh, leg, and ankle in the lower limb and on the chest and arm in upper limb. Subcutaneous plane is opened to prepare a facial tunnel, and pedicle graft is gently negotiated to reach the site of insertion. Throughout the procedure, due care is observed to avoid hematoma and tearing of omentum.

The Various Surgical Uses of Omentum

Revascularization of Ischemic Extremities

Peripheral vascular disease (synonymous with chronic occlusive diseases)
Occlusive:

> Buerger's disease
> Atherosclerosis
> Diabetic

Vaso-spasmodic:
> Raynaud's disease
> Early stage Buerger's disease

Surgical treatment of peripheral vascular diseases especially Buerger's disease remains a challenge. Though in recent years the concept of Buerger's disease as a distinct entity has been questioned in Western countries, but in South East Asian countries, especially in India, it is very common in comparison to atherosclerosis, the latter forming only 10 % of cases of peripheral vascular disease.

The pathological process in Buerger's disease (also called as thromboangiitis obliterans) involves inflammatory reaction in the arterial wall with involvement of the vein and nerves, leading to thrombosis and obliteration of the arteries. As a consequence, the surgical reconstructive procedures are technically difficult and often unsuccessful.

Patients with end-stage Buerger's disease present with severe pain intermittent claudication which may progress to

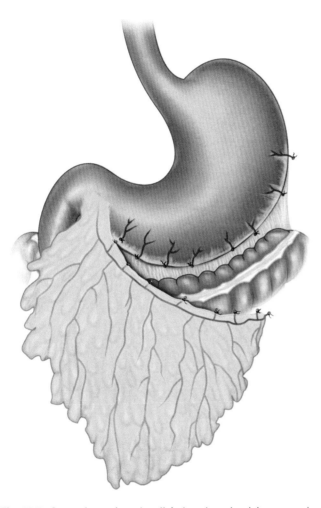

Fig. 42.3 Omental vessels and pedicle based on the right gastroepiploic artery

Fig. 42.4 Showing designing of omental pedicle by cotton tape

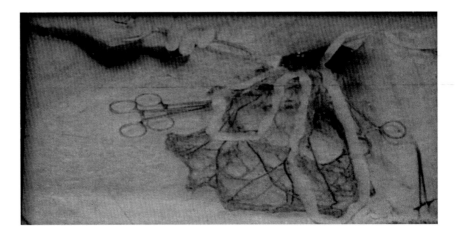

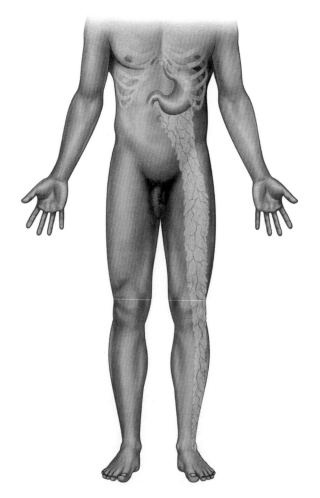

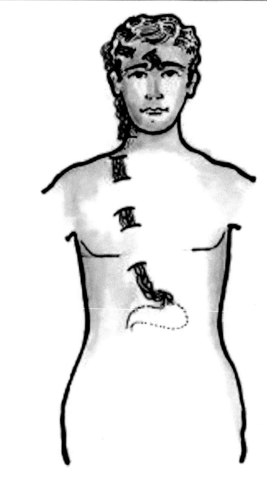

Fig. 42.6 Pedicle omentum brought to the forehead

Fig. 42.5 Omental pedicle attached only to the stomach lengthened reaching up to ankle

rest pain, ulceration (pre-gangrenous), and gangrene of the digit. Investigations are directed to note the level of obstruction and vasospasm which include mainly arteriography and Doppler studies.

Standard treatment consists of conservative approach including abstaining from tobacco. Operative intervention includes sympathectomy in early cases where there is vasospasm element and in late cases amputations, as reported in text book of surgery amputation has to be done eventually [12].

Numerous operative procedures have been attempted in the past as alternative to amputation, but none of these procedures has led to satisfactory long-term results. Direct reconstructive surgery like bypass grafting is not feasible due to poor distal runoff caused by multiple occlusions in the small peripheral vessels. Hence, a salvage of limbs affected by Buerger's disease has been a dilemma for surgeons.

The ability of the omentum to serve as a source of arterial supply has been used for revascularization of ischemic extremities. For patients in imminent danger of amputation, the omental transfer may achieve optimum revascularization to save the limbs.

Basically, the omentum is a highly vascular organ with rich source of angiogenic factors that provide the growth of blood vessels into whatever tissue it is placed close to. Biological anastomosis on its own occurs between the omental arteriolar network and capillaries of ischemic tissue in 3 days, thus filling the original vessels [6].

We have used omental transfer for end-stage Buerger's disease since 1980. Eight hundred cases with imminent gangrene where sympathectomy had already been tried comprised the case material. The results have been most gratifying. All the limbs became warm (100%). Rest pain was relieved in 96% and ulcers healed in 90% of cases. Postoperative improvements in angiographic and color Doppler findings were noted. Angiograms showed omental capillaries anastomosing with original vessel capillaries and retrograde filling the vessel like bypass (Figs. 42.7 and 42.8).

Color Doppler study is simple and gives good information of the arterial vessels of extremities showing flow and level of blocks which are usually multiple (Fig. 42.9). Postoperative follow-up showed increased blood flow and filling of the arteries (Fig. 42.10).

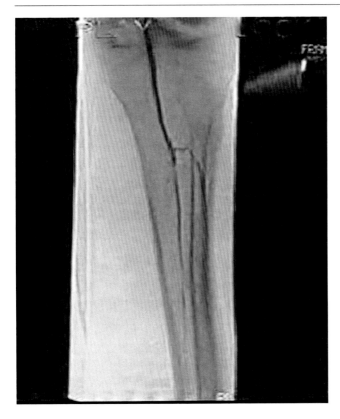

Fig. 42.7 Preoperative arteriogram showing block in the anterior and posterior tibial arteries

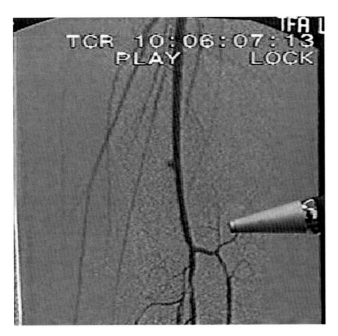

Fig. 42.8 Postoperative arteriogram of the same patient as in Fig. 42.7, showing anastomosis of the omental capillaries with retrograde filling of the tibial vessels

In one of our largest series of long-term follow-up [13], good results were seen in 85 % patients followed for 15 years (Kaplan–Meier Curve 20 years Fig. 42.11). Many other centers have reported encouraging results in patients undergoing omentopexy for limb salvage in end-stage Buerger's disease [14–17].

Several workers have used this technique for limb salvage in atherosclerosis and diabetic patients with good results; Casten and Alday [5] showed marked increase in collateral circulation, atherosclerotic limbs with 70 % improvement rate, remarkable healing, and limb salvage.

The mechanism of the effectiveness of the omental transfer is that omental vessels develop new capillaries, which make biological anastomosis within the capillaries of ischemic muscle tissue, filling retrograde original artery like bypass (Figs. 42.7 and 42.8).

Vineberg and Lwin [6], in an experimental study, have shown that the omental graft forms anastomotic capillary channels with the surrounding tissue within 3 days and arteriolar-sized channels within 8 days. The omental vessels seem to have an unlimited capacity to increase in size and at a rapid rate due to omnipotent stem cells.

With these properties of the omentum, the omental graft develops the natural blood supply to the limb which may even be superior to what may be possible, by the direct reconstructive surgery in chronic ischemic limbs, where direct arterial surgery is not possible.

The omental transfer seems to be the answer toward replenishment of the limb nutrition.

Improvement of Lymphatic Drainage

The omentum, besides having arteries and veins, also has lymphatics and has been used in the lymphatic edematous tissues of extremities.

Goldsmith and De los Santos [4] demonstrated the formation of lymphatic new connections between the tissues of extremity and omentum in dogs. Based on these observations, these workers placed a long pedicle of omentum in the subcutaneous tissues of edematous limb anticipating formation of anastomosis channels between the omental lymphatic vessels and the lymphatic of the lymph edematous tissues. The clinical results, however, have not been encouraging.

Reconstructive Surgical Procedure to Salvage Chronic or Acute Ischemic Hand and Tissues

The omentum has been used as a source of free tissue transfer by anastomosing through microsurgical technique, the omental vessels to vessels in the vicinity of the defect.

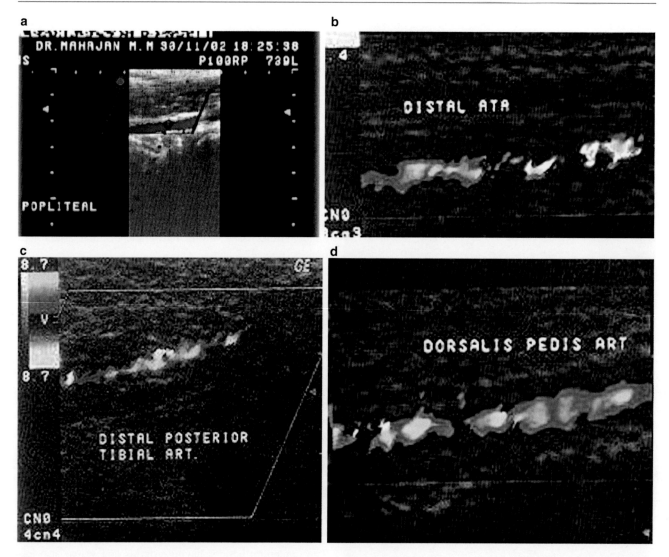

Fig. 42.9 Color Doppler study (preoperative) showing reduced peak systolic velocity with reduced to no flow in diastole in (**a**) popliteal, (**b**) anterior tibial, (**c**) posterior tibial, and (**d**) dorsalis pedis arteries

Its beneficial characteristics include thinness, marked vascular, and plasticity.

The omentum also constitutes a readily available and virtually limitless source of both arterial and venous microconduits. The omentum may be used to fill in soft tissue defects. For example, a gastroepiploic vessel may be used to reconstitute the superficial arch of the hand for hand salvage in chronic or acute ischemic conditions.

Excellent results have been reported in treatment of large skull defects by anastomosing the free omental graft to the superficial temporal and occipital vessels.

With further development and refinement of microvascular surgical technique, the free vascular omental grafts may be used virtually in all parts of the human body, from the scalp to the great toe.

Large decubitus ulcers have been managed by omental transposition. In superimposed spilt thickness, skin graft

omentum may be used to close wall defect from extensive resections for malignant tumors. This may be achieved by transposition of the omentum on a vascular pedicle. The full thickness or split thickness skin graft offers reconstruction by epithelial coverage.

Revascularization of Ischemic Conditions in the Eye

There are many situations where direct revascularization is not possible, and surgeon feels helpless to lose these ischemic tissues and organs, the eye being one of them. The eye is a special organ; ischemic disease of the eye leads to blindness.

Broadly, the eye has two chambers. The anterior chamber consists of the cornea and lens, of which treatment is well

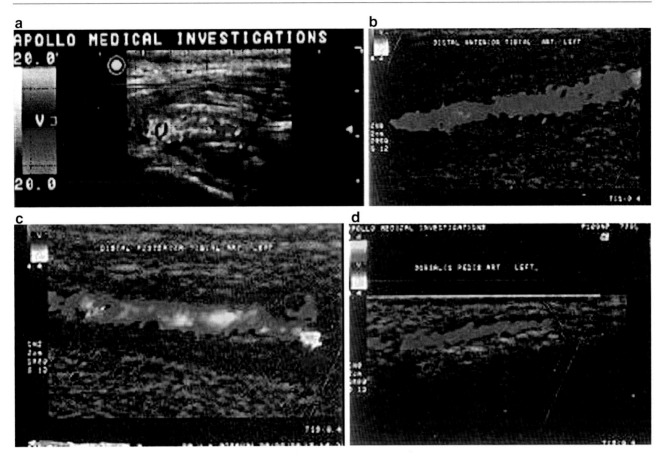

Fig. 42.10 Color Doppler study (postoperative) in the same patient as in Fig. 42.9, showing increased peak systolic velocities with significant forward diastolic flow in (**a**) popliteal, (**b**) anterior tibial, (**c**) posterior tibial, and (**d**) dorsalis pedis arteries

Fig. 42.11 Kaplan–Meier curve demonstrating survival of the limbs in relation to time in months

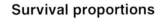

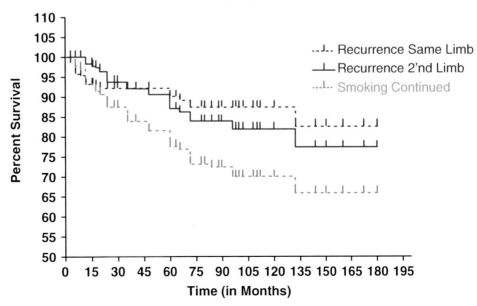

established. It is in the diseases of the posterior chamber that the surgeon feels helpless.

Diseases like retinal ischemic disease lead to degeneration of the retinal epithelium, converting rods, and cones in bony corpuscles in conditions like retinitis pigmentosa, age-related macular degeneration, optic atrophy, etc. Various treatments have been tried to increase vascularity of retina. Medical treatments include drugs like antioxidants, ribo, etc.

Newer surgical procedures described in various retinal surgical techniques are not widely accepted due to technical difficulties, complications, and poor long-term results. Heckenlively and Silver [18] went on to declare that treatments for ocular-only forms of RP are currently unavailable. As there is no medical treatment of these diseases, ophthalmologist helplessly sees patients going blind. For a long time, research has been going on in several countries to revascularize retinas, including the development of artificial retinal chip (Humayun et al. [19]), but none have succeeded.

Retinal artery originates intracranially. Its extracranial part, covered by dura, however, does not supply rods and cones, which are nourished by choroidal capillaries, branches of posterior short colliery artery. To revascularize rods and cones, we have to bypass posterior short ciliary artery (Fig. 42.12). The direct reconstructive surgery is not feasible at posterior short ciliary artery; this leads to search for alternative techniques. Figure 42.12 is showing blood vessels of retina and choroidal capillaries which are branches of posterior short ciliary artery.

Goldsmith et al. [20], in an experimental study, demonstrated that intact omentum can be successfully transposed to the eye of the dog, with evidence of vascular connection developing between the omentum and intraocular vascular channels.

With the experimental evidence and our 25 years of clinical experience in limb revascularization, we modified Agarwal technique for pedicle omental transplant into eye. Lengthened omentum is brought out of the abdomen at xiphisternum, and subcutaneous tunnel is created on the chest, neck, and mid-forehead (Fig. 42.6). In the eye, conjunctiva is reflected, and a tunnel is made subconjunctively to the forehead incision in both the eyes. Through these tunnels, strips of the omentum are passed and then placed posteriorly round the optic nerve in the eyeball near the posterior short ciliary artery. No attempt of anastomosis is made between eye vessels and omentum. This procedure resulted in choroidal revascularization, as the omental vessels encouraged development of new capillaries which cross-anastomosed between omental and posterior short colliery artery, which in turn filled choroidal vessels in a retrograde manner (Fig. 42.13). Visual acuity improved in 12 weeks from preoperative 6/18 to 6/6 postoperatively. Field of vision also improved from 10 to 12°.

Indocyanine green angiograms postoperative showed increase in choroidal vasculature at posterior pole, suggestive of increased vascularity of choroid (Fig. 42.14). Further loss of vision was checked in all cases. Vision and field increased in cases that had preoperative vision up to 6/60.

This was pioneering work in omental transplant in the eye, never previously tried in the world. As it is the first series of long-term results in the world ever published [21], it will prove to be a breakthrough in medical science.

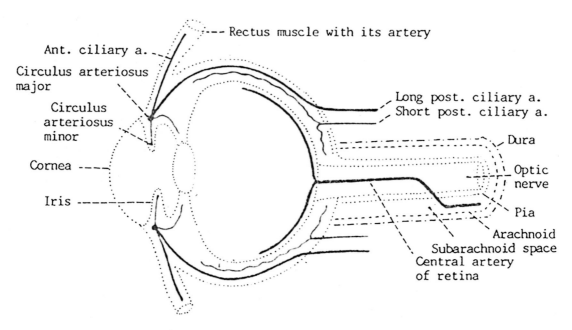

Fig. 42.12 Showing blood vessels of retina and choroidal capillaries which are branch of posterior short ciliary

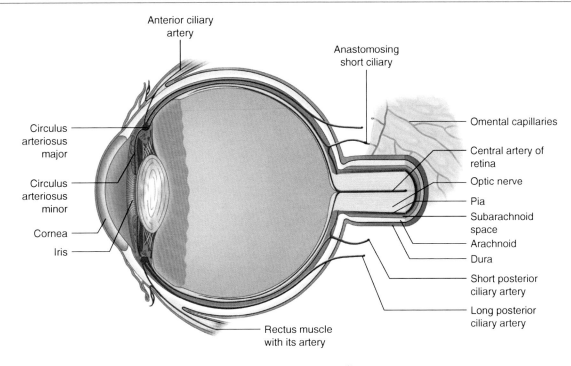

Fig. 42.13 Omentum throwing capillaries, which anastomose with posterior short ciliary

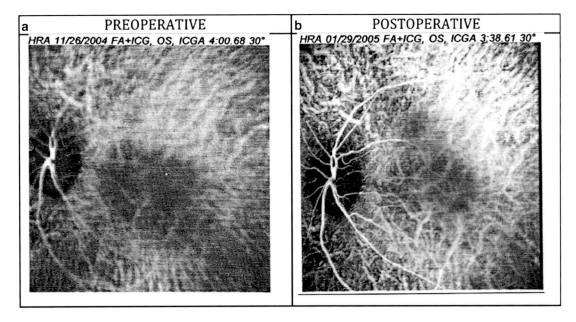

Fig. 42.14 Indocyanine green angiograms (ICG) showing choroidal vasculature at macula preoperatively (**a**) and 3 months postoperatively (**b**) showing increased choroidal vasculature at posterior pole sugges- tive of increased vascularity of choroid (both ICG angiogram were taken after 4 min of dye injection)

Revascularization of Myocardium (Heart)

Shaughnessy [2] was the first scientist to demonstrate that a pedicle omental graft placed in the myocardium developed vascular connections with the myocardial vessels, and this procedure was later popularized by Vineberg and Lwin [6].

However, with the advent of coronary artery surgery, this has now become a historical curiosity.

However, in cases where aorta coronary bypass surgery is not feasible or re-do transmyocardial revascularization has been tried, based on experimental study of Sen et al. [22]. This was not popular due to poor results, as outer 1/12 myocardium is not vascularized. In an experimental study, we combined transmyocardial revascularization with pedicle omentopexy [23]. This revascularized the outer myocardium was targeted following the principle of developing vessels from the omentum, and is recommended in complicated cases where aorta coronary bypass surgery or re-do surgery is not feasible.

Use in Gastrointestinal Surgery

Every abdominal surgeon has instinctively used the omentum as a "wrap around" to provide reinforcement for difficult bowel closures. The value of omental wrapping is especially effective as a cover for extraperitoneal anastomosis, such as for the esophagus or rectum where the absence of serosa is associated with an increased tendency for anastomosis breakdown. McLacblin et al. [24], in canine studies, found a high rate of leak with the increased dead space surrounding the anastomosis, which significantly decreased with an omental pedicle graft filling the pelvic region.

Role of Omental Graft in Urogenital Surgery

Repair of vesicovaginal fistula earlier had a notoriously high failure rate, which has been improved upon to a large extent by interposition of a pedicle omentum graft between the repaired organs [25]. Turner-Warwick [3] recommended wrapping of the kidney with pedicle omentum after procedure such as pyelolithotomy or nephrolithotomy (especially in solitary kidney). It was thought that in these patients, re-exploration for recurrent stones will be easier if it becomes necessary. Tiptaft et al. [26] used omental wrapping of the ureter in retroperitoneal fibrosis. The omental wrapping of the released ureter obviates recurrence of fibrosis and stricture formation.

The omentum has been used for cystoplasty in experimental animals, where the pedicle omentum adhered rapidly to the bladder wall, and the luminal surface of the patch was covered with the transitional epithelium within 15 days.

Turner-Warwick [27] has also recommended the use of pedicle omental graft around the area of excision and anastomosis for traumatic posterior urethral stricture.

It is recommended that trans-abdominal VVF repairs be performed with an interposition flap regardless of the appearance of healthy surrounding tissues and etiology.

Principles of surgical repair of VVF include optimal tissue condition (adequate vascular supply and freedom from infection, inflammation, necrosis, and malignancy); option of complete excision of fistulous tract, a tension-free, watertight, multilayered closure with avoidance of overlapping suture lines; interposition of healthy vascularized tissue between the bladder and vaginal suture lines; and continuous postoperative bladder drainage. Trans-abdominal repair described by O'Conor adheres to these guiding principles. All these criteria are aptly fulfilled by the omentum.

The omentum which is usually used for interposition has an abundant vascular supply and lymphatic drainage. It provides the suture lines with a vascular graft, replacement tissue, and a mechanism for absorption of debris increasing the chance of success of the repair [2]. After healing, the omentum retains its suppleness and maintains a plane of separation, should reoperation be necessary.

Use in Thoracic Surgical Procedures

Omental grafts have been used to repair bronchopleural fistulas, and esophageal perforations to reinforce esophagogastric anastomosis have shown satisfactory results for esophageal graft protection and for repair of chest wall defect.

For Revascularization of the Central Nervous System

Recently there has been an increasing interest in using the omentum for the purpose of revascularization of the central nervous system, as an extensive new source of blood to the brain and spinal cord.

Use of the Omentum in Spleen Trauma

Spleen lacerations may be sutured over the omentum, and the latter may well be exercising a hemostatic effect. Morrison reported that the omentum had provided a new blood supply to a detached uterine fibroid, and on the same basis, the implant of spleen (after splenectomy for trauma) may be desirable. For the transplanted spleen tissue to have the protective function, when splenectomy becomes inevitable, autotransplantation by the omentum can be done, keeping in mind its limited protective value.

Conclusion

Certain special attributes of the omentum favor its innumerable applications in day-to-day surgical practices. Basically, it is a highly vascular organ with rich source of angiogenic factors that provide the growth of blood vessels into whatever tissue it is placed close to. The potent lymphatic system of the omentum can absorb enormous amounts of fluids causing edema and remove metabolic waste and toxic substances.

Recent studies have revealed that the omentum, apart from being a great source of various growth factors, is full of omnipotent stem cell having power to migrate. CD34+ cell population of human omentum could be responsible for the clinical benefit of omental transplantation by promoting angiogenesis and synthesizing angiogenic growth to facilitate revascularization of injured tissue. In other words nature has provided minibank of omnipotent cells in the form of the omentum.

Morrison [1] has rightly named it as "the policeman of the abdomen." By extra-abdominal mobilization, the omentum can be used in all parts of the body from the scalp to the toe. The policeman of the abdomen can become the border security force.

Omental transplant's greatest therapeutic use is in limb salvage of chronic ischemic limbs. As millions of limbs are amputated, due to diabetes and atherosclerosis in Western countries and Buerger's disease in Asian countries, either due to failure or non-feasibility of direct reconstructive surgery, mental transplant shows a new ray of hope.

We have used omental transfer for end-stage Buerger's disease since year 1980 and for limb salvage in 800 cases with imminent gangrene where sympathectomy had already failed. The results have been most gratifying. During the long-term follow-up, the results continued to be excellent in 70 %, good in 16 %, and poor in 4 %.

Several workers have used this technique for limb salvage in Buerger's disease [5, 8, 13–17]. Casten and Alday [5] showed marked increase in collateral circulation, atherosclerotic limbs with 70 % improvement rate, remarkable healing, and limb salvage.

We found that our described technique of pedicled omental transfer to the periphery of critically ischemic limbs (stages III and IV) in Buerger's disease provides extremely good limb salvage results.

This technique is easy to perform and gives good results in a population of patients who have no other therapeutic option except amputation. We achieved an 85 % limb salvage rate (in follow-up of up to 15 years) and thereby significantly reduced morbidity in these patients.

Omentopexy is thus recommended as the choice of treatment in patients with end-stage Buerger's disease.

References

1. Morrison R. Remarks on some functions of the omentum. Br J Med. 1906;1:76.
2. Shaughnessy L. An experimental method of providing a collateral circulation to the heart. Br J Surg. 1936;23:665.
3. Turner-Warwick R. The use of omental pedical graft in urinary tract reconstruction. J Urol. 1976;116:341.
4. Goldsmith HS, De los Santos R. Omental transposition for the treatment of chronic lymphedema. Rev Surg. 1966;23:303.
5. Casten DF, Alday ES. Omental transfer for revascularisation of the extremities. Surg Gynecol Obstet. 1971;132:301.
6. Vineberg A, Lwin MM. Fostering a natural artery bypass for disseminated coronary artery disease by pericoronory omental strips. Surg Gynecol Obstet. 1973;137:565.
7. Carter DC, Jenkins DHR, Whitfield HN. Omental re-inforcement of intestinal anastomosis and experimental study in the rabbit. Br J Surg. 1972;59:129.
8. Agarwal VK, Agarwal S. Omental allograft: its role in revascularization of ischemic limbs with special reference to the Buerger's disease—a clinical and experimental study. In: Masutomo A, DeBakey ME, Kondo J, editors. Advances cardiovascular surgery. New York: Elsevier; 1991. p. 89–96.
9. Solvason N, Kearney JF. The human fetal omentum: a site of B cell generation. J Exp Med. 1992;175(2):397–404.
10. Solvoson N, Chen X, Shu F, Kearney JF. The fetal omentum in mice and human. A site enriched for precursor of Cd5 B cells early in development. Ann N Y Acad Sci. 1992;651:10–20.
11. García-Gómez I, et al. Angiogenic capacity of human omental cells. Neurol Res. 2005;27(8):807–11.
12. Murie JA. Short practice of surgery. 23rd ed. London: Arnold; 2000.
13. Agarwal VK. Long term results of omental transplantation in chronic occlusive arterial disease (Buerger's disease) and retinal avascular diseases (retinitis pigmentosa). Int Surg. 2007;92:174–83.
14. Hoshino S, Nakayama K, Igari T, Honda K. Long term results of omental transplantation for chronic occlusive arterial diseases. Int Surg. 1983;68:47–50.
15. Talwar S, Jain S, Parwal R, Laddha BL, Prashad P. Pedical omental transfer for limb salvage in Buerger's disease. Int J Cardiol. 2002;72:127–32.
16. Nishimura A, Sano F, Nakanishi Y. Omental transplantation for relief of limb ischaemia. Surg Forum. 1977;28:213–5.
17. Hoshino S, Hamada O, Iwaya F, Takahira H, Honda K. Omental transplantation for chronic occlusive arterial diseases. Int Surg. 1979;64:21–9.
18. Heckenlively JR, Silver J. Management and treatment of retinitis pigmentosa. In: Heckenlively JR, editor. Retinitis pigmentosa. London: J.B. Lippincott; 1988. p. 90–106.
19. Humayun MS, Weiland JD, De Juan Jr E. Artificial vision. In: Peyman GA, Meffer SA, Conway MD, et al., editors. Viteroretinal surgical techniques. London: Martin Dunitz; 2001, p. 579–82.
20. Goldsmith HS, Chen WF, Palena PV. Intact omentum for ocular vascularization. Invest Opthalmol. 1975;14:163–5.
21. Agarwal VK, Hardia PS. Pedicle omental transplant. In: Catlin RB, editor. Retinal degeneration: causes, diagnosis and treatment. Nova Science; 2009. 978-1-60741-007-2.
22. Sen PK, et al. Transmyocardial acupuncture: a new approach to myocardial revascularization. J Thorac Cardiovas Surg. 1965;50:181–9.
23. Agarwal VK. Myocardial revascularization by pedicled omentopexy and transmyocardial acupuncture an experimental study in dogs. Saudi Heart J. 1996;7(1):49–54.
24. McLacblin AD, Olsson IS, Pill DF. Anterior anastomosis of the rectosigmoid colon: an experimental study. Surgery. 1976;800:306.
25. Kiricuta I, Goldstein AMB. The repair of extensive vesico-vaginal fistula with pedicled omentum: review of 27 cases. J Urol. 1972;104:724.
26. Tiptaft RC, Costello AJ, Paris AMI. The long term follow up of retroperitoneal fibrosis. Br J Urol. 1982;54:630.
27. Turner-Warwick R. Complex traumatic posterior urethral strictures. J Urol. 1977;118:564.

Hyperbaric Oxygen Therapy for Critical Limb Ischemia

Raymond C. Shields

The earliest known use of a pressurized container or chamber for therapeutic purposes dates back to 1662, by a British clergyman, Henshaw. More than 250 years later, the application of oxygen, in a mixed gas, under pressure was found to improve and speed recovery from decompression illness, a sudden damaging release of inert gases into tissues, notably by Alfred R. Behnke, US Navy physician scientist, and Louis A. Shaw, a physiologist in the 1930s. This experience with decompression illness led to additional applications. Modern clinical and scientific use of hyperbaric oxygen started in 1955 as an adjunct to cardiac surgery. Dutch cardiac surgeon, Ite Boerema, found that ischemic time was significantly increased while operating in a hyperbaric oxygen chamber adapted operating room [1]. This approach was later supplanted by the development of extracorporeal circulation devices or cardiopulmonary bypass machines [2]. Since these early foundational works, hyperbaric oxygen therapy (HBO) is now an important component of comprehensive treatment of diabetic foot wounds, compromised surgical grafts, and acute ischemic conditions.

Hyperbaric oxygen therapy is defined as the administration of greater than atmospheric pressure while breathing 100 % oxygen. Under conditions of normal perfusion at rest, tissues extract 5–6 mL of oxygen per deciliter of blood. Based on Henry's law (partial pressure and concentration of gas dissolved in a liquid is determined by the partial pressure of the gas on the surface of that liquid) at sea level while breathing air, the plasma oxygen concentration is 0.3 mL/deciliter. At sea level this increases fivefold to 1.5 mL/deciliter with administration of 100 % oxygen. At 3 atmospheres of pressure, the dissolved plasma oxygen content approximates 6 mL/deciliter—allowing for sufficient oxygenation of resting tissues regardless of the oxygen-hemoglobin content [3]. An alternative way to consider this is at sea level or 1 atmosphere of pressure, on room air (i.e., 21 % oxygen), the partial pressure of oxygen is 160 mmHg. At 3 atmospheres of pressure (ATA) while breathing 100 % oxygen, the partial pressure of oxygen is up to 2280 mmHg in the alveolus. At the tissue level, such as with muscle and subcutaneous tissue, the partial pressure of oxygen at 2 atmospheres of compression while breathing 100 % oxygen approximates 300 mmHg, compared to 30 mmHg with air at sea level. Also important is the expansion of the effective diffusion radius of oxygen from arterioles to the surrounding tissues with hyperbaric oxygen, which is increased more than threefold at 3 ATA [4].

Hyperbaric oxygen is administered in a pressure-certified chamber, large enough to hold at least one patient. The level of pressure applied is 2–3 ATA with 100 % oxygen breathed comfortably for 90–120 min, depending on the indication for treatment, once or twice daily.

Critical limb ischemia (CLI) represents an end-stage complication of severe peripheral arterial disease, and it should be considered a medical emergency. It is commonly the result of severe multilevel arterial occlusive disease with associated presentation of limb pain at rest and/or a hypoxic wound or threatened tissue.

Below are important physiological considerations in reference to the potential application of HBO in the management of critical limb ischemia.

Physiologic Mechanisms

Ischemia-Reperfusion Injury

Ischemia-reperfusion (IR) injury occurs when an acute interruption of tissue perfusion of nutrients and oxygen results in tissue injury. Then the restoration of circulation creates an inflammatory and oxidative stress to the then already compromised tissue, thereby rendering it subject to further

R.C. Shields, MD (✉)
Department of Medicine, College of Medicine, Mayo Clinic, Rochester, MN, USA

Division of Cardiovascular Diseases, and Preventive, Occupational, and Aerospace Medicine, Mayo clinic, Rochester, MN, USA

© Springer International Publishing Switzerland 2017
R.S. Dieter et al. (eds.), *Critical Limb Ischemia*, DOI 10.1007/978-3-319-31991-9_43

damage. On the cellular level, the reduced provision of metabolic substrates and oxygen results in reduced adenosine triphosphate (ATP) production and ultimately cell death. Free radicals or reactive species generation in this compromised tissue leads to microvascular disruption, extracellular tissue extravasation, inflammatory mediator generation, and recruitment of neutrophils. Neutrophils then serve as an additional source of damaging reactive species [5]. Neutrophils depend on a CD-18 surface protein complex and its upregulation to adhere to the endothelium, as another component of the microcirculatory disruption with IR injury [6]. HBO not only reduces the number of neutrophils attached to venule endothelium in association with IR injury, but also the polymerization of CD-18 is inhibited in experimental models, suggesting another mechanism for the positive effects of HBO on IR injury [7, 8]. Nitric oxide (·NO) is an important regulator of neutrophil-endothelial adhesion. Reduced·NO, as it occurs with IR injury, is associated with increased expression of cell adhesion molecules, thereby increasing adherence of neutrophils [9]. HBO induces upregulation of endothelial nitric oxide synthase (eNOS) and increased NO production with resultant reduction in tissue injury due to IR injury [10].

Remarkably, hyperoxygenation without HBO during reperfusion after initial ischemic injury can lead to worse reperfusion injury. Mickel et al. found that mortality was increased in laboratory animals following global brain ischemia then reperfusion and provision of 100 % oxygen at sea level compared to controls receiving room air. This also correlated with increased reactive species-mediated lipid peroxidation [11]. Despite these findings, hyperoxygenation with HBO, postischemia, and tissue preservation is instead improved. Takahashi et al. found enhanced neurological recovery with HBO administered after complete global cerebral ischemia versus room air without HBO in a canine model. Similar findings are noted in other animal models [12–14]. Improvement with HBO occurs despite suspected production of free radicals with HBO. This is thought to be due to a protective effect, exhibited by a reduction in lipid peroxidation with HBO [15, 16].

Vasoconstriction

Vasoconstriction is an established physiologic response to hyperoxygenation, although, under HBO conditions——without degradation in tissue oxygenation [17, 18]. The vasoconstriction under HBO conditions may also counteract the reflex vasodilatation and subsequent transudation due to injury. With a reduction in arterial inflow and maintenance of venous outflow, there is thought to be a net reduction in extracellular tissue edema through a shift in transcapillary flow and perhaps cellular oxygen-dependent mechanisms. Strauss et al. found a reduction in muscle tissue necrosis

with HBO in an experimental compartment syndrome, theoretically due to a reduction in the partial edema barrier to tissue oxygenation [19]. This is an important aspect in the management of acute ischemic limb conditions with improvement in microcirculation via reduction in interstitial pressure [20, 21].

Neovascularization

Tissue hypoxia has been demonstrated in the midst of wounds, which is a stimulus for angiogenesis. Hyperbaric oxygen therapy stimulates angiogenesis by increasing the oxygen gradient and increasing wound levels of vascular endothelial growth factors (VEGF) [22, 23]. Upregulation of cytokines such as TNF-alpha, as a part in angiogenesis, was also demonstrated in an experimental wound ischemia model and in healthy humans [24, 25]. Increased endothelial progenitor cell release into circulation, via nitric oxide bone marrow mechanisms, also seems to be stimulated by HBO, thereby leading to improved ischemic wound healing and closure rates [26, 27].

Enhanced Wound-Healing Mechanisms

Local hypoxia when encountered with wounds or tissue injury contributes to poor wound healing [28]. Clearance of local infection by the immune system is an important component of wound healing. Bacterial killing by leukocytes is more effective at higher tissue oxygen levels that can be achieved with HBO. Leukocyte killing is substantially reduced at tissue oxygen levels of less than 40 mmHg [29–31]. Collagen deposition by fibroblasts in the wound bed is also influenced by local oxygen tensions [32]. Basic fibroblast growth factor (bFGF) production and fibroblast proliferation are enhanced under HBO conditions which is important in the later phases of wound healing [33].

With these physiologic considerations in mind, the utility of hyperbaric oxygen therapy in the management of certain ischemic conditions will be reviewed.

Ischemic Clinical Conditions

Acute Crush Injury

Crush injuries occupy a substantial portion of trauma center admissions. These acute traumatic injuries include damage to multiple tissues that can be complicated by tissue hypoxia, edema, reperfusion injury, and necrosis. Monies-Chass et al. noted prevention of gangrenous degeneration of acutely ischemic limbs in seven healthy subjects that maintained severely ischemic limb changes, despite standard vascular repair [21]. HBO is also suspected to be beneficial in the management of especially early clinical cases compartment syndrome [34, 35]. Garcia-Covarrubias et al. conducted a systematic literature review on the management of crush injury and found eight of nine articles of at least five patients (total of 150 patients) showed a benefit with HBO [36]. This has principally been proposed due to the edema reduction and perhaps mitigation of the self-perpetuating ischemia-edema cycle. Bouachour et al. completed a randomized controlled double-blind trial of 36 acute crush injury patients, within 24 h of initial evaluation and surgery, with half receiving HBO and the control group receiving normal air. The two groups were comparable in the level of trauma and demographics. Although the time of healing and length of hospitalization were similar between the groups, complete healing was achieved in 17/18 in the HBO group compared to 10/18 in the control group ($p<0.01$). New surgical procedures (including amputation) were necessary in 1/18 in the HBO group vs. 6/18 in the control group ($p<0.05$). For patients older than 40 years of age, in matched subgroup analysis with severe (grade III) soft-tissue injury, wound healing was achieved in seven (87.5 %) in the HBO group vs. three patients (30 %) in the control group ($p<0.05$) [37].

Zonis et al. also found HBO to be beneficial in achieving limb salvage in a case series of pediatric patients with severe extremity crush injuries that failed to improve following initial attempts at surgical revascularization [38].

Compromised Grafts and Flaps

There are considerable experimental data indicating the efficacy of HBO for ischemic grafts or flaps. Much of the rationale for HBO in these conditions is based on the prior outlined physiologic mechanisms [39–41]. There is one clinical prospective randomized trial of HBO for skin grafts that showed improved graft healing in the HBO group compared to the control group. However, the rate of failure in the control group is considered to be higher than expected in current practice, and this trial was not specifically evaluating ischemic grafts [42]. Comprehensive reviews of the application of HBO in the management of flaps and grafts have previously been conducted. The current recommendations for HBO in the management of compromised grafts are based, in part, on case series and the substantial evidence with diabetic foot wounds [21, 43–45].

Critical Limb Ischemia

Given the end-stage nature and complexity of CLI, currently available medical, surgical, and endovascular management strategies remain disappointing. Limb loss and mortality rates with the diagnosis of CLI are 25 % at 1 year [46, 47]. Even after revascularization, the amputation-free survival is reduced to 34 % at 5 years [48]. A single-center retrospective review of 112 patients who required infrainguinal bypass for limb salvage revealed that only 14 % had preferred outcomes of long-term symptom relief, maintenance of functional status, uncomplicated wound healing, and no recurrence or repeat operation [49]. Martini et al. found the mortality rate to be 23.2 % at 24 months, particularly in elderly patients, with critical limb ischemia, but a multidisciplinary approach including HBO may be beneficial when revascularization is not possible [50]. The current American Heart Association guidelines for CLI management do not include HBO as an option. The Inter-Society Consensus for the Management of Peripheral Arterial Disease (TASC II) outlines that HBO reduced the risk of major amputation in patients with diabetic wounds and may be considered for select patients with ischemic ulcers who have not responded to or are not suitable candidates for revascularization [46, 51]. However, criteria for this select group of patients were not provided. Grolman et al. found that transcutaneous oxygen measurements (TCOM) are helpful in predicting response to HBO in patients with CLI [52]. This has also been supported by the works of others utilizing a suggested algorithmic approach for the application of HBO in ischemic wound management (Fig. 43.1). In-chamber limb TCOM testing has also been important in predicting response to HBO. Fife and colleagues found that for diabetic foot wounds, that a TCOM value of <100 mmHg on 100 % oxygen at 2 ATA, only 14 % benefited from HBO compared to a TCOM of >200 mmHg; 84 % showed benefit with HBO [53]. Faglia et al. found that a cutoff of 34 mmHg on normobaric room air for diabetics with CLI was predictive of the need for further revascularization [54].

Prospective clinical trials of HBO for CLI are very limited. Alternatively, HBO is suspected to beneficial for more acute phases of limb ischemia, for example, with acute traumatic injury. The recurring theme in the reports reviewed above is the need for at least minimal arterial perfusion in order for HBO to be effective. In the acute injury state, it remains challenging to ascertain which case is best suited for HBO, even when surgical options are exhausted. In some cases it may be speculated that there is residual subclinical arterial perfusion, and the interstitial pressures, in the case of ischemia-related edema, have not yet exceeded microvascular perfusion pressures, thereby allowing an opportunity for improvement with HBO. This area needs further investigation in a prospective trial.

Currently, there are no specific recommended treatment guidelines for HBO in treating CLI, and it may not be reimbursed by insurance or Medicare health-care coverage in the USA. Typically 2–2.4 ATA pressure on 100 % oxygen for 90 min for 10–20 sessions conducted once or twice a day would be considered.

Hyperbaric Ischemic Wound TcPO₂ Algorithm

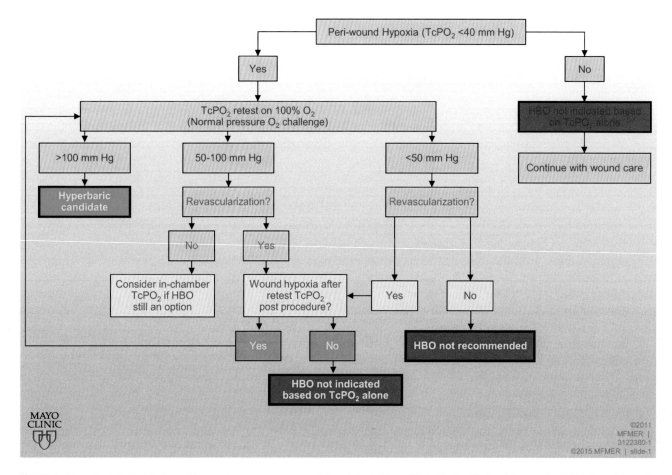

Fig. 43.1 Hyperbaric ischemic wound transcutaneous oxygen algorithm. Adapted from Dick Clarke, National Baromedical Services, Inc., with permission

The multilevel arterial occlusive disease that is often found with CLI likely limits the application of HBO for this condition. However, HBO is potentially beneficial in limiting the level of amputation and supporting the amputated site [55, 56].

Diabetes mellitus is an independent and potent risk factor for peripheral arterial disease (PAD) [57]. Diabetics tend to have more tibial vessel atherosclerotic disease involvement and are at an increased risk for limb amputation and death compared to nondiabetics with PAD [58, 59]. In addition, diabetics with PAD are more likely to present with ischemic wounds and gangrene than nondiabetics [60]. Faglia et al. found that adjunctive HBO (average of 38 ± 8 daily 90 min sessions) resulted in significantly reduced major amputations of predominately Wagner-IV diabetic and presumed ischemic wounds in the treated vs. nontreated group [55].

Although a significant reduction in major amputation rates in the diabetic foot wound patient is attributed to dedicated multidisciplinary medical teams and adjunctive hyperbaric oxygen therapy, these results have not been shown specifically in diabetics with critical limb ischemia [61].

Future Directions

CLI remains a challenging area for the clinician with limited confirmed modalities for preservation of patient's limbs and functionality. Future opportunities to improve outcomes in these patients are likely to include cell-based angiogenesis. HBO stimulates endothelial progenitor cell (EPC) proliferation and mobilization via ·NO-dependent mechanisms in the bone marrow and thereby increases circulating EPC.

This along with stimulation of VEGF formation, the most specific angiogenic growth factor, in ischemic wounds by HBO is an intriguing area of ongoing research [62]. Wang et al. recently reported a meta-analysis of autologous bone marrow cell therapy trials and found a suggested benefit in patients with severe arterial occlusive disease and unsuitability for revascularization. There was a significant reduction in pain, and amputation-free survival was improved in the stem-cell therapy group [63]. This approach remains preliminary and it is uncertain how applicable this is to CLI.

Conclusion

CLI is a complex end-stage peripheral arterial disease manifestation that is associated with a high risk for limb loss and death. Surgical and endovascular revascularization, when possible, are the primary means of management, but the results remain limited and disappointing. The physiological benefits of HBO, including EPC mobilization, are hoped to provide opportunity for further research and considerations for clinical trials toward improved patient management.

HBO is not a primary therapy for limb ischemia but is instead adjunctive. Addressing appropriate care needs, including proper wound management, pain management, off-loading, debridement as necessary, and maintenance of reasonable arterial perfusion, seems collectively important in the management of limb ischemia and its potential complications [64]. HBO is thought to be cost-effective compared to limb amputation for patients with diabetic foot ulcers. Certainly this technology needs to be appropriately applied to render the best patient outcomes [65, 66]. Serious complications, such as oxygen toxicity, pulmonary edema, and decompression injury, associated with HBO are fortunately rare with appropriate screening in a certified facility with trained staff. More common side effects such as claustrophobia and middle-ear barotrauma are generally manageable if not averted with attentive care.

There is supportive data for the application of HBO in other ischemic conditions such as acute crush injury and compromised grafts/flaps. Further investigations are necessary to better define the role and application of HBO, as well as the efficacy in the management of CLI. In the interim, much is being learned about the mechanisms of hyperoxia in the preservation of tissues threatened by ischemia.

References

1. Boerema I, Meyne NG, Brummelkamp WH, Bouma S, Mensch MH, Kamermans F, et al. Life without blood. Ned Tijdschr Geneeskd. 1960;104:949–54.
2. Haux GFK. History of hyperbaric chambers. Flagstaff: Best Publishing Company; 2000.
3. Tibbles PM, Edelsberg JS. Hyperbaric-oxygen therapy. N Engl J Med. 1996;334(25):1642–8.
4. Saltzman HA. Rational normobaric and hyperbaric oxygen therapy. Ann Intern Med. 1967;67(4):843.
5. Carden DL, Granger DN. Pathophysiology of ischaemia-reperfusion injury. J Pathol. 2000;190(3):255–66.
6. Jones SR, Carpin KM, Woodward SM, Khiabani KT, Stephenson LL, Wang WZ, et al. Hyperbaric oxygen inhibits ischemia-reperfusion-induced neutrophil CD18 polarization by a nitric oxide mechanism. Plast Reconstr Surg. 2010;126(2):403–11.
7. Zamboni WA, Roth AC, Russell RC, Graham B, Suchy H, Kucan JO. Morphologic analysis of the microcirculation during reperfusion of ischemic skeletal muscle and the effect of hyperbaric oxygen. Plast Reconstr Surg. 1993;91(6):1110–23.
8. Khiabani KT, Bellister SA, Skaggs SS, Stephenson LL, Nataraj C, Wang WZ, et al. Reperfusion-induced neutrophil CD18 polarization: effect of hyperbaric oxygen. J Surg Res. 2008;150(1):11–6.
9. Lefer AM, Lefer DJ. The role of nitric oxide and cell adhesion molecules on the microcirculation in ischaemia-reperfusion. Cardiovasc Res. 1996;32(4):743–51.
10. Buras JA, Stahl GL, Svoboda KKH, Reenstra WR. Hyperbaric oxygen downregulates ICAM-1 expression induced by hypoxia and hypoglycemia: the role of NOS. Am J Physiol Cell Physiol. 2000;278(2):C292–302.
11. Mickel HS, Vaishnav YN, Kempski O, von Lubitz D, Weiss JF, Feuerstein G. Breathing 100% oxygen after global brain ischemia in Mongolian Gerbils results in increased lipid peroxidation and increased mortality. Stroke. 1987;18(2):426–30.
12. Mink RB, Dutka AJ. Hyperbaric oxygen after global cerebral ischemia in rabbits reduces brain vascular permeability and blood flow. Stroke. 1995;26(12):2307–12.
13. Reitan JA, Kien ND, Thorup S, Corkill G. Hyperbaric oxygen increases survival following carotid ligation in gerbils. Stroke. 1990;21(1):119–23.
14. Takahashi M, Iwatsuki N, Ono K, Tajima T, Akama M, Koga Y. Hyperbaric oxygen therapy accelerates neurologic recovery after 15-minute complete global cerebral ischemia in dogs. Crit Care Med. 1992;20(11):1588–94.
15. Thom SR. Antagonism of carbon monoxide-mediated brain lipid peroxidation by hyperbaric oxygen. Toxicol Appl Pharmacol. 1990;105(2):340–4.
16. Chen Q, Banick PD, Thom SR. Functional inhibition of rat polymorphonuclear leukocyte B2 integrins by hyperbaric oxygen is associated with impaired cGMP synthesis. J Pharmacol Exp Ther. 1996;276(3):929–33.
17. Demchenko IT, Zhilyaev SY, Moskvin AN, Krivchenko AI, Piantadosi CA, Allen BW. Baroreflex-mediated cardiovascular responses to hyperbaric oxygen. J Appl Physiol. 2013;115(6):819–28.
18. Weaver LK, Howe S, Snow GL, Deru K. Arterial and pulmonary arterial hemodynamics and oxygen delivery/extraction in normal humans exposed to hyperbaric air and oxygen. J Appl Physiol. 2009;107(1):336–45.
19. Strauss MB, Hargens AR, Gershuni DH, Greenberg DA, Crenshaw AG, Hart GB, et al. Reduction of skeletal muscle necrosis using intermittent hyperbaric oxygen in a model compartment syndrome. J Bone Joint Surg Am. 1983;65(5):656–62.
20. Nylander G, Lewis D, Nordstrom H, Larsson J. Reduction of postischemic edema with hyperbaric oxygen. Plast Reconstr Surg. 1985;76(4):596–603.
21. Monies-Chass I, Hashmonai M, Hoere D, Kaufman T, Steiner E, Schramek A. Hyperbaric oxygen treatment as an adjuvant to reconstructive vascular surgery in trauma. Injury. 1977;8(4):274–7.
22. Sheikh AY, Gibson JJ, Rollins MD, Hopf HW, Hussain Z, Hunt TK. Effect of hyperoxia on vascular endothelial growth factor levels in a wound model. Arch Surg. 2000;135(11):1293–7.

23. Hopf HW, Gibson JJ, Angeles AP, Constant JS, Feng JJ, Rollins MD, et al. Hyperoxia and angiogenesis. Wound Repair Regen. 2005;13(6):558–64.

24. Sander AL, Henrich D, Muth CM, Marzi I, Barker JH, Frank JM. In vivo effect of hyperbaric oxygen on wound angiogenesis and epithelialization. Wound Repair Regen. 2009;17(2):179–84.

25. Fildissis G, Venetsanou K, Myrianthefs P, Karatzas S, Zidianakis V, Baltopoulos G. Whole blood pro-inflammatory cytokines and adhesion molecules post-lipopolysaccharides exposure in hyperbaric conditions. Eur Cytokine Netw. 2004;15(3):217–21.

26. Goldstein LJ, Gallagher KA, Bauer SM, Bauer RJ, Baireddy V, Liu Z-J, et al. Endothelial progenitor cell release into circulation is triggered by hyperoxia-induced increases in bone marrow nitric oxide. Stem Cells. 2006;24(10):2309–18.

27. Kivisaari J, Niinikoski J. Effects of hyperbaric oxygenation and prolonged hypoxia on the healing of open wounds. Acta Chir Scand. 1975;141(1):14–9.

28. Wutschert R, Bounameaux H. Determination of amputation level in ischemic limbs. Reappraisal of the measurement of TcPo2. Diabetes Care. 1997;20(8):1315–8.

29. Smith BM, Desvigne LD, Slade JB, Dooley JW, Warren DC. Transcutaneous oxygen measurements predict healing of leg wounds with hyperbaric therapy. Wound Repair Regen. 1996; 4(2):224–9.

30. Rollins MD, Gibson JJ, Hunt TK, Hopf HW. Wound oxygen levels during hyperbaric oxygen treatment in healing wounds. Undersea Hyperb Med. 2006;33(1):17–25.

31. Hohn DC, MacKay RD, Halliday B, Hunt TK. Effect of O2 tension on microbicidal function of leukocytes in wounds and in vitro. Surg Forum. 1976;27(62):18–20.

32. Jonsson K, Jensen JA, Goodson 3rd WH, Scheuenstuhl H, West J, Hopf HW, et al. Tissue oxygenation, anemia, and perfusion in relation to wound healing in surgical patients. Ann Surg. 1991;214(5):605–13.

33. Kang TS, Gorti GK, Quan SY, Ho M, Koch RJ. Effect of hyperbaric oxygen on the growth factor profile of fibroblasts. Arch Facial Plast Surg. 2004;6(1):31–5.

34. Strauss MB, Hart GB. Hyperbaric oxygen and the skeletal muscle-compartment syndrome. Contemp Orthop. 1989;18:167–74.

35. Strauss MB. The effect of hyperbaric oxygen in crush injuries and skeletal muscle-compartment syndromes. Undersea Hyperb Med. 2012;39(4):847–55.

36. Garcia-Covarrubias L, McSwain Jr NE, Van Meter K, Bell RM. Adjuvant hyperbaric oxygen therapy in the management of crush injury and traumatic ischemia: an evidence-based approach. Am Surg. 2005;71(2):144–51.

37. Bouachour G, Cronier P, Gouello JP, Toulemonde JL, Talha A, Alquier P. Hyperbaric oxygen therapy in the management of crush injuries: a randomized double-blind placebo-controlled clinical trial. J Trauma. 1996;41(2):333–9.

38. Zonis Z, Weisz G, Ramon Y, Bar Joseph G, Torem S, Melamed Y, et al. Salvage of the severely injured limb in children: a multidisciplinary approach. Pediatr Emerg Care. 1995;11(3):176–8.

39. Stevens DM, Koller WA, Weiss DD, Bianchi DA. Survival of normothermic microvascular flaps after prolonged secondary ischemia: effects of hyperbaric oxygen. Otolaryngol Head Neck Surg. 1996;115(4):360–4;115.

40. Kaelin CMIM, Myers RA, Manson PN, Hoopes JE. The effects of hyperbaric oxygen on free flaps in rats. Arch Surg. 1990;125(5): 607–9.

41. Hong JP, Kwon H, Chung YK, Jung SH. The effect of hyperbaric oxygen on ischemia-reperfusion injury: an experimental study in a rat musculocutaneous flap. Ann Plast Surg. 2003;51(5):478–87.

42. Perrins DJD. Influence of hyperbaric oxygen on the survival of split skin grafts. Lancet. 1967;1:868–71.

43. Thom S. Hyperbaric oxygen—its mechanisms and efficacy. Plast Reconstr Surg. 2011;127 Suppl 1:131S–41S.

44. Friedman HI, Fitzmaurice M, Lefaivre JF, Vecchiolla T, Clarke D. An evidence-based appraisal of the use of hyperbaric oxygen on flaps and grafts. Plast Reconstr Surg. 2006;117(7 Suppl): 175S–90S.

45. Baynosa RC, Zamboni WA. The effect of hyperbaric oxygen on compromised grafts and flaps. Undersea Hyperb Med. 2012; 39(4):857–65.

46. Norgren L, Hiatt WR, Dormandy JA, Nehler MR, Harris KA, Fowkes FG. Inter-Society Consensus for the Management of Peripheral Arterial Disease (TASC II). J Vasc Surg. 2007;45(Suppl S):S5–67.

47. Varu VN, Hogg ME, Kibbe MR. Critical limb ischemia. J Vasc Surg. 2010;51(1):230–41.

48. Adam DJ, Beard JD, Cleveland T, Bell J, Bradbury AW, Forbes JF, et al. Bypass versus angioplasty in severe ischaemia of the leg (BASIL): multicentre, randomised controlled trial. Lancet. 2005;366(9501):1925–34.

49. Nicoloff AD, Taylor Jr LM, McLafferty RB, Moneta GL, Porter JM. Patient recovery after infrainguinal bypass grafting for limb salvage. J Vasc Surg. 1998;27(2):256–63. discussion 64-6.

50. Martini R, Andreozzi GM, Deri A, Cordova R, Zulian P, Scarpazza O, et al. Amputation rate and mortality in elderly patients with critical limb ischemia not suitable for revascularization. Aging Clin Exp Res. 2012;24(3 Suppl):24–7.

51. Rooke TW, Hirsch AT, Misra S, Sidawy AN, Beckman JA, Findeiss L, et al. Management of patients with peripheral artery disease (compilation of 2005 and 2011 ACCF/AHA Guideline Recommendations): a report of the American College of Cardiology Foundation/American Heart Association Task Force on Practice Guidelines. J Am Coll Cardiol. 2013;61(14):1555–70.

52. Grolman RE, Wilkerson DK, Taylor J, Allinson P, Zatina MA. Transcutaneous oxygen measurements predict a beneficial response to hyperbaric oxygen therapy in patients with nonhealing wounds and critical limb ischemia. Am Surg. 2001;67(11):1072–9. discussion 80.

53. Fife CE, Buyukcakir C, Otto GH, Sheffield PJ, Warriner RA, Love TL, et al. The predictive value of transcutaneous oxygen tension measurement in diabetic lower extremity ulcers treated with hyperbaric oxygen therapy: a retrospective analysis of 1144 patients. Wound Repair Regen. 2002;10(4):198–207.

54. Faglia E, Clerici G, Caminiti M, Quarantiello A, Curci V, Morabito A. Predictive values of transcutaneous oxygen tension for above-the-ankle amputation in diabetic patients with critical limb ischemia. Eur J Vasc Endovasc Surg. 2007;33(6):731–6.

55. Faglia E, Favales F, Aldeghi A, Calia P, Quarantiello A, Oriani G, et al. Adjunctive systemic hyperbaric oxygen therapy in treatment of severe prevalently ischemic diabetic foot ulcer. A randomized study. Diabetes Care. 1996;19(12):1338–43.

56. Heyboer 3rd M, Grant WD, Byrne J, Pons P, Morgan M, Iqbal B, Wojcik SM. Hyperbaric oxygen for the treatment of nonhealing arterial insufficiency ulcers. Wound Repair Regen. 2014;22(3): 351–5.

57. Pyorala K, Laakso M, Uusitupa M. Diabetes and atherosclerosis: an epidemiologic view. Diabetes Metab Rev. 1987;3(2):463–524.

58. Haltmayer M, Mueller T, Horvath W, Luft C, Poelz W, Haidinger D. Impact of atherosclerotic risk factors on the anatomical distribution of peripheral arterial disease. Int Angiol. 2001; 20:200–7.

59. Faglia E, Clerici G, Clerissi J, Gabrielli L, Losa S, Mantero M, et al. Long-term prognosis of diabetic patients with critical limb ischemia: a population-based cohort study. Diabetes Care. 2009;32(5):822–7.

60. Jude EB, Eleftheriadou I, Tentolouris N. Peripheral arterial disease in diabetes—a review. Diabet Med. 2010;27(1):4–14.

61. Faglia E, Favales F, Aldeghi A, Calia P, Quarantiello A, Barbano P, et al. Change in major amputation rate in a center dedicated to diabetic foot care during the 1980s: prognostic determinants for major amputation. J Diabet Complicat. 1998;12(2):96–102.

62. Gallagher KA, Goldstein LJ, Thom SR, Velazquez OC. Hyperbaric oxygen and bone marrow-derived endothelial progenitor cells in diabetic wound healing. Vascular. 2006;14(6):328–37.

63. Wang ZX, Li D, Cao JX, Liu YS, Wang M, Zhang XY, Li JL, Wang HB, Liu JL, Xu BL. Efficacy of autologous bone marrow mononuclear cell therapy in patients with peripheral arterial disease. J Atheroscler Thromb. 2014;21(11):1183–96.

64. HW Hopf MK, D Shapshak. In: TS Neuman and SR Thom, editor. Physiology and medicine of hyperbaric oxygen therapy. Philadelphia: Saunders Elsevier; 2008. p. 203–28.

65. Cianci P, Hunt TK. Long term results of aggressive management of diabetic foot ulcers suggest significant cost effectiveness. Wound Repair Regen. 1997;5:141–6.

66. Chuck AW, Hailey D, Jacobs P, Perry DC. Cost-effectiveness and budget impact of adjunctive hyperbaric oxygen therapy for diabetic foot ulcers. Int J Technol Assess Health Care. 2008;24(2):178–83.

Gene and Cell Therapy for Critical Limb Ischemia

44

Surovi Hazarika and Brian H. Annex

Introduction

Peripheral arterial disease (PAD) is caused by atherosclerosis that results in narrowing and frequently complete occlusions of one or more arteries that supply the lower extremities. PAD affects ~8.5 million Americans at or over the age of 40 [1]. The two major clinical manifestations of PAD are intermittent claudication (IC) and critical limb ischemia (CLI). Intermittent claudication is defined by the presence of leg pain/cramping with walking that relieves with rest. CLI is defined as pain present at rest, with or without ischemic ulcers or gangrene, classified as Rutherford-Becker Class 4–6 or Fontaine Class III and IV. Patients with CLI are quite different than those with IC. The 1-year mortality rate in patients with CLI is approximately 25 %, and the overall amputation rate over 1 year is approximately 30 % [2]. While medical therapies to limit complications from atherosclerosis reduce general cardiovascular mortality in patients with CLI, at present there is no definitive medical therapy for CLI. Newer medications such as Praxilene (a metabolic enhancer and a 5-HT2 receptor antagonist) and Alprostadil (a prostaglandin E1 analogue) have been recently approved for use in Europe in patients with PAD to improve blood flow to the ischemic limb. However, mixed results from the clinic studies indicate that these drugs need further long-term evaluation to establish their role in PAD.

The primary clinical goal of treatment in critical limb ischemia is to relieve ischemic pain, promote wound healing, and reduce limb loss. Currently, these are commonly achieved with endovascular and/or surgical revascularization. However, many patients with CLI are not suitable candidates for revascularization based on their vessel anatomy, or the procedure is often unsuccessful due to graft failure and/or stent thrombosis or restenosis. Currently, there is no specific medical treatment directed at improving blood flow distal to vessel occlusion in CLI. To address this relative lack of specific medical therapy, current investigational approaches involve promotion of therapeutic angiogenesis in the limb distal to the occlusion site. Angiogenesis is the growth and proliferation of blood vessels from an existing vascular structure, with the potential to enhance tissue perfusion distal to a vessel occlusion. This chapter summarizes key approaches to therapeutic angiogenesis and clinical studies using genetic and cellular approaches to promote angiogenesis in CLI.

Angiogenesis

In the setting of an occlusion(s) in the artery(ies) that provides blood flow to the leg, perfusion becomes dependent on the growth of new blood vessels or neovascularization which is a physiological process that occurs as an adaptation to ischemia. The process of neovascularization can involve some or all of the processes of angiogenesis, arteriogenesis, and vasculogenesis [3–5].

Angiogenesis is the process of formation of new capillaries (vessels 8–12 μm in diameter) from preexisting blood vessels induced by the proliferation, differentiation, and migration of endothelial cells in response to stimuli such as hypoxia, ischemia, mechanical stretch, and inflammation. This process is regulated by a complex interaction of pro- and antiangiogenic growth factors, local tissue environment, and genetic factors (Fig. 44.1). Harnessing this physiological process using pharmacological and/or genetic modulation to enhance formation of new blood vessels distal to an arterial occlusion is known as therapeutic angiogenesis.

S. Hazarika, MBBS, PhD • B.H. Annex, MD (✉)
Division of Cardiovascular Medicine, University of Virginia, 1215 Lane Rd, Hospital Extension Building 4th floor, Charlottesville, VA 22908, USA

© Springer International Publishing Switzerland 2017
R.S. Dieter et al. (eds.), *Critical Limb Ischemia*, DOI 10.1007/978-3-319-31991-9_44

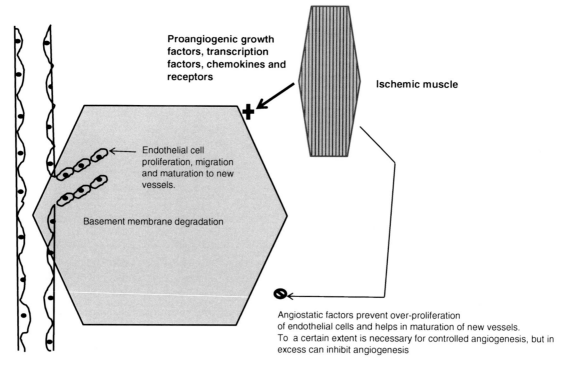

Fig. 44.1 Overview of angiogenesis. Signals from ischemic muscle result in release of pro-angiogenic transcription factors, growth factors, chemokines, and their receptors. These cumulatively results in basement membrane degradation, endothelial cell proliferation, migration, and maturation into new vessels, resulting in the process of angiogene-sis. This process is under complex regulation by simultaneous effects of angiostatic factors, which prevent uncontrolled endothelial cell prolif-eration and help in the formation of more mature and functional vessels. However, impairing this balance in favor of more angiostatic factors results in impaired angiogenesis

Angiogenesis and Peripheral Arterial Disease

In PAD, tissue ischemia should lead to activation of hypoxia-inducible factor 1-alpha, a transcription factor that leads to downstream transcription of several pro-angiogenic growth factors and growth factor receptors, which cumulatively work to initiate endothelial cell sprouting, differentiation, and pro-liferation, thereby initiating the process of angiogenesis. Ischemia-induced angiogenesis can enhance tissue perfusion by providing a larger capillary surface area for blood flow in the microcirculation and thereby enhanced O2 delivery and also by reducing the peripheral resistance to blood flow.

It is highly likely that functional performance in patients with PAD is related to the amount of blood flow to leg mus-cle with exercise. Though measures such as the ankle-brachial blood pressure index (ABI) have not been able to predict functional capacity in PAD, we showed that in human subjects with PAD (intermittent claudication), lower capillary density in the ischemic tissue (calf muscle) corre-lates with worse functional performance [6]. Supervised exercise training has been shown to be the most effective treatment for patients with intermittent claudication to

improve functional capacity and peak walking time. In patients with PAD who undergo supervised exercise train-ing, angiogenesis in the ischemic calf muscles precedes changes in functional capacity. In addition, improvement in functional capacity was noted without an appreciable increase in blood flow [7], indicating a role of microcircula-tion in enhancing muscle performance independent of mac-rovascular measurable blood flow.

Approaches to Therapeutic Angiogenesis

The primary objective for therapeutic angiogenesis is to cre-ate a "pro-angiogenic" microenvironment in the ischemic tissue. Several different approaches have been under investi-gation to achieve this pro-angiogenic milieu. These involve direct injection of growth factors into ischemic tissue, gene therapy to promote pro-angiogenic growth factors in isch-emic tissue, and stem/progenitor cell therapy to promote angiogenesis in the ischemic tissue.

Earlier studies investigated effects of direct injection of recombinant growth factors to ischemic tissue. However, direct protein therapy has significant limitations due to dif-ficulty in routes of delivery, limited uptake by muscle cells, and short half -life of proteins. As such, gene therapy and cell therapy now are currently the focus of investigations in therapeutic angiogenesis.

Gene Therapy

Gene therapy involves insertion of genetic material to target cells or tissues to achieve sustained expression of the therapeutic protein of interest, with the aim to correct dysfunctional cellular processes underlying a disease. The origin of gene therapy dates back to 1960s, when the first evidence for

uptake and expression of exogenous DNA in mammalian cells was obtained [8]. The advantages of gene therapy over protein delivery include prolonged and more controlled expression of the transgene products compared to transient expression and rapid degradation of proteins.

Modes of Delivery for Gene Therapy

Current techniques in delivering the gene of interest to cells/tissues include utilizing viral and nonviral vectors (Fig. 44.2). Viruses have the inherent capability to infect host cells and

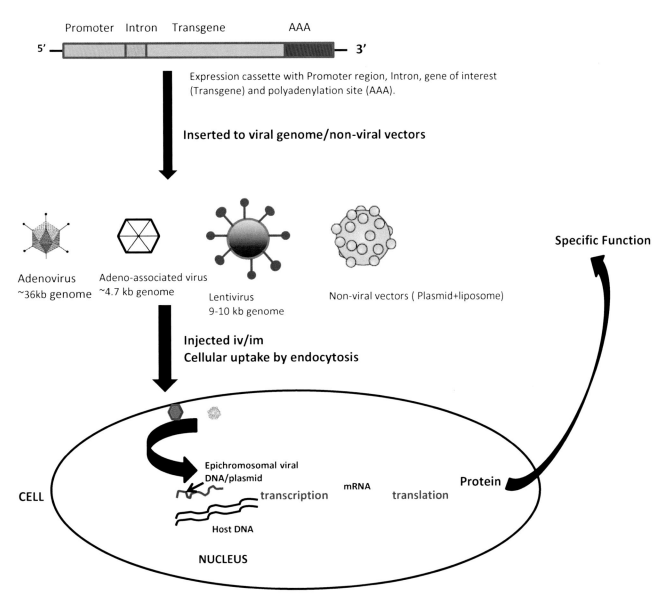

Fig. 44.2 Overview of gene therapy. Therapeutic transgene of interest is packaged into an expression cassette consisting of a promoter at the 5′ site and a polyadenylated sequence at 3′ site. The expression cassette is then inserted into viral vectors or nonviral vectors plasmids (packaged with liposomes). The vectors are then injected intramuscularly or intravenously Cellular uptake occurs by endocytosis, either receptor-

mediated (viral vectors) or by liposome fusion in case of nonviral vectors. (In specific cases, alternate delivery using direct mechanical forces (electroporation) can cause direct cellular incorporation of plasmids.) The epichromosomal viral/plasmid DNA then undergoes transcription followed by translation, ultimately resulting in expression of the transgene protein, with resultant intended function of the protein

insert their genetic material. This property of viruses is utilized to achieve high transfection efficiency to deliver a target gene. The genetic material to be transferred is packaged into viral vectors with defective replication, but preserved ability to incorporate its genome into the host genome. This enables insertion of the transgene into cells without the vector virus replicating and infecting the host. The most common viral vectors used for gene therapy are different viral and nonviral gene delivery system including naked or plasmid DNA, which is inserted into cells using physical or chemical forces. Physical forces include electroporation, microinjection, particle bombardment, ultrasound bubbles, and hydrodynamic delivery. Chemical techniques include use of lipids or polymers capable of binding DNA and facilitating its transfer across the plasma membrane. Nonviral vectors have the advantage of low immunogenicity and therefore more flexibility for repeat dosing, but usually have low efficiencies and can lead to cellular toxicity. Viral vectors have the advantage of high transfection efficiency, but have high immunogenicity and have potential for insertion mutagenesis. *Lentivirus* (retrovirus that can infect both dividing and nondividing cells and can enter cells through intact cell membrane by membrane fusion) have the ability to provide high levels of gene expression. Adeno-associated viruses (AAV) are emerging as perhaps the most promising vector for gene therapy. AAV serotype 9 is well known to have selectivity for skeletal muscle, and we recently described the potential for even greater selectivity to ischemic skeletal muscle [9].

Gene Therapy in Critical Limb Ischemia

The primary goal of gene therapy in CLI is to promote therapeutic angiogenesis. Table 44.1 summarizes the different growth factors, transcription factors, and chemokines which have been tested till date to promote angiogenesis, in both clinical and preclinical settings. The most common pro-angiogenic growth factors or growth factor enhancers investigated in clinical trials include vascular endothelial growth factor (VEGF), fibroblast growth factor (FGF), hepatocyte growth factor (HGF), and HIF-1 alpha. Table 44.2 summarizes the key clinical trials of pro-angiogenic growth factors in patients with critical limb ischemia.

Table 44.1 Factors with angiogenic potential

Growth factors	VEGF A–E, PLGF, FGF-1, 2, 3, 5, angiopoietin-1 and 2, HGF, PDGF, GM-CSF, neurotrophin, IGF-1 and 2
Chemokines	MCP-1
Transcription factors	HIF-α, EGR-1, Prox-1

VEGF vascular endothelial growth factor, *PLGF* placenta growth factor, *FGF* fibroblast growth factor, *HGF* hepatocyte growth factor, *PDGF* placenta-derived growth factor, *GM-CSF* granulocyte-macrophage colony-stimulating factor, *IGF* insulin-like growth factor, *MCP* monocyte chemoattractant protein, *HIF* hypoxia-inducible factor, *EGR* early growth response protein, *Prox* prospero homeobox

Table 44.2 Clinical trials of growth factors in CLI

Reference	Year	Study type	Gene	Vector	Route of delivery	Improvements in
Isner et al. [10]	1996	Phase I	VEGF	Plasmid	Intra-arterial	Collateral vessels and distal flow
Baumgartner et al. [11]	1998	Phase I	VEGF$_{165}$	Plasmid	Intramuscular	Distal flow, ulcer healing
Simovic et al. [12]	2001	Phase I	VEGF$_{165}$	Plasmid	Intramuscular	Symptom score, neurological exam, ABI, collaterals
Kim et al. [13]	2004	Phase I	VEGF$_{165}$	Plasmid	Intramuscular	Collaterals
Makinen et al. [14]	2002	Phase II	VEGF	Adenovirus	Intramuscular	Vascularity
Kusumanto et al. [15]	2006	Phase II	VEGF$_{165}$	Plasmid	Intramuscular	Ulcer healing
						Hemodynamics
Comerota et al. [16]	2001	Phase I	FGF-1	Plasmid	Intramuscular	Pain
						Ulcer healing
						ABPI
						Transcutaneous oxygen pressure
Nikol et al. [17]	2008	Phase II	FGF-1	Plasmid	Intramuscular	Risk of amputation
Belch et al. [18]	2011	Phase III	FGF-1	Plasmid	Intramuscular	No benefit
Morishita et al. [19]	2004	Phase I	HGF	Plasmid	Intramuscular	Pain, ABI, ulcer size
Powell et al. [20]	2008	Phase II	HGF	Plasmid	Intramuscular	Transcutaneous oxygen pressure
Powell et al. [21]	2010	Phase II	HGF	Plasmid	Intramuscular	Rest pain
Shigematsu et al. [22]	2010	Phase III	HGF	Plasmid	Intramuscular	Rest pain, ulcer size, QOL
Rajagopalan et al. [23]	2007	Phase I	HIF-1α	Adenovirus	Intramuscular	Rest pain, ulcer size

VEGF vascular endothelial growth factor, *FGF* fibroblast growth factor, *HGF* hepatocyte growth factor, *HIF-1α* hypoxia-inducible transcription factor-1α

Vascular Endothelial Growth Factor

The vascular endothelial growth factor family is the most well-characterized family of angiogenic growth factors, first identified in 1983 by Senger and Colleagues [24]. VEGF family consists of VEGF-A, VEGF-B, VEGF-C, VEGF-D, VEGF-E, and PLGF, which share a secretory signal sequence and binds to VEGF receptors 1, 2, and 3 with different affinities. VEGF-A has five different isoforms identified in humans, namely, VEGF-121, 145, 165,189, and 206, and VEGF 189 and 206 have extensive heparin-binding ability and are primarily matrix bound. VEGF 121 and 165 do not bind heparin and are primarily found in circulation [25, 26]. Knockout mice of all three VEGF receptors are lethal [27–30], indicating a coordinated role of signaling via all three VEGF receptors during developmental vasculogenesis. Recent reports have described that not all VEGF-A is angiogenic as indeed an antiangiogenic form has been identified in cancers and may be important in PAD [31].

Clinical Trials with VEGF Gene Therapy

Primary VEGF isoforms used in clinical trials to date has been VEGF 121 and VEGF 165, though approaches to increase all VEGF transcripts do exist. Several preclinical trials with VEGF gene therapy showed promising results in preclinical models of PAD [32–34].

Following the preclinical studies, Isner et al. did the first clinical trial using VEGF in humans in 1996 [10]. A patient was given phVEGF 165 intra-arterially to the distal popliteal artery using the hydrogel polymer coating of an angioplasty balloon. Digital subtraction angiography 4 weeks after gene therapy showed an increase in collateral vessels which persisted at 12 weeks follow-up. In addition, intra-arterial Doppler-flow studies also showed increased resting and maximum flows. In 1998, Baumgarther et al. administered phVGEF 165 by direct intramuscular injection into ischemic limbs of patients with CLI [35]. This study showed an increase in ankle-brachial index (ABI) and increased collateral vessels as evidenced by contrast angiography or MRA in the VEGF-treated patients. In a subsequent study done by Simvoic et al. [12] with phVEGF165 in patients with CLI, intramuscular injection of phVEGF165 resulted in increased ABI, reduced symptoms, and improved neurological sensory and motor functions, indicating a role of VEGF165 in chronic ischemic neuropathy. Kim et al. [13] injected plasmid DNA containing VEGF 165 gene (pCK) intramuscularly into patients with CLI and noted reduced pain, improved ulcer healing, improved ABI, and increased collaterals at 6 months follow-up.

The first phase II clinical study of VEGF 165 gene therapy was published by Makinen et al. in 2002 [14]. In a randomized, placebo-controlled, double-blinded study, patients received either ad-VEGF or VEGF-plasmid versus ringers lactate for controls. Injections were given via an intra-arterial catheter during PTA. Primary endpoint measured was vascularity, as assessed by digital subtraction angiography (DSA). DSA measured vascularity significantly increased compared to that in controls in both forms of VEGF treatment. Kusumanto and coworkers published a phase II study of VEGF gene therapy in patients with diabetes and CLI [15]. This was a double-blinded placebo-controlled study where VEGF gene carrying plasmid (phVEGF 165) or placebo (0.9 % NaCl) was administered intramuscularly to 54 diabetic patients with CLI. The primary endpoint studied was amputation rate at 100 days, and secondary endpoints were a 15 % or more increase in ABI/toe brachial index, clinical improvement, and safety. There was no improvement in the primary endpoint with VEGF therapy, but hemodynamic improvements and improvement in ulcer healing were noted.

Fibroblast Growth Factor

Fibroblast growth factors (FGF) are a family of heparin-binding angiogenic growth factors with 22 structurally related proteins [36]. Several members of the FGF family have been shown to regulate developmental and various cellular pathways. FGF signaling also plays a significant role in angiogenesis. In particular, FGF-1 and FGF-2 have been the focus of therapies for promoting angiogenesis [17, 18, 37, 38].

Clinical Trials with FGF Gene Therapy

The first phase I clinical trial using FGF gene therapy was published in 2002 by Comerota et al. in 2002 [16]. In this study, a naked plasmid vector encoding FGF-1 (NV1FGF) was administered intramuscularly to the ischemic limbs of patients with CLI. The primary objective of this study was to evaluate the safety and tolerance of increasing and repeated (two) doses of NV1FGF. The secondary objectives were to determine the biologic activity of NV1FGF on hemodynamic and clinical parameters associated with improved perfusion. At 12 months follow-up, there NV-1FGF was found to be well tolerated. A significant improvement in ABI was noted posttreatment, and significant reduction in pain and aggregate ulcer size was noted, associated with an increased transcutaneous oxygen pressure compared with baseline pretreatment values. These encouraging results lead to the first phase II clinical trial with FGF in patients with CLI [17]. In this double-blinded, randomized placebo-controlled trial, investigators injected NV1FGF or placebo intramuscularly in ischemic limbs of patients with CLI. There was no significant improvement in ulcer healing, but the use of NV1FGF significantly reduced the risk of all amputations and major amputations compared to placebo. Following this, a phase III trial, TAMARIS, was published in 2011 [18]. In this study, 525 patients unsuitable for revascularization were randomly assigned to placebo or naked DNA plasmid with gene encoding FGF-1 (NV1FGF1) delivered intramuscularly. After 1-year follow-up, there was no difference in the primary endpoint to time to major amputation or death. Peripheral edema was the most commonly noted adverse effect.

Hepatocyte Growth Factor

Hepatocyte growth factor is (HGF, also known as scatter factor) is a powerful mitogen or motility factor in different cells, acting through the tyrosine kinase receptor encoded by the MET proto-oncogene [39, 40].

Clinical Trials with HGF Therapy

The first phase I clinical study using HGF in PAD was published by Morishita et al. in 2004 [19]. This study investigated the safety and efficiency of HGF plasmid DNA in patients with CLI. HGF plasmid DNA was injected intramuscularly into the ischemic hind limbs of six patients with CLI. After 12 weeks follow-up, no significant complications or adverse effects were detected. Specifically, no edema was observed with HGF treatment as opposed to all other gene therapy trials. A reduction in analogue pain scale, increase in ankle pressure index, and reduced ulcer size were noted, warranting more clinical trials. Following this, phase II clinical studies of HGF administration in patients with CLI showed that intramuscular injection of HGF plasmid was safe and well tolerated [20, 21]. There were significant improvement in transcutaneous oxygen pressure [20] and decreased rest pain [21] compared to placebo.

Subsequently, HGF was investigated in a multicenter, randomized, double-blind placebo-controlled trial [22]. Placebo or HGF plasmid was injected to ischemic limbs of patients with CLI. After 12 weeks follow-up, there was improvement in rest pain and reduction of ulcer size in the HGF group, and HGF plasmid group also had improved quality of life. There were no major safety problems. An ongoing phase IIB pilot study is evaluating the feasibility and tolerability of HGF plasmid therapy in CLI.

HIF-1 α

Hypoxia-inducible factor 1 (HIF-1) is a heterodimeric transcription factor that plays a key role in cellular adaptation/response to ischemia or hypoxia. HIF-1 heterodimer consists of constitutively expressed subunit HIF-1β and oxygen-regulated subunit HIF-1α [41, 42]. Under normoxic conditions, HIF-1α undergoes rapid proteosomal degradation, while under hypoxic conditions, HIF-1α stabilizes, accumulates, and dimerizes with HIF-1β [43]. This heterodimer then translocates to the nucleus and binds to hypoxia response elements (HRE), which initiates transcription of several hundreds of genes that encodes proteins involved in angiogenesis, vascular remodeling, and mobilization of circulating angiogenic cells. This makes HIF-1α an attractive therapeutic target to modulate angiogenesis. However, it is pertinent to consider that HIF-1α overexpression to promote angiogenesis has the potential for success only in situations where endogenous activation is submaximal.

Clinical Trials with HIF-1α Therapy

A phase I trial using a constitutively active form of HIF-1α was published in 2007 by Rajagopalan et al. [23]. This included two studies: a randomized, double-blinded, placebo-controlled study and an open-label extension study. In total, 34 no-option patients with critical limb ischemia received HIF-1α adenoviral particles. No serious adverse events were attributable to study treatment. At 1 year, limb status observations in HIF-1α patients included complete rest pain resolution in 14 of 32 patients and complete ulcer healing in five of 18 patients, and the therapy was well tolerated, with the most common adverse events reported being peripheral edema. Though not in CLI, HIF-1α was unable to promote therapeutic angiogenesis in patients with IC [44].

Summary of Gene Therapy for Angiogenesis

Despite promising results from preclinical studies and some small-scale phase I and phase II clinical trials, gene therapy to promote angiogenesis still remains an investigational approach in patients with CLI. Further research in this area is ongoing and will need continued efforts in identification of systems to improve gene delivery and to produce enhanced and sustained expression. In addition, incorporation of systems biology knowledge and perhaps combined delivery of mixed growth factors and/or delivery of growth factors with cell therapy need to be considered as opposed to single gene therapy approach. In addition, the potential for gene therapy as an adjunctive therapy to surgical/endovascular therapies to promote neovascularization in areas distal to surgical/endovascular revascularization needs to be considered. Finally, gene therapy also holds the potential to be used in conjunction with surgical and endovascular therapies to limit graft failure and to limit in-stent restenosis.

Cell Therapy for Therapeutic Angiogenesis

The discovery of stem cells has opened new possibilities for treating old diseases. Although the first identified source of stem cells was embryonic tissue, clinical use of this source is complicated due to ethical issues, complications from unlimited potential of these cells to differentiate (potential for tumors), and immune reaction due to their allogenic origin. A more usable source of stem cells originates from adult tissue. Most mature adult tissue contains pluripotent cells that have the ability to differentiate into different adult cell types based on the microenvironmental cues. In addition, adult tissue also contains committed stem cells or progenitor cells, which can be activated by environmental stimuli to differentiate into specific cell populations. This concept of tissue regeneration using stem cells or progenitor cells has led to many studies investigating the role of cell therapy in critical limb ischemia.

Advantages of Cell Therapy Over Gene Therapy

The advantage of cell therapy over administration of a specific growth factor is that cell therapy can produce an array of cytokines as opposed to a single cytokine. In addition, stem cells can enhance angiogenesis by homing and differentiating into endothelial cells at sites of ischemia and/or by differentiation into supporting cells with paracrine effect on proliferation and budding of endothelial cells during angiogenesis. Cell therapy therefore has the potential to be a more efficient and durable treatment for therapeutic angiogenesis.

Modes of Cell Therapy

Currently, three different modes of delivery for cell therapy are under investigation (Fig. 44.3):

1. Direct intramuscular or intra-arterial injection of bone marrow-derived mononuclear cells (BMMNCs)
2. Direct intramuscular injection of cytokine-mobilized and apheresed peripheral mononuclear cells (PBMNC)
3. Mobilization of self stem cells to sites of ischemia

Clinical Trials of Cell Therapy in Patients with CLI

Bone marrow-derived mononuclear cells or peripheral blood mononuclear cells contain a small fraction of endothelial progenitor cells (EPCs) that can incorporate into the vascular network to form new capillaries. However, a definitive way to identify these cells has not been established. At present, different surface markers are used to identify and sort these endothelial progenitor cells, although the surface markers selected are not uniform across different studies. The commonly used surface markers to identify endothelial progenitor cells include

CD 34, CD133, and KDR (VEGF-/receptor 2). In addition to EPCs, BMMNCs also has cells of monocyte/macrophage lineage that contribute to angiogenesis by secreting angiogenic cytokines and matrix metalloproteinases. Other BM-derived cells such as pericytes can contribute to angiogenesis by stabilizing new endothelial networks.

Several clinical trials have established safety, feasibility, and efficacy of intramuscular injection of bone marrow-derived stem cells into ischemic limbs in patients with critical limb ischemia (Table 44.3). Cumulatively, these studies have shown that intramuscular delivery of bone marrow-derived stem cells is clinically safe with no major adverse events and helps in improvements in rest pain, vascular quality of life questionnaire score, and limb salvage and increases ABI and transcutaneous oxygen levels.

Another approach to cell therapy is mobilization of bone marrow stem cells to the periphery using cytokine injection and harvesting mobilized mononuclear cells, which are then apheresed and concentrated. These cells are then transplanted to ischemic tissue using intramuscular or intra-arterial injections. This avoids the need for bone marrow aspiration, but may provide lesser number of cells and expose tissue to potential hazards of cytokine injections. Several clinical trials using apheresed peripheral blood mononuclear cells in patients with critical limb ischemia are summarized in Table 44.3. In summary, these studies showed improved ABI, improved wound healing, and increased formation of collaterals in response to treatment with PBMNCs.

A third method of cell therapy is mobilization of self stem cells from the bone marrow to peripheral sites of ischemia using injection of cytokines. Several studies have shown that granulocyte colony-stimulating factor given intramuscularly is a relatively safe procedure and effectively mobilizes stem cells from bone marrow to peripheral blood, which then homes in ischemic tissue in response to specific chemotactic factors expressed in severely ischemic tissue. While conceptually this method seems simpler, the lack of arterial beds in the ischemic tissue and the relative lack of blood flow may affect delivery of adequate number of cells needed for effective neovascularization. A few small clinical trials have shown that this method of cell therapy results in significant increase in ABI, rest pain, limb salvage, and healing of limb ulcers [63, 64].

Summary of Cell Therapy for Angiogenesis

While stem cell therapy in patients with critical limb ischemia has been proven to be safe, feasible, and effective in smaller clinical trials, it is yet to reach its full potential as very few randomized and/or controlled trials have been completed using cell therapy [45, 49, 54, 58–60, 62, 63, 65, 66].

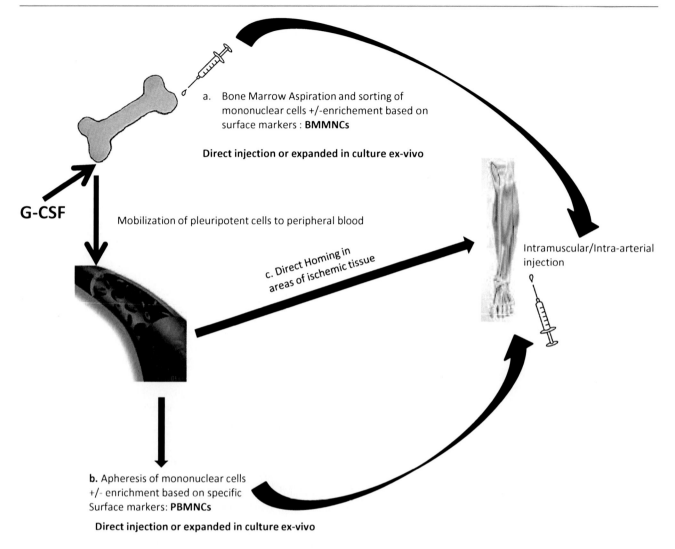

G-CSF

a. Bone Marrow Aspiration and sorting of mononuclear cells +/-enrichement based on surface markers : **BMMNCs**

Direct injection or expanded in culture ex-vivo

Mobilization of pleuripotent cells to peripheral blood

c. Direct Homing in areas of ischemic tissue

Intramuscular/Intra-arterial injection

b. Apheresis of mononuclear cells +/- enrichment based on specific Surface markers: **PBMNCs**

Direct injection or expanded in culture ex-vivo

Fig. 44.3 Methods of cell therapy: (**a**) direct aspiration from bone marrow and sorting of mononuclear cells based on specific cell surface markers—bone marrow-derived mononuclear cells (BMMNC); (**b**) treatment of bone marrow with granulocyte colony-stimulating factor (G-CSF), mobilization of cells to peripheral blood, collection of peripheral blood, and apheresis based on specific cell surface markers, periph-eral blood-derived mononuclear cells (PBMNC); and (**c**) treatment of bone marrow with granulocyte colony-stimulating factor (G-CSF), mobilization of cells to peripheral blood, direct homing of cells to isch-emic tissue based on increased adhesion molecules expressed in isch-emic tissue, and/or increased vascular permeability in ischemic tissue

In addition, the cumulative interpretation of the existing clinical trials is complicated due to multiple variables including stem cell lineage, routes of delivery, dose of delivery, and duration of follow-up. In addition, the clinical trials thus far have been done in patients with critical ischemia that are not can-didates for revascularization. It is yet to be determined if stem cell therapy at earlier stages of the disease can prevent progression to critical limb ischemia. As such, larger and randomized clinical trials with more standardized methods of stem cell selection, delivery, and in vitro tracking are needed to establish cell therapy as a standard therapy for vascular regeneration.

Table 44.3 Clinical trials of cell therapy in CLI

Reference	Disease	Source of cells/cell preparation	Route of administration/average no. of cells	Results
Tateishi-Yuyama et al. [45]	CLI	BMMNC: no further fractionation	Intramuscular/3.7×10^{10}	Improved ABI and TcO2
				Increased pain-free walking time
				Increased collateral by angiography
Nizankowski et al. [46]	CLI	BMMNC: cell enriched for CD34 and AC 133 +ve cells	Intramuscular	Increased laser Doppler flux
				Increased ABI and TcO2
				Improved ischemic ulcers
				Improved symptoms
Kajiguchi et al. [47]	CLI	BMMNC/PBMNC(1): no further fractionation	Intramuscular/$4 \times 110^{6} – 7 \times 10^{7}$	No change in ABI
				Increased TcO2
				Improved subjective symptoms
Saigawa et al. [48]	CLI	BMMNC: no further fractionation	Intramuscular/6×10^{7}/kg	Increased ABI and TcO2
				Increased vessel formation by digital angiography
Huang et al. [49]	CLI	PBMNC; G-CSF stimulation and apheresis on day 5	Intramuscular/3×10^{9}	Increased laser Doppler flux, increased ABI, increased collaterals by angiography, improved ulcer healing
Kawamura et al. [50]	CLI	PBMNC; G-CSF stimulation and apheresis	Intramuscular/1.9×10^{8}	Improved subjective symptoms, improved thermography, improvement in 3D-CT
Isida et al. [51]	CLI	PBMNC; G-CSF stimulation and apheresis	Intramuscular/3.9×10^{10}	Improved ulcer healing, increased ABI, increased TCO2, enhanced acetylcholine mediated dilatation, no change in nitroprusside-mediated dilatation
Lenk et al. [52]	CLI	PBMNC: circulating progenitor cells, G-CSF stimulation, and MNC cultured	Intra-arterial/3.9×10^{7}	Increased peak walking time, increased ABI, TcO2, increased adenosine dilatation, increased acetylcholine dilatation
Miyamoto et al. [53]	CLI	BMMNC and EPCs	Intramuscular/3.5×10^{9}	Improved ABI, pain-free walking time
Powell et al. [54]	CLI	BMMNC: enriched for CD90 +ve and CD45 +ve cells	Intramuscular/$136 \pm 41 \times 10^{6}$	Improved wound healing
Benoit et al. [55]	CLI	BMMNC, no further fractionation	Intramuscular	Reduced amputation rate
Lu et al. [56]	CLI	BMMSC cultured and expanded (based on CD29, 71, 90, 105, 34, and 45 +ve cells) and BMMNC	Intramuscular	Improved ulcer healing, increased pain-free walking time, improved TCO2
Powell et al. [57]	CLI	BMMNC: cultured and expanded, enriched for CD90+ and CD 14+ cells	Intramuscular/$35–295 \times 10^{6}$	Decreased major amputation, improved would healing
Idei et al. [58]	CLI	BMMNC: no further fractionation	Intramuscular/1.8×10^{9}	Decreased major amputation
Iafrati et al. [59]	CLI	BM-aspirate concentrate	Intramuscular	Decreased major amputation, improved rest pain
Walter et al. [60]	CLI	BMMNC: enriched for CD34+, CD45+, and CD133+ cells	Intra-arterial	Decreased ulcer healing
Murphy et al. [61]	CLI	BMMNC: enriched for CD34+, CD133+, and KDR +ve cells	Intramuscular $1.3–2 \times 10^{9}$	Increased perfusion index by PET-CT, improved rest pain, increased first toe pressure
Losordo et al. [62]	CLI	PBMNC; GCS-F stimulation and mobilization of BM cells, apheresis, and enriched for CD 34+ cells	Intramuscular/1×10^{5} cells/kg (low dose) 1×10^{5} cells/kg (high dose)	Favorable trend toward reduced amputation

BMMNC bone marrow-derived mononuclear cells, *PBMNC* peripheral blood-derived mononuclear cells, *BMMSC* bone marrow-derived mesenchymal stem cells

References

1. Go AS, et al. Heart disease and stroke statistics—2014 update: a report from the American Heart Association. Circulation. 2014;129(3):e28–292.
2. Norgren L, et al. Inter-Society Consensus for the Management of Peripheral Arterial Disease (TASC II). J Vasc Surg. 2007;45 Suppl S:S5–67.
3. Annex BH. Therapeutic angiogenesis for critical limb ischaemia. Nat Rev Cardiol. 2013;10(7):387–96.
4. Carmeliet P. Angiogenesis in life, disease and medicine. Nature. 2005;438(7070):932–6.
5. Ferrara N, Kerbel RS. Angiogenesis as a therapeutic target. Nature. 2005;438(7070):967–74.
6. Robbins JL, et al. Relationship between leg muscle capillary density and peak hyperemic blood flow with endurance capacity in peripheral artery disease. J Appl Physiol. 1985;111(1):81–6.
7. Duscha BD, et al. Angiogenesis in skeletal muscle precede improvements in peak oxygen uptake in peripheral artery disease patients. Arterioscler Thromb Vasc Biol. 2011;31(11):2742–8.
8. Strohman RC. Gene therapy. Nature. 1992;355(6362):667.
9. Katwal AB, et al. Adeno-associated virus serotype 9 efficiently targets ischemic skeletal muscle following systemic delivery. Gene Ther. 2013;20(9):930–8.
10. Isner JM, et al. Clinical evidence of angiogenesis after arterial gene transfer of phVEGF165 in patient with ischaemic limb. Lancet. 1996;348(9024):370–4.
11. Baumgartner I, et al. Constitutive expression of phVEGF165 after intramuscular gene transfer promotes collateral vessel development in patients with critical limb ischemia. Circulation. 1998;97(12):1114–23.
12. Simovic D, et al. Improvement in chronic ischemic neuropathy after intramuscular phVEGF165 gene transfer in patients with critical limb ischemia. Arch Neurol. 2001;58(5):761–8.
13. Kim HJ, et al. Vascular endothelial growth factor-induced angiogenic gene therapy in patients with peripheral artery disease. Exp Mol Med. 2004;36(4):336–44.
14. Makinen K, et al. Increased vascularity detected by digital subtraction angiography after VEGF gene transfer to human lower limb artery: a randomized, placebo-controlled, double-blinded phase II study. Mol Ther. 2002;6(1):127–33.
15. Kusumanto YH, et al. Treatment with intramuscular vascular endothelial growth factor gene compared with placebo for patients with diabetes mellitus and critical limb ischemia: a double-blind randomized trial. Hum Gene Ther. 2006;17(6):683–91.
16. Comerota AJ, et al. Naked plasmid DNA encoding fibroblast growth factor type 1 for the treatment of end-stage unreconstructible lower extremity ischemia: preliminary results of a phase I trial. J Vasc Surg. 2002;35(5):930–6.
17. Nikol S, et al. Therapeutic angiogenesis with intramuscular NV1FGF improves amputation-free survival in patients with critical limb ischemia. Mol Ther. 2008;16(5):972–8.
18. Belch J, et al. Effect of fibroblast growth factor NV1FGF on amputation and death: a randomised placebo-controlled trial of gene therapy in critical limb ischaemia. Lancet. 2011;377(9781):1929–37.
19. Morishita R, et al. Safety evaluation of clinical gene therapy using hepatocyte growth factor to treat peripheral arterial disease. Hypertension. 2004;44(2):203–9.
20. Powell RJ, et al. Results of a double-blind, placebo-controlled study to assess the safety of intramuscular injection of hepatocyte growth factor plasmid to improve limb perfusion in patients with critical limb ischemia. Circulation. 2008;118(1):58–65.
21. Powell RJ, et al. Safety and efficacy of patient specific intramuscular injection of HGF plasmid gene therapy on limb perfusion and wound healing in patients with ischemic lower extremity ulceration: results of the HGF-0205 trial. J Vasc Surg. 2010;52(6):1525–30.
22. Shigematsu H, et al. Randomized, double-blind, placebo-controlled clinical trial of hepatocyte growth factor plasmid for critical limb ischemia. Gene Ther. 2010;17(9):1152–61.
23. Rajagopalan S, et al. Use of a constitutively active hypoxia-inducible factor-1 alpha transgene as a therapeutic strategy in no-option critical limb ischemia patients: phase I dose-escalation experience. Circulation. 2007;115(10):1234–43.
24. Senger DR, et al. Tumor cells secrete a vascular permeability factor that promotes accumulation of ascites fluid. Science. 1983;219(4587):983–5.
25. Ferrara N, Davis-Smyth T. The biology of vascular endothelial growth factor. Endocr Rev. 1997;18(1):4–25.
26. Ferrara N, Keyt B. Vascular endothelial growth factor: basic biology and clinical implications. EXS. 1997;79:209–32.
27. Ferrara N, et al. Heterozygous embryonic lethality induced by targeted inactivation of the VEGF gene. Nature. 1996;380(6573):439–42.
28. Fong GH, et al. Role of the Flt-1 receptor tyrosine kinase in regulating the assembly of vascular endothelium. Nature. 1995;376(6535):66–70.
29. Shalaby F, et al. Failure of blood-island formation and vasculogenesis in Flk-1-deficient mice. Nature. 1995;376(6535):62–6.
30. Taipale J, et al. Vascular endothelial growth factor receptor-3. Curr Top Microbiol Immunol. 1999;237:85–96.
31. Dokun AO, Annex BH. The VEGF165b "ICE-o-form" puts a chill on the VEGF story. Circ Res. 2011;109(3):246–7.
32. Mohler 3rd ER, et al. Adenoviral-mediated gene transfer of vascular endothelial growth factor in critical limb ischemia: safety results from a phase I trial. Vasc Med. 2003;8(1):9–13.
33. Hopkins SP, et al. Controlled delivery of vascular endothelial growth factor promotes neovascularization and maintains limb function in a rabbit model of ischemia. J Vasc Surg. 1998;27(5):886–94. discussion 895.
34. Li Y, et al. In mice with type 2 diabetes, a vascular endothelial growth factor (VEGF)-activating transcription factor modulates VEGF signaling and induces therapeutic angiogenesis after hindlimb ischemia. Diabetes. 2007;56(3):656–65.
35. Baumgartner I, Isner JM. Stimulation of peripheral angiogenesis by vascular endothelial growth factor (VEGF). Vasa. 1998;27(4):201–6.
36. Presta M, et al. Fibroblast growth factor/fibroblast growth factor receptor system in angiogenesis. Cytokine Growth Factor Rev. 2005;16(2):159–78.
37. Nabel EG, et al. Recombinant fibroblast growth factor-1 promotes intimal hyperplasia and angiogenesis in arteries in vivo. Nature. 1993;362(6423):844–6.
38. Williams D, Davenport K, Tan Y. Angiogenesis with recombinant fibroblast growth factor-2 for claudication. Lancet. 2003;361(9353):256. author reply 256.
39. Bussolino F, et al. Hepatocyte growth factor is a potent angiogenic factor which stimulates endothelial cell motility and growth. J Cell Biol. 1992;119(3):629–41.
40. Nakamura Y, et al. Hepatocyte growth factor is a novel member of the endothelium-specific growth factors: additive stimulatory effect of hepatocyte growth factor with basic fibroblast growth factor but not with vascular endothelial growth factor. J Hypertens. 1996;14(9):1067–72.
41. Wang GL, et al. Hypoxia-inducible factor 1 is a basic-helix-loop-helix-PAS heterodimer regulated by cellular O2 tension. Proc Natl Acad Sci U S A. 1995;92(12):5510–4.
42. Wang GL, Semenza GL. Purification and characterization of hypoxia-inducible factor 1. J Biol Chem. 1995;270(3):1230–7.
43. Jaakkola P, et al. Targeting of HIF-alpha to the von Hippel-Lindau ubiquitylation complex by O2-regulated prolyl hydroxylation. Science. 2001;292(5516):468–72.

44. Creager MA, et al. Effect of hypoxia-inducible factor-1 alpha gene therapy on walking performance in patients with intermittent claudication. Circulation. 2011;124(16):1765–73.

45. Tateishi-Yuyama E, et al. Therapeutic angiogenesis for patients with limb ischaemia by autologous transplantation of bone-marrow cells: a pilot study and a randomised controlled trial. Lancet. 2002;360(9331):427–35.

46. Nizankowski R, et al. The treatment of advanced chronic lower limb ischaemia with marrow stem cell autotransplantation. Kardiol Pol. 2005;63(4):351–60. discussion 361.

47. Kajiguchi M, et al. Safety and efficacy of autologous progenitor cell transplantation for therapeutic angiogenesis in patients with critical limb ischemia. Circ J. 2007;71(2):196–201.

48. Saigawa T, et al. Clinical application of bone marrow implantation in patients with arteriosclerosis obliterans, and the association between efficacy and the number of implanted bone marrow cells. Circ J. 2004;68(12):1189–93.

49. Huang P, et al. Autologous transplantation of granulocyte colony-stimulating factor-mobilized peripheral blood mononuclear cells improves critical limb ischemia in diabetes. Diabetes Care. 2005;28(9):2155–60.

50. Kawamura A, et al. Clinical study of therapeutic angiogenesis by autologous peripheral blood stem cell (PBSC) transplantation in 92 patients with critically ischemic limbs. J Artif Organs. 2006;9(4):226–33.

51. Ishida A, et al. Autologous peripheral blood mononuclear cell implantation for patients with peripheral arterial disease improves limb ischemia. Circ J. 2005;69(10):1260–5.

52. Lenk K, et al. Therapeutical potential of blood-derived progenitor cells in patients with peripheral arterial occlusive disease and critical limb ischaemia. Eur Heart J. 2005;26(18):1903–9.

53. Miyamoto M, et al. Therapeutic angiogenesis by autologous bone marrow cell implantation for refractory chronic peripheral arterial disease using assessment of neovascularization by 99mTc-tetrofosmin (TF) perfusion scintigraphy. Cell Transplant. 2004;13(4):429–37.

54. Powell RJ, et al. Interim analysis results from the RESTORE-CLI, a randomized, double-blind multicenter phase II trial comparing expanded autologous bone marrow-derived tissue repair cells and placebo in patients with critical limb ischemia. J Vasc Surg. 2011;54(4):1032–41.

55. Benoit E, et al. The role of amputation as an outcome measure in cellular therapy for critical limb ischemia: implications for clinical trial design. J Transl Med. 2011;9:165.

56. Lu D, et al. Comparison of bone marrow mesenchymal stem cells with bone marrow-derived mononuclear cells for treatment of diabetic critical limb ischemia and foot ulcer: a double-blind, randomized, controlled trial. Diabetes Res Clin Pract. 2011;92(1):26–36.

57. Powell RJ, et al. Cellular therapy with Ixmyelocel-T to treat critical limb ischemia: the randomized, double-blind, placebo-controlled RESTORE-CLI trial. Mol Ther. 2012;20(6):1280–6.

58. Idei N, et al. Autologous bone-marrow mononuclear cell implantation reduces long-term major amputation risk in patients with critical limb ischemia: a comparison of atherosclerotic peripheral arterial disease and Buerger disease. Circ Cardiovasc Interv. 2011;4(1):15–25.

59. Iafrati MD, et al. Early results and lessons learned from a multicenter, randomized, double-blind trial of bone marrow aspirate concentrate in critical limb ischemia. J Vasc Surg. 2011;54(6):1650–8.

60. Walter DH, et al. Intraarterial administration of bone marrow mononuclear cells in patients with critical limb ischemia: a randomized-start, placebo-controlled pilot trial (PROVASA). Circ Cardiovasc Interv. 2011;4(1):26–37.

61. Murphy MP, et al. Autologous bone marrow mononuclear cell therapy is safe and promotes amputation-free survival in patients with critical limb ischemia. J Vasc Surg. 2011;53(6):1565–74-e1.

62. Losordo DW, et al. A randomized, controlled pilot study of autologous CD34+ cell therapy for critical limb ischemia. Circ Cardiovasc Interv. 2012;5(6):821–30.

63. Arai M, et al. Granulocyte colony-stimulating factor: a noninvasive regeneration therapy for treating atherosclerotic peripheral artery disease. Circ J. 2006;70(9):1093–8.

64. van Royen N, et al. START Trial: a pilot study on STimulation of ARTeriogenesis using subcutaneous application of granulocyte-macrophage colony-stimulating factor as a new treatment for peripheral vascular disease. Circulation. 2005;112(7):1040–6.

65. Bartsch T, et al. Transplantation of autologous mononuclear bone marrow stem cells in patients with peripheral arterial disease (the TAM-PAD study). Clin Res Cardiol. 2007;96(12):891–9.

66. Cobellis G, et al. Long-term effects of repeated autologous transplantation of bone marrow cells in patients affected by peripheral arterial disease. Bone Marrow Transplant. 2008;42(10):667–72.

Rodney M. Stuck, Coleen Napolitano, Daniel Miller,
and Francis J. Rottier

The number of cases of diabetes diagnosed internationally is rapidly growing and is expected to reach 366 million by the year 2025 [1]. The annual incidence for diabetic foot ulceration is between 1 and 7 % with a lifetime risk of 15–25 % in patients with diabetes. Diabetic foot ulcers (DFU) are thought to develop from atherosclerosis, peripheral neuropathy, or a combination of these two disorders [2, 3]. Additionally, problems such as foot deformity, callus formation, motor imbalance, and trauma play a role in ulcer formation [4, 5]. Approximately 15 % of diabetic foot ulcers result in amputation and contribute to more than 85 % of all diabetes-related amputations.

Patients with foot ulcerations perceive themselves as disabled as those patients with a lower limb amputation [6]. Several studies have shown a relationship of diabetic foot ulcers to mortality in patients with diabetes. Reportedly, the 5-year mortality rates for patients affected by diabetic foot ulcers are near 50 % [7]. Clearly, a diabetic foot ulcer is a marker of disease severity.

As this chapter evolves, wound assessment, vascularity/tissue nutrition, local care, compression and off-loading, debridement, advanced therapies, and surgical care will all be discussed.

Ulcer Evaluation and Classification

Finding the initial cause for ulceration is critical for the wound resolution. A history of recurrent wounds with prior difficulties, infection, and the impact on patient mobility is critical to providing care for the patient. Once vascularity and sensation have been assessed, the wound is evaluated for its relation to musculoskeletal deformity and local callus formation [6]. The ulceration is measured for size (including length, width, and depth) as well as inspection with a probe to evaluate for sinus tracts or a probe-to-bone finding. The wound margins are evaluated for undermining necrosis, purulence, and percent of granulation tissue. Pain and malodor are also assessed.

The clinician must also be aware of cellulitis and gangrene, osteomyelitis or related Charcot foot deformity. Ankle mobility is important to assess especially for chronic and recurrent forefoot ulcerations.

The most well-established diabetic foot ulcer rating systems are those developed by Wagner [8], Armstrong, and Lavery (University of Texas) [9] (Table 45.1). While the Wagner system is the most simplistic and easy to use, the University of Texas system better defines ulcer depth, infection, and ischemia (Table 45.2).

R.M. Stuck, DPM (✉) • C. Napolitano, DPM • F.J. Rottier, DPM
Department of Orthopaedic Surgery and Rehabilitation,
Loyola University Stritch School of Medicine, 2160 S. First Ave,
Maywood, IL 60153, USA

Hines Veterans Administration Hospital, Hines, IL, USA

D. Miller, DPM
Podiatry, St. Joseph Medical Center, Kansas City, MO, USA

Table 45.1 Wagner classification—modified [8]

(The premise being that all feet up to a Grade 4 can be converted back to a Grade 0 foot.)

Foot grade	Lesion type
0	No open wound
1	Superficial ulceration in epidermis to dermis
2	Deep ulcer to tendon or joint capsule
3	Deep ulceration with abscess, osteomyelitis, or joint sepsis
4	Localized gangrene—forefoot or locally on heel
5	Gangrene of foot—unsalvageable state

© Springer International Publishing Switzerland 2017
R.S. Dieter et al. (eds.), *Critical Limb Ischemia*, DOI 10.1007/978-3-319-31991-9_45

Table 45.2 University of Texas Diabetic Wound Classification-modified [9]—helps to differentiate infected and ischemic wounds

Wound grade	Depth			
	0	1	2	3
A	Pre-ulcer	Superficial wound	Tendon/capsule—no infection	Bone/joint—no infection
B	Closed with cellulitis	Superficial wound, cellulitis	Tendon/capsule, cellulitis	Bone/joint—infected
C	Closed with ischemia	Superficial wound, ischemic	Tendon/capsule, ischemic	Bone/joint, ischemic
D	Closed, B + C	Superficial, B + C	Tendon/capsule, B + C	Bone/joint, B + C

Treatment of foot ulcerations involves management of arterial disease, providing an appropriate wound healing environment, infection control, wound protection, and advanced wound therapies should the wound fail to improve.

Vascularity and Tissue Nutrition

As ischemia may be a factor in foot ulceration development and nonhealing, when pulses are absent, assessment of blood flow is pursued. Doppler ultrasonography is commonly utilized to determine whether adequate perfusion exists in the extremity to heal the foot ulceration. The ischemic index is a ratio of the systolic Doppler pressure at the ankle to the brachial systolic pressure. An ischemic index of 0.5 or greater is thought to be necessary to support wound healing. An ankle-brachial index of 0.45 in the patient with diabetes has been considered adequate for healing as long as the systolic pressure at the ankle was 70 mmHg or higher. These values are falsely elevated and non-predictive, in at least 15 % of patients with peripheral arterial disease. This is primarily due to the non-compressibility of calcified peripheral arteries. Other forms of noninvasive vascular testing can be considered when ABIs are unreliable. This would include the use of transcutaneous partial pressure of oxygen (TcPO2), measurement of skin perfusion pressure (SPP), and the toe brachial index (TBI) [10]. A vascular laboratory can measure toe pressures as an indicator of arterial inflow to the foot. The arteries of the hallux are less commonly found to be calcified than the vessels of the leg and at the level of the ankle [11–14]. The accepted threshold for toe pressure is at least 30 mmHg. Consultation with a vascular specialist should be obtained for patients who do not have adequate inflow demonstrated on these exams.

For nonhealing wounds, the review of nutritional status is obtained by measuring the serum albumin and the total lymphocyte count (TLC). The serum albumin should be at least 3.0 gm/dL and the total lymphocyte count should be greater than 1500. A serum albumin level of 3.5 g/dL or less indicates malnutrition. Serum prealbumin levels can also be considered when nutritional competence is border line. Prealbumin levels are thought to be a better measure when determining the effects of nutritional supplementation due to its short half-life. Normal prealbumin levels range from 6 to 35 mg/dL. The TLC is calculated by multiplying the white blood cell count by the percent of lymphocytes in the differential. When these values are suboptimal, consultation with a nutritionist is helpful to assist with optimizing the patient before definitive amputation. Surgery in stabilized patients with malnutrition or immunodeficiency should be delayed until these issues can adequately be addressed. When infection or gangrene requires urgent surgery, the goal should be to eradicate infection and eliminate necrotic tissue to viable margins. Deep tissue or bone cultures are taken to direct antibiotic therapy while the patient's nutrition and vascularity are optimized [15–18]. Patients with severe renal disease may never achieve desirable nutritional parameters. Local wound care attempts may still be pursued, but at known higher risk for failure.

Poor glycemic control has been identified as a risk factor associated with a higher frequency of amputation [19, 20]. Hyperglycemia will deactivate macrophages and lymphocytes and may impair wound healing. There is also a higher risk of urinary tract and respiratory infections when glucose levels are uncontrolled. Ideal management involves maintenance of glucose levels below 200 mg/dL [18]. Caution must be taken in managing the ulcerated patient's glucose with calorie reduction. This may lead to significant protein depletion and subsequent wound failure. If the patient's BMI is normal, 25 cal/kg is required to maintain adequate nutrition and avoid negative nitrogen balance.

The combined wound healing parameters of vascular inflow and nutritional status have been shown to significantly affect healing rates for pedal wounds. Optimizing the patient's nutritional parameters and achieving adequate tissue perfusion will limit the risk of wound complications and failure.

Local Wound Care

Acute vs Chronic Ulceration

Ulcers can be classified as acute or chronic. Acute ulcerations usually heal within a short period of time. A chronic ulcer is one that has failed to proceed through an orderly and timely process to produce anatomic and functional integrity or proceeded through the repair process without establishing or maintaining a sustained anatomic and functional result within 3 months [21]. The exact factors that contribute to producing a chronic wound are not known but likely involve both local and systemic factors. It is important to understand the normal healing process of Hemostasis/Inflammatory phase, Proliferative phase, and the Remodeling phase whether you are treating an acute or chronic wound. Factors that can adversely affect healing such as vascular disease, uncontrolled or poorly controlled metabolic disorders, malnutrition, pressure relief, and edema control have already been addressed and will not be repeated. Discussion here will focus on topical wound care management and topical wound care dressings.

Topical Therapies

The application of combining substances in the topical care of wounds has been recorded back to 2000 BCE. The Ancient Egyptians had specific details on how to clean the wound and prepare the wound for application of the topical compounding substance [22, 23]. Traditionally topical wound care had been directed at creating a dry wound. Winter is credited with recognizing the importance of a moist wound environment for more rapid wound healing [24, 25]. The primary goal of any wound care is to facilitate resolution of a wound by creating an environment ideal for wound healing. A wound dressing alone will not heal a wound. A wound dressing has ideal components which include the removal of excessive exudate, maintain a moist wound environment, protect against contaminants, cause no pain or trauma with dressing changes, leave no debris within the wound, and provide thermal insulation [24]. Wound characteristics should be evaluated and your choice of wound dressing should match the wound.

Antimicrobial topical agents have been utilized to reduce the microbial bioburden of the wound. Iodine, honey, and/or silver has been the most commonly utilized antimicrobial products and has been used topically or incorporated into various wound dressing products. Iodine has been used for over 100 years without any bacteria resistance. Free iodine combines irreversibly with tyrosine residues of protein to result in oxidase reaction that adversely affected normal cellular metabolism. The use of iodine has declined due to the potential for toxic effects to human fibroblast. Newer versions of iodine-containing products have a sustained delivery of bactericidal concentrations to moist wounds without apparent tissue damage [26]. The newer products also have properties that can absorb up to seven times its weight in exudate. Iodine-containing products are not recommended if there is an allergy to iodine or if the patient is on lithium.

Honey has beneficial antimicrobial effects related to the osmotic effect produced by the high sugar content and the presence of an enzyme that produces hydrogen peroxide. Different honeys have not exhibited the same antimicrobial effect. Medical-grade honey is recommended and has unidentified non-peroxide factors that exert an even higher antimicrobial activity. Medical-grade honey is resistant to denaturing by heat or light and still be effective if diluted [27]. Honey products should not be used if there is an allergy to bee venom.

Topical agents with silver have been utilized in wound care for over 100 years. The effectiveness of silver products varies from bacteriostatic to bactericidal. The bactericidal effect of silver is directly proportional to the silver ions in the wound exudate. The mechanism of action includes the ability of the positively charged silver ion to attract the negatively charge cell wall and enter the bacterial cell. The interaction of the silver ion and bacterial thiol damages/ blocks the cell wall, membranes, respiratory enzymes, and ribonucleoproteins [28]. Silver dressing should not be used in persons who may have an allergic reaction to metal and should not be used with enzymatic debriding agents. Prolonged use of silver is not recommended as it may be toxic to keratinocytes and fibroblasts. Although silver dressings have been the subject of case series, there have no reported results from a well-designed clinical trial [26]. Bergin and Wright failed to locate any clinical study pertaining to the use of silver dressing for the treatment of foot ulcers that would qualify for the Cochrane systematic review criteria [29].

Topical antimicrobial agents have a potential role in wound care but do not replace the need for sharp debridement of a wound bed to remove necrotic tissue and bacteria/ biofilm. Steed et al. found that wounds without debridement had a 75% nonhealing rate, while wounds treated with debridement had a 20% nonhealing rate [30]. Moist to dry dressings for wound coverage and debridement is no longer universally accepted as a gold standard for diabetic wound care. The use of moist to dry dressings should be reserved for grossly contaminated wounds and when removal of necrotic tissue must be performed faster than use of autolytic or enzymatic measures. A moist to dry dressing does not permit selective debridement of only necrotic tissue as it can leave gauze fibers within the wound and can be painful when changed, and the moisture of the dressing may evaporate too quickly to maintain a moist wound environment [24, 31].

Enzymatic agents have been utilized for wound debridement. Collagenase is an exopeptidase and is derived from *Clostridium histolyticum*. Collagenase specifically digests the denatured collagen on the wound base [32]. This enzymatic agent can be deactivated by such elements as pH, heat, silver, peroxide, and some antibiotics.

A biological debriding agent is medicinal maggots. Maggot therapy is regulated by the FDA for the debridement of wounds. Maggots are applied to the wound bed, 5–10 larva/cm^2, in a maggot-confined dressing which secures the maggots within the wound bed. The dressing has a porous net overlying the maggots and then an absorptive out layer for exudate. Medicinal maggots are left on the wound for up to 72 h. Although maggot therapy has been proven effective in wound debridement of necrotic tissue, pain can be associated with this debridement method. Contraindications for the use of maggots include bleeding disorders, deep tunneling wounds, and ischemia [33].

Other debriding methods include autolytic debridement. The autolytic debriding agents are used to help address the moisture imbalances, allowing the enzymes within the wound to digest damaged extracellular matrix and necrotic tissue. The debridement process by the use of autolytic agents is a slow process. Hydrogels and hydrocolloids are examples of autolytic debriding agents. (Surgical debridement will be addressed later in this chapter.)

The hydrogels are an insoluble hydrophilic polymer, a three-dimensional structure containing either polyethylene oxide or carboxymethyl cellulose and 90 % water. The high water content permits the hydrogel to donate moisture [22, 25, 34]. Hydrogel products come in sheets, gels, or gauzes. The use of hydrogels should be reserved for a noninfected wound since most have no antimicrobial properties. Hydrogels should be used on wounds with minimal exudate.

Hydrocolloid products are autolytic debriding agents. Hydrocolloids have a hydrophilic polymer inner layer and a water-resistant outer layer. Unlike hydrogels, the hydrocolloid dressing absorbs the exudate. The wound exudate interacts with the inner layer as it is absorbed and forms a gel that conforms to the wound base. The gel prevents the disruption of the wound base with dressing changes. The gel material that forms over the wound can vary in color from yellow to light brown and should not be mistaken for pus. The hydrocolloids are to be used in wounds with low to moderate exudate. Dressing changes can vary depending on the wound exudate but may be left in place up to 7 days or when fluid leaks. The wound environment under the hydrocolloid dressing is acidic (pH 5). This acidic environment has been shown to inhibit *Pseudomonas aeruginosa* and *Staphylococcus aureus* [35]. Some hydrocolloid products have odor-controlling properties. The hydrocolloid dressing can also assist in shear/friction protection.

Foam dressings assist in shear protection and cushioning over boney prominences while providing thermal insulation. Foam dressings are for wounds with moderate to heavy exudate. The foam dressings have a highly absorptive hydrophilic polyurethane or silastic inner membrane and a hydrophobic outer film layer [36, 37]. The outer film of the dressing provides a barrier to water and bacteria. Some foam products have adhesive borders but most require a secondary dressing. Variations of the foam products include cavity filling or spreadable versions. Caution should be used not to fill cavity more than 50 % with foam as expansion of the foam may prevent wound from contracting.

A very highly absorptive wound care product is the calcium alginates. A calcium alginate product is a biodegradable dressing that is derived from brown seaweed. Alginate products may be used on high exudating wounds. The alginates can absorb 20 times its weight in exudate. The interaction of the calcium ions of the alginate and sodium ions from the exudate forms a soluble gel that provides the moist wound environment. The absorptive ability of the alginate across the entire wound, "lateral wicking," can lead to periwound maceration if the alginate overlaps the adjacent skin [38]. Active release of the calcium ion of the alginate can assist with hemostasis. Alginates may assist in antimicrobial activity by bacteria from the wound exudate becoming trapped in the dense fibers of the alginate [39]. Alginates are available in sheet and rope versions and can be used in wound sinus or tunneling wounds. The alginates do require a secondary dressing. The time frame for dressing changes would be directly proportional to the amount of exudate. Although alginate dressing product is reported to be biodegradable, residual product in a wound can result in inflammation and pain.

Bioengineered products have been developed to assist in the healing of chronic wounds. Delay in the proliferative and remodeling phase is when the use of these products is traditionally warranted. Included in the advanced bioengineered products are the collagen products. Collagen is the major protein of the extracellular matrix. The collagen dressings absorb excess matrix metalloproteinases (MMPs) that can lead to a chronic wound, to degrade the collagen of the product thus protecting the patient's collagen within the wound. The degradation process of the collagen in the wound dressing also protects other growth factors from degradation. The different collagen products have various types of collagen, denatured (gelatin) and/or native (Type 1) [40]. The collagen difference determines which of the MMP the product is targeting. Collagen products are usually derived from ovine, bovine, porcine, or equine so allergic reactions are possible (Fig. 45.1).

Other advances in bioengineered wound care have been the production and use of skin substitutes and biologic cellular therapies and membranes [41]. These products are developed to facilitate wound healing with as many key features of skin as possible including but not limited to growth factors, cytokines, and human keratinocytes. Products vary as to whether they have inductive or conductive properties. These products are effective in providing a wound environment to facilitate healing, but these products are also associated with high manufacturing costs.

A wound care product does not heal a wound. There is no single wound care product designed to be utilized from

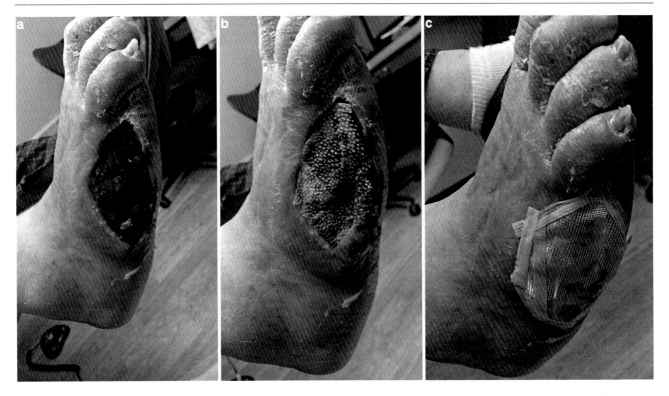

Fig. 45.1 Application of ovine forestomach dressing to lateral ray amputation wound. Note non-adherent dressing over this with Steri-Strip application for stability. This type of dressing is changed every 3–5 days. This product is a collagen base that will absorb MMPs to promote healing

wound origin to complete wound repair. The wound care provider needs to understand that wound healing is a dynamic process. The wound care specialist must be prepared to adapt the wound care plan to accommodate the changing wound needs.

Compression Therapy

Compression therapy is widely considered a first-line efficacious treatment in the management of ulceration of the lower extremity. Multiple studies have indicated the superiority of compression therapy versus standard wound care in the treatment of foot and leg ulceration, provided the etiology of the wound is clear and that confounding factors such as nutrition and various comorbidities are properly addressed by the clinician. Compression therapy relieves edema and stasis of the lower extremity by reducing distention of the superficial venous system and assisting the calf muscle pump. Compression may also help stimulate healthier granulation tissues within wounds and decrease presence of pro-inflammatory cytokines in wound exudates [24, 42]. Prior to the initiation of compression therapy, baseline noninvasive vascular studies should be considered to ensure adequate circulation to the involved limb with interventional cardiology or vascular surgery consultation if needed.

Gravity is a significant contributor to ulceration of the lower extremities as it leads to increased hydrostatic pressures within the venous system thereby creating a venous component even to wounds that may not be entirely venous in origin. Compression therapy at its basic tenants exists to combat these hydrostatic pressure increases. The exact mechanisms of the pathogenesis of ulceration remain unclear, but proposed theories include the fibrin cuff theory (pericapillary fibrin cuffs reduce local oxygenation to tissues), white cell trapping (trapped WBCs activate in tissues releasing cytokines with local tissue destruction), and growth factor trapping (growth factors inhibited by molecules which have undergone extravasation due to venous hypertension) [44, 45].

In an increasingly crowded commercial market, there are terms the clinician must be familiar with to help delineate appropriate treatment and appreciate differences when examining literature. Compression bandages are subdivided into three basic categories: inelastic, short stretch, or elastic. An inelastic bandage is a rigid wrap with a maximal stretch of 0–10 %, whereas the short-stretch bandage may extend from 10 to 100 %. Bandages with a stretch greater than 100 % are termed elastic [43]. Short-stretch bandages have been shown to be more effective in reducing venous volume and venous filling time when patients are standing, as well as generate larger-pressure amplitudes during exercise which makes them particularly effective for ambulating patients [46]. Short-stretch bandages also have the advantage of having decreases in pressure when the patient is not standing which can make them safer in patients with peripheral arterial occlusive disease and diabetes. The main disadvantage to a short-stretch dressing is that they have a tendency to loosen and can lose up to 50% of their initial interface compression within the first few hours of wear and tend to slide down the leg [46]. Elastic bandages have the advantage of being more easily molded and sustain compression better than inelastic materials. Elastic bandages typically are also more user friendly and can be applied by the patient or their relatives, whereas short-stretch or inelastic bandages tend to require a more experienced healthcare provider to apply the dressing appropriately.

Many of these compressive wraps have now been integrated into multilayered compression systems aimed at integrating the benefits of the different types of wraps while avoiding some of their disadvantages. There are now commercially available four-layer compression wrap systems that generally follow a composition of an initial contact layer that is usually made of orthopedic-style padded wool. The second component of the bandage of the four-layer bandage is most commonly a short-stretch bandage followed by an elastic third layer. The fourth component is commonly an intermediate stretch bandage that often has adhesive properties so that the bandage adheres to itself to maintain wrap integrity and compression. The four-layer bandage is advantageous in that it allows for high-pressure amplitudes during ambulation but allows a decrease in compressive pressure when the patient is supine. This trait makes the four-layer compressive dressing ideal for patients with chronic venous insufficiency without concurrent peripheral vascular disease, but also means that it must be used carefully in patients who do have PVD [46]. The four-layer bandage has also been shown to have the smallest decrease in pressure after 2 days of wear compared to other multilayered bandaging styles although RCT comparing four-layer bandaging systems with a multilayered bandaging has shown similar healing rates of venous leg ulcers (55% vs. 57% at 1 year) with both systems. Studies have also shown superiority of the four-layer bandage over patients treated with adhesive single-layer bandages [45].

Previous literature has shown the essential component to any limb compression therapy is the maintenance of pressure between 20 and 40 mmHG of pressure. Despite adequate compression, not all patients will heal with compression, with success rates ranging from 70 to 85% at 1 year of therapy [47]. Studies have evaluated patient populations to attempt to predict which patients will heal with compression therapy and have found that there are two predictive factors, namely, the age and size of the wound at initial presentation to the clinician. Wounds present less than 6 months and with a size smaller than 5 cm^2 at initial presentation have been found to carry a positive predictive value of 93–95% of healing with compression therapy at 24 weeks versus larger wounds with chronic duration [47]. Once wounds are healed, there is level 1A evidence for compression hosiery (30–40 mmHG) showing prevention of recurrence of ulceration [48]. This finding suggests that in patients without significant PVD, strong compression devices should be prescribed for daily use to maintain a healed limb.

In summary, compression therapy is indicated for lower extremity wounds and is very likely to assist with wound closure, particularly in smaller wounds of recent onset provided other patient comorbidities have been addressed. Compression must be used with caution in the setting of peripheral vascular disease.

Off-Loading of Wounds

Biomechanical factors play a significant role in the development and persistence of lower extremity ulceration. Elevated plantar pressures significantly raise the potential for foot ulceration in patients with peripheral neuropathy, with studies showing that neuropathic patients with high barefoot peak pressures have three to four times the risk of development of foot ulceration compared to those with normal or low plantar foot pressure [49]. Reduction of these increased foot pressures is the driving principle of off-loading plantar foot ulcerations and leads to a reduction in time to wound closure [49, 50]. Increased plantar pressures in these patients tend to result from foot deformity, reduced soft-tissue quality, decreased joint mobility, and ankle equinus (i.e., Achilles contracture).

Increased plantar pressures increase ulceration risk but the pressure thresholds for causing ulceration and healing ulcerations are unknown. Shear forces cause microseparation between skin layers and damage tissues and must be considered as ulcerations often develop underneath calluses which are influenced by shear [50]. Regular foot callus removal has been shown to reduce plantar foot pressures [51]. Furthermore, patient lifestyle, activity level, and compliance are also factors in predicting clinical outcome. Studies show that diabetics spend twice as much time standing instead of walking per day and that number of steps taken per day can help discriminate between ulcerated and ulcer-free patients [49]. Patient compliance with this therapy cannot be understated, and studies consistently show more effective healing rates with nonremovable off-loading treatments versus removable modalities, with some studies showing patient adherence to wearing removable prescribed off-loading footwear as low as 25% [49, 51].

According to the 2007 International Working Group on the Diabetic foot guidelines, total contact casting (TCC) should be the first choice treatment line for management of neuropathic foot ulceration. Total contact casting works by helping to disperse plantar pressures evenly across the plantar foot as well as divert some pressure into the cast wall and lower leg and is particularly useful for patients with midfoot ulceration and Charcot neuroarthropathy collapse [50]. Meta-analysis showed average time to healing ulceration decreased from 184 days to 44 days with the use of total contact casting. An additional benefit to the TCC is that they cannot be removed by the patient. Studies have shown that patients off-loaded with removable cast boots walk without them 72 % of the time [50, 52]. If TCC is not available, below-knee walking boots are recommended but should be made irremovable to aid in patient compliance with therapy (instant total contact casting) [49, 51, 52]. Instant total contact casting (iTCC) has been demonstrated in randomized controlled trials to have similar wound healing rates as traditional TCC casting [52]. Total contact casts are not without risk and can lead to other ulcerations and a risk for DVT.

Forefoot off-loading shoes, half shoes, and cast shoes have limited evidence to support their usage but are recommended when below the knee devices are contraindicated. These shoes have been shown to reduce forefoot pressures but not as significantly as TCC or iTCC [52]. Forefoot off-loading style shoes should be avoided with midfoot or rearfoot ulceration as they inherently increase pressures at these locations [53]. Customized insoles have also been shown to reduce peak plantar pressures by up to 30 % and may help reduce shear by stabilizing the foot [49, 50].

Despite evidence that TCC is a "gold-standard" treatment modality for neuropathic foot ulceration, a recent nationwide survey found that less than 2 % of polled centers use TCC as a primary off-loading method for diabetic neuropathic foot ulceration [52]. Such low usage of the modality may be secondary to lack of trained technicians, lack of reimbursement, immobility for the patient, and inconvenience [49, 50, 52]. Currently, evidence supports the usage of total contact casting or instant total contact casting for the treatment of neuropathic foot ulceration for reduction of pressure to the plantar foot. The safety, medical history, and mobility of each patient must be assessed to determine what off-loading modality is best for their situation.

Advanced Therapies

Hyperbaric oxygen therapy has been shown to provide healing benefits when combined with other wound care therapies. Several studies have shown long-standing healing in limb salvage for patients including this therapy in their treatment regimen [54, 55]. Guidelines for usage are in Table 45.3:

Other advanced therapy modalities include skin substitute, negative pressure wound therapy (NPWT), and

Table 45.3 Guidelines for hyperbaric oxygen therapy, referral for wound therapy

Diabetic foot/ankle ulceration
Wagner Grade 3 ulcer or higher
Failed standard wound care after 30+ days
Must be reassessed on 30-day intervals of care
Must discontinue therapy if no improvement at each 30-day interval

application of wound growth factors. Due to cost these modalities have often been considered as "final options." Efforts have been made to develop an appropriate time for using these interventions to reduce the chronicity of ulcerations and to limit those ulcer progressions to osteomyelitis and amputation.

Margolis et al. performed a meta-analysis including 622 patients all treated with standard off-loading and wound products. Healing rates were 24.2 % at 12 weeks and 30.9 % at 20 weeks [56]. Sheehan et al. evaluated wound percent area reduction (PAR) in size from baseline to 4 weeks. Sheehan found that wounds healing greater than 53 % at the 4-week marker had a 58 % healing rate at 4 weeks, whereas those with a PAR are less than 53 % at 4 weeks at a 9 % healing rate [57]. These findings were confirmed by Snyder et al. who found that the 50 % PAR marker at 4 weeks was strongly associated with healing by 12 weeks [58]. So, assessment of wound size and a calculation of percent area reduction is a valuable tool in assessing wound healing potential for the foot ulceration. As importantly, Lavery and Armstrong showed that ulceration presence increased the risk of infection by 2193 times versus no ulcer presence. Also, wound present for >30 days had an odd ratio of 4.7 to become infected [59]. Clearly, these wounds need to be closed to limit the risk of infection and reduce the potential for hospitalization.

Over the last 10 years, the most common products utilized for wound healing have included Becaplermin Gel and living skin equivalents that are applied to wounds on a weekly basis. The bioengineered alternative tissue (BAT) market is exploding. New products in this arena include amniotic membrane products. Currently these are available in dehydrated form (DHAM) containing both amnion and chorion or in cryopreserved form available either as amnion or chorion. Wound healing rates at 12–20 weeks may surpass 80 %.

BATs are a valuable treatment for our ulcerated patients that fail to heal 50 % in the first 4 weeks when treated as outlined above. The alternative tissues are readily available and can be applied in an outpatient setting. They don't require an operating room for application and polyneuropathy typically negates any anesthetic need. Without anesthetic, the cardiovascular risk to this patient population is minimized. Additionally, there is no donor site to heal as would be present with split thickness graft harvesting and application.

Cost plays into this as a single OR experience may cost over $4000 for a split thickness graft. Depending on the type applied, several BAT applications could be performed for the same expense. A cost analysis comparing these treatments has not been done nor has a randomized trial comparing BATs versus split thickness skin grafting. Skin grafting can be an effective therapy and donor site morbidity may not be significant [9]. However, due to the cardiovascular risk associated with any surgical procedure, skin graft therapies may be better reserved for the patient failing to improve with BAT therapy. There may be a point in wound size where STSG application becomes more economical. The cost vs patient cardiovascular risk needs to be balanced with larger wounds as the cost of clinical application of a more expensive BAT may not be covered under current payer rules in the ambulatory clinical set-

ting. Currently, about 80% of the wounds the authors treat are small enough to be covered by BATs that will be reimbursed using 2015 guidelines for clinical care (depending on the product applied to the ulceration). BAT therapy examples are many and are shown in Figs. 45.2–45.4.

Negative pressure (NPWT) has also been advocated as a wound therapy and may have value in maintaining a proper wound environment while limiting fluid collections at the site of the wound leading to a better healing environment [60]. These devices are contraindicated in infected or necrotic wounds. Currently, electrical corded, battery-powered, and mechanical suction devices are available for use (Fig. 45.5). The device must be changed every 3–7 days increasing the intensity of care. Because they rely on suction, if the vacuum seal is lost, the dressing must be replaced.

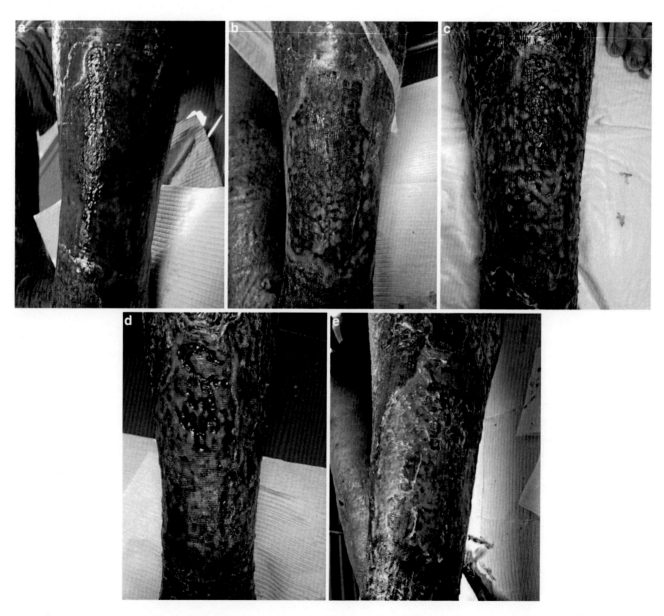

Fig. 45.2 Venous leg ulcer not progressing with local care and compression therapies treated over 4 weeks with weekly application of dehydrated amniotic membrane powder (DHAM) and multilayer compression dressings. Note near-complete healing from (**a**) to (**e**)

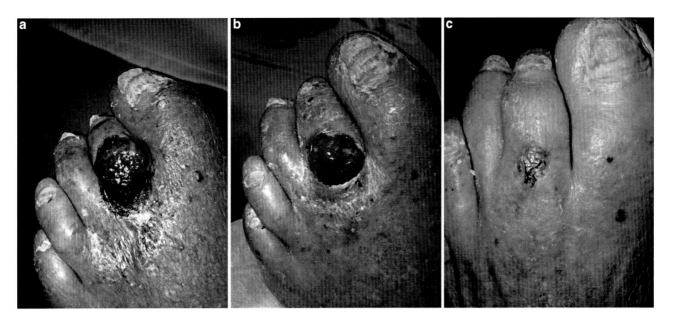

Fig. 45.3 Hypergranular second toe ulcer (**a**) that had failed to heal with local care and surgical shoe was treated with two injections of amniotic membrane graft reconstituted with saline. Note the healing at two weeks (**b**) and four weeks (**c**) after the first injection

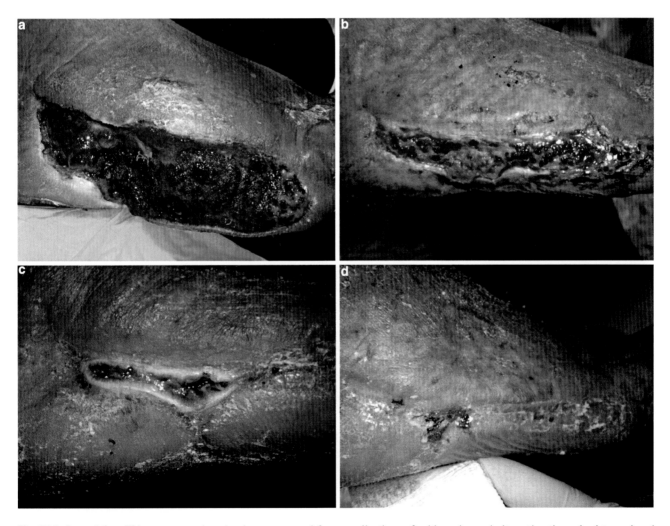

Fig. 45.4 Lateral foot fifth ray amputation site that was treated for 4 weeks with normal postoperative care and negative pressure wound therapy. This wound had a clean base but closed less than 10 % in the prior 4 weeks. With (**a**) being the starting point, weekly applications of a bioengineered alternative tissue lead to a closed wound over eight applications with multilayer compression therapy. Healing progression is noted at two weeks (**b**), six weeks (**c**) and eight weeks (**d**)

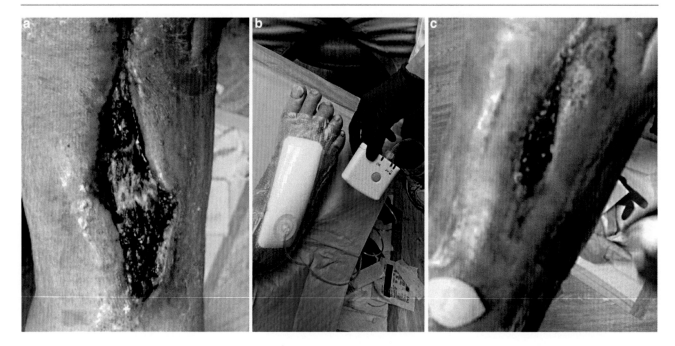

Fig. 45.5 Negative pressure wound therapy. (**a**) Initial wound that had progressed only 20 % in prior 4 weeks. (**b**) Battery powered, disposable VAC replaced weekly. (**c**) After 3 weeks of VAC therapy, marked improvement in wound base. Wound healed after 5 weeks of therapy

Debridement

Nonhealing wounds are frequently found to have local ischemia, necrotic tissue, and heavy bacterial loads. The chronic inflammation in these wounds leads to increased production of inflammatory cytokines and matrix metalloproteinase (MMPs).

Surgical debridement may be helpful in converting the chronic wound into an acute wound to help control infection, reduce inflammation, and remove necrotic and infected tissue. Excisional debridement of wounds is performed as needed to address necrotic or fibrous tissue. While there is no clear evidence that superficial wound debridement speeds wound healing, the practice seems intuitive and should be utilized for nonviable tissue. The author's group has a saying, "Biopsy what you culture and culture what you biopsy." Ulcerated tissue, especially when it is not healing or is not on a typical pressure point, should be biopsied to evaluate for malignancy. Bone biopsy is also a routine for those wounds that probe to bone. Both of these can be done in the office using local anesthetic if needed. Typical ulcer debridement steps are shown in Fig. 45.6.

Achilles Procedures for Recalcitrant Plantar Forefoot Ulceration

When patients have a forefoot ulcer that cannot be closed (or maintained closed), the Achilles should be evaluated for contracture. When this is identified, either Achilles lengthening or gastroc recession should be considered. The Hoke triple hemisection technique is performed through three percutaneous incisions along the central Achilles (see Fig. 45.7) as drawn by Sanders. Alternatively, the gastroc slip of the Achilles is isolated and released. Both of these procedures require immobilization 24 h/day for the first 4 weeks and then protected weight bearing in a cast boot for 2 additional weeks. Both procedures are valuable in gaining remission of these ulcers. Our own study of 20 patients undergoing gastroc recession showed 90 % remission of ulcers at 2-year follow-up.

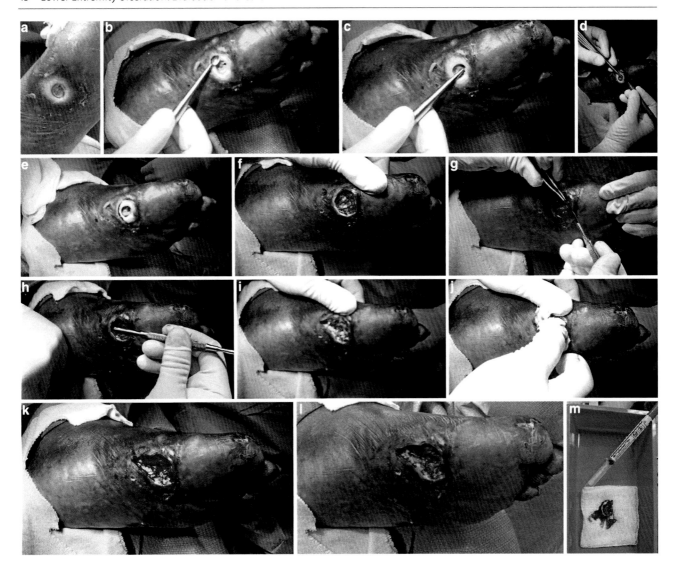

Fig. 45.6 Ulcer debridement of medial arch fibrotic ulceration. (**a–e**) Show undermining of the ulcer edge with marking of the amount of undermining so that the overlying tissue could be resected. (**f–h**) Show debridement of further fibrotic structures in the base of the wound as well as gentle probing to assess for any sinus tract. (**i–k**) Show obtaining hemostasis with l showing marks from silver nitrate application to bleeder sites. (**l**) Shows one-week follow-up, while (**k**) shows reminder to culture and biopsy the local tissues with such an extensive clinical debridement. Resection of the overlying ulcer tissue in undermined ulcers is not always needed but may lead to more rapid healing and easier management. (**m**) Reminds the reader that the best practice is to submit a pathologic and microbiologic specimen with the culture material

Arthroplasty or Amputation

Occasionally the patient with chronic ulceration requires excision of a bony prominence or amputation of a part that has become nonviable and fails to heal. Amputation or resection of the bone may be the best option for many of these patients' quality of life. Surveys have shown that patients with ulcer-ations perceive their quality of life to be quite similar to those people with an amputation and possibly worse [6]. Keeping in mind those patients with foot ulcerations have a 5-year mortality rate of 37–55 %, the rate associated at 5 years with lower extremity amputation ranges from 50 to 76 %. Foot ulceration is indeed a marker of disease severity. (See Amputation Chap. 52).

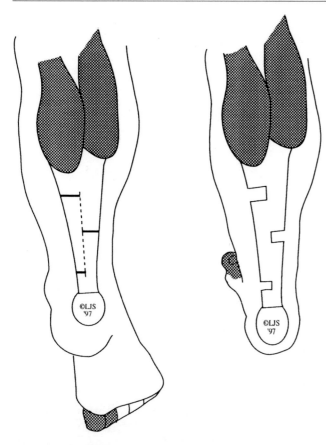

Fig. 45.7 Hoke triple hemisection lengthening of the Achilles for forefoot ulceration (Courtesy of Lee J. Sanders, DPM)

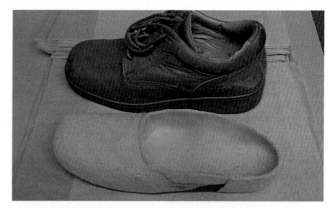

Fig. 45.8 Inlay depth shoe with deep toe box. Note the dual density of materials for insole to allow for improved shock absorption and friction reduction. This insole also has a forefoot filler for a transmetatarsal amputation

Long-Term Care

Once our patient's wound is closed (in remission), the patient needs prescription footwear to limit the risk of re-ulceration. This is a shoe with a deeper toe box and a multi-density insole to relieve pressure and friction (Fig. 45.8). Additionally, the patient needs regular clinical visits to assess for keratosis and foot conditions that may lead to new ulceration.

Summary

The complications associated with limb loss in the diabetic patient are quite high as are the treatments of diabetic foot infection. The described methods for evaluation and treatment of foot ulceration will help with early assessment, restoration of tissue nutrition, and protection of the limb to aid in healing. Long-term care of the extremity after healing through regular foot care and protective measures with therapeutic shoes is imperative for the long-term preservation of the patient's limb and restoration of quality of life.

References

1. Reiber GE, Ledoux WR. Epidemiology of diabetic foot ulcers and amputations: evidence for prevention. In: Williams R, Herman W, Kinmonth AL, Wareham NJ, editors. The evidence base for diabetes care. Hoboken, NJ: John Wiley; 2002. p. 641–65.
2. Boulton AJ, Kirsner RS, Vilekyte L. Clinical practice. Neuropathic diabetic foot ulcers. N Engl J Med. 2004;351(1):48–55.
3. Boulton AJ, Vilekyte L, Ragnarson-Tennvall G, Apelgvist J. The global burden of diabetic fool disease. Lancet. 2005;366(9498):1719–24.
4. Sanders LJ. Diabetes mellitus: prevention of amputation. J Am Podiatric Med Assoc. 1994;84(7):322–8.
5. Lavery LA, Armstrong DG, Wunderlich RP, et al. Diabetic foot syndrome evaluating the prevalence and incidence of foot pathology in Mexican American and non-Hispanic Whites from a diabetes disease management cohort. Diabetes Care. 2003;26(5):1435–8.
6. Willrich A, Pinzur M, McNeil M, Juknelis D, Lavery L. Health related quality of life cognitive function, and depression in diabetic patients with foot ulcer or amputation. A preliminary study. Foot Ankle Int. 2005;26(2):128–34.
7. Iverson MM, Tell GS, Riise T, et al. History of foot ulcer increases mortality among individuals with diabetes: ten-year follow-up of the Nord-Trondelag Health Study, Norway. Diabetes Care. 2009;32(12):2193–9.
8. Wagner FW. The dysvascular foot: a system for diagnosis and treatment. Foot Ankle. 1981;2:64–122.
9. Lavery LA, Armstrong DG, Harkless LB. Classification of diabetic foot wounds. J Foot Ankle Surg. 1996;35:528–31.
10. Lo T, Sample R, Moore P, et al. Prediction of wound healing outcome using skin perfusion pressure and transcutaneous oximetry: a single-center experience in 100 patients. Wounds. 2009;21(11):310–6.
11. Pahlsson HI, Wahlberg E, Olofsson P, Swedenborg J. The toe pole test for evaluation of arterial insufficiency in diabetic patients. Eur J Endovasc Surg. 1999;18:133–7.
12. Carter SA, Tate RB. The value of toe pulse waves in determination of risks for limb amputation and death in patients with peripheral arterial disease and skin ulcers or gangrene. J Vasc Surg. 2001; 33:708–14.
13. Ubbink DT, Tulevski II, de Graaff JC, Legemate DA, Jacobs JHM. Optimisation of the non-invasive assessment of critical limb

ischaemia requiring invasive treatment. Eur J Endovasc Surg. 2000;19:131–7.

14. Misuri A, Lucertini G, Nanni A, et al. Predictive value of transcutaneous oximetry for selection of the amputation level. J Cardiovasc Surg. 2000;41(1):83–7.

15. Dickhaut SC, Delee JC, Page CP. Nutrition status: importance in predicting wound healing after amputation. J Bone Joint Surg Am. 1984;64:71–5.

16. Haydock DA, Hill GL. Improved wound healing response in surgical patients receiving intravenous nutrition. Br J Surg. 1987; 74:320–3.

17. Jensen JE, Jensen TG, Smith TK, et al. Nutrition in orthopaedic surgery. J Bone Joint Surg Am. 1982;64:1263–72.

18. Mowat AG, Baum J. Chemotaxis of polymorphonuclear leukocytes from patients with diabetes mellitus. N Engl J Med. 1971;248:621–7.

19. Miyajima S, Shirai A, Yamamoto S, et al. Risk factors for major limb amputation in diabetic foot gangrene patients. Diabetes Res Clin Pract. 2006;71:272–9.

20. Imran S, Ali R, Mahboob G. Frequency of lower extremity amputation in diabetics with reference to glycemic control and wagner's grades. J Coll Physicians Surg. 2006;16(2):124–7.

21. Werdin M, et al. Evidence-based management strategies for treatment of chronic wounds. Eplasty. 2009;9:e19. PMCID: PMC 2691645.

22. Ovington L. Advances in wound dressings. Clin Dermatol. 2007;5:33–8.

23. Hess CT. Part 2 Skin and wound care products. In: Clincal guide skin & wound care, 6th ed. Lippincott: Williams & Wilkins. 2008; p 166.

24. Fonder M, et al. Treating the chronic wound: a practical approach to wound care of non healing wounds and wound care dressings. J Am Acad Dermatol. 2008;58(2):185–206.

25. Veves A, Giurini J, LoGerfo L. Local care of diabetic foot ulcers: assessments, dressings, and topical treatments. In: The diabetic foot. 3rd ed. Humana Press; 2012. p. 289–306.

26. Lipsky B, Hoey C. Topical antimicrobial therapy for treating chronic wounds. Clin Pract. 2009;49:1541–9.

27. Bradshaw C. An *in vitro* comparison of the antimicrobial activity of honey, iodine and silver wound dressings. Biosci Horiz. 2011;4(1):61–70.

28. Castellano JJ, Shafi SM, Ko F, et al. Comparative evaluation of silver containing antimicrobial dressings and drugs. Int Wound J. 2007;4:114–22.

29. Bergin SM, Wraight P. Silver based wound dressings and topical agents for treating diabetic foot ulcers. Cochrane Database of Syst Rev. 2006.

30. Steed DL, et al. Effects of extensive debridement and treatment on the healing of diabetic foot ulcers. Diabetic Ulcer Study Group J Am Coll Surg. 1996;183:61–4.

31. Hakakian C, Suzuki K. What you should know about emerging wound care dressings. Podiatry Today. 2014;27(8):52–8.

32. Hess CT. Part 2 Skin and wound care products. In: Clincal guide skin & wound care, 6th ed. Lippincott Williams & Wilkins, 2008; p 549.

33. Sherman RA, et al. Maggott Therapy in Biotherapy-History, Principles and Practice: a practical guide to the diagnosis and treatment of disease using living organisms. 2013 Springer, pp 5–31.

34. McCulloch JM, Kloth LC. Dressing and Skin Substitutes. In: Wound Healing: Evidence-Based Management, 4th ed. FA Davis Company; 2010. pp 180–201.

35. Varghese MC, et al. Local environment of chronic wounds under synthetic dressings. Arch Dermatol. 1986;122:52–7.

36. Sarabahi S, Tiwari VK. Dressings and topical agents in wound care. In: Principles and Practice of Wound Care. Jaypee Brothers Medical Publishers; 2012. pp 79–85.

37. O'Connell SC, et al. Management of patients with dermatologic problems. In: Brunner, Suddarth, editors. Textbook of medical-surgical nursing. 12th ed. Lippincott Williams & Wilkins; 2010. p. 1679.

38. Agren MS. Four alginate dressings in the treatment of partial thickness wounds: a comparative experimental study. Br J Plast Surg. 1996;49:129–34.

39. Thomas S. Alginate dressing in surgery and wound management: Part 3. J Wound Care. 2009;9:163–6.

40. Lanza R, Lange R, Vacanti J. Basic biology of wound repair. In: Principles of tissue engineering, 3rd ed. Elsevier, Inc; 2011. pp 1150–1166.

41. Kamolz LP, Lumenta DP. The use of dermal substitutes in dermato-surgery. In: Dermal replacements in general, burn, plastic surgery. In: Tissue engineering in clinical practice. Springer; 2013. pp 130–138.

42. Velasco M. Diagnostic and treatment of leg ulcers. Actas Dermosifiliogr. 2011;102(10):780–90.

43. Partsch H. Compression therapy in leg ulcers. Rev Vasc Med. 2013;1:9–14.

44. Gohel M, Poskitt K. Chronic ulceration of the leg. Surgery. 2013;31(5):224–8.

45. Nelson A, Prescott R, Harper D, Gibson B, Brown D, Vaughan Ruckley C. A factorial, randomized trial of pentoxifylline or placebo, four-layer or single-layer compression, and knitted viscose or hydrocolloid dressings for venous ulcers. J Vasc Surg. 2007;45(1):134–41.

46. Hafner J, Botonakis I, Burg G. A comparison of multilayer bandage systems during rest, exercise, and over two days of wear time. Arch Dermatol. 2000;136:857–63.

47. Margolis D, Berlin J, Strom B. Which venous leg ulcers will heal with limb compression bandages? Am J Med. 2000;109:15–9.

48. Coleridge-Smith P. Leg ulcer treatment. J Vasc Surg. 2009;49(3):804–8.

49. Bus S. Priorities in offloading the diabetic foot. Diabetes Metab Res Rev. 2012;28 Suppl 1:54–9.

50. McCartan B, Rosenblum B. Offloading of the diabetic foot: orthotic and pedorthic strategies. Clin Podiatr Med Surg. 2014;31:71–88.

51. Bus S, van Deursen R, Armstrong D, Caravaggi C, Hlavacek P, Bakker K, et al. The effectiveness of footwear and offloading interventions to prevent and heal foot ulcers and reduce plantar pressure in diabetes: a systematic review. Diabetes Metab Res Rev. 2008;24 Suppl 1:S162–80.

52. Wu S, Jenson J, Weber A, Robinson D, Armstrong D. Use of pressure offloading devices in diabetic foot ulcers: do we practice what we preach? Diabetes Care. 2008;31(11):2118–9.

53. Bus S, van Deursen R, Kanade R, Wissink M, Manning E, van Baal J, et al. Plantar pressure relief in the diabetic foot using forefoot offloading shoes. Gait Posture. 2009;29:618–22.

54. Faglia E, Favales F, Aldeghi A, et al. Adjunctive system hyperbaric oxygen therapy in treatment of severe prevalently ischemic diabetic foot ulcer: a randomized study. Diabetes Care. 1996;19(2):1338–43.

55. Abidia A, et al. The role of hyperbaric oxygen therapy in ischaemic diabetic lower extremity ulcers: a double-blind, randomized-controlled trial. Eur J Vasc Endovasc Surg. 2003;25(6):513–8.

56. Margolis DJ, Allen-Taylor L, Hoffstad O, et al. Diabetic neuropathic foot ulcers: the association of wound size, wound duration, and wound grade on healing. Diabetes Care. 2002;25(10):1835–9.

57. Sheehan P, Jones P, Caselli A, et al. Percent change in wound area of diabetic foot ulcers over a 4-week period is a robust predictor of complete healing in a 12 week prospective trial. Diabetes Care. 2003;26(6):1879–82.

58. Synder R, Cardinal M, Dauphinee D, et al. A post-hoc analysis of reduction in diabetic foot ulcer size at 4 weeks as a predictor of healing by 12 weeks. Ostomy Wound Manage. 2010;56(3):44–50.

59. Lavery LA, Armstrong DG, Wunderlich RP, et al. Risk factors for foot infections in individuals with diabetes. Diabetes Care. 2006;29(6):1288–93.

60. Blume OA, Walther J, Payne W, et al. Comparison of negative pressure wound therapy using vacuum-assisted closure with advanced moist wound therapy in the treatment of diabetic foot ulcers: multicenter randomized controlled trial. Diabetes Care. 2008;31(4):631–6.

Diagnosis and Management of Wound Infections

46

Alfredo J. Mena Lora, Jesica A. Herrick, Bradley Recht, and Ivette Murphy-Aguilu

Introduction

Throughout history, wound infections have had an important impact on public health. No story provides greater illustration of the importance of wound infections than statistics from historic conflicts. Prior to the development of effective antimicrobials, early amputation was considered the most effective way to treat wound infections [1], and battlefield wound infections historically had an estimated mortality as high as 38–62% [2]. Historians estimate that prior to World War II, more victims of war died of infectious causes than of battle-related injuries [3, 4].

Though the development of antibiotics improved survival of those with infected wounds, wound infections continue to be a major problem in the modern era. Alarmingly, reports from current war zones show a high rate of wound colonization with multidrug-resistant (MDR) pathogens [5, 6]. As the frequency of MDR organisms continues to increase in battlefield wounds, these wounds may become progressively more difficult to treat.

Compared to acute traumatic wounds in young healthy soldiers, chronic wounds in patients with multiple comorbidities may present a larger and more costly medical challenge. A primary risk factor for lower extremity wounds is diabetes; patients with diabetes have a 25% lifetime risk of developing

A.J.M. Lora, MD
Department of Medicine, Section of Infectious Diseases, University of Illinois at Chicago, Chicago, IL, USA

J.A. Herrick, MD, MS
Department of Medicine; Section of Infectious Diseases, Immunology, and International Medicine, University of Illinois at Chicago, Chicago, IL, USA

B. Recht, MD
Department of Internal Medicine, Jesse Brown VA, Chicago, IL, USA

I. Murphy-Aguilu, DO (✉)
Infectious Disease, Alexian Brothers Medical Center, Elk Grove Village, Chicago, IL, USA

an ulcer, and half of those ulcers will become infected [7]. Diabetic wound infections have been shown to increase the risk for hospitalization and lower extremity amputation by 55- and 150-fold, respectively [7]. Due to increasing rates of diabetes, increased obesity in the population, and a longer life span of patients with diabetes, it is expected that lower extremity wounds will become an increasingly burdensome public health problem in the coming years [8].

Infection of a skin ulcer has been shown to lead to decreased healing, increased treatment costs, and increased morbidity for patients. One study found that subjects with postsurgical wound infections had a twofold increase in the average number of hospitalization days compared to uninfected patients [9]. Increased hospitalization days, decreased healing, and increased need for therapeutic interventions have all been associated with increased costs [10].

Clinical Manifestations of the Infected Wound

Given the morbidity associated with wound infections, it is extremely important to accurately and promptly identify an infected wound. Additionally, we must also consider the clinical impact of overtreating the *uninfected* wound. By treating uninfected ulcers, we unnecessarily place patients at risk for complications such as *Clostridium difficile*-associated diarrhea, development of antibiotic resistance, and an increased cost of care due to the expense of unnecessary antimicrobials. Not only are these outcomes potentially problematic to the individual; they are also costly to the health-care system as a whole.

The Wound Infection Continuum

One of the most important concepts to understand in the pathogenesis of wound infections is that of microbial con-

© Springer International Publishing Switzerland 2017
R.S. Dieter et al. (eds.), *Critical Limb Ischemia*, DOI 10.1007/978-3-319-31991-9_46

Fig. 46.1 The wound infection continuum, starting with contamination and leading to infection

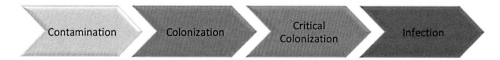

Contamination → Colonization → Critical Colonization → Infection

tamination/colonization and the subsequent path to infection. *Wound contamination* is defined as the presence of nonreplicating organisms in a wound. Sources for organisms present in a contaminated wound include environmental sources, normal skin flora, or endogenous sources (gastrointestinal, genitourinary, etc.) [11]. Wound contamination is the first step in what is known as the wound infection continuum [11, 12]. It is the interaction between these bacteria and the host's immune system that can lead to infection [13, 14].

The next stage in the wound infection continuum is *wound colonization*. A wound is defined as colonized when the microorganisms present are dividing and multiplying, but are not causing injury to the host tissue [13–15]. Exposed tissue in acute or chronic wounds provides an excellent environment for pathogens to proliferate [16].

Critical colonization is a term first defined by E. Davis in 1996 as "multiplication of organisms without invasion but interfering with wound healing." However, this definition lacked either a clear clinical or microbiological meaning [17]. Later it was redefined as the inability of the wound to maintain a balance between increasing "bioburden" of bacterial replication and the host immune system [18]. Some studies have suggested that a bacterial load >10^5 colony-forming units (CFU) per gram of tissue may provide a quantitative estimate of the point of critical colonization, above which colony count infection becomes increasingly likely. However, this is a controversial subject, and definitive proof about the presence of a specific colony count associated with critical colonization is lacking.

Several studies have suggested that it may not be the bacterial load but rather the presence of a particular species of bacteria or a specific host response to colonization that define the concept of critical colonization [19]. Regardless, the process of critical colonization and its clinical significance warrant further investigation as this process may represent an opportunity for early intervention and healing as well as potentially decreased need for systemic antimicrobials [11].

While the concept and definition of critical colonization remain an ongoing discussion among wound care experts, there is little scientific evidence to support impaired wound healing based on bacterial burden or critical colonization alone [8, 11, 13, 17]. Most experts do agree that there are instances in which a wound may not display overt or classic signs of infection but instead display secondary signs that signal the presence of a subclinical infection. These signs include delayed healing, friable granulation tissue, increased serous drainage, or increased pain. Early antimicrobial therapy may be warranted in the setting of these secondary signs of infection, but clear guidelines for when to initiate treatment in patients with secondary signs of infection are lacking [8, 11] (Fig. 46.1).

Wound infection represents the final stage of the infection continuum. An acute or chronic wound can progress to infection after colonization occurs and when the right conditions are present for tissue invasion. An infected wound is defined as invasion of microorganisms within the wound area, leading to cell injury, tissue damage, and inflammation [20].

Clinical Spectrum of Skin and Soft-Tissue Infections

Understanding the anatomy of skin structures and the various clinical manifestations of skin infections can be helpful in determining likely pathogens for a given patient. Infectious syndromes involving skin and soft-tissue structures can be caused by a variety of organisms, but certain syndromes are highly associated with specific pathogens. This may help the clinician predict the pathogen and select appropriate empiric therapy (Fig. 46.2).

Erysipelas is defined as infection of the superficial layers of the dermis without subcutaneous involvement. Erysipelas can travel through lymphatic tissue and spread quickly. Erysipelas is typically caused by *Streptococci*. In contrast, cellulitis is an infection of the skin and underlying connective tissue. *Streptococcus pyogenes* can play an important role in both erysipelas and cellulitis. Large studies have shown that *Streptococci* may be the most common cause of cellulitis [21, 22]. *Staphylococcus aureus* (including MRSA) plays an important role as well and is more common in the setting of cellulitis with purulence [23].

Impetigo (easily identifiable due to the characteristic associated honey-colored exudate) and ecthyma are both infections of the superficial dermis. Ecthyma is an ulcerative pyoderma of the skin that extends into the deeper tissues. Ecthyma is typically referred to as a deeper form of impetigo. Both impetigo and ecthyma are commonly caused by *Staphylococcal* and *Streptococcal* spp. Similarly, furuncles and carbuncles (both forms of cutaneous abscesses) involve these same structures and pathogens.

Diabetic infections can involve multiple tissue planes and are typically polymicrobial. Highly pathogenic organisms such as *Pseudomonas* spp. can be involved in these infections. Though this association is well known, the contribution of this organism to underlying pathology of diabetic foot infections has recently been questioned. A recent randomized controlled trial challenged the idea that empiric antimicrobials that cover *Pseudomonas* species are necessary in diabetic foot infections

Fig. 46.2 The layers of skin structure and the skin and soft-tissue infections associated with each level

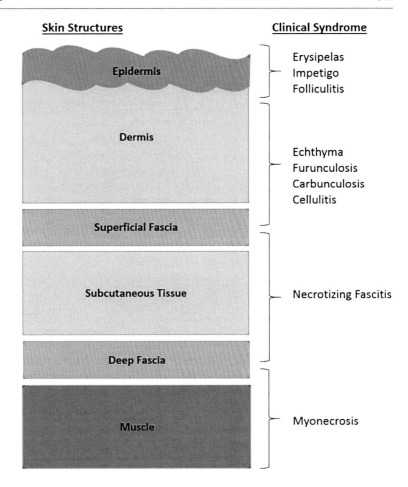

[24]. Given the difficulty in obtaining and interpreting appropriate culture samples for microbiologic diagnosis in wound infections, it is always prudent to monitor patients closely once therapy has been initiated.

Surgical site infections can involve superficial incisional tissues, deep incisional tissues, or deep organ spaces. These infections can be caused by typical causative organisms involved in skin infections or by normal flora of the organs involved in specific procedures. Finally, vascular surgical wounds or ischemic wounds can have a variety of organisms. Postoperative infectious complications from vascular surgery cause significant morbidity and are common [25]. Infected anatomical sites and risk of infection are typically dependent on the degree of hypoxia in the affected tissues [25]. A case series of vascular cases from Sri Lanka demonstrated that *Pseudomonas* was involved in many of its infections [26] (Table 46.1).

Microbiology of Wound Infections

Wound infections have a complex microbiology that is dependent on interactions between the host and their environment. Understanding the microbiology of infected wounds is of importance for clinicians in order to properly identify infected wounds, accurately interpret microbiologic data, and make appropriate medical decisions regarding patient care.

Organisms can colonize wounds from a variety of sources. Normal skin flora, largely composed of Gram-positive organisms, is the most common source of colonization in wounds. Organisms from other mucosal surfaces and anatomical compartments (e.g., Gram-negative organisms from the gastrointestinal tract or upper airway) can also migrate to the wound. Finally, the environment can play a key role, as organisms from the environment can be introduced into a wound through direct contact [16].

Endogenous Sources

The skin microbiota consists mostly of Gram-positive bacteria such as *Staphylococcus epidermidis*, other coagulase-negative *Staphylococci*, and *Propionibacterium acnes*. These bacteria coexist with human beings in a delicate balance of natural immune barriers and bacterial properties that confer a propensity toward survival and persistence rather than aggressive virulence and host-damaging properties [27]. However, these organisms can easily migrate to deeper tissues when

Table 46.1 Skin and soft-tissue infection syndromes [6, 24]

Syndrome	Anatomy	Microbiology
Erysipelas	Epidermis	Group A *Streptococcus*
Cellulitis	Dermis	Group A *Streptococcus* Group G *Streptococcus* S. *aureus*
Furuncles	Epidermis	S. *aureus*
Carbuncles	Epidermis, dermis	S. *aureus*
Diabetic foot infection	Epidermis, dermis, fascia, bone	Polymicrobial
Surgical site infection	Epidermis, dermis, fascia, deep organs	S. *aureus*, *Streptococci*, anaerobes
Vascular surgery and ischemic limbs	Multiple tissue planes, depends on level of tissue hypoxia	S. *aureus*, *Streptococci*, anaerobes

natural skin barriers are compromised, and in that setting, skin commensals can play a pathogenic role [28, 29]. As evidence for their contribution to the pathology of wound infections, the resistance pattern of skin commensals has been linked with overall mortality [30].

Other endogenous sources of importance are the oral, genital, and gastrointestinal mucosa. A large study of surgical wounds showed that the predominant organisms in abdominal infections were primarily endogenous gastrointestinal organisms including *E. coli*, *Streptococcus* species, *Bacteroides*, *Peptostreptococcus*, and *Clostridium* species [31]. Similarly, a study of decubitus ulcers in children showed the presence of enteric pathogens as well as *Pseudomonas* [32].

Exogenous Sources

The environment can play an important role in the colonization of wound infections. Once only diagnosed in patients with contact with health care, the so-called hospital-acquired multidrug-resistant pathogens have now spread to the community. A study assessing the prevalence of MDR organisms in diabetics and nondiabetics showed that the prevalence of these organisms can be as high as 63% [33]. Animals have been shown to serve as a reservoir of drug-resistant organisms, and contact with animals can be associated with subsequent transmission of MDR organisms to the community [34]. Infection control measures have decreased the burden of transmission of MDR organisms in the hospital setting [35], but colonization through exogenous contamination remains a problem both in the hospital setting and in the community.

Anaerobes

Due to the difficulty in isolating anaerobic bacteria, the role of anaerobes in wound infections has been neglected in the past by the scientific community [9, 16, 29]. However, multiple recent studies have consistently shown that anaerobic

organisms may play a major role in the microbiology of contaminated and infected wounds [28, 29, 36]. Microbiologic data from over half a dozen studies demonstrated that anaerobes were present in about 38% of wounds [16]. Hence, the presence of anaerobic organisms should always be considered as contributing to the pathology of infected and noninfected wounds.

Variables Affecting Microbial Proliferation

An acute or chronic wound that has been colonized with bacteria can progress to infection when the right conditions are present for tissue invasion and bacterial replication. Factors that favor the development of wound infection include tissue hypoxia and patient comorbidities.

Tissue Oxygenation and Bacterial Growth

Perhaps the most important factor affecting the transition from colonization to infection is tissue perfusion. A hypoxic environment allows for increased microbial growth, as oxygen is a key component of oxidative reactions in polymorphonuclear leukocytes [37]. Chronic nonhealing ulcers are frequently hypoxic and therefore are more susceptible to infection than well-perfused tissues [38]. Surgical wounds in anatomical sites that have excellent tissue perfusion typically heal rapidly and have less likelihood of infection [39]. Studies have shown that wounds will likely heal adequately if tissue oxygen tension is above 40 mmHg; however, when perfusion fell to levels of less than 20 mmHg, healing was found to be less likely and infection more common [39].

Comorbidities

Comorbidities present in the host may contribute both to colonization and subsequent infection of the wound. Comorbidities that cause decreased perfusion or alteration in the innate or acquired immune system may increase the risk of wound infections and also lead to impaired wound healing in the event of infection. Recently debrided or amputated tissue has been shown to have decreased concentration of antibiotics compared to serum levels, demonstrating an important mechanism by which poor perfusion leads to impaired wound healing [40].

Foot infections have been shown to be the most common cause of hospitalization among patients with diabetes [8]. Large observational studies show that peripheral artery disease (PAD) plays a key role in diabetic foot infections, as almost half of the patients enrolled in these studies had evidence of such [8]. Other comorbidities that lead to PAD can therefore predispose patients to wound infections and decreased healing.

Diagnosis of Wound Infections

Diagnosis of wound infections is based primarily on clinical signs and symptoms (Table 46.2). Most studies relating to diagnosis of wound infections have been conducted on patients with diabetic foot wounds. In 1994, Cutting and Harding first identified criteria to diagnose an infected wound, which included the classic signs of inflammation: erythema, warmth, pain, and edema [41]. The current Infectious Disease Society of America (IDSA) guidelines for diabetic foot infections recommend diagnosing a diabetic foot infection based on the presence of at least two of these classic signs or symptoms of inflammation in addition to purulence from the wound [2, 42].

However, it is necessary to take into account all of the clinical features of an individual patient's presentation to make appropriate clinical decisions, as the classic signs of infection may be absent in some patients with an infected wound [28]. In particular, patients with limb ischemia may lack erythema and warmth, and those with peripheral neuropathy may not present with pain. In these circumstances, the presence of secondary signs of infection such as an increase in nonpurulent secretions, friable granulation tissue, foul odor, undermining of the wound edges, or delayed wound healing can be helpful in making the diagnosis of a wound infection [41].

Once a wound has been identified as infected, it can then be further defined as mild, moderate, or severe. Determining the severity of a wound infection can help determine how best to manage the patient. The IDSA and the International Working Group of the Diabetic Foot (IWGDF) have developed a classification for determining the severity of a diabetic foot infection (Table 46.3). Per this classification system, mild infection involves only the skin and subcutaneous tissue, with a limited area (if any) of surrounding erythema. A moderate infection is defined as either a superficial infection involving a larger area (>2 cm) of the skin surrounding the ulcer or an infection that involves deeper structures (i.e., an abscess, osteomyelitis, fasciitis). Finally, a severe infection is any local infection associated with two or more of the following SIRS criteria: a leukocyte count >12,000/μL or <4000/μL or >10 % immature (band) forms, temperature >38 °C or less than 36 °C, heart rate of more than 90 beats per minute, respiratory rate of more than 20 breaths per minute, or arterial carbon dioxide tension ($PaCO_2$) of less than 32 mmHg [43]. Patients with severe infections require hospitalization, while those with mild infection can typically be managed as outpatients. In regard to those with moderate infections, many can be managed as an outpatient, with the exception of those with critical ischemia [8].

Although the IDSA/IWGDF classification system has primarily been validated in patients with diabetes and may not be applicable to other patient populations, it is likely that all patients with a wound infection would at least benefit from a determination of the severity of their wound and a strategy of intensifying care based on the severity level of the wound.

When to Obtain a Culture

As described previously, all chronic wounds are at the very least colonized with bacteria. For this reason, it is imperative that wounds are not routinely cultured unless there is suspicion for infection.

Most wounds that are clinically believed to be infected should be cultured. The sole exception would be in the case of a mild infection in an antibiotic naïve individual with low risk for MRSA infection. In that setting, a wound culture

Table 46.2 Clinical signs of wound infections

Classic	Secondary	Systemic
Erythema	Malodor	Tachycardia
New or increased pain/tenderness	Friable granulation tissue	Fever/chills
Purulence	Delayed healing	Hypotension
Swelling or induration	Increased nonpurulent secretions	Delirium
	Discoloration	
	Pocketing at base of wound	

Table 46.3 IDSA classification system for diabetic foot ulcers [6]

Infection severity	Signs/symptoms
Uninfected	No signs or symptoms of infection
Infected	At least two of the following: • Pain/tenderness • Erythema • Warmth • Swelling or induration • Purulent discharge
Mild infection	• Local infection: involves only the skin and subcutaneous tissue • Erythema >0.5 cm to <2 cm around ulcer • No other etiology for inflammatory response of the skin (thrombosis, venous stasis, gout, etc.)
Moderate infection	• Local infection with • Erythema >2 cm or • Involving deeper structures than the skin and • No systemic inflammatory response signs
Severe infection	Local infection with signs of SIRS; at least two of the following: • Temp >38 °C or <36 • Heart rate >90 beats/min • Respiratory rate >20 breaths/min or $PaCO_2$ <32 mmHg • White blood cell count >12,000 or <4000 or >10 % bands

may be unnecessary as these types of infections are invariably caused by *Streptococci* or *Staphylococci*, and an empiric regimen covering these organisms is typically a sufficient therapy [8]. In all other cases of presumed wound infection, however, wound culture should be obtained. Whenever possible, culture samples should be obtained prior to the initiation of antimicrobial therapy [8].

What Type of Wound Culture to Obtain

Obtaining an adequate sample from an infected wound may be challenging. Potential types of samples include superficial swabs, deep tissue cultures, sterile needle aspiration, tissue biopsy, and others.

Superficial wound swabs have been shown to have an extremely poor ability to identify the true pathogens responsible for a wound infection. In particular, if a wound has not been properly debrided, the swab may be contaminated by normal skin flora, and anaerobic or fastidious aerobic organisms may fail to grow. A meta-analysis demonstrated that superficial wound swabs had a sensitivity as low as 49 % and a specificity of 62 % to identify the causative organisms of an infection; these cultures were therefore deemed incapable of directing antimicrobial therapy [44]. Because these samples may confuse clinicians and expose the patient to unnecessarily broad antimicrobials, it is generally recommended to limit the use of wound swabs to infection control purposes and possibly to help identify future empiric regimens if the patient decompensates.

Compared to superficial wound swabs, deep tissue cultures may be more likely to identify the truly invasive and

pathogenic organism in any given case [16]. If a significant amount of fluid is present, for example, in the case of an intact abscess, an alternative method is needle aspiration which has been shown to have good sensitivity for the diagnosis of skin and soft-tissue infections [45].

The clinician may obtain valuable information from superficial or deep samples, but ultimately proper management will require close observation to assess for clinical improvement. Due to these limitations, investigators are studying the use of novel PCR- and molecular-based techniques for bacteriologic diagnoses in wound infections [46].

How to Obtain a Culture

Culture samples should be obtained only after the wound has been cleansed and debrided. If the wound is open, whenever possible the tissue sample should be obtained from the debrided base. The samples should then be sent to the laboratory in a sterile and properly labeled container for aerobic and anaerobic culture [8, 16]. Regardless of the specimen type obtained, prompt transportation to the laboratory is essential to increase the likelihood of isolating all microorganisms, in particular anaerobic bacteria.

Quantitative Significance of Colonies

As early as 1964 a study showed that an increased (>10^6 CFU/mL) bacterial load of wound cultures may be related to the progression of wound ulcers and infection [47]. Since that original study, the pendulum has swung on both sides, but the overall weight evidence demonstrates that higher CFUs are associated with increased rates of infection and inadequate wound healing. Recent studies continue to confirm this observation, with one study showing that a bacterial concentration over 10^4 CFU must be reached to cause infection in lower extremity wounds [48].

Other Diagnostic Studies

A comprehensive evaluation of the patient with a suspected wound infection is essential. This includes examination of the patient as a whole, not just focusing on the wound or affected limb. Signs and symptoms such as tachycardia, altered mentation, hypotension, or fever may be present and are suggestive of a systemic illness that warrants more aggressive care. Additionally, the work-up should include a complete blood count with differential to evaluate for a leukocytosis or a neutrophilia, erythrocyte sedimentation rate (ESR), and a C-reactive protein level (CRP). Recently, several prospective studies have shown the promising role of procalcitonin (PCT) as an indicator of bacterial infection in diabetic foot infections [8]. Jafari et al. [49] showed that PCT could help distinguish between uninfected and infected ulcers. However, PCT was found to be highest in severe diabetic foot infections, but only slightly increased in mild infections. For that reason, the highest sensitivity in distinguishing uninfected ulcers from infected ulcers was by combining PCT with another marker such as ESR or CRP [19]. If a patient appears systemically ill or is classified as having a severe infection, blood cultures should be obtained in addition to tissue culture prior to the initiation of broad-spectrum antibiotics.

Treatment

General Approach to Antibiotic Therapy

In the era of increasing antimicrobial resistance and multidrug-resistant organisms, it is imperative to exercise judicious use of antibiotics to both minimize the emergence of drug resistance and the risk to patients of adverse side effects. Whenever feasible, antibiotic therapy should be guided by microbiologic culture with antibiotic susceptibility testing. Empiric choices of antibiotics should be directed against the most common pathogens and narrowed accordingly when further microbiologic information is available.

It is important to note that not all wound infections require the use of systemic antibiotics. If the infection appears mild and there are no clinical signs of sepsis as defined by the SIRS criteria [43], then the patient may not require systemic antibiotic therapy; in this setting, local wound care or an incision and drainage (if there is evidence of localized, purulent infection) may suffice.

Conventional teaching has historically stated that a bactericidal antibiotic is preferred over a bacteriostatic antibiotic. A bactericidal antibiotic is defined as one that kills bacteria. In contrast, a bacteriostatic organism suppresses the growth of bacteria in order to allow the host's immune system to kill bacteria [50]. Although conventional wisdom has favored the use of bactericidal bacteria, for most infections outcomes using bacteriostatic versus bactericidal antibiotics are similar. Generally, it is recommended to choose a bactericidal antibiotic for infections likely to have an impaired contribution from the host immune system either due to a neutropenic or immunocompromised patient or in the setting of infections such as osteomyelitis where the immune system has impaired access to the site of infection. In all other cases, bacteriostatic and bactericidal antibiotics are likely to have similar outcomes [50, 51].

The initial choice between oral and parenteral antibiotics should be based on the clinical presentation of the patient. If the patient is defined as having a severe infection according to the IDSA/IWGDF, parenteral antibiotics are recommended. When signs of sepsis are absent, oral regimens are acceptable.

The specific choice of antibiotics will depend on the clinical history and the presentation of the patient. As discussed earlier in the chapter, *Staphylococcus aureus* and *Streptococcal* spp. are the most common microbiologic cause of infections. Accordingly, initial antibiotic therapy should be directed against these most common etiologic bacteria. Ideally, appropriate culture samples will be obtained prior to antibiotic initiation and therapy can be tapered when culture results are available.

Staphylococcus aureus

MRSA
Choosing an antibiotic that is effective against methicillin-resistant *Staphylococcus aureus* (MRSA) is recommended pending microbiologic data to further guide therapeutic decisions. Studies have shown high rates of MRSA (ranging from 15 to 74 %) in community-acquired, purulent skin and soft-tissue infections in the USA [52]. The "best" antibiotic with which to treat MRSA wound infections is not clear. A systematic review to assess for the best choice of antibiotic to treat MRSA-infected nonsurgical wounds was unable to find any difference in outcomes between those treated with vancomycin versus daptomycin [53]. The IDSA recommendations for MRSA skin and soft-tissue infections (SSTIs) suggest oral clindamycin, Bactrim, or a tetracycline (doxycycline or minocycline) for mild infections where systemic antibiotic therapy is indicated. Linezolid is available in both oral and intravenous formations but remains expensive. For more serious infections, intravenous therapy with vancomycin, daptomycin, linezolid, or ceftaroline is recommended [23]. In summary, the choice of antibiotic for MRSA disease is an interplay between disease severity, patient profile (allergies, interacting medications, comorbidities, etc.), and clinician experience (Table 46.4).

Table 46.4 Antibiotics for methicillin-resistant *Staphylococcus aureus* [24]

Antibiotic	Dose (adults)	Dose (children)	Adverse effects	Comment
Vancomycin	30 mg/kg/day in two divided doses IV	40 mg/kg/day in four divided doses IV	Nephrotoxicity Ototoxicity Red man syndrome	Drug of choice in PCN allergic patients
Daptomycin	4 mg/kg every 24 h IV	n/a	Rhabdomyolysis	Bactericidal
Linezolid	600 mg every 12 h IV or 600 mg bid po	10 mg/kg every 12 h IV or po for children <12 years	Possible serotonin syndrome when combined with SSRIs	Bacteriostatic
Clindamycin	600 mg every 8 h IV or 300–450 mg qid po	25–40 mg/kg/day in three divided doses IV or 30–40 mg/kg/day in three divided doses po		Bacteriostatic; potential of cross-resistance and emergence of resistance in erythromycin-resistant strains; inducible resistance in MRSA
Ceftaroline	600 mg bid IV	n/a		Bactericidal
Doxycycline, minocycline	100 mg bid po	Not recommended for age <8		Bacteriostatic
Trimethoprim-sulfamethoxazole	1–2 double-strength tablets BID	8–12 mg/kg/day (based on trimethoprim component) in either four divided doses IV or two divided doses po	Sulfa allergy Renal toxicity	Bactericidal

PCN penicillin, *SSRI* selective serotonin reuptake inhibitors

MSSA

If microbiologic data reveals methicillin-susceptible *Staphylococcus aureus* (MSSA), then a first-generation cephalosporin (cefalexin or cefazolin) or an antistaphylococcal semisynthetic penicillin is indicated (nafcillin, oxacillin, or dicloxacillin).

Penicillin or any of its derivatives is acceptable when microbiologic testing shows evidence of streptococcal disease (either group A *Streptococci* such as *Streptococcus pyogenes* or beta-hemolytic *Streptococci*) (Table 46.5).

Gram-Negative Infections

For Gram-negative infections, the main antibiotic coverage considerations include whether the patient is at risk for infection with *Pseudomonas aeruginosa* and if the patient has risk factors for multidrug-resistant (MDR) Gram-negative infections.

For *Pseudomonas aeruginosa*, the choice of antibiotic should ultimately be based on local antibiotic-resistant patterns. Options include piperacillin-tazobactam, a third-/fourth-generation cephalosporin with antipseudomonal activity (ceftazidime, cefepime), or a carbapenem (ertapenem is the only carbapenem without activity against *P. aeruginosa*). Fluoroquinolones are an attractive therapeutic choice given their high oral bioavailability. Unfortunately, however, resistance rates of *Pseudomonas aeruginosa* to fluoroquinolones in the USA have been found to be as high as 25 % [54]. Thus, the use of fluoroquinolones to treat *Pseudomonas* infections is only recommended in isolates that have been shown to be susceptible to fluoroquinolones (Table 46.6).

Multidrug-resistant (MDR) Gram-negative infections are an increasing global health concern. Surveillance data from the USA showed rising rates between 2003 and 2009 [55], and data from other countries show similar trends. For extended-spectrum beta-lactamase-producing (ESBL) Gram-negative infections, the bacteria will not be inhibited by commonly used, broad-spectrum Gram-negative drugs such as piperacillin-tazobactam. Third-/fourth-generation cephalosporins only have potential efficacy in treating ESBL organisms when the minimum inhibitory concentration is less than or equal to 1 [56–58]. The drug of choice for ESBL infections is a carbapenem (ertapenem, imipenem, meropenem, or doripenem).

Recent years have seen increased rates of infection with carbapenem-resistant *Enterobacteriaceae* CRE), which are highly drug resistant. For CRE infections, drugs such as colistin (polymyxin E), tigecycline, or aminoglycosides are usually necessary. Given the high toxicity of these agents, infectious disease consultation is recommended for their use.

Anaerobic infections are a less common but potentially life-threatening cause of wound infections. A number of the antibiotics discussed previously also have excellent anaerobic bacterial coverage, notably clindamycin, piperacillin-tazobactam, and the carbapenems. If an anaerobic infection is suspected, it may be warranted to add an antibiotic with anaerobic coverage.

Table 46.5 Antibiotics for use in methicillin-susceptible *Staphylococcus aureus* [24]

Antibiotic	Dose (adult)	Dose (pediatric)	Adverse effects	Comments
Cefazolin	1 g every 8 h IV	50 mg/kg/day in three divided doses		Can be given to PCN allergic patients[a]
Cephalexin	500 mg qid po	25–50 mg/kg/day four divided doses po		Can be given to PCN allergic patients[a]
Nafcillin or oxacillin	1–2 g every 4 h IV	100–150 mg/kg/day in four divided doses	Bone marrow suppression Interstitial nephritis	Parenteral drug of choice
Dicloxacillin	500 mg qid po	25–50 mg/kg/day in four divided doses po		Oral drug of choice
Clindamycin	600 mg every 8 h IV or 300–450 mg qid po	25–40 mg/kg/day in three divided doses IV or 30–40 mg/kg/day in three divided doses po		Bacteriostatic; potential of cross-resistance and emergence of resistance in erythromycin-resistant strains; inducible resistance in MRSA
Doxycycline, Minocycline	100 mg bid po	Not recommended for age <8		Bacteriostatic
Trimethoprim-sulfamethoxazole	1–2 double-strength tablets BID	8–12 mg/kg/day (based on trimethoprim component) in either four divided doses IV or two divided doses po	Sulfa allergy Renal toxicity	Bactericidal

[a]Except in those with immediate hypersensitivity (anaphylaxis); *PCN* penicillin

Table 46.6 Antibiotics for Gram-negative infections [24]

Antibiotic	Dose (adults)	Dose (pediatrics)	Adverse effects	Comments
Piperacillin-tazobactam	3.375 mg every 8 h[a]	300–400 mg/kg/day every 4–6 h		Higher dosages for *Pseudomonas*
Cephalosporins 1. Ceftazidime 2. Cefepime	1. 1–2 g IV/IM every 8 h 2. 2 g IV every 8–12 h	1. 30–50 mg/kg IV every 8 h 2. 50 mg/kg/dose IV every 12 h		Can be given to PCN allergic patients[b]
Carbapenems 1. Ertapenem 2. Doripenem 3. Meropenem 4. Imipenem-cilastatin	1. 1 g IV/IM once daily 2. 500 mg IV every 8 h 3. 2 g IV every 8 h 4. 500 mg IV every 6 h	1. 15 mg/kg IV/IM twice a day 3. 40 mg/kg IV every 8 h 4. 15–25 mg/kg/dose IV every 6 h		Inactive against *Pseudomonas* Safety/efficacy in children not established

[a]For antipseudomonal dosing, piperacillin-tazobactam must be either given 4.5 g every 6 h if infused over a 30 min period or 3.375 g every 8 h if infused over a 4 h period

[b]For those without history of immediate hypersensitivity reaction (anaphylaxis)

Topical Antibiotics and Antiseptics

Topical antiseptic and antibiotic preparations are often used in clinical practice to aid in the treatment of wound infections. Several substances have been investigated, including cadexomer-iodine, povidone-iodine preparations, honey, chlorhexidine, and silver-impregnated wound dressings. However, the majority of studies investigating these treatments suffer from a small size and various biases. A Cochrane review of these modalities in the treatment of venous ulcerations was inconclusive; the authors could not recommend for or against their routine use [59].

Osteomyelitis

Treatment of infections involving the bone is one of the most challenging aspects of the care of patients with wounds due to critical limb ischemia. The presence of osteomyelitis increases the likelihood of hospitalization and lower extremity amputation [7, 8, 60] and lengthens the recommended duration of antibiotic therapy and treatment costs [8]. Osteomyelitis of the foot and ankle is responsible for approximately 75,000 hospitalizations in the USA each year, and the economic burden of this disease process is tremendous [61].

Osteomyelitis typically occurs due to contiguous spread from a superficial wound [8, 62]. This infection has been primarily studied in patients with diabetes, because they have a high lifetime risk of developing a foot wound, and osteomyelitis complicates between 15 and 60 % of infected wounds in individuals with diabetes [7, 8, 63, 64].

Microbiology of Osteomyelitis

Superficial wound infections, especially in the setting of diabetes, are typically polymicrobial. In contrast, studies evaluating the yield of bone biopsies in patients with osteomyelitis found that 93–98 % of patients were infected with a single organism [65, 66].

Infecting organisms for osteomyelitis are similar to those of superficial wound infections and include *S. aureus*, *S. epidermidis*, *Streptococcus* spp., *Enterococcus* spp., *E. coli*, *Klebsiella pneumonia*, *Proteus* spp., *Acinetobacter* spp., and *Pseudomonas aeruginosa* [8, 65, 67–69]. Anaerobic organisms are rare in osteomyelitis, possibly due to a high rate of surgical debridement in these cases. Anaerobes have been found to represent 3–9 % of cultured organisms in various case series [67, 68].

Clinical and Laboratory Diagnosis of Osteomyelitis

Diagnosis of osteomyelitis can be challenging, as many patients are asymptomatic, the presence of vascular disease or neuropathy can mask infectious symptoms, and noninfectious chronic osteopathy can cause a similar presentation as osteomyelitis [63, 65]. Osteomyelitis should be suspected in any patient with recurrent wounds or wounds that do not respond to empiric antibiotic therapy [7, 8]. Classic signs of superficial wound infection such as fever, erythema, and increased leukocyte count are not associated with an increased likelihood of bone infection [8, 63, 65]. Purulent exudates, which can be useful to diagnose superficial wound infections, are found in less than 15 % of cases of osteomyelitis [70].

Many studies, primarily in patients with underlying diabetes, have assessed the utility of the physical exam in diagnosing osteomyelitis in individuals with a wound. Any wound with visible bone or a positive probe-to-bone (PTB) test (where a sterile, blunt, stainless steel probe is used to examine the wound for the presence of palpable bone at the base of the wound) is likely to be complicated by osteomyelitis. Several recent studies examining the likelihood ratios of the PTB test have shown that a positive test makes osteomyelitis highly likely, but a negative PTB test does not have adequate negative likelihood ratio to exclude the diagnosis [8, 63, 64, 70]. The presence of an ulcer area >2 cm on exam also increases the likelihood of osteomyelitis [63].

The combination of physical exam findings and laboratory testing may lead to a greater ability to distinguish between osteomyelitis and a superficial wound. A recent retrospective case-control study found that the presence of an ulcer depth >3 mm and ESR >60 mm/h or CRP >3.2 mg/dL had 100 % sensitivity and 55–60 % specificity for diagnosis of underlying osteomyelitis [60].

The gold standard test for diagnosis of osteomyelitis is culture and histology from a percutaneous bone biopsy sample obtained without traversal of an open wound [8, 67, 68].

Histologic changes suggestive of osteomyelitis include focal necrosis, intramedullary fibrosis, bone marrow edema, and infiltration of inflammatory cells [60, 62]. Culture of the bone from a biopsy sample allows for identification of the responsible organisms and provides antibiotic susceptibility data to guide therapy. The yield of bone culture in the literature has been reported to have a sensitivity from 50 to 100 % [66]. Although soft-tissue cultures are frequently used in clinical practice, most studies have shown that these cultures do not correlate well with bone biopsies [67–69, 71]. Indeed, the concordance between soft-tissue swabs and bone biopsies has been found to be 17–30 % in various studies [8, 68, 69]. Superficial and bone cultures appear to correlate better when *Staphylococcus aureus* is isolated, but even then concordance occurs in only 43–50 % of cultures.

Despite the documented utility of bone biopsy in guiding care of patients with osteomyelitis, many practitioners prefer to avoid biopsy due to the invasive nature of this test. Current Infectious Disease Society of America guidelines for treatment of diabetic foot osteomyelitis recommend bone biopsy for everyone in whom the diagnosis of osteomyelitis is considered, but also state that biopsy is most strongly indicated when there is uncertainty about the diagnosis of osteomyelitis, poor culture data from soft-tissue specimens, failure to respond to empiric antibiotic therapy, and mid-foot or hind-foot lesions (which are more difficult to treat, frequently lead to a high-level amputation, and often yield a good bone specimen) [8]. Obtaining accurate culture results through bone biopsy specimens has been associated with an increase rate of treatment success in patients with osteomyelitis [72].

Prebiopsy antibiotic exposure and fear that antibiotics will render cultures ineffective are often cited as a primary reason for the low proportion of osteomyelitis cases that undergo bone biopsy in clinical practice [66]. If possible, a 2-week period of antibiotics is recommended prior to obtaining a biopsy. However, two recent retrospective reviews found that prebiopsy antibiotics did not alter the diagnostic yield of bone biopsy [66, 67], suggesting that antibiotic use should not exclude the possibility of obtaining an adequate bone biopsy sample.

Radiographic Diagnosis of Osteomyelitis

A multitude of imaging tests has been studied for diagnosis of osteomyelitis (Table 46.7). Plain radiography is one of the most common imaging tests used for diagnosis of osteomyelitis due to wide availability and low cost [73]. Findings on plain radiographs that are suggestive of osteomyelitis include periosteal reaction, sclerosis, and cortical erosion [8, 63]. However, the utility of this test is limited by the fact that radiographic changes do not manifest until 2–4 weeks after

Table 46.7 Accuracy of imaging modalities for osteomyelitis

Imaging modality[a]	Sensitivity (%)	Specificity (%)
Plain radiography	22–75	33–100
99mTc-MDP bone scan	50–100	0–100
WBC scan	33–97	29–85
MRI	77–100	40–100

[a]References [61, 64, 65, 75]

the onset of infection and by a low sensitivity and specificity compared to other imaging modalities (see Table 46.7) [61, 64, 74, 75]. Due to these limitations, plain radiography is typically used to identify bony abnormalities in individuals with a superficial wound, but is not the test of choice for diagnosis of osteomyelitis.

A large number of nuclear medicine scans have been evaluated for their utility in diagnosing osteomyelitis including conventional bone scans (99mTc-MDP), labeled leukocyte (with 99mTc or 111In), and anti-granulocyte Fab fragment or monoclonal antibody scans. Various studies evaluating the utility of these tests have shown that the principal limitation is low specificity as inflammation of any cause can lead to increased uptake of the tracer substance into the bone [64, 65, 75]. Because they are labor intensive and less specific, nuclear medicine scans are typically reserved for patients for whom other imaging tests, such as MRI, are contraindicated [8].

Many studies have shown MRI to have the greatest accuracy in diagnosing osteomyelitis compared to other imaging modalities [61, 62, 64, 75]. Studies have shown that MRI is both sensitive and specific for the diagnosis of osteomyelitis [61, 64, 75]. Diagnostic findings of osteomyelitis on MRI include decreased signal intensity on T1-weighted images with increased signal intensity in the same area on fat-suppressed T2-weighted or short tau inversion recovery images [61].

A recent retrospective review compared MRI findings to histology results in 16 patients with neuropathic and ischemic ulcers who also underwent bone biopsy [62]. This study found that noncontrast MRI did not identify any cases of osteomyelitis in the setting of ischemic ulcers that had not been revascularized and that post-revascularization MRI also demonstrated low sensitivity (27.3%). Although this study raises concerns about the utility of MRI in patients with ischemia, the study included a very small number of patients and further studies should be performed.

Many newer imaging tests, including combined fluorodeoxyglucose-positron emission tomography/computed tomography and single-photon emission CT (SPECT/CT), have been investigated for utility in diagnosing osteomyelitis [74, 76–79]. Currently, however, these tests do not have sufficient data to recommend them as tests of choice for osteomyelitis.

Treatment of Osteomyelitis

Conventional wisdom has long held that surgical debridement of all infected bone following revascularization (if indicated) leads to the best outcome in treatment of osteomyelitis [8, 80–82]. Several recent studies demonstrating good outcomes with medical management alone have challenged this conception [80, 83–85], but these studies were all small and retrospective in design. Unfortunately, there are no studies that directly compare surgical to nonsurgical treatment. Currently, there is no available data to help decide between a surgical or medical strategy for treatment of osteomyelitis or to identify which patients may be at higher risk for failure of medical therapy [86]. Given this dearth of data, current guidelines recommend considering surgical options in all patients, but specify that patients without an ideal surgical target, who do not want surgery or are poor surgical candidates, or who have a limited area of osteomyelitis confined to the forefoot may be considered good candidates for medication-only therapy [8]. Patients in whom bone resection may be indicated include those with persistent sepsis, progressive bony deterioration despite antimicrobial therapy, bony destruction that has compromised the mechanics of the foot, or those who cannot tolerate prolonged antibiotics [8, 81, 82]. In patients with limb ischemia and osteomyelitis, there is a substantial body of evidence that revascularization improves rates of limb salvage, although the timing of these procedures in relation to bone debridement or resection is controversial [82].

In the absence of studies examining the optimal treatment duration for osteomyelitis, treatment durations have been determined based on expert recommendations [86]. In general, if the patient has received adequate bone resection with bone margins free of residual infection, a 2–5-day course of therapy postresection is considered adequate. If bone margins show residual infected bone, then patients can be treated with a 4–6-week course of therapy; patients who do not undergo resection typically require at least 3 months of antibiotic therapy [8]. However, length of therapy is also dependent on patient response to close clinical follow-up, and lack of improvement of superficial infection, worsening infection on imaging studies, or lack of improvement in inflammatory markers can all signal the need for increasing the duration of antimicrobial therapy [81].

Table 46.8 Culture-guided therapy for osteomyelitis

Organism	Recommended antibiotic (preferred regimens are bolded)
Anaerobe	**1. Clindamycin, 600 mg IV every 6 h** **2. Ticarcillin/clavulanate, 3.1 g IV every 4 h** 3. Cefotetan, 2 g IV every 12 h 4. Metronidazole 500 mg IV every 6 h
Enterobacteriaceae (fluoroquinolone resistant)	**1. Ticarcillin/clavulanate, 3.1 g IV every 4 h** **2. Piperacillin/tazobactam 3.375 g IV every 6 h** 3. Ceftriaxone, 2 g IV every 24 h
Enterobacteriaceae (fluoroquinolone sensitive)	**1. Ciprofloxacin 400 mg IV every 8–12 h** 2. Ceftriaxone, 2 g IV every 24 h
Pseudomonas	**1. Cefepime, 2 g IV every 8–12 h PLUS ciprofloxacin, 400 mg IV every 8–12 h** **2. Piperacillin/tazobactam 3.375 g IV every 6 h PLUS ciprofloxacin, 400 mg IV every 8–12 h** **3. Ciprofloxacin, 400 mg IV every 8–12 h** 4. Imipenem/cilastatin, 1 g IV every 8 h PLUS an aminoglycoside 5. Ceftazidime 2 g IV every 8 h
MRSA	**1. Vancomycin 1 g every 12 h** **2. Linezolid 600 mg every 12 h** 3. Trimethoprim/sulfamethoxazole, one double-strength tablet every 12 h 4. Minocycline 200 mg orally then 100 mg daily 5. Levofloxacin 750 mg IV daily plus rifampin 600 mg IV every 12 h 6. Daptomycin 6–10 mg/kg/day
MSSA	**1. Nafcillin or oxacillin, 1–2 g IV every 4 h** **2. Cefazolin 1–1.5 g IV every 6 h** 3. Ceftriaxone, 2 g IV every 24 h 4. Vancomycin 1 g IV every 12 h 5. Clindamycin 600 mg IV every 6 h
Streptococcus spp.	**1. Penicillin G, 2 to 4 million units IV every 4 h** 2. Ceftriaxone, 2 g IV every 24 h 3. Clindamycin 600 mg IV every 6 h 4. Ampicillin 2 g IV every 6 h
Enterococcus	**1. Penicillin G, 2 to 4 million units IV every 4 h PLUS gentamicin** **2. Vancomycin 1 g IV every 12 h**

Patients likely benefit from parenteral antibiotics for the treatment of osteomyelitis. However, a short course of parenteral antibiotics followed by a highly bioavailable oral regimen has been shown to be as effective as a long-term parenteral course [8, 80, 81].

No data have shown superiority of any empiric antibiotic regimen for the treatment of osteomyelitis. In the absence of culture data, treatment with broad-spectrum empiric antibiotics is recommended [8, 86] (Table 46.8). Although individual regimens have not been shown to be superior, therapy directed by results of bone culture has been associated with improved outcomes [8, 80, 85]. Unless the patient has signs of sepsis or severe infection, in the majority of cases, antibiotic therapy should be withheld until cultures can be obtained [2]. Table 46.8 lists the recommended initial antibiotic choice based on cultured organism [8, 81, 87–89].

Adjunctive therapies such as hyperbaric oxygen, growth factors, and negative pressure therapy have not been shown to improve outcomes in patients with osteomyelitis and are not currently recommended [8, 88]. Antibiotic-impregnated cement spacers and, more recently, bioabsorbable vehicles impregnated with antibiotics have been shown to be useful in patients with osteomyelitis who have undergone extensive debridement. Although the specific indications for use have not yet been determined, these therapies are likely underutilized, and they are likely to become increasingly important in the treatment of osteomyelitis in the future [8, 82, 90, 91].

References

1. Murray CK, Hinkle MK, Yun HC. History of infections associated with combat-related injuries. J Trauma. 2008;64:S221–31.
2. Wangensteen OH, Wangensteen SD. Military surgeons and surgery, old and new: an instructive chapter in management of contaminated wounds. Surgery. 1967;62:1102–24.
3. Mathiasen H. Bugs and battles during the American Civil War. Am J Med. 2012;125:111.
4. Smallman-Raynor MR, Cliff AD. Impact of infectious diseases on war. Infect Dis Clin N Am. 2004;18:341–68.
5. Calhoun JH, Murray CK, Manring MM. Multidrug-resistant organisms in military wounds from Iraq and Afghanistan. Clin Orthop Relat Res. 2008;466:1356–62.
6. Koole K, Ellerbroek PM, Lagendijk R, Leenen LP, Ekkelenkamp MB. Colonization of Libyan civil war casualties with multidrug-resistant bacteria. Clin Microbiol Infect. 2013;19:E285–7.

7. Lavery LA, Peters EJ, Armstrong DG, Wendel CS, Murdoch DP, Lipsky BA. Risk factors for developing osteomyelitis in patients with diabetic foot wounds. Diabetes Res Clin Pract. 2009;83:347–52.

8. Lipsky BA, Berendt AR, Cornia PB, et al. 2012 Infectious Diseases Society of America clinical practice guideline for the diagnosis and treatment of diabetic foot infections. Clin Infect Dis. 2012;54:e132–73.

9. Johnson JT, Yu VL. Role of anaerobic bacteria in postoperative wound infections following oncologic surgery of the head and neck. Ann Otol Rhinol Laryngol Suppl. 1991;154:46–8.

10. Zoutman D, McDonald S, Vethanayagan D. Total and attributable costs of surgical-wound infections at a Canadian tertiary-care center. Infect Control Hosp Epidemiol. 1998;19:254–9.

11. Kingsley A. The wound infection continuum and its application to clinical practice. Ostomy Wound Manage. 2003;49:1–7.

12. Bryant RA, Nix DP. Acute and chronic wounds: current management concepts. 4th ed. St. Louis, MO: Elsevier/Mosby; 2012.

13. Cutting KF, White RJ, Mahoney P, Harding KG. Clinical identification of wound infection: a Delphi approach, European Wound Management Association: Position Statement 2005.

14. Gardner SE, Frantz RA. Wound bioburden and infection-related complications in diabetic foot ulcers. Biol Res Nurs. 2008;10:44–53.

15. Glanze WD. Mosby's dictionary of medicine, nursing and health professions. 9th ed. St Louis, MO: Elsevier Health Sciences; 2012.

16. Bowler PG, Duerden BI, Armstrong DG. Wound microbiology and associated approaches to wound management. Clin Microbiol Rev. 2001;14:244–69.

17. Thomas JG, Cutting KF, Ruiz J, Leaper D, Synder RJ, Wolcott R. Advancing Your Practice: Understanding Wound Infection and the Role of Biofilm. Malvern, PA; 2008.

18. White RJ, Cutting K, Kingsley A. Topical antimicrobials in the control of wound bioburden. Ostomy Wound Manage. 2006;52:26–58.

19. Gardner SE, Frantz RA, Doebbeling BN. The validity of the clinical signs and symptoms used to identify localized chronic wound infection. Wound Repair Regen. 2001;9:178–86.

20. Mooney J. Illustrated dictionary of podiatry and foot science. Edinburgh, New York: Churchill Livingstone; 2009.

21. Jeng A, Beheshti M, Li J, Nathan R. The role of beta-hemolytic streptococci in causing diffuse, nonculturable cellulitis: a prospective investigation. Medicine (Baltimore). 2010;89:217–26.

22. Karppelin M, Siljander T, Vuopio-Varkila J, et al. Factors predisposing to acute and recurrent bacterial non-necrotizing cellulitis in hospitalized patients: a prospective case-control study. Clin Microbiol Infect. 2010;16:729–34.

23. Stevens DL, Bisno AL, Chambers HF, et al. Practice guidelines for the diagnosis and management of skin and soft tissue infections: 2014 update by the Infectious Diseases Society of America. Clin Infect Dis. 2014;59:e10–52.

24. Lipsky BA, Armstrong DG, Citron DM, Tice AD, Morgenstern DE, Abramson MA. Ertapenem versus piperacillin/tazobactam for diabetic foot infections (SIDESTEP): prospective, randomised, controlled, double-blinded, multicentre trial. Lancet. 2005;366:1695–703.

25. Daryapeyma A, Ostlund O, Wahlgren CM. Healthcare-associated infections after lower extremity revascularization. Eur J Vasc Endovasc Surg. 2014;48:72–7.

26. Ratnayake A, Samarasinghe B, Bala M. Outcomes of popliteal vascular injuries at Sri Lankan war-front military hospital: case series of 44 cases. Injury. 2014;45:879–84.

27. Christensen GJ, Bruggemann H. Bacterial skin commensals and their role as host guardians. Benefic Microbes. 2014;5:201–15.

28. Bowler PG, Davies BJ. The microbiology of infected and noninfected leg ulcers. Int J Dermatol. 1999;38:573–8.

29. Brook I, Frazier EH. Aerobic and anaerobic bacteriology of wounds and cutaneous abscesses. Arch Surg. 1990;125:1445–51.

30. Obolski U, Alon D, Hadany L, Stein GY. Resistance profiles of coagulase-negative staphylococci contaminating blood cultures predict pathogen resistance and patient mortality. J Antimicrob Chemother. 2014.

31. Brook I. A 12 year study of aerobic and anaerobic bacteria in intra-abdominal and postsurgical abdominal wound infections. Surg Gynecol Obstet. 1989;169:387–92.

32. Brook I. Microbiological studies of decubitus ulcers in children. J Pediatr Surg. 1991;26:207–9.

33. Trivedi U, Parameswaran S, Armstrong A, et al. Prevalence of multiple antibiotic resistant infections in diabetic versus nondiabetic wounds. J Pathog. 2014;2014:173053.

34. Verkade E, Kluytmans-van den Bergh M, van Benthem B, et al. Transmission of methicillin-resistant *Staphylococcus aureus* CC398 from livestock veterinarians to their household members. PLoS One. 2014;9, e100823.

35. Landelle C, Marimuthu K, Harbarth S. Infection control measures to decrease the burden of antimicrobial resistance in the critical care setting. Curr Opin Crit Care. 2014;20(5):499–506.

36. Summanen PH, Talan DA, Strong C, et al. Bacteriology of skin and soft-tissue infections: comparison of infections in intravenous drug users and individuals with no history of intravenous drug use. Clin Infect Dis. 1995;20 Suppl 2:S279–82.

37. Hohn DC, MacKay RD, Halliday B, Hunt TK. Effect of O_2 tension on microbicidal function of leukocytes in wounds and in vitro. Surg Forum. 1976;27:18–20.

38. Niinikoski J, Gottrup F, Hunt TK. The role of oxygen in wound repair. Petersfield: Wrightson Biomedical Publishing Ltd; 1991.

39. Hunt TK, Hopf HW. Wound healing and wound infection. What surgeons and anesthesiologists can do. Surg Clin North Am. 1997;77:587–606.

40. Seabrook GR, Edmiston CE, Schmitt DD, Krepel C, Bandyk DF, Towne JB. Comparison of serum and tissue antibiotic levels in diabetes-related foot infections. Surgery. 1991;110:671–6. discussion 6–7.

41. Cutting KF, White R. Defined and refined: criteria for identifying wound infection revisited. Br J Community Nurs. 2004;9:S6–15.

42. Hunt TK. Surgical wound infections: an overview. Am J Med. 1981;70:712–8.

43. Bone RC, Balk RA, Cerra FB, et al. Definitions for sepsis and organ failure and guidelines for the use of innovative therapies in sepsis. The ACCP/SCCM Consensus Conference Committee. American College of Chest Physicians/Society of Critical Care Medicine. Chest. 1992;101:1644–55.

44. Chakraborti C, Le C, Yanofsky A. Sensitivity of superficial cultures in lower extremity wounds. J Hosp Med. 2010;5:415–20.

45. Lee PC, Turnidge J, McDonald PJ. Fine-needle aspiration biopsy in diagnosis of soft tissue infections. J Clin Microbiol. 1985;22:80–3.

46. Dunyach-Remy C, Cadiere A, Richard JL, et al. Polymerase chain reaction-denaturing gradient gel electrophoresis (PCR-DGGE): a promising tool to diagnose bacterial infections in diabetic foot ulcers. Diabetes Metab. 2014;40(6):476–80.

47. Bendy Jr RH, Nuccio PA, Wolfe E, et al. Relationship of quantitative wound bacterial counts to healing of decubiti: effect of topical gentamicin. Antimicrob Agents Chemother (Bethesda). 1964;10:147–55.

48. Breidenbach WC, Trager S. Quantitative culture technique and infection in complex wounds of the extremities closed with free flaps. Plast Reconstr Surg. 1995;95:860–5.

49. Jonaidi Jafari N, Safaee Firouzabadi M, Izadi M, Safaee Firouzabadi MS, Saburi A. Can procalcitonin be an accurate diagnostic marker for the classification of diabetic foot ulcers? Int J Endocrinol Metab. 2014;12, e13376.

50. Gallagher JC, MacDougall C. Antibiotics, simplified. Sudbury: Jones and Bartlett Publishers; 2009.

51. Finberg RW, Moellering RC, Tally FP, et al. The importance of bactericidal drugs: future directions in infectious disease. Clin Infect Dis. 2004;39:1314–20.

52. Moran GJ, Krishnadasan A, Gorwitz RJ, et al. Methicillin-resistant *S. aureus* infections among patients in the emergency department. N Engl J Med. 2006;355:666–74.

53. Gurusamy KS, Koti R, Toon CD, Wilson P, Davidson BR. Antibiotic therapy for the treatment of methicillin-resistant *Staphylococcus aureus* (MRSA) in non surgical wounds. Cochrane Database Syst Rev. 2013;11, CD010427.

54. Master RN, Clark RB, Karlowsky JA, Ramirez J, Bordon JM. Analysis of resistance, cross-resistance and antimicrobial combinations for *Pseudomonas aeruginosa* isolates from 1997 to 2009. Int J Antimicrob Agents. 2011;38:291–5.

55. Pillar CM, Brown NP, Sahm DF et al. Trends towards increased resistance among clinically important gram-negative pathogens in the US; results from 10 years of TRUST surveillance (1999–2009). Abstract C2-696, Interscience Conference on Antimicrobial Agents and Chemotherapy. Boston, MA; 2010.

56. Bin C, Hui W, Renyuan Z, et al. Outcome of cephalosporin treatment of bacteremia due to CTX-M-type extended-spectrum beta-lactamase-producing *Escherichia coli*. Diagn Microbiol Infect Dis. 2006;56:351–7.

57. Labombardi VJ, Rojtman A, Tran K. Use of cefepime for the treatment of infections caused by extended spectrum beta-lactamase-producing *Klebsiella pneumoniae* and *Escherichia coli*. Diagn Microbiol Infect Dis. 2006;56:313–5.

58. Lee NY, Lee CC, Huang WH, Tsui KC, Hsueh PR, Ko WC. Cefepime therapy for monomicrobial bacteremia caused by cefepime-susceptible extended-spectrum beta-lactamase-producing Enterobacteriaceae: MIC matters. Clin Infect Dis. 2013;56:488–95.

59. O'Meara S, Al-Kurdi D, Ologun Y, Ovington LG, Martyn-St James M, Richardson R. Antibiotics and antiseptics for venous leg ulcers. Cochrane Database Syst Rev. 2013;12, CD003557.

60. Fleischer AE, Didyk AA, Woods JB, Burns SE, Wrobel JS, Armstrong DG. Combined clinical and laboratory testing improves diagnostic accuracy for osteomyelitis in the diabetic foot. J Foot Ankle Surg. 2009;48:39–46.

61. Kapoor A, Page S, Lavalley M, Gale DR, Felson DT. Magnetic resonance imaging for diagnosing foot osteomyelitis: a meta-analysis. Arch Intern Med. 2007;167:125–32.

62. Fujii M, Armsrong DG, Terashi H. Efficacy of magnetic resonance imaging in diagnosing diabetic foot osteomyelitis in the presence of ischemia. J Foot Ankle Surg. 2013;52:717–23.

63. Butalia S, Palda VA, Sargeant RJ, Detsky AS, Mourad O. Does this patient with diabetes have osteomyelitis of the lower extremity? JAMA. 2008;299:806–13.

64. Dinh MT, Abad CL, Safdar N. Diagnostic accuracy of the physical examination and imaging tests for osteomyelitis underlying diabetic foot ulcers: meta-analysis. Clin Infect Dis. 2008;47:519–27.

65. Ertugrul MB, Baktiroglu S, Salman S, et al. The diagnosis of osteomyelitis of the foot in diabetes: microbiological examination vs. magnetic resonance imaging and labelled leucocyte scanning. Diabet Med. 2006;23:649–53.

66. Marschall J, Bhavan KP, Olsen MA, Fraser VJ, Wright NM, Warren DK. The impact of prebiopsy antibiotics on pathogen recovery in hematogenous vertebral osteomyelitis. Clin Infect Dis. 2011;52:867–72.

67. Khatri G, Wagner DK, Sohnle PG. Effect of bone biopsy in guiding antimicrobial therapy for osteomyelitis complicating open wounds. Am J Med Sci. 2001;321:367–71.

68. Senneville E, Melliez H, Beltrand E, et al. Culture of percutaneous bone biopsy specimens for diagnosis of diabetic foot osteomyelitis: concordance with ulcer swab cultures. Clin Infect Dis. 2006;42:57–62.

69. Zuluaga AF, Galvis W, Jaimes F, Vesga O. Lack of microbiological concordance between bone and non-bone specimens in chronic osteomyelitis: an observational study. BMC Infect Dis. 2002;2:8.

70. Morales Lozano R, Gonzalez Fernandez ML, Martinez Hernandez D, Beneit Montesinos JV, Guisado Jimenez S, Gonzalez Jurado MA. Validating the probe-to-bone test and other tests for diagnos-

71. Malone M, Bowling FL, Gannass A, Jude EB, Boulton AJ. Deep wound cultures correlate well with bone biopsy culture in diabetic foot osteomyelitis. Diabetes Metab Res Rev. 2013;29:546–50.

72. Howard CB, Einhorn M, Dagan R, Yagupski P, Porat S. Fine-needle bone biopsy to diagnose osteomyelitis. J Bone Joint Surg (Br). 1994;76:311–4.

73. Sanverdi SE, Ergen BF, Oznur A. Current challenges in imaging of the diabetic foot. Diabet Foot Ankle. 2012;3, 18754.

74. Erdman WA, Buethe J, Bhore R, et al. Indexing severity of diabetic foot infection with 99mTc-WBC SPECT/CT hybrid imaging. Diabetes Care. 2012;35:1826–31.

75. Capriotti G, Chianelli M, Signore A. Nuclear medicine imaging of diabetic foot infection: results of meta-analysis. Nucl Med Commun. 2006;27:757–64.

76. Basu S, Chryssikos T, Houseni M, et al. Potential role of FDG PET in the setting of diabetic neuro-osteoarthropathy: can it differentiate uncomplicated Charcot's neuroarthropathy from osteomyelitis and soft-tissue infection? Nucl Med Commun. 2007;28:465–72.

77. Heiba SI, Kolker D, Mocherla B, et al. The optimized evaluation of diabetic foot infection by dual isotope SPECT/CT imaging protocol. J Foot Ankle Surg. 2010;49:529–36.

78. Keidar Z, Militianu D, Melamed E, Bar-Shalom R, Israel O. The diabetic foot: initial experience with 18F-FDG PET/CT. J Nucl Med. 2005;46:444–9.

79. Nawaz A, Torigian DA, Siegelman ES, Basu S, Chryssikos T, Alavi A. Diagnostic performance of FDG-PET, MRI, and plain film radiography (PFR) for the diagnosis of osteomyelitis in the diabetic foot. Mol Imaging Biol. 2010;12:335–42.

80. Widatalla AH, Mahadi SE, Shawer MA, Mahmoud SM, Abdelmageed AE, Ahmed ME. Diabetic foot infections with osteomyelitis: efficacy of combined surgical and medical treatment. Diabet Foot Ankle. 2012;3, 18809.

81. Hatzenbuehler J, Pulling TJ. Diagnosis and management of osteomyelitis. Am Fam Physician. 2011;84:1027–33.

82. Sagray BA, Malhotra S, Steinberg JS. Current therapies for diabetic foot infections and osteomyelitis. Clin Podiatr Med Surg. 2014;31:57–70.

83. Game FL, Jeffcoate WJ. Primarily non-surgical management of osteomyelitis of the foot in diabetes. Diabetologia. 2008;51:962–7.

84. Ulcay A, Karakas A, Mutluoglu M, Uzun G, Turhan V, Ay H. Antibiotherapy with and without bone debridement in diabetic foot osteomyelitis: a retrospective cohort study. Pak J Med Sci. 2014;30:28–31.

85. Senneville E, Lombart A, Beltrand E, et al. Outcome of diabetic foot osteomyelitis treated nonsurgically: a retrospective cohort study. Diabetes Care. 2008;31:637–42.

86. Berendt AR, Peters EJ, Bakker K, et al. Diabetic foot osteomyelitis: a progress report on diagnosis and a systematic review of treatment. Diabetes Metab Res Rev. 2008;24 Suppl 1:S145–61.

87. Kasper DL, Fauci AS, Harrison TR. Harrison's infectious diseases. 2nd ed. New York: McGraw-Hill Medical; 2013.

88. Blanes JI, Representatives of Spanish Society of Surgeons, Representatives of Spanish Society of Angiology and Vascular Surgery, et al. Consensus document on treatment of infections in diabetic foot. Rev Esp Quimioter. 2011;24:233–62.

89. Lima AL, Oliveira PR, Carvalho VC, Cimerman S, Savio E, Diretrizes Panamericanas para el Tratamiento de las Osteomielitis e Infecciones de Tejidos Blandos Group. Recommendations for the treatment of osteomyelitis. Braz J Infect Dis. 2014;18(5):526–34.

90. Melamed EA, Peled E. Antibiotic impregnated cement spacer for salvage of diabetic osteomyelitis. Foot Ankle Int. 2012;33:213–9.

91. Zalavras CG, Patzakis MJ, Holtom P. Local antibiotic therapy in the treatment of open fractures and osteomyelitis. Clin Orthop Relat Res. 2004;427:86–93.

Wound Care: Maggot Debridement Therapy

Taku Maeda and Chu Kimura

Introduction

For thousands of years, people have cleaned and disinfected wounds with the larvae (maggots) of certain dipteran flies, such as the greenbottle fly *Lucilia sericata*, a practice referred to now as maggot debridement therapy (MDT). Ancient paintings as far apart as Central America and Australia show such use. In more modern times, the inspector general of the medical department of Napoleon's army, Baron D. J. Larrey, was the first to describe the benefits of MDT in writing. In 1931, William Baer, a consultant orthopedic surgeon at Johns Hopkins Hospital in Baltimore, reported the effectiveness of MDT for chronic osteomyelitis [1]. However, with the discovery of antibiotics and subsequent development of various other treatments to promote wound healing, MDT gradually fell out of favor. Its popularity started to rise again in the late 1980s when medicinal larvae were reintroduced to combat issues with antibiotic resistance and the failure of modern wound care to heal many types of chronic infected wounds [2].

It was not until the early twenty-first century that MDT was officially approved as a treatment by the US Food and Drug Administration (FDA). According to the FDA, the indications for MDT are for "debriding non-healing necrotic skin and soft tissue wounds, including pressure ulcers, and non-healing traumatic of post-surgical wounds." (http://www.accessdata.fda.gov/cdrh_docs/pdf10/K102827.pdf). MDT is now a widely accepted practice that has three primary effects: debridement, disinfection, and growth stimulation [3]. Although ischemia has been considered a relative contraindication for larval therapy [4], a number of recent studies have reported its effectiveness for critical limb ischemia (CLI) [5, 6]. This extension of the applications of MDT is supported by laboratory studies suggesting that maggot excretions/secretions may play a role in wound healing by stimulating angiogenesis [7].

Effects of Larval Secretions

Although the mechanisms of MDT are not yet fully understood, what is apparent is that necrotic tissue is selectively eliminated through the action of proteolytic enzymes in maggot saliva, and bacteria present in the wound are destroyed by maggot secretions, which include an antimicrobial peptide [8, 9]. While the efficacy of MDT for debridement has been proven in randomized clinical trials [10], the evidence for antimicrobial activity from the use of maggots comes mainly from laboratory studies [11].

Larval Secretions Disrupt Bacterial Biofilms

Tough, protective biofilms formed by microcolonies of bacteria can contribute to the chronicity of wounds [12] as many topical treatments and systemic antibiotics are ineffective against them. Yet, a promising way forward has been found in that the secretions of larvae used in MDT have been demonstrated to disrupt even established biofilms and break them down [13–15]. These secretions can also prevent the biofilms from forming.

Of particular promise is the recent finding that chymotrypsin derived from larval secretions functioned to disrupt the protein-dependent mechanisms underlying biofilm formation. In fact, recombinant chymotrypsin showed optimal effect for *Staphylococcus epidermidis* 5179-R1, on both nascent and established biofilms [16]. A DNAse component of the secretions may also play a role.

T. Maeda, Doctor (✉) • C. Kimura, Doctor
Plastic and Reconstructive Surgery, Hakodate General Central Hospital, 33-2, Honmachi, Hakodate City, Hokkaido, Japan

© Springer International Publishing Switzerland 2017
R.S. Dieter et al. (eds.), *Critical Limb Ischemia*, DOI 10.1007/978-3-319-31991-9_47

Larval Secretions Inhibit Inflammatory Processes

Tissue healing requires activation of the complement system, a system which is crucial to activating the inflammatory response to injury. Prolonged inflammation that can contribute to further tissue damage [17, 18] can sometimes occur due to abnormal complement system activation. Larval secretions have been shown to break down several inappropriate complement components, helping to alleviate this abnormal activation [19]. They can also—in a dose-dependent manner—increase anti-inflammatory cytokines (e.g., interleukin-10) and decrease pro-inflammatory cytokines (e.g., interleukin-12 and tumor necrosis factor-alpha, TNF-α) [20, 21].

Larval Secretions Affect Fibroblast Migration, Angiogenesis, and Growth Factor Production

Larval secretions also contain serine protease activity. In two-dimensional and three-dimensional cultures, this activity can significantly affect the motogenesis of fibroblasts [22, 23]. Larval secretions may also exert pro-angiogenic effects. In an ex vivo model of wound healing, increased phosphotyrosine expression at the migrating cell front suggested that the secretions activate the PI3K/AKT1 protein kinase pathway that probably mediates fibroblast motogenesis [24]. PI3K itself was activated by several pro-angiogenic factors [24].

In 2010, Bexfield et al. demonstrated for the first time that the amino acid-like compounds, amino acids L-histidine, 3-guanidinopropionic acid, and L-valinol, present in maggot excretions/secretions, may contribute to wound healing by stimulating angiogenesis [7]. Other studies have also demonstrated the pro-angiogenic activity of the secretions. Three days after applying dried extracts of *L. sericata* larvae to dermal excision wounds, Zhang et al. observed a significant increase in the upregulation of vascular endothelial growth factor (VEGF) expression [25]. Van der Plas et al. also reported enhanced production of VEGF and other growth factors by monocytes and macrophages with larval secretion treatment [21]. Moreover, alongside low levels of pro-inflammatory cytokines such as TNF-α, these growth factors mediate endothelial cell migration and proliferation, both of which are essential processes for angiogenesis [26]. Taken together, the evidence to date indicates that larval secretions not only stimulate the migration of fibroblast and keratinocytes but also exert pro-angiogenic effects and increase the production of growth factors.

Maggot

MDT makes use of sterile maggots, either fly larvae or immature flies. The flies most often used for maggot therapy are "blow flies" (family Calliphoridae); the species most commonly used is *L. sericata*. The maggots are bred and grown in the laboratory setting and are therefore safe to use with patients. They innately attach themselves only to necrotic tissue. Even if they were to leave the confines of the wound, they would not transform into adults and fly away.

Practical Considerations and Use (Fig. 47.1)

1. It is important to attach a hydrogel wound dressing to the tissue surrounding the wound. This prevents the maggots leaving the confines of the wound, by acting as a barrier around the edges, and prevents the exudate from causing dermatitis.
2. With a fine brush, maggots measuring 1–2 mm in length are placed on the wound. Before MDT is started, the maggots are usually maintained asleep under cold temperatures. Sleeping maggots can be placed on the wound easily. Typically, the "dosage" is 5–10 larvae/cm^2 for a necrotic ulcer.
3. A special dressing with a mesh is then applied to the wound containing the maggots. It is important to dress the wound securely enough to prevent the maggots from leaving the wound. Exudate from the wound passes to the outside through the mesh, where it is absorbed by a gauze dressing added to the special dressing.
4. Maggots are removed 2–3 days after placement, when they are fully grown to about 10 mm.
5. This is one treatment cycle. The treatment is usually repeated continuously for about 2–4 weeks. Another procedure using a "biobag," where the larvae are contained in a bag, is another option [27].

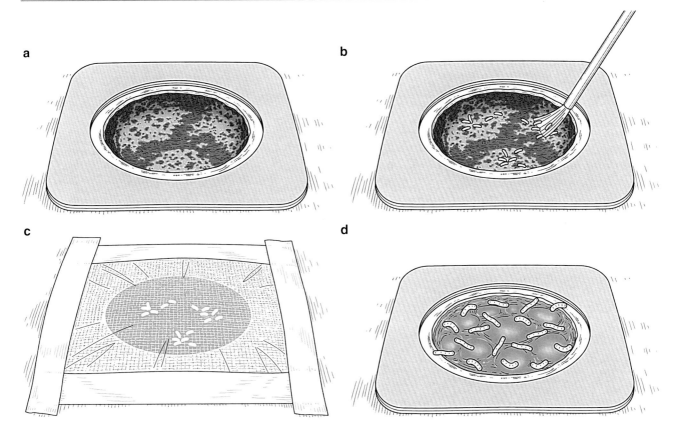

Fig. 47.1 Schema of the procedure in maggot debridement therapy. (**a**) The dressing is attached around the wound; (**b**) maggots are placed on the ischemic wound with a fine brush; (**c**) the wound with maggots placed on it is covered with a special dressing with a mesh; and (**d**) maggots are removed 2–3 days later, when they are fully grown to about 10 mm in length

MDT for CLI

CLI, the most advanced form of peripheral arterial disease, is defined as the presence of chronic ischemic rest pain, ulcer, or gangrene attributable to objectively proven arterial occlusive disease [28]. Management aims to relieve the ischemic pain, heal the ulcer, prevent limb loss, improve function and quality of life, and prolong survival. The mainstay of CLI therapy is revascularization. However, when revascularization is not technically feasible or when all previous revascularization attempts have failed, additional and supplementary therapy should be considered. Hyperbaric therapy, spinal cord stimulation [29], and intermittent pneumatic compression [30] have been variously proposed.

It had been thought that MDT is contraindicated for ischemic ulcer [4], but an increasing number of recent reports have documented its effectiveness for the treatment of these ulcers [5, 31]. Figure 47.2 illustrates a case of successful treatment of MDT for CLI. To evaluate the ischemic stage of an ischemic ulcer, skin perfusion pressure (SPP) is gaining popularity. SPP is the perfusion pressure at the level of the skin and serves as an index of peripheral circulation in the skin and subcutaneous tissue; in this noninvasive measurement, laser Doppler measures the blood pressure at the capillary level [32]. Therefore, an increase in SPP indicates increased blood supply at the skin level and improved peripheral circulation. A recent report described an increase in SPP after MDT for CLI(6) in the clinical setting. Thus, taking together the abovementioned laboratory findings and the elevation of SPP seen clinically with MDT, it would seem that MDT can improve local perfusion in patients with CLI. This would make ischemic ulcer a good candidate for MDT. However, since the number of reports exploring the effectiveness of MDT for CLI is still limited, more clinical data should be accumulated and the efficacy and safety of MDT for CLI needs to be properly assessed in future trials.

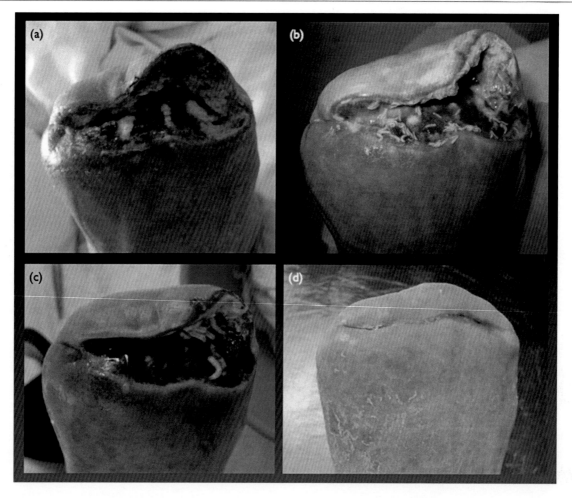

Fig. 47.2 Clinical course of a 78-year-old man with a severe ulcer on the left foot who received maggot debridement therapy [6]. (**a**) Condition 2 months after modified transmetatarsal amputation; (**b**) maggots placed on the ischemic wound; (**c**) 2 days after initial maggot placement; and (**d**) 6 months after maggot debridement therapy. From Maeda TM et al. Increase in skin perfusion pressure after maggot debridement therapy for critical limb ischemia. Clin Exp Dermatol. 2014:911–914. © 2014 British Association of Dermatologists, reprinted with permission from John Wiley and Sons

References

1. Baer WS. The classic: the treatment of chronic osteomyelitis with the maggot (larva of the blow fly). 1931. Clin Orthop Relat Res. 2011;469(4):920–44.
2. Sherman RA, Pechter EA. Maggot therapy: a review of the therapeutic applications of fly larvae in human medicine, especially for treating osteomyelitis. Med Vet Entomol. 1988;2(3):225–30.
3. Sherman RA. Mechanisms of maggot-induced wound healing: what do we know, and where do we go from here? Evid Based Complement Alternat Med. 2014;2014:592419.
4. Sherman RA. Maggot therapy for foot and leg wounds. Int J Low Extrem Wounds. 2002;1(2):135–42.
5. Nordstrom A, Hansson C, Karlstrom L. Larval therapy as a palliative treatment for severe arteriosclerotic gangrene on the feet. Clin Exp Dermatol. 2009;34(8):e683–5.
6. Maeda TM, Kimura CK, Takahashi KT, Ichimura KI. Increase in skin perfusion pressure after maggot debridement therapy for critical limb ischaemia. Clin Exp Dermatol. 2014;39(8):911–4.

7. Bexfield A, Bond AE, Morgan C, Wagstaff J, Newton RP, Ratcliffe NA, et al. Amino acid derivatives from Lucilia sericata excretions/secretions may contribute to the beneficial effects of maggot therapy via increased angiogenesis. Br J Dermatol. 2010;162(3):554–62.
8. Mumcuoglu KY, Miller J, Mumcuoglu M, Friger M, Tarshis M. Destruction of bacteria in the digestive tract of the maggot of Lucilia sericata (Diptera: Calliphoridae). J Med Entomol. 2001;38(2):161–6.
9. Mumcuoglu KY. Clinical applications for maggots in wound care. Am J Clin Dermatol. 2001;2(4):219–27.
10. Dumville JC, Worthy G, Bland JM, Cullum N, Dowson C, Iglesias C, et al. Larval therapy for leg ulcers (VenUS II): randomised controlled trial. BMJ. 2009;338:b773.
11. Cazander G, Pritchard DI, Nigam Y, Jung W, Nibbering PH. Multiple actions of Lucilia sericata larvae in hard-to-heal wounds: larval secretions contain molecules that accelerate wound healing, reduce chronic inflammation and inhibit bacterial infection. Bioessays. 2013;35(12):1083–92.
12. Leaper DJ, Schultz G, Carville K, Fletcher J, Swanson T, Drake R. Extending the TIME concept: what have we learned in the past 10 years?(*). Int Wound J. 2012;9 Suppl 2:1–19.

13. James GA, Swogger E, Wolcott R, Pulcini E, Secor P, Sestrich J, et al. Biofilms in chronic wounds. Wound Repair Regen. 2008;16(1):37–44.
14. Cazander G, van de Veerdonk MC, Vandenbroucke-Grauls CM, Schreurs MW, Jukema GN. Maggot excretions inhibit biofilm formation on biomaterials. Clin Orthop Relat Res. 2010;468(10):2789–96.
15. Harris LG, Bexfield A, Nigam Y, Rohde H, Ratcliffe NA, Mack D. Disruption of Staphylococcus epidermidis biofilms by medicinal maggot Lucilia sericata excretions/secretions. Int J Artif Organs. 2009;32(9):555–64.
16. Harris LG, Nigam Y, Sawyer J, Mack D, Pritchard DI. Lucilia sericata chymotrypsin disrupts protein adhesin-mediated staphylococcal biofilm formation. Appl Environ Microbiol. 2013;79(4):1393–5.
17. Trouw LA, Daha MR. Role of complement in innate immunity and host defense. Immunol Lett. 2011;138(1):35–7.
18. Markiewski MM, Lambris JD. The role of complement in inflammatory diseases from behind the scenes into the spotlight. Am J Pathol. 2007;171(3):715–27.
19. Cazander G, Schreurs MW, Renwarin L, Dorresteijn C, Hamann D, Jukema GN. Maggot excretions affect the human complement system. Wound Repair Regen. 2012;20(6):879–86.
20. van der Plas MJ, van der Does AM, Baldry M, Dogterom-Ballering HC, van Gulpen C, van Dissel JT, et al. Maggot excretions/secretions inhibit multiple neutrophil pro-inflammatory responses. Microbes Infect/Inst Pasteur. 2007;9(4):507–14.
21. van der Plas MJ, van Dissel JT, Nibbering PH. Maggot secretions skew monocyte-macrophage differentiation away from a pro-inflammatory to a pro-angiogenic type. PloS one. 2009;4(11), e8071.
22. Horobin AJ, Shakesheff KM, Pritchard DI. Maggots and wound healing: an investigation of the effects of secretions from Lucilia sericata larvae upon the migration of human dermal fibroblasts over a fibronectin-coated surface. Wound Repair Regen. 2005;13(4):422–33.
23. Horobin AJ, Shakesheff KM, Pritchard DI. Promotion of human dermal fibroblast migration, matrix remodelling and modification of fibroblast morphology within a novel 3D model by Lucilia sericata larval secretions. J Invest Dermatol. 2006;126(6):1410–8.
24. Wang SY, Wang K, Xin Y, Lv DC. Maggot excretions/secretions induces human microvascular endothelial cell migration through AKT1. Mol Biol Rep. 2010;37(6):2719–25.
25. Zhang Z, Wang S, Diao Y, Zhang J, Lv D. Fatty acid extracts from Lucilia sericata larvae promote murine cutaneous wound healing by angiogenic activity. Lipids Health Dis. 2010;9:24.
26. Sunderkotter C, Steinbrink K, Goebeler M, Bhardwaj R, Sorg C. Macrophages and angiogenesis. J Leukoc Biol. 1994;55(3):410–22.
27. Grassberger M, Fleischmann W. The biobag – a new device for the application of medicinal maggots. Dermatology. 2002;204(4):306.
28. Becker F, Robert-Ebadi H, Ricco JB, Setacci C, Cao P, de Donato G, et al. Chapter I: Definitions, epidemiology, clinical presentation and prognosis. Eur J Vasc Endovasc Surg. 2011;42 Suppl 2:S4–12.
29. Ubbink DT, Vermeulen H. Spinal cord stimulation for non-reconstructable chronic critical leg ischaemia. Cochrane Database Syst Rev. 2013;2, CD004001.
30. Kavros SJ, Delis KT, Turner NS, Voll AE, Liedl DA, Gloviczki P, et al. Improving limb salvage in critical ischemia with intermittent pneumatic compression: a controlled study with 18-month follow-up. J Vasc Surg. 2008;47(3):543–9.
31. Igari K, Toyofuku T, Uchiyama H, Koizumi S, Yonekura K, Kudo T, et al. Maggot debridement therapy for peripheral arterial disease. Ann Vasc Dis. 2013;6(2):145–9.
32. Malvezzi L, Castronuovo Jr JJ, Swayne LC, Cone D, Trivino JZ. The correlation between three methods of skin perfusion pressure measurement: radionuclide washout, laser Doppler flow, and photoplethysmography. J Vasc Surg. 1992;15(5):823–9. Discussion 9–30.

Medical Therapy for Critical Limb Ischemia

48

Gianluca Rigatelli, Sara R. Shah, Amsa Arshad, Nisa Arshad, and Thach Nguyen

Background

Critical limb ischemia (CLI) is defined as the combination of evidence of ischemia together with any conditions of rest pain, nonhealing ulcers, or gangrene in the lower extremities. CLI leads to an amputation rate of 14–20% and a death rate of 25% within the first year and 50% within 5 years.

The aims of management in patients with CLI are to relieve ischemic pain, heal ulcers, prevent limb loss, reduce mortality, and improve function and quality of life [1, 2].

Management

Current recommendations state that all patients with CLI must receive antiplatelet therapy, stop smoking, and be screened and treated for hyperlipidemia, along with hypertension (HTN) and diabetes mellitus (DM), in addition to modification of lifestyle (Table 48.1).

G. Rigatelli, MD, PhD
Cardiovascular Diagnosis and Endoluminal Interventions Unit, Rovigo General Hospital, viale Tre Martiri, Rovigo 45100, Italy

S.R. Shah
Department of Cardiology, Community Hospital, Munster, IN 46321, USA

A. Arshad, MD • N. Arshad, MD
Cardiology, St. Mary's Medical Center, 1500 S Lake Ave, Hobart, IN 46342, USA

T. Nguyen, MD (✉)
Cardiology, Cardiovascular Clinics, 200 E 86th Place, Merrillville, IN 46410, USA

Table 48.1 Management of CLI

Antiplatelet therapy
ASA 81 mg
Lipid control
Initiate statin therapy regardless of lipid levels.
Blood pressure control
Systolic blood pressure <120 mmHg
Diastolic blood pressure <80 mmHg
Glycemic control
HbA1C <7%

Lifestyle Modification

Smoking

The degree of damage caused by smoking is directly related to the amount of tobacco consumed. When CLI is identified in a critical clinical setting, smoking cessation is an important modifiable behavior that may impact subsequent vascular or endovascular interventions. Patients with CLI must refrain from smoking. Smoking cessation improves walking distance, doubles the 5-year survival rate [3], and reduces the incidence of postoperative complications [4]. More than 75% of patients presenting with CLI have tried and failed to quit smoking. Up to 25% of patients will try to follow clinical advice to stop smoking, but more than 75% of them will fail in less than 3 months [5]. With medical advice alone, approximately 5% of patients will have long-term success in quitting. However, the urgency of management for CLI prevents smoking cessation from having time to take effect.

Hyperlipidemia

Increasing concentrations of each of the lipid components—cholesterol, low-density lipoprotein (LDL), triglyceride, and lipoprotein (a)—have shown to be independent factors for acceleration of CLI [6]. So treatment with statins helps to prevent plaque instability and thrombosis due to their pleiotropic effects, such as improvement of endothelial function, reduction of inflammation, and stabilization of atherosclerotic

© Springer International Publishing Switzerland 2017
R.S. Dieter et al. (eds.), *Critical Limb Ischemia*, DOI 10.1007/978-3-319-31991-9_48

plaques [7]. In a retrospective review for CLI patients undergoing endovascular interventions (highlighted below), statin use was associated with significantly higher rates of patency, limb salvage, and overall survival [8]. Perioperative statin treatment in statin-naive patients reduces atrial fibrillation, MI, and duration of hospital stay [9].

Evidence-Based Medicine: Effect of Statins on Endovascular Interventions for Critical Limb Ischemia [8]

This is a retrospective review of 646 patients, 319 receiving statin therapy and 327 without, who underwent an endovascular intervention for CLI. The statin group had significantly higher rates of DM, coronary artery disease (CAD), congestive heart failure (CHF), previous myocardial infarction (MI), and coronary artery bypass grafting (CABG) ($P<0.05$). The two groups had similar lesion length, location, lesion type, TransAtlantic Inter-Society Consensus (TASC) classification, and primary procedure. At 24 months, the statin-treated group had higher rates of primary patency (43% vs 33%; $P=0.007$), secondary patency (66% vs 51%; $P=0.001$), limb salvage (83% vs 62%; $P=0.001$), and overall survival (77% vs 62%; $P=0.038$). Therefore, statin therapy was proven to be beneficial with improved limb salvage and mortality in patients undergoing endovascular intervention for CLI [8].

Hypertension

Control of blood pressure remains an important intervention for cardiovascular (CV) primary prevention and also has been established as one of the principal improvements in stroke and PAD reduction. Current HTN guidelines advocate aggressive treatment in patients with atherosclerosis. The angiotensin-converting enzyme inhibitor (ACEI) ramipril (10 mg/day) has been shown to increase pain-free walking distance, maximum walking time, and Walking Improvement Questionnaire scores in a small randomized placebo-controlled study [9]. This has been replicated in a larger study where ramipril 10 mg/day increased the mean of pain-free walking time by 92% (87 s) and the maximum walking time by 139% (193 s) [10]. Calcium channel blockers are protective against all-cause, CV, and cerebrovascular disease mortality [11].

Critical Thinking: Beta-Blockers in CLI

There is currently no evidence that beta-blockers (BB) adversely affect walking distance in patients with CLI. Two meta-analyses of studies involving patients with mild and moderate lower-limb ischemia did not confirm that BBs were associated with exacerbation of PAD symptoms [12, 13]. As a result of these trials, beta-1-specific BBs are now commonly prescribed for the treatment of HTN in PAD patients. The clinical value of administering perioperative beta-blockers was shown to be associated with significant reductions of perioperative myocardial ischemia and infarction in various surgical settings [14, 15]. In patients undergoing vascular surgery or major amputation, with low to intermediate cardiac risk, preoperative targeted beta-blockade alone is more effective in preventing cardiac morbidity than selective cardiac stress testing and non-targeted beta-blockade [16].

Diabetes Mellitus

DM is independently associated with the development of PAD and its progression to CLI. DM has also been shown to be an independent risk factor for amputation and increased complications in CLI patients. In the STENO-2 study, 160 diabetics were randomly assigned to either intensified or conventional therapy (i.e., control of blood glucose, statins, antithrombotic therapy, blood pressure control). On follow-up, intensive therapy was associated with significantly reduced risks of all-cause death and CV death [17]. In the United Kingdom Prospective Diabetes Study, therapy was associated with risk reductions for microvascular disease, MI, and death from any cause as well as for any diabetes-related endpoint [18]. On the contrary, in the Action in Diabetes and Vascular Disease: Preterax and Diamicron MR Controlled Evaluation (ADVANCE) trial, the rates of microvascular complications were improved by intensive diabetes therapy during a follow-up of 5 years [19]. However, this treatment did not lower macrovascular complications or cardiovascular deaths. The benefits of tight diabetes control on functional lower-limb outcomes such as limb salvage or freedom from repeated revascularization in CLI patients has not been determined.

Medical Therapy

Antithrombotic Agents

There is a direct clinical benefit of antiplatelet therapy for primary CV prevention; however, there is currently no convincing data showing a delay or reduction of the progression in lower-limb disease. The Clopidogrel versus Aspirin in Patients at Risk of Ischemic Events trial (CAPRIE) confirmed that the combined risk of death from vascular causes, MI, and stroke was significantly lower with clopidogrel (75 mg/day) than compared with aspirin (325 mg/day). These benefits were most pronounced in patients with PAD [20]. The Antithrombotic Trialists' Collaboration meta-analysis found a 23% reduction in serious vascular events within 42 trials [21]. However, there was no significant reduction of CV events in patients with PAD. In a subsequent analysis, which included study data on various antiplatelet drugs such as aspirin, clopidogrel, ticlopidine, and dipyridamole, the group reported a 23% risk reduction of CV events in patients with PAD [22]. Low-dose aspirin (75–325 mg) is similarly effective as a higher dose in PAD patients. However, higher doses of aspirin will result in increased bleeding rates and very low doses (<75 mg) are not effective. The daily dose of clopidogrel for secondary prevention in PAD patients is 75 mg. Compared to aspirin alone, dual antiplatelet therapy (DAT) was associated with a lower rate of a composite of index graft occlusion or revascularization, above-ankle amputation of the affected limb, or death, without increasing bleeding risks [23].

Evidence-Based Medicine: Antiplatelet Therapy for CLI

Two RCTs analyzed whether or not antiplatelet therapy may improve patency rates subsequent to lower-limb endovascular therapy. In the first study, a total of 199 patients undergoing angioplasty of the femoropopliteal segment were randomized to three groups: dipyridamole (75 mg) plus aspirin (330 mg), dipyridamole (75 mg) plus aspirin (100 mg), or placebo. Patients from both dipyridamole arms showed higher patency rates as compared to those on placebo [24]. In the second study, of patients randomized to placebo or aspirin (50 mg) plus dipyridamole (400 mg) after peripheral vascular angioplasty, there were no significant differences in primary patency [25]. The Coronary Artery Spasm in Patients with Acute Coronary Syndrome (CASPAR) study randomized a total of 425 patients undergoing below-the-knee bypass grafting to either aspirin (75–100 mg/day) alone or aspirin (75–100 mg/day) plus clopidogrel (75 mg/day) [26]. Unfortunately, the combination of clopidogrel plus aspirin did not improve lower-limb or systemic outcomes.

Anticoagulants

Evidence of the effects of warfarin in patients with atherosclerosis comes mainly from trials of patients with coronary artery disease (CAD). Two meta-analyses demonstrated that warfarin at both moderate- and high-intensity levels reduces the risk of death, MI, or stroke, but this is counteracted by an increased rate of bleeding [27, 28]. In a study comparing the efficacy of warfarin (with a target international normalized ratio of 3.0–4.5) with aspirin (80 mg) on infra-inguinal graft patency in patients with PAD, a similar number of graft occlusions occurred in each group [29]. On the other hand, the risk of bleeding was almost doubled in the oral anticoagulation group. A Cochrane systematic review examined the use of heparin products for intermittent claudication [30]. The use of heparins was not associated with a significant difference in CV events compared with placebo. Therefore, the use of warfarin and heparin is not recommended in patients with intermittent claudication.

Antithrombotic Agents After Bypass or Angioplasty and Stenting

Antiplatelet agents have a beneficial effect on graft or stent patency. The relative risk of infra-inguinal graft occlusion in patients treated with aspirin was 0.78 in one meta-analysis [31].

A recent Cochrane review demonstrated that antiplatelet agents improved graft patency rates to a greater extent in patients with prosthetic grafts compared to those with venous grafts [32]. From the same review, it was also concluded that there was no statistically significant improvement in survival or CV events in those treated with aspirin following bypass surgery. Henceforth, aspirin is recommended for patients undergoing lower-limb angioplasty. Belch et al. [22] investigated the use of adjuvant combination clopidogrel and aspirin therapy following below-knee bypass graft surgery. They found that, in the population as a whole, the combination did not show an improvement in the composite primary endpoint of index graft occlusion or revascularization, above-ankle amputation, or death compared with aspirin alone. However, the combination did improve outcome in a subgroup analysis of patients with prosthetic grafts, without significantly increasing major bleeding rates. The evidence for use of adjuvant anticoagulation has been summarized in a recent Cochrane review [33]. It was concluded that patients undergoing infrainguinal venous grafts are more likely to benefit from vitamin K antagonists such as warfarin than platelet inhibitors; this difference is not seen in those with artificial grafts.

Claudication Relief

Prostanoids

Prostanoids act by preventing platelet and leukocyte activation and protect the vascular endothelium. A recent systematic review and meta-analysis of the use of prostanoids for CLI included 20 RCTs with a total of 2724 participants [34]. The trials investigated intravenous prostaglandin (PG) E1, intra-arterial PGE1, intravenous iloprost, low-dose iloprost infusion, oral iloprost, intravenous prostacyclin (PGI2), lipoecraprost, and ciprostene. The comparators were placebo and other pharmacological agents. The findings of the meta-analysis showed that prostanoids when compared with placebo appeared to have some efficacy for treating rest pain (RR 1.32, 95 % CI 1.10–1.57) and ulcer healing (RR 1.54, 95 % CI 1.22–1.96). There was no statistically significant effect on the number of amputations and mortality when prostanoids were examined as a group, but iloprost showed favorable results in reducing major (above-/below-knee) amputations (RR 0.69, 95 % CI 0.52–0.93). Therefore, there is no conclusive evidence based on a high-quality meta-analysis of homogeneous long-term RCTs, regarding efficacy and safety of different prostanoids in patients with CLI, and further high-quality trials are required.

Pentoxifylline

It has been reported that pentoxifylline (Trental, Sanofi, Paris France) improves blood flow by increasing blood cell deformity and decreasing viscosity. In one study, pentoxifylline 600 mg given intravenously twice daily to patients with CLI was associated with reduced pain scores [35]. However, no significant benefit was demonstrated in another study of the same dosing regimen [36]. Therefore, there is currently a lack of consistent evidence to recommend the use of pentoxifylline for the treatment of CLI.

Cilostazol

Cilostazol (Pletal by Otsuka, Tokyo, Japan) is used to treat the symptoms of intermittent claudication, but its use for CLI is less well studied. In a small study of the effect of cilostazol treatment on skin perfusion pressure in severely ischemic limbs, it was found that the drug improved microvascular circulation [37]. However, there is no strong evidence that cilostazol improves clinical outcomes in patients with CLI. In a retrospective analysis of data from 618 patients who underwent endovascular stenting for CLI (356 of whom were treated with cilostazol at the discretion of the surgeon), 5-year outcomes were compared between those who were prescribed cilostazol and those who were not. Treatment with cilostazol was associated with higher rates of amputation-free survival and limb salvage but not overall survival or freedom from repeat revascularization [38]. In the absence of RCTs in patients with CLI, there is insufficient evidence to recommend the use of cilostazol in this patient group.

Naftidrofuryl

A recent Cochrane review of intravenous administration of naftidrofuryl included eight trials with a total of 269 participants [39]. The trials were generally of low quality, and the duration of treatment was short. A number of endpoints were studied and showed statistically nonsignificant trends toward reduction in pain and necrosis scores. Therefore, there is currently insufficient evidence to support the use of the drug for treatment of CLI.

Pain Relief

Opiate analgesia is one of the main medications in treating resistant pain in CLI patients with no other options. A slow-release opiate such as morphine seems a good option. Opiates can be supplemented by nonsteroidal anti-inflammatory drugs if these are not contraindicated. About 20–30 % of patients with CLI have non-revascularized disease; phantom limb pain may complicate major amputation. In this situation, amitriptyline hydrochloride and carbamazepine are well known to help. Propionyl-L-carnitine (PLC) has been shown to be efficacious in improving pain-free walking distance in PAD with claudication; it also exerts favorable effects on the arterial wall and on

endothelial function. In a recent series, it has been demonstrated to improve microcirculation (postischemic hyperemia, TcPO2 and TcPCO2 production). PLC also enhances endothelium-dependent dilation and reduces analgesic consumption and pain perception [40]. Gabapentin 300 mg twice a day is a useful adjuvant in the management of CLI and leads to significant reductions in pain scores and improves night pain for most patients [41].

Spinal Cord Stimulation (SCS)

Electrical neuromodulation is defined as a therapeutic modality that aims to restore functions of the nervous system or modulate neural structures involved in the dysfunction of organ systems. Patients with CLI and PAD are eligible for SCS when they experience disabling pain, resulting from ischemia. This pain should be considered therapeutically refractory to standard treatment intended to decrease metabolic demand or following revascularization procedures. Several studies have demonstrated the beneficial effect of SCS on CLI and PAD by improving the quality of life of this group of severely disabled patients, without adversely influencing mortality and morbidity. The SCS implantation technique is relatively simple. An epidural electrode is implanted under local anesthesia (supervised by the anesthetist) with the tip at T10-11 T1, covering the painful area with paresthesia by external stimulation (pulse width 210, rate 85 Hz) and connecting this electrode to a subcutaneously implanted pulse generator. All patients should be therapeutically refractory (medication and revascularization) to become eligible for SCS. Ulcers on the extremities should be minimal. In PAD the majority of the patients show significant reduction in pain, and more than half of the patients show improvement of circulatory indices, as shown by Doppler, thermography, and oximetry studies. Limb salvage studies show variable results depending on the stage of the trophic changes [42].

Hyperbaric Therapy

There is no proven benefit of hyperbaric oxygen in CLI. A Cochrane review of the effect of hyperbaric oxygen on ulcer healing in patients with DM concluded that the therapy increased the rate of ulcer healing at 6 weeks but not at 1 year, and there was no significant difference in the risk of major amputation [43]. The TASC II guidelines advocate considering hyperbaric oxygen in selected patients who have not responded to revascularization [44].

Gene Therapy

In the last 10 years, there has been a great deal of research into the usefulness of growth factors and gene transfer to promote angiogenesis and improve blood flow for the treatment of CLI. A number of Phase I clinical trials and long-term follow-up studies have evaluated the safety and potential efficacy of a variety of growth factors including hepatocyte growth factor (HGF) [45], vascular endothelial growth factor (VEGF) [46], and FGF1 [47], or a combination of growth factors [48]. The majority of these studies have shown that the treatments are safe, and in some, there was an indication of potential benefit. A few small RCTs of HGF have demonstrated improvements in pain scores and toe–brachial index compared with placebo [49, 50]. In a larger RCT ($n = 104$), it was found that HGF was not associated with significant differences in ankle–brachial or toe–brachial index, pain relief, or wound healing compared with placebo, although these were secondary endpoints [51]. Further large RCTs are needed to evaluate their efficacy.

Cell Therapy

Stem-cell therapy has been identified as a potential new treatment option to induce angiogenesis, and this possibility has been investigated in a number of trials. A meta-analysis of trials involving patients with PAD has shown that autologous stem-cell therapy was effective in improving a variety of parameters [52]. A number of pilot studies have been performed specifically in patients with CLI. The majority of these studies used granulocyte colony-stimulating factor to mobilize peripheral blood mononuclear cells [53], endothelial progenitor cells [54], or CD34+ cells [55], which are subsequently injected intramuscularly. In the majority of studies, it has been shown that the techniques are safe, and there is some indication that they may be effective in improving tissue perfusion and reducing amputation rates. In older patients the treatment seems to increase the rate of AMI, heart failure, and mesenteric thrombosis [56].

References

1. Davies A. The practical management of claudication. BMJ. 2000;321(7266):911–2.
2. Murabito JM, Evans JC, Nieto K, Larson MG, Levy D, Wilson PW. Prevalence and clinical correlates of peripheral arterial disease in the Framingham Offspring Study. Am Heart J. 2002;143(6):961–5.
3. Faulkner K, House A, Castleden W. The effect of cessation of smoking on the accumulative survival rates of patients with symptomatic peripheral vascular disease. Med J Aust. 1983;1:217–9.
4. Mills E, Eyawo O, Lockhart I, Kelly S, Wu P, Ebbert J. Smoking cessation reduces postoperative complications: a systematic review and meta-analysis. Am J Med. 2011;124:144–54.
5. Fiore MC. Methods used to quit smoking in the United States. Do cessation programs help? JAMA. 1990;263(20):2760–5.
6. Grundy SM, Cleeman JI, Merz CN, Brewer Jr HB, Clark LT, Hunninghake DB, et al. Implications of recent clinical trials for National Cholesterol Education Program Adult Treatment Panel III guidelines. Circulation. 2004;110(2):227–39.
7. Backer G, Ambrosioni E, Borch-Johnsen K, Brotons C, Cifkova R, Dallongeville J, et al. European guidelines on cardiovascular disease prevention in clinical practice. Third Joint Task Force of European and other Societies on Cardiovascular Disease Prevention in Clinical Practice (constituted by representatives of eight societies and by invited experts). Atherosclerosis. 2004;173(2):381–91.
8. Aiello FA, et al. Statin therapy is associated with superior clinical outcomes after endovascular treatment of critical limb ischemia. J Vasc Surg. 2012;55:371–80.
9. Chopra V, Wesorick DH, Sussman JB, Greene T, Rogers M, Froehlich JB, et al. Effect of perioperative statins on death, myocardial infarction, atrial fibrillation, and length of stay: a systematic review and meta-analysis. Arch Surg. 2012;147(2):181–9.
10. Ahimastos AA, Lawler A, Reid CM, Blombery PA, Kingwell BA. Brief communication: ramipril markedly improves walking ability in patients with peripheral arterial disease: a randomized trial. Ann Intern Med. 2006;144:660–4.
11. Ahimastos A, Walker P, Askew C, et al. Ramipril therapy in patients with intermittent claudication: a randomised, double-blind, placebo-controlled trial. JAMA. 2013;309:453–60.
12. Li X, Li J, Nguyen T, et al. Effect of statins and calcium channel blockers on all-cause mortality and cardiovascular and cerebrovascular disease mortality in 958 Chinese hospitalised patients with peripheral arterial disease after 13 months of follow-up. J Health Sci. 2007;53:226–33.
13. Paravastu SC, Mendonca DA, da Silva A. Beta blockers for peripheral arterial disease. Eur J Vasc Endovasc Surg. 2009;38(1):66–70.
14. Radack K, Deck C. Beta-adrenergic blocker therapy does not worsen intermittent claudication in subjects with peripheral arterial disease. A meta-analysis of randomized controlled trials. Arch Intern Med. 1991;151(9):1769–76.
15. Poldermans D, Bax JJ, Boersma E, De Hert S, Eeckhout E, Fowkes G, et al. Guidelines for pre-operative cardiac risk assessment and perioperative cardiac management in noncardiac surgery. Eur Heart J. 2009;30(22):2769–812.
16. Paravastu S, Mendonca D, Silva AD. Beta blockers for peripheral arterial disease. Cochrane Database Syst Rev. 2010;3.
17. de Virgilio C, Yaghoubian A, Nguyen A, Lewis RJ, Dauphine C, Sarkisyan G, et al. Peripheral vascular surgery using targeted beta blockade reduces perioperative cardiac event rate. J Am Coll Surg. 2009;208(1):14–20.
18. Peacock I, Donnelly R. The UK Prospective Diabetes Study (UKPDS): clinical and therapeutic implications for type 2 diabetes. Br J Clin Pharmacol. 1999;48(5):643–8.
19. Holman RR, Paul SK, Bethel MA, Matthews DR, Neil HA. 10-year follow-up of intensive glucose control in type 2 diabetes. N Engl J Med. 2008;359(15):1577–89.
20. CAPRIE Steering Committee. A randomised, blinded, trial of clopidogrel versus aspirin in patients at risk of ischemic events (CAPRIE). Lancet. 1996;3489(9038):1329–39.
21. Antiplatelet Trialists' Collaboration. Collaborative meta-analysis of randomised trials of antiplatelet therapy for prevention of death, myocardial infarction, and stroke in high risk patients. BMJ. 2002;324(7329):71–86.
22. Clagett GP, Sobel M, Jackson MR, Lip GY, Tangelder M, Verhaeghe R. Antithrombotic therapy in peripheral arterial occlusive disease. The Seventh ACCP Conference on Antithrombotic and Thrombolytic Therapy. Chest. 2004;126 Suppl 3:609S–26S.

23. Poredos P, Jezovnik MK. Antiplatelet and antithrombotic treatment of patients with peripheral arterial disease. Int Angiol. 2010;29(1):20–6.

24. Dorffler-Melly J, Koopman MM, Prins MH, Buller HR. Antiplatelet and anticoagulant drugs for prevention of restenosis/reocclusion following peripheral endovascular treatment. Cochrane Database Syst Rev. 2005;1, CD002071.

25. Study group on pharmacological treatment after PTA. Platelet inhibition with ASA/dipyridamole after percutaneous balloon angioplasty in patients with symptomatic lower limb arterial disease. A prospective double-blind trial. Study group on pharmacological treatment after PTA. Eur J Vasc Surg. 1994;8(1):83–8.

26. Belch JJ, Dormandy J, Biasi GM, Cairols M, Diehm C, Eikelboom B, et al. Results of the randomized, placebo-controlled clopidogrel and acetylsalicylic acid in bypass surgery for peripheral arterial disease (CASPAR) trial. J Vasc Surg. 2010;52(4):825–33.

27. Anand SS, Yusuf S. Oral anticoagulant therapy in patients with coronary artery disease: a meta-analysis. JAMA. 1999;282:2058–67.

28. Anand SS, Yusuf S. Oral anticoagulants in patients with coronary artery disease. J Am Coll Cardiol. 2003;41(4 Suppl. S):62S–9S.

29. Dutch Bypass Oral anticoagulants or Aspirin (BOA) Study Group. Efficacy of oral anticoagulants compared with aspirin after infrainguinal bypass surgery (The Dutch Bypass Oral Anticoagulants or Aspirin Study): a randomised trial. Lancet. 2000;355:346–51.

30. Cosmi B, Conti E, Coccheri S. Anticoagulants (heparin, low molecular weight heparin and oral anticoagulants) for intermittent claudication. Cochrane Database Syst Rev. 2001;CD001999.

31. Tangelder MJ, Lawson JA, Algra A, Eikelboom BC. Systematic review of randomized controlled trials of aspirin and oral anticoagulants in the prevention of graft occlusion and ischemic events after infrainguinal bypass surgery. J Vasc Surg [Meta-Analysis]. 1999;30:701–9.

32. Brown J, Lethaby A, Maxwell H, Wawrzyniak AJ, Prins MH. Antiplatelet agents for preventing thrombosis after peripheral arterial bypass surgery. Cochrane Database Syst Rev. 2008;CD000535.

33. Geraghty AJ, Welch K. Antithrombotic agents for preventing thrombosis after infrainguinal arterial bypass surgery. Cochrane Database Syst Rev. 2011;CD000536.

34. Ruffolo AJ, Romano M, Ciapponi A. Prostanoids for critical limb ischaemia. Cochrane Database Syst Rev. 2010;CD006544.

35. The European Study Group. Intravenous pentoxifylline for the treatment of chronic critical limb ischaemia. Eur J Vasc Endovasc Surg. 1995;9:426–36.

36. Norwegian Pentoxifylline Multicenter Trial Group. Efficacy and clinical tolerance of parenteral pentoxifylline in the treatment of critical lower limb ischemia. A placebo controlled multicenter study. Int Angiol. 1996;15:75–80.

37. Miyashita Y, Saito S, Miyamoto A, Iida O, Nanto S. Cilostazol increases skin perfusion pressure in severely ischemic limbs. Angiology. 2011;62:15–7.

38. Soga Y, Iida O, Hirano K, et al. Impact of cilostazol after endovascular treatment for infrainguinal disease in patients with critical limb ischemia. J Vasc Surg. 2011;54:1659–67.

39. Smith FB, Bradbury A, Fowkes G. Intravenous naftidrofuryl for critical limb ischaemia. Cochrane Database Syst Rev. 2012;7, CD002070.

40. De Marchi S, Zecchetto S, Rigoni A, Prior M, Fondrieschi L, Scuro A, et al. Propionyl-L-carnitine improves endothelial function, microcirculation and pain management in critical limb ischemia. Cardiovasc Drugs Ther. 2012;26(5):401–8.

41. Morris-Stiff G, Lewis MH. Gabapentin (Neurontin) improves pain scores of patients with critical limb ischaemia: an observational study. Int J Surg. 2010;8(3):212–5.

42. De Vries J, De Jongste MJ, Spincemaille G, Staal MJ. Spinal cord stimulation for ischemic heart disease and peripheral vascular disease. Adv Tech Stand Neurosurg. 2007;32:63–89.

43. Kranke P, Bennett M, Martyn-St James M, Schnabel A, Debus S. Hyperbaric oxygen therapy for chronic wounds. Cochrane Database Syst Rev. 2012;4, CD004123.

44. Harris KA, Fowkes FGR. Inter-Society Consensus for the Management of Peripheral Arterial Disease (TASC II). Eur J Vasc Endovasc Surg. 2007;33(Suppl 1).

45. Shigematsu H, Yasuda K, Sasajima T, et al. Transfection of human HGF plasmid DNA improves limb salvage in Buerger's disease patients with critical limb ischemia. Int Angiol. 2011;30:140–9.

46. Morishita R, Makino H, Aoki M, et al. Phase I/IIa clinical trial of therapeutic angiogenesis using hepatocyte growth factor gene transfer to treat critical limb ischemia. Arterioscler Thromb Vasc Biol. 2011;31:713–20.

47. Muona K, Makinen K, Hedman M, Manninen H, Yla-Herttuala S. 10-Year safety follow-up in patients with local VEGF gene transfer to ischemic lower limb. Gene Ther. 2012;19:392–5.

48. Niebuhr A, Henry T, Goldman J, et al. Long-term safety of intramuscular gene transfer of non-viral FGF1 for peripheral artery disease. Gene Ther. 2012;19:264–70.

49. Anghel A, Taranu G, Seclaman E, et al. Safety of vascular endothelial and hepatocyte growth factor gene therapy in patients with critical limb ischemia. Curr Neurovasc Res. 2011;8:183–9.

50. Powell RJ, Goodney P, Mendelsohn FO, Moen EK, Annex BH. Safety and efficacy of patient specific intramuscular injection of HGF plasmid gene therapy on limb perfusion and wound healing in patients with ischemic lower extremity ulceration: results of the HGF-0205 trial. J Vasc Surg. 2010;52:1525–30.

51. Shigematsu H, Yasuda K, Iwai T, et al. Randomized, double-blind, placebo-controlled clinical trial of hepatocyte growth factor plasmid for critical limb ischemia. Gene Ther. 2010;17:1152–61.

52. Fadini GP, Agostini C, Avogaro A. Autologous stem cell therapy for peripheral arterial disease meta-analysis and systematic review of the literature. Atherosclerosis. 2010;209:10–7.

53. Ozturk A, Kucukardali Y, Tangi F, et al. Therapeutical potential of autologous peripheral blood mononuclear cell transplantation in patients with type 2 diabetic critical limb ischemia. J Diabetes Complications. 2012;26:29–33.

54. Lara-Hernandez R, Lozano-Vilardell P, Blanes P, Torreguitart-Mirada N, Galmes A, Besalduch J. Safety and efficacy of therapeutic angiogenesis as a novel treatment in patients with critical limb ischemia. Ann Vasc Surg. 2010;24:287–94.

55. Kawamoto A, Katayama M, Handa N, et al. Intramuscular transplantation of G-CSF-mobilized CD34(+) cells in patients with critical limb ischemia: a phase I/IIa, multicenter, single blinded, dose-escalation clinical trial. Stem Cells. 2009;27:2857–64.

56. Gabr H, Hedayet A, Imam U, Nasser M. Limb salvage using intramuscular injection of unfractionated autologous bone marrow mononuclear cells in critical limb ischemia: a prospective pilot clinical trial. Exp Clin Transplant. 2011;9:197–202.

Endocrine Considerations in Critical Limb Ischemia

Ioanna Eleftheriadou, Nicholas Tentolouris, and Edward B. Jude

Introduction

Peripheral arterial disease (PAD) is a chronic atherosclerotic process characterized by narrowing or occlusion of the arteries resulting in a gradual reduction of blood supply to the lower limbs. Patients with PAD may be asymptomatic or may develop symptoms of intermittent claudication (IC) or symptoms of critical limb ischemia (CLI), characterized by pain in the lower limbs at rest, ischemic ulceration, or gangrene. CLI refers to the end stage of PAD that occurs when arterial occlusive lesions impair blood flow to such an extent that the nutrient requirements of the tissues cannot be met and the lower limb is at risk [1].

Diabetic patients with PAD are at high risk of increased morbidity and mortality from cardiovascular diseases. Considering that over 350 million people suffer from diabetes mellitus (DM) worldwide and that diabetic patients are at an excess risk of developing PAD, the implications of the problem are enormous [2].

The importance of macrovascular disease in the lower limbs in patients with DM is several-fold. PAD is a manifestation of systemic atherosclerosis and is associated with substantial morbidity and mortality from PAD itself and other atherosclerotic diseases, such as cardiovascular and cerebrovascular disease [3–6]. CLI represents a severe form of PAD and as expected, the incidence of cardiovascular and cerebrovascular disease is higher than in patients with milder

disease. PAD in patients with DM may be asymptomatic until it reaches the advanced stage of CLI [5–7]. Atherosclerosis of the lower limbs sets in at an earlier age in diabetic individuals and progresses more rapidly than in non-diabetic patients. It is usually more severe and diffuse in extent, making revascularization procedures more technically challenging and demanding than in patients without DM [3]. Moreover, the outcome after revascularization procedures is poorer and many patients end up with a major amputation [5, 6, 8].

CLI is the most severe manifestation of PAD and a very severe medical condition with poor prognosis and major impact on patients' quality of life. CLI is characterized by high burden of co-morbidities and can result in limb loss, disability, or even death if not treated promptly [5, 6]. The pathway in reducing lower limb amputation starts with a comprehensive understanding of CLI, particularly early detection and appropriate management.

Epidemiology

The true incidence of PAD and CLI in diabetic patients is difficult to estimate and can be erroneous due to several reasons. A significant number of patients with PAD are asymptomatic because presence of peripheral neuropathy may mask the symptoms of IC [7]. Furthermore, the method used to diagnose PAD and CLI [symptoms of IC, palpation of peripheral pulses, ankle-brachial index (ABI), toe pressures, and transcutaneous oxygen pressure (TcPO$_2$)], as well as the criteria used for the classification of CLI (Fontaine classification or Rutherford classification [9]) has a major influence on statistics in large epidemiological studies. Moreover, the definition of CLI has changed over the last decades, with less severe ischemia of the lower limbs being classified as CLI [1]. It is also important to bear in mind that studies addressing the selected population of patients with DM and CLI are still limited and most data are from subgroup analysis of PAD studies.

I. Eleftheriadou, MD, PhD
Internal Medicine, 1st Department of Propaedeutic and Internal Medicine, Laiko General Hospital, Medical School, University of Athens, Goudi, Athens, Greece

N. Tentolouris, MD
Internal Medicine and Diabetes, 1st Department of Propaedeutic and Internal Medicine, Laiko General Hospital, Medical School, University of Athens, Goudi, Athens, Greece

E.B. Jude, MBBS, MD (✉)
Diabetes and Endocrinology, Tameside Hospital NHS Foundation Trust, Fountain St., Ashton-Under-Lyne, Lancashire 0LG9RW, UK

© Springer International Publishing Switzerland 2017
R.S. Dieter et al. (eds.), *Critical Limb Ischemia*, DOI 10.1007/978-3-319-31991-9_49

Large population-based studies have shown that the prevalence of PAD is higher in diabetic patients compared with non-diabetic individuals. The Framingham study showed that there was a 3.5- and 8.6-fold excess risk among men and women, respectively, of developing PAD in patients with DM [10]. With respect to CLI, diabetic patients with PAD have a fourfold increased risk of developing CLI in comparison with non-diabetic individuals with PAD [11].

The incidence of CLI has been estimated to be approximately 500–1000 per million every year in a European or North American population [11]. The prevalence of CLI, on the other hand, in individuals 60–90 years old has been estimated to be approximately 0.5–1.2 %, but figures are inconsistent among different studies [1]. The true incidence and prevalence of CLI in diabetic patients are difficult to assess, since most CLI study populations consist of both diabetic and non-diabetic patients, while the proportion of diabetic participants varies from 35 to 80 % [1].

The natural course of CLI if left untreated is difficult to determine, since most patients with CLI receive some type of revascularization. If an exclusively conservative approach is applied in patients with CLI, irrespective of DM status, almost 50 % will end up with major amputation within 1 year [12]. However, diabetic patients with CLI appear to be at increased risk of death in comparison with non-diabetic individuals with CLI and have over 50 % mortality at 6 months if revascularization is not performed [12]. Nevertheless, although not all studies have reached similar conclusions, it seems that even when revascularization is performed in suitable patients, those with DM have higher amputation and mortality rates in comparison with non-diabetic individuals [13–16].

In a cohort of 564 diabetic patients with CLI endovascular procedure was performed in 74 % of the patients, surgical revascularization in 21, and 5 % of the patients were found unsuitable for revascularization and were treated with prostanoids [17, 18]. Major amputation rate within 30 days after intervention was only 4.1 %, while during the 6 years follow-up period 13 % of all patients underwent amputation, 8 % in the group treated with percutaneous transluminal angioplasty (PTA), 21 % in the group treated with bypass grafting (BG), and 59 % in the group no suitable for revascularization. Almost half of the patients died during the follow-up period [17]. Interestingly, amputated patients who had previously undergone revascularization had significantly longer survival than amputated patients who had not previously had revascularization [19]. Moreover, almost half of the participants developed CLI in the contralateral limb over a 6-year period [20]. However, the level of amputation was lower in the contralateral limb probably due to increased patient awareness and immediate management.

Most studies have shown that the 2-year mortality rates in diabetic patients with ischemic or neuro-ischemic foot ulcers or after amputation are up to 30–50 %, while the 5-year mortality rates reach up to 50–70 % [21]. It should be noted that ulcer infection is an extremely problematic issue and in combination with ischemia is associated with increased amputation risk. Presence of advanced infection and ischemia is the cause of lower limb amputations in 25–50 % of diabetic patients [21, 22].

Pathogenesis of Macrovascular and Microvascular Disease in Diabetes Mellitus

Atherosclerosis in DM has various biologic and clinical differences from the disease in non-diabetic patients [3]. Vascular disease in DM affects both microcirculation and macrocirculation [5, 6, 22, 23].

Microvascular disease is characterized by involvement of blood vessels at the level of the arterioles and capillaries [5, 6]. Microvascular changes in DM include thickening of the basement membrane, endothelial dysfunction, and impaired vasodilatation, leading to impaired response to stress and trauma when an increased nutritional circulation is needed [5]. DM impairs endothelial function through hyperglycemia, excess circulating free fatty acids, and insulin resistance and results in inhibition of endothelial nitric oxide (NO) synthase and impaired NO-mediated dilatation [24]. In addition to reducing NO and prostacyclin, DM increases endothelin-I and angiotensin-II, which are potent vasoconstrictors [24]. Microvascular dysfunction due to diabetic neuropathy and loss of vessel auto-regulation is characterized by opening of the arterio-venous shunts, altered vascular resistance, and permeability that result in impaired capillary circulation and functional ischemia [21–23]. The abnormal distribution of blood flow at the capillary level is found in diabetic patients even in the absence of PAD, but is more pronounced in the presence of PAD [23]. Functional ischemia and skin microcirculation are further impaired by the altered hemorheology and the pro-thrombotic environment that prevails in DM [23]. Thus, although PAD is the underlying and main defect in diabetic patients with CLI, the impaired capillary circulation and the reduction in total blood flow induce a series of local responses in the microcirculation that may contribute to ischemic rest pain and foot ulceration.

Macrovascular disease is characterized by involvement of large- and medium-sized vessels. PAD in diabetic patients involves predominantly the medium-sized arteries and is due to the abnormal metabolic state that prevails in DM leading to vascular inflammation and alteration in several cell types [6]. The most important metabolic aberrations are chronic hyperglycemia, insulin resistance, dyslipidemia, and hypercoagulability, which render the arteries susceptible to atherosclerosis [6].

Hyperglycemia is a major risk factor in the pathogenesis of atherosclerosis in DM and accelerates the atherosclerotic process through several mechanisms. One of them is the non-enzymatic glycosylation of proteins and lipids that interfere with their normal function [6]. Glycosylation of low density lipoprotein (LDL) leads to functional alterations in LDL clearance and in increased susceptibility to oxidation which is strongly associated with the development of atherosclerosis. Glycosylated proteins interact with advanced glycosylated end products receptor (RAGE) on several cells such as endothelial cells, smooth muscle cells, and monocytes-derived macrophages resulting in increased oxidative stress, pro-inflammatory responses, and smooth muscle cell proliferation and migration. Elevated levels of glucose also promote protein kinase C (PKC) system that is involved in the transcription of various growth factors and in signal transduction in response to growth factors [6]. Furthermore, hyperglycemia increases intracellular concentration of glucose in platelets as its uptake is non-insulin dependent leading to decreased production of platelet-derived NO and excess production of oxygen free radicals [25]. Calcium homeostasis regulating platelet shape, secretion, aggregation, and thromboxane production also gets disturbed in DM [26]. Platelet expression of receptor proteins for von Willebrand factor and fibrin products is increased in DM, which could be the result of decreased production of the antiaggregants NO and prostacyclin, and increased production of fibrinogen and platelet activators such as thrombin and von Willebrand factor [27]. This increase in intrinsic platelet activity contributes to the state of enhanced thrombotic potential.

Moreover, patients with DM have impaired fibrinolytic activity [3]. Also, there are increased circulating levels of procoagulants such as tissue factor, factor VII, and decreased levels of anticoagulants such as antithrombin-III and Protein C, thus favoring a tendency to coagulation, impaired fibrinolysis, and persistence of thrombi [28].

DM is characterized by a chronic low-grade inflammatory state and patients with impaired glucose regulation have elevated levels of C-reactive protein (CRP), which is strongly associated with PAD development [3, 4]. CRP has been shown to inhibit endothelial NO synthase and stimulate the production of procoagulant tissue factor, leukocyte adhesion molecules, chemotactic substances, and plasminogen activator inhibitor (PAI)-1 and thus contributing to a thrombotic environment and an abnormal regulation of the vascular tone [3, 4].

In brief, some of the cellular events in the process of atherosclerosis are as follows: DM augments the process of atheroma formation. The migration of T-lymphocytes into the intima, their activation, and secretion of cytokines is enhanced. Monocytes ingest oxidized LDL molecules on reaching the subendothelial space and become foam cells which lead to fatty streak formation, the precursors of the atheroma. The atheromatous plaque so formed is unstable as diabetic endothelial cells secrete cytokines which inhibit production of collagen by smooth muscle cells [25]. They also secrete metalloproteinases which break down the collagen in the fibrous cap of atheromas, leading to a tendency to plaque rupture and thrombus formation [29]. Endothelial cells produce increased amounts of tissue factor, a major procoagulant factor. Medial vascular smooth muscle cells migration into the intimal fatty streak lesion is enhanced. These cells then produce extracellular matrix, further aggravating atheroma formation.

CLI represents the end stage of PAD and is a state of arterial insufficiency, where lower limb perfusion is excessively reduced and nutrient supply and blood flow in the microcirculation is severely disturbed [1, 23]. The severity of CLI is related to the efficiency of collateral vessel formation as an adaptive response to ischemia. The development of new blood vessels from the pre-existing capillary network is called angiogenesis, while arteriogenesis is the formation of collateral vessels based on the growth of pre-existing arterioles and vasculogenesis is the de novo formation of new blood vessels by recruitment of precursor cell (endothelial progenitor cells, EPCs) from the bone marrow [30, 31]. Neovascularization has been described to be impaired in diabetic patients [30, 32, 33]. Thus, in patients with DM the formation of functional collateral circulation is decreased or even absent and they may present with CLI even in the absence of severe arterial obstruction of the large vessels [34].

The relative poor prognosis of CLI in patients with DM is most likely related to underlying multi-factorial pathophysiologic mechanisms, such as the association with peripheral and autonomic neuropathy and changes in microcirculation, the difficult to treat diffuse and distal distribution of arterial obstructive lesions, as well as the susceptibility to infection and the abnormal inflammation responses.

Risk Factors for CLI in Diabetes Mellitus

CLI is the end stage of chronic atherosclerotic disease of the lower limbs. Patients with CLI share the same traditional risk factors as patients with atherosclerosis in other vascular beds. The cardiovascular risk factors most strongly associated with CLI are DM, smoking, age>65 years, dyslipidemia, and chronic renal disease [1, 3, 11]. Notably, diabetic patients with PAD have a fourfold increased risk in progressing to CLI in comparison with non-diabetic individuals with PAD [11].

As far as the increased predisposition to the development of PAD in diabetic patients, various risk factors have been described. Many studies have attempted to resolve this complicated issue by comparing diabetic patients with PAD to non-diabetic patients with PAD and between diabetic patients with and without PAD [10, 35–39].

Duration and degree of hyperglycemia is associated with an increased risk for PAD independently of other factors [4, 22, 35]. More specifically, every 1 % increase in HbA1c has been found to increase the risk of PAD by 28 % [4]. Increasing age also correlates strongly with PAD in patients with DM [36]. The Framingham Offspring Study reported that for each 10 years of age, the odds of PAD increased 2.6-fold [37]. Male gender has been found to correlate with increased PAD risk, whereas diabetic women have more often PAD compared to non-diabetic women of similar age [38]. The UK Prospective Diabetes Study (UKPDS) found that increased systolic blood pressure was an independent risk factor for PAD and each 10 mmHg increase in systolic blood pressure was associated with a 25 % increased risk for PAD [35].

Profile of CLI in Diabetes Mellitus

The pattern of lower limb atherosclerotic obstructive lesions differs between diabetic and non-diabetic patients [8, 40]. Diabetic patients with CLI commonly show involvement of the arteries below the knee, especially at the tibial and peroneal arteries, unlike non-diabetic individuals who show mainly involvement of the iliac and femoral arteries [34, 41–43]. Moreover, in diabetic patients arterial obstructions are more commonly symmetrical and multi-segmental even in the collateral vessels. Non-diabetic patients with atherosclerosis usually present with single, unilateral, and proximal arterial stenosis [34, 42, 43]. Furthermore, calcification in patients with DM is diffuse, circumferential, and found in the tunica media of the arterial wall, while in patients without DM calcification is usually focal, eccentric, and found in the sub-intimal space [34]. The typical characteristics of diabetic macrovascular disease make revascularization procedures more technically challenging and demanding than in patients without DM.

Clinical Presentation of CLI in Diabetes Mellitus

Up to 75 % of diabetic patients with PAD are initially asymptomatic [22]. Eventually many patients develop symptomatic PAD that manifests as IC and progresses to CLI [7]. However, it should be emphasized that the natural history of PAD does not always follow a course of disease through standardized clinical stages. It has been reported that 5–10 % of patients with asymptomatic PAD or with IC will progress to CLI within 5 years, while 1–3 % of individuals with PAD are diagnosed with CLI at initial presentation [11]. Patients with DM are at even greater risk of PAD progression [7]. Notably, diabetic patients with decreased pain perception due to peripheral neuropathy may delay the recognition of PAD and may be diagnosed when revascularization is not an option [7,

21]. A number of studies have reported that 30–50 % of diabetic patients with foot ulcers have already gangrene at the first investigation [22].

CLI is characterized by the presence of ischemic rest pain, ischemic ulceration, and gangrene and is a limb-threatening condition. Ischemic rest pain of the lower limbs is described as burning pain mostly in the toes or the foot that most typically occurs at night when the patient is in bed and the extremities at the horizontal position; hanging the foot out of bed increases perfusion and usually relieves pain [1]. Notably, presence of rest pain depends on pain perception which is reduced or abolished in the presence of peripheral neuropathy [3]. It is important that all diabetic patients and especially those with foot ulcers are examined for the presence of peripheral neuropathy [44, 45]. The prevalence of peripheral neuropathy is 30–50 % among diabetic patients [46], while rest pain is absent in about 50 % of ischemic ulcer [34]. CLI may also present with loss of hair of the lower limbs, nail dystrophy, and loss of subcutaneous tissue leading to a shiny appearance of the skin and pallor at elevation of the feet [6].

However, every burning and aching sensation in the lower limb of diabetic patients should not be mistakenly diagnosed as CLI. Patients with DM often suffer from painful diabetic neuropathy and present with symptoms that are difficult to be distinguished from atypical ischemic rest pain. Almost 40–50 % of the patients with peripheral neuropathy have painful symptoms starting in the toes and extend proximally to involve the calves in a stocking distribution that usually worsen at night [47]. Unlike ischemic rest pain, patients with neuropathic pain do not find comfort by hanging the feet out of bed and they describe reduction in painful symptoms during walking.

Foot ulcers in diabetic patients are divided into three broad categories: neuropathic, ischemic, or neuro-ischemic [23]. Ischemic ulcers are usually seen in the toes and around the edges of the foot and have an irregular necrotic base, while neuropathic ulcers are found in the sole of the foot and are deep with surrounding callus formation [3]. It is important to bear in mind that in DM both peripheral neuropathy and PAD are major risk factors for foot ulceration. In a study by Moulik et al. in 185 diabetic patients with recent-onset full-thickness foot wounds, 45 % of the ulcers were neuropathic, 24 % ischemic, and 16 % neuro-ischemic [48]. Most studies suggest that PAD is present in up to 50 % of the diabetic patients with foot ulcer [21, 49, 50].

Furthermore, every foot ulcer should be examined for the presence of infection. Diagnosis of infection is based on local signs and symptoms of inflammation, such as warmth, redness, swelling, pain, bad odor, or purulent exudation [22]. Infected ischemic ulcers are a medical emergency and should be treated preferably within 24 h [50].

Summarizing, the diagnosis of CLI is mainly clinical based on the presence of rest pain, ulceration, and gangrene attributable to objectively proven PAD. However, patients with DM may commonly present with peripheral neuropathy and thus decreased pain perception and absence of ischemic rest pain. On the other hand, diabetic patients often present with neuropathic and infected diabetic foot ulcers even in the absence of PAD. Hence, especially in diabetic patients, the presence of ulceration and trophic changes of the lower limbs do not definitely imply that CLI is present. Nevertheless, all diabetic patients with foot ulcers should undergo vascular evaluation for the exclusion of PAD [22, 50].

Diagnosis of CLI in Diabetes Mellitus

The diagnosis of CLI is particularly challenging in patients with DM due to several reasons.

Palpation of peripheral pulses should be performed in all patients, although absence of pulses is unreliable for detection of PAD. The dorsalis pedis and tibialis posterior pulse may be absent congenitally in about 10 % of the population [5, 51]. Inspection of the foot may reveal findings of chronic ischemia in the periphery such as pallor on limb elevation and dependent rubor, ulceration, and distal gangrene that are all suggestive of CLI [5, 6].

Diagnosis criteria and definition of CLI have changed over the last decades. The TransAtlantic Inter-Society Consensus (TASC II) for the management of PAD in 2007 states that although the diagnosis of CLI is mainly clinical based on the presence of chronic rest pain, ulceration or gangrene attributable to proven PAD, it should be supported by objective tests [11]. The non-invasive hemodynamic tests most commonly used are measurement of ankle and toe systolic pressures and TcPO$_2$. For patients with ischemic rest pain in the lower limbs CLI is suggested when ankle systolic pressure is <50 mmHg and/or toe pressure <30 mmHg. For patients with ischemic ulceration or gangrene, CLI is suggested by ankle systolic pressures <70 mmHg and/or toe pressures <50 mmHg [11]. The former TASC for the management of PAD in 2000 included measurement of TcPO$_2$ as a diagnostic tool for the evaluation of CLI, with supine forefoot TcPO$_2$ values <30–50 mmHg in the presence of ischemic rest pain, ulceration, or gangrene being suggestive of CLI [52].

Diagnosis of CLI in diabetic patients based on hemodynamic tests is presented in Table 49.1.

ABI is a sensitive, specific, and reproducible screening tool for the assessment of PAD and the initial evaluation of CLI and should be measured in both lower limbs [9, 43]. ABI values <0.9 indicate presence of PAD, values <0.4 presence of CLI, while values >1.3 indicate presence of medial arterial calcification [3, 44]. ABI values <0.6 or ankle systolic pressures <50–80 mmHg are associated with poor healing in patients with foot ulcers [21, 22, 50].

Table 49.1 Diagnosis of CLI in diabetic patients based on hemodynamic tests

Hemodynamic measurements		Interpretation
ABI	>1.30	Medial arterial calcification
	0.91–1.30	Normal
	0.70–0.90	Mild obstruction
	0.40–0.69	Moderate obstruction
	<0.40	CLI
Ankle systolic pressures		
with ischemic rest pain	<50 mmHg	CLI
with ischemic ulceration or gangrene	<70 mmHg	CLI
Toe systolic pressures		
with ischemic rest pain	<30 mmHg	CLI
with ischemic ulceration or gangrene	<50 mmHg	CLI
TcPO$_2$	<30–50 mmHg	CLI

CLI critical limb ischemia, *ABI* ankle-brachial index, *TcPO2* transcutaneous oxygen pressure

The measurement of ankle pressures in patients with DM is sometimes impeded by the occlusion of tibial arteries, especially in patient with CLI, or by rigid or incompressible arteries, with pressures >250 mmHg [17, 21, 22, 51, 53, 54]. Interestingly, ankle and toe systolic pressures measurements may not be assessable in almost half of the patients with DM and CLI [17, 55, 56].

Medial arterial calcification (Mönckeberg's sclerosis) of the lower limbs has been reported to be more frequent in patients with DM and end-stage renal disease and usually correlates with the presence of peripheral neuropathy [53, 54]. In one study up to 50 % of diabetic patients with CLI had calcified arteries of the lower limbs [18]. Presence of arterial calcification may lead to either inability to obtain the ankle systolic blood pressures or to artificially elevated values that may mask the presence of arterial insufficiency [34, 43, 53, 57]. Thus, an ankle systolic pressure ≥70 mmHg or an ABI value 0.9–1.3 should not rule out the presence of PAD and CLI in patients with DM and should be interpreted with caution, since ankle systolic pressures may be overestimated due to medial arterial calcification [22, 43, 51, 53, 55].

Notably, in one study arterial calcification, defined as ABI values >1.3 in CLI patients, was associated significantly with major amputation but not with increased mortality during follow-up [58]. Almost half of the study participants (47 %) had DM and ABI values >1.3 were associated with the presence of DM and renal insufficiency. The authors suggest that high ABI values should be considered an indicator of poor prognosis in patients with CLI.

Another study in CLI patients reported that although arterial calcification, assessed angiographically, was significantly associated with DM and hemodialysis, it was not associated with ankle systolic pressures and ABI [59]. The authors suggest that their finding could be explained by the presence of systemic calcification in patients with CLI and that the artificial elevation of ankle systolic pressure due to tibial calcification could be canceled by the artificial elevation of brachial systolic pressure due to calcified brachial arteries.

In patients where arterial calcification is present or suspected, measurement of great toe systolic blood pressures using a strain gauge sensor or a photoplethysmography is clearly recommended, since the vessels of the toes are not generally affected by media sclerosis [3, 44, 57]. However, a number of diabetic patients with CLI have toe ulcers or amputated toes that make the toe systolic pressures measurement impossible [22, 43, 55, 57]. Toe-brachial index (TBI) values <0.7 indicate presence of PAD, while toe systolic pressures <30 mmHg are associated with poor healing in patients with foot ulcers [22, 50].

Determination of $TcPO_2$ may help assess CLI and local microcirculation and has a high prognostic value in predicting ulcer healing and amputations [1, 3, 21, 60] (Table 49.2). Notably, each 1 mmHg increase of $TcPO_2$ has been found to reduce the risk of above-the-ankle amputation by 10 % in diabetic patients with CLI [56]. $TcPO_2$ values <30 mmHg have been associated with poor ulcer healing, while $TcPO_2$ values >50 mmHg with fairly good prognosis [3, 21, 50]. $TcPO_2$ is a very useful and reliable test for the assessment of blood supply in tissues that can be used not only as a screening tool to select patients with CLI, but also to select the level of amputation and to evaluate the outcome of endovascular procedures [34, 61]. More specifically, after a successful revascularization procedure $TcPO_2$ increases and reaches a peak 4 weeks after angioplasty [62]. Presence of edema, cellulitis, hyperkeratosis, or abundant subcutaneous fat may alter $TcPO_2$ levels, but $TcPO_2$ measurement is feasible in almost all patients [43, 57].

Color duplex ultrasound is recommended as the first-line imaging modality and has good sensitivity for detecting high-grade stenosis in below-knee arteries both in diabetic and non-diabetic patients [54, 57, 63–65]. Moreover, color duplex imaging provides both hemodynamic and anatomical information of vascular lesions [51, 54, 57]. However, color duplex imaging is more difficult to perform, more time-consuming and needs extensive experience from the examiner in patients with DM [51, 64]. Newer diagnostic modalities, such as magnetic resonance angiography (MRA) and computer tomography angiography (CTA), are increasingly being used and should be offered to patients before considering revascularization [57, 63]. MRA is recommended to diagnose anatomical location and severity of stenosis in patients with PAD, as well as to select patients for revascularization procedures [9, 57, 63, 65]. When MRA is contraindicated, CTA can be performed. Disadvantages of CTA are the need of radiation exposure, the risk of contrast induced nephropathy, and the interference of arterial calcification with image quality [9, 57, 63, 65]. However, gadolinium use for MRA has been reported to cause nephrogenic systemic sclerosis in patients with impaired renal function [57]. It should be noted that the data about the efficiency of MRA and CTA in patients with CLI and DM are limited. Digital subtraction angiography (DSA) remains the gold standard against which all other imaging modalities should be compared and should be used when a vascular intervention is planned [3, 5, 57].

All non-invasive and invasive diagnostic modalities have their own strengths and weaknesses and none is satisfactory as a single tool for the diagnosis of CLI. Information gained from several diagnostic methods should be combined and interpreted together with the clinical presentation to make appropriate decisions for the management of each individual patient.

Management

The primary goals of the management of diabetic patients with CLI are to relieve ischemic rest pain, heal foot ulceration, prevent amputation and cardiovascular morbidity and prolong survival [11]. Due to multi-factorial pathophysiologic mechanisms underlying diabetic CLI and the complex nature of treatment in such high-risk patients, a multidisciplinary approach is warranted and ultimately a revascularization procedure [21, 22, 50, 63, 66]. However, at present there is a lack of robust evidence to guide definite treatment strategies.

Lifestyle modification and medical treatment for cardiovascular risk factor control, as well as for pain relief are of great importance. Less well established is the role of medical management for treating symptoms of CLI and complications of lower limb hypo-perfusion. It should also be emphasized that diabetic patients with CLI usually present significant co-morbidities, such as coronary artery disease, cerebrovascular disease, carotid disease, and renal disease. Thus, screening of these patients for co-existing co-morbidities and appropriate management according to current guidelines is also important [9, 65, 67]. Appropriate foot care, sufficient footwear, debridement of foot ulcers, non-adherent dressings, and aggressive treatment of infections with antibiotics are essential for preventing amputation [3, 66, 68–70]. It is important to bear in mind that most of the following recommendations apply to patients with PAD in general and are extrapolated to the subgroup of patients with CLI.

Table 49.2. *CLI* critical limb ischemia, *DM* diabetes mellitus, *PAD* peripheral arterial disease, *IC* intermittent claudication, *ABI* ankle-brachial index, *TcPO₂* transcutaneous oxygen pressure, *MRA* magnetic resonance angiography, *CTA* computer tomography angiography, *DSA* digital subtraction angiography. *ABI values 0.9–1.3 should not rule out the presence of CLI in diabetic patients due to frequent presence of arterial calcification

---

All patients with DM should have their feet evaluated at least annually.

If PAD is present evaluation should be performed every 2-3 months

and in case of history of ulcer or amputation every 1-2 months.

History:

symptoms of PAD (IC, ischemic rest pain, foot ulcer or gangrene)

General inspection of the foot:

hair loss, thickened toenail, loss of subcutaneous tissue, pallor at elevation,

ulceration, gangrene, signs of infection

Neurological assessment:

10-g monofilament and one of the following:

- vibration perception using a 128-Hz tuning fork

- pinprick sensation

- ankle reflexes

- vibration perception threshold using a biothesiometer

Palpation of foot pulses
including posterior tibial and dorsalis pedis arteries

ABI measurement*
if ABI > 1.3 or ABI > 0.9 but high suspicious of arterial calcification or CLI

Systolic toe pressure measurements

TcPO₂ measurement:

assessment of ischemia and wound healing potential,

necessity and success of revascularization,

selection of amputation level

Colour duplex ultrasound as a first line imaging modality:
detection of anatomic localization and severity of arterial stenosis

---

MRA
or CTA if MRA is contraindicated:
selection of candidates for revascularization

DSA:
if revascularization is planned

CLI critical limb ischemia, *DM* diabetes mellitus, *PAD* peripheral arterial disease, *IC* intermittent claudication, *ABI* ankle-brachial index, *TcPO 2* transcutaneous oxygen pressure, MRA magnetic resonance angiography, *CTA* computer tomography angiography, *DSA* digital subtraction angiography

*ABI values 0.9–1.3 should not rule out the presence of *CLI* in diabetic patients due to frequent presence of arterial calcification

Lifestyle Modifications

Cigarette smoking is the single most important risk factor for the development of atherosclerosis and the amount and duration of smoking exposure correlate with the severity of atherosclerotic disease, the rate of lower limb amputation, and recurrence after revascularization as well as with mortality rate [3, 67, 71]. Smoking cessation may halt the progression of disease and is a cornerstone in the management of CLI [3, 67].

Although physical activity is usually recommended in patients with atherosclerotic disease, patients with CLI are at increased risk for ulcer development or worsening of already existing wounds and exercise is contraindicated until revascularization is provided [67].

Cardiovascular Risk Factors Modifications

Glycemic Control

Current guidelines from the American Diabetes Association (ADA) recommend a target glycosylated hemoglobin (HbA1c) level <7% in patients with DM in order to prevent microvascular complications and even long-term macrovascular complications, if implemented soon after the diagnosis of DM [45]. More stringent HbA1c goal (<6.5%) or less stringent HbA1c goal (<8%) may be appropriate for individual patients based on age, co-morbidities, life expectancy, and treatment's adverse events such as hypoglycemia. However, it should be noted that no specific recommendation is available for patients with CLI due to the lack of randomized clinical trials [45, 71].

Most large randomized controlled and epidemiological trials have shown that intensified glycemic control was associated with reduction of microvascular complications of DM (retinopathy, nephropathy, and neuropathy) [45, 67]. The association between intensified glycemic control and macrovascular complications of DM is, however, less clear [45, 67]. So far, there is no conclusive evidence to suggest that optimal DM control lowers risk of PAD and its progression to CLI [71–73]. However, there are some data that suggest that pre-procedural higher fasting glucose levels are associated with decreased vessel patency, while higher HbA1c levels are associated with higher major amputation rates after endovascular procedures in diabetic patients with CLI [74, 75].

The use of medications which improve insulin resistance could be in favor of other hypoglycemic agents, since insulin resistance is a risk factor for PAD. However, although metformin may be associated with reduced risk for cardiovascular events [45], it has not been found superior to sulfonylureas or insulin in the prevention of PAD in diabetic patients [72]. In the PROactive study only patients without PAD at baseline benefited from treatment with pioglitazone [76]. As far

as the data regarding the association of insulin treatment at the time of revascularization with limb prognosis, the results of the studies are inconclusive. One study reported that insulin treatment was associated with poor lower limb prognosis in the subgroup of patients with DM and CLI [77], while another study found no association between insulin treatment and major amputation risk [78].

Dyslipidemia

Aggressive management of dyslipidemia with statins in diabetic patients with CLI is warranted and the primary aim is LDL-cholesterol levels <100 mg/dL or even lower (<70 mg/dL), although no overall consensus exist regarding the optimal target LDL-cholesterol level in this high-risk group of patients [4, 9, 45, 65, 67]. Large randomized controlled trials have established that treatment of high-risk patients with statins is associated with reduced all-cause and cardiovascular mortality and reduced risk for major cardiovascular events [79–82].

Very recently two observational cohort studies were published about the association of statin treatment on mortality in patients with CLI [83, 84]. Westin et al. reported that therapy with statins (simvastatin and atorvastatin were the most commonly administered agents) was associated with reduced 1-year rate of major cardiovascular and cerebrovascular events (defined as death, myocardial infarction, or stroke), reduced 1-year mortality rate, and lower 1-year rate of major amputation or death [83]. Of the total 380 patients with CLI who participated in the study, 232 patients (61%) had DM, while 295 patients (78%) underwent endovascular revascularization, and 38 patients (10%) surgical revascularization. Moreover, statin treatment was associated with improved lesion patency at 1 year in patients who underwent infrapopliteal angioplasty.

Suckow et al. examined data from 2067 patients who underwent infrainguinal BG, of whom 1389 patients (67%) had CLI and 983 patients (48%) had DM [84]. CLI patients on statin therapy had higher 5-year survival rates in comparison with CLI patients who were not on statin treatment (60% vs. 51%). However, statin treatment was not associated with lower major amputation rates or lower graft occlusion rates at 1 year in CLI patients.

Hypertension Control

Optimal control of hypertension to 140/80 mmHg has been shown to reduce cardiovascular morbidity and mortality in patients with DM, although no specific treatment goal exists regarding the selected population of patients with CLI [45].

Long-term tight blood pressure control was associated with a 50% lower risk for PAD in the United Kingdom Prospective Diabetes Study (UKPDS) with no difference between the primary medications (captopril and atenolol) used for the management of hypertension [85]. The Heart

Outcomes Prevention Evaluation (HOPE) study showed that ramipril, an angiotensin-converting enzyme (ACE) inhibitor, decreased the rates of myocardial infarction, stroke, and cardiovascular death in diabetic patients with cardiovascular disease [86]. The reduction of cardiovascular morbidity and mortality in the subgroup of patients with PAD was 25 %. Interestingly, the trial showed that the cardiovascular benefits of ramipril treatment were independent of blood pressure lowering.

Treatment with beta blockers has been previously discouraged in patients with PAD due to the possible inhibition of smooth muscle relaxation in blood vessels by β2-receptor blockade. However, two meta-analyses of studies in patients with PAD concluded that beta blockade was not associated with worsening symptoms in patients with IC [87, 88]. Hence, since diabetic patients with CLI often present with concomitant coronary artery disease, treatment with beta blockers, especially selective β1-receptor blockers, is not contraindicated [65, 67, 71]. Moreover, beta blockers are recommended in patients who undergo surgical revascularization, since beta blockade has been associated with reduced risk of cardiovascular morbidity in high-risk patients during and after vascular surgery [65, 67].

Although it is well known that acute lowering of blood pressure is contraindicated in patients with CLI and could lead to limb loss, there have been no reports on exacerbation of symptoms after hypertension control in this group of patients [71].

Anti-Platelet Agents

Anti-platelet agents are of benefit in diabetic patients at increased cardiovascular risk [45]. Treatment with aspirin, at doses 75–162 mg/day, has been shown to be effective as a secondary prevention in reducing cardiovascular morbidity and mortality in patients with DM [45, 89]. The most effective dose of aspirin remains to be determined, but higher doses of aspirin did not show any additional benefit over a dose of 75 mg and were associated with higher bleeding rates [45, 67]. Patients with aspirin allergy should receive clopidogrel at doses 75 mg/day, although the 2003 ADA consensus statement on PAD suggested that diabetic patients with PAD may benefit more by taking clopidogrel based primarily on the results of the Clopidogrel vs. Aspirin in Patients at Risk of Ischemic Events (CAPRIE) study [3, 90].

In the CAPRIE study, treatment with clopidogrel was associated with 24 % reduction in the relative risk for myocardial infarction, ischemic stroke, or vascular death compared with aspirin treatment in the subgroup of patients who had PAD at baseline (about one-third of the PAD population had DM) [90]. However, no data were reported separately in patients with CLI in this study.

Ticlopidine, another anti-platelet thienopyridine agent, has been shown to improve clinical outcomes in patients with PAD but is not recommended because of adverse effects (neutropenia and increased risk for thrombotic thrombocytopenic purpura) [67].

It has been suggested that long-term treatment with anti-platelet agents reduce progression of femoral atherosclerosis and improve patency rates after revascularization procedures [11, 65, 67, 71]. Dual anti-platelet therapy is not recommended at present for patients with PAD undergoing endovascular intervention with or without stenting, while for patients undergoing below-knee BG with prosthetic grafts dual therapy with aspirin and clopidogrel for 1 year is suggested, although high quality evidence is lacking [65, 71, 91].

Nevertheless, no data exist so far about the efficacy of anti-platelet agents in improving outcomes in patients with CLI and reducing its progression towards lower limb amputation [11].

Medical management of cardiovascular risk factors in diabetic patients with CLI is presented in Table 49.3.

Vaso-Active Drugs: Prostanoids

Prostanoids like iloprost prevent platelet activation, adhesion, and aggregation and have vasodilatory and antithrombotic effects [5, 11, 71]. Although no high quality evidence is available, especially in patients with DM, there are some studies and a meta-analysis that have reported beneficial effects of prostanoids treatment in patients with CLI [9, 71]. More specifically, iloprost has been found to improve rest pain and improve ulcer healing, as well as to prevent limb loss and increase survival [92–94]. At present parenteral iloprost is recommended in patients with CLI for whom revascularization is not an option or has failed [11, 34, 67, 95, 96].

Drugs of Possible Benefit

Cilostazol is a selective phosphodiesterase-III inhibitor that inhibits platelet aggregation and induces vasodilatation [5]. Treatment with cilostazol increases pain-free and maximal walking distances in diabetic patients with IC [97] and is recommended in patients with PAD and IC [3, 5, 7, 91]. However, no significant advantage has been found in patients with CLI.

Treatment with pentoxifylline, a hemorheological agent with anti-platelet action, may benefit patients with CLI and improve rest pain [98]. However, most studies have reported inconclusive results and at present data are insufficient to justify pentoxifylline for the management of CLI [11, 67, 71, 91].

Table 49.3 Medical management of cardiovascular risk factors in diabetic patients with CLI

Treatment	Goals	Agents	Outcomes
Glycemic control	HbA1c <7%	Insulin-sensitizing agents are preferred	Reduced microvascular complications.
	HbA1c <6.5% or <8% for selected individual patients[a]		May be associated with reduced cardiovascular morbidity and mortality.
			May be associated with improved outcomes after endovascular procedures.
Lipid lowering	LDL-cholesterol <100 mg/dL (or even <70 mg/dL)	Statins	Reduced cardiovascular morbidity and mortality.
			May be associated with improved outcomes after revascularization procedures and limb salvage.
Blood pressure control	<140/80 mmHg	ACE inhibitors are preferred.	Reduced cardiovascular morbidity and mortality.
		Beta blockers are not contraindicated.	
		β1-receptor blockers are recommended in patients with coronary artery disease and those who undergo surgical revascularization.	
Anti-platelet agents	–	Aspirin (75–162 mg/day) or clopidogrel (75 mg/day).	Reduced cardiovascular morbidity and mortality.
		Dual therapy for patients undergoing below-knee BG with prosthetic graft is preferred.	May be associated with improved outcomes after revascularization procedures.

CLI critical limb ischemia, *HbA1c* glycosylated hemoglobin, *LDL-cholesterol* low density lipoprotein, *ACE* angiotensin-converting enzyme, *BG* bypass grafting

[a]Individualization should be based on patient's age, co-morbidities, life expectancy, and treatment's adverse events

Pain Control

Pain management in patients with CLI is ultimately achieved by reperfusion of the lower limb after the revascularization procedure. However, until the revascularization is scheduled or in cases where a revascularization procedure is not possible, pain relief can be achieved with acetaminophen, paracetamol, and non-steroidal anti-inflammatory medications. If complete pain relief is not achieved, opioids can be administered. Antidepressant agents could also be used for pain relief [11, 34, 63].

Management of Foot Ulceration

The frequent participation of multiple factors that lead to diabetic foot ulceration emphasizes the need for a multidisciplinary approach in the management of diabetic foot wounds [22, 45, 50, 66, 70]. The mainstay of management of diabetic foot ulcers is standard wound care with extensive and regular debridement of the wound, followed by non-adherent dressings that maintain a moist wound environment, protect from infections and promote tissue regeneration [3]. Plantar pressure offloading with therapeutic footwear and removable or non-removable contact casts is also of major importance [3, 66, 70]. Immediate identification and control of infection remains a top priority with empirical broad spectrum antibiotic treatments and drainage [3, 68–70]. Patient education in the area of foot care and skin hygiene is also essential and should be provided to all patients [45].

Revascularization Procedures

Revascularization is ultimately the elective treatment for CLI. The revascularization procedures currently available are PTA, conventional balloon angioplasty or angioplasty with stenting, and the surgical revascularization by means of BG using autologous vein or endarterectomy for localized lesions [99, 100]. The number of revascularization procedures for PAD is about 8- to 16-fold higher in diabetic compared to non-diabetic patients, while distal revascularization procedures are also performed more often in diabetic patients [3].

In view of the distal and diffuse multilevel nature of the disease and the presence of arterial calcification in patients with DM, the procedures are technically difficult to perform. The distal run off tends to be poor and the collateral vessel formation inadequate and hence the primary patency rates after endovascular procedures are lower than in patients without DM [101, 102]. However, secondary patency and 1-year limb survival rates have been reported similar in patients with and without DM [102, 103]. Moreover, newer drug-eluting balloon angioplasty has been associated with lower re-stenosis rates in comparison with conventional PTA in diabetic patients with CLI [104].

Revascularization appears to be possible in the large majority of cases if patients are referred promptly to a vascular multidisciplinary vascular team [66, 100, 105]. Indeed, in a cohort of 344 diabetic patients with CLI hospitalized in a specialized and multidisciplinary Diabetic Foot Centre, over

96% of the patients were eligible to undergo endovascular or surgical revascularization [106].

The choice of a procedure depends on several factors like site and length of the atherosclerotic lesion, distal run off, availability of suitable veins, life expectancy and surgical risk due to associated co-morbidities such as cardiovascular, cerebrovascular and renal disease [100, 107–110]. Extensive and diffuse aorto-iliac occlusive disease, lesions of the common femoral artery and long lesions (>15 cm) of the superficial femoral artery are often managed with surgical revascularization (BG or endarterectomy) [100, 101, 110]. Short lesions of the iliac artery, superficial femoral artery, and most infrapopliteal lesions are amenable to endovascular revascularization [101, 108, 110]. Furthermore, endovascular procedures can be used as an adjunct to surgical intervention or as a temporary bridge to definite treatment when patients are not stable enough to undergo major surgery [102].

Due to the improvement of endovascular techniques over the last decade, endovascular treatment is gaining acceptance as the first-choice treatment in patients with CLI by most experts, with similar results with surgical intervention, but with less complication rates [21, 22, 34, 105, 111]. However, a recent published systematic review of the effectiveness of revascularization procedures in patients with DM, PAD, and foot ulceration concluded that there is insufficient data to recommend endovascular over surgical treatment and emphasized the need for standardized reporting of disease severity and outcome [112]. PTA and BG using autologous vein were the most commonly used techniques with similar outcomes and same rate for mortality and major complications. The selection of one treatment over the other was mainly based on morphological distribution of occlusive lesions and local availability and expertise [112]. In the absence of randomized controlled trials that compare endovascular and surgical revascularization in diabetic patients with CLI, the decision depends on the individual patient and the expertise of the center and the surgeon [22, 50, 99].

Regular follow-up after revascularization procedures is mandatory to achieve optimal primary and secondary patency rates and best medical treatment [101, 113].

Outcomes

Graft occlusion after peripheral revascularization procedures is higher and limb salvage rates are suggested to be lower in patients with DM [3, 8, 15, 114]. Presence of peripheral neuropathy that may decrease pain perception and result in more advanced disease at presentation, as well as infection is associated with lower limb salvage rates in diabetic patients. Peri-operative morbidity has also been reported higher in diabetic than in non-diabetic patients [115, 116], while survival of diabetic patients following revascularization procedures has been reported lower than

that in non-diabetic patients [8, 13, 14, 117]. However, most recent studies suggest that patency rates, limb salvage rates, and survival after aggressive revascularization procedures for CLI are similar in diabetic and non-diabetic patients [116, 118–121].

According to the recently published meta-analysis of the International Working Group on the Diabetic Foot, peri-operative major systemic complication rate was about 10%, with similar rates among patients who underwent endovascular or surgical treatment, but it is important to bear in mind that this percentage is most likely related to the poor general health status of the patients and not to the revascularization procedure alone [112]. The 1-year limb salvage rate was 78% following PTA and 85% following BG. Ulcer healing rate was >60% at 1 year following revascularization procedures. Major amputations were performed in <5% of patients 30 days after intervention, while the 2-year amputation rates were 8.9% and 17.3% following PTA and BG, respectively [112]. Notably, aggressive revascularization of as many vessels as possible has been associated with increased limb salvage and ulcer healing rates in diabetic patients with CLI [101]. Peri-operative mortality following revascularization procedures was relatively low (0.5% for PTA and 1.4% for BG), but 1-year and 5-year mortality rates were high, around 10% and 50% respectively [112]. Moreover, revascularization procedures have been reported to improve quality of life and glycemic control in patients with DM and CLI [122, 123].

Amputation

All patients with CLI should be assessed by a multidisciplinary team before treatment decisions are made and major amputation should not be offered to patients until all options for revascularization have been discussed in a multidisciplinary team [50, 63].

However, amputation may be the first treatment approach in some patients [11, 96]. These are the patients who are severely frail to undergo revascularization due to overwhelming life-threatening infection and sepsis or patients with excessive tissue loss and severe functional impairment where revascularization will not result in limb salvage. Patients at increased surgical risk due to severe co-morbidities or short life expectancy (<6–12 months) are also candidates for primary amputation [3, 11, 22, 50, 96].

Therapies of Possible Benefit in Patients Unsuitable for Revascularization

Lumbar Sympathectomy

Lumbar sympathectomy, chemical or surgical, has been shown to have favorable effects in patients with CLI when revascularization procedure is not an option. Most studies report pain relief and enhanced ulcer healing, although no reduction in amputation rate and mortality has been observed [96, 110]. It should be noted, however, that presence of diabetic peripheral neuropathy reduces pain perception, and hence limits the indications of lumbar sympathectomy in diabetic patients. No high quality evidence is available about the effect of lumbar sympathectomy in patients with DM and CLI and at present lumbar sympathectomy is performed in research settings [96].

Spinal Cord Stimulation

Spinal cord stimulation is a technique where the dorsal columns of the spinal cord are activated by an implanted pacemaker in the epidural space [6]. Although some small studies with diabetic patients with CLI have reported beneficial results in pain relief and blood flow of the lower limbs [124, 125], a meta-analysis of randomized studies that included patients with inoperable CLI did not show favorable effects on limb salvage rate or mortality [126]. Moreover, presence of autonomic neuropathy in diabetic patients may be associated with unsuccessful results of spinal cord stimulation treatment and unsatisfactory pain relief [127]. Thus, at present there is insufficient evidence to recommend spinal cord stimulation in diabetic patients with CLI [110].

Novel Therapies for CLI

Therapeutic angiogenesis, the development of new blood vessel from a pre-existing capillary network, represents a novel approach to increase blood flow and provide oxygen and nutrients to ischemic tissues by induction of a collateral vascular network [128]. These therapies are of particular interest in patients with DM, in whom the process of collateral vessel formation driven by angiogenesis is reduced. Three modes of angiogenesis are emerging; the first is the topical (in the muscles or in the arteries of the lower limbs) administration of recombinant growth factors, the second is incorporation of genes encoding angiogenic growth factors into a vector (virus or plasmid) to deliver DNA to human cells and the third is the topical or systematic administration of EPCs [128, 129]. Topical, rather than intravenous administration of these factors is preferred because systemic toxicity is low and higher concentrations are achieved locally [129].

Angiogenic growth factors that have been administered in patients with PAD are vascular endothelial growth factor (VEGF), basic fibroblast growth factor (bFGF), hepatocyte growth factor (HGF), and nerve growth factor (NGF) [129]. No randomized controlled trials are available about the effect of growth factor treatment in patients with DM and CLI and at present recombinant growth factors are not recommended for CLI management.

Intramuscular administration of HGF gene resulted in pain relief and improvement in limb perfusion in patients with CLI, but no reduction of major amputation and mortality rate was observed [130]. VEGF gene administered at the angioplasty site during endovascular procedure in patients with CLI was associated with increased vascularity and improvements in limb perfusion [131], but intramuscular VEGF gene treatment did not result in amputation rate reduction [132]. The only gene therapy at present that has resulted in reduction in major amputation rate and in pain relief in patients with CLI was intramuscular administration of fibroblast growth factor 1 (FGF-1) gene [133, 134]. Although pilot studies with several gene-based therapies have reported promising findings, only a few patients with DM were included and we still have to wait for randomized controlled trials before gaining confidence on the efficacy and safety of these treatments in diabetic patients with CLI. Hence, gene therapy is still confined to research settings [67, 71, 110].

Human bone marrow cells contain stem cells that have the potential for differentiation into a variety of tissues, including endothelium. A meta-analysis of studies about the efficiency of autologous peripheral blood mononuclear cells (PB-MNCs) or bone marrow mononuclear cells (BM-MNCs) transplantation in patients with PAD demonstrated that administration of stem cells improved pain, ulcer healing, and amputation rate, and it was safe and well tolerated [135]. Intramuscular administration of stem cells was more effective than intrarterial administration. In diabetic patients with CLI, intramuscular injections of autologous PB-MNCs or BM-MNCs into the ischemic lower limb resulted in pain relief, improved blood flow, ulcer healing and limb survival according to several studies, while no major adverse events were observed [136–142]. Combined intramuscular administration of BM-MNCs and VEGF gene in diabetic patients with CLI has also shown favorable results [143]. A recent study comparing the effects of autologous PB-MNCs or BM-MNCs transplantation with endovascular procedures in diabetic patients with CLI demonstrated that limb salvage at 6 and 12 months after treatment did not differ significantly between the two treatment arms, while control patients underwent more often amputation [140]. Moreover, there was greater ulcer healing in the group of patients who received stem cells.

Although several studies with cell-based therapies have shown beneficial results in diabetic patients with CLI, clinical experience is limited and larger studies are needed to confirm these preliminary promising findings [67, 71]. Moreover, cell types used, amount of cells administered and administration route varies among different studies and data are insufficient so far to recommend cell-based therapies in clinical practice [67]. However, they could serve as a treatment option in patients not amenable to revascularization procedures due to morphological distribution of the atherosclerotic disease or high surgical risk.

Table 49.4 Proposed protocol for the management of CLI in diabetic patients

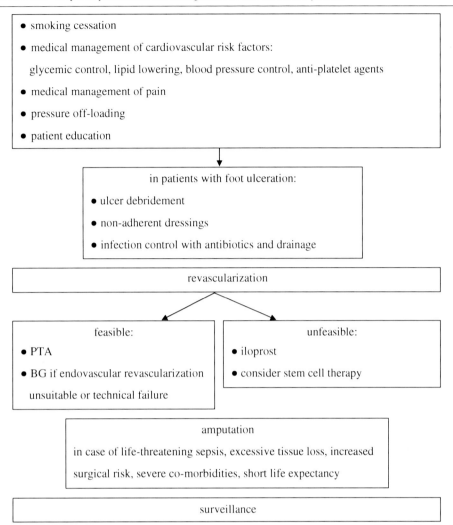

- smoking cessation
- medical management of cardiovascular risk factors:
  glycemic control, lipid lowering, blood pressure control, anti-platelet agents
- medical management of pain
- pressure off-loading
- patient education

in patients with foot ulceration:
- ulcer debridement
- non-adherent dressings
- infection control with antibiotics and drainage

revascularization

feasible:
- PTA
- BG if endovascular revascularization unsuitable or technical failure

unfeasible:
- iloprost
- consider stem cell therapy

amputation

in case of life-threatening sepsis, excessive tissue loss, increased surgical risk, severe co-morbidities, short life expectancy

surveillance

CLI critical limb ischemia, P *TA* percutaneous transluminal angioplasty, *B G* bypass grafting

CLI Prognosis

The overall management of CLI has changed over the last decade and diabetic patients with CLI are offered a multidisciplinary management with modification of the cardiovascular risk factor profile, appropriate medical treatment and revascularization options when possible that could result in improved global prognosis [66, 144–147]. Indeed, some studies have reported that a multidisciplinary and aggressive approach of diabetic patients with CLI resulted in low amputation rates and probably in reduced mortality rates [144–148].

Summary

Patients with DM are prone to develop PAD. CLI represents the most severe form of PAD and poses a major threat to both lower limb and life of the affected patient. Due to multifactorial pathophysiologic mechanisms underlying diabetic CLI and the complex nature of treatment, a multidisciplinary management is warranted (Table 49.4). Medical management of cardiovascular risk factors plays an important role for secondary prevention of cardiovascular disease and for pain relief in patients not suitable for revascularization. The cornerstone of CLI management is revascularization and should be attempted without delay in diabetic patients presenting with CLI. Early, aggressive management of the risk factors and timely referral for revascularization might improve outcomes in diabetic patients with CLI. Therapeutic angiogenesis represents a novel and promising therapeutic adjunct in the management of CLI and is likely to increase treatment options in the future.

References

1. Becker F, Robert-Ebadi H, Ricco JB, Setacci C, Cao P, de Donato G, et al. Chapter I: definitions, epidemiology, clinical presentation and prognosis. Eur J Vasc Endovasc Surg. 2011;42 Suppl 2:S4–12.
2. Whiting DR, Guariguata L, Weil C, Shaw J. IDF diabetes atlas: global estimates of the prevalence of diabetes for 2011 and 2030. Diabetes Res Clin Pract. 2011;94:311–21.
3. American Diabetes Association. Peripheral arterial disease in people with diabetes. Diabetes Care. 2003;26:3333–41.
4. Marso SP, Hiatt WR. Peripheral arterial disease in patients with diabetes. J Am Coll Cardiol. 2006;47:921–9.
5. Jude EB, Eleftheriadou I, Tentolouris N. Peripheral arterial disease in diabetes—a review. Diabet Med. 2010;27:4–14.
6. Mascarenhas JV, Albayati MA, Shearman CP, Jude EB. Peripheral arterial disease. Endocrinol Metab Clin North Am. 2014;43:149–66.
7. Jude EB. Intermittent claudication in the patient with diabetes. Br J Diabetes Vasc Dis. 2004;4:238–42.
8. Jude EB, Oyibo SO, Chalmers N, Boulton AJ. Peripheral arterial disease in diabetic and nondiabetic patients: a comparison of severity and outcome. Diabetes Care. 2001;24:1433–7.
9. Hirsch AT, Haskal ZJ, Hertzer NR, Bakal CW, Creager MA, Halperin JL, et al. ACC/AHA 2005 guidelines for the management of patients with peripheral arterial disease (lower extremity, renal, mesenteric, and abdominal aortic): executive summary a collaborative report from the American Association for Vascular Surgery/Society for Vascular Surgery, Society for Cardiovascular Angiography and Interventions, Society for Vascular Medicine and Biology, Society of Interventional Radiology, and the ACC/AHA Task Force on Practice Guidelines (Writing Committee to Develop Guidelines for the Management of Patients With Peripheral Arterial Disease) endorsed by the American Association of Cardiovascular and Pulmonary Rehabilitation; National Heart, Lung, and Blood Institute; Society for Vascular Nursing; TransAtlantic Inter-Society Consensus; and Vascular Disease Foundation. J Am Coll Cardiol. 2006;47:1239–312.
10. Kannel WB, McGee DL. Update on some epidemiologic features of intermittent claudication: the Framingham Study. J Am Geriatr Soc. 1985;33:13–8.
11. Norgren L, Hiatt WR, Dormandy JA, Nehler MR, Harris KA, Fowkes FG. Inter-Society Consensus for the Management of Peripheral Arterial Disease (TASC II). J Vasc Surg. 2007;45(Suppl S):S5–67.
12. Lepantalo M, Matzke S. Outcome of unreconstructed chronic critical leg ischaemia. Eur J Vasc Endovasc Surg. 1996;11:153–7.
13. Malmstedt J, Leander K, Wahlberg E, Karlstrom L, Alfredsson L, Swedenborg J. Outcome after leg bypass surgery for critical limb ischemia is poor in patients with diabetes: a population-based cohort study. Diabetes Care. 2008;31:887–92.
14. Liang KW, Kuo HN, Lee WL, Liu TJ, Lin WW, Tsao CR, et al. Different mid-term prognostic predictors of major adverse events in diabetic and nondiabetic peripheral artery disease presenting with critical limb ischemia. Angiology. 2016;67(3):287–91.
15. Suzuki K, Iida O, Yamauchi Y, Nakano M, Soga Y, Kawasaki D, et al. Impact of diabetes mellitus on critical limb ischemia with

below the knee disease: Japan below-the-knee artery treatment subanalysis. Angiology. 2013 [Epub ahead of print].
16. Tentolouris N, Al-Sabbagh S, Walker MG, Boulton AJ, Jude EB. Mortality in diabetic and nondiabetic patients after amputations performed from 1990 to 1995: a 5-year follow-up study. Diabetes Care. 2004;27:1598–604.
17. Faglia E, Clerici G, Clerissi J, Gabrielli L, Losa S, Mantero M, et al. Long-term prognosis of diabetic patients with critical limb ischemia: a population-based cohort study. Diabetes Care. 2009;32:822–7.
18. Faglia E, Clerici G, Clerissi J, Gabrielli L, Losa S, Mantero M, et al. Early and five-year amputation and survival rate of diabetic patients with critical limb ischemia: data of a cohort study of 564 patients. Eur J Vasc Endovasc Surg. 2006;32:484–90.
19. Faglia E, Clerici G, Caminiti M, Curci V, Clerissi J, Losa S, et al. Mortality after major amputation in diabetic patients with critical limb ischemia who did and did not undergo previous peripheral revascularization data of a cohort study of 564 consecutive diabetic patients. J Diabetes Complications. 2010;24:265–9.
20. Faglia E, Clerici G, Mantero M, Caminiti M, Quarantiello A, Curci V, et al. Incidence of critical limb ischemia and amputation outcome in contralateral limb in diabetic patients hospitalized for unilateral critical limb ischemia during 1999–2003 and followed-up until 2005. Diabetes Res Clin Pract. 2007;77:445–50.
21. Apelqvist JA, Lepantalo MJ. The ulcerated leg: when to revascularize. Diabetes Metab Res Rev. 2012;28 Suppl 1:30–5.
22. Lepantalo M, Apelqvist J, Setacci C, Ricco JB, de Donato G, Becker F, et al. Chapter V: diabetic foot. Eur J Vasc Endovasc Surg. 2011;42 Suppl 2:S60–74.
23. Jorneskog G. Why critical limb ischemia criteria are not applicable to diabetic foot and what the consequences are. Scand J Surg. 2012;101:114–8.
24. Stratmann B, Tschoepe D. Atherogenesis and atherothrombosis—focus on diabetes mellitus. Best Pract Res Clin Endocrinol Metab. 2009;23:291–303.
25. Beckman JA, Creager MA, Libby P. Diabetes and atherosclerosis: epidemiology, pathophysiology, and management. JAMA. 2002;287:2570–81.
26. Li Y, Woo V, Bose R. Platelet hyperactivity and abnormal Ca(2+) homeostasis in diabetes mellitus. Am J Physiol Heart Circ Physiol. 2001;280:H1480–9.
27. Vinik AI, Erbas T, Park TS, Nolan R, Pittenger GL. Platelet dysfunction in type 2 diabetes. Diabetes Care. 2001;24:1476–85.
28. Carr ME. Diabetes mellitus: a hypercoagulable state. J Diabetes Complications. 2001;15:44–54.
29. Uemura S, Matsushita H, Li W, Glassford AJ, Asagami T, Lee KH, et al. Diabetes mellitus enhances vascular matrix metalloproteinase activity: role of oxidative stress. Circ Res. 2001;88:1291–8.
30. Chen MC, Sheu JJ, Wang PW, Chen CY, Kuo MC, Hsieh CJ, et al. Complications impaired endothelial progenitor cell function in Type 2 diabetic patients with or without critical leg ischaemia: implication for impaired neovascularization in diabetes. Diabet Med. 2009;26:134–41.
31. Waltenberger J. Impaired collateral vessel development in diabetes: potential cellular mechanisms and therapeutic implications. Cardiovasc Res. 2001;49:554–60.
32. Ruiter MS, van Golde JM, Schaper NC, Stehouwer CD, Huijberts MS. Diabetes impairs arteriogenesis in the peripheral circulation: review of molecular mechanisms. Clin Sci (Lond). 2010;119:225–38.
33. Fadini GP, Sartore S, Agostini C, Avogaro A. Significance of endothelial progenitor cells in subjects with diabetes. Diabetes Care. 2007;30:1305–13.
34. Graziani L. Comprehensive approach to management of critical limb ischemia. Curr Treat Options Cardiovasc Med. 2014;16:332.

35. Adler AI, Stevens RJ, Neil A, Stratton IM, Boulton AJ, Holman RR. UKPDS 59: hyperglycemia and other potentially modifiable risk factors for peripheral vascular disease in type 2 diabetes. Diabetes Care. 2002;25:894–9.

36. Walters DP, Gatling W, Mullee MA, Hill RD. The prevalence, detection, and epidemiological correlates of peripheral vascular disease: a comparison of diabetic and non-diabetic subjects in an English community. Diabet Med. 1992;9:710–5.

37. Murabito JM, Evans JC, Nieto K, Larson MG, Levy D, Wilson PW. Prevalence and clinical correlates of peripheral arterial disease in the Framingham Offspring Study. Am Heart J. 2002;143:961–5.

38. Abbott RD, Brand FN, Kannel WB. Epidemiology of some peripheral arterial findings in diabetic men and women: experiences from the Framingham Study. Am J Med. 1990;88:376–81.

39. Melton 3rd LJ, Macken KM, Palumbo PJ, Elveback LR. Incidence and prevalence of clinical peripheral vascular disease in a population-based cohort of diabetic patients. Diabetes Care. 1980;3:650–4.

40. van der Feen C, Neijens FS, Kanters SD, Mali WP, Stolk RP, Banga JD. Angiographic distribution of lower extremity atherosclerosis in patients with and without diabetes. Diabet Med. 2002;19:366–70.

41. Ciavarella A, Silletti A, Mustacchio A, Gargiulo M, Galaverni MC, Stella A, et al. Angiographic evaluation of the anatomic pattern of arterial obstructions in diabetic patients with critical limb ischaemia. Diabete Metab. 1993;19:586–9.

42. Graziani L, Silvestro A, Bertone V, Manara E, Andreini R, Sigala A, et al. Vascular involvement in diabetic subjects with ischemic foot ulcer: a new morphologic categorization of disease severity. Eur J Vasc Endovasc Surg. 2007;33:453–60.

43. Faglia E. Characteristics of peripheral arterial disease and its relevance to the diabetic population. Int J Low Extrem Wounds. 2011;10:152–66.

44. Boulton AJ, Armstrong DG, Albert SF, Frykberg RG, Hellman R, Kirkman MS, et al. Comprehensive foot examination and risk assessment: a report of the task force of the foot care interest group of the American Diabetes Association, with endorsement by the American Association of Clinical Endocrinologists. Diabetes Care. 2008;31:1679–85.

45. American Diabetes Association. Standards of medical care in diabetes—2014. Diabetes Care. 2014;37 Suppl 1:S14–80.

46. Boulton AJ, Malik RA, Arezzo JC, Sosenko JM. Diabetic somatic neuropathies. Diabetes Care. 2004;27:1458–86.

47. Tesfaye S, Vileikyte L, Rayman G, Sindrup S, Perkins B, Baconja M, et al. Painful diabetic peripheral neuropathy: consensus recommendations on diagnosis, assessment and management. Diabetes Metab Res Rev. 2011;27(7):629–38.

48. Moulik PK, Mtonga R, Gill GV. Amputation and mortality in new-onset diabetic foot ulcers stratified by etiology. Diabetes Care. 2003;26:491–4.

49. Prompers L, Huijberts M, Apelqvist J, Jude E, Piaggesi A, Bakker K, et al. High prevalence of ischaemia, infection and serious comorbidity in patients with diabetic foot disease in Europe. Baseline results from the Eurodiale study. Diabetologia. 2007;50:18–25.

50. Schaper NC, Andros G, Apelqvist J, Bakker K, Lammer J, Lepantalo M, et al. Specific guidelines for the diagnosis and treatment of peripheral arterial disease in a patient with diabetes and ulceration of the foot 2011. Diabetes Metab Res Rev. 2012;28 Suppl 1:236–7.

51. Venermo M, Vikatmaa P, Terasaki H, Sugano N. Vascular laboratory for critical limb ischaemia. Scand J Surg. 2012;101:86–93.

52. Dormandy JA, Rutherford RB. Management of peripheral arterial disease (PAD). TASC Working Group. TransAtlantic Inter-Society Consensus (TASC). J Vasc Surg. 2000;31:S1–296.

53. Potier L, Abi Khalil C, Mohammedi K, Roussel R. Use and utility of ankle brachial index in patients with diabetes. Eur J Vasc Endovasc Surg. 2011;41:110–6.

54. Dyet JF, Nicholson AA, Ettles DF. Vascular imaging and intervention in peripheral arteries in the diabetic patient. Diabetes Metab Res Rev. 2000;16 Suppl 1:S16–22.

55. Faglia E, Clerici G, Caminiti M, Quarantiello A, Curci V, Somalvico F. Evaluation of feasibility of ankle pressure and foot oximetry values for the detection of critical limb ischemia in diabetic patients. Vasc Endovascular Surg. 2010;44:184–9.

56. Faglia E, Clerici G, Caminiti M, Quarantiello A, Curci V, Morabito A. Predictive values of transcutaneous oxygen tension for above-the-ankle amputation in diabetic patients with critical limb ischemia. Eur J Vasc Endovasc Surg. 2007;33:731–6.

57. Cao P, Eckstein HH, De Rango P, Setacci C, Ricco JB, de Donato G, et al. Chapter II: diagnostic methods. Eur J Vasc Endovasc Surg. 2011;42 Suppl 2:S13–32.

58. Silvestro A, Diehm N, Savolainen H, Do DD, Vogelea J, Mahler F, et al. Falsely high ankle-brachial index predicts major amputation in critical limb ischemia. Vasc Med. 2006;11:69–74.

59. Takahara M, Kaneto H, Iida O, Katakami N, Matsuoka TA, Ikeda M, et al. Association of diabetes and hemodialysis with ankle pressure and ankle-brachial index in Japanese patients with critical limb ischemia. Diabetes Care. 2012;35:2000–4.

60. Khodabandehlou T, Vimeux M, Le Devehat C. Measurements of transcutaneous oxygen pressure and changes in blood rheology as markers of prognosis of critically ischemic limb in diabetes mellitus patients. Int J Low Extrem Wounds. 2003;2:13–8.

61. Redlich U, Xiong YY, Pech M, Tautenhahn J, Halloul Z, Lobmann R, et al. Superiority of transcutaneous oxygen tension measurements in predicting limb salvage after below-the-knee angioplasty: a prospective trial in diabetic patients with critical limb ischemia. Cardiovasc Intervent Radiol. 2011;34:271–9.

62. Caselli A, Latini V, Lapenna A, Di Carlo S, Pirozzi F, Benvenuto A, et al. Transcutaneous oxygen tension monitoring after successful revascularization in diabetic patients with ischaemic foot ulcers. Diabet Med. 2005;22:460–5.

63. National Institute for Health and Care Excellence [Internet]. Lower limb peripheral arterial disease: diagnosis and management. 2012. Available from: http://www.nice.org.uk/guidance/cg147/resources/guidance-lower-limb-peripheral-arterial-disease-diagnosis-and-management-pdf

64. Marti X, Romera A, Vila R, Cairols MA. Role of ultrasound arterial mapping in planning therapeutic options for critical ischemia of lower limbs in diabetic patients. Ann Vasc Surg. 2012;26:1071–6.

65. Tendera M, Aboyans V, Bartelink ML, Baumgartner I, Clement D, Collet JP, et al. ESC guidelines on the diagnosis and treatment of peripheral artery diseases: document covering atherosclerotic disease of extracranial carotid and vertebral, mesenteric, renal, upper and lower extremity arteries: the Task Force on the Diagnosis and Treatment of Peripheral Artery Diseases of the European Society of Cardiology (ESC). Eur Heart J. 2011;32:2851–906.

66. Sumpio BE, Armstrong DG, Lavery LA, Andros G. The role of interdisciplinary team approach in the management of the diabetic foot: a joint statement from the Society for Vascular Surgery and the American Podiatric Medical Association. J Vasc Surg. 2010;51:1504–6.

67. Diehm N, Schmidli J, Setacci C, Ricco JB, de Donato G, Becker F, et al. Chapter III: management of cardiovascular risk factors and medical therapy. Eur J Vasc Endovasc Surg. 2011;42 Suppl 2:S33–42.

68. Caravaggi C, Ferraresi R, Bassetti M, Sganzaroli AB, Galenda P, Fattori S, et al. Management of ischemic diabetic foot. J Cardiovasc Surg (Torino). 2013;54:737–54.

69. Edmonds M. Modern treatment of infection and ischaemia to reduce major amputation in the diabetic foot. Curr Pharm Des. 2013;19:5008–15.

70. Forsythe RO, Hinchliffe RJ. Management of peripheral arterial disease and the diabetic foot. J Cardiovasc Surg (Torino). 2014;55:195–206.

71. Lambert MA, Belch JJ. Medical management of critical limb ischaemia: where do we stand today? J Intern Med. 2013;274:295–307.

72. Holman RR, Paul SK, Bethel MA, Matthews DR, Neil HA. 10-year follow-up of intensive glucose control in type 2 diabetes. N Engl J Med. 2008;359:1577–89.

73. Camafort M, Alvarez-Rodriguez LR, Munoz-Torrero JF, Sahuquillo JC, Lopez-Jimenez L, Coll R, et al. Glucose control and outcome in patients with stable diabetes and previous coronary, cerebrovascular or peripheral artery disease. Findings from the FRENA Registry. Diabet Med. 2011;28:73–80.

74. Singh S, Armstrong EJ, Sherif W, Alvandi B, Westin GG, Singh GD, et al. Association of elevated fasting glucose with lower patency and increased major adverse limb events among patients with diabetes undergoing infrapopliteal balloon angioplasty. Vasc Med. 2014;19:307–14.

75. Takahara M, Kaneto H, Iida O, Gorogawa S, Katakami N, Matsuoka TA, et al. The influence of glycemic control on the prognosis of Japanese patients undergoing percutaneous transluminal angioplasty for critical limb ischemia. Diabetes Care. 2010;33:2538–42.

76. Dormandy JA, Betteridge DJ, Schernthaner G, Pirags V, Norgren L. Impact of peripheral arterial disease in patients with diabetes—results from PROactive (PROactive 11). Atherosclerosis. 2009;202:272–81.

77. Dosluoglu HH, Lall P, Nader ND, Harris LM, Dryjski ML. Insulin use is associated with poor limb salvage and survival in diabetic patients with chronic limb ischemia. J Vasc Surg. 2010;51:1178–89. discussion 88–9.

78. Takahara M, Kaneto H, Iida O, Katakami N, Sakamoto F, Matsuoka TA, et al. No association of diabetic duration or insulin use with the prognosis of critical limb ischemia after endovascular therapy. J Atheroscler Thromb. 2011;18:1102–9.

79. Pyorala K, Pedersen TR, Kjekshus J, Faergeman O, Olsson AG, Thorgeirsson G. Cholesterol lowering with simvastatin improves prognosis of diabetic patients with coronary heart disease. A subgroup analysis of the Scandinavian Simvastatin Survival Study (4S). Diabetes Care. 1997;20:614–20.

80. Heart Protection Study Collaborative Group. MRC/BHF Heart Protection Study of cholesterol lowering with simvastatin in 20,536 high-risk individuals: a randomised placebo-controlled trial. Lancet. 2002;360:7–22.

81. Colhoun HM, Betteridge DJ, Durrington PN, Hitman GA, Neil HA, Livingstone SJ, et al. Primary prevention of cardiovascular disease with atorvastatin in type 2 diabetes in the Collaborative Atorvastatin Diabetes Study (CARDS): multicentre randomised placebo-controlled trial. Lancet. 2004;364:685–96.

82. Aung PP, Maxwell HG, Jepson RG, Price JF, Leng GC. Lipid-lowering for peripheral arterial disease of the lower limb. Cochrane Database Syst Rev. 2007;(4):CD000123.

83. Westin GG, Armstrong EJ, Bang H, Yeo KK, Anderson D, Dawson DL, et al. Association between statin medications and mortality, major adverse cardiovascular event, and amputation-free survival in patients with critical limb ischemia. J Am Coll Cardiol. 2014;63:682–90.

84. Suckow BD, Kraiss LW, Schanzer A, Stone DH, Kalish J, DeMartino RR, et al. Statin therapy after infrainguinal bypass surgery for critical limb ischemia is associated with improved 5-year survival. J Vasc Surg. 2014.

85. Holman RR, Paul SK, Bethel MA, Neil HA, Matthews DR. Long-term follow-up after tight control of blood pressure in type 2 diabetes. N Engl J Med. 2008;359:1565–76.

86. Heart Outcomes Prevention Evaluation Study Investigators. Effects of ramipril on cardiovascular and microvascular outcomes in people with diabetes mellitus: results of the HOPE study and MICRO-HOPE substudy. Lancet. 2000;355:253–9.

87. Radack K, Deck C. Beta-adrenergic blocker therapy does not worsen intermittent claudication in subjects with peripheral arterial disease. A meta-analysis of randomized controlled trials. Arch Intern Med. 1991;151:1769–76.

88. Paravastu SC, Mendonca DA, da Silva A. Beta blockers for peripheral arterial disease. Eur J Vasc Endovasc Surg. 2009;38:66–70.

89. Baigent C, Blackwell L, Collins R, Emberson J, Godwin J, Peto R, et al. Aspirin in the primary and secondary prevention of vascular disease: collaborative meta-analysis of individual participant data from randomised trials. Lancet. 2009;373:1849–60.

90. CAPRIE Steering Committee. A randomised, blinded, trial of clopidogrel versus aspirin in patients at risk of ischaemic events (CAPRIE). Lancet. 1996;348:1329–39.

91. Alonso-Coello P, Bellmunt S, McGorrian C, Anand SS, Guzman R, Criqui MH, et al. Antithrombotic therapy in peripheral artery disease: Antithrombotic Therapy and Prevention of Thrombosis, 9th ed: American College of Chest Physicians Evidence-Based Clinical Practice Guidelines. Chest. 2012;141:e669S–90S.

92. Duthois S, Cailleux N, Benosman B, Levesque H. Tolerance of iloprost and results of treatment of chronic severe lower limb ischaemia in diabetic patients. A retrospective study of 64 consecutive cases. Diabetes Metab. 2003;29:36–43.

93. Altstaedt HO, Berzewski B, Breddin HK, Brockhaus W, Bruhn HD, Cachovan M, et al. Treatment of patients with peripheral arterial occlusive disease Fontaine stage IV with intravenous iloprost and PGE1: a randomized open controlled study. Prostaglandins Leukot Essent Fatty Acids. 1993;49:573–8.

94. Loosemore TM, Chalmers TC, Dormandy JA. A meta-analysis of randomized placebo control trials in Fontaine stages III and IV peripheral occlusive arterial disease. Int Angiol. 1994;13:133–42.

95. Weck M, Slesaczeck T, Rietzsch H, Munch D, Nanning T, Paetzold H, et al. Noninvasive management of the diabetic foot with critical limb ischemia: current options and future perspectives. Ther Adv Endocrinol Metab. 2011;2:247–55.

96. Rumenapf G, Morbach S. What can i do with a patient with diabetes and critically impaired limb perfusion who cannot be revascularized? Int J Low Extrem Wounds. 2014;13(4):378–89.

97. Rendell M, Cariski AT, Hittel N, Zhang P. Cilostazol treatment of claudication in diabetic patients. Curr Med Res Opin. 2002;18:479–87.

98. The European Study Group. Intravenous pentoxifylline for the treatment of chronic critical limb ischaemia. Eur J Vasc Endovasc Surg. 1995;9:426–36.

99. Conte MS. Diabetic revascularization: endovascular versus open bypass—do we have the answer? Semin Vasc Surg. 2012;25:108–14.

100. Albayati MA, Shearman CP. Peripheral arterial disease and bypass surgery in the diabetic lower limb. Med Clin North Am. 2013;97:821–34.

101. Georgakarakos E, Papanas N, Papadaki E, Georgiadis GS, Maltezos E, Lazarides MK. Endovascular treatment of critical ischemia in the diabetic foot: new thresholds, new anatomies. Angiology. 2013;64:583–91.

102. Pedrajas FG, Cafasso DE, Schneider PA. Endovascular therapy: is it effective in the diabetic limb? Semin Vasc Surg. 2012;25:93–101.

103. DeRubertis BG, Pierce M, Ryer EJ, Trocciola S, Kent KC, Faries PL. Reduced primary patency rate in diabetic patients after percutaneous intervention results from more frequent presentation with limb-threatening ischemia. J Vasc Surg. 2008;47:101–8.

104. Liistro F, Porto I, Angioli P, Grotti S, Ricci L, Ducci K, et al. Drug-eluting balloon in peripheral intervention for below the knee angioplasty evaluation (DEBATE-BTK): a randomized trial in

diabetic patients with critical limb ischemia. Circulation. 2013; 128:615–21.

105. Peeters P, Verbist J, Keirse K, Callaert J, Deloose K, Bosiers M. Endovascular procedures and new insights in diabetic limb salvage. J Cardiovasc Surg (Torino). 2012;53:31–7.

106. Faglia E, Clerici G, Losa S, Tavano D, Caminiti M, Miramonti M, et al. Limb revascularization feasibility in diabetic patients with critical limb ischemia: results from a cohort of 344 consecutive unselected diabetic patients evaluated in 2009. Diabetes Res Clin Pract. 2012;95:364–71.

107. Manzi M, Palena L, Cester G. Endovascular techniques for limb salvage in diabetics with crural and pedal disease. J Cardiovasc Surg (Torino). 2011;52:485–92.

108. Tenna AS, Watson A, Stansby G. Revascularization for critical limb ischemia in diabetes: surgery or angioplasty? Angiology. 2014;65:272–3.

109. Setacci C, Sirignano P, Galzerano G, Mazzitelli G, Sauro L, de Donato G, et al. Endovascular first as "preliminary approach" for critical limb ischemia and diabetic foot. J Cardiovasc Surg (Torino). 2013;54:679–84.

110. Setacci C, de Donato G, Teraa M, Moll FL, Ricco JB, Becker F, et al. Chapter IV: treatment of critical limb ischaemia. Eur J Vasc Endovasc Surg. 2011;42 Suppl 2:S43–59.

111. Lepantalo M. The path from art to evidence in treating critical limb ischaemia—reflections on 35 years' experience. Scand J Surg. 2012;101:78–85.

112. Hinchliffe RJ, Andros G, Apelqvist J, Bakker K, Friederichs S, Lammer J, et al. A systematic review of the effectiveness of revascularization of the ulcerated foot in patients with diabetes and peripheral arterial disease. Diabetes Metab Res Rev. 2012;28 Suppl 1:179–217.

113. Arvela E, Dick F. Surveillance after distal revascularization for critical limb ischaemia. Scand J Surg. 2012;101:119–24.

114. da Silva AF, Desgranges P, Holdsworth J, Harris PL, McCollum P, Jones SM, et al. The management and outcome of critical limb ischaemia in diabetic patients: results of a national survey. Audit Committee of the Vascular Surgical Society of Great Britain and Ireland. Diabet Med. 1996;13:726–8.

115. Wallaert JB, Nolan BW, Adams J, Stanley AC, Eldrup-Jorgensen J, Cronenwett JL, et al. The impact of diabetes on postoperative outcomes following lower-extremity bypass surgery. J Vasc Surg. 2012;56:1317–23.

116. Lazaris AM, Tsiamis AC, Fishwick G, Bolia A, Bell PR. Clinical outcome of primary infrainguinal subintimal angioplasty in diabetic patients with critical lower limb ischemia. J Endovasc Ther. 2004;11:447–53.

117. Wolfle KD, Bruijnen H, Loeprecht H, Rumenapf G, Schweiger H, Grabitz K, et al. Graft patency and clinical outcome of femorodistal arterial reconstruction in diabetic and non-diabetic patients: results of a multicentre comparative analysis. Eur J Vasc Endovasc Surg. 2003;25:229–34.

118. Ballotta E, Toniato A, Piatto G, Mazzalai F, Da Giau G. Lower extremity arterial reconstruction for critical limb ischemia in diabetes. J Vasc Surg. 2014;59:708–19.

119. An JH, Jang YM, Song KH, Kim SK, Park SW, Jung HG, et al. Outcome of percutaneous transluminal angioplasty in diabetic patients with critical limb ischaemia. Exp Clin Endocrinol Diabetes. 2014;122:50–4.

120. Awad S, Karkos CD, Serrachino-Inglott F, Cooper NJ, Butterfield JS, Ashleigh R, et al. The impact of diabetes on current revascularisation practice and clinical outcome in patients with critical lower limb ischaemia. Eur J Vasc Endovasc Surg. 2006;32: 51–9.

121. Panneton JM, Gloviczki P, Bower TC, Rhodes JM, Canton LG, Toomey BJ. Pedal bypass for limb salvage: impact of diabetes on long-term outcome. Ann Vasc Surg. 2000;14:640–7.

122. Tolva VS, Casana R, Lonati L, Invitti C, Bertoni GB, Bianchi PG, et al. Percutaneous transluminal angioplasty improves glucose control and quality of life in patients with critical limb ischemia. Eur Rev Med Pharmacol Sci. 2012;16:2082–7.

123. Engelhardt M, Bruijnen H, Scharmer C, Jezdinsky N, Wolfle K. Improvement of quality of life six months after infrageniculate bypass surgery: diabetic patients benefit less than non-diabetic patients. Eur J Vasc Endovasc Surg. 2006;32:182–7.

124. Petrakis IE, Sciacca V. Epidural spinal cord electrical stimulation in diabetic critical lower limb ischemia. J Diabetes Complications. 1999;13:293–9.

125. Petrakis IE, Sciacca V. Spinal cord stimulation in diabetic lower limb critical ischaemia: transcutaneous oxygen measurement as predictor for treatment success. Eur J Vasc Endovasc Surg. 2000;19:587–92.

126. Klomp HM, Steyerberg EW, Habbema JD, van Urk H. What is the evidence on efficacy of spinal cord stimulation in (subgroups of) patients with critical limb ischemia? Ann Vasc Surg. 2009;23: 355–63.

127. Petrakis IE, Sciacca V. Does autonomic neuropathy influence spinal cord stimulation therapy success in diabetic patients with critical lower limb ischemia? Surg Neurol. 2000;53:182–8. discussion 8–9.

128. Baltzis D, Eleftheriadou I, Veves A. Pathogenesis and treatment of impaired wound healing in diabetes mellitus: new insights. Adv Ther. 2014;31:817–36.

129. Papanas N, Maltezos E. Advances in treating the ischaemic diabetic foot. Curr Vasc Pharmacol. 2008;6:23–8.

130. Powell RJ, Goodney P, Mendelsohn FO, Moen EK, Annex BH. Safety and efficacy of patient specific intramuscular injection of HGF plasmid gene therapy on limb perfusion and wound healing in patients with ischemic lower extremity ulceration: results of the HGF-0205 trial. J Vasc Surg. 2010;52:1525–30.

131. Makinen K, Manninen H, Hedman M, Matsi P, Mussalo H, Alhava E, et al. Increased vascularity detected by digital subtraction angiography after VEGF gene transfer to human lower limb artery: a randomized, placebo-controlled, double-blinded phase II study. Mol Ther. 2002;6:127–33.

132. Kusumanto YH, van Weel V, Mulder NH, Smit AJ, van den Dungen JJ, Hooymans JM, et al. Treatment with intramuscular vascular endothelial growth factor gene compared with placebo for patients with diabetes mellitus and critical limb ischemia: a double-blind randomized trial. Hum Gene Ther. 2006;17:683–91.

133. Nikol S, Baumgartner I, Van Belle E, Diehm C, Visona A, Capogrossi MC, et al. Therapeutic angiogenesis with intramuscular NV1FGF improves amputation-free survival in patients with critical limb ischemia. Mol Ther. 2008;16:972–8.

134. Comerota AJ, Throm RC, Miller KA, Henry T, Chronos N, Laird J, et al. Naked plasmid DNA encoding fibroblast growth factor type 1 for the treatment of end-stage unreconstructible lower extremity ischemia: preliminary results of a phase I trial. J Vasc Surg. 2002;35:930–6.

135. Fadini GP, Agostini C, Avogaro A. Autologous stem cell therapy for peripheral arterial disease meta-analysis and systematic review of the literature. Atherosclerosis. 2010;209:10–7.

136. Ruiz-Salmeron R, de la Cuesta-Diaz A, Constantino-Bermejo M, Perez-Camacho I, Marcos-Sanchez F, Hmadcha A, et al. Angiographic demonstration of neoangiogenesis after intra-arterial infusion of autologous bone marrow mononuclear cells in diabetic patients with critical limb ischemia. Cell Transplant. 2011;20:1629–39.

137. Subrammaniyan R, Amalorpavanathan J, Shankar R, Rajkumar M, Baskar S, Manjunath S, et al. Our experience of application of autologous bone marrow stem cells in critical limb ischemia in six diabetic patients—a five-year follow-up. J Stem Cells Regen Med. 2011;7:97.

138. Kirana S, Stratmann B, Prante C, Prohaska W, Koerperich H, Lammers D, et al. Autologous stem cell therapy in the treatment of limb ischaemia induced chronic tissue ulcers of diabetic foot patients. Int J Clin Pract. 2012;66:384–93.

139. Mohammadzadeh L, Samedanifard SH, Keshavarzi A, Alimoghaddam K, Larijani B, Ghavamzadeh A, et al. Therapeutic outcomes of transplanting autologous granulocyte colony-stimulating factor-mobilised peripheral mononuclear cells in diabetic patients with critical limb ischaemia. Exp Clin Endocrinol Diabetes. 2013;121:48–53.

140. Dubsky M, Jirkovska A, Bem R, Fejfarova V, Pagacova L, Sixta B, et al. Both autologous bone marrow mononuclear cell and peripheral blood progenitor cell therapies similarly improve ischaemia in patients with diabetic foot in comparison with control treatment. Diabetes Metab Res Rev. 2013;29:369–76.

141. Ozturk A, Kucukardali Y, Tangi F, Erikci A, Uzun G, Bashekim C, et al. Therapeutical potential of autologous peripheral blood mononuclear cell transplantation in patients with type 2 diabetic critical limb ischemia. J Diabetes Complications. 2012;26:29–33.

142. Huang P, Li S, Han M, Xiao Z, Yang R, Han ZC. Autologous transplantation of granulocyte colony-stimulating factor-mobilized peripheral blood mononuclear cells improves critical limb ischemia in diabetes. Diabetes Care. 2005;28:2155–60.

143. Skora J, Barc P, Pupka A, Dawiskiba T, Korta K, Albert M, et al. Transplantation of autologous bone marrow mononuclear cells with VEGF gene improves diabetic critical limb ischaemia. Endokrynol Pol. 2013;64:129–38.

144. Scatena A, Petruzzi P, Ferrari M, Rizzo L, Cicorelli A, Berchiolli R, et al. Outcomes of three years of teamwork on critical limb ischemia in patients with diabetes and foot lesions. Int J Low Extrem Wounds. 2012;11:113–9.

145. Zayed H, Halawa M, Maillardet L, Sidhu PS, Edmonds M, Rashid H. Improving limb salvage rate in diabetic patients with critical leg ischaemia using a multidisciplinary approach. Int J Clin Pract. 2009;63:855–8.

146. Aragon-Sanchez J, Maynar-Moliner M, Pulido-Duque JM, Rabellino M, Gonzalez G, Zander T. The role of a specialized approach for patients with diabetes, critical ischaemia and foot ulcers not previously considered for proactive management. Diabet Med. 2011;28:1249–52.

147. Uccioli L, Gandini R, Giurato L, Fabiano S, Pampana E, Spallone V, et al. Long-term outcomes of diabetic patients with critical limb ischemia followed in a tertiary referral diabetic foot clinic. Diabetes Care. 2010;33:977–82.

148. Liistro F, Angioli P, Grotti S, Brandini R, Porto I, Ricci L, et al. Impact of critical limb ischemia on long-term cardiac mortality in diabetic patients undergoing percutaneous coronary revascularization. Diabetes Care. 2013;36:1495–500.

Renal Considerations in Critical Limb Ischemia

50

Pranav Sandilya Garimella, Amit M. Kakkar,
and Prakash Muthusami

Introduction

Peripheral artery disease (PAD) and its consequent critical limb ischemia (CLI) are commonly seen with increasing age in the general population. PAD patients present on a spectrum ranging from intermittent claudication to CLI, which is the most devastating outcome with high rates of mortality and morbidity including limb loss. The current TransAtlantic Inter-Society Consensus (TASCII) guidelines define CLI as a complex devastating syndrome that manifests as (1) ischemic rest pain, (2) ulcers, or (3) gangrene, attributable to arterial occlusive disease (Table 50.1). Persons with chronic kidney disease (CKD) especially those with end-stage renal disease (ESRD) on dialysis have significantly higher rates and severity of disease compared to age-matched population controls. Over- and above-traditional PAD risk factors like diabetes, hypercholesterolemia, smoking, and age, persons with kidney disease have a unique set of conditions including uremic stress, chronic inflammation, hypoalbuminemia, and a predisposition to vascular calcification which may accelerate the natural progression of PAD. Patients with CKD often develop CLI with poorer outcomes despite therapy. Both endovascular and open surgical procedures in CKD are associated with higher rates of loss of patency, infections, and amputations when compared to non-CKD persons. However, any revascularization procedure for CLI in patients with kidney disease is associated with improved outcomes compared to nonrevascularization. This chapter reviews the epidemiology, disease burden, risk factors, clinical features, and therapeutic options and outcomes of CLI in persons with kidney disease and dialysis. We will also discuss hemodialysis access-related steal syndromes, a form of limb ischemia unique to persons on dialysis.

Epidemiology of PAD and CLI in Patients with Kidney Disease

Patients with CKD are more likely to develop atherosclerotic cardiovascular disease than the general population with preserved kidney function [1, 2]. Data from the National Health and Nutrition Examination Survey (NHANES 1999–2000) showed that 24 % of persons with stage 3 CKD or greater (creatinine clearance of <60 mL/min/1.73 m^2) had PAD as defined by an ankle-brachial index (ABI) <0.9 [2]. This was a sixfold higher prevalence rate compared to persons with a creatinine clearance of >60 mL/min/1.73 m^2 (4 %). Given that recent data show an increasing prevalence of PAD globally [3], it is likely that the CKD-specific rates of PAD are going to be higher as well. Depending on the definition and the population studied, the exact prevalence of PAD varies even among persons with kidney disease. When only clinical symptoms and signs are considered, prevalence rates of approximately 25 % have been reported in ESRD patients [4, 5]. Rates however increase to nearly 35 % when reduced ABI is also considered as a diagnostic criterion [6]. These studies, however, likely still underrepresent the true burden of disease as claims data from the United States Renal Data System (USRDS) shows that nearly 46 % of prevalent dialysis patients in the USA have a code associated with PAD [7].

P.S. Garimella, MD, MPH (✉)
Division of Nephrology, Tufts Medical Center,
800 Washington Street, Box 391, Boston, MA 02111, USA

A.M. Kakkar, MD
Department of Medicine, Albert Einstein College of Medicine,
Bronx, NY 10461, USA

Division of Cardiology, Jacobi Medical Center, Bronx,
NY 10461, USA

P. Muthusami, MD
Division of Diagnostic Imaging, The Hospital for Sick Children,
Toronto, ON, Canada

© Springer International Publishing Switzerland 2017
R.S. Dieter et al. (eds.), *Critical Limb Ischemia*, DOI 10.1007/978-3-319-31991-9_50

Table 50.1 TransAtlantic Inter-Society Consensus (TASC) II definition of CLI

Category	Description	Findings		Noninvasive
		Sensory loss	Motor weakness	
Viable	Limb not threatened	None	None	Doppler signal present
Threatened				
Marginal	Salvageable	None or minimal	None	No Doppler signal
Immediate	Salvageable	Above toes ± rest pain	Mild to moderate	No Doppler signal
Irreversible	Major tissue loss, probable permanent nerve damage	Diffuse	Paralysis, may see rigors	No arterial or venous Doppler signal

Table 50.2 Risk factors for PAD in kidney disease

Traditional PAD risk factors	Risk factors unique to kidney disease
Male sex	Chronic inflammation
Age	Oxidative stress
Hypertension	Hypoalbuminemia
Diabetes	Hyper homocysteinemia
Smoking	Albuminuria
Obesity	
Dyslipidemia	

Unfortunately, there is very little data on the epidemiology of CLI among persons with kidney disease. Considering nontraumatic amputations to be a surrogate for CLI, the prevalence was approximately 4.3/100 persons per year for all ESRD patients with rates as high as 13.8/100 persons per year for diabetic ESRD patients [8]. These rates however likely underrepresent the true burden of disease as they fail to account for persons who do not receive treatment, those undergoing revascularization procedures for CLI, or those who die of other causes before receiving treatment. In the above referenced study, the authors reported high mortality rates of nearly 50–60 % in those undergoing nontraumatic amputations [8]. Long-term survival after revascularization surgery in ESRD patients is quite poor as well, being approximately 25 % at 5 years [9].

Traditional and Novel Risk Factors for PAD in Kidney Disease

Traditional cardiovascular risk factors, such as smoking, hypertension, diabetes, dyslipidemia, and older age, are more prevalent in patients with CKD than in the general population and contribute to increasing atherosclerosis and progression of PAD [4, 10, 11]. There are several nontraditional risk factors unique to patients with kidney disease that have been associated with the development of PAD (Table 50.2) [12]. In advanced CKD, the chronic inflammatory state induced by uremia and oxidative stresses in these patients can lead to hypoalbuminemia which is known to be associated with PAD [10]. Hypoalbuminemia [13, 14] and lipoprotein-a (Lp-a) are also known to be associated with PAD in dialysis patients [11]. Whether arterial stiffness and abnormalities in calcium, phosphorus, vitamin, and parathyroid hormone contribute to PAD in this population is yet unclear. Finally, a reduction in glomerular function is itself a risk factor for the development of PAD, with risk increasing with decreasing glomerular filtration rate (GFR) [15]. Albuminuria, a marker of diffuse vascular endothelial damage, has also been shown to be independently associated with the risk of developing PAD [16–18]. Specific associations of these biomarkers with progression to CLI in patients with CKD are yet unknown.

Symptoms of Limb Ischemia in Patients with Kidney Disease

A clinical diagnosis of early PAD is often difficult to make in persons with kidney disease. Intermittent claudication, defined as muscle fatigue, discomfort, cramping, or pain that is reproducibly induced by exercise and relieved by rest, is often considered to be the most easily recognized ischemic symptom in persons with PAD. However, this classic claudication is infrequently present (<10–15 % of cases) in individuals with significant PAD, and this is likely also true in patients with CKD and PAD [19]. Low levels of physical activity in patients with CKD, especially those on dialysis, may in part contribute to a delay in this diagnosis. In addition, non-PAD leg symptoms are frequent in dialysis patients due to comorbid neuropathy, pruritis, restless leg syndrome, and arthritis. As a result, most patients with kidney disease who are evaluated for PAD manifest signs of CLI including rest pain, non-healing ulcers, and gangrene.

Diagnosis of CLI in CKD

Contrast-based studies like conventional catheter angiography, computerized tomography angiography (CTA), and magnetic resonance angiography (MRA) in contrast to physiologic studies (ABI, toe-brachial index, and transcutaneous oxygen tension studies) or duplex ultrasound studies should be reserved for use when invasive treatments are planned. The accuracy of arterial imaging techniques has not been tested in advanced CKD populations, even though these are the very patient groups in whom the risk for contrast-induced nephrotoxicity is highest. Both computed tomography and magnetic resonance angiography have excellent accuracy in detecting lower limb PAD [20].

Treatment Options for CLI

Revascularization: The Conundrum

Given the high co-prevalence of PAD and CKD, it is important to understand how treatment decisions for one condition may affect the other. Patients with CKD already face exceedingly high mortality, and kidney disease may be worsened by limb-saving interventions. For those who have advanced CKD but are not yet dialysis dependent, revascularization either percutaneously or surgically may lead to ESRD. Physicians and patients often face this dilemma of what is more life changing for the patient—permanent dialysis or a limb amputation and prosthesis. Indeed, either outcome is suboptimal, but the risk-benefit ratio must be discussed explicitly prior to proceeding or withholding therapy for CLI.

Even in CKD patients with CLI, selecting the subpopulation that will benefit from lower limb revascularization is challenging. Complications from CLI are among the major causes of mortality in dialysis patients and survival is reduced after major amputation [21]. Several factors contribute to these poor outcomes. First, early detection of PAD may be missed due to lack of symptoms. ESRD patients may be physically inactive and therefore not have a history of classic claudication. If known at an early stage, therapies could be implemented to prevent progression of PAD to CLI. Second, the use of the ABI to diagnose PAD in CKD and ESRD has also been questioned due to the high prevalence of vascular calcification which may result in false negative tests. Finally, CKD persons have a high burden of associated cardiovascular morbidities resulting in a high threshold for the treatment of anything less than severely disabling CLI.

Patients with CLI who at baseline are non-ambulatory and have a short life expectancy can be considered for primary amputation or endovascular revascularization. Ambulatory patients with a life expectancy >2 years and those who are good surgical candidates should undergo bypass [33]. Actual treatment algorithms show considerable practice variations. Some centers advocate primary amputation in patients with ESRD citing dismal outcomes with revascularization and limb sparing procedures [22], while some have recommended avoiding surgeries altogether, on the basis of data pointing toward poor outcomes with both surgical bypass and amputation [23]. Yet others have supported early endovascular and surgical revascularization in the ESRD population [24, 25]. Clearly, there is a lack of consensus among practitioners and this highlights the need for including CKD patients in large trials of CLI therapy.

Endovascular Revascularization for CLI in CKD

The endovascular approach is typically chosen due to its rapidity, minimal invasiveness, and lack of complications associated with surgical wound healing. Unfortunately, patients who are generally considered unsuitable for surgery are also often poor candidates for endovascular procedures, because of the high incidence of outflow lesions and because of accelerated vascular calcifications. Recent technical and device advances have also resulted in centers performing infrapopliteal/outflow lesion angioplasties in the CKD population [26]. The decision to perform endovascular revascularization in CKD is complicated by the occurrence of contrast nephropathy (see Risk of Contrast-Based Imaging Studies in Special Considerations section below). Complete vascular assessment of lesion anatomy, location, and contrast load needed allow designing an individualized strategic plan which includes optimization of catheter manipulation as well as contrast doses during endovascular interventions. Successful procedural outcomes and improved long-term patency vary directly with lesion location and categorization as classified by the TASCII guidelines. A retrospective study that evaluated 535 patients undergoing endovascular therapy for superficial femoral artery (SFA) disease found significantly worse tibial runoff and limb salvage rates in the GFR $\leq$60 mL/min/1.73 m^2 group compared to those with better kidney function [27]. Over 50 % of the patients in the GFR <60 mL/min/1.73 m^2 group had manifestations of CLI at the time of endovascular therapy. The factors associated with poor limb salvage were tissue loss at presentation, presence of diabetes, congestive heart failure, embolization at time of intervention, 0 or 1 vessel tibial runoff, and progression of distal disease at follow up. Another study on 107 dialysis patients reported a technical success of 96 %, with limb salvage rates at 1, 2, 3, and 4 years of 86 %, 84 %, 84 % and 62 %, respectively. Similarly, good primary patency rates were also reported in studies that evaluated iliac-femoropopliteal [24] and infrapopliteal [28] angioplasties in ESRD patients.

Certain clinical and angiographic features may promote improved long-term outcomes and greater freedom from amputation after endovascular therapy. Unfortunately, the existing literature is scant in this regard. In one small case series of 55 diabetic patients on hemodialysis who underwent an endovascular revascularization for CLI, the clinical presentation was noted, including classification of ulcers using the Wagner criteria (Table 50.3) [29]. Forty-six limbs were classified as Wagner grades 4 or 5 upon presentation.

Table 50.3 Wagner classification of diabetic ulcers

Grade	Denomination	Gross description
0	Foot at risk	Thick calluses, bone deformities, clawed toes, and prominent metatarsal head
1	Superficial ulcers	Total destruction of the thickness of the skin
2	Deep ulcers	Infected, penetrates through skin, fat, and ligaments. No bone involvement
3	Abscessed deep ulcers	Limited necrosis in the toes or the foot, osteitis, or osteomyelitis may be present
4	Limited gangrene	Limited necrosis of the forefoot
5	Extensive gangrene	Necrosis of the complete foot with system effects

Patients presenting with rest pain did not require amputation. Those with healing ulcers showed similar rates of limb loss at 12 months, approaching 60 % compared to those without ulcers. These and other emerging data show improved amputation-free survival and rates of limb salvage with revascularization in persons with CLI at all levels of renal impairment [30]. A feature typically seen in advanced kidney disease is heavy calcification of the distal vessels, which tend to be smaller in caliber (Fig. 50.1), and multilevel disease (Fig. 50.2), including SFA and popliteal arteries. As a result, surgical bypass targets may be limited. With the evolution of endovascular techniques, more dedicated devices and equipment have become available to deal with infrapopliteal disease. Chronic total occlusions, CTOs, are a common feature. Lesion length varies inversely with the likelihood of successful recanalization. Adventitial calcium may prevent guide wire reentry when attempting an extraluminal recanalization. To facilitate lesion crossing, newer wires are available with heavier tips (up to 20 gms) which are better able to pierce the proximal or distal lesion caps. These caps tend to be heavily calcified and fibrotic and present the initial challenge with true lumen crossing. Newer hydrophilic, or polymer-coated, wires are lubricious enough to find and navigate microchannels. Access from a retrograde approach via the dorsalis pedis artery, which can be accessed using ultrasound guidance, may facilitate true lumen crossing. Using an antegrade approach via a direct SFA puncture or retrograde approach via dorsalis pedis artery, may allow for greater maneuverability of balloons, or support catheters. Some novel reentry devices incorporate intravascular ultrasound imaging; however, their utility in the treatment of patients with advanced CKD needs to be established.

Balloon angioplasty with a residual lesion <30 % remains the gold standard definition of success for peripheral vascular interventions. However, the restenosis rates remain high and peripheral artery stenting has been adapted from the experience in the coronary world with hopes of overcoming the restenosis problem, for which diabetes is a known risk factor. Stents used in peripheral interventions may be self-expanding nitinol, balloon expandable, bare metal, or drug eluting. Stenting however remains controversial due to the concerns that stents can fracture with lower extremity movements and may also eliminate future bypass targets and injure collaterals. In the short term, dual antiplatelet therapy may be necessary to prevent occlusion. This is of concern in patients with CKD and ESRD who may be at increased risk for bleeding complications. However, if significant lesion recoil occurs after deflation of the balloon, a stent may be the only viable solution to keep the artery open and more importantly keep inline flow adequate. Most trials of endovascular stenting for CLI treatment did not recruit significant numbers of CKD and ESRD patients. Also, a common contraindication to stenting in trials was lack of vessel runoff or only one vessel runoff with 50 % lesion present, both of which are common in persons with advanced kidney disease.

Access site complications may also be higher in patients with eGFR <60 mL/min/1.73 m² due to non-compressibility of vessels and/or tortuous anatomy. However, access site complications have decreased in recent times due to more meticulous arterial access and use of adjunctive aids such as fluoroscopy and ultrasound to localize the artery. Additionally, 4Fr micropuncture kits can be used that allow for contrast injection to ensure optimal arteriotomy access at the mid-femoral head. Still, this population frequently has difficult anatomy that stratifies them into a higher risk subset.

Surgical Revascularization for CLI in CKD

Although initial results of endovascular treatment suggested a similar benefit and lower cost over surgical revascularization [31], long-term follow-up has shown that a surgical approach may be associated with improved overall survival and amputation-free survival when the patient survives beyond 2 years [32]. Thus, current AHA/ACC guidelines have recommended that surgical revascularization should be considered as first-line revascularization therapy in persons with a life expectancy greater than 2 years [33]. However, whether this is true in persons with CKD is unclear, and there is a need to study surgical interventions prospectively given high rates of adverse events after revascularization procedures in persons with advanced CKD. The dismal survival of

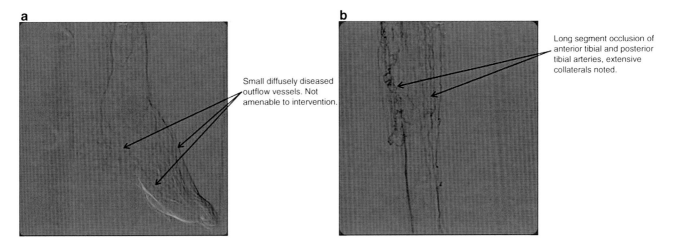

Fig. 50.1 A 61-year-old female with a history of coronary artery disease, coronary artery bypass grafting, ESRD on dialysis, diabetes, human immunodeficiency virus infection on retroviral therapy presenting with non-healing ulcer of the left first toe. (**a**) Diffuse small vessel disease at foot with heavy calcification. (**b**) Leg angiogram showing occluded anterior tibial, posterior tibial, and peroneal arteries

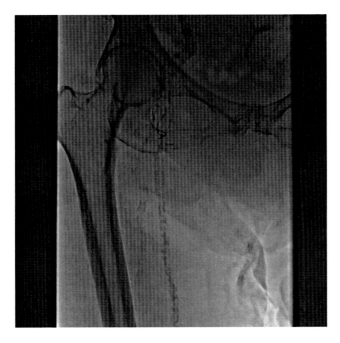

Fig. 50.2 Fluoroscopy showing heavily calcified superficial femoral artery and profunda arteries in an elderly female with long-standing diabetes

persons with advanced CKD and ESRD who also have PAD means that there is little information on long-term graft patency in the few who undergo revascularization. A recent meta-analysis of 28 studies reported pooled estimates of 50, 66, and 23 % for primary patency, limb salvage, and mortality, respectively, at 5 years in dialysis patients undergoing infrainguinal arterial reconstruction [9].

Analysis of retrospective data suggest that patients receiving dialysis, but not those with earlier stages of CKD, are more likely to experience lower extremity amputation after a surgical revascularization [34]. Comorbidities, most commonly cardiac disease, are associated with a high mortality rate and should likely be taken into consideration when treatment decisions are made for this population. It seems likely that high postprocedure adverse event rates have shaped treatment practices for CLI. Although data suggests that patients with CLI and eGFR <60 mL/min/1.73 m² are less likely to undergo a revascularization procedure compared with those with better kidney function, nevertheless, for all groups, including those with CKD, patients who underwent revascularization experienced lower mortality rates than these other groups [35].

Currently available data suggests that the option of surgical revascularization for CLI in the presence of advanced CKD and especially ESRD should be offered if it would lead to a significant increase in quality of life and, if offered, should be with the caveat of increased intraoperative and postoperative complications, irrespective of anatomical vascular outcomes.

Special Considerations in the Treatment of PAD and CLI Among Persons with CKD

Drug Dose Adjustment

Anti-platelet agents are recommended for prevention of secondary cardiovascular disease (CVD) events in persons with PAD, even though their benefit in treating symptomatic claudication is unclear. The current AHA/ACC PAD guidelines recommend low-dose aspirin or clopidogrel in persons with symptomatic PAD to reduce adverse CVD events [33, 36]. The benefit of clopidogrel in CKD patients may not be to the same degree as in those with normal renal function [37]. This may in part be explained by increased platelet reactivity leading to resistance in persons with CKD [38]. There is no added benefit of warfarin for preventing CVD events compared to anti-platelet agents alone in persons with PAD [39]. This should be kept in mind given the increased bleeding risk seen in patients with advanced kidney disease receiving warfarin therapy for atrial fibrillation.

Cilostazol, a phosphodiesterase-3 inhibitor, has achieved a Class IA guideline-based recommendation to be the first-line medical therapy individuals with lifestyle-limiting claudication [20]. Among dialysis patients, there is emerging data to suggest that cilostazol may also improve patency after lower limb percutaneous transluminal angioplasty [40, 41]. It is however contraindicated in heart failure patients and thus must be used with caution in the ESRD population which has a significant prevalence of heart failure [42, 43]. Caution is also likely reasonable in individuals with significant CKD and in dialysis patients due to the high protein binding of cilostazol and impaired excretion when creatinine clearance is <25 mL/min. This would primarily help to lower adverse event rates (headache, tachycardia, or loose bowel movements).

Risk of Contrast-Based Imaging Studies

Contrast-induced nephropathy (CIN) is a known complication, especially in the setting of coronary and peripheral revascularization procedures. While the overall incidence of CIN is believed to be between 3 and 5 %, persons with diabetes and those with CKD have a higher risk of developing CIN [44, 45]. The use of both noninvasive (CTA and MRA) and invasive conventional angiography should usually be reserved for patients in whom severe claudication or CLI is not responsive to non-invasive therapies. In persons with CKD, the KDIGO guidelines recommend the use of the lowest possible dose of a low-osmolar or iso-osmolar contrast agent and volume expansion to prevent the occurrence of CIN [46]. The use of N-acetyl cysteine has not conclusively shown to reduce CIN even among diabetics and patients with underlying CKD [47]. The risk of gadolinium-induced nephrogenic systemic fibrosis limits the utility of contrast-enhanced MRA in individuals with PAD on dialysis [48]. In general, contrast-based diagnostic imaging studies are avoided in patients with eGFR <30 mL/min/1.73 m^2 unless an intervention is planned as the risks may outweigh the benefits. In this regard, there is a growing role for and interest in non-contrast techniques for MRA for pre-procedural lesion assessment, including phase contrast MRA, balanced steady-state free precession, and arterial spin labeling.

Pre- and Post-Kidney Transplant Care

Given the increased risk for CVD in persons with CKD, it is not uncommon to assess for underlying PAD during pretransplant evaluation. There are however no recommendations for the routine screening of transplant recipients. Since the presence of PAD at time of transplantation is associated with diminished graft and patient survival in addition to the need for amputations [49, 50], Doppler studies may be useful in patients with diabetes, a history of claudication, or poor peripheral pulses on examination [51].

Patients with a kidney transplant are at increased risk of both CIN and wound infections due to use of immunosuppressive medications. Sirolimus, a mammalian target of rapamycin (mTOR) inhibitor, commonly used to prevent allograft rejection impairs wound healing. Patients with kidney transplants needing amputations, revascularizations, or large debridement may need to have the immunosuppression changed to agents like tacrolimus to prevent postoperative complications [52].

Dialysis Access-Associated Steal Syndrome

Dialysis access-associated steal syndrome (DAASS) is a condition wherein persons with arteriovenous fistulae (AVF) and sometimes AV grafts (AVG) develop signs and symptoms of limb ischemia distal to the access site as a result of decreased perfusion. Some authors have suggested that the name distal hypoperfusion ischemic syndrome (DHIS) is more appropriate given that retrograde flow causing "steal" can be demonstrated often with AVF, although true clinical symptoms are not always seen in these cases. Depending on the location and associated risk factors, the incidence of DAASS ranges from 1 to 15 % with upper limb vascular access and can be as high as 36 % after lower limb vascular access procedures [53, 54].

DAASS is more common in persons with upper-arm (brachial) AVF which have high flows and may cause "true" stealing of blood from the distal hand arteries. However, even in the absence of a high-flow AVF, patients who develop symptoms have also been shown to have increased arterial occlusive lesions proximal or distal to the arteriovenous anastomoses. In addition, the presence of poor arterial circulation (distal arteriopathy) downstream of the AVF due to diabetes and vascular calcification also increases the risk of developing symptomatic steal syndrome. A number of patient-associated risk factors have been associated to increase the likelihood of developing DAASS after access creation in dialysis patients (Table 50.4).

Clinical features of DAASS are those of distal hypoperfusion and may occur independent of dialysis treatment. These include pain, numbness, coldness, and sometimes cyanosis of extremities. In more advanced cases, ulcers of fingers and gangrene of the fingertips may be seen. Different classification systems have been proposed to categorize severity of symptoms ranging from mild/no symptoms to gangrene and tissue loss [55, 56].

The overall goal of treating DAASS is dual: first to relieve symptoms of ischemia and prevent ulcers and gangrene in the limb and second to ensure long-term patency of the dialysis access. This can be achieved either via percutaneous

Table 50.4 Risk factors for symptomatic DAASS

Patient specific risk factors	Limb vasculature specific risk factors
Older age	Proximal (brachial) AVF
Female gender	Proximal AVF compared to graft
Diabetes	High-flow AVF
Hypertension	Presence of multiple arterial stenoses
Coronary artery disease	Distal arteriopathy
Smoking	Multiple AVF creations

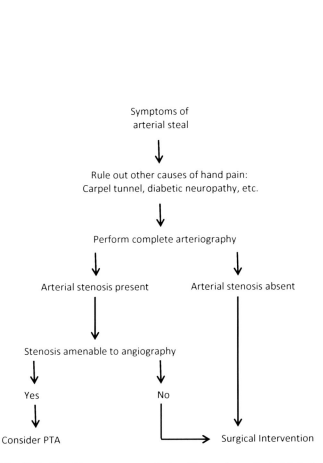

Fig. 50.3 Algorithm to manage patients with symptoms of arterial steal (From Asif et al. Am J Kidney Dis. 2006 Jul;48(1):88–97. Reprinted with permission from Elsevier)

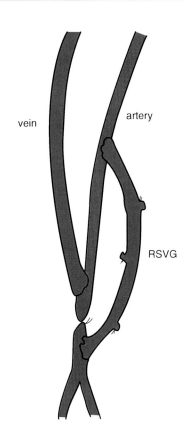

Fig. 50.4 Schematic representation of DRIL. The artery is ligated distally to the access anastomosis, and a vein bypass is inserted from proximal of the anastomosis to distal of the ligation. It is recommended that construction of the proximal anastomosis should be a reasonable distance (>5 cm) proximal to the access to prevent diastolic retrograde flow, and thereby recurrence of steal syndrome, within the bypass. *RSVG* reverse saphenous vein graft (From Mwipatayi et al. Curr Surg. 2006 Mar-Apr;63(2):130–5. Reprinted with permission from Elsevier)

approach which has been gaining significance or by surgical revascularization. Knowledge regarding treatment of DAASS is limited to analysis of patient registries and published case series. To date no clinical trials have been performed to evaluate optimal strategies to treat DAASS.

Arterial inflow stenosis is often the culprit lesion in a majority of DAASS-related symptoms (ranging from 25–83 % depending on the case series), and a thorough evaluation of the arterial tree proximal to the anastomosis should be performed. When present, treatment of stenosis is important to prevent thrombosis of the AVF or graft [57]. Asif and colleagues have proposed a simple algorithm to the approach

and treatment of suspected extremity ischemia in the setting of symptoms suggestive of DAASS (Fig. 50.3) [58]. In the absence of a stenosis proximal to the AVF/AVG or when the stenosis is not amenable to percutaneous interventions, surgical intervention should be considered.

Banding reduces the vessel caliber and decreases flow through the AV access and is thus often reserved for patients with high-flow AVF to avoid thrombosis in those with low access flows. An alternative procedure known as revision using distal inflow (RUDI) technique has also emerged which used a graft between radial and ulnar arteries to treat steal associated with high flow AVF [59]. The distal revascularization-interval ligation procedure (DRIL) has been used successfully for the treatment of DAASS since its introduction in 1988 [60]. The DRIL procedure involves the ligation of the artery distal to the anastomosis, thus reducing retrograde flow. When the access involved is a brachial AVF, a vein graft is used to connect the proximal artery above the anastomosis to a more distal artery (Fig. 50.4) [61]. When the steal is due to a radial AVF and there is adequate perfusion from the ulnar and palmar arteries, a distal radial artery ligation (DRAL) is sufficient without the need for the interpositioned vein graft [62]. Further details of these procedures and other revascularization techniques including the proximal arteriovenous anastomoses (PAVA) [63] and the newer minimally invasive limited ligation endoluminal assisted revision (MILLER) procedure [64] have been described in detail elsewhere [57, 65, 66].

References

1. Sarnak MJ, Levey AS, Schoolwerth AC, Coresh J, Culleton B, Hamm LL, et al. Kidney disease as a risk factor for development of cardiovascular disease: a statement from the American Heart Association Councils on Kidney in Cardiovascular Disease, High Blood Pressure Research, Clinical Cardiology, and Epidemiology and Prevention. Hypertension. 2003;42(5):1050–65.
2. O'Hare AM, Glidden DV, Fox CS, Hsu CY. High prevalence of peripheral arterial disease in persons with renal insufficiency: results from the National Health and Nutrition Examination Survey 1999–2000. Circulation. 2004;109(3):320–3.
3. Fowkes FG, Rudan D, Rudan I, Aboyans V, Denenberg JO, McDermott MM, et al. Comparison of global estimates of prevalence and risk factors for peripheral artery disease in 2000 and 2010: a systematic review and analysis. Lancet. 2013;382(9901):1329–40.
4. Rajagopalan S, Dellegrottaglie S, Furniss AL, Gillespie BW, Satayathum S, Lameire N, et al. Peripheral arterial disease in patients with end-stage renal disease: observations from the Dialysis Outcomes and Practice Patterns Study (DOPPS). Circulation. 2006;114(18):1914–22.
5. Cheung AK, Sarnak MJ, Yan G, Dwyer JT, Heyka RJ, Rocco MV, et al. Atherosclerotic cardiovascular disease risks in chronic hemodialysis patients. Kidney Int. 2000;58(1):353–62.
6. Testa A, Ottavioli JN. Ankle-arm blood pressure index (AABPI) in hemodialysis patients. Arch Mal Coeur Vaiss. 1998;91(8):963–5.
7. US Renal Data System. USRDS 2010 annual data report: atlas of chronic kidney disease and end-stage renal disease in the United States. Bethesda: National Institutes of Health, National Institute of Diabetes and Digestive and Kidney Diseases; 2010.
8. Eggers PW, Gohdes D, Pugh J. Nontraumatic lower extremity amputations in the Medicare end-stage renal disease population. Kidney Int. 1999;56(4):1524–33.
9. Albers M, Romiti M, De Luccia N, Brochado-Neto FC, Nishimoto I, Pereira CA. An updated meta-analysis of infrainguinal arterial reconstruction in patients with end-stage renal disease. J Vasc Surg. 2007;45(3):536–42.
10. O'Hare AM, Hsu CY, Bacchetti P, Johansen KL. Peripheral vascular disease risk factors among patients undergoing hemodialysis. J Am Soc Nephrol. 2002;13(2):497–503.
11. Jaar BG, Plantinga LC, Astor BC, Fink NE, Longenecker C, Tracy RP, et al. Novel and traditional cardiovascular risk factors for peripheral arterial disease in incident-dialysis patients. Adv Chronic Kidney Dis. 2007;14(3):304–13.
12. Chen J, Mohler 3rd ER, Xie D, Shlipak MG, Townsend RR, Appel LJ, et al. Risk factors for peripheral arterial disease among patients with chronic kidney disease. Am J Cardiol. 2012;110(1):136–41.
13. Chuang FR, Fang JT, Chen JB, Lin CL, Chen HY, Lee CN, et al. Hyperhomocysteinemia and the prevalence of symptomatic atherosclerotic vascular disease in Taiwanese chronic hemodialysis patients: a retrospective study. Ren Fail. 2003;25(5):765–74.
14. Manns BJ, Burgess ED, Hyndman ME, Parsons HG, Schaefer JP, Scott-Douglas NW. Hyperhomocysteinemia and the prevalence of atherosclerotic vascular disease in patients with end-stage renal disease. Am J Kidney Dis. 1999;34(4):669–77.
15. Wattanakit K, Folsom AR, Selvin E, Coresh J, Hirsch AT, Weatherley BD. Kidney function and risk of peripheral arterial disease: results from the Atherosclerosis Risk in Communities (ARIC) Study. J Am Soc Nephrol. 2007;18(2):629–36.
16. Baber U, Mann D, Shimbo D, Woodward M, Olin JW, Muntner P. Combined role of reduced estimated glomerular filtration rate and microalbuminuria on the prevalence of peripheral arterial disease. Am J Cardiol. 2009;104(10):1446–51.
17. Wattanakit K, Folsom AR, Criqui MH, Kramer HJ, Cushman M, Shea S, et al. Albuminuria and peripheral arterial disease: results from the multi-ethnic study of atherosclerosis (MESA). Atherosclerosis. 2008; 201(1):212–6.
18. Wu CK, Yang CY, Tsai CT, Chiu FC, Huang YT, Lee JK, et al. Association of low glomerular filtration rate and albuminuria with peripheral arterial disease: the National Health and Nutrition Examination Survey, 1999–2004. Atherosclerosis. 2009;209(1):230–4.
19. Lash JP, Go AS, Appel LJ, He J, Ojo A, Rahman M, et al. Chronic Renal Insufficiency Cohort (CRIC) Study: baseline characteristics and associations with kidney function. Clin J Am Soc Nephrol. 2009;4(8):1302–11.
20. Koelemay MJ, Lijmer JG, Stoker J, Legemate DA, Bossuyt PM. Magnetic resonance angiography for the evaluation of lower extremity arterial disease: a meta-analysis. JAMA. 2001;285(10): 1338–45.
21. Koch M, Trapp R, Kulas W, Grabensee B. Critical limb ischaemia as a main cause of death in patients with end-stage renal disease: a single-centre study. Nephrol Dial Transplant. 2004;19(10):2547–52.
22. Edwards JM, Taylor Jr LM, Porter JM. Limb salvage in end-stage renal disease (ESRD). Comparison of modern results in patients with and without ESRD. Arch Surg. 1988;123(9):1164–8.
23. Isiklar MH, Kulbaski M, MacDonald MJ, Lumsden AB. Infrainguinal bypass in end-stage renal disease: when is it justified? Semin Vasc Surg. 1997;10(1):42–8.
24. Kumada Y, Aoyama T, Ishii H, Tanaka M, Kawamura Y, Takahashi H, et al. Long-term outcome of percutaneous transluminal angioplasty in chronic haemodialysis patients with peripheral arterial disease. Nephrol Dial Transplant. 2008;23(12):3996–4001.
25. Mills JL, Gahtan V, Fujitani RM, Taylor SM, Bandyk DF. The utility and durability of vein bypass grafts originating from the popliteal artery for limb salvage. Am J Surg. 1994;168(6):646–50. discussion 50–1.
26. Graziani L, Silvestro A, Bertone V, Manara E, Alicandri A, Parrinello G, et al. Percutaneous transluminal angioplasty is feasible and effective in patients on chronic dialysis with severe peripheral artery disease. Nephrol Dial Transplant. 2007;22(4):1144–9.
27. Bakken AM, Protack CD, Saad WE, Hart JP, Rhodes JM, Waldman DL, et al. Impact of chronic kidney disease on outcomes of superficial femoral artery endoluminal interventions. Ann Vasc Surg. 2009;23(5):560–8.
28. Brosi P, Baumgartner I, Silvestro A, Do DD, Mahler F, Triller J, et al. Below-the-knee angioplasty in patients with end-stage renal disease. J Endovasc Ther. 2005;12(6):704–13.

29. Calhoun JH, Cantrell J, Cobos J, Lacy J, Valdez RR, Hokanson J, et al. Treatment of diabetic foot infections: Wagner classification, therapy, and outcome. Foot Ankle. 1988;9(3):101–6.

30. Ortmann J, Gahl B, Diehm N, Dick F, Traupe T, Baumgartner I. Survival benefits of revascularization in patients with critical limb ischemia and renal insufficiency. J Vasc Surg. 2012;56(3):737–45.e1.

31. Adam DJ, Beard JD, Cleveland T, Bell J, Bradbury AW, Forbes JF, et al. Bypass versus angioplasty in severe ischaemia of the leg (BASIL): multicentre, randomised controlled trial. Lancet. 2005;366(9501):1925–34.

32. Bradbury AW, Adam DJ, Bell J, Forbes JF, Fowkes FG, Gillespie I, et al. Bypass versus Angioplasty in Severe Ischaemia of the Leg (BASIL) trial: an intention-to-treat analysis of amputation-free and overall survival in patients randomized to a bypass surgery-first or a balloon angioplasty-first revascularization strategy. J Vasc Surg. 2010;51(5 Suppl):5S–17.

33. Rooke TW, Hirsch AT, Misra S, Sidawy AN, Beckman JA, Findeiss LK, et al. 2011 ACCF/AHA focused update of the guideline for the management of patients with peripheral artery disease (updating the 2005 guideline): a report of the American College of Cardiology Foundation/American Heart Association Task Force on Practice Guidelines. Circulation. 2011;124(18):2020–45.

34. O'Hare AM, Sidawy AN, Feinglass J, Merine KM, Daley J, Khuri S, et al. Influence of renal insufficiency on limb loss and mortality after initial lower extremity surgical revascularization. J Vasc Surg. 2004;39(4):709–16.

35. O'Hare AM, Bertenthal D, Sidawy AN, Shlipak MG, Sen S, Chren MM. Renal insufficiency and use of revascularization among a national cohort of men with advanced lower extremity peripheral arterial disease. Clin J Am Soc Nephrol. 2006;1(2):297–304.

36. Hirsch AT, Haskal ZJ, Hertzer NR, Bakal CW, Creager MA, Halperin JL, et al. ACC/AHA 2005 Practice Guidelines for the management of patients with peripheral arterial disease (lower extremity, renal, mesenteric, and abdominal aortic): a collaborative report from the American Association for Vascular Surgery/Society for Vascular Surgery, Society for Cardiovascular Angiography and Interventions, Society for Vascular Medicine and Biology, Society of Interventional Radiology, and the ACC/AHA Task Force on Practice Guidelines (Writing Committee to Develop Guidelines for the Management of Patients With Peripheral Arterial Disease): endorsed by the American Association of Cardiovascular and Pulmonary Rehabilitation; National Heart, Lung, and Blood Institute; Society for Vascular Nursing; TransAtlantic Inter-Society Consensus; and Vascular Disease Foundation. Circulation. 2006;113(11):e463–654.

37. Best PJ, Steinhubl SR, Berger PB, Dasgupta A, Brennan DM, Szczech LA, et al. The efficacy and safety of short- and long-term dual antiplatelet therapy in patients with mild or moderate chronic kidney disease: results from the Clopidogrel for the Reduction of Events During Observation (CREDO) trial. Am Heart J. 2008;155(4):687–93.

38. Angiolillo DJ, Bernardo E, Capodanno D, Vivas D, Sabate M, Ferreiro JL, et al. Impact of chronic kidney disease on platelet function profiles in diabetes mellitus patients with coronary artery disease taking dual antiplatelet therapy. J Am Coll Cardiol. 2010;55(11):1139–46.

39. Anand S, Yusuf S, Xie C, Pogue J, Eikelboom J, Budaj A, et al. Oral anticoagulant and antiplatelet therapy and peripheral arterial disease. N Engl J Med. 2007;357(3):217–27.

40. Ishii H, Kumada Y, Toriyama T, Aoyama T, Takahashi H, Tanaka M, et al. Effects of oral cilostazol 100 mg BID on long-term patency after percutaneous transluminal angioplasty in patients with femoropopliteal disease undergoing hemodialysis: a retrospective chart review in Japanese patients. Clin Ther. 2010;32(1):24–33.

41. Ishii H, Kumada Y, Toriyama T, Aoyama T, Takahashi H, Yamada S, et al. Cilostazol improves long-term patency after percutaneous

transluminal angioplasty in hemodialysis patients with peripheral artery disease. Clin J Am Soc Nephrol. 2008;3(4):1034–40.

42. Harnett JD, Foley RN, Kent GM, Barre PE, Murray D, Parfrey PS. Congestive heart failure in dialysis patients: prevalence, incidence, prognosis and risk factors. Kidney Int. 1995;47(3):884–90.

43. Stack AG, Bloembergen WE. A cross-sectional study of the prevalence and clinical correlates of congestive heart failure among incident US dialysis patients. Am J Kidney Dis. 2001;38(5):992–1000.

44. Tommaso CL. Contrast-induced nephrotoxicity in patients undergoing cardiac catheterization. Catheter Cardiovasc Diagn. 1994;31(4):316–21.

45. Rihal CS, Textor SC, Grill DE, Berger PB, Ting HH, Best PJ, et al. Incidence and prognostic importance of acute renal failure after percutaneous coronary intervention. Circulation. 2002;105(19):2259–64.

46. KDIGO clinical practice guideline for the management of blood pressure in chronic kidney disease. Kidney Int Suppl. 2012;2:337–414.

47. Act Investigators. Acetylcysteine for prevention of renal outcomes in patients undergoing coronary and peripheral vascular angiography: main results from the randomized Acetylcysteine for Contrast-induced nephropathy Trial (ACT). Circulation. 2011;124(11):1250–9.

48. Agarwal R, Brunelli SM, Williams K, Mitchell MD, Feldman HI, Umscheid CA. Gadolinium-based contrast agents and nephrogenic systemic fibrosis: a systematic review and meta-analysis. Nephrol Dial Transplant. 2009;24(3):856–63.

49. Sung RS, Althoen M, Howell TA, Merion RM. Peripheral vascular occlusive disease in renal transplant recipients: risk factors and impact on kidney allograft survival. Transplantation. 2000;70(7):1049–54.

50. Snyder JJ, Kasiske BL, Maclean R. Peripheral arterial disease and renal transplantation. J Am Soc Nephrol. 2006;17(7):2056–68.

51. Kasiske BL, Cangro CB, Hariharan S, Hricik DE, Kerman RH, Roth D, et al. The evaluation of renal transplantation candidates: clinical practice guidelines. Am J Transplant Off J Am Soc Transplant Am Soc Transplant Surg. 2001;1 Suppl 2:3–95.

52. Dean PG, Lund WJ, Larson TS, Prieto M, Nyberg SL, Ishitani MB, et al. Wound-healing complications after kidney transplantation: a prospective, randomized comparison of sirolimus and tacrolimus. Transplantation. 2004;77(10):1555–61.

53. Taylor SM, Eaves GL, Weatherford DA, McAlhany Jr JC, Russell HE, Langan 3rd EM. Results and complications of arteriovenous access dialysis grafts in the lower extremity: a five year review. Am Surg. 1996;62(3):188–91.

54. Morsy AH, Kulbaski M, Chen C, Isiklar H, Lumsden AB. Incidence and characteristics of patients with hand ischemia after a hemodialysis access procedure. J Surg Res. 1998;74(1):8–10.

55. Tordoir JH, Dammers R, van der Sande FM. Upper extremity ischemia and hemodialysis vascular access. Eur J Vasc Endovasc Surg. 2004;27(1):1–5.

56. Sidawy AN, Gray R, Besarab A, Henry M, Ascher E, Silva Jr M, et al. Recommended standards for reports dealing with arteriovenous hemodialysis accesses. J Vasc Surg. 2002;35(3):603–10.

57. Leon C, Asif A. Arteriovenous access and hand pain: the distal hypoperfusion ischemic syndrome. Clin J Am Soc Nephrol. 2007;2(1):175–83.

58. Asif A, Leon C, Merrill D, Bhimani B, Ellis R, Ladino M, et al. Arterial steal syndrome: a modest proposal for an old paradigm. Am J Kidney Dis. 2006;48(1):88–97.

59. Minion DJ, Moore E, Endean E. Revision using distal inflow: a novel approach to dialysis-associated steal syndrome. Ann Vasc Surg. 2005;19(5):625–8.

60. Schanzer H, Schwartz M, Harrington E, Haimov M. Treatment of ischemia due to "steal" by arteriovenous fistula with distal artery ligation and revascularization. J Vasc Surg. 1988;7(6):770–3.

61. Mwipatayi BP, Bowles T, Balakrishnan S, Callaghan J, Haluszkiewicz E, Sieunarine K. Ischemic steal syndrome: a case series and review of current management. Curr Surg. 2006;63(2):130–5.

62. Bussell JA, Abbott JA, Lim RC. A radial steal syndrome with arteriovenous fistula for hemodialysis. Studies in seven patients. Ann Intern Med. 1971;75(3):387–94.

63. Zanow J, Kruger U, Scholz H. Proximalization of the arterial inflow: a new technique to treat access-related ischemia. J Vasc Surg. 2006;43(6):1216–21. discussion 21.

64. Goel N, Miller GA, Jotwani MC, Licht J, Schur I, Arnold WP. Minimally Invasive Limited Ligation Endoluminal-assisted Revision (MILLER) for treatment of dialysis access-associated steal syndrome. Kidney Int. 2006;70(4):765–70.

65. Scali ST, Huber TS. Treatment strategies for access-related hand ischemia. Semin Vasc Surg. 2011;24(2):128–36.

66. Mickley V. Steal syndrome: strategies to preserve vascular access and extremity. Nephrol Dial Transplant. 2008;23(1):19–24.

Upper Extremity Amputation

51

Nikola Babovic and Brian T. Carlsen

Introduction

Although significantly less common than vascular insufficiency in the lower extremities, heart, and other organs, processes leading to inadequate vascular flow in the upper extremity carry significant morbidity [1]. This is largely due to the functional importance of the upper extremity to human life. It is most commonly caused by chronic progressive disease, which can usually be treated medically at first and eventually necessitating surgical management.

Limb ischemia in the upper extremity has many causes, including but not limited to acute arterial/venous injury, iatrogenic events, chronic processes (occlusive, spastic, or combined), or congenital malformations. The end result is a spectrum of decreased flow of blood and nutrition to tissues. Vascular insufficiency causes intermittent or chronic symptoms of pain, sensory changes, or ulceration [2]. Critical limb ischemia can be simply defined as ischemia causing cell death and necrosis which leads to or necessitates amputation. In the setting of acute arterial injury, arterial reconstruction is indicated in an attempt to restore flow and prevent tissue necrosis. In this chapter, we will address only management of critical limb ischemia through amputation. Amputation is indicated when revascularization has failed to restore adequate tissue perfusion and necrosis has ensued.

In the setting of vascular insufficiency requiring amputation in the upper extremity, functional rehabilitation with early return to activities of daily living is the primary goal, with secondary goals being:

1. Preservation of functional length as allowed by remaining vascular flow
2. Durable skin coverage
3. Preservation of sensibility
4. Prevention of neuroma
5. Early prosthetic fitting, when applicable
6. Minimize convalescence
7. Early return to activity and work
8. Prevention of secondary complications

Understanding the patient's own personal goals and motivation is paramount to creating a successful treatment plan. In the case of a traumatic amputation or mangled extremity, a well-planned amputation may be favorable to a replantation when considering technical demands of the operation, potential complications, postoperative rehabilitation, time lost from work, and ultimate functional needs and outcomes for that particular patient. For nonurgent amputation in the case of chronic disease, a lengthy discussion with the patient must be had to understand attitude, functional/work needs, and commitment to treatment for that particular patient. Return to normal activities and work is a primary consideration and the surgeon must be mindful of the patient's work, hobbies, and personal desires. There is often a balance between definitive amputation at a level of known tissue viability and preserving marginal tissue. While preserving tissue is important, some patients may be better served by early definitive surgery that enables a quicker return to work and activities. Cold intolerance is a common consequence of amputation, especially after digital loss. While symptoms can persist years later, they generally improve over time [3, 4].

N. Babovic, MD
Orthopaedic Surgery, Allegheny Health Network,
Pittsburgh, PA, USA

B.T. Carlsen, MD (✉)
Orthopedic and Plastic Surgery, Mayo Clinic,
Rochester, MN, USA

Limb Salvage and Replantation

No hand is so badly crippled that, if it is painless, has sensation, and strong prehension, it is [not] far better than any prosthesis.
Norman Kirk, 1944 [5]

© Springer International Publishing Switzerland 2017
R.S. Dieter et al. (eds.), *Critical Limb Ischemia*, DOI 10.1007/978-3-319-31991-9_51

Dr. Kirk's statement in 1944 is as true today as it was then. For the hand surgeon, limb salvage and hand preservation are common considerations, typically presenting after severe trauma. Salvage of a functional hand may require revascularization, nerve repair, skeletal fixation, tendon repair, and/or soft tissue coverage. The goal of these procedures is to restore a pain-free, sensate hand that is capable of some sort of prehension. It is important to consider the minimum requirement that can allow prehension. This is possible with a single movable digit and some sort of post. This could mean a preserved thumb and just enough residual hand ("mitten hand") or a thumb post and (a) movable finger(s) that can oppose. Therefore, the greatest value is placed on thumb reconstruction, even if it requires replantation of a finger in the thumb position (Fig. 51.1) or pollicization of a neighboring digit (Fig. 51.2). The thumb's importance is recognized by work-related injury compensation where 40 % of the hand function and 25 % of total body function is attributed to the thumb.

Reattachment or replantation of the amputated part(s) often provides the best available reconstructive option. Indications for replantation include the following [6]:

- Thumb
- Multiple digits
- Hand amputation through palm
- Hand amputation (distal wrist)
- Any part in a child
- More proximal arm (sharp only)
- Finger distal to sublimis insertion (zone I)

while contraindications include the following:

- Single digits proximal to flexor digitorum superficialis insertion (zone II)
- Severely crushed or mangled parts
- Multiple-level amputations
- Replantation in patients with multiple trauma or severe medical problems (relative contraindication)

Digits are quite tolerant of ischemia with successful revascularization reported after 33 h of warm ischemia [7] and 94 h of cold ischemia [8]. To protect the amputated part (and prevent cold injury), it should be cleansed, wrapped in moist sterile gauze, and placed in a water and airtight bag or container, which is then placed on ice. The patient and amputated part should be transferred to a level-1 trauma center with microsurgical and hand surgery expertise. Even with sharp, guillotine amputations, there is a zone of injury and modest skeletal shortening facilitates reattachment. This can be achieved by joint fusion if the amputation transections a joint, which is relatively common (Fig. 51.3). Although crush and avulsion injuries can make reattachment more challenging, these are not absolute contraindications for replantation and the digits should be considered for reattachment, excluding other contraindications. The sequence of repair is determined surgeon preference. The author's preference typically begins with skeletal fixation, followed by tendon preparation, arterial repair, nerve repair, tendon repair, vein repair, and (loose) skin approximation. The dressing and splint are kept bulky and non-constrictive and allow for examination of the digit. Monitoring the part can be a challenge, especially if the part becomes macerated [9].

Hand salvage and length preservation can make a tremendous difference in the patient's final functional outcome. The use of spare parts for reattachment or soft tissue coverage as a fillet flap must be considered. Often the spare parts are ischemic and there will not be an opportunity for use beyond the initial operation. Again, the guiding principles are the restoration of prehension for hand injuries and maintaining length for more proximal injuries. One consideration, when using a fillet flap for residual limb coverage, is to include innervated skeletal muscle that can be used acutely for targeted muscle reinnervation for prosthetic control (Fig. 51.4). However, when considering the inclusion of muscle, one must consider the ischemia time of the tissue, as the metabolic demand of skeletal muscle is relatively high and, additionally, there may be a risk of myoglobinuria.

Multiple Digit/Partial Hand Amputation

Digits threatened by vascular compromise can present significant difficulties, specifically with patient rehabilitation and disability (Fig. 51.5). Whether a single or multiple digits are to be amputated, an analysis of retained function must be made to employ the most appropriate surgical plan. Inevitably, any loss of tissue will lead to decreased function (most commonly grip strength). Interestingly, the level of amputation does not always correlate with patient disability [10]. However, it is important to recognize that amputation is irreversible. When in doubt, it is better to leave a digit that may offer some unforeseeable function as it can always be removed later with little morbidity.

A multitude of various surgical options exist for digital amputation, ranging from simple guillotine amputation to complex reconstruction and tissue transfers. Preservation of length, soft tissue coverage, and functional sensibility are the core concepts in digital and partial hand amputations [11–15]. Postoperatively, the residual finger and/or hand is often hypersensitive. Directed hand therapy is often helpful to "desensitize" the remaining digit(s). Cold intolerance is also common, especially, when the remaining tissues may have insufficient circulation. This can be debilitating, especially in colder climates. While cold intolerance subsides with time, many patients will struggle long term. Some individuals

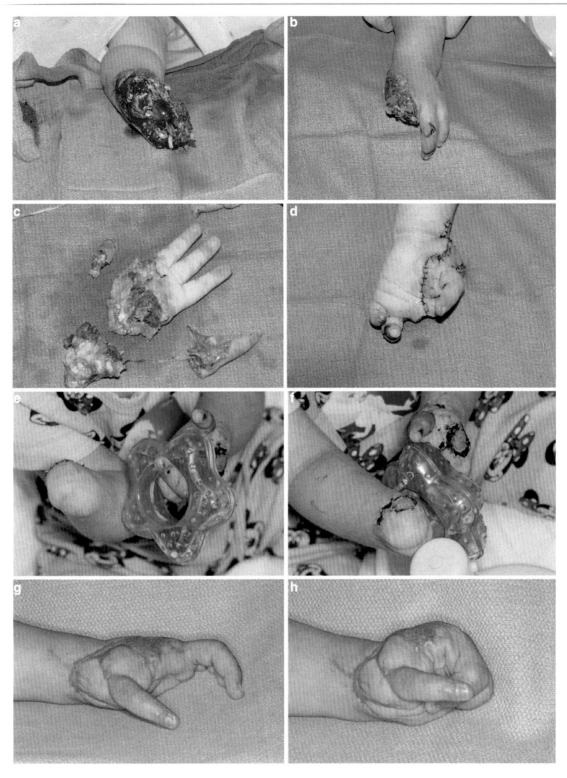

Fig. 51.1 Shown is an infant child with severe lawn-mower injury to bilateral hands. The right hand was amputated at the radiocarpal joint (**a**). On the left, the radial half of the hand was amputated which included the thumb to the level of the carpometacarpal joint (**b**). The largest amputated part belonged to the contralateral index, middle, and ring finger (**c**). The middle finger was fashioned to reconstruct the left thumb, while fillet flaps were used of the neighboring digits to provide (incomplete) skin coverage (**d**). The patient was able to use the neo-thumb for pinch and grasp activity even in the early postoperative period (**e**) while the contralateral extremity served as a useful "helper hand" after revision amputation (**f**). Follow-up at 12 weeks demonstrates completely healed wounds with grafted areas and good motion of the neo-thumb (**g**, **h**). From Chim H, et al. Challenges in replantation of complex amputations. Semin Plast Surg, 2013. 27(4): p. 182–9. Reprinted with permission from Thieme

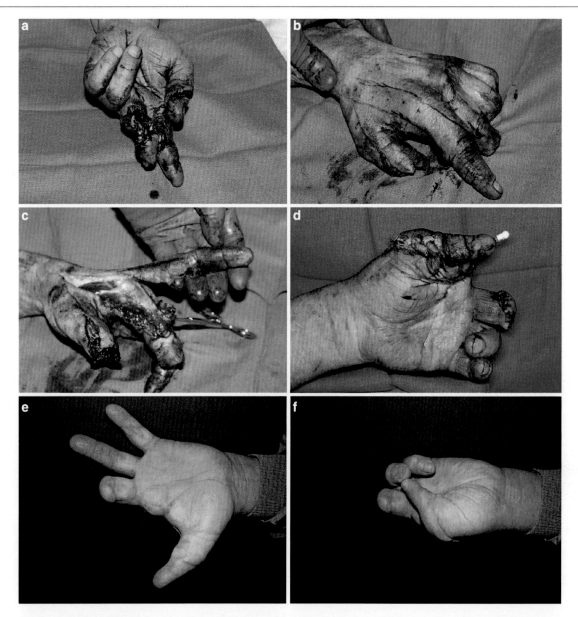

Fig. 51.2 Shown is the left hand of a middle-aged man who sustained a mangling table saw injury. The thumb was dysvascular and included a sagittal injury. The index finger was also dysvascular with two-level injury to the neurovascular bundles (**a**). The index finger was used for thumb reconstruction via pollicization, while maintaining integrity of the dorsal veins and extensor mechanism and microsurgical arterial revascularization and flexor tendon reconstruction (**b–d**). Later follow-up demonstrated good healing with protective sensation and functional motion (**e, f**)

may find it necessary to change work and/or living environments to avoid exposure to cold [3].

It should be highlighted that the thumb receives special attention due to its functional importance. It is estimated that the thumb comprises 40–50 % of overall hand function. Every effort should be made preserve the thumb. When this is not possible, thumb reconstruction should be considered. Advanced reconstructive techniques such as pollicization of a neighboring digit and toe-to-thumb transfers, can be employed, if possible and appropriate, to regain function [16, 17].

Regarding digit amputation, classically, greater value is placed on the central digits (middle and ring finger) in comparison to the border digits (index and small finger). It is easier to compensate for the loss of a border digit both functionally and cosmetically. A three-finger hand can actually look remarkably normal (Fig. 51.2) and functionally compensated. However, the loss of hand span (width) does present a loss of pronosupination strength due to loss of the lever arm length [15]. Loss of a central digit leaves a gap in the hand that is very noticeable and presents a functional problem with use of the hand as a cup or scoop. Narrowing the

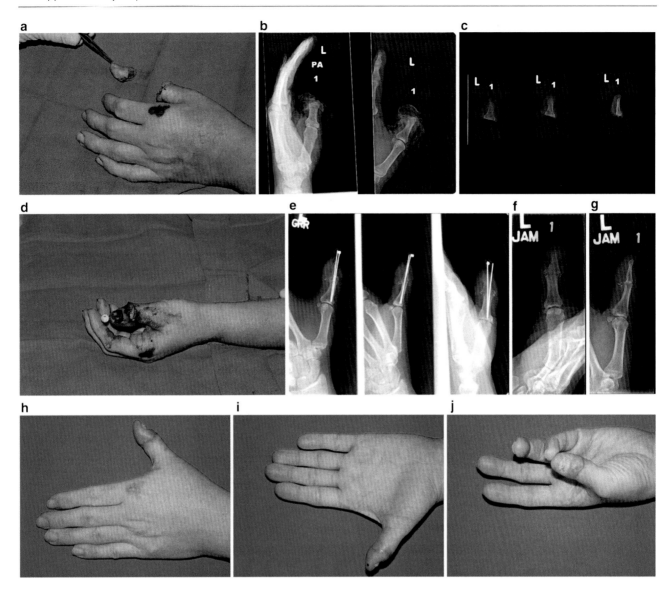

Fig. 51.3 43-year-old female with left thumb amputation through the interphalangeal (IP) joint (**a–c**). Modest skeletal shortening is performed and replantation (**d**) at the joint level and the joint is fused acutely with K-wires (**e**). K-wires are removed at 6 weeks after radio-graphic union (**f, g**). Skin and bone are healed at 12 weeks (**h, i**). Fusion at the IP joint is well-compensated in the thumb due to the mobility of the trapeziometacarpal joint (**j**)

resultant space after central digit loss can be accomplished by ray resection with intermetacarpal ligament repair (Fig. 51.6) or ray transposition as described by Carroll and others [18, 19].

Wrist Disarticulation

Amputation at the level of the wrist causing loss of the entire hand significantly decreases the overall function of the upper extremity secondary to loss of grip and intrinsic function of the hand. Creating wrist-level prosthetics is difficult and options are limited. Every option to preserve the hand must be entertained.

Conversely, as a salvage procedure, amputation at this level provides several distinct advantages, and is usually preferred to a slightly more proximal level. If the distal radioulnar joint can be preserved with an intact pronator, full forearm rotation is maintained and this will improve the capability of the amputee. Maintaining length of the forearm allows the patient to use the extremity for reach and in conjunction with the contralateral extremity, functioning as a "helper hand" (Fig. 51.1). Retention of the distal radial flare also provides a wide base for prosthetic mounting and improves prosthetic fitting, suspension, and control. Prosthetists often prefer a more proximal (*trans*radial) amputation to wrist disarticulation. The primary reason is that the myoelectric controls and battery can be fit inside the

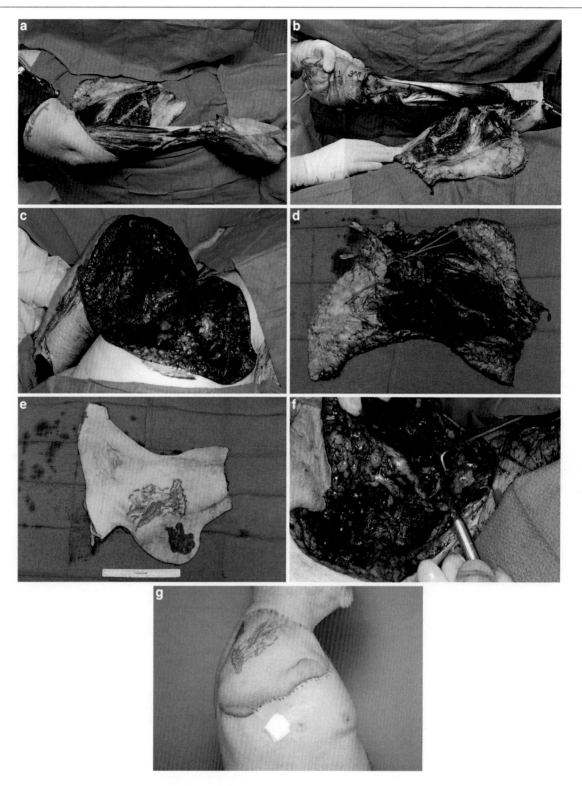

Fig. 51.4 73-year-old male with recurrent poorly differentiated sarcoma involving right the proximal humerus. Prior to oncologic resection, a radial forearm flap is harvested neurotized flexor muscle mass with median and ulnar nerves (**a**, **b**). Oncologic resection is then performed (**c**), and the flap is harvested just before the specimen is rendered ischemic (**d**, **e**). The median and ulnar nerves are coapted to the transected brachial plexus (TMR) to provide intuitive myoelectric signals for intuitive prosthetic control (**f**). His healing flap is shown 1 month postoperative (**g**)

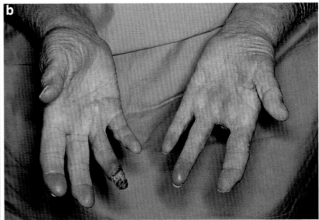

Fig. 51.5 50-year-old female with diabetic nephropathy and vasculopathy with bilateral hand ischemia (**a**, **b**)

prosthetic without resulting in a forearm of inappropriate length. In the authors' opinion, however, this prosthetic advantage is outweighed by the advantages of added length and function without a prosthetic. In addition, we have had success working with prosthetists to fit our wrist-level amputees (Fig. 51.7). However, the best approach is not rigid but rather a collaborative approach between surgeon, patient, and prosthetist [20].

For a wrist disarticulation, the skin flaps are usually planned such that the palmar flap is longer than the dorsal flap due to differences in palmar and dorsal skin quality. Plan the incision so that the final closure minimizes/avoids incision lines on weight-bearing surfaces (i.e., distal end of distal radius/ulna). The superficial veins are ligated. The dorsal sensory branch of the ulnar nerve and superficial branch of the radial nerve are ligated proximally to minimize chance of neuroma formation. The radial and ulnar artery and nerve are ligated and allowed to retract into the forearm. The flexor and extensor tendons are transected as proximal as possible and allowed to retract into the forearm. When the carpus is disarticulated from the distal radius and ulna, care is taken not to disrupt the distal radioulnar joint and triangular fibrocartilage. The volar and radial radiocarpal ligaments are resected and the radial and ulnar styloid processes should be rounded off with a rasp. Finally, the skin flaps and incision lines are closed in a manner that provides adequate padding at the end of the limb and well-placed closure lines.

At the surgeon's discretion, more proximal ligation of the radial, median, and ulnar nerves may be performed at this point by way of a separate proximal incision as described by Louis [21] to help prevent neuroma formation. Retention of the carpal bones (i.e., transcarpal amputation) has shown no added benefit compared to a wrist disarticulation procedure.

Hand prosthetics can be utilized to recreate the motions of wrist flexion/extension as well as finger function [22]. Although historically, simple designs such as hook or pincer grasp have been most successful secondary to simplicity,

new horizons such as targeted muscle reinnervation show promise for functionally superior prosthetics in the future [23, 24].

Transradial Amputation

The transradial amputation (forearm amputation, below elbow amputation) is the most common major (proximal to hand) upper extremity amputation (Fig. 51.8). Obvious advantages to performing an amputation at this level in the upper extremity are preservation of motion at the shoulder and elbow, as well as superior prosthetic acceptance rates. It has been reported to have the highest rate of prosthetic acceptance and use among all upper extremity amputation levels, which can be explained by the ability to retain pronation/supination while recreating a cosmetic hand and restoring at least some hand function [24–26].

Amputations carried out at any level of the forearm are technically similar but function allowed to the amputee is dictated by length of the limb. Preservation of forearm rotation is achieved when greater than 50 % of forearm length is maintained. Even with only 5 cm of ulnar length, the elbow joint can remain intact and a satisfactory prosthesis can be fitted while maintaining elbow motion. This is much preferred to an elbow disarticulation despite the lack of pronation-supination associated with amputation at this level. In cases where 5 cm of ulna cannot be preserved, preserving the residual ulna may still be beneficial as it can aid in prosthetic fitting and is a good weight-bearing surface. It is important to note, however, that when a very proximal amputation is carried out (i.e., proximal to the bicipital tuberosity or with removal of radius), it is recommended to reattach the biceps tendon to the ulna to facilitate prosthetic fitting as well as provide improved elbow flexion. Equal limb lengths usually can be easily created with prosthetics for transradial amputees.

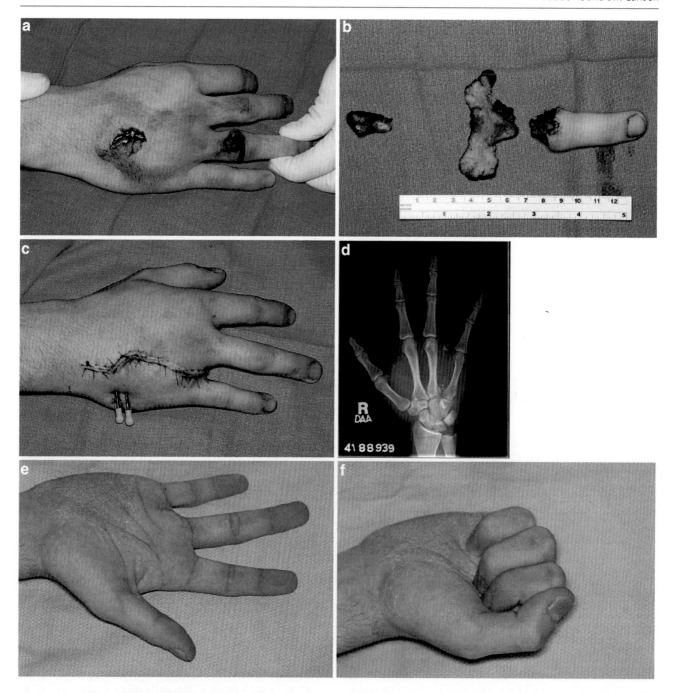

Fig. 51.6 25-year-old male sustained a gunshot wound to the right hand with skeletal destruction of the metacarpal, proximal phalanx, and joint of the ring finger (**a**). Definitive treatment is accomplished with ray resection and web space closure with intermetacarpal liga-ment repair and K-wire fixation (**b**). Motion is preserved without mal-rotation or scissoring of the neighboring digits (**c, d**). Postoperative appearance demonstrates acceptable closure of the webspace and good function (**e, f**)

Typically, and as allowed by soft tissues, equal length volar and dorsal skin flaps are created to allow adequate closure at the level of bony resection. Superficial veins are ligated and divided. Radial and ulnar arteries are identified, securely ligated, and divided. Depending on the level of amputation, either the tendons or muscle bellies are divided at a length appropriate for tenodesis or myodesis, respec-tively. Muscle and tendon length are maintained to provide soft tissue coverage over the end of the bone. The median, radial, and ulnar nerves should be divided proximal to the level of the bone cuts. Management of the nerve endings is an important consideration. Classical teaching is to divide the nerves as high as possible and allow them to retract (i.e., "traction neurectomy"); however, this can leave the end of

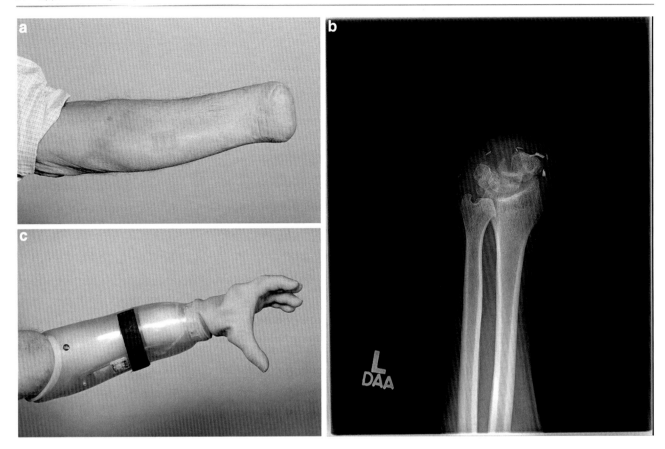

Fig. 51.7 60-year-old male sustained bilateral hand loss after farm injury. The left hand was amputated at the midcarpal joint (**a**, **b**), maintaining length for function without a prosthesis, yet enabling fit and use of a myoelectric hand prosthetic (**c**)

the limb insensate and could limit future reconstruction options (transplantation, targeted muscle reinnervation). On the other hand, leaving the nerves too long can result in painful neuroma at the end of the limb. Therefore, a balance must be sought and the nerves divided at a level proximal enough such that if a neuroma develops, it will not interfere with prosthetic wear. Giving the nerve a "target" may be beneficial in neuroma prevention. This can be performed through a separate incision as described by Louis [21]. The bone is transected and bone ends are smoothed with a rasp. Some authors advocate that for transradial amputation, resection of 5–8 cm of bone should always be performed in order to create a robust soft tissue envelope for bony coverage [27]. Additionally, with removal of the DRUJ, soft tissue interposition between the distal ends of the radius and ulna may improve stability and decrease painful convergence.

One rarely indicated option to restore some pincer grasp function for patients with distal forearm amputation or wrist disarticulation is the Krukenberg procedure [28]. Described in 1917 by German army surgeon Hermann Krukenberg, the procedure is used to create a pincer mechanism between the radius and ulna, powered by pronator teres [29]. It is often

rejected due to its unfavorable cosmetic appearance and is most often used for blind bilateral amputees who lack the visual feedback to function a prosthetic device effectively and in developing countries where access to prosthetic rehabilitation is limited.

Elbow Disarticulation

When proximal ulna cannot be preserved, elbow disarticulation must be considered. While carrying multiple disadvantages when compared to transradial amputation, preservation of the distal humeral condyles provides the benefits of a long lever arm and snug-fitting prosthesis. This in turn leads to more effective transmission of humeral rotation to the prosthesis when compared to a more proximal transhumeral amputation.

Soft tissues allowing, equal anterior and posterior soft tissue flaps are created and are reflected over the humeral condyles. Beginning anteriorly, the brachial artery and forearm veins are ligated. The superficial sensory nerves (medial brachial and antebrachial as well as lateral antebrachial) are

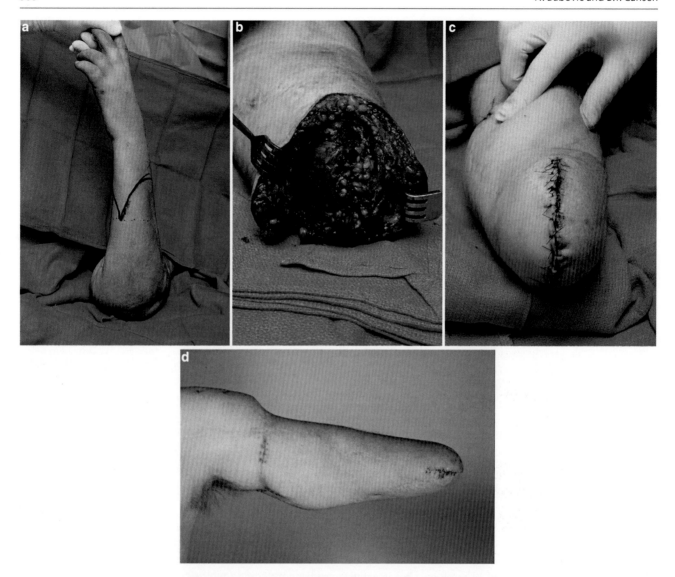

Fig. 51.8 Transradial amputation is performed for functionless, painful hand (**a**). Myodesis is performed for soft tissue coverage of the residual radius and ulna (**b**). Skin closure (**c**) and postoperative appearance (**d**) are shown

divided as proximally as possible. The median, ulnar, and radial nerves are divided proximally and allowed to retract under muscle or are used for targeted innervation. The biceps tendon and brachialis muscle are divided and tagged for subsequent tenodesis with the triceps tendon. The forearm flexor and extensor musculature is then divided or detached from its origin, the joint capsule is fully incised, and the triceps muscle is divided and fixed to the elbow flexors to complete the amputation.

While maintaining humeral length and the metaphyseal flare of the distal humeral condyles allows for a mechani-cally superior prosthesis, cosmesis may not be ideal due to a change in position of the elbow joint once prosthesis has been fitted. This limb length discrepancy can also present a functional obstacle for prosthetic use and functional posi-tioning. In some instances, this may be corrected with an immediate or delayed humeral shortening osteotomy. Preservation of the condyles together with humeral shorten-ing osteotomy provides functional advantages over initial transhumeral amputation. In addition to improved prosthetic fit, the condylar flare provides a notch or shelf to allow car-riage of a strap (i.e., grocery bag, hand bag).

Transhumeral Amputation

Amputations at the level of the elbow should aim to preserve as much length as possible. At least 5–7 cm of the humerus should be maintained for prosthesis suspension and acceptance. Ideally, amputation 3–5 cm proximal to the elbow joint allows for the best functional outcome. Skin grafting or free tissue transfer should be considered in cases where humeral length may be maintained by adjuvant methods. Latissimus dorsi, parascapular, and other free tissue transfers have been successfully used to preserve amputation length and facilitate salvage of humeral length (Fig. 51.9). The deltoid muscle should be preserved even in very proximal transhumeral amputations, to preserve stability and control of the shoulder joint. It is also important to salvage the humeral head whenever possible. Without retention or reconstruction of the insertions of the pectoralis major, latissimus dorsi, and deltoid, however, the functional result will be the same as that of a shoulder disarticulation with regard to prosthetic use. For this reason, if the humeral head is retained to improve the cosmetic appearance of the shoulder and to potentially aid in force transmission.

Soft tissues allowing, equal medial and lateral skin flaps are created and are reflected proximally. The brachial artery and vein are ligated. The median, radial, and ulnar nerves are either proximally divided and allowed to retract under musculature or are used for targeted muscle reinnervation. The flexor and extensor muscles are transected just distal to the level of intended bone resection. The bone is then transected at the desired level. Flexor and extensor musculature can be used to create a covering for the residual bone followed by skin closure.

Prosthetic rejection rates are high among transhumeral amputees [30–32]. There are multiple factors that contribute to prosthetic rejection which are magnified with proximal amputation, discomfort, poor fit, and poor function. The more proximal the amputation, the more function the individual needs from the prosthesis. However, the more proximal the amputation, the less control (short lever arm, limited muscle availability) is needed for the prosthesis. It is this subgroup of amputees that can benefit the most from adjunctive reconstruction such as skeletal lengthening and targeted muscle reinnervation, discussed below.

Shoulder Disarticulation

Shoulder disarticulation is very morbid, is rarely performed, and is usually the result of substantial trauma or tumor (Fig. 51.4). In the elective setting, reconstruction can be more effectively planned toward prosthetic fitting, and certain anatomy can be preferentially preserved. The clavicle and scapula are important for prosthetic suspension and should be preserved. The distal branches of the brachial plexus can be used for TMR.

Soft tissue allowing, shoulder musculature such as deltoid and overlying skin should be preserved for closure. Approaching anteriorly, pectoralis muscle and deltoid are detached from the humerus. The axillary vessels are ligated. The median, radial, ulnar, musculocutaneous nerves are identified, transected, and allowed to retract. The fate of these nerves should be carefully planned, and they can either be cut short and allowed to retract or skillfully kept long and buried in the muscle for later use with TMR. The anterior and posterior musculature is detached to reveal the short external rotators, subscapularis, and anterior joint capsule, which are also detached from their insertion on the humerus. Preserved muscle (usually deltoid) is used to create a contoured shoulder with good cosmesis and one that can support/power and prosthesis.

Forequarter amputation is a more radical amputation involving removal of the entire shoulder girdle (including scapula) and is usually reserved for cases of aggressive or metastatic malignancy to the upper extremity. Functionally, it is similar to shoulder disarticulation with the disadvantage of lack of clavicle and scapula for prosthetic suspension.

Targeted Muscle Reinnervation

The loss of one or both upper extremities is an extremely morbid and debilitating condition. Past and current prosthesis have a limited ability to restore the complex function of the upper extremity through cable-controlled and myoelectric designs. The most common modern prostheses utilize EMG signals in residual limb musculature to control specific prosthesis functions. These devices are often slow and nonintuitive, can only function to recreate simple motions and actions, and are of limited utility for high-level amputations. Rapid advances in the field of targeted muscle reinnervation (TMR) may allow for more complex and intuitive control of prosthetics which will allow for restoration of greater function.

In 2004, Kuiken et al. introduced the concept of targeted reinnervation (TR) in a case report of a patient with bilateral shoulder disarticulation injury [33]. TR utilizes nonfunctional muscles (distal muscular attachment is missing) as amplifiers for nonfunctional nerves that are present as neuromas. TR can provide signals to these muscles to provide intuitive prosthetic function, for example, radial nerve innervation to a segment of the pectoralis major muscle, providing

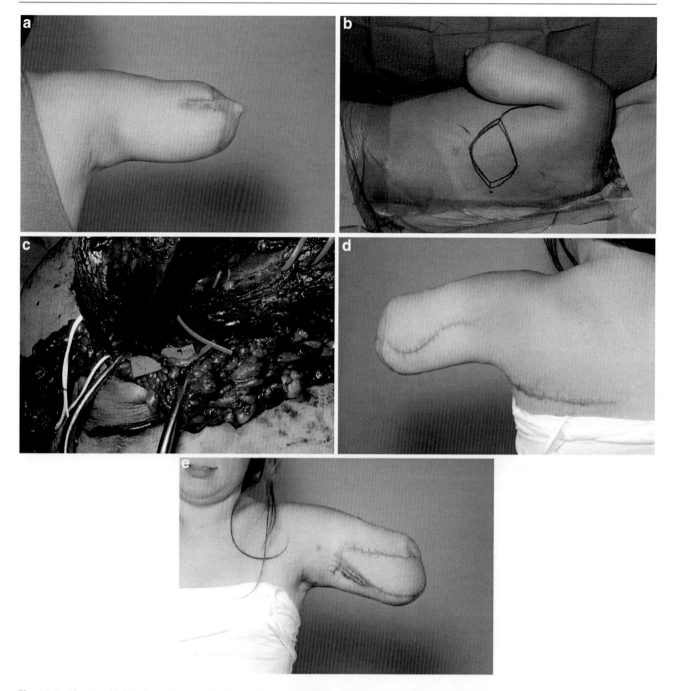

Fig. 51.9 12-year-old female presented with traumatic transhumeral amputation, unstable scar, and skeletal overgrowth (**a**). Skeletal length is maintained and the residual limb is covered with a pedicled latissimus dorsi musculocutaneous flap (**b**). TMR is performed which included ulnar nerve transfer to the thoracodorsal nerve (**c**) resulting in six separate and myoelectric signals for intuitive prosthetic control. Early postoperative appearance is shown (**d**, **e**)

a new and intuitive signal for myoelectric control of hand opening function of the prosthesis. TR for motor control is called targeted muscle reinnervation or TMR. TMR has been used for patients with amputations at the shoulder disarticu-

lation and *trans*humeral level and has implications for amputations at other levels.

Individuals with transhumeral amputation should have intact biceps and triceps muscle function before consideration of TMR [34]. Conventional control of a myoelectric prosthetic for these individuals is with one triceps signal and one biceps signal. This provides intuitive control of elbow flexion and extension, but control of forearm rotation (pro-supination), and hand open and close actions is not intuitive and requires a "switch" between modes on the device. Continuous switching between modes is cumbersome and nonintuitive and requires too much cognitive oversight. The median, ulnar, and radial nerves in these individuals are typically present as nonfunctional neuromas at the end of the limb. Since there are two heads to the biceps, one can be sacrificed as a recipient signal amplifier without sacrificing the intuitive elbow flexion signal that is provided by the remaining biceps muscle with native innervation via the musculocutaneous nerve. Typically, the median nerve is transferred to the short head of the biceps muscle to provide an intuitive signal for hand close or pronation. If the brachialis muscle is present, the ulnar nerve can be transferred to its motor branch to provide an additional intuitive signal for hand close, or other prosthetic hand function. The radial nerve is approached posteriorly and typically transferred to the lateral head of the triceps muscle providing an intuitive signal for hand opening or supination for the prosthetic. Native innervation of the long head of the triceps is preserved so that intuitive elbow extension remains intact.

Targeted muscle reinnervation (TMR) can also be helpful for individuals with amputation at the shoulder disarticulation level [33, 35] (Fig. 51.10). In this case, the procedure is more complex and requires signals for elbow control in addition to wrist and hand. At this level, the following transected and nonfunctional nerves are transferred: musculocutaneous, radial, median, and ulnar. These nerves are then coapted to the isolated motor segments of the pectoralis major muscle (three segments) and the pectoralis minor muscle. Other shoulder girdle muscles that are nonfunctional and present are also potential recipients and candidates for nerve transfer (i.e., latissimus dorsi and serratus anterior muscles). When performing this procedure, it is important to thin the skin overlying the muscle, thus removing subcutaneous fat in order to maximize the strength of the EMG signal. With the overlying skin thinned and denervated, a fascinating and serendipitous finding was discovered in that the transferred nerve reinnervated the overlying skin and thus provided the possibility to experience "hand" sensation in the reinnervated chest wall skin. Some have referred to this as targeted sensory reinnervation, or TSR.

Prior to proceeding with)TMR surgery, it is important to rule out any proximal nerve injury, such as a brachial plexus injury that could have occurred at the time of a traumatic amputation. Strong and intact biceps and triceps function with localized Tinel's signs for the residual median, ulnar, and radial nerves are sufficient to proceed to surgery and in this case, no further investigation is required. The locations for each nerve's Tinel's sign should be noted. If the Tinel's sign is at the distal end of the limb, this is a good sign that the nerve will have plenty of length to reach its target. If the Tinel's sign is proximal, there may not be sufficient length to reach the target muscle. In this case, the surgeon should be prepared for nerve grafting to reach the target. We have been successful using nerve graft to reach the muscle target. However, since the target muscle is otherwise completely denervated, the nerve graft should be short enough so that the target is reached with regeneration through the graft before denervation-induced muscle atrophy occurs. It is important that the target muscle does not have any native innervation as this will certainly overpower the nerve transfer and the desired signal will not be evident. Finally, a proximally based, adipofascial flap is designed to minimize the tissue between the muscles and overlying skin and, after nerve transfer, is interposed between the muscle heads to separate their EMG signals.

Since TMR is a relatively new procedure, the literature is lacking in terms of outcomes. A report published functional outcomes after TMR for three shoulder disarticulation amputees and three transhumeral amputees [36]. Reported outcomes on these six patients were very positive with improved function following the procedure as reported by the Box and Blocks Test, Clothespin Relocation Test, and Assessment of Motor and Process Skills Test. The authors also note improved function in more complicated tasks with the ability to simultaneously control two joints at a time and subjective improvements in the ease of performing activities of daily living. In 2012, researchers from the same institution reported a comparison of TR and transplantation with a comparative discussion based on the level of amputation, function, and cost [37]. The authors insightfully state that TR and transplantation are complementary, rather than competitive, procedures. Finally, TR has not been considered for individuals with more distal amputations. For patients with transradial and distal amputation, the extrinsic muscles are present and should be amenable to myoelectric control. Intrinsic hand muscles are, of course, absent. A transfer of the recurrent motor portion of the median nerve or motor component of the ulnar nerve could theoretically be transferred in a manner similar to TMR at the forearm level. However, the current level of prosthetic function is not sophisticated enough to make use of the refined hand function signals that could result from this transfer.

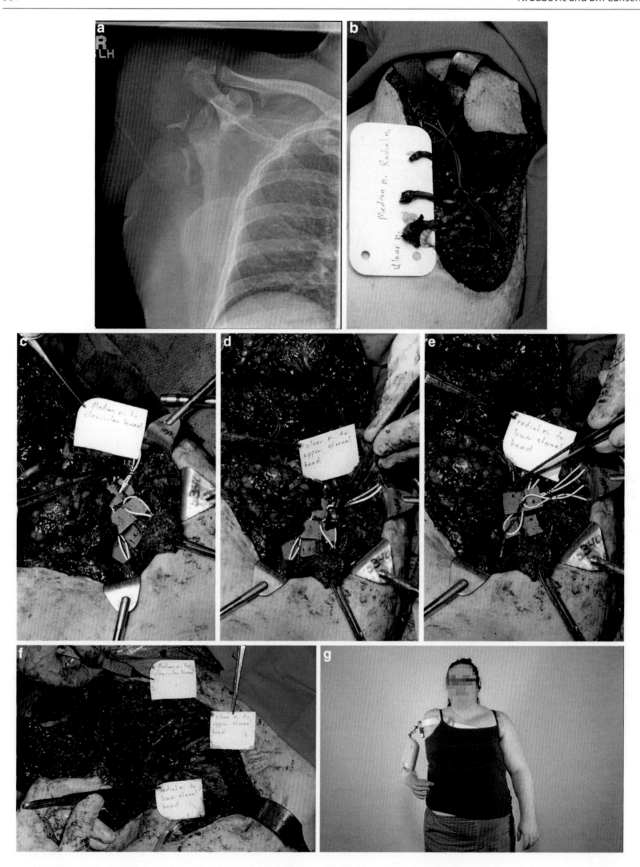

Fig. 51.10 39-year-old female sustained traumatic shoulder disarticulation (**a**) with intuitive residual biceps and triceps innervation. Brachial plexus explored and median, ulnar, and radial nerves are identified (**b**). Coaptation (TMR) is performed to the three heads of the pectoralis major muscle (**c–f**) with five resultant intuitive myoelectric signals (**g**)

References

1. Fuchs JC. The pathology of upper-extremity arterial disease. Hand Clin. 1993;9(1):1–4.
2. van Gils W et al. Sensibility of the stump in adults with an acquired major upper extremity amputation. Arch Phys Med Rehabil. 2013;94(11):2179–85.
3. Carlsson IK, Dahlin LB. Self-reported cold sensitivity in patients with traumatic hand injuries or hand-arm vibration syndrome: an eight year follow up. BMC Musculoskelet Disord. 2014;15:83.
4. Carlsson IK, Rosen B, Dahlin LB. Self-reported cold sensitivity in normal subjects and in patients with traumatic hand injuries or hand-arm vibration syndrome. BMC Musculoskelet Disord. 2010;11:89.
5. Kirk NT. Amputations, a monograph volume III, Lewis' practice of surgery. Hagerstown: W. F. Prior Co., Inc; 1943.
6. Pederson WC. Replantation. Plast Reconstr Surg. 2001;107(3): 823–41.
7. Chiu HY, Chen MT. Revascularization of digits after thirty-three hours of warm ischemia time: a case report. J Hand Surg [Am]. 1984;9A(1):63–7.
8. Wei FC et al. Three successful digital replantations in a patient after 84, 86, and 94 hours of cold ischemia time. Plast Reconstr Surg. 1988;82(2):346–50.
9. Jones NF, Gupta R. Postoperative monitoring of pediatric toe-to-hand transfers with differential pulse oximetry. J Hand Surg [Am]. 2001;26(3):525–9.
10. Giladi AM et al. Measuring outcomes and determining long-term disability after revision amputation for treatment of traumatic finger and thumb amputation injuries. Plast Reconstr Surg. 2014; 134(5):746e–55e.
11. Chim H et al. Challenges in replantation of complex amputations. Semin Plast Surg. 2013;27(4):182–9.
12. Yabe T et al. Treatment of fingertip amputation: comparison of results between microsurgical replantation and pocket principle. J Reconstr Microsurg. 2012;28(4):221–6.
13. Wang K et al. A systematic review of outcomes of revision amputation treatment for fingertip amputations. Hand (N Y). 2013;8(2):139–45.
14. Alper N, Sood A, Granick MS. Composite graft repair for distal fingertip amputation. Eplasty. 2013;13:ic32.
15. Moran SL, Berger RA. Biomechanics and hand trauma: what you need. Hand Clin. 2003;19(1):17–31.
16. Lin PY et al. A systematic review of outcomes of toe-to-thumb transfers for isolated traumatic thumb amputation. Hand (N Y). 2011;6(3):235–43.
17. Agarwal JP et al. Selected outcomes of thumb replantation after isolated thumb amputation injury. J Hand Surg [Am]. 2010;35(9): 1485–90.
18. Carroll RE. Transposition of the index finger to replace the middle finger. Clin Orthop. 1959;15:27–34.
19. Posner MA. Ray transposition for central digital loss. J Hand Surg [Am]. 1979;4(3):242–57.
20. Carlsen BT, Prigge P, Peterson J. Upper extremity limb loss: functional restoration from prosthesis and targeted reinnervation to transplantation. J Hand Ther. 2014;27(2):106–13. quiz 114.
21. Louis DS, Hunter LY, Keating TM. Painful neuromas in long below-elbow amputees. Arch Surg. 1980;115(6):742–4.
22. Pasquina PF et al. Advances in amputee care. Arch Phys Med Rehabil. 2006;87(3 Suppl 1):S34–43. quiz S44–5.
23. Tager G, Nast-Kolb D. Amputation and prosthesis management of the upper extremity. Unfallchirurg. 2000;103(11):977–92.
24. Cayci C, Carlsen BT, Saint-Cyr M. Optimizing functional and aesthetic outcomes of upper limb soft tissue reconstruction. Hand Clin. 2014;30(2):225–38.
25. Burger H et al. Validation of the orthotics and prosthetics user survey upper extremity functional status module in people with unilateral upper limb amputation. J Rehabil Med. 2008;40(5):393–9.
26. Baumgartner RF. Upper extremity amputation and prosthetics. J Rehabil Res Dev. 2001;38(4):7–10.
27. Meier 3rd RH, Melton D. Ideal functional outcomes for amputation levels. Phys Med Rehabil Clin N Am. 2014;25(1):199–212.
28. Kleeman LT, Shafritz AB. The Krukenberg procedure. J Hand Surg [Am]. 2013;38(1):173–5.
29. Krukenberg H. Uber plastische umvertung von armamputationsstumpfen. Stuttgart: Ferdinand Enke; 1917.
30. Biddiss E, Chau T. Upper-limb prosthetics: critical factors in device abandonment. Am J Phys Med Rehabil. 2007;86(12):977–87.
31. Dillingham TR et al. Use and satisfaction with prosthetic devices among persons with trauma-related amputations: a long-term outcome study. Am J Phys Med Rehabil. 2001;80(8):563–71.
32. Wright TW, Hagen AD, Wood MB. Prosthetic usage in major upper extremity amputations. J Hand Surg [Am]. 1995;20(4):619–22.
33. Kuiken TA et al. The use of targeted muscle reinnervation for improved myoelectric prosthesis control in a bilateral shoulder disarticulation amputee. Prosthet Orthot Int. 2004;28(3):245–53.
34. Dumanian GA et al. Targeted reinnervation for transhumeral amputees: current surgical technique and update on results. Plast Reconstr Surg. 2009;124(3):863–9.
35. Hijjawi JB et al. Improved myoelectric prosthesis control accomplished using multiple nerve transfers. Plast Reconstr Surg. 2006;118(7):1573–8.
36. Miller LA et al. Improved myoelectric prosthesis control using targeted reinnervation surgery: a case series. IEEE Trans Neural Syst Rehabil Eng. 2008;16(1):46–50.
37. Agnew SP et al. Limb transplantation and targeted reinnervation: a practical comparison. J Reconstr Microsurg. 2012;28(1):63–8.

Rodney M. Stuck, Coleen Napolitano,
and Francis J. Rottier

Introduction

When pedal amputation becomes necessary, functional foot and ankle amputation is the goal for the limb salvage surgeon. Half of the lower extremity amputations performed lie within the foot and ankle. Simply providing soft tissue coverage over an open pedal wound does not necessarily create a functional amputation. As this discussion evolves, review of infection control, tissue nutrition, anesthetic concerns, and functional amputation levels will be reviewed.

Clinical Roles

Once the patient develops non-reconstructable soft tissue loss or irreparable vascular insufficiency, amputation becomes the patient's next step toward rehabilitation and recovery. Helping the patient through this transition is both a medical team and family effort for the patient [1]. These two groups play an integral role in both physical and emotional support as well as the medical and psychological well-being of the patient through this entire process. While the foot and ankle surgeon stabilizes infection and plans for functional amputation, the vascular interventionalist will assure adequate blood flow is present and the medical staff will stabilize systemic disease and administer antibiotic therapy, and psychiatry/psychology may provide a role for counseling. Physical therapy is necessary to aid with gait assistance pre- and postoperatively and a physiatrist may be of assistance to aid with mobility as well. Once the patient has closure of the residual limb, a pedorthotist or prosthetist

R.M. Stuck, DPM (✉) • C. Napolitano, DPM • F.J. Rottier, DPM
Podiatry Division, Department of Orthopaedic Surgery and
Rehabilitation, Loyola University Stritch School of Medicine,
2160 S. First Ave, Maywood, IL 60153, USA

Hines Veterans Administration, Hines, IL, USA

may be invaluable in helping choose appropriate footwear accommodation and protection for the residual foot. Family or caregiver participation in this entire process is critical for the best outcomes. Clearly, the transition through the process of amputation is a team effort that involves medical staff and family working toward the recovery of their shared patient and loved one.

Amputation Level Selection

There are many factors involved in selecting the appropriate amputation level. At times the surgeon may choose the biologic amputation level, which is the most distal level the foot can heal. Although this level may sometimes be appropriate, the residual limb may not withstand the activities of daily living. Education of the patient, family, and medical staff regarding functional amputation levels will help ensure that a durable level is chosen at which the patient is best able to perform their activities of daily living [2–4]. Occasionally these choices must be made in the face of a nonambulatory patient, and the team must decide whether local salvage should be chosen or would proximal amputation (such as a through-knee amputation) be more beneficial for the long-term health of the patient. Sepsis and medical instability of the patient may also influence the amputation level decision. When the patient is too unstable for any surgical care, a freezer boot may be applied to the limb. While this provides a physiologic amputation of the limb that may be lifesaving, the process also commits the patient to an above-knee amputation.

Care must be taken to protect the contralateral foot during the process of surgery and recovery. Regular checks of the contralateral limb should be incorporated in the postoperative assessment of the patient. Should the patient wear prescription footwear, this should be worn during any physical therapy, and care should be taken to make sure that the contralateral foot does not rest against the end of the bed or on a wheelchair foot plate for extended periods of time as ulceration or soft tissue injury may occur. The ultimate goal is to maximize quality of life and preserve a functional level of independence. Utilizing this team approach, our patients can often reach a reasonable level of postoperative function.

Decision Making

The most common amputation levels within the foot are digital (distal and proximal), toe and metatarsal, transmetatarsal (TMA), Lisfranc, Chopart, and ankle disarticulation. Each of these amputations may be left open to heal on their own or may be utilized as stepping-stones to a more proximal amputation due to persisting infection or mechanical considerations. The statistics for pedal amputation show that revisions are more frequent when amputations are performed within the foot. This fact is not unexpected. It is quite common for a patient to have an open amputation of a toe, metatarsal, or even a midfoot/hind foot disarticulation to eradicate severe infection or gangrene. Once the patient has recovered from their sepsis and soft tissue infection is controlled, a decision on wound closure or amputation level can be made. Care can be taken to make sure that the patients have control of their infection, adequate tissue nutrition, and an appropriate choice for amputation level leading to the best function.

Osteomyelitis can be a limiting factor in salvage of the forefoot and midfoot. Early resection of metatarsal heads or the local bone that is infected for biopsy and culture in the care process can lead to accurate early decisions on antibiotic therapy. This in turn may improve the rate of cure and more distal salvage of the infected limb by reducing soft tissue destruction from infection. Consideration may be given to taking a "clearance fragment" of the bone at the most proximal level of amputation [5]. This specimen is sent for pathologic and microbiologic assessment to make sure that all of the infection has been resected. Should these fragments not be infection-free, consideration must be given to an extended course of antibiotics, unless further revision amputation removes the remainder of the affected bone. Certainly culture-driven antibiotic therapy with infectious disease consultation, as needed, will lead to the best potential outcome.

Vascular Perfusion

Amputation flaps predominately heal by collateral circulation. Due to this phenomenon, arteriography is rarely useful as diagnostic tool to predict amputation healing. Doppler ultrasonography is commonly utilized to determine whether adequate perfusion exists in the extremity prior to performing an amputation. The ischemic index is a ratio of the Doppler pressure at the anatomic level of concern compared to the brachial systolic pressure. An ischemic index of 0.5 or greater at the surgical site is thought to be necessary to support wound healing. An ankle-brachial index (ABI) of 0.45 in the patient with diabetes has been considered adequate for healing as long as the systolic pressure at the ankle was 70 mmHg or higher [6]. These values are falsely elevated, and non-predictive, in at least 15 % of patients with peripheral arterial disease. This is primarily due to the non-compressibility of calcified peripheral arteries [7]. Other forms of noninvasive vascular testing can be considered when ABIs are unreliable. This would include the use of transcutaneous partial pressure of oxygen (TcPO2) [8–10], measurement of skin perfusion pressure (SPP), and the toe brachial index (TBI) [11–14]. The vascular laboratory can measure toe pressures as an indicator of arterial inflow to the foot. The arteries of the hallux are less commonly found to be calcified than the vessels of the leg and at the level of the ankle. The accepted threshold for toe pressure is 50 mmHg. Consultation with a vascular specialist should be obtained for patients who do not have adequate inflow demonstrated on these exams.

Nutrition and Immunocompetence

Preoperative review of nutritional status is obtained by measuring the serum albumin and the total lymphocyte count (TLC). The serum albumin should be at least 3.0 gm/dL and the total lymphocyte count should be greater than 1500. A serum albumin level of 3.5 g/dL or less indicates malnutrition [15]. Serum prealbumin levels can also be considered when nutritional competence is borderline. Prealbumin levels are thought to be a better measure when determining the effects of nutritional supplementation due to its short half-life. Normal prealbumin levels range from 6 to 35 mg/dL [16]. The TLC is calculated by multiplying the white blood cell count by the percent of lymphocytes in the differential. When these values are suboptimal, consultation with a nutritionist is helpful to assist with optimizing the patient before definitive amputation. Surgery in stabilized patients with malnutrition or immunodeficiency should be delayed until these issues can adequately be addressed. When infection or gangrene dictates urgent surgery, the goal should be to eradicate infection and eliminate necrotic tissue to viable margins. An open amputation at the most distal viable level, followed by open wound care, should be performed until wound healing potential can be optimized [15, 17–19]. Patients with severe renal disease may never achieve desirable nutritional parameters. Distal salvage attempts may still be pursued, but at known higher risk for failure.

Poor glycemic control has been identified as a risk factor associated with a higher frequency of amputation [20, 21]. Hyperglycemia will deactivate macrophages and lymphocytes and may impair wound healing. There is also a higher risk of urinary tract and respiratory infections when glucose levels are uncontrolled. Ideal management involves maintenance of glucose levels below 200 mg/dL [22]. Caution must be taken in managing the perioperative patient's glucose with calorie reduction. This may lead to significant protein depletion and subsequent wound failure. If the patient's BMI is normal, 25 cal/kg is required to maintain adequate nutrition and avoid negative nitrogen balance.

The combined wound healing parameters of vascular inflow and nutritional status have been shown to significantly affect healing rates for pedal amputations. Optimizing the patient's nutritional parameters and achieving adequate perfusion will limit the risk of wound complications and failure.

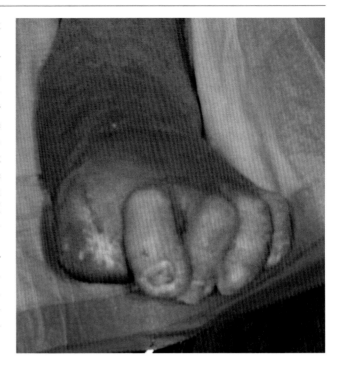

Fig. 52.1 Claw toe formation after great toe amputation

Anesthetic Considerations

Many of the patients that require surgical care for amputation have significant cardiovascular disease. Recurrent anesthetic exposures may be detrimental to such patients. All pedal amputations can be performed under local anesthesia with monitored care (MAC) or under a regional block with sedation. Regional blocks can be quite successful with sedation and provide a comfortable option for the patient. Care must be taken to assure that anesthesia is provided at the level of the tourniquet. Tourniquets at the ankle, calf, and thigh may be used, but care must be taken not to place these over areas of cellulitis/abscess or at a level of vascular repair. Elevation of the extremity for three minutes prior to tourniquet inflation is preferred to exsanguination of the infected extremity as compression of the soft tissues from distal to proximal may spread infection. Spinal anesthetics are contraindicated in the septic patient due to the risk of seeding the spinal fluid during the procedure.

Mechanical Considerations

Peripheral neuropathy affects many of the diabetics who require peripheral amputation [22]. Significant motor imbalance with overpowering of the posterior leg compartment is not uncommon. Neuropathy can lead to nonfunctional intrinsic muscles within the foot as well as a weakened anterior motor compartment of the lower limb. This imbalance can lead to significant contractures postamputation

(Fig. 52.1). The potential for imbalance at each of the amputation levels will be addressed through discussion of these amputation levels.

Internal Amputation/Arthroplasty of the Forefoot

Occasionally, forefoot infection may be well localized to an immediate infected area of ulceration. Soft tissue infection may be controlled with antibiotic therapy, and there is no ascending cellulitis or lymphangitis. There is minimal soft tissue necrosis in the area. This site may or may not be associated with a significant bony prominence. Additionally, the patient has no systemic signs of infection. Such findings are often present and associated with focal osteomyelitis at a metatarsal head or phalanx. Local resection of that metatarsal head or portion of the phalanx may be performed [23]. The microbiologic specimen and pathologic specimen are taken and sent for assessment. Depending on the resection of the bone, this procedure may be curative or may require a longer course of antibiotics. The wound may be closed or may be packed open and treated much like an ulceration leading to closure of the wound with wound care. This internal amputation of the bone may allow for preservation of the soft tissues and lead to a stable digit over time [24]. Digital surgery, such as this, functions much like hammertoe surgery and may lead to a long-term cure for local infection

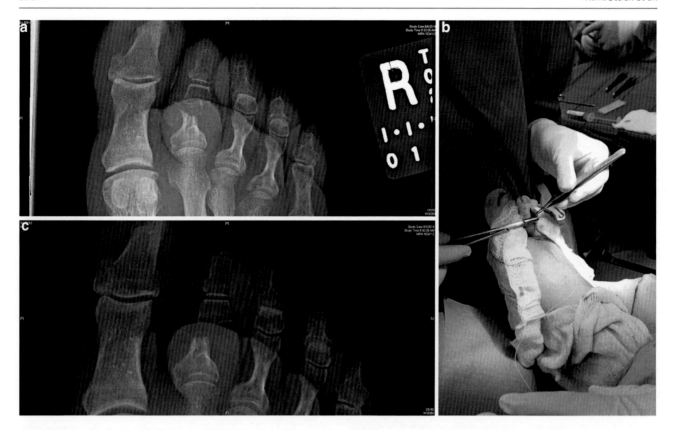

Fig. 52.2 (**a**) Osteomyelitis of the second IPJ after oral abx therapy for ulcer at PIPJ dorsally, (**b**) resection of the PIPJ, and (**c**) resolution of osteomyelitis after 6 weeks of culture-driven antibiotic therapy. The toe remains closed after 6 months

(Fig. 52.2). Metatarsal head resections function much like a ray amputation. Transfer ulceration to an adjacent metatarsal head is possible. Prevention may be possible with prescription footwear, accommodative insoles, and frequent clinical follow-up. When ulceration persists, pan metatarsal head resection [25, 26] and/or posterior compartment lengthening such as an Achilles lengthening or gastrocnemius recession may be needed.

Toe Amputations

Sizer and Wheelock [27] described toe amputations and their healing outcomes. They reviewed 692 toe amputations. When pulses were palpable, nearly 98 % healed; but, if pulses were not palpable, the failure rate was 11 %. Attempts to predict toe amputation healing with vascular studies have not been fully successful.

The anatomy of the toe limits amputation to either proximal or distal levels. The wing and sling mechanism allows flexion of the toes at the distal interphalangeal joint (DIPJ) and toe extension occurs through a lifting mechanism at the base of the proximal phalanx. Excision of a portion of the distal phalanx may allow for a stable digit with good motor

balance. Resection through the PIPJ in the neuropathic patient may, however, result in extension deformity of the toe. Extension can lead to irritation of the residual toe from footwear with the possibility of new ulceration. The unsalvageable toe is best resected through its base or disarticulation at the metatarsal phalangeal joint (MPJ). Preservation of the MPJ maintains the plantar plate and joint intrinsic muscle capsule attachments and may limit proximal retraction of the plantar fat pad of the forefoot. Whether or not this absolutely reduces the risk of ulceration at the metatarsal heads has yet to be determined. If the toe is disarticulated at the MPJ, and the wound is to be left open for drainage, the cartilage of the metatarsal head is resected to allow granulation over the residual metatarsal [28]. This resection is not absolutely necessary if wound closure is performed. Due to the cartilage avascularity, the authors will typically resect the cartilage.

Incisions for toe amputations create flaps dorsal to plantar or medial to lateral. Plantar flaps have more durable skin and are preferred when healthy tissue is available. Side-to-side flaps are of value if proximal incision is necessary over the foot dorsally or plantarly to allow drainage of infection. Hallux amputation has the most elevated risk of complications with new ulcers developing at adjacent metatarsal heads as well as increased hammertoe formation on the residual foot.

Fig. 52.3 Postoperative appearance of toe amputation terminal Syme procedure. (**a**) dorsal view of great toe after distal tuft amputation, (**b**) plantar view of great toe after tuft amputation plantar flap utilized here

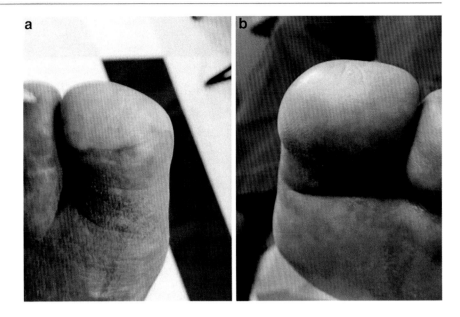

Terminal Syme Toe Amputation

Nail bed and distal tip ulceration from osteomyelitis or gangrene may occasionally be managed with bone biopsy and culture-driven antibiotic therapy [29]. When this is not feasible, amputation is needed (Fig. 52.3).

Authors' Preferred Method

A plantar flap is used when possible. A transverse incision is created just behind the toenail. A distal arm of the incision is placed on the medial and lateral margins of the toenail along the sides of the toe. This incision meets over the distal tuft of the toe. The encompassed portions of the distal phalanx, nail, and associated nail bed are excised. After irrigation, the plantar flap is sewn to the dorsal margin with nonabsorbable suture. A nonadherent dressing is applied and postoperative ambulation, when permitted, is in a surgical shoe. Complications include wound dehiscence/necrosis and infection.

Toe Amputation: Authors' Preferred Method

A fish-mouth or flapped incision is placed at the base of the toe (Figs. 52.4 and 52.5). The incision should be of full thickness to the bone. The soft tissues are reflected from the proximal phalanx at a periosteal level. Once the flair of the base of the phalanx is identified, a power saw or bone-cutting forceps is used to transect the bone. A rasp or rongeur may be used to smooth the cut end of the bone. After irrigation,

the skin is closed with a nonabsorbable suture. Alternatively, the toe may be disarticulated at the base of the MPJ and closure, when possible, is the same.

A nonadherent dressing is used to support the wound. Ambulation, when allowed, is in a surgical shoe.

Wound complications after toe amputation include dehiscence, soft tissue necrosis, and infection [30]. These complications, depending on severity, may require further surgical care or local wound care and antibiotic therapy. If revision is necessary and no other impairments are identified, a ray amputation or midfoot amputation may be necessary. Mechanical complications can develop with time. Contracture of adjacent digits, dislocation or transverse plane deformity of residual toes, as well as new plantar foot ulcers may develop.

Ray Amputation

A toe and metatarsal amputation may be utilized as a definitive amputation procedure or as an incision and drainage for management of infection. Isolated ray amputations have an elevated risk of new ulceration developing at an adjacent metatarsal head [28]. The risk of re-ulceration at an adjacent metatarsal is higher with the first ray than with lateral ray resections [31].

Authors' Preferred Method for Ray Amputation

Although the first and fifth rays have better soft tissue mobility for wound closure, a similar approach is taken for most ray amputations. A medial-to-lateral fish-mouth or wedge resection

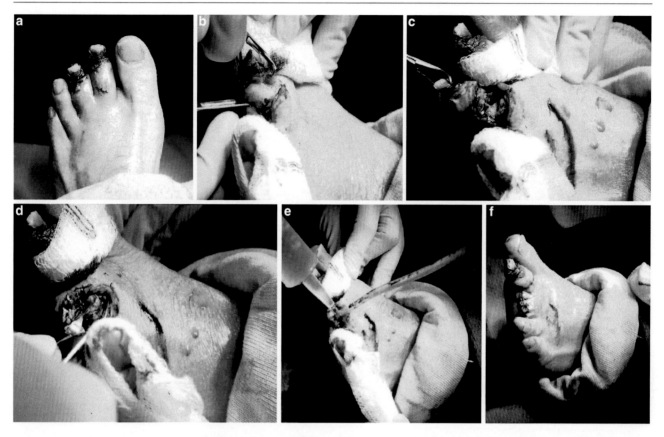

Fig. 52.4 Toe amputation surgery. (**a**) gangrene limited to digit, (**b**) dorsal-to-plantar flaps created full thickness, (**c**) the toe is disarticulated at the PIPJ, (**d**) the head of the proximal phalanx is resected, (**e**) the wound is irrigated, and (**f**) the wound is closed with nonabsorbable suture

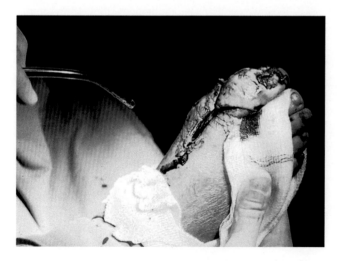

Fig. 52.5 A medial-to-lateral flap created for a great toe amputation

of the toe and metatarsal head is performed in a full-thickness fashion (Fig. 52.6). Typically, the metatarsal is transected at a level of healthy tissue and the metatarsal is not excised in total. The cut end of the metatarsal is beveled plantarly to avoid irritation of the plantar soft tissues. All bone edges are rasped smooth and cultures are obtained followed by irrigation.

Adjacent metatarsal phalangeal joints are inspected for infection and debrided/resected as indicated. Tendons are gently retracted and sectioned at the level of the wound. The wound may be closed when there is no deep soft tissue infection. If there is gross contamination, these wounds are best treated with open wound care for a minimum of 3–5 days. Initial dressing changes are performed at 24–48 h. When significant drainage is expected, earlier dressing changes and wound care may be necessary to limit the risk of wound maceration. Once soft tissue infection is controlled, ambulation may be allowed in a surgical shoe or walking boot.

Early wound complications are managed with wound care and debridement as well as antibiotic therapy or revision amputation. Most of the ray resection complications occur, however, after the patient has healed and returned to weight bearing. The patient's new weight-bearing pattern may result in transfer pressure at adjacent metatarsal heads leading to development of a plantar hyperkeratotic lesion. These lesions require pressure reduction and paring to limit their risk of progression ulceration. This pressure reduction can be managed through footwear and insoles. More severe cases may require Achilles tendon lengthening or gastrocnemius recession to aid in pressure reduction (Fig. 52.7).

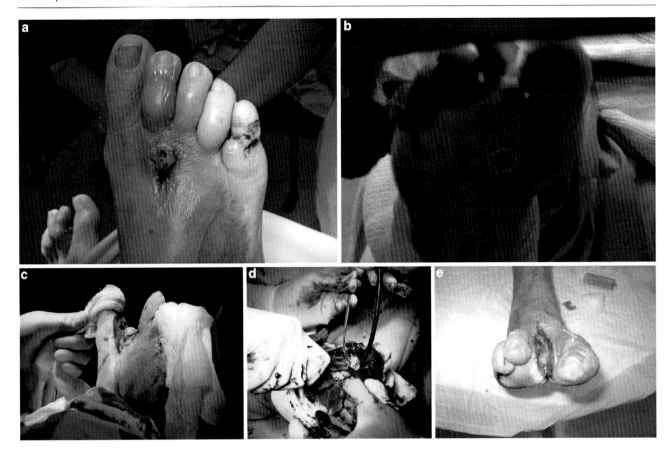

Fig. 52.6 Patient with chronic osteomyelitis requiring second ray amputation. (**a**) Dorsal sinus tract to second MPJ, (**b**) nonhealing plantar foot ulceration, (**c**) dorsal-to-plantar wedge resection of the toe and soft tissue at the MPJ level, (**d**) resection of the metatarsal with a bone-cutting forceps, (**e**) note healing and granulation at 2 weeks' post-op. Consideration might be given to a delayed primary closure of this wound once infection is completely resolved

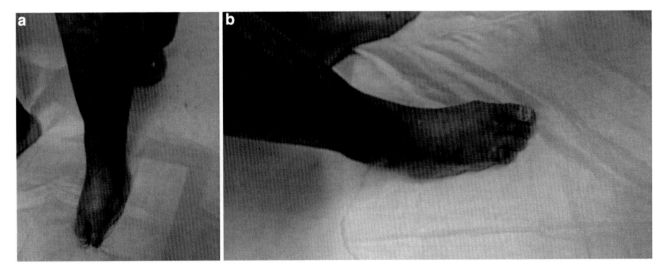

Fig. 52.7 Patient with multiple toe and metatarsal amputations bilateral has required Achilles lengthening and midfoot osteotomy to maintain function without ulcerating. He has prescription footwear but rarely uses them. He has remained ulcer-free for 3 years. (**a**) dorsal view of left foot and (**b**) dorsal view of right foot

Pan metatarsal head resection to remove the remaining metatarsal heads may be of value to aid in load redistribution of the forefoot.

Transmetatarsal Amputation

McKittrick popularized the transmetatarsal amputation in 1949 as an alternative to leg amputation [32]. He developed three basic indications for this amputation:

1. Gangrene of one or more toes with minimal extension onto the foot
2. Stabilized infection or open forefoot wound of the foot
3. Recurrent ulcerations in a neuropathic forefoot

When a patient is healed at this amputation level, the patient is able to ambulate without a prosthesis or brace. An accommodative insole with forefoot filler is valuable to limit the risk of re-ulceration of the foot [33].

Authors' Preferred Method

Bony landmarks for the first and fifth metatarsal heads and bases are marked and noted. The desired level of bone resection is identified as well. Incisional lines are then drawn extending distally along the first and fifth metatarsal shafts to the base of the great and fifth toe and then curved across the plantar skin in the sulcus area. The dorsal section is curved across the dorsal metatarsal shafts. This creates a shorter dorsal and longer plantar flap. The scalpel is held perpendicular to the skin and the incisions are made full thickness on the dorsal aspect of the foot and this is extended transversely across the foot and back to the base of the predetermined level on the fifth metatarsal. The incision is deepened to the level of the metatarsals and a dorsal flap is created. Vessels are identified and ligated or coagulated. A key elevator, osteotome, or new scalpel is used to reflect the soft tissues and periosteum from the dorsal aspect of the metatarsal on the flap so that the flap is reflected proximally. The plantar incision is then carried distally toward the base of the toes and across the sulcus area developing a full-thickness myocutaneous flap. A power saw is then utilized to transect the metatarsals at the predetermined level creating a bony parabola from medial-to-lateral as well as a dorsal-distal to plantar-proximal angulation of approximately 15° from the weight-bearing surface. The distal portions of the metatarsals at the osteotomy site are then elevated dorsally through the osteotomy site. A mayo scissor, key elevator, or knife is used to transect the soft tissue attachments on the inferior side of the metatarsals. This is followed distally to the level of the plantar incision and the forefoot is removed from the wound.

The flaps are inspected and debrided of any further diseased tissue. Flexor tendons and extensor tendons are grasped and excised under minimal tension. The flaps are trimmed of redundant skin and the wound is closed in a layered fashion. Consideration may be given to releasing or deflating the tourniquet prior to wound closure to allow for ligation or coagulation of transected vessels. A drain may be utilized as well if dead space is noted. Should the patient have identified equinus, a Hoke triple hemisection [34]. Achilles lengthening or a gastrocnemius recession should be performed. Care is taken to close the amputation wound and use clean surgical instruments for the posterior lengthening procedure.

A nonadherent dressing is applied in layers and a posterior splint is applied. Drains, when used, are removed within the first 48 h. Sutures are removed after 14–21 days, and the patient is maintained in a short leg cast for 4–6 weeks. Accommodative footwear is prescribed for ambulation.

Sanders described a modification of the plantar incision to accommodate for ulcer excision or prior ray amputation. A V-shaped excision of the wound or ulcer site is performed allowing a T-type closure of the plantar flap. This allows primary repair/closure of the midfoot wound in one procedure [35] (Fig. 52.8).

Lisfranc Amputation

The Lisfranc amputation is dynamically less stable than the transmetatarsal amputation as the insertion of the peroneus longus and brevis tendons is released. Equinus and varus are complications of the surgery. Short-term complications include wound dehiscence and recurrent infection. The long-term complications of midfoot amputations include a 25 % risk of distal lateral stump ulceration and equinovarus [36]. These complications may be treated with further posterior Achilles lengthening and/or tibialis anterior transfer to the central portion of the dorsal midfoot to diminish the amount of varus moment on the residual foot.

Authors' Preferred Technique

Similar flaps are created as with the transmetatarsal amputation. The tarsal metatarsal joint is disarticulated at the first metatarsal. A power saw is utilized from medial to lateral transecting the base of the second metatarsal leaving this intact. The third and fourth metatarsal tarsal joints are disarticulated, and a portion of the fifth metatarsal base is left in place as well and transected with a power saw. When this is possible, this maintains the peroneal tendon attachments that help limit varus foot contracture. Closure is performed in a manner similar to that in the transmetatarsal amputation.

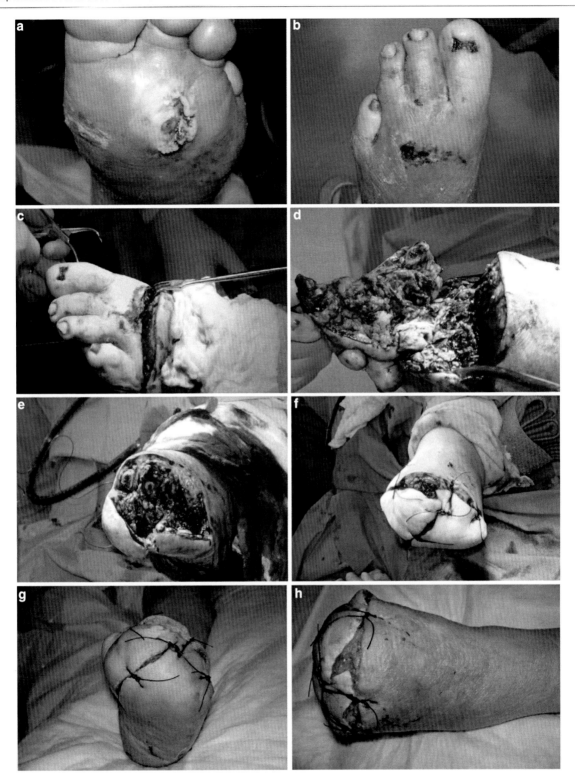

Fig. 52.8 (**a** and **b**) Plantar ulceration with forefoot osteomyelitis with plan for midfoot amputation; (**c**) dorsal foot incision for exposure of dorsal metatarsal shafts; (**d**) after metatarsal osteotomy, the plantar soft tissues are released from the inferior margin of the metatarsal shafts proximal to distal to the level of the distal plantar flap incision; (**e** and **f**) the flaps is trimmed to allow closure using Sander's technique; (**g** and **h**) the plantar flap is healing well at 10 days postoperatively—the closure was loose due to concerns for infection and tension on the wound margins

A posterior lengthening with a gastrocnemius recession or Achilles lengthening is typically performed with this procedure as well due to the motor imbalance created by the surgery.

Chopart Amputation

Chopart amputation is a disarticulation of the talonavicular and calcaneal cuboid joints. This level of amputation is valuable for resolution of significant forefoot infection and soft tissue loss prior to definitive ankle disarticulation amputation or transtibial amputation. Occasionally, patients are amputated at this level when they are severely ill with sepsis, and a guillotine amputation is performed at this level. After surgery, they granulate and contract this wound during their medical recovery. Cartilage may be debrided from the calcaneus and talus to help foster this granulation. A percutaneous Achilles release will help manage the equinus. Such a limb may tolerate low levels of ambulation and transferring for the patient, but the risk of equinus and stump ulceration is high.

This level may function much like a midfoot amputation if muscle balancing at the amputation can be restored. As the amputation leaves only the attachment of the Achilles tendon intact on the residual foot, motor rebalancing of the foot is important. Bowker [37] and Marquardt [38] have made recommendations to help maintain motor balance and limit the equinus development long associated with this amputation level. A 2-cm section of the Achilles tendon is resected from the Achilles from a separate incision. During the procedure, vertical slots are created in the talar head for the tibialis anterior tendon and the extensor hallucis longus tendon. A vertical slot is created in the anterior calcaneus for the extensor digitorum longus tendon. The plantar margin of the calcaneus is rongeured smooth, and then each of the tendons is anchored to the plantar capsule or fascia stabilizing the respective tendons in the grooves.

Some authors have recommended arthrodesis of the subtalar and ankle joints to improve hindfoot stability and prevent equinus. This recommendation must be weighed with the expectation of successful arthrodesis and additional incisions in an already compromised patient.

Authors' Preferred Method

Attention is directed first to the posterior ankle. This is maintained clean from the foot wound. A longitudinal incision is placed along the Achilles tendon and deepened to the tendon sheath. The sheath is opened and a 2-cm portion of tendon is resected. The sheath is closed, as is the overlying skin. A dressing is placed at this site and attention is directed to the foot.

A plantar flap is planned with a small amount of fish-mouth-like creation at the level of the talonavicular (TN) and calcaneal cuboid (CC) joints. The dorsal incision is made to the level of the extensor tendons. These tendons are protected and sectioned 1 to 2 cm distal to the incision to maintain length. The TN and CC joints are disarticulated, and a scalpel or mayo scissor is used to release the plantar soft tissues from the distal tarsal metatarsal structures removing the infected or dysvascular forefoot. The flaps are inspected for any nonviable tissue and this is resected if needed. The wound is irrigated and then the plantar margin of the calcaneus is rongeured smooth. Vertical slots are cut or rongeured with two placed in the talar neck and one in the calcaneus. The tibialis anterior, extensor hallucis longus, and extensor digitorum longus are placed into these slots from medial to lateral, respectively. The tendons are anchored with suture to the plantar capsule or fascia. The ankle will now be positioned at neutral or in some dorsiflexion. The plantar flap is then closed. The wound is dressed and the patient is placed in a splint or cast to maintain this position. The first dressing change is typically at 5 days. The casting is maintained for 6 weeks (Fig. 52.9).

The patient will require an AFO with forefoot filler for ambulation. Occasionally, a prosthesis is required for stability.

Syme's Ankle Disarticulation Amputation

Syme's amputation was first described by Syme in 1843 and is considered a partial foot amputation. The load-bearing surface of the Syme's is physiologic through the distal tibia and the heel pad, which is meant to bear direct load. Because the calcaneus and talus have been excised, there is sufficient space created beneath the residual limb for a prosthetic foot that aids in propulsive ambulation. Boyd and Pirogoff amputations [39] have been promoted as an alternative to the Syme's amputation; however, these amputations rely on satisfactory fusion of a portion of calcaneus to the tibia followed by AFO use leading to a less propulsive gait. The amputation used to be performed in two stages: The first procedure disarticulated the ankle and secured the heel pad. The second stage removed the medial and lateral dog-ears of the ankle with resection of the malleoli, too. This procedure is now typically accomplished in one stage.

Several reviews of Syme's procedure have shown its durability. In a review by Pinzur et al. [40], 88% of Syme's amputees healed if their ABI was greater than 0.5 or TCPO2 was greater the 20 mmHg, and their serum albumin was 2.5 gm/dL or better. Smokers healed the amputation as well as nonsmokers but had three times the infection rate. Approximately 30% of the patients were dead at 57.1 months. All but two became prosthetic users.

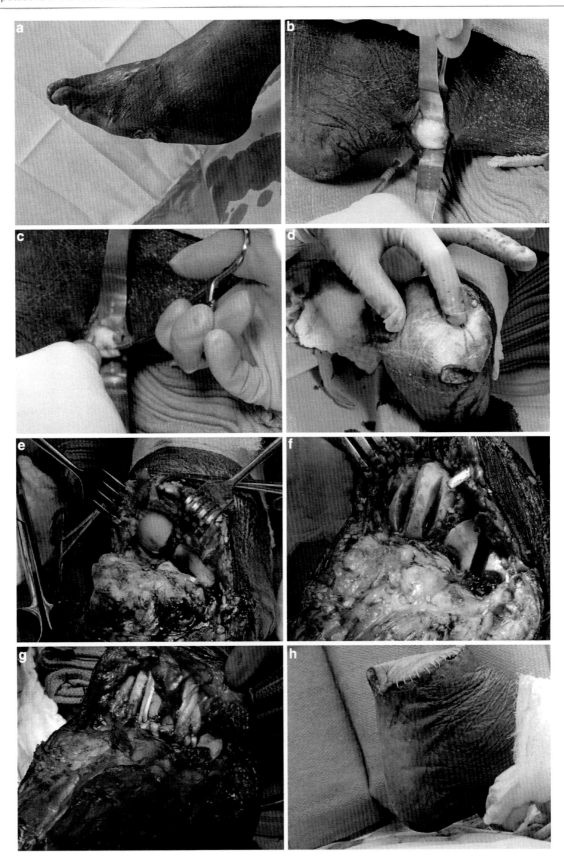

Fig. 52.9 Chopart amputation: (**a**) Multiple sites of gangrene and forefoot osteomyelitis; (**b** and **c**) Achilles wedge resection; (**d**) resection of forefoot and creation of plantar flap to cover the amputation site; (**e, f** and **g**) cuboid and talar head are identified and vertical slots are placed in the talar head and the cuboid for placement of tendons as described; and (**h**) the flap is closed and good position is noted

Authors' Preferred Method

Once sufficient anesthesia has been achieved, the lower leg and residual foot are prepared and draped aseptically. An anterior incision is made at the level of the ankle mortise from the anterior aspect of the medial malleolus to the anterior aspect of the fibula. This incision is deepened to the ankle mortise and the anterior tibial artery and associated veins are tied with absorbable suture. A medial incision is then extended plantarly. The lateral incision is extended plantarly as well in a stirrup fashion around the anterior heel pad to the level of the calcaneus. A bone hook is placed in the talar dome and distal distraction is applied. The collateral ligaments in the ankle are released on either side of the talus allowing anterior dislocation of the talus within the ankle mortise.

The soft tissues are released along the calcaneus and the soft tissue attachments of the posterior heel are visualized. Care is taken to release soft tissue from the posterior calcaneus to limit the chance of "buttonholing" through the posterior calcaneal skin. The remainder of the calcaneus is released and the foot is removed from the operative field. Soft tissues are released from the medial and lateral malleoli, while care is taken to protect the posterior medial soft tissues as the tibial artery resides in this area. The medial and lateral malleoli are then transected with a power saw, and the flares are rongeured and rasped smooth. The cartilage of the distal tibia is left intact centrally, and the posterior and anterior margins may be rongeured or rasped smooth. The wound is thoroughly irrigated. The Achilles may be attached to the posterior tibia with large absorbable suture through drill holes. At the anterior margin, the plantar fascia is sewn into the anterior ankle joint capsule with large absorbable suture as well. This provides secure attachment for the heel pad. A medium suction drain is placed from this wound and exits proximal anterior-laterally. Subcutaneous closure is performed with 2-0 absorbable suture and the skin closed with 3-0 nylon sutures or staples (Fig. 52.10).

The patient is placed in a soft dressing and a posterior splint or short leg cast. The drain is pulled within 24–48 h and antibiotics are discontinued after 24 h. With a stable surgical wound, the patient may be placed in a fiberglass cast with a walking heel after 3 weeks. At 6 weeks a fiberglass cast with a medial window, which is closed with loop and pile strapping, may be utilized. The soft tissue size of the lower level stabilizes after 12 weeks and the patient is fitted for a prosthesis (Fig. 52.11).

Calcanectomy

Partial or total calcanectomy has been utilized to aid closure of recalcitrant heel ulcerations [41–44]. This is done either through a straight longitudinal incision or with a hurricane-shaped incision as described by Fisher [45]. This incision has proximal and distal arms that take the shape of the meteorological symbol for hurricanes.

The author's outcome experience with total calcanectomy has been poor but partial calcanectomy has been quite valuable for limb salvage. Once healed, the patient may be able to return to inlay depth shoes or high-top shoes. Occasionally, an AFO may be required with a heel filler.

Authors' Preferred Technique

The patient is placed either prone or in a lateral decubitus position. A longitudinal incision is made to the bone posteriorly. Subperiosteal dissection of the medial and lateral calcaneus is performed until adequate soft tissue envelope exists for closure. A power saw or osteotomy is utilized to resect the posterior calcaneus with a bevel from dorsal proximal to plantar distal. Bone cultures are taken as indicated. After irrigation, consideration may be given to posterior reattachment of the Achilles tendon if the site is free of infection. Closure of the skin is performed with 3-0 nylon or staples. A drain may be valuable due to the vascularity of the calcaneus. The drain is removed within 48 h. The patient is placed in a posterior splint followed by casting for 3–6 weeks (Fig. 52.12).

Wounds that cannot be completely closed may be treated with open wound care or negative pressure applications to closure. Footwear is prescribed as needed and described earlier.

Long-Term Care

Once the residual limb has healed, the patient will need long-term foot care. Chronic care and foot assessments are associated with improved preservation of limbs. At the time of follow-up, the patients are evaluated for nail and skin pathologies as well as the need for prescription footwear, bracing, and prosthetic needs. Long-term care is essential to educate patients and their caregivers as well as provide early identity of any risk factors or early warnings for pathology of the feet [46, 47].

Summary

Pedal amputation, whether it is a digit or ankle disarticulation, permanently changes the patient's perspective on ambulation and mandates that the patient have close follow-up for foot care and prescription footwear. Prevention of reamputation is only possible through a cooperative effort of the medical care team, the patient, and the patient's caregiver.

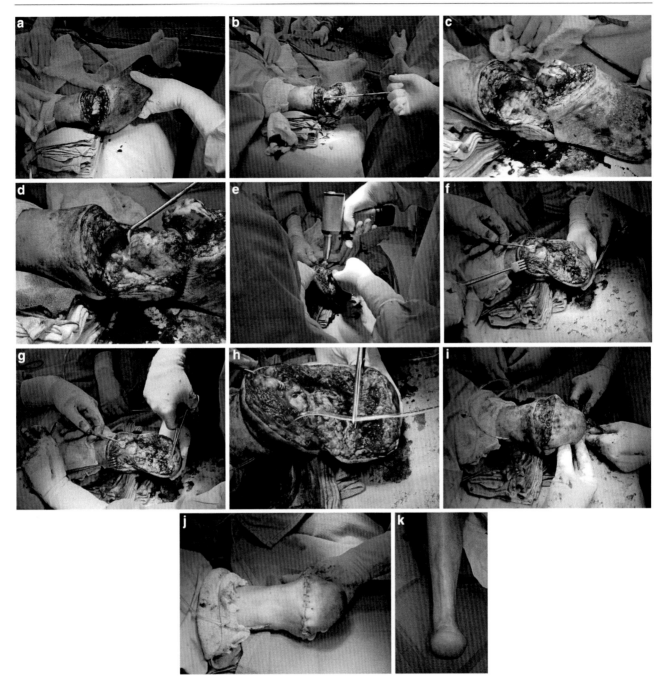

Fig. 52.10 Syme's ankle disarticulation process (**a**) An anterior ankle incision is placed just to the side of each malleolus at the joint level; (**b**, **c** and **d**) a bone hook is used to distract the talus distally while the collateral ankle ligaments and soft tissue are released from the calcaneus allowing removal of the calcaneus from the wound; (**e**) the malleoli are resected at the joint level with a power saw while the anterior and posterior tibial margins are rongeured smooth; (**f** and **g**) drill holes are placed along the posterior tibia and the Achilles is sutured into the posterior tibia; (**h** and **i**) the drain is placed and deep closure with absorbable suture is performed; (**j**) wound closure; and (**k**) eight weeks postamputation

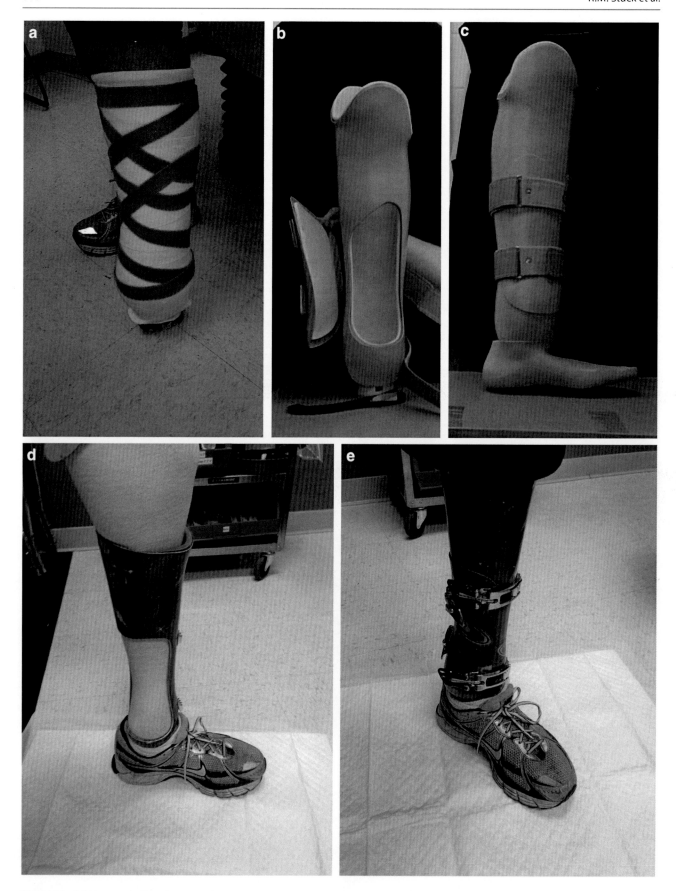

Fig. 52.11 (**a**) Temporary fiberglass cast with rubber bumper for ambulation when wound is stable; (**b**) Canadian Syme's prosthesis with medial window that is open; (**c**) prosthesis with cosmetic foot and window closure; (**d** and **e**) custom prosthesis with fabric laminated cover

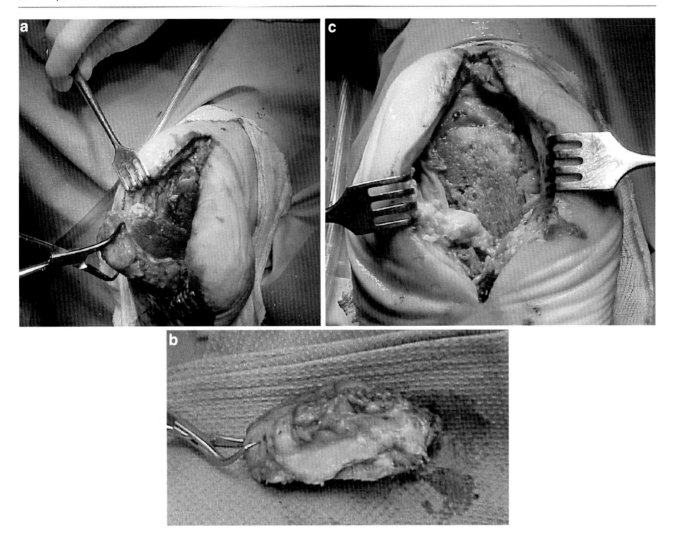

Fig. 52.12 (**a**) The vertical incision is placed at the posterior heel and incised to the level of the calcaneus. The soft tissues are reflected medial and lateral on the calcaneus; (**b**) the calcaneus is resected with an osteotome and the remaining bone is smoothed; (**c**) the sufficient bone is resected to allow closure of the posterior heel without tension

References

1. Osterman H. The process of amputation and rehabilitation. Clin Podiatr Med Surg. 1997;14(4):585–97.
2. Pinzur M, Gold J, Schwartz D, et al. Energy demands for walking in dysvascular amputees as related to level of amputation. Orthopedics. 1992;15:9.
3. Fisher SV, Gullickson G. Energy cost of amputation in health and disability: a literature review. Arch Phys Med Rehabil. 1978; 59:124–33.
4. Pinzur MS, Gold J, Schwartz D, et al. Energy demands for walking in dysvascular amputees related to the level of amputation. Orthopaedics. 1992;15:1033–7.
5. Atway S, Nerone VS, Springer KD, Woodruff DM. Rate of residual osteomyelitis after partial foot amputation in diabetic patients: a standardized method for evaluating bone margins with intraoperative culture. J Foot Ankle Surg. 2012;51(6):749–52.
6. Wagner F. Transcutaneous Doppler ultrasound in the prediction of healing and the selection of surgical level for dysvascular lesions of the toes and forefoot. Clin Orthop. 1979;142:110–4.
7. Pinzur MS, Sage R, Stuck R, et al. Transcutaneous oxygen as a predictor of wound healing in amputations of the foot and ankle. Foot Ankle. 1992;13:271–2.
8. Adera HM, James K, Castonuovo JJ. Prediction of amputation wound healing with skin perfusion pressure. J Vasc Surg. 1995;21:823–9.
9. Ameli FM, Byrne P, Provan JL. Selection of amputation level and prediction of healing using transcutaneous tissue oxygen tension (TcPo2). J Cardiovasc Surg. 1989;30:220–4.
10. Bacharach JM, Rooke TW, Osmundson PJ, et al. Predictive value of transcutaneous oxygen pressure and amputation success by use of supine and elevation measurements. J Vasc Surg. 1992;15:558–63.
11. Lo T, Sample R, Moore P, et al. Prediction of wound healing outcome using skin perfusion pressure and transcutaneous oximetry: a single-center experience in 100 patients. Wounds. 2009;21(11): 310–6.

12. Pahlsson HI, Wahlberg E, Olofsson P, Swedenborg J. The toe pole test for evaluation of arterial insufficiency in diabetic patients. Eur J Endovasc Surg. 1999;18:133–7.

13. Carter SA, Tate RB. The value of toe pulse waves in determination of risks for limb amputation and death in patients with peripheral arterial disease and skin ulcers or gangrene. J Vasc Surg. 2001;33:708–14.

14. Misuri A, Lucertini G, Nanni A, et al. Predictive value of transcutaneous oximetry for selection of the amputation level. J Cardiovasc Surg. 2000;41(1):83–7.

15. Dickhaut SC, Delee JC, Page CP. Nutrition status: importance in predicting wound healing after amputation. J Bone Joint Surg Am. 1984;64:71–5.

16. Yu GV, Schinke TL, Mezaros A. Syme's amputation: a retrospective review of 10 cases. Clin Podiatr Med Surg N Am. 2005; 22:395–427.

17. Haydock DA, Hill GL. Improved wound healing response in surgical patients receiving intravenous nutrition. Br J Surg. 1987; 74:320–3.

18. Jensen JE, Jensen TG, Smith TK, et al. Nutrition in orthopaedic surgery. J Bone Joint Surg Am. 1982;64:1263–72.

19. Mowat AG, Baum J. Chemotaxis of polymorphonuclear leukocytes from patients with diabetes mellitus. N Engl J Med. 1971;248: 621–7.

20. Miyajima S, Shirai A, Yamamoto S, et al. Risk factors for major limb amputation in diabetic foot gangrene patients. Diabetes Res Clin Pract. 2006;71:272–9.

21. Imran S, Ali R, Mahboob G. Frequency of lower extremity amputation in diabetics with reference to glycemic control and wagner's grades. J Coll Physicians Surg. 2006;16(2):124–7.

22. Stuck RM, Sage R, Pinzur M, et al. Amputations in the diabetic foot. Clin Podiatr Med Surg. 1995;12:141–55.

23. Faglia E, Clerici G, Caminiti M, et al. Feasibility and effectiveness of internal pedal amputation of phalanx or metatarsal head in diabetic patients with forefoot osteomyelitis. J Foot Ankle Surg. 2012;51(5):593–8.

24. Rosenblum B, et al. Preventing loss of the great toe with the hallux interphalangeal joint arthoplasty. J Foot Surg. 1994;33:557.

25. Petrov O, et al. Recurrence of plantar ulceration following panmetatarsal head resection. J Foot Surg. 1996;35:573–7.

26. Jacobs R. Hoffman procedure in the ulcerated diabetic neuropathic foot. J Foot Surg. 1982;3:142–9.

27. Sizer J, Wheelock F. Digital amputations in diabetic patients. Surgery. 1972;72:980.

28. Gianfortune P, Pulla R, Sage R. Ray resection in the insensitive or dysvascular foot: a critical review. J Foot Surg. 1985;24:103–7.

29. Boffeli TJ, Abben KW, Hyllengren SB. In-office distal Symes lesser toe amputation: a safe, reliable and cost effective treatment of diabetesrelated tip of toe ulcers complicated by osteomyelitis. J Foot

Ankle Surg. 2014;53(6):720–6. doi:10.1053/j.jfas.2014.04.020. Epub 2014 Jul 22.

30. Chu YJ, Li XW, Wang PH, et al. Clinical outcomes of toe amputation in patients with type 2 diabetes in Tianjin. China Int Wound J. 2016;13(2):175–81. doi:10.1111/iwj.12249. Epub 2014 Mar 14.

31. Borkosky SL, Roukis TS. Incidence of re-amputation following partial first ray amputation associated with diabetes mellitus and peripheral sensory neuropathy: a systematic review. Diabet Foot Ankle. 2012; 3. doi:10.3402/dfa.v3i0.12169. Epub 2012 Jan 20.

32. McKittrick L, McKittick J, Risely T. Transmetatarsal amputation for infection of gangrene in patients with diabetes mellitus. Ann Surg. 1949;130:826.

33. Sanders LJ, Dunlap G. Transmetatarsal amputation: a successful approach to limb salvage. J Am Podiatr Med Assoc. 1992;82:129.

34. Hoke M. An operation for the correction of extremely relaxed foot. J Bone Joint Surg. 1931;13:773.

35. Sanders LJ. Amputations in the diabetic foot. Clin Podiatr Med Surg. 1987;4:481.

36. Pinzur M, Kaminsky M, Sage R, et al. Amputations at the middle level of the foot. J Bone Joint Surg. 1986;68A:1061–4.

37. Bowker JH. Partial foot amputations and disarticulations: surgical aspects. JPO. 2007;19(3S):62–76.

38. Marquardt E. Die Chopart-Exartikulation mit tenomyoplastik. Z Orthop. 1973;111:584–6.

39. Nather A, Wong KL, Lim AS, et al. The modified Pirogoff's amputation in treating diabetic foot infections: surgical technique and case series. Diabet Foot Ankle. 2014;3:5.

40. Pinzur MS, Stuck RM, Sage R, Hunt N, Rabinovich Z. Syme ankle disarticulation in patients with diabetes. J Bone Joint Surg Am. 2003;85(A9):1667–72.

41. Smith DG, Stuck RM, Ketner L, Sage RM, Pinzur MS. Partial calcanectomy for the treatment of a large ulceration of the heel and calcaneal osteomyelitis. An amputation of the back of the foot. J Bone Joint Surg Am. 1992;74(4):571–6.

42. Van Riet A, Harake R, Stuyck J. Partial calcanectomy: a procedure to cherish or to reject? Foot Ankle Surg. 2012;18(1):25–9.

43. Faglia E, Clerici G, Caminiti M, Vincenzo C, Cetta F. Heel ulcer and blood glow: the importance of the angiosome concept. Int J Low Extrem Wounds. 2013;12(3):226–30.

44. Schade VL. Partial or total calcanectomy as an alternative to below-the-knee amputation for limb salvage: a systematic review. J Am Podiatr Med Assoc. 2012;102(5):396–405.

45. Fisher TK, Armstrong DG. Partial calcanectomy in high-risk patients with diabetes: use and utility of a "hurricane" incisional approach. Eplasty. 2010;10:e17.

46. Sanders LJ. Diabetes mellitus: prevention of amputation. J Am Podiatr Assoc. 1994;84:322–8.

47. Robbins JM, Ober S, et al. Long-term aftercare and prevention of further amputation. Clin Podiatr Med Surg. 1997;14:4.

Major Amputation of the Lower Extremity for Critical Limb Ischemia

Ryan P. Ter Louw, Benjamin J. Brown, and Christopher E. Attinger

Introduction

Critical limb ischemia is a common problem in the US healthcare system with over 35,000 lower extremity amputations that occur each year. The prevalence of peripheral vascular disease has increased over the past 10 years. Thus, limb salvage has become a multidisciplinary approach with surgeons, hospitalists, physical therapists, prosthetists, and many others to optimize patient outcomes. The acuity of limb ischemia requires efficient communication between multiple teams to provide the appropriate care for each patient. When considering amputation, long-term function should be at the forefront of surgical planning.

Preoperative Evaluation

A thorough yet efficient history should be obtained upon presentation to the hospital, as "time is tissue" in limb ischemia. Special attention should be paid to known heart disease, diabetes, heart failure, end-stage renal disease, peripheral arterial disease, and any interventions related to such. Comorbidities should be acutely managed in a multidisciplinary approach to optimize surgical outcomes. Preoperative cardiac risk stratification is recommended for all patients with a known cardiac history who face amputation. In the diabetic patient, blood glucose management below 200 mg/dL has been shown to significantly decrease perioperative complications and surgical dehiscence rates [1]. Inherited or medication-induced coagulopathy should be noted and corrected.

A focused vascular exam should begin with palpation and Doppler evaluation of femoral, popliteal, anterior/posterior tibial, and peroneal arteries. Patients with a history of bypass should be evaluated for graft patency. Abdominal exam should focus on identification of abdominal aortic aneurysms and auscultation for bruits. Skin perfusion may also be assessed by temperature, as there is often a transition in an ischemic limb. The level where there is a clear demarcation between warm and cool tissue should be noted. If the patient complains of ischemic pain, the level at which the pain ceases should also be demarcated. Both temperature change and pain often coincide. The lack of hair on the distal limb may also suggest the chronicity of peripheral vascular disease.

The vascular surgeon plays a critical role in the decision for limb salvage versus amputation. A preoperative angiogram should be obtained to evaluate potential bypass targets and endovascular interventions. Even in renal transplant patients, good studies can be obtained with minimal dye (<10 cc of dye). Review of previous angiograms or Doppler exams is also helpful in noting acute change and progression of disease. The presence and caliber of diseased or collateral vessels are paramount in determining the level of amputation that is most likely to heal.

Limb ischemia is frequently accompanied by soft tissue infections and osteomyelitis. This particular subset of patients typically has a history of multiple hospitalizations and surgical interventions, increasing their likelihood of carrying multi-drug-resistant organisms. Thus, the antibiotic dosing and management in this patient population is complex and regimens should be culture directed. At the senior author's institution, infectious disease is routinely consulted to aid in preoperative and, perhaps more importantly, postoperative antibiotic management.

R.P. Ter Louw, MD
Department of Plastic Surgery, Medstar Georgetown University Hospital, Washington, DC 20007, USA

B.J. Brown, MD
Plastic Surgery, Gulf Coast Plastic Surgery, Pensacola, FL 32503, USA

C.E. Attinger, MD (✉)
Department of Plastic Surgery, Medstar Georgetown University Hospital, Washington, DC 20007, USA

© Springer International Publishing Switzerland 2017
R.S. Dieter et al. (eds.), *Critical Limb Ischemia*, DOI 10.1007/978-3-319-31991-9_53

Indications

Primary amputation in limb ischemia is neither the patient's nor the provider's preferred method of treatment. However, there are several clinical circumstances in which amputation should be strongly considered. The most important factor is to realistically assess the patient's ultimate functional goal as well as the quality of function the patient will enjoy with a salvaged versus amputated limb. For example, a patient who wants to be able to live at home and carry out the acts of daily living might be very satisfied with a partial mid-foot and hindfoot amputation, while a more active patient may elect a below-knee amputation to be able to do what he/she wants to do. The decision then to salvage or amputate depends upon the resources available to the provider. Centers equipped for vascular bypass as well as angiography, intraoperative angiography and intervention, pedicled and microsurgical flaps, and external fixation or suspension have far more tools at their disposal for attempt limb salvage procedures than centers that do not have some of these options.

Previous literature suggests decreased life expectancy after amputation secondary to restricted mobility and the relative increased cardiovascular demand with ambulation with a prosthesis. However, the mechanism of increased risk of cardiovascular events in amputees has not been well studied [2]. Salvage of a nonfunctional foot can lead to deconditioning because of limited ambulation and can be a constant drain both on the patient's physiologic and health-care resources. Pell et al. showed that quality of life in amputees is associated with mobility and function, rather than length of lower extremity [3]. After reviewing our outcomes of 294 below-knee amputations at a major limb salvage center, 78 % of patients were ambulatory postoperatively [4]. With proper surgical technique, intensive rehabilitation, and the advancement of prosthetic technology, amputees have very good functional outcomes and quality of life.

Indications for Amputation

- Significant soft tissue ischemia/loss without a bypass target and no possible endovascular intervention
- The inability to reconstruct a functional foot that has a low risk of recurrent breakdown
- Osteomyelitis refractory to debridement and antibiotics
- Stable or progressive dry gangrene whose removal leads to a nonfunctioning limb
- Ascending infection or signs of sepsis
- Patient's level of activity and functional preference

Technique

Surgical planning in the setting of acute limb ischemia should be directed in optimizing long-term patient function. The level of amputation is multifactorial and depends upon the soft tissue availability, blood flow, infection status, and rehabilitation options as well as the available resources of the reconstruction team. In this chapter, below-knee amputation (BKA), BKA using the ERTL technique, knee disarticulation (KD), and above-knee amputation (AKA) will be discussed.

Preoperative medical management is of equal importance to surgical technique. Diabetes, end-stage renal disease, coronary artery disease, coagulopathy, and chronic anemia are associated with increased surgical complications and should be optimized. Patients with ESRD should have their potassium level checked on the day of surgery and dialyzed appropriately. Beta-blockers should be taken the morning of surgery and perioperative antibiotics should be current and re-dosed as needed.

The level of anesthesia may vary based on the planned procedure. The senior author prefers epidural anesthesia that can be kept in postoperatively. If it is started up to 48 h before surgery, it may help improve postoperative pain control. In this comorbid patient population, every attempt should be made to lower the risk due to anesthesia. However, a recent study by Lin et al. compared the 30-day mortality of general anesthesia to regional blocks following below-knee amputation. Their review of 156 patients revealed no difference in 30-day mortality between general anesthesia or spinal anesthesia [5]. In our recent experience, local injection of EXPAREL, a 72 h liposomal bupivacaine (Pacira, Parsippany, New Jersey), at the operation of the definitive amputation, also appears to provide improved postoperative pain control and aids in the transition of intravenous narcotics to oral pain control regimens.

The senior author prefers that amputations performed in the setting of infection should be done in two stages. The initial drainage amputation if the foot is involved is an ankle disarticulation. If the ankle is involved, a guillotine amputation is planned above the infection. The completion amputation is then performed at least 2–3 days afterward with negative pressure therapy dressing covering the amputated stump in the interim. Two-stage below-knee amputation for ischemic and infectious causes has been shown to have decreased reoperation rates [6]. It allows for limited cross contamination from the wound as well as tissue demarcation if there is suspected progression of soft tissue ischemia. In two-stage operations where massive edema is present in the leg, a lymphedema wrap is applied to the residual limb post-drainage amputation to decrease the edema and make the tissue more pliable for the definitive amputation.

The advent of fluorescent angiography is an additional tool in determining the level of soft tissue viability in amputation. The SPY (Novadaq, Vancouver, Canada) system has been commercially used for the evaluation of mastectomy flap viability in the setting of breast reconstruction. We have also utilized this technology at our institution for cases in which lower extremity soft tissue viability is uncertain. Intraoperative injection of 3–5 mL of indocyanine green allows for real-time identification of vascularized cutaneous angiosomes. This technology is currently being investigated in the planning of both the design of incisions and the level of amputation.

It also critical that the patient meets with a prosthetist pre-operatively so that the patient fully understands what is about to occur. The prosthetist can give invaluable feedback to the surgeon so that the ideal residual limb can be designed. If possible, it is also very valuable if they can meet with another amputee who has gone through what the patient is about to experience. This pre-amputation consultation is invaluable not only in allaying the fears of the patient but also ensuring the most functional outcome.

Below-Knee Amputation

Bickel popularized the use of the superficial posterior compartment myocutaneous flap in 1943. Burgess later modified it by recommending that the deep posterior compartment be removed to limit unnecessary bulk in the posterior flap and limit the amount of remaining tissue that is dependent on presumably diseased posterior tibial and peroneal arteries [7]. Interestingly, in popliteal or trifurcation disease, the sural arteries that feed the gastrocnemius muscles are usually spared and provide the necessary blood flow to the posterior flap. This is reflected in our series of 294 flaps where the ratio of BKA to AKA was 4:1 with a 2 % eventual conversion rate from BKA to AKA. Our institution uses a superficial posterior compartment myocutaneous flap in which the superficial posterior compartment provides vascularized and durable coverage of the tibial osteotomy (Fig. 53.1). Tenodesis and myodesis of the superficial posterior compartment have several functions. Gastrocnemius muscles continue to function as knee flexors and thus maintain bulk and prevent atrophy. A second benefit of the PMF is preventing a suture line and future scar over the distal stump. A final benefit is that the musculature still functions as a venous pump preventing lower leg edema.

The componentry below the socket in the average below-knee prosthesis requires at least 8 inches clearance from the ground. In addition, preserving extra length is critical as it allows increased leverage and it provides additional tissue for an adequate revision BKA should it ever be required. After consulting with the prosthetist, the senior author plans each BKA with a tibial osteotomy at 15–18 cm from tibial tubercle if there is adequate distal soft tissue. Otherwise the amputation is done no shorter than 12 cm from the tibial tubercle. The leg is elevated and the thigh tourniquet is inflated provided there is no counter-indication (e.g., recent femoral popliteal bypass). Coban is used to isolate the distal drainage wound or foot to prevent contamination of the field and proximal clean tissue.

An anterior skin incision is drawn 1 cm longer than the planned tibial osteotomy site, encompassing two-third the circumference of the leg. Medially and laterally the skin incision is carried inferiorly with a slight anterior slant toward the ankle (Fig. 53.2). The dissection of the anterior compartment is performed with electrocautery. Special attention is paid to preserve the lateral compartment that may be used for myodesis later. The anterior tibial artery is identified and suture ligated. Both peroneal nerves and saphenous nerve are marked and saved for future injection with local anesthesia and divsion under traction.

The tibia is exposed and the planned osteotomy is verified at preplanned distance. An army-navy retractor is passed posterior to the tibia and the osteotomy is made perpendicular to the longitudinal axis of the tibia. The fibular osteotomy is approximately 1 cm shorter with a bevel slightly oriented from lateral to medial (Fig. 53.3).

After both osteotomies, a bone hook into the open end of distal tibia provides anterior retraction to expose the deep posterior compartment. A 10 blade is used to sharply dissect the deep posterior compartment off the distal tibia and fibula (Fig. 53.4). The distal leg is then cut at a distance that guarantees sufficient distance to fold the posterior flap anteriorly to close the remaining leg. After removing the distal leg, the deep posterior compartment is dissected off of the superficial compartment (Fig. 53.5) and removed with careful ligation of the peroneal and posterior tibial perforators to the superficial posterior department. The posterior tibial and peroneal arteries are tied off, and the deep peroneal nerve and posterior tibial nerves are preserved for later injection with anesthetic subsequent proximal division under traction.

The anterior half of the tibial cortex is then beveled for about 1 cm using a sagittal saw (Fig. 53.6). The bevel is then sanded down by brushing the sagittal saw over that area. Three holes are drilled into the anterior tibia from the anterior cortex into the medullary canal and will be used for future tenodesis (Fig. 53.7).

Irrigation is performed followed by changing of surgeon's outer gloves. New sterile drapes are placed and a clean table and set of instrumentation is used. Tourniquet is let down and hemostasis is obtained. Saphenous, tibial, and both peroneal

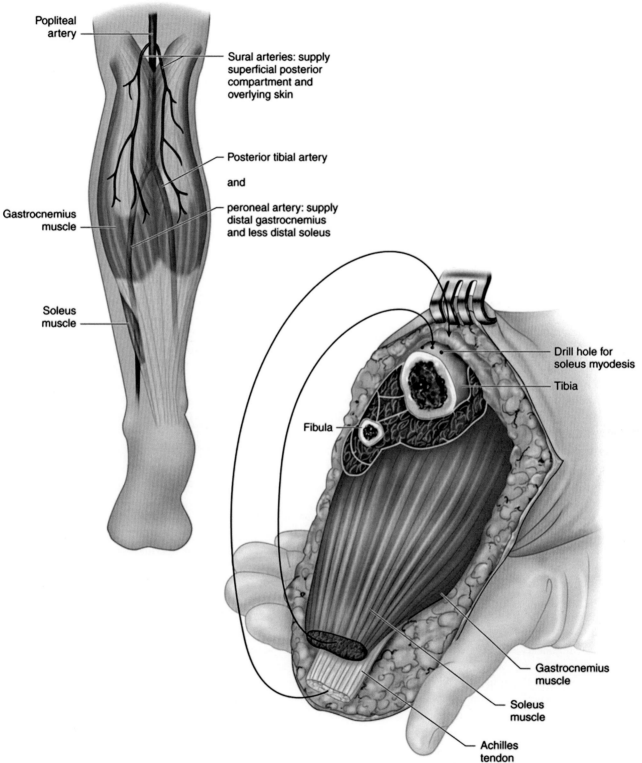

Myocutaneous flap blood supply

Popliteal artery

Sural arteries: supply superficial posterior compartment and overlying skin

Posterior tibial artery

and

peroneal artery: supply distal gastrocnemius and less distal soleus

Gastrocnemius muscle

Soleus muscle

Drill hole for soleus myodesis

Tibia

Fibula

Gastrocnemius muscle

Soleus muscle

Achilles tendon

Fig. 53.1 Posterior flap design for BKA: Note that the flap is dependent on the sural arteries that are usually spared in patients with vascular disease. This drawing does not show that the anterior portion of the tibia has to be beveled to prevent distal anterior bulk at the distal suture line. From Brown BJ, Iorio ML, Hill L, Carlisle B, Attinger CE. Below-knee amputation with a vascularized fibular graft and headless compression screw. Plast Reconstr Surg. 2013 Feb;131(2):323–7. Reprinted with permission from Wolters Kluwer Health, Inc

nerves are placed under traction, injected with a long-acting anesthetic and cut with number 10 blade, allowing them to retract into the proximal muscle groups. The posterior flap is then swung up to the level of the anterior portion of the tibia, and a semilunar line is drawn on the soleus muscle to mark that level (Fig. 53.8a). One or two JP drains are placed along the base of the flap. The soleus muscle is then incised along the drawn line with a number 10 blade down to Achilles tendon at a beveled angle (Fig. 53.8b) so that when the posterior flap is rotated forward, the distal soleus fascia tendinous can

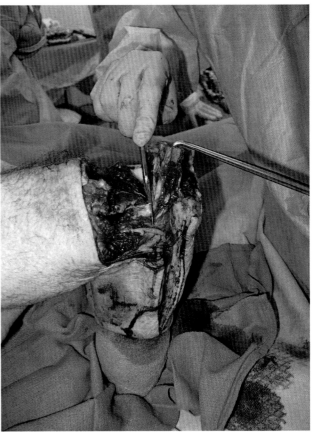

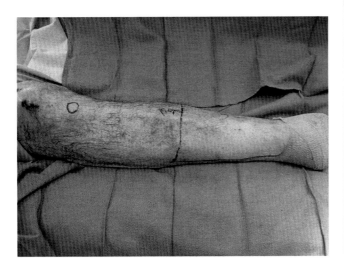

Fig. 53.2 An anterior skin incision is drawn 1 cm longer than the planned tibial osteotomy site, encompassing two-third the circumference of the leg. Medially and laterally the skin incision is carried inferiorly with a slight anterior slant toward the ankle

Fig. 53.4 After both osteotomies, a bone hook into the open end of distal tibia provides anterior retraction to expose the deep posterior compartment. A 10 blade is used to sharply dissect the deep posterior compartment off the distal tibia and fibula

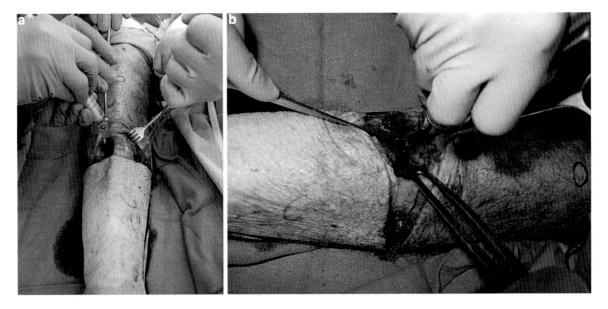

Fig. 53.3 Osteotomy of tibia (**a**) and fibula (**b**). The fibular cut is 1 cm shorter than the tibia and is done carefully not to damage the peroneal artery and nerves

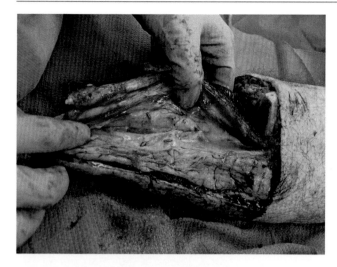

Fig. 53.5 The deep posterior compartment is dissected off of the superficial compartment tying off the posterior and peroneal perforators to the soleus muscle

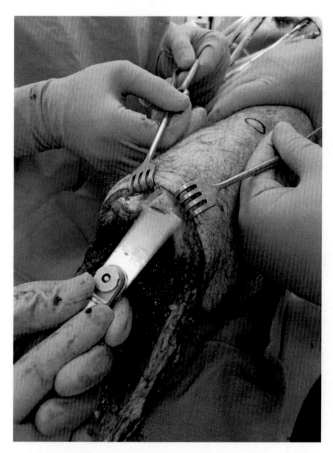

Fig. 53.6 The anterior half of the tibial cortex is then beveled for about 1 cm using a sagittal saw. The bevel is then sanded down by lightly brushing the sagittal saw over the cut area

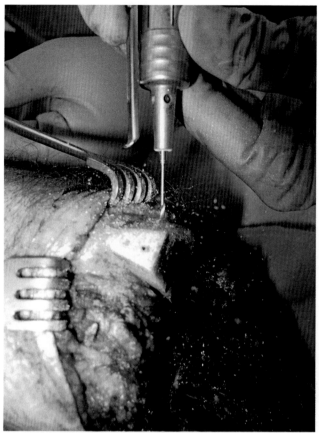

Fig. 53.7 Three holes are drilled into the anterior tibia from the anterior cortex into the medullary canal to tenodese the soleus muscle portion of the Achilles tendon

0 PDS suture (Fig. 53.8c). The skin and subcutaneous tissue is then dissected off the distal anterior tibial fascia for a distance of about 1 cm (Fig. 53.8d).

The Achilles tendon is then cut 1 cm distal to the distal end of the soleus tenodesis (Fig. 53.9a). The Achilles is then sewn to the anterior tibial fascia with a running back and forth 2-0 prolene (Fig. 53.9b). Skin is closed with vertical mattress 2-0 prolene and skin staples to ensure good skin edge eversion (Fig. 53.10). Dog ears, if present at the medial and lateral edge of the closure, are contoured to aid in optimal fitting of prosthesis. The wound is then dressed and the leg is placed in a knee immobilizer to protect it and prevent future knee contracture. The skin clips are removed at 1 week and the stitches at 4 weeks.

Evidence comparing PMF versus skew or sagittal flaps shows no significant differences although the level of evidence is poor [8]. In our hands however, the PMF provides sufficient vascularized soft tissue coverage over the tibial osteotomy to allow us to successfully perform below-knee amputations in 80% of all patients who presented with an ischemic or a nonviable or nonfunctional foot. This 80% underestimates the success of this flap because if the patient

be sewn into the anterior tibial cortex. The distal soleus muscle is then rotated forward, and the fascia tendinous layer is sewn into the three previously drilled holes in the tibia with

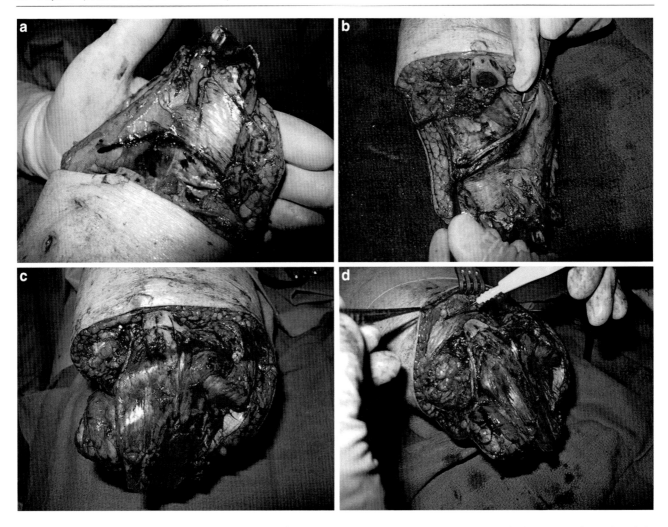

Fig. 53.8 The posterior flap is then swung up to the level of the anterior portion of the tibia and a *semilunar line* is drawn on the soleus muscle to mark that level (**a**). The soleus muscle is then incised along the drawn line with a 10 blade down to Achilles tendon at a beveled angle (**b**). The distal soleus muscle is then rotated forward, and the fascia-tendinous layer is sewn into the three previously drilled holes in the tibia with 0 PDS suture (**c**). The skin and subcutaneous tissue is then dissected off the distal anterior tibial fascia (**d**)

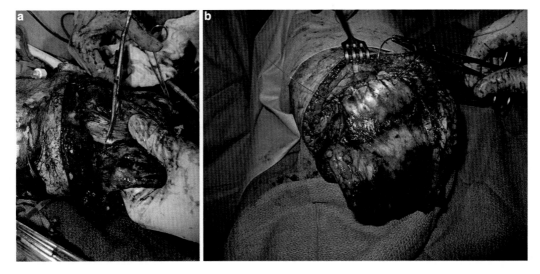

Fig. 53.9 The Achilles tendon is then cut 1 cm distal to the distal end of the soleus tenodesis (**a**). The Achilles is then sewn to the anterior tibial fascia with a running back and forth 2-0 prolene (**b**)

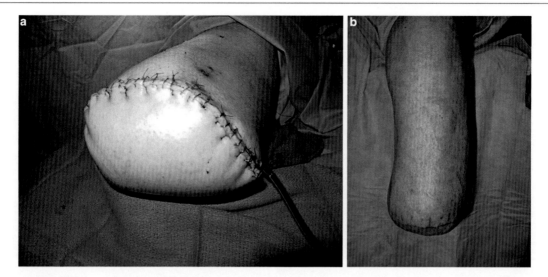

Fig. 53.10 The skin is closed and dog ears are removed so that the distal leg is well tapered (**a**). The stump should look tapered at and ready to fit into a prosthetic socket when the stitches are removed at 4 weeks (**b**)

was a nonambulator, the patient received a through-knee or AKA amputation. In addition, only 2 % of the below-knee amputations had to undergo a higher-level amputation [4]. This is the highest rate of BKA versus AKA in the literature suggesting that the vascular supply to the PMF may be superior to that of other flap designs.

BKA Using the ERTL Technique

Alternatively an ERTL modification to the BKA can be performed in patients who have the capacity of being very physically active. The ERTL modification for below-knee amputation involves a fibula vascularized bone graft between the tibia and fibula to promote distal bony fusion between the two to better transfer torque to the artificial ankle [9]. It also allows the distal stump to be end bearing when not wearing a prosthesis.

The initial surgical technique and markings are identical up to the planning of the fibular osteotomy. The first of two fibular osteotomies is marked distal to the tibial osteotomy (approx. 1.5–2 cm) so that the distance is equal to the width between the medial cortex of the fibula and the lateral cortex of the tibia (Fig. 53.11a). The fibula and the vessels are tied off at the level of the distal fibular osteotomy. After the distal fibular osteotomy, the distal leg is removed (Fig. 53.11b) in similar fashion as described above.

The proximal fibulotomy is performed after reconfirming the bone graft length is equal to the interosseous distance. Great care is taken to avoid traumatizing the peroneal artery and venae comitantes to maintain the vascularization of the bone graft. We recommend a lateral approach to the fibular osteotomy with care when meeting the medial fibular cortex so as not to damage the peroneal artery (Fig. 53.11c).

The lateral cortex of the tibia and medial cortex of the fibula are then burred down to aid in bony fusion and stable contact. The vascularized fibular bone graft (Fig. 53.12a) is then interposed between the distal fibula and tibia (Fig. 53.12b) and fixated with fine wires or screws (Fig. 53.12c). The closure is same as described above for the normal BKA.

If a screw is chosen, then our preference is for a headless compression screw (Fig. 53.13) to minimize chances of the screw having to be removed at a later date [9]. A bone clamp is used to prevent spinning of vascularized bone graft, while a K-wire is driven from lateral fibula to medial tibia. A cannulated 4.2-mm drill bit is passed from the tibia to the fibula through all four cortices. The countersink 5.5-mm drill bit is used to increase the diameter of the medial tibial cortex to aid in burying the head of the compression screw. We currently use the 5.5-mm Large Qwix Fixation and positioning screw (Integra LifeSciences, Plainsboro, NJ). When placing the headless compression screw, overtightening must be avoided to prevent accidental fracture of the medial tibial cortex. The result should be an excellent fusion at 2–3 months of the fibular strut with the distal fibula and tibia (Fig. 53.14).

Through-Knee Amputation

Knee disarticulations (KDs) account for less than 2 % of lower extremity amputations in the United States. Though the indications are few, the advantages of KDs over above-knee amputations include lower metabolic demand of ambulation, longer lever arm with intact insertion of thigh adductors, and decreased length and weight of prosthesis. A knee disarticulation is also an end-bearing amputation and provides a better counterbalance for nonambulatory patients while they transfer [10].

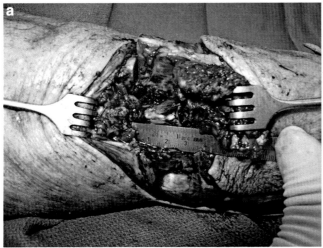
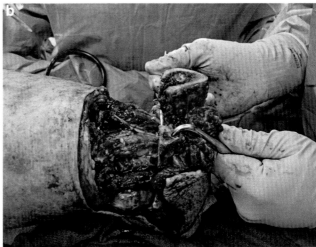
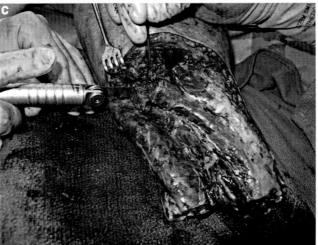

Fig. 53.11 The first of two fibular osteotomies is marked distal to the tibial osteotomy (approx. 1.5–2 cm) so that the distance is equal to the width between the medial cortex of the fibula and the lateral cortex of the tibia (**a**). The distal fibula is cut at that mark taking care to avoid traumatizing the distal peroneal artery and venae comitantes to maintain the vascularization of the bone graft, and the lower leg is then removed (**b**). The proximal fibulotomy is then performed without damaging the medial peroneal neurovascular bundle after reconfirming the bone graft length is equal to the interosseous distance (**c**)

It is important to discuss with the prosthetist if the femoral heal needs to be shaved down for a better fitting. If the prosthetist does not need to have the femoral head shaved down or if the patient is a nonambulator, the TKA should be done without shaving the femoral head. This allows for a quicker and more bloodless procedure. Otherwise, one can decrease the size of the femoral head by shaving it on all sides much like in a total knee replacement. Great care is taken to preserve the cruciates and posterior capsule in either case as the patella is brought down anteriorly to become end bearing and is held in its position by attaching the distal patellar tendon to the cruciates and posterior capsule. If the femoral head is shaved down, the same should be done to the posterior surface of patella for bone fusion to occur.

The tibial tubercle and joint line are identified. The incision is marked outlining a posterior compartment myocutaneous cutaneous flap to allow for tension-free closure. A sterile tourniquet is placed and inflated above the knee and an incision line is drawn two-thirds of the way around at a level just proximal to the tibial tubercle, leaving a posterior flap of about 10 cm to help close the wound (Fig. 53.15a). The incision is carried sharply into the knee joint and along the posterior flap (Fig. 53.15b). Attention is paid to preserve the cruciate ligaments' femoral attachment and posterior capsule. The distal leg is then removed leaving the posterior flap with the proximal soleus and gastrocnemius attached (Fig. 53.15c). The popliteal artery and vein are tied off at the level of the joint line. Both the peroneal and popliteal nerves are identified, are injected with long-lasting anesthetic placed on traction, and are then cut so they can retract into the proximal deeper tissue. The proximal soleus muscle is then removed as it may have lost its blood supply when tying off the popliteal artery.

If the distal femoral head is to be debulked, it is shaved down on all sides in a box-like fashion so that it is less bulky

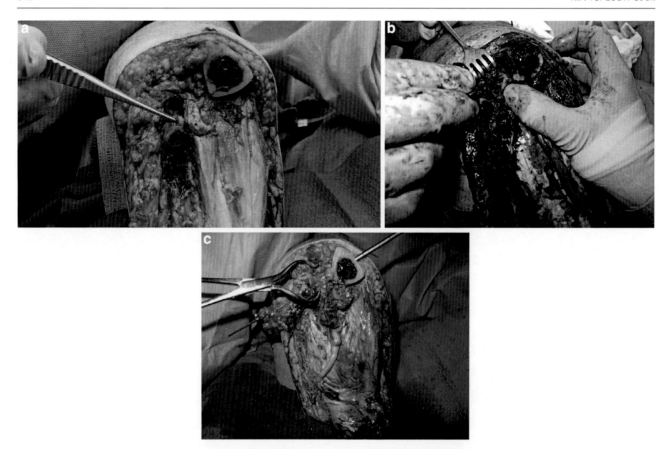

Fig. 53.12 The vessels are tied off at the level of the distal fibular osteotomy and preserved at the site of the proximal osteotomy (**a**). The vascularized fibular bone graft is then interposed between the distal fibula (**b**) and tibia and fixated with wires or screws (**c**)

for the prosthesis. To shave the distal femur down, all sides are sawed back about 0.5–1 cm (anterior, medial, superior, posterior, and lateral articular surface) to remove all cartilage and make the distal femur square (Fig. 53.16). Great care is taken to preserve the anterior and posterior cruciate ligament femoral attachments. The patella is identified and rotated anteriorly to expose the posterior articulating surface. A sagittal saw is used to shave the cartilaginous surface and bevel (Fig. 53.17a). For nonambulators, this step of bone cuts in both the patella and femur is skipped, and one can proceed directly to the tenodesis of the patellar tendon to the cruciates and posterior capsule. This avoids the risk of additional bleeding that the bone cuts might cause.

The patella is rotated up so the posterior aspect of its surface is exposed and the distal patellar tendon sutures are placed into the posterior capsule and remnant of the cruciate ligament (Fig. 53.17b). The assistant should hold the patellar cap in place while the surgeon ties the sutures. The shaved surface of the patella should be in direct contact with the shaved end of the femur. In the process, the patella is fixed in an anterior position so that it remains in direct contact with the distal anterior femoral head (Fig. 53.17c). Subsequent myodesis of the quadriceps and hamstrings is performed with 2-0 polydiaxone suture to provide complete muscle

coverage of the distal femur after a Jackson-Pratt drain has been placed. Skin closure is completed with interrupted vertical mattress 2-0 prolene suture. The area between each stitch is stapled to maximize wound edge eversion. The staples are removed before discharge, and the drain is removed when output is below 30 mL per day. Weight bearing on the residual limb is discouraged until all incisions have healed and sutures have been removed, which typically occurs around 4–6 weeks postoperatively (Fig. 53.18).

Above-Knee Amputation

Above-knee amputation should also be directed at optimizing functional outcome. The average above-knee amputation prosthesis usually requires at least 11 cm from the joint line to distal femur for adequate knee componentry. A two-stage amputation is still recommended in the setting of infection in the lower leg or foot. When planning for an above-knee amputation, initial drainage amputation is typically a knee disarticulation.

A sterile tourniquet is placed as proximal as possible. An anterior point is marked at 11 cm proximal to the joint line. Corresponding points are then marked at 11 cm medially and

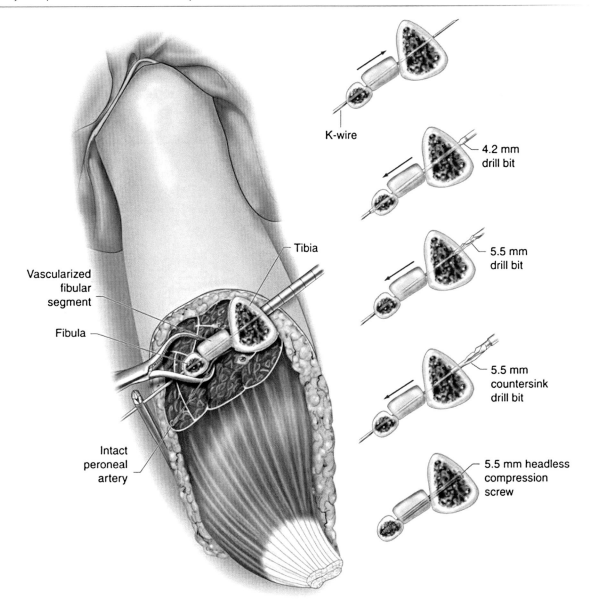

Fig. 53.13 A drawing shows how to apply a headless screw for optimal fusion of the fibula with the tibia [9]. From Brown BJ, Iorio ML, Hill L, Carlisle B, Attinger CE. Below-knee amputation with a vascularized fibular graft and headless compression screw. Plast Reconstr Surg. 2013 Feb;131(2):323–7. Reprinted with permission from Wolters Kluwer Health, Inc

laterally and an anterior and posterior U-shaped clamshell incision with the 11 cm mark as its base is designed. The anterior flap should extend just short of the patella, while the posterior flap goes to the proximal popliteal fossa. Tourniquet is inflated and skin incision is made with a 10 blade. Electrocautery is used to carry dissection down the fascia, with close attention medially to identify and suture ligate the saphenous vein and nerve. At the level of the fascia, the adductor muscles and hamstrings are identified and preserved at length. Each muscle is tagged with 2-0 PDS. The remaining musculature can be amputated at similar length to the designed skin flap edges. Posteriorly, care is taken to identify the popliteal artery, vein, sciatic, and peroneal nerve.

Anteriorly, the femur then is exposed and dissected circumferentially. The femoral osteotomy is performed in a transverse plane with slight bevel from lateral (shorter) to medial (longer) with the mid-point of the bevel at 11 cm from the joint line. Care is taken to not disrupt the marrow. Holes are then drilled medially, laterally, and anteriorly for eventual myodesis. The femoral artery and veins are suture ligated at the level of the bone cut. The sciatic and peroneal nerves are injected with long-lasting anesthetic, placed on traction and cut proximally at the level of the bone cut. Alternatively, one can do a neurorrhaphy between the tibial and peroneal nerves using a nerve sleeve to short-circuit possible phantom paint.

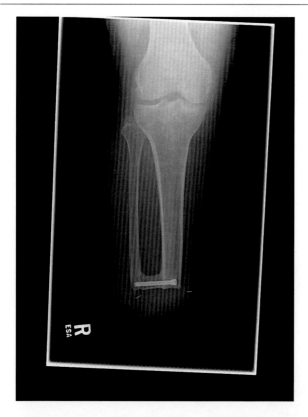

Fig. 53.14 X-ray of an ERTL using a headless screw. Note the fusion of the fibular strut with the fibula and tibia

Myodesis is critical for achieving maximal range of motion of the residual limb. It also maintains muscle bulk that is critical for long-term prosthetic fitting. The previously tagged adductors are sewn in medially, the midline of the quadriceps is attached to the femur anteriorly, and the hamstring is sewn into the posterior medial and lateral holes. The distal ends of each muscle group are attached to one another to reinforce the myodesis. This provides durable padding over femoral osteotomy. A 10 French drain is placed laterally. The anterior and distal fasciocutaneous flaps are then separated from the underlying muscle groups for approximately 5 cm to allow for good contour and minimal tension of the final closure. The skin is closed with interrupted vertical mattress 2-0 prolene sutures and staples to achieve adequate edge eversion.

Postoperative Care

Postoperative care is a critical component in major lower extremity amputations. Pain control immediately following surgery typically involves intravenous narcotics via patient-controlled analgesia (PCA). Intraoperative use of long-lasting local anesthesia is strongly recommended into identifiable nerves. Alternatively, epidurals can last for up to 5 days and are extremely effective when they work.

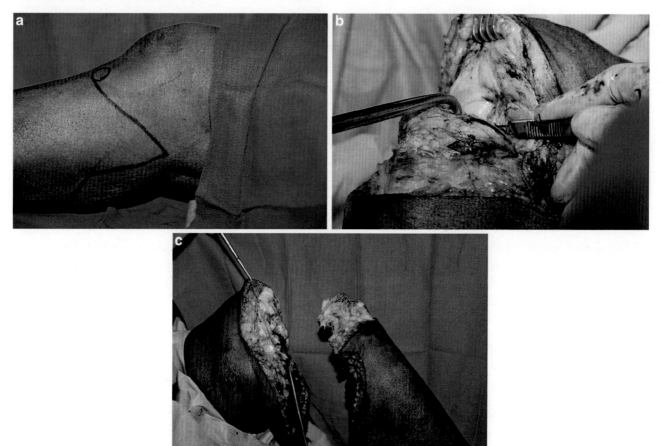

Fig. 53.15 For a knee disarticulation, an incision line is drawn two-thirds of the way around at a level just proximal to the tibial tubercle (**a**), the knee is disarticulated at the knee joint (**b**), leaving a posterior flap of about 10 cm to help close the wound (**c**)

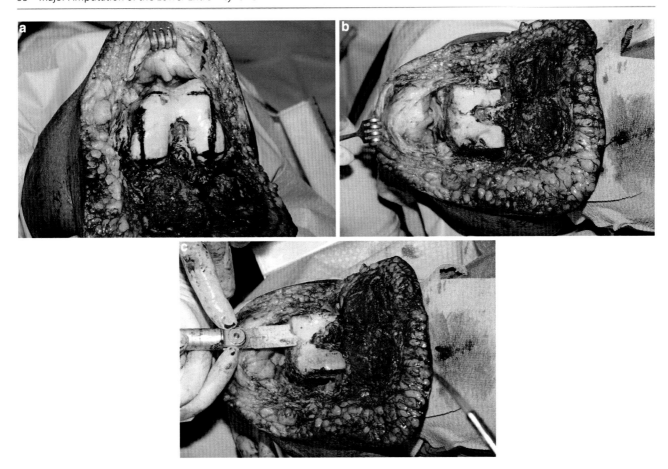

Fig. 53.16 If the distal femoral head is to be debulked, it is shaved down on all sides in a box-like fashion so that it is less bulky for the prosthesis. The *square* is drawn on the distal femoral head (**a**). The sides, *top*, and *bottom* have been shaved down (**b**). The anterior portion is now being shaved off while taking great care to preserve the proximal cruciates and the posterior capsule (**c**)

After lower extremity amputation, there is a significant disturbance in the patient's sense of balance as their center of gravity has been altered significantly. Nursing care and physical therapy play an important role in protecting the patient as they learn to transfer. Falls after amputation can be devastating and frequently lead to reoperation. Nearly one in five amputees will require amputation revisions due to postoperative falls. Thus, it is important to protect the residual limb. A knee immobilizer is placed immediately after each below-knee amputation to both protect the distal stump and prevent knee contracture until the patient is ready for a prosthesis.

Gentle compression in the immediate postoperative period aids with swelling but should be balanced when there is a question of possible ischemia. Compression should be avoided in patients with severe ischemic disease. The dressing is removed on day two to evaluate for signs of hematoma and ischemia. Drains should be observed and output recorded. Once the amount is less than 30 mL daily, the drain may safely be removed. Surgical staples are removed the day of discharge and the sutures are typically removed at 4 weeks in clinic.

Rehabilitation

The rehabilitation process begins immediately in the hospital. We typically keep each patient 4–5 days for inpatient pain control and evaluation by physical therapy. Physical therapy assesses each patient's strength and ability to transfer safely. Physical therapy determines the amount of assistance needed and recommends acute, subacute, or home-based rehabilitation. Our strong preference is an acute rehabilitation facility, and it is important to have a center that is familiar and trained in caring for amputees. The medical complexity and need for frequent follow-up underscore the importance of open communication and a multidisciplinary approach.

The prosthetist now becomes the most important component in caring for amputees. After the surgical incision has completely healed and the sutures have been removed, the fitting of the prosthesis may begin. Patients should be educated on the care of the residual limb, compression devices, and the progression from initial prosthetic fitting to final prosthesis. We advocate for fitting and ambulation as soon as it is safe for the patient. This prevents further deconditioning and promotes

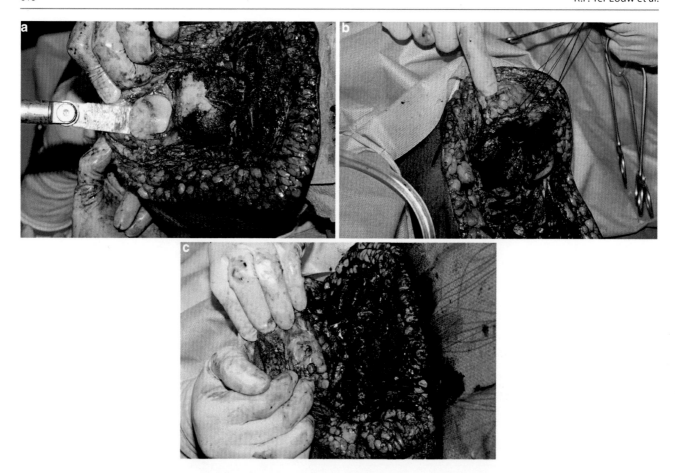

Fig. 53.17 The patella is rotated up so the posterior aspect of its surface is exposed and the undersurface of the patella is shaved down so that it has a better chance of fusing with the distal femoral head (**a**). The distal patellar tendon sutures are placed into the posterior capsule and remnant of the cruciate ligament (**b**). The assistant should then hold the patellar cap in place while the surgeon ties the sutures. In the process, the patella is rotated down so that is in direct contact with the distal anterior femoral head (**c**)

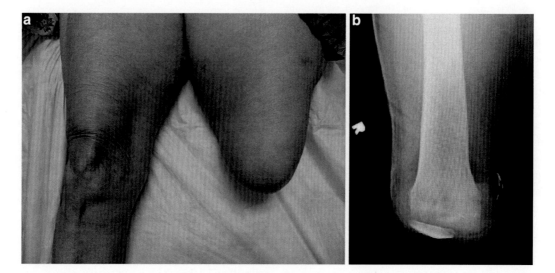

Fig. 53.18 The disarticulation is healed (**a**) and the X-ray shows fusion of the patella with the distal femur (**b**)

their return to normal functional status. Rehabilitation is recommended immediately after receiving the prosthesis to aid in teaching and preventing injuries from falls.

Follow-Up

Reoperation following amputation is unfortunate but it is relatively common occurring in up to 30 % of amputations. Trauma, dehiscence, infection, wound healing, and ischemia all contribute to high reoperation rates. Follow-up is recommended in the 2- and 4-week interval. At 2 weeks, the residual limb can be examined for signs of infection, dehiscence, or progressive ischemia. The 4-week visit typically involves the removal of sutures and arrangement of prosthetic fitting. If the postoperative course is uneventful, we aim to have each patient ambulating at 6–12 weeks.

Economic Cost

The economic cost of peripheral vascular disease and diabetes in the lower extremity is increasing. Inpatient hospitalization, surgery, clinic visits and prostheses all contribute to significant expenses. Over 35,000 lower extremity amputations occur each year in the United States with an estimated hospital cost of $8.3 billion [11]. A recent study by Yin et al. estimated that the average hospital stay alone for the diabetic lower extremity amputation is estimated at $17,103 [12]. Apelqvist et al. estimated the total cost of healing a lower extremity ulcer was $6664 by primary healing with local wound care vs. $44,790 by amputation. Greater than 60 % of the total cost for each ulcer were inpatient expenses [13].

The average BKA prosthesis can approach $20,000 while that of AKA prosthesis nearly $60,000. The prosthesis is changed on average every 5 years. Multiple studies have focused on the economic analysis of lower extremity salvage and have shown that a multidisciplinary approach with preventive healthcare can decrease the number of major amputations by 62–80 % [14, 15].

However, the important lesson is to keep function in mind when making the decision to salvage a limb or amputate a limb. If the resulting function of the salvaged limb does or will not meet the patient's physical needs, then a major amputation should be performed. It has to be done with the same amount of care and attention to detail and function as would have been done for limb salvage because the surgeon is actually creating a new, albeit shorter, limb. Focusing on myodesis and tenodesis ensures that the residual muscles remain functional

and that the residual limb does not loose mobility and strength. The closure should have a smooth tapered design so that the patient can start wearing prosthesis as soon as the stitches are removed and the prosthesis is ready. Our duty as amputation surgeons is to give the patient the best possible leg to return to as active a lifestyle as he or she may desire.

References

1. Endara M, Masden D, Goldstein J, Gondek S, Steinberg J, Attinger C. The role of chronic and perioperative glucose management in high-risk surgical closures. Plast Reconstr Surg. 2013;132(4): 996–1004.
2. Naschitz JE, Lenger R. Why traumatic leg amputees are at increased risk for cardiovascular diseases. QJM. 2008;101(4):251–9.
3. Pell JP, Donnan PT, Fowkes FGR, Ruckley CV. Quality of life following lower limb amputation for peripheral arterial disease. Eur J Vasc Surg. 1993;7(4):448–51.
4. Brown BJ, Iorio ML, Klement M, Conti Mica MR, El-Amraoui A, O'halloran P, et al. Outcomes after 294 transtibial amputations with the posterior myocutaneous flap. Int J Low Extrem Wounds. 2014;13(1):33–40.
5. Lin R, Hingorani A, Marks N, Ascher E, Jimenez R, McIntyre T, et al. Effects of anesthesia versus regional nerve block on major leg amputation mortality rate. Vascular. 2013;21(2):83–6. doi:10.1177/1708538113478718. Epub 22 Mar 2013.
6. Fisher Jr DF, Clagett GP, Fry RE, Humble TH, Fry WJ. One-stage versus two-stage amputation for wet gangrene of the lower extremity: a randomized study. J Vasc Surg. 1988;8(4):428–33.
7. Burgess EM, Romano RL, Zettl JH, Schrock Jr RD. Amputations of the leg for peripheral vascular insufficiency. J Bone Joint Surg Am. 1971;53(5):874–90.
8. Tisi PV, Than MM. Type of incision for below knee amputations. Cochrane Database Syst Rev. 2014;8:4.
9. Brown BJ, Iorio ML, Hill L, Carlisle B, Attinger CE. Below-knee amputation with a vascularized fibular graft and headless compression screw. Plast Reconstr Surg. 2013;131(2):323–7.
10. Albino FP, Seidel R, Brown BJ, Crone CG, Attinger CE. Through knee amputation: technique modifications and surgical outcomes. Arch Plast Surg. 2014;41(5):562–70. doi:10.5999/aps.2014.41.5.562.
11. HCUP Nationwide Inpatient Sample (NIS). Healthcare Cost and Utilization Project (HCUP). Rockville, MD: Agency for Healthcare Research and Quality; 2009.
12. Yin H, Radican L, Kong SX. A study of regional variation in the inpatient cost of lower extremity amputation among patients with diabetes in the United States. J Med Econ. 2013;16(6):820–7. doi:10.3111/13696998.2013.801349. Epub 15 May 2013.
13. Apelqvist J, Ragnarson-Tennvall G, Persson U, Larsson J. Diabetic foot ulcers in a multidisciplinary setting. An economic analysis of primary healing and healing with amputation. J Intern Med. 1994;235(5):463–71.
14. Sanders LJ, Robbins JM, Edmonds ME. History of the team approach to amputation prevention: pioneers and milestones. J Vasc Surg. 2010;52(3 Suppl):3S–16S.
15. Driver VR, Fabbi M, Lavery LA, Gibbons G. The costs of diabetic foot: the economic case for the limb salvage team. J Vasc Surg. 2010;52 Suppl 3:17S–22.

Extremity Replantation or Transplantation

Raymond A. Dieter, Jr., George B. Kuzycz, and Raymond A. Dieter, III

Major traumatic episodes usually involve the chest and abdomen. As such, many of these result in death or prolonged recovery periods prior to rehabilitation of the individual. Concomitant to these torso and head injuries, extremity trauma may also occur simultaneously. When such injuries do take place, the orthopedists are usually consulted to manage the injured arm or leg fracture or soft tissue "injury."

We have seen a number of these major traumatized individuals for treatment of their crushed, devascularized, or, even, transected extremity. Usually, when the lesion is more central, we have been requested to consult and to provide patient care. But when the injury involves the digits or hand, the hand surgeon or orthopedist has been the primary responsible operating surgeon. Whether the injury is proximal—near the trunk—or distal and involving the hand or foot, care of the patient and the traumatized or amputated tissue is a major surgical and postsurgical medical care project. Certainly, amputation may be the ultimate result in extremity ischemia.

In our experience, the most difficult patients to treat and care for are those who have a major crush injury. These injuries cause tissue trauma that many times are beyond salvage. The tissue is crushed and macerated and lacks reconstructionable or usable potentially viable structures for salvage and preservation of the arm, leg, and the individual. This is most apparent when a portion of the torso is also involved in these major crush injuries. Frequently, the combination of extremity and torso injuries has made debridement, resection, and replantation in these patients virtually impossible. Most of these incidents have been seen with garbage truck, fork lift, and similar heavy crushing machinery.

The type of injury most amenable to surgical reconstruction usually is the sharper more "clean-cut" injury with little adjacent tissue damage. Accidents which provide knife-like transection of tissue allow the surgeon to more readily locate, identify, debride, and then properly anastomose the involved tissues. These situations lend themselves to a greater chance of a functional and viable extremity or portion of an extremity then with the crushing or crush-amputation injury.

History

Historically, the amputated fingertip, distal phalanx, or the entire digit was the first to be replanted. With the advent of microsurgery 50 years ago, the reattachment success rate was increased and thus the salvage rate improved. Function and sensation were enhanced with restoration of circulation (arterial and venous), bone stabilization, tendon repair, nerve connection, and skin closure. Attention to the preoperative, operative, and postoperative care has all led to improved function [1].

Simultaneously, larger amputated structures were being replanted in an effort to provide a functional and viable arm or leg. In the early 1960s, replantation of the arm was attempted and accomplished by a number of surgical programs throughout the USA. In January 1963, a 15-year-old Eskimo male accidentally caused the amputation of his right arm just below the shoulder while playing a game with friends using a commercial washing machine. The arm had been amputated just below the shoulder, due to the rotary motion of the machine. Feeling he would bleed massively, all automobile speed limits were broken by me when the ER nurse contacted me. On my arrival, the boy was reading a comic book in no distress at the nurse's desk. Ten minutes later another boy brought the arm wrapped in a towel to me

R.A. Dieter, Jr., MD, MS (✉)
Northwestern Medicine, At Central DuPage Hospital, Winfield, IL, USA

International College of Surgeons, Cardiothoracic and Vascular Surgery, Glen Ellyn, IL, USA

G.B. Kuzycz, MD
Thoracic and Cardiovascular Surgery, Cadence Hospital of Northwestern System, Winfield, IL 60190, USA

R.A. Dieter, III, MD
Division of Cardiothoracic Surgery, The University of Tennessee Medical Center, Knoxville, TN 37920, USA

© Springer International Publishing Switzerland 2017
R.S. Dieter et al. (eds.), *Critical Limb Ischemia*, DOI 10.1007/978-3-319-31991-9_54

at the hospital outpatient clinic. After laboratory, blood typing, proper surgical preparation, and repair of the nasal injuries while using a pHisoHex prep, the mangled arm was reattached focusing primarily on the vascular supply. Following several hours of surgery, we then elected to remove the arm due to its condition and close the upper arm stump approximately 4–6 inches below the shoulder. Later, after consultation with other centers, the consensus was that the brachial plexus twisting and avulsion along with the mangled multiply fractured distal arm wounds incurred by the arm would not have allowed function in the future, even if viable, and that no replantation and that arm removal was the best option. His wounds healed well and he was referred for outpatient physical therapy and rehabilitation.

Unfortunately, functionality of these extremities was and remains a major concern for the treating physician and the patient. Viability did not guarantee usability of the replanted extremity nor was the patient free from complications and further health risks. Later, when Professor Harold Haley and I attended a trauma meeting in San Antonio, two patients were presented. One had an upper arm amputation without replantation. He was happy, outgoing, and employed. The other had a surviving upper arm replantation without return of function. He was depressed, withdrawn, and not working—thus a concern as to whether the arm should have been reattached was expressed.

Some time later, we then encountered the near-total amputation of a leg except for a few inches of skin. He represents a viable replant but with minimal function. After reconstructive boney, muscular, vascular, and neural component surgery, his leg was viable. But a decade later, he requested amputation of the near-functionless but viable extremity due to multiple problems, including infection, with the replanted extremity.

Initial Trauma Care

With experience over the years, physicians and surgeons learned more about the multiple aspects of extremity amputation and salvage reattachment. The factors concerning preoperative preparation, surgery, and postsurgical care all became of importance if one wished to salvage the amputated extremity or a part thereof of the body Table 54.1.

As listed above, a number of factors concerning the incident, its location, the cause, and the condition of the injured patient are all relevant to the possible salvage and replantation of an extremity. Obviously, the part amputated must be salvageable and potentially viable without undue risk of life while obtaining a viable replant. The harmed individual must be potentially salvageable and transportable to a facility where the amputated part and amputee may receive appropriate care without undue delay. Infection potential and time delay must be managed appropriately and safely.

Table 54.1 Factors influencing survival of an amputated extremity

Site of accident
Type of injury
Location of injury
Condition of individual
Condition of amputated structure
Preop management
Cleanliness
Antibiotics
Stability of patient
Ancillary injuries
Operative management
Anesthetic
Tissue condition
Surgical repair
Maintenance of vitals
Postoperative care
Maintenance of vitals
Possible ICU
Stabilization of patient and extremity
Monitoring extremity
Factors influencing survival of an amputated extremity
Antibiotic consideration
Protection of reimplanted denervated amputated tissue
Long-term care
Patient participation
Rehabilitation program

At the treating facility, evaluation of the tissue for crush, mangling, or inappropriate contamination with infectious or noxious agents will be performed. Antibiotic and resuscitation steps will be initiated. Simultaneously, determination as to the patient's acute and possibly chronic health condition will be taken into consideration. Checking for other major ancillary injuries will be important—especially of the cranial, thoracic, and abdominopelvic organs. Cleanliness and patient temperature concerns will be important determinants in the decision process.

In surgery, appropriate anesthesia and multisystem monitoring will be maintained before, during, and after the reattachment. Blood loss, body and extremity temperature, heart rate, and urine volume will require consideration. Certainly the ability to locate and label appropriate structures will require adequate time after boney stabilization. Tendon, neural, and vascular (venous and arterial) anastomoses will follow with appropriate identification and surgical techniques [1]. The closure of skin over the exposed structures without tension will aid in tissue survival and avoidance of infection. All of this care will require a long period of anesthesia, maintenance of vitals, and multiple personnel—including surgical specialties or subspecialties.

Postoperatively, depending on the condition of the patient and the amputated structure, the use of the intensive care facilities and staff may be necessary. Laboratory, vital signs, and patient-extremity monitoring will all be of value. Complete blood count (CBC), electrolyte, x-ray, and urine volume will be followed as appropriate. Patient alertness and responsiveness will affect one's evaluation as well as color and temperature of the amputated tissue replanted. With time, dietary and ambulatory options will be advanced. With more stabilization, short-term physical and occupational rehab programs will be initiated and the longer programs introduced. Reasonable early onset of such programs will aide in the eventual rehab of the patient.

Personnel Involvement

As presented above, the number and type of personnel involved in the patient's care vary from the local accident scene to the long-term post-discharge rehab staff. At the scene of the trauma, there may be only the patient, a few bystanders, or a crowd. Many times the paramedics or emergency personnel will arrive at the scene and monitor the situation. With our first patient, he and his friends walked to the clinic. Later, two friends carried the arm in to the clinic.

At the hospital, the emergency staff (nurses, LPNs, secretaries, transport team, and physicians) will all become involved (Table 54.2). Diagnostic personnel including x-ray and laboratory individuals will perform necessary testing. The surgical team then provides the necessary anesthesia; nurses; orthopedists; general, vascular, neural, or hand surgeons as well as circulators; and other OR staff. Then the patient is transferred to the recovery, regular ward, or intensive care staff for 24 h care depending on the patient's condition and level of amputation (Table 54.3). After stability, the regular floor or ward staff and

Table 54.2 Personnel involved in patient care

Site of injury
Friends
Crowd
Paramedics
Hospital
Emergency room staff
Preoperative staff
Surgical staff
Multiple specialties
Anesthesia
Postoperative
Intensive care
Nursing
Physical therapy
Post discharge
Physical therapy
Occupational therapy
Continued medical/nursing care

Table 54.3 Types of extremity amputation

Digits—most frequent
Fingers
Toes
Joint level
Ankle
Wrist
Major extremity
Arm
Elbow and below
Upper arm—below shoulder
Leg
Below knee
Below hip

inpatient physical or occupational therapy programs will be initiated. The long-term posthospital rehabilitation program and staff will then follow, as well as the posthospital medical staff, to monitor for complications and possible need for repeat interventions.

Upper Extremity Replantation

The most common amputations encountered involve the digits of either the upper or lower extremity. These are a frequent occurrence and commonly are seen by the hand surgeon or the microsurgeon. When the amputated tissue is salvageable and the site of potential reimplant usable, the reconstruction is frequently undertaken—especially if this is the thumb or larger digit (index and long). In a 2014 review of 326 patients who had 680 injuries from Sweden, 350 fingers and 88 thumbs were replanted with a survival rate of 91% for fingers and 86% for thumbs [2]. Most such injuries were due to saws (22%), machines (20%), and wood splints (cutters) (20%). Direct anastomosis (30%) or vein grafts (70%) were benefitted by microsurgical techniques. 59% of these injuries were classified as major and 28% as severe. 10% of the patients required retirement status thereafter and only 13 of their patients had amputation above the wrist.

Multiple digit, hand, or wrist amputations all present their individual complexities and success stories (Table 54.4). Each level has a different and significant technical challenge. Certainly, caring for four or five separate amputations or a transpalmar lesion presents challenges not seen at the wrist with regard to the neurovascular anastomosis. No amputation injury is looked at as minor, but as one moves from the digit to the hand or wrist, certainly the potential for significant disability increases—especially as the complexity and tissue volume at risk increases. Successful replantations have been reported despite an occasional risk of thrombosis [3].

Table 54.4 Some considerations in patients with traumatic amputations

Survival
Patient
Extremity
Future function
Sensation
Touch
Temperature
Flexion-contraction
Infections
Initial
Repeated
Tissue reconstruction
Thrombosis/vascular compromise
Tendon/bone
Amputation
Initial
Future
Psychologic

Table 54.5 Some indications or contraindications for upper extremity replantation

Indications	Possible contraindications
Thumb amputation	Crush
Children	Prolonged warm ischemia
Wrist or palm	Patient's general health
Multiple digits	Patient's coexisting major injuries
Sharp amputation	Psychologic or rehab concerns
	Avulsion injuries such as brachial plexus
	Multilevel amputations

Moving above the wrist to the elbow, to the upper arm, or below the shoulder, one encounters more and different concerns. Replantations at these levels are less common and trauma occurrence fortunately is less. Various authors have reported success with upper arm replantation, as well as the difficulties that may be encountered [4–7]. Outlined below are some of these difficulties that the patient and treating team may encounter.

Certainly the anatomic union of bone, tendon, nerve, vascular, and skin structures may be accomplished in these unfortunate individuals. Not only do they have the acute episode of injury and surgery to survive, but they also must accept a prolonged period of disability with the hopes of future function and minimal secondary complications.

Crush injuries and prolonged ischemia times (often 8–10 h) are less conducive to successful grafting. Reperfusion injury has been minimized in major amputations by cross-limb vascular shunting to reduce ischemic injury [8]. Other innovative procedures may include cross-arm replantation for traumatic bilateral upper extremity amputation or bone shortening procedures [7, 9].

Major amputations in children have presented separate distinct concerns since the first successful replantation of a complete amputation of the arm in a 12-year-old boy in 1962 [10]. Our previously mentioned case of an unsuccessful replantation of a badly mangled arm followed in less than a year. We felt the revision amputation was probably best for the long-term functional and psychologic concerns of an individual in the arctic. Beris et al. reported on the use of microsurgical techniques, free tissue transfer, vascularized bone transfers,

nerve grafts, and toe to thumb transfers with 86 % replantation success and/or reconstructive procedures at 96 % [11].

Some authors have outlined indications and contraindications to upper extremity replantation. We have already mentioned some areas of consideration for patients who have experienced upper extremity amputation. Table 54.5 outlines some of these concerns or situations. A viable replantation does not necessarily imply a "successful" replantation. Functionality and viability of the reattached tissue is the real test of success. Movement of digits, touch sensation, temperature perception, flexibility of joints or lack of repeated surgeries and complications are strong success evaluators. Various authors have devised tables or charts to define these concerns and stratified such issues. When considering the individual for prolonged and possible multiple surgeries, a number of clinical factors have been reviewed by Larson et al. Most of these factors are only relative contraindications such as occupation, crush vs. guillotine, injury level, contamination, multilevel, and self-inflicted injuries [12]. Even postoperative concerns may vary in actual importance such as anticoagulation or not, smoking, and implantation without digital vein repair [13]. Strict postoperative routines have been developed by some surgeons and not by others [14].

Rehabilitation of these unfortunate patients may require long recovery periods as well as following an intense rehab program. Such a program actually may start at the initial injury setting and definitely by the surgical procedure. When the patient's condition is not permissive, cold preservation of the amputated site for up to 25 or 48 h or longer may provide salvage of the extremity [13].

Following surgery, wound and splint care in association with early protected motion and assisted flexion starts in the first week. Weekly programs and strengthening exercises begin. Definitive reconstruction after 6 months may be of value in certain patients [15]. Long-term results of these patient catastrophes have been shown after 15 years to be positive by Gulgonin and Ozer with function and usage [16].

Lower Extremity

Injuries to the lower extremities are quite frequent and usually occur in the younger individual. We have seen a number of these patients with major lower extremity trauma. Many of these patients have had crushing, cutting, or tearing injuries. The attempt to repair has often been limited due to concomitant torso injuries. Consequently, the safest procedure was amputation with patient survival being the final goal. Amputation or near-total amputation in our area has usually occurred in the severely traumatized individual from high-speed motorcycle or auto accidents. Thus preservation of life has been paramount and amputation the safest. Snowmobile accidents, especially when hitting a fence or wire, have led to major vascular, neural, and soft tissue repair with avoidance of amputation due to the cutting-type injury.

Replantation of lower extremities has not experienced the same enthusiasm or success as have upper extremity replants. Complications of surgical repair are common. There are certain guidelines that may lend assistance in decision making and include (1) preservation of the knee when possible and (2) consideration of heel and sole replantation while great toe salvage programs may be iffy. If limb replantation is considered then ischemia time minimization and boney stabilization is paramount, followed by definitive wound coverage [17]. Unfortunately, soft tissue necrosis may occur in 90 % of these patients. But, with persistence, the goal of returning to work may be accomplished in most injured patients.

Some unusual and successful stories do exist regarding lower limb replantation. Fang et al. reported a literature review of 13 patients who had bilateral successful replantation of lower limb amputations [18]. Daigeler et al. reported on orthotopic (same leg) and heterotopic (opposite leg) replant results [19]. An even more unusual replantation result was reported by Pei of four-limb replantation in one patient [20].

Extremity Transplantation

Transplantation of tissues from one individual to another has been performed for nearly a century. In our area in 1935, blood was withdrawn from one individual and injected directly into another individual using the same syringe without crossmatch for successful treatment of meningitis. Also, while I was a resident, pediatric renal transplantation was initiated in our training programs, in the 1960s.

During the mid-1960s, we began working with cardiopulmonary bypass utilizing profound hypothermia and marked hemodilution while studying the metabolic aspects of such [21]. Simultaneously, we were performing heart transplantation studies in the dog and calf. By 1968 and 1969, we were able to initiate a human heart and lung transplant program after the world's first such cardiac transplant procedure in South Africa.

Transplantation programs continued to develop with additional transplantation research leading to bilateral lung, liver, pancreas, and small bowel transplants for the benefit of the patient. Subsequent to this, on 23 September 1998, the first human hand transplantation was performed in Lyon, France, as reported by Jean-Michel Dubernard et al. [22]. They further reported that the rapidity and quality of nerve regrowth were surprising and probably related to a clean-cut amputation in the donor, use of the Wisconsin IV preservative solution, and ischemic time of only 12.5 h. Antirejection therapy to combat rejection was the main obstacle encountered, as discussed extensively by them.

Morrison presented a history of transplantation beginning with Cosmos and Damien (died 287 AD) for "transplantation" of a leg of a Moor to a church worker after amputation for a cancerous growth [23]. A painting from 590 AD shows replantation of four legs of a horse. The Italian Leonardo Fioravanti reattached successfully an amputated nose after he urinated on it to wash away the sand in 1570. In 1814, Balfour reattached an amputated carpenter's finger. Canine vascular limb surgery by Carrel in 1912 earned the Nobel Prize. And Malt, in 1962, reattached an above-elbow amputation.

Of interest, after our efforts at reattachment surgery, cardiac bypass surgery, and injuries to the hand and nerves, we then asked Ethicon suture company to construct 9-0 and 10-0 suture in the early 1980s for the necessary microvascular and nerve reconstructions in these complicated patients. Surgeons readily adopted small suture and microvascular or microneural reconstruction—including the use of magnification. Simultaneously, additional reports of hand transplantation and the International Registry of Hand and Composite Tissue Transplantation report have been published [24, 25]. Subsequent transplants, including double-hand transplantation, have also been reported by Dubernard et al. [26]. Acute skin rejection, a prime concern, along with the antirejection immunosuppressive protocol was also simultaneously presented.

One of the presumed attributes of these transplant procedures' success is ascribed to the sharp transection of the tissues by the scalpel. This same postulate was recently presented at the International College of Surgeons Annual Meeting in Annapolis by Dr. Sergio Canavero of Italy on 12 June 2015. He presented the concept of sharp transection of the spinal cord followed by spinal cord reconnection and successful ambulation of dogs with four functional extremities and also head transplants in mice. He postulates, for the same reason, the possibility of brain-head transplants in the human or repair of the traumatized spinal cord or paraplegic patient [27]. Some individuals, for example, with single or double upper extremity amputation theoretically may be candidates for hand-arm transplantation. When the patient has a functional thumb or finger remaining on one arm and an opposite upper extremity functional prosthesis, the consideration for further surgery and a functional hand may be outweighed by the required process for the patient to accomplish the transplant. Preoperative testings, surgical and anesthetic considerations, postoperative care, time required to evaluate the results, and additional antirejection therapy present a challenge to the stable and functional patient. Thus, many patients with single or double amputation may avoid the risks and discomfort of upper extremity transplantation.

Transplantation or replantation of major extremities—arm or leg—is technically possible but practically may not be a viable option in many situations at this time. With time and gathering of further knowledge, the future presents us a challenge for the benefit of our patients.

References

1. Beris AE, Lykissas MG, Koromilias AV, Mitsionis GI, Vekris MD, Kostas-Agnantis IP. Digit and hand replantation. Arch Orthop Trauma Surg. 2010;130(9):1141–7.
2. Rosberg H-E. Disability and health after replantation or revascularization in the upper extremity in a population in southern Sweden - a retrospective long time follow up. BMC Musculoskelet Disord. 2014;15:73. http://www.biomedcentral.com/1471-2474/15/73.
3. Visnjic MM, Kovacevic PT, Paunkovic LM, Milenkovic SS. Single centre experience of the upper limb replantation and revascularisation. Folia Med (Plovdiv). 2004;46(4):32–6.
4. Cavadas PC. Salvage of replanted upper extremities with major soft-tissue complications. J Plast Reconstr Aesthet Surg. 2007;60(7):769–75.
5. Matsuda M, Kato N, Hosoi M. The problems in replantation of limbs amputated through the upper arm region. J Trauma. 1981;21(5):403–6.
6. D'Addato M, Pedrini L, Bertoni M, Stella A, Vitacchiano G, Sardella C, et al. Traumatic amputation of the upper limb: replantation of the arm. J Trauma. 1989;29(6):876–9.
7. Axelrod TS, Buchler V. Severe complex injuries to the upper extremity: revascularization and replantation. J Hand Surg Am. 1991;16(4):574–84.
8. Lee YC, Lee JW. Cross-limb vascular shunting for major limb replantation. Ann Plast Surg. 2009;62(2):139–43.
9. Liang K, Zhong G, Yin J, Xiang Z, Cen S, Huang F. Cross-arm replantation for traumatic bilateral upper extremity amputations: a case report. Arch Orthop Trauma Surg. 2011;131(2):157–61.
10. Beris AE, Soucacos PN, Malizo KN, Mitsionis GJ, Soucaros PK. Major limb replantation in children. Micosurgery. 1994;15(7): C-474–8.
11. Beris AE, Soucacos PH, Malizos KN. Microsurgery in children. Clin Orthop Relat Res. 1995;314:112–21.
12. Larson JV, Kung TA, Cederna PS, Sears ED, Urbanchek MG, Langhals NB. Clincial factors associated with replantation after traumatic major upper extremity amputation. Plast Reconstr Surg. 2013;132(4):911–9.
13. Prucz RB, Friedrich JB. Upper extremity replantation: current concepts. Plast Reconstr Surg. 2014;133(2):333–42.
14. DP H, Chin SH. Wrist level and proximal-upper extremity replantation. Hand Clin. 2007;23:13–21.
15. Papanastasiou S. Rehabilitation of the replanted upper extremity. Plast Reconstr Surg. 2002;109(3):978–81.
16. Gulgonen A, Ozer K. Long-term results of major upper extremity replantations. J Hand Surg (Eur). 2011;37(3):225–32.
17. Cavodas PC, Thione A. Lower limb replantation. In: Salyapongse AN et al., editors. Extremity replantation: a comprehensive clinical guide. New York: Springer; 2015. p. 145–59. doi:10.1007/978-1-4899-7516-4_12.
18. Fang J-L, Yang C-S, Tang H-C, Changchien C-H, Lai Y-Y. Successful replantation of amputated bilateral lower limbs. Plast Reconstr Surg. 2012;129(1):215c–7c.
19. Daigeler A, Fansa H, Schneider W. Orthotopic and heterotopic lower leg reimplantation. Evaluation of seven patients. J Bone Joint Surg. 2003;85-B:554–8.
20. Pei GX, Kunde L, Churwen C, Dengshong Z, Fuyi W, Songto W, et al. Replantation of four severed limbs in one patient. Injury. 1997;28(1):73–6.
21. Dieter Jr RA. Metabolic aspects of total body perfusion using profound hypothermia with marked hemodilution (Master of Science Thesis). Chicago: Univ IL Medical Center; 1966.
22. Dubernard J-M, Owens E, Lefrancois N, Petruzzo P, Martin X, Dawahra M, et al. First human hand transplantation case report. Transpl Int. 2000;13 Suppl I:5521–4.
23. Morrison WA. The history of extremity replantation. In: Saylyapongse AN, et al., editors. Extremity replantation: a comprehensive clinical guide. New York: Springer; 2015. p. 1–8. doi:10.1007/978-1-4899-7516-4_1.
24. Lanzetta M, Petruzzo P, Dubernard JM, Margreiter R, Schwind F, Breidenbach W, et al. Second report (1998–2006) of the International Registry of Hand and Composite Tissue Transplantation. Transpl Immunol. 2007;18(1):1–6. Epub 9 Apr 2007.
25. Kaufman CL, Blair B, Murphy E, Breidenbach WB. A new option for amputees: transplantation of the hand. J Rehabil Res Dev. 2009;46(3):395–404.
26. Dubernard JM, Petruzzo P, Lanzetta M, Parmitier H, Martin X, Dawahra M, et al. Functional results of the first human double-hand transplantation. Ann Surg. 2003;238(1):128–36.
27. Canavero S. Human brain-head transplantation. Oral presentation. Int Coll Surg—US Section Annual Meeting. Annapolis, MD. 12 June 2015.

The Importance of a Multidisciplinary Approach to Leg Ulcers

Albeir Mousa, Mehiar El Hamdani, Raymond A. Dieter, Jr.,
Aravinda Nanjundappa, Mohamed A. Rahman,
David J. Leehey, Raymond A. Dieter, III, James S. Walter,
Scott T. Sayers, Sanjay Singh, Morgan M. Meyer,
Amit S. Dayal, Amir Darki, and Robert S. Dieter

Introduction

Although intentionally brief, this chapter is to remind the clinician that the treatment of the patient with critical limb ischemia (CLI) is inherently multidisciplinary (Fig. 55.1). Depending on the type of lesion and the etiology, one, two, or more consultants will be required.

Arterial disease is the etiology of only about 50 % of foot ulcerations. The remainder is due to a variety of causes, including neuropathic/neuroischemic, rheumatological disorders, venous stasis disease, trauma, nutritional, etc.

Above the foot ulcers, the role of venous pathology contributing to the ulcer exceeds that of arterial insufficiency [1]. Furthermore, the complexity of the microcirculation and nutritional factors in the development and nonhealing of ulcerations highlights the complexity of these lesions.

It is naïve for the clinician to believe that they can act in isolation when caring for most of these patients. Accurate imaging, wound care, and risk factor modification are all required for the optimization of the limb and patient. Frequently, these patients will require the coordinate involvement of primary care and medical specialties—including endocrinology, nephrology, and rheumatology. Many patients

A. Mousa, MD, MPH, MBA
Surgery, Charleston Area Medical Center,
WVU Physicians of Charleston, Charleston, WV, USA

M. El Hamdani, MD
Medicine, Marshall University School of Medicine,
Huntington, WV, USA

R.A. Dieter, Jr., MD, MS
Northwestern Medicine, At Central DuPage Hospital,
Winfield, IL, USA

International College of Surgeons, Cardiothoracic
and Vascular Surgery, Glen Ellyn, IL, USA

A. Nanjundappa, MD, RVT
Medicine and Surgery, West Virginia University, Charleston,
WV, USA

M.A. Rahman, MD
Medicine, Nephrology, Hines VA Hospital, Loyola University,
Hines, IL, USA

D.J. Leehey, MD
Medicine, Loyola University Medical Center and Hines VA,
Maywood, IL, USA

R.A. Dieter, III, MD
Division of Cardiothoracic Surgery, The University of Tennessee
Medical Center, Knoxville, TN, USA

J.S. Walter, PhD
Research Service, Hines VA Hospital, Hines, IL, USA

S.T. Sayers, PhD
Department of Thoracic and Cardiovascular Surgery, Loyola
University Medical Center, Maywood, IL, USA

S. Singh, MS, PhD
Research Service, Edward Hines Jr., VA Hospital, Hines, IL, USA

M.M. Meyer, MD
Internal Medicine, Illinois State Medical Society,
Lombard, IL, USA

A.S. Dayal, MD
Medicine, Edward Hines Jr., Veterans Affair Hospital,
Hines, IL, USA

A. Darki, MD, MSc
Medicine, Cardiology, Loyola University Medical Center,
Maywood, IL 60153, USA

R.S. Dieter, MD, RVT (✉)
Medicine, Cardiology, Vascular and Endovascular Medicine,
Loyola University Medical Center, Maywood, IL, USA

© Springer International Publishing Switzerland 2017
R.S. Dieter et al. (eds.), *Critical Limb Ischemia*, DOI 10.1007/978-3-319-31991-9_55

Fig. 55.1 Multidisciplinary
approach to critical limb
ischemia

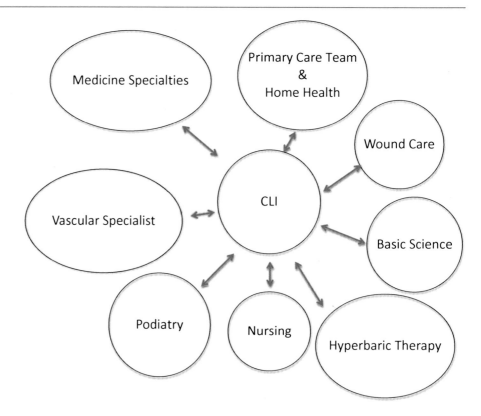

will require endovascular or surgical revascularization. Endovascular therapies have epitomized the overlap of a therapy offered by different disciplines. Rather than interdepartmental conflicts, working together enhances patient care and creates a collaborative learning environment that benefits all. Critical limb ischemia is one end of the spectrum of cardiovascular disease—an extreme with incredibly sick patients. Rather than focusing on our differences, combined programs recognize our common grounds so that these patients are appropriately recognized and treated.

Definition, Incidence, and Epidemiology of Critical Limb Ischemia

Critical limb ischemia may develop consequent to a number of acute or chronic processes including trauma, vascular, or malignant processes that endanger the viability of the extremity. Chronic limb ischemia contributes to significant morbidity and mortality; it is estimated to account for more than 400,000 hospitalizations in the United States every year. It also carries a 20 % annual mortality [2]. The various degrees of limb ischemia—acute, subacute, or chronic—are a growing problem in United States secondary to an increase in the aging population who have many comorbidities such as diabetes mellitus, hypertension, atherosclerosis, and end-stage renal disease. The afflicted require appropriate and timely intervention to salvage the patient and the extremity after appropriate pre-intervention review.

Multidisciplinary Approach for Treating Patients with CLI Secondary to Obstructive Arterial Disease

Ideal therapy for peripheral arterial occlusive disease is yet to be determined. Standard surgical therapy has been bypass for those patients who have tissue loss or rest pain. However, since the advent of endovascular therapy, minimally invasive therapy has been replacing open revascularization in most institutions. These interventions are only advised after initial noninterventional diagnostic approaches, treatment of any underlying processes (such as infection, edema, wound care, nutritional status, etc.), and appropriate consideration and treatment of non-arterial contributors to the CLI.

In a comparative study between open surgical revascularization and endovascular therapies for femoropopliteal occlusive disease in patients with no previous intervention, surgical bypass for the primary treatment of claudication showed improved freedom from restenosis and symptom relief despite treatment of more extensive disease, but was associated with increased length of stay and wound infection. Medical therapy with statins has shown improved freedom from restenosis and symptom recurrence overall [3].

Yet the only randomized controlled study comparing the bypass versus the angioplasty in patients with CLI is the "Bypass versus Angioplasty in Severe Ischemia of the Leg" [4]. This study concluded that there is no initial difference between angioplasty and open surgery arms regarding the amputation-free survival or overall survival. However after 2 years, patients with surgery did better than angioplasty. Secondary analysis of the same study indicated that both failed endovascular and prosthetic bypass grafts were predictors of failure after intervention. This further points out the need to justify initial intervention and whether it should be delayed or performed as well as the need for further study.

In a retrospective study to evaluate the efficacy of endovascular therapies in recurrent femoropopliteal occlusive disease, this study concluded that second-time femoropopliteal angioplasty/stenting has excellent technical success but limited midterm primary and secondary patency. Early failure of the initial endovascular intervention strongly predicts poor outcome and in this cohort was more significant than comorbidities, anatomic factors, or procedural characteristics. These data suggest that after early endovascular failure, alternatives to a continued endoluminal strategy should be adopted [5]. Although endovascular therapy allows for a less invasive approach, the clinician must be open minded to surgical revascularization when symptoms warrant.

Flush ostial occlusion of the SFA may contribute to significant challenge to the vascular specialist; Hayes et al. found that a combined femoral endarterectomy and endovascular femoral-popliteal stent grafting provides a viable option for revascularization of flush SFA occlusions utilizing only a minimal groin incision [6]. This highlights the necessity to approach revascularization in an open-minded, multidisciplinary approach.

According to the Trans-Atlantic Inter-Society Consensus (TASC) II guidelines, lesions can be classified according to their complexity. These provide a common recommendation to confer endovascular treatment to TASC II A and B lesions. With increasing experience, there is an ongoing expansion of the indications and utilization of endovascular therapies in TASC II C and D. Sidhu et al. evaluated 120 patients with TASC II C/D lesions intervened upon and found the technical success was 91 %. Primary patency at 6 and 12 months was 90 % and 73 %. Secondary patency at 6 and 12 months was 94 % and 85 %. The long-term amputation-free survival was 90 % with limb salvage rate of 98 % at 1 year. The authors concluded that endovascular treatment for TASC C/D lesions is a safe procedure and may be considered an alternative to bypass, especially in high-risk patients [7]. Once again, this highlights the necessity to look at patients in a cross-disciplinary manner to optimize patient care.

Chronic Venous Ulceration

The prevalence of chronic venous ulcers (CVU) is underestimated. It affects more than 600,000 people annually in the United States. In the general population, the prevalence of CVU is estimated to be 2 % and increasing, as it is more common in the population >65 years [8]. In addition, it contributes to a significant socioeconomic burden in our society as it accrues treatment costs of US$2.5–5 billion per year [8, 9].

Risk factors for CVU include age, heredity, female sex, and obesity [10]. The underlying pathophysiology of CVU is a complex interplay between many pathological factors such as chronic DVTs, venous hypertension (valvular dysfunction and varicosities), chronic dermal inflammation with subsequent lipodermatosclerosis, and cellular dysfunction secondary to cytokine and matrix metalloproteinase (MMP) activation [10].

Besides compression and elevation, the main therapy to treat venous hypertension is multidisciplinary. Patients require elevation, wound care, compression stockings, or Unna boots; some require venous ablation and nutritional support. For example, one of our patients was admitted to the hospital 6 times due to recurrent infected ulceration. Once she accepted periodic leg elevation and night time elevation of the foot of the bed, the ulcers never recurred.

Additionally, venous ablation helps with wound care and reduction in ulcer recurrence [11]. The long-term corner stone element of treating CVU is elevation and to maintain compression therapy to reduce venous stasis. The ESCHAR trial showed that superficial venous surgery and compression is equivalent to compression alone for wound healing but superior regarding CVU recurrence. In CVU, combined therapy achieved a 24-week healing rate of 65 % and 12-month recurrence rate of 12 % ($p < 0.0001$) [12]. The same authors in another trial reported that superficial venous surgery also resulted in a significant hemodynamic benefit for limbs with CVU despite coexistent deep reflux and residual saphenous reflux being common [13]. Others have related CVU to an increase in the compartment pressure. Within a 4-year period, 58 patients with 70 CVU were evaluated with superficial venous ablation plus subcutaneous fasciotomy, and it was found that this approach can expedite ulcer healing and decrease recurrence especially in patients without the postphlebitic syndrome [14]. Further, negative pressure wound therapy (NPWT) may play a role in wound healing, stimulation, and possibly preparing the ulcers for the next treatment therapy such as artificial or autogenous skin graft [15].

Diabetic Ulcers/Diabetic Neuropathy

There is no doubt that diabetes mellitus with its possible complications is a major contributor to leg and foot ulcer formation. The natural history of diabetic neuropathy is a progressive and irreversible loss of sensitivity in the feet. As such, it is crucial to remember the multidisciplinary approach to the diabetic patient—to involve podiatry, endocrinology, and other disciplines, highlighting the fact that diabetic foot ulcers are the consequence of multiple factors including peripheral neuropathy, decreased blood supply, and high plantar pressures. [16].

Basic Science

Whatever the reasons for the development of the leg ulcer, continued study into causes and treatments is necessary. For example, better dietary treatment of diabetes and atherosclerotic risk factors is a cornerstone to nutritional support. The role of gene therapy and growth factors for angiogenesis and wound healing is evolving. It is through basic science and benchtop/translational research that we have a better understanding of how to treat our patients, ultimately in a less invasive and more efficient manner.

In conclusion, it is only through a multidisciplinary approach to the patient and the wound that the ulceration will be adequately healed and associated mortality reduced.

References

1. Serra R, et al. Low molecular weight heparin improves healing of chronic venous ulcers especially in the elderly. Int Wound J. 2013;12:150–3.
2. Conrad MF, et al. Intermediate results of percutaneous endovascular therapy of femoropopliteal occlusive disease: a contemporary series. J Vasc Surg. 2006;44(4):762–9.
3. Siracuse JJ, et al. Long-term results for primary bypass versus primary angioplasty/stent for intermittent claudication due to superficial femoral artery occlusive disease. J Vasc Surg. 2012;55:1001–7.
4. Conte MS. Bypass versus angioplasty in severe ischaemia of the leg (BASIL) and the (hoped for) dawn of evidence-based treatment for advanced limb ischemia. J Vasc Surg. 2010;51(5):69S–75S.
5. Robinson 3rd WP, et al. Results of second-time angioplasty and stenting for femoropopliteal occlusive disease and factors affecting outcomes. J Vasc Surg. 2011;53(3):651–7.
6. Hayes Jr DJ, Dougherty MJ, Calligaro KD. Management of flush superficial femoral artery occlusions with combined open femoral endarterectomy and endovascular femoral-popliteal angioplasty and stent-grafting. Ann Vasc Surg. 2011;25(4):559.e19–23.
7. Sidhu R, et al. Subintimal angioplasty for advanced lower extremity ischemia due to TASC II C and D lesions of the superficial femoral artery. Vasc Endovascular Surg. 2010;44(8):633–7.
8. McDaniel JC, Roy S, Wilgus TA. Neutrophil activity in chronic venous leg ulcers—a target for therapy? Wound Repair Regen. 2013;21(3):339–51.
9. Serra R, et al. Doxycycline speeds up healing of chronic venous ulcers. Int Wound J. 2013;12:179–84.
10. Raffetto JD. Inflammation in chronic venous ulcers. Phlebology. 2013;28(1):61–7.
11. Sufian S, Lakhanpal S, Marquez J. Superficial vein ablation for the treatment of primary chronic venous ulcers. Phlebology. 2011;26(7):301–6.
12. Barwell JR, et al. Comparison of surgery and compression with compression alone in chronic venous ulceration (ESCHAR study): randomised controlled trial. Lancet. 2004;363(9424):1854–9.
13. Gohel MS, et al. Randomized clinical trial of compression plus surgery versus compression alone in chronic venous ulceration (ESCHAR study)—haemodynamic and anatomical changes. Br J Surg. 2005;92(3):291–7.
14. Christenson JT, Prins C, Gemayel G. Subcutaneous fasciotomy and eradication of superficial venous reflux for chronic and recurrent venous ulcers: mid-term results. Phlebology. 2011;26(5):197–202.
15. Kieser DC, et al. Negative pressure wound therapy as an adjunct to compression for healing chronic venous ulcers. J Wound Care. 2011;20(1):35–7.
16. Kavitha KV, et al. Choice of wound care in diabetic foot ulcer: a practical approach. World J Diabetes. 2014;5(4):546–56.

Appropriate Endpoints for Chronic Limb Ischemia

56

Dustin Y. Yoon, Alejandro Garza, and Heron E. Rodriguez

Introduction

Chronic limb ischemia due to peripheral arterial disease (PAD) remains one of the most common yet challenging clinical issues encountered by vascular specialists. The manifestations of chronic limb ischemia vary in its spectrum, and it remains a challenge for clinicians to quantify the extent of local and systemic disease, degree of impairment, treatment plan and postoperative surveillance and outcomes. The traditional methods of assessing outcomes and quality of care in patients with limb ischemia are ambiguous and lack comprehensiveness. Limb salvage, 30-day mortality, and patency rates are finite and only represent a small fraction of "successful" and meaningful endpoints. Because of the chronicity of chronic limb ischemia and the need for continual surveillance and monitoring, there are both short- and long-term endpoints in anatomic, physiologic, and functional outcomes (Table 56.1).

Anatomical Endpoints

There is significant heterogeneity in the vascular literature regarding the clinical response to endovascular and surgical therapy. The revised Society for Vascular Surgery Lower Extremity Ischemia Reporting Standards [1] accentuates the need for uniform and cogent criteria in evaluating "successful" outcomes for limb ischemia. Critical limb ischemia is categorized according to the following symptoms: asymptomatic disease; mild, moderate, or severe claudication; ischemic rest pain; and minor or major tissue loss. The most

commonly used measurement of clinical response combines clinical and noninvasive testing in examining the resolution of symptoms, such as an increase in the Rutherford scale with an increase in the ankle-brachial index (ABI) of 0.15 or greater. The revised guidelines, however, still lack the functional outcomes of interventions and should be used only as part of a comprehensive evaluation.

Technical Success Measure

Most vascular interventionalists would generally agree that the technical success of an intervention is the presence of antegrade flow through a treated lesion at the conclusion of a procedure. This can be measured semi-objectively through palpation of distal pulses and Doppler flow, duplex scanning, angioscopy, and most frequently completion angiography. Angiography is typically the simplest, most effective, and widely used measure of technical success. Unlike Doppler flow, intraoperative duplex scanning, and angioscopy, angiography can rapidly evaluate the conduit, tunnel, proximal and distal anastomoses, and outflow for graft-threatening lesions with relatively

Table 56.1 Endpoints for chronic limb ischemia

Anatomical endpoints
Angiographic success
Technical success: visual inspection, palpable pulse, and Doppler flow
Graft patency: primary, assisted primary, and secondary
Target lesion revascularization
Physiological endpoints
Ankle-brachial index and toe pressures
Transcutaneous oxygen measurements
Functional endpoints
Wound healing
Amputation-free survival
Return to ambulation
Quality-of-life questionnaires

D.Y. Yoon, MD • H.E. Rodriguez, MD (✉)
Division of Vascular Surgery, Northwestern University Feinberg School of Medicine, Chicago, IL 60626, USA

A. Garza, MD
Division of Plastic Surgery, Northwestern University Feinberg School of Medicine, Chicago, IL, USA

© Springer International Publishing Switzerland 2017
R.S. Dieter et al. (eds.), *Critical Limb Ischemia*, DOI 10.1007/978-3-319-31991-9_56

minimal contrast, time, and increased user-friendliness. Mills et al. prospectively evaluated 214 consecutive infrainguinal bypass grafts (209 reversed vein and five PTFE) with the use of visual inspection, pulse palpation, Doppler flow patterns, and completion angiography. Their group identified 8 % significant lesions requiring revision with angiography, with a higher incidence in tibial than popliteal reconstructions [2].

Graft Patency

Graft patency, although with a wide range of definitions, is an objectively measured outcome. It is described as primary, assisted primary, or secondary patency rates. Primary patency describes a continuously patent graft without any intervention to itself directly. This definition varies in the endovascular literature since the native artery was patent before treatment; thus, most include recurrent stenosis in this patency rate, which is usually 50 % restenosis [3]. Other reported measures of primary patency have included duplex ultrasound-obtained velocity ratios >2.4 or ABI decreases >0.15 [4]. Assisted primary patency describes patency after an intervention, whether endovascular or open, to maintain patency without an occlusive event. Stenotic lesions found after primary intervention and treated by endovascular means have the same low morbidity as those "de novo" lesions treated with primary endovascular therapy [5]. Lastly, secondary patency describes an occluded graft or vessel in which patency was restored after successful reintervention. Thus, overall, primary patency reflects the durability and technical success of the initial bypass graft or endovascular procedure, assisted primary patency reflects the impact of surveillance and appropriate reintervention before occlusion, and secondary patency reflects the timing of intervention and efforts of the surgeon in restoring patency after occlusion. The use of patency rates in terms of successful outcomes should be used with caution, however, as it does not correlate well with limb preservation. For example, Smith et al. [6] found that 10 % of patients who underwent lower extremity bypass did not improve clinically despite having a patent graft at 1 year postoperatively.

Target Lesion Revascularization

Target lesion revascularization (TLR) is typically used to define a reintervention performed on a recurrent lesion within 5 mm of the lesion treated during the index procedure. Similarly, target vessel revascularization characterizes any repeat intervention on the same vessel as the index procedure. Although the concept of TLR was first used to assess the safety, efficacy, and durability of percutaneous interventions, it has been shown to be a surrogate endpoint of patency with no direct correlation with healing, function, and limb preservation. It can also overestimate the efficacy of the

index reintervention since patients may elect not to undergo surgery for mild symptoms, such as claudication. Thus, the usage of TLR as an endpoint is typically less accurate than patency rates.

Physiological Endpoints

Physiologic testing is another objective method of obtaining changes in outcomes. Noninvasive testing, such as the ankle-brachial index (ABI) and toe pressures, has become the preferred method of monitoring progression of disease and revascularization procedures for restenosis. It can provide information about new or existing lesions; it may predict the ability of ischemic ulcers to heal and provides guidance for the optimal level of amputation.

Ankle-Brachial Index (ABI)

Measurement of the ABI is the simplest and preferred noninvasive method of detecting lower extremity arterial occlusive disease and its progression. The standard deviation for the ABI is approximately 0.07, so differences of twice this deviation (0.15) represent a significant and clinical difference [7]. The ABI has been validated against angiography in the detection of stenoses greater than 50 % [8]. It has also been correlated with an increase in mortality, regardless of whether leg symptoms are present [9].

Transcutaneous Oxygen Measurements (tcPO2)

Measurement in transcutaneous oxygen (tcPO2) is a noninvasive method of determining the partial pressure of oxygen transcutaneously. A small sensor is placed on the skin, and by heating the sensor and skin to 44 °C, local hyperemia results in decreased flow resistance and vasodilation of capillary blood. Several studies have shown that tcPO2 levels have an accuracy of 87–100 % in wound healing [10]. Increases in tcPO2 levels greater than 30 mmHg following lower extremity revascularization are predictive of successful clinical outcomes [11]. In terms of selecting the optimal level of amputation, direct comparisons between segmental pressures, and skin blood flow, tcPO2 levels have been the most accurate predictor of wound healing [12] (Table 56.2).

Functional Endpoints

The traditional methods of assessing outcomes and quality of care in patients with CLI (such as survival and limb salvage) are increasingly noted to be inadequate. Instead,

Table 56.2 Wound healing by noninvasive studies

Study	Threshold (mmHg)	Wound healing (%)	
		Below threshold	Above threshold
SPP	40	10	69
TcPO2	30	14	63
TP	30	12	67
AP	80	11	45

Adapted from Yamada T, et al.: Clinical reliability and utility of skin perfusion pressure measurement in ischemic limbs—comparison with other noninvasive diagnostic methods. *J Vasc Surg.* 2008;47:318, with permission from Elsevier

SPP skin perfusion pressure, *TcPO2* transcutaneous oxygen pressure, *TP* toe pressure, *AP* ankle pressure

functional outcomes, such as maintenance of ambulatory status and independent living status, achievement of healed wound status, avoidance of repeat hospitalizations, and interventions, are being proposed as more meaningful parameters in these patients [13]. The key outcome events for CLI patients are survival, limb preservation, avoidance of reinterventions, and quality of life [14]. Patient-oriented outcome endpoints, such as health-related quality of life and functional status, are essential in defining optimal treatment options for the population of patients with CLI [15].

Wound Healing

Wound healing, which is the time required to achieve complete epithelialization of all lesions, is a major challenge after endovascular or open revascularization [16]. Chung et al. [16] determined that the baseline lesion severity predicted wound healing rather than graft patency and other clinical characteristics (serum albumin level and duration of symptoms). Although most patients with CLI treated with the optimal revascularization procedure healed all wounds and retained their functional status, a significant minority did not heal their wounds and lost ambulatory capacity and independent living status. One-fourth of patients did not achieve wound healing at 1 year of follow-up, 19 % had lost ambulatory function, and 5 % had lost independent living status.

Goshima et al. [17] attempted to define the expenditure of effort, complications, and difficulties encountered by the patient and the surgical team to achieve limb salvage in the early and intermediate postoperative period. They analyzed three specific, nontraditional outcomes measures: (1) reoperation within 3 months, (2) readmission in the first 6 months after the index revascularization, and (3) time to complete wound healing. Hospital readmissions within 6 months were required in 49.3 % of patients. Less than half of those patients presenting with ischemic tissue loss achieved complete wound healing within a 3-month period. In this study, diabetes proved to be the dominant risk factor for the prolonged wound healing. The pathophysiologic relationship between

diabetes and impaired wound healing is complex, but vascular, neuropathic, immunogenic, and biochemical abnormalities all contribute to a diminished capacity for tissue repair [18]. Diabetic patients, particularly those with renal failure, often suffer nonhealing wounds despite patent, functional bypass grafts. Numerous studies have suggested that the presence of renal failure interferes with wound healing. In the present report, although renal failure was a major risk factor for repeat operation and readmissions, it was not a major risk factor for prolonged wound healing. In a study published by Johnson et al. [19], failure of foot salvage in renal failure patients was related to poor wound healing, such as ongoing ischemia or uncontrollable infection, despite a functional graft. These patients may ultimately require major limb amputation despite ongoing graft patency [20]. Elderly patients with preoperative ambulatory impairment, dementia, and end-stage renal disease often achieved very little improvement in their functional performance after successful revascularization, regardless of whether the treatment was percutaneous or open bypass [21].

Conte and authors [14] state that patients with CLI and nonhealing wounds incur pain, disability, and extensive treatments that may be dramatically relieved by effective revascularization. Wound healing is an important measure of clinical success, but is fraught with difficulties as a clinical trial endpoint. They suggested that wound care guidelines should be established by protocol to provide uniform care for all subjects in a trial where healing is an endpoint. Ulcers should be photographed at baseline; 3, 6, and 12 months posttreatment; and prior to revascularization or major amputation. An independent core laboratory should review the size of ischemic ulcers at baseline and an independent observer (physician) should confirm the complete healing of the target ulcers posttreatment. The duration of complete healing as confirmed by the outside observer should be at least 2 weeks.

Limb-threatening ischemia frequently results in chronic ischemic ulcers, or areas of gangrene, the healing of which is one of the goals of limb salvage surgery. If healing of wounds and preservation of ambulation do not accompany the preservation of ischemic limbs by revascularization, then successful limb salvage has little meaning in functional terms [22].

Amputation-Free Survival

Outcome measures such as survival or amputation-free survival (AFS) have also been widely used [13]. AFS is defined as the time between initial revascularization and either major amputation or death and is also known as cumulative palliation.

The primary goal of revascularization in advanced limb ischemia is preservation of a functional limb in a surviving patient. Thus, AFS is a critical outcome measure and an appropriate endpoint for randomized controlled trials [23]. In the Bypass versus Angioplasty in Severe Ischemia of the Leg (BASIL) trial [23], the authors studied survival and complications comparing the two limb revascularization strategies. A key limitation of AFS as a primary endpoint was that most events occurred within the first 2 years, and two-thirds were mortality events that were unlikely related to the ischemic leg of interest. The use of AFS as the primary endpoint is that it ignores clinical events that are of major importance to the patient and directly attributable to the initial procedure, namely, reinterventions. The difficulty with reinterventions, as pointed out by the BASIL authors, is the challenge of incorporating the magnitude and frequency of these events into an integrated outcome measure and the influence of surgical decision-making on the timing and need for secondary procedures. Established approaches for surveillance and reintervention of vein grafts on one hand and the lack of any consensus in this regard for endovascular therapies on the other further confound comparison of open vs. endovascular treatment. These issues notwithstanding studies comparing revascularization strategies should measure and report on reintervention-free survival, as well as the magnitude and number of reinterventions per limb saved [23].

Limb revascularization procedures have inherent risks including mortality, but they are not intended to improve survival. Therefore, endpoints that correlate limb-related outcomes and patient survival over time such as AFS are compromised as measures of effectiveness for revascularization. Patient selection factors (comorbidities and demographics) which are strongly associated with survival will greatly influence such endpoints. It is crucial to consider both limb-specific and survival-related endpoints, especially in nonrandomized comparisons [14].

Return to Ambulation

Limb salvage surgery aims to maintain patient ambulatory status and, more importantly, potential for independent living. Patient mobility strongly correlates with perception of health and is preferable to primary amputation in the financial cost as well [22].

A retrospective analysis by Abou-Zamzam et al. [22] examined the goals of maintaining independent living and ambulation in those undergoing revascularization procedures for limb salvage. The study demonstrated that lower extremity revascularization resulted in satisfactory functional outcomes consisting of independent living and ambulation in more than 96% of surviving patients evaluated at 6 months after surgery. Not surprisingly, preoperative living status and ability to ambulate were the most important factors predictive of functional outcome. The operative mortality rate was acceptably low at 2.7%, but the postoperative survival rate was 48% at 5 years after surgery, emphasizing morbidity of the patient undergoing surgery.

Patients who are nonambulatory or nursing home residents with renal insufficiency before the occurrence of limb-threatening ischemia experience little improvement in functional status after successful revascularization and have poor long-term survival rates.

Taylor et al. [24] retrospectively evaluated similar functional outcomes at 5 years in 1000 patients undergoing surgical revascularization for CLI. Ambulatory and living status were evaluated and correlated with traditional outcome measures of graft patency, limb salvage, and survival. Not surprisingly, 5-year overall graft patency (72.4%) and limb salvage (72.1%) were excellent, with a low 5-year survival (41.9%). Independent ambulatory (70.6%) and living status (81.3%) were maintained postoperatively, but with preoperative impaired ambulatory status at presentation and dementia, these factors were predictive of poor functional outcomes. The anatomic location and type of reconstruction did not predict functional outcomes, nor did other associated comorbidities such as age, diabetes, history of coronary artery disease, or renal failure.

Chung and colleagues [16] showed in their infrainguinal bypass group that approximately 20% of patients did not return to their preoperative level of ambulation and 5% of patients did not return to independent living status 6 months postoperatively. There was a correlation between lesion severity and ambulatory status at 1 month: patients who presented with mild pedal necrosis were more likely to ambulate at 6 months than those who presented with severe pedal necrosis. It was not surprising that more severe pedal necrosis at baseline inversely correlated with subsequent ambulatory function.

While reintervention and amputation are clinical events indicative of revascularization failure, the approach to surveillance and objective findings of hemodynamic failure drive the decision to perform reintervention. These events thus link only indirectly to the sustained effectiveness of the original procedure [14]. Differences in criteria for reintervention can greatly influence clinical endpoints while masking important differences in therapeutic benefit. Conversely, long-term hemodynamic success may not be required in all patients to achieve meaningful clinical benefit in CLI. In either case, some measure of sustained hemodynamic improvement is intrinsically important in the evaluation of limb revascularization procedures. No single efficacy endpoint captures the full impact of revascularization in CLI. It is necessary to assess efficacy of revascularization at both limb and patient levels, and this is incompletely measured by clinical events such as amputation or reintervention [14].

Limb salvage will continue to be the overriding goal for most patients referred for vascular therapy, but amputation clearly better serves a subset of patients with CLI. Unfortunately, it is not always clear ahead of time which patients will benefit from primary amputation vs. attempted limb salvage with revascularization [15].

Nehler et al. [21] demonstrated that at 1 year after amputation, 65 % of below-knee amputees were ambulatory, with approximately half of these only ambulatory indoors. Only 29 % of above-knee amputees were ambulatory, with two-thirds of these only ambulatory indoors. Thus, for patients to have any hope of returning to ambulatory status, preserving the knee joint is critical. Although the goal of amputation is generally to rehabilitate the patients to ambulate with prosthesis, many amputees never reach independent ambulatory status [15].

Quality-of-Life Questionnaires

Quality of life (QOL) is an important outcome measure for interventions designed to improve health and overall well-being. In the assessment of patients with lower limb ischemia, outcomes examining ABIs, walking distance, amputation, and death have only recently been augmented by QOL measures. Over recent years, a wide variety of different assessment tools have been used, including, but not limited to, Short Form-36 (SF-36), the Nottingham Health Profile, and the Sickness Impact Profile. Recently, many centers have suggested that the SF-36 be used as a standard instrument in vascular studies, although it has been recommended that this should be accompanied by a disease-specific measure [25].

Generalized questionnaires, such as the Short Form-36 (SF-36) and Nottingham Health Profile (NHP), are advantageous in assessing overall quality of life and are applicable across multiple disease states. The SF-36 addresses eight health concepts: vitality, physical functioning, pain, general health perceptions, physical, emotional and social role funcitoning and mental health. The NHP covers six types of experience that illness may affect: pain, physical mobility, sleep, emotional reactions, energy, and social isolation [20]. The disadvantage of generic questionnaires is that they are less able to detect small changes related to treatment of specific disease states [25].

In any quality-of-life questionnaire, validity is the most important attribute: it must measure what it is supposed to measure [26]. It should also detect those components of QOL relevant to vascular disease [27]. Patient assessment of quality of life is an important element of functional outcome assessment inconsistently defined in patients undergoing interventions for CLI [15]. A major weakness of health-related quality-of-life questionnaire studies is that they rely on patient perceptions rather than objectively measuring performance [15]. QOL is more often used in claudication, since it is difficult to obtain CLI patients due to the severity of their illnesses.

Society for Vascular Surgery's Objective Performance Goals

Using aggregate data from randomized trials of lower extremity bypass, the Society for Vascular Surgery developed objective performance goals (OPGs) in order to standardize the measurement of outcomes after lower extremity revascularization [14]. Although initially thought to serve as objective outcome measures of new catheter-based therapies, OPGs have been validated in everyday vascular surgery practice and have been recommended as outcome measurements for quality improvement initiatives as well as clinical trials [28]. The SVS OPGs include safety goals like major adverse limb event (MALE) and major adverse cardiac event (MACE) as well as efficacy goals like limb salvage and amputation-free survival.

Society for Vascular Surgery's Objective Performance Goals for the Evaluation for Critical Limb Ischemia

Safety OPGs at 30 days

Major adverse limb event (MALE): amputation, major reintervention defined as placement of a new bypass graft, use of thrombectomy or thrombolysis, and major surgical revision

Major adverse cardiac event (MACE): MI, stroke, or death

Efficacy OPGs at 1 year

Freedom from MALE or postoperative death
Limb salvage
Survival
Amputation-free survival
Freedom from reintervention, amputation, or restenosis
Freedom from reintervention or amputation

Adapted from [14] with permission from Elsevier

Conclusion

Technological advancements in the percutaneous treatment of peripheral arterial disease have enabled vascular interventionalists to treat successfully more complex arterial lesions [29]. Because of these improvements, multiple approaches to limb salvage for patients with CLI have been widely adopted by different medical disciplines [30]. Several reports have challenged the adequacy of traditional markers of success for interventions in patients with CLI. Although 70–90 % of patients enjoy primary-assisted graft patency and limb salvage at 1–3 years [31–33], only a minority will obtain the ideal result of a single operative procedure, complete wound healing, resolution of pain, limb preservation, and return to full functional status [17, 34].

The management of patients with critical limb ischemia (CLI) remains complex, with several factors contributing to the treatment decision-making process. The "success" of vascular interventions has been measured solely in terms of mortality, graft patency, and limb salvage rates. However, these traditional measurements underestimate patient morbidity and fail to consider the entire spectrum of treatment that is required to restore patients to their premorbid state [17]. Beyond just mortality, other measures such as QOL, functional status, and resources utilized are critical measures for assessing the effectiveness of vascular care [23].

Outcomes research in CLI is entering a new phase where patient-oriented outcomes are replacing traditional surgeon-oriented or lesion-oriented outcomes. A number of questionnaires and objective functional assessments are available, but the optimal method of assessing interventions for critical limb ischemia is not yet defined. This will become increasingly important from a public health standpoint as the population of patients with critical limb ischemia and the number of treatment options for this disease continue to grow [26].

Endpoints can be divided into anatomic, physiological, or functional and either physician or patient reported. Anatomic outcomes are surrogates of clinical success and very poor tools when evaluating the efficacy of intervention in chronic limb ischemia. Physiologic and functional outcomes need to be reported more often in the literature since this will provide a more complete assessment of revascularization success in chronic limb ischemia patients. Comprehensive evaluation of chronic limb ischemia requires total integration of the anatomic, physiologic, and functional outcomes.

References

1. Rutherford RB, Baker JD, Ernst C, Johnston KW, Porter JM, Ahn S, et al. Recommended standards for reports dealing with lower extremity ischemia: revised version. J Vasc Surg. 1997;26(3):517–38.
2. Mills JL, Fujitani RM, Taylor SM. Contribution of routine intraoperative completion arteriography to early infrainguinal bypass patency. Am J Surg. 1992;164(5):506–10. discussion 10-1.
3. Lazaris AM, Tsiamis AC, Fishwick G, Bolia A, Bell PR. Clinical outcome of primary infrainguinal subintimal angioplasty in diabetic patients with critical lower limb ischemia. J Endovasc Ther. 2004;11(4):447–53.
4. Myers KA. Reporting standards and statistics for evaluating intervention. Cardiovasc Surg. 1995;3(5):455–61.
5. DeRubertis BG, Pierce M, Chaer RA, Rhee SJ, Benjeloun R, Ryer EJ, et al. Lesion severity and treatment complexity are associated with outcome after percutaneous infra-inguinal intervention. J Vasc Surg. 2007;46(4):709–16.
6. Simons JP, et al. Failure to achieve clinical improvement despite graft patency in patients undergoing infrainguinal lower extremity bypass for critical limb ischemia. J Vasc Surg. 2010;51:1419–24.
7. Baker JD, Dix DE. Variability of Doppler ankle pressures with arterial occlusive disease: an evaluation of ankle index and brachial-ankle pressure gradient. Surgery. 1981;89(1):134–7.
8. Lijmer JG, Hunink MG, van den Dungen JJ, Loonstra J, Smit AJ. ROC analysis of noninvasive tests for peripheral arterial disease. Ultrasound Med Biol. 1996;22(4):391–8.
9. Feringa HH, Bax JJ, van Waning VH, Boersma E, Elhendy A, Schouten O, et al. The long-term prognostic value of the resting and postexercise ankle-brachial index. Arch Intern Med. 2006;166(5):529–35.
10. Ballard JL, Eke CC, Bunt TJ, Killeen JD. A prospective evaluation of transcutaneous oxygen measurements in the management of diabetic foot problems. J Vasc Surg. 1995;22(4):485–90. discussion 90-2.
11. Bunt TJ, Holloway GA. TcPO2 as an accurate predictor of therapy in limb salvage. Ann Vasc Surg. 1996;10(3):224–7.
12. Malone JM, Anderson GG, Lalka SG, Hagaman RM, Henry R, McIntyre KE, et al. Prospective comparison of noninvasive techniques for amputation level selection. Am J Surg. 1987;154(2):179–84.
13. Cronenwett JL, Johnston KW. Rutherford's vascular surgery. In: York JW, Taylor SM, editors. Decision making for revascularization, vol. 2. 8th ed. Philadelphia: Saunders; 2014. p. 1686.
14. Conte MS, Geraghty PJ, Bradbury AW, Hevelone ND, Lipsitz SR, Moneta GL, et al. Suggested objective performance goals and clinical trial design for evaluating catheter-based treatment of critical limb ischemia. J Vasc Surg. 2009;50(6):1462-73.e1-3.
15. Landry GJ. Functional outcome of critical limb ischemia. J Vasc Surg. 2007;45:141A–8A.
16. Chung J, Bartelson BB, Hiatt WR, Peyton BD, McLafferty RB, Hopley CW, et al. Wound healing and functional outcomes after infrainguinal bypass with reversed saphenous vein for critical limb ischemia. J Vasc Surg. 2006;43:1183–90.
17. Goshima KR, et al. A new look at outcomes after infrainguinal bypass surgery: traditional reporting standards systematically underestimate the expenditure of effort required to attain limb salvage. J Vasc Surg. 2004;29:330–5.
18. Greenhalgh DG. Wound healing and diabetes mellitus. Clin Plast Surg. 2003;30:37–45.
19. Johnson BL, Glickman MH, Bandyk DF, Esses GE. Failure of foot salvage in patients with end-stage renal disease after surgical revascularization. J Vasc Surg. 1995;22:280–5.
20. Edwards JM, Taylor LM, Porter JM. Limb salvage in end-stage renal disease. Comparison of modern results in patients with and without ESRD. Arch Surg. 1988;123:1164–8.
21. Nehler MR, et al. Functional outcome in a contemporary series of major lower extremity amputations. J Vasc Surg. 2003;38:704–8.
22. Abou-Zamzam Jr AM, Lee RW, Moneta GL, Taylor Jr LM, Porter JM. Functional outcome after infrainguinal bypass for limb salvage. J Vasc Surg. 1997;25:287–95.
23. Conte MS. Bypass versus Angioplasty in Severe Ischaemia of the Leg (BASIL) and the (hoped for) dawn of evidence-based treatment for advanced limb ischemia. J Vasc Surg. 2010;51(5S):69S–75S.
24. Taylor SM, Kalbaugh CA, Blackhurst DW, Cass AL, Trent EA, Langan EM, et al. Determinants of functional outcome after

revascularization for critical limb ischemia: an analysis of 1000 consecutive vascular interventions. J Vasc Surg. 2006;44:747–56.

25. Litwin MS. Health-related quality of life. In: Penson DF, Wei JT, editors. Clinical research methods for surgeons. Totowa, NJ: Human Press; 2006. p. 237–53.

26. Morgan MBF, et al. Developing the vascular quality of life questionnaire: a new disease-specific quality of life measure for use in lower limb ischemia. J Vasc Surg. 2001;33:679–87.

27. Beattie DK, Golledge J, Greenhalgh RM, Davies AH. Quality of life assessment in vascular disease: towards a consensus. Eur J Vasc Endovasc Surg. 1997;13:9–13.

28. Goodney PP, Schanzer A, Demartino RR, Nolan BW, Hevelone ND, Conte MS, et al. Validation of the Society for Vascular Surgery's objective performance goals for critical limb ischemia in everyday vascular surgery practice. J Vasc Surg. 2011;54(1):100-8.e4.

29. Kalbaugh CA, et al. One-year prospective quality-of-life outcomes in patients treated with angioplasty for symptomatic peripheral arterial disease. J Vasc Surg. 2006;44:296–302.

30. Veith FJ, Gupta SK, Wengerter KR, Goldsmith J, Rivers SP, Bakal CW, et al. Changing arteriosclerotic disease patterns and management strategies in lower-limb-threatening ischemia. Ann Surg. 1994;212:402–14.

31. Feinglass J, Pearce WH, Martin GJ, Gibbs J, Cowper D, Sorensen M, et al. Postoperative and amputation-free survival outcomes after femorodistal bypass grafting surgery: findings from the Department of Veterans Affairs National Surgical Quality Improvement Program. J Vasc Surg. 2001;34:283–90.

32. Chew DK, Conte MS, Donaldson MC, Whittemore AD, Mannick JA, Belkin M. Autogenous composite vein bypass graft for infrainguinal arterial reconstruction. J Vasc Surg. 2001;33:259–64.

33. Taylor Jr LM, Hamre D, Dalman RL, Porter JM. Limb salvage vs amputation for critical ischemia. The role of vascular surgery. Arch Surg. 1991;126:1251–7.

34. Nicoloff AD, Taylor Jr LM, McLafferty RB, Moneta GL, Porter JM. Patient recovery after infrainguinal bypass grafting for limb salvage. J Vasc Surg. 1998;27:256–63.

Economic Burden of Chronic Critical Limb Ischemia

Taishi Hirai, Benjamin Ross Weber, John P. Pacanowski, Jr., Miguel F. Montero Baker, and Raymond A. Dieter, IV

Resources Utilized for Treatment of Critical Limb Ischemia

Diagnosis of critical limb ischemia (CLI) is important given the high morbidity and mortality associated with the disease [1]. Once the diagnosis is confirmed, the goals of treatment are to relieve ischemic pain, heal ischemic ulcers, prevent limb loss, improve patient function and quality of life, and prolong survival. Revascularization, whether by surgical bypass or endovascular treatment, should be offered to patients with CLI if the procedure can be tolerated.

Consideration of cost-effectiveness in the management of CLI is important for two reasons. First, care for these patients is costly and laborious [2]. Second, with an aging population in the USA as well as an increasing incidence of diabetes, the incidence of CLI is expected to increase [3].

Multiple resources are utilized for treatment of critical limb ischemia. After confirmatory testing for CLI, the patient needs to be optimized for modifiable risk factors such as smoking cessation, lifestyle modification, and pharmacotherapy [1]. Revascularization, either surgical bypass or percutaneous intervention, is considered first-line therapy if a patient is a suitable candidate. Wound care is utilized along with medical therapy if the patient is stable with uncomplicated tissue loss. Amputation should be performed if a limb is deemed unsalvageable. In addition, rehabilitation and limb prosthesis are necessary in amputees [2]. Management of amputees requires prolonged, longitudinal care. Marston et al. reported a subset of patients with CLI with uncomplicated tissue loss who underwent medical management [4]. Ulcer healing was slow, with only 25% healed at 6 months and slightly more than 50% at 1 year. According to a recent report, independent predictors for increased health-care service utilization include older age, female gender, care at the private hospital, longer length of hospitalization, African American race, highest income quartile, and undergoing amputation or debridement [5].

Medications for Treatment of Critical Limb Ischemia

The goals of treatment for peripheral artery disease are to prevent future major coronary and cerebrovascular events and improve leg symptoms [6]. Risk factor modifications, including smoking cessation, exercise, statins, and antihypertensive medications, are known to improve symptoms in peripheral vascular disease. Smoking cessation, blood pressure control, blood sugar control, weight loss, and antiplatelet therapy are important to prevent future vascular events [6].

More specifically, these medical treatment options have also been demonstrated to be effective in the subpopulation with critical limb ischemia (CLI). Shanzer et al. demonstrated the effect of statin use on survival in critical limb ischemia patients [3]. Performing a propensity score matching comparison using the PREVENT III trial population, the investigators found survival advantage at 1 year of 86% vs. 81% (Hazard ratio 0.71; CI 0.52–0.90; $p = 0.001$) in patients who were on statins. Chung et al. demonstrated that despite existing guidelines recommending optimization of atherosclerotic risk factors such as statins, antihypertensive medications, and antiplatelet agents, less than one-third of patients with CLI presented with their risk factors optimally managed [7]. Underscoring the importance of optimal medical management in this patient population, suboptimal medical management at presentation

T. Hirai, MD
Division of Cardiology, Department of Medicine, Stritch School of Medicine, Loyola University Medical Center, Loyola University Chicago, Maywood, IL 60153, USA

B.R. Weber, MD (✉)
Internal Medicine, University of Chicago, Chicago, IL 60637, USA

J.P. Pacanowski, Jr., MD • M.F. Montero Baker, MD
Vascular Surgery, Pima Vascular, Tucson, AZ 85718, USA

R.A. Dieter, IV, BA
Health Science Center, University of Tennessee, College of Medicine, Memphis, TN 37931, USA

© Springer International Publishing Switzerland 2017
R.S. Dieter et al. (eds.), *Critical Limb Ischemia*, DOI 10.1007/978-3-319-31991-9_57

was an independent predictor of major amputation or death (hazard ratio 8.54; CI 2.05–35.65).

Cost of Treatment for Chronic Critical Limb Ischemia (Endovascular vs. Surgery)

The introduction of endovascular treatment for peripheral vascular disease has led to widespread adoption of minimally invasive percutaneous interventions in the treatment of CLI. Although there are many reported benefits to such an approach compared to traditional bypass surgery, questions remain about their long-term durability and rates of re-intervention [8]. There have been multiple efforts to compare the cost-effectiveness of these two strategies.

The BASIL trial was a randomized controlled trial conducted in the UK that compared outcome of bypass surgery (BSX) and balloon angioplasty (BAP) in patients with severe limb ischemia. The trial showed that in the medium term (1 year), the outcomes after two strategies were broadly similar for amputation free survival (BSX 68 % vs. BAP 71 %). In the cost-effectiveness analysis of the BASIL trial, the mean cost of inpatient hospital treatment during the first 12 months in patients assigned to bypass first strategy was approximately $36,638 (£23,332), compared to approximately $27,364 (£17,419) for angioplasty first [9]. Using the data from BASIL trial, Forbes et al. compared the effect on hospital cost and health-related quality of life (HRQOL) of the BSX first and BAP first strategies [10]. During the first year from randomization, the mean cost of inpatient hospital treatment was $8469 higher in BSX first treatment strategy (BSX $34,378 vs. BAP $25,909). The main difference in costs between the two strategies was related to length of hospital stay, including the greater requirement for patients undergoing BSX to be cared within high dependency units and intensive therapy units. Owing to increased costs subsequently incurred by the BAP patients, the difference decreased to $5521 at the end of follow-up.

Stoner et al. developed cost-efficacy analysis comparing 183 BSX cases to 198 BAP cases. Although the initial cost for BSX was significantly higher compared to BAP cases (BSX $13,277 vs. BAP $7176), the cost-savings of endovascular therapy was ultimately lost at 1 year secondary to subsequent intervention in CLI patients [11].

Finally, Barshes et al. performed a detailed simulation of patient-oriented outcome comparing six strategies: (1) local wound care, (2) primary amputation, (3) bypass with surgical revision, (4) bypass with endovascular revisions, (5) purely endovascular, and (6) endovascular first and bypass for failure. In this study, surgical bypass with endovascular revision as needed was most cost-effective when compared to other management strategies for CLI with tissue loss [2].

In conclusion, there is conflicting evidence providing economic inferences about the relative merits of endovascular

and open surgical approaches to the treatment of CLI [8]. Although endovascular procedures appear less costly in the short term, long-term comparison between catheter-based procedure and open revascularization remains uncertain. Additional research is needed to investigate these uncertainties of cost-effectiveness in CLI.

Cost of Amputation for Chronic Critical Limb Ischemia

Peacock et al. assessed the incidence of ischemic amputation using all inpatient hospital discharge claims in Minnesota from 2005 to 2008 [12]. They reported age-adjusted annual incidence of lower limb ischemic amputation was 20 per 100,000. This was more than half the annual stroke mortality (38.3 per 100,000). The median inflation-adjusted direct inpatient hospital charge was $35,893, which was comparable to the charge for coronary heart disease ($33,321) and was almost twice as high as the inpatient hospital charge for stroke and transient ischemic attack ($17,831).

Cost of Wound Care for Chronic Critical Limb Ischemia

In the cost-effectiveness analysis performed by Barshes et al., the cost of local wound care was estimated to be $21,029/year [2]. The cost for inpatient rehabilitation and/or home health nursing was estimated to be $12,048/year, and cost for residence in nursing home was estimated to be $67,878/year.

Conclusions

Chronic critical limb ischemia is a significant atherosclerotic disease with significant medical and functional consequences. The economic burden of critical limb ischemia is considerable. Although endovascular therapy appears less costly in the short term compared to surgical therapy, long-term comparison remains uncertain. Further research is necessary to investigate cost-effectiveness of various treatment strategies.

References

1. Varu VN, Hogg ME, Kibbe MR. Critical limb ischemia. J Vasc Surg. 2010;51(1):230–41.
2. Barshes NR, Chambers JD, Cohen J, Belkin M. Model to Optimize Healthcare Value in Ischemic Extremities 1 (MOVIE) study collaborators. Cost-effectiveness in the contemporary management of critical limb ischemia with tissue loss. J Vasc Surg. 2012;56(4):1015–24.e1.
3. Schanzer A, Hevelone N, Owens CD, Beckman JA, Belkin M, Conte MS. Statins are independently associated with reduced mortality in patients undergoing infrainguinal bypass graft surgery for critical limb ischemia. J Vasc Surg. 2008;47(4):774–81.

4. Marston WA, Davies SW, Armstrong B, Farber MA, Mendes RC, Fulton JJ, et al. Natural history of limbs with arterial insufficiency and chronic ulceration treated without revascularization. J Vasc Surg. 2006;44(1):108–14.

5. Davies MG. Critical limb ischemia: epidemiology. Methodist Debakey Cardiovasc J. 2012;8(4):10–4.

6. Hankey GJ, Norman PE, Eikelboom JW. Medical treatment of peripheral arterial disease. JAMA. 2006;295(5):547–53.

7. Chung J, Timaran DA, Modrall JG, Ahn C, Timaran CH, Kirkwood ML, et al. Optimal medical therapy predicts amputation-free survival in chronic critical limb ischemia. J Vasc Surg. 2013;58(4):972–80.

8. Moriarty JP, Murad MH, Shah ND, Prasad C, Montori VM, Erwin PJ, et al. A systematic review of lower extremity arterial revascularization economic analyses. J Vasc Surg. 2011;54(4):1131–44.e1.

9. Adam DJ, Beard JD, Cleveland T, Bell J, Bradbury AW, Forbes JF, et al. Bypass versus Angioplasty in Severe Ischaemia of the Leg (BASIL): multicentre, randomised controlled trial. Lancet. 2005;366(9501):1925–34.

10. Forbes JF, Adam DJ, Bell J, Fowkes FG, Gillespie I, Raab GM, et al. Bypass versus Angioplasty in Severe Ischaemia of the Leg (BASIL) trial: Health-related quality of life outcomes, resource utilization, and cost-effectiveness analysis. J Vasc Surg. 2010;51 Suppl 5:43S–51S.

11. Stoner MC, Defreitas DJ, Manwaring MM, Carter JJ, Parker FM, Powell CS. Cost per day of patency: understanding the impact of patency and reintervention in a sustainable model of healthcare. J Vasc Surg. 2008;48(6):1489–96.

12. Peacock JM, Keo HH, Duval S, Baumgartner I, Oldenburg NC, Jaff MR, et al. The incidence and health economic burden of ischemic amputation in Minnesota, 2005–2008. Prev Chronic Dis. 2011;8(6):A141.

The Long-Term Care of Patients with Critical Limb Ischemia (CLI)

Larry J. Diaz-Sandoval

Introduction

Critical limb ischemia (CLI) is synonymous with "end-stage" peripheral artery disease (PAD) and ultimately develops when the capillary beds are inadequately perfused and unable to sustain tissue viability. Several clinical and noninvasive criteria have been used to determine which CLI patients would benefit from revascularization. These include Rutherford categories 4–6, systolic ankle pressure <50 mmHg, non-pulsatile plethysmographic tracing, and/or transcutaneous oxygen pressure <30 mmHg [1, 2]. The European Consensus Conference has also included the need for analgesia for more than 2 weeks as part of the definition [3]. Anatomically, CLI is characterized by multilevel and multivessel infrainguinal and tibial arterial stenoses and occlusions that create a severe imbalance between supply and demand of oxygen in the affected tissues, compromising its viability and threatening limb loss. Although CLI encompasses <5 % of all cases of PAD, its prognosis is poor. The 1-year mortality and major amputation rates range from 20 to 50 % [4–6]. Under less severe circumstances, compensatory mechanisms such as angiogenesis and arteriogenesis [7] are sufficient to overcome the increased demand imposed by the lack of adequate tissue perfusion; however, in patients with CLI, these mechanisms have been exhausted and/or are defective. Inadequate perfusion of the skin and surrounding tissues leads to endothelial dysfunction, chronic inflammation [8], and muscle damage [9–11]. The clinical manifestations of these molecular changes are ischemic rest pain, non-healing ulcerations, and gangrene. A staggering 20–25 % of patients with CLI will undergo primary amputation, 50–60 % undergo revascularization (surgical and/or

endovascular), and 25 % are treated medically [12]. The 5-year mortality rate for populations with CLI is 60 % [13]. Among CLI patients who do not undergo revascularization, approximately 40 % will undergo a major amputation within 6 months and 20 % will die [8]. Observational studies indicate that only about 50 % will be alive without a major amputation at 1 year, 25 % will have died, and 25 % will have required a major amputation. PAD is usually a manifestation of systemic atherosclerosis and is associated with substantial morbidity and mortality both from PAD itself and other atherosclerotic diseases such as myocardial infarction (MI) and stroke. Significant coronary artery disease has been demonstrated in 60–80 % of patients with PAD [14], and hemodynamically significant carotid artery stenoses (by duplex ultrasound) have been demonstrated in 12–25 % [15–17]. The increased risk of MI, stroke, and cardiovascular mortality in patients with PAD is explained by the diffuse nature of the atherosclerotic process, which expands across most, if not all, arterial beds. The annual overall major cardiovascular event rate (MI, ischemic stroke, and vascular death) is approximately 5–7 %. The risk of MI is increased by 20–60 %, whereas the risk of death from coronary artery disease is increased two- to sixfold. The presence of PAD is associated with a 40 % increase in the risk of stroke [18–22].

CLI represents the "point of no return" in the clinical spectrum of the patient with PAD. Medical management has a role in the treatment of risk factors for secondary prevention of cardiovascular disease end points, which are highly prevalent among these patients. However, the role of medical management in treating the symptoms and complications of severe limb hypoperfusion is less well established. Surgery and more recently percutaneous endovascular treatments have become the mainstays of management of CLI, but pharmacological agents can have a role as adjuncts or alternatives in patients who are unsuitable for revascularization or those who have suboptimal results. Newer techniques such as the use of growth factors, gene therapy, and stem cells are being investigated. Management of novel risk factors and new

L.J. Diaz-Sandoval, MD (✉)
Department of Medicine, Metro Health Hospital, Michigan State University, Wyoming, MI, USA

© Springer International Publishing Switzerland 2017
R.S. Dieter et al. (eds.), *Critical Limb Ischemia*, DOI 10.1007/978-3-319-31991-9_58

applications of technology such as spinal cord stimulators are being studied, and the findings of these studies are likely to increase treatment options in the future.

Treatment of CLI

The treatment of patients with CLI is rather complex and the issue is further complicated by the current paradigm. Although the purpose of this chapter is to discuss the long-term care of the patient with CLI, it must be emphasized that the contemporary management of CLI should include a combination of endovascular and surgical revascularization as the mainstay of therapy, complemented by a host of noninterventional therapies. This newly proposed, combined

approach should be delivered in a "continuum of care" model, represented by a *chain* whereby patient care is carried by each one of its *links* or team members. One of the greatest weaknesses, perhaps the "Achilles heel" of our current approach to CLI, is the reigning "disjointment" of the pieces that should conform to the "CLI continuum of care." In this proposed multidisciplinary approach (see Fig. 58.1), the patient first enters "the chain" through any of its constituent links. The first member of the team sees and evaluates the patient and then proceeds with a simultaneous referral to the remainder of the team. In this model, the patient is evaluated by the primary care physician (sometimes an endocrinologist), an infectious disease specialist, a wound care specialist, a podiatrist, occasionally an orthotics specialist as well as a "vascular rehabilitation specialist," and, last but not least,

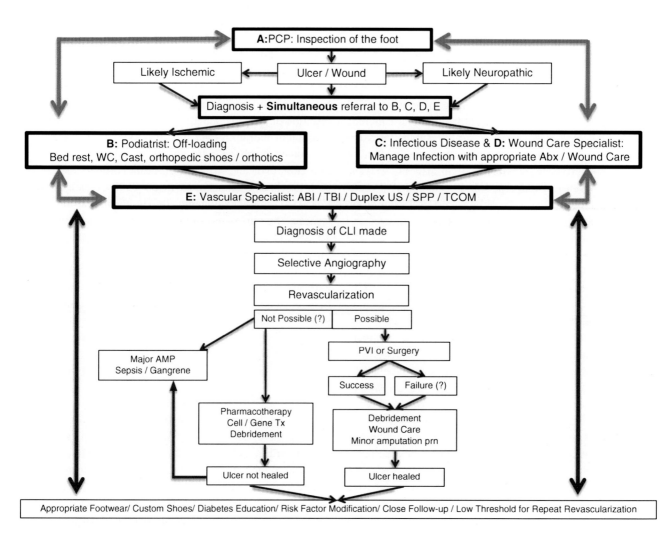

Fig. 58.1 The CLI continuum of care. The figure shows a proposed "chain" model of care for the patient with CLI. The diagnosis is made by any of the members of the team (located in the *dark boxes*). Once this is done, the patient is simultaneously referred to all of the other members of the team, each of which has specific tasks (some of which overlap). The patient ultimately undergoes adequate noninvasive testing, angiography, and revascularization, as well as risk factor modifica-

tion, wound care, and medical therapy. In the minority of cases where revascularization is either not possible or unsuccessful, the patient undergoes minor or major amputation, but is kept in the continuum of care with close follow-up and surveillance by members of the team. At the first signal of decline, stalled progress or recurrence, prompt referral for repeat testing, and revascularization should occur the vascular specialist (either a vascular surgeon with endovascular training and experience, an interventional cardiologist, or an interventional radiologist). The patient then undergoes a series of noninvasive vascular tests in order to diagnose the extent of disease, to plan the therapeutic revascularization strategy, and to serve as baseline for future surveillance studies. Once the patient undergoes complete revascularization (in many instances, this could require up to three or four interventions in the threatened limb), the continuum of care perpetuates. The patient should continue to be followed by all the members of the team to ensure complete healing. Each member should participate in the follow-up and surveillance and should keep a high index of suspicion and an aggressive approach with prompt referral for repeat revascularization, which is of paramount importance since these patients live on a very delicate balance where perfusion is barely able to keep the metabolic needs of "healed" tissue, but will become insufficient if there is another insult to the skin barrier. The currently working system is not designed to function in this manner. Generally, the patient is only referred to the vascular specialist after months of failed wound therapy or repetitive visits to the podiatrist for serial debridements. Only after these traditional modalities have failed is the patient referred to the vascular specialist, in many instances too late. Another weakness of this approach has been the traditional referral to specialists who are not trained in the latest revascularization techniques, and these patients frequently undergo amputations without even to have undergone an angiographic evaluation. In the best of scenarios, the patient is properly referred to a vascular specialist, undergoes appropriate noninvasive and invasive testing, and finally receives adequate revascularization therapy. Among these (unfortunately the minority), only a very small fraction returns for follow-up with the vascular specialist or with any of the other members of the team. Many times they do follow-up with a "wound clinic" which is not affiliated with the system where the vascular specialist performed the intervention and therefore is not familiar with the latest techniques and advances. Thanks to the disjointment, there is no communication of the progress of the patient, and many times when the patient comes back, the situation is worse than it was at the first encounter. Overall, there is a widespread lack of knowledge and attachment to the old ways that needs to be overcome. Unfortunately, data-driven clinical studies to evaluate strategies for surveillance, use, and duration of antiplatelets, anticoagulants, and other risk factor-modifying agents, as well as the use of noninvasive testing, and indications for repeat revascularization in these patients do not exist. Current data has been derived from retrospective studies, with inconsistent reporting standards leading to a paucity of evidence, especially following endovascular revascularization in CLI [23].

Noninterventional therapies have a role as primary treatment in patients who have failed to improve symptoms (despite revascularization) and in patients who are unsuitable or unfit for revascularization, as adjuvant treatment after revascularization procedures, and to reduce the incidence of cardiovascular events.

The goals and pillars of CLI treatment are:

(a) Medical: pain control, reduction of major adverse cardiovascular events, and improvement in quality of life.
(b) Interventional: limb salvage, wound healing, maintenance of ambulatory status (fostering independence and psychological well-being) [11, 24].
(c) Surveillance: close follow-up and monitoring after delivery of treatment and even after healing. At first sign of recurrence or evidence of stalled progress, the patient should once again enter the CLI continuum of care.

The medical goals are tasks that should be led by the primary care physician and endocrinologists. The interventional goals require the active participation of podiatrists, wound care and infectious disease specialists, vascular specialists, and vascular rehabilitation and orthotics specialists. The surveillance goals should be a task of all the members of the team.

Noninterventional therapies for the management of CLI comprise the use of preventive measures, wound care, pharmacotherapy (primary, to treat CLI, and adjuvant, to reduce major adverse cardiovascular events and to improve post-interventional outcomes), biotherapies (cell and gene therapy), and mechanical therapies designed to achieve the goals aforementioned. The stakeholders involved are the patients and the members of the CLI continuum of care, all of whom represent an integral part, a link of the chain that has to be in place in order to improve outcomes.

Prevention

Preventive measures should constitute the cornerstone of managing patients with CLI, especially among patients without tissue loss. Primary prevention efforts should be directed at measures to avoid skin breakdowns. These include skin moisture, adequate footwear/orthotics, adequate toenail care, and education on preventing foot trauma/falls. The role of the primary care physician and podiatrist is primordial at this junction. The patients need to be educated on being proactive and inspecting their feet daily and to contact the team if there is evidence of any new skin breakdown or any change in preexisting wounds. Secondary prevention is of paramount importance and should address smoking cessation, blood pressure and glycemic control, lipid lowering, and antiplatelet agents. Unfortunately, many patients with CLI do not receive and/or do not follow intensive risk factor modification.

Wound Care

Meticulous wound care is critical for patients with CLI and tissue loss. Underlying infection should be treated and necrotic tissue debrided. Antibiotic therapy should target cultured microbial agents within infected wounds. Topical therapies with recombinant growth factors and hyperbaric oxygen are being investigated [25]. If there are wounds present, the wound care specialist (or clinic), the infectious disease specialist, and the vascular specialist should be primarily involved. The repetitive debridement and application of topical therapies without urgently involving the vascular specialist tends to be the norm in current practice in the United States and Latin America. Once again, the simultaneous participation of several members of the team represents one of the cornerstones of a successful strategy to manage the patient with CLI and should be the direction we start to follow. All members of the team should be involved intimately with the CLI patient from the time of diagnosis until complete wound healing has occurred (median time from revascularization to complete wound healing is approximately 190 days) [26, 27]. Female patients tend to have poorer wound healing compared to their male counterparts [28].

Pharmacotherapy

Risk factor modification and optimization of medical therapy is an effort that should be directed by the primary care physician (endocrinologist), the vascular specialist, and the patient (who has to be accountable and "buy in") in order for the program to be successful. There are no medical therapies specifically approved for the treatment of CLI in the United States. Primary pharmacotherapy with cilostazol, prostaglandins, pentoxifylline, and novel agents may play a role. Adjuvant pharmacotherapy is directed to achieve secondary prevention of myocardial infarction and stroke, as well as to improve outcomes after revascularization procedures. These include aggressive medical management of comorbidities such as diabetes, hypertension, and hyperlipidemia.

Cilostazol (Primary and Adjuvant)
Cilostazol is approved in Japan for the management of CLI, including ulceration and pain.

There are no prospective trials evaluating the benefit of cilostazol in CLI. While objective prospective data for the use of cilostazol in CLI are limited, case studies demonstrate successful wound healing in both upper and lower extremity

arterial wounds associated with CLI [29, 30]. Similar to its role in intermittent claudication (IC), the mechanisms by which cilostazol improves tissue perfusion and wound healing in CLI remain elusive. Cilostazol has been shown to improve skin perfusion pressure, suggesting a role in improving microvascular function [31]. In addition, patients with CLI successfully treated with endovascular intervention may benefit from adjunctive cilostazol, as shown by Soga et al. [32], who demonstrated improvement in amputation-free survival (AFS) and limb salvage in patients treated with cilostazol compared with placebo (47.7% vs. 32.7%; $p<0.01$), as well as reduction in binary restenosis, reocclusion, and TLR in patients with infrapopliteal disease treated with angioplasty (PTA) [33].

Pentoxifylline (Primary)
Intravenous pentoxifylline has been compared to placebo in two studies of patients with CLI with conflicting results, as one trial showed improvement in rest pain [34], while the other did not [35]. No further investigations have been performed, and there are no trials investigating the use of the available oral pentoxifylline preparations in patients with CLI.

Prostanoids (Primary)
PGE-1, prostacyclin, iloprost, lipoecaprost, and ciprostene have been studied in CLI. The use of intravenous PGE-1 or iloprost for 7–28 days in patients with CLI currently has an ACC/AHA level IIB recommendation based on level A evidence for the efficacy and safety of the therapy, with the caveat that small numbers of patients are likely to benefit. However, oral iloprost was found to be ineffective and, as such, there is a class III recommendation against use of this agent in CLI [24, 36]. In a recent Cochrane systematic review of 20 trials, a small but statistically significant benefit was seen for prostanoids. This review suggests prostaglandins are generally effective at improving rest pain (RR 1.32, 95% CI 1.10, 1.57) and ulcer healing (RR 1.54, 95% CI 1.22, 1.96). However, the effect on amputations and mortality was not significant [11, 24, 37]. Both low- and high-dose oral iloprost compared with placebo failed to demonstrate significant effects on pain relief, ulcer healing, major amputations, and mortality.

Ace Inhibitors (Ace-I) and Statins (Adjuvant)
In a prospective observational study of 553 consecutive patients with diabetes and CLI undergoing revascularization, therapy with Ace-I and statins was recorded. At 2 years, the life expectancy was improved among patients receiving combined therapy with Ace-I and statins; however, there was no improvement among patients treated with either agent alone [38]. Another retrospective study of patients with CLI undergoing below-the-knee interventions determined that

treatment with statins did not affect overall survival, cardio-vascular death, AFS, limb salvage, or repeat revasculariza-tion at 4 years [39]. However, in another study, amputation rates at 12 months post-PTA improved from 21.1% in patients receiving aspirin alone to 11.1% when lovastatin was used in conjunction with aspirin [40]. These findings could be interpreted in several ways. It could be construed that statins alone do not confer protection against major end points, but used in combination with other therapies, they do exert a protective role. It could also be argued that the type and dose of statins used in these studies were not adequate, which is a consequence of the retrospective nature of the analyses.

Antiplatelets and Statins (Adjuvant)

All patients with PAD and CLI should be considered for anti-platelet therapy to reduce the incidence of cardiovascular events and for their beneficial effect on graft and stent patency. The relative risk of infrainguinal graft occlusion in patients treated with aspirin was 0.78 in one meta-analysis [41]. A recent Cochrane review demonstrated that antiplate-let agents improved graft patency rates to a greater extent in patients with prosthetic grafts compared with those with venous grafts [42]. The use of aspirin is recommended in patients undergoing lower limb PTA [43]. The use of adju-vant dual antiplatelet therapy (DAPT) with clopidogrel and aspirin following below-the-knee bypass graft surgery did not show an improvement in the composite primary end point of index graft occlusion or revascularization, above-ankle amputation, or death compared with aspirin alone. However, the combination did improve outcomes in a sub-group analysis of patients with prosthetic grafts, without sig-nificantly increasing major bleeding rates [44]. A post hoc analysis of the PREVENT III cohort examined the effective-ness of medical therapy including beta blockers, statins, and acetylsalicylic acid in 1404 patients with CLI. The use of statins was associated with a statistically significant survival advantage at 1 year (HR 0.67; 95% CI 0.51–0.90; $p=0.001$) [45]. The daily use of aspirin and statins was associated with a nearly 50% reduction in restenosis (42% vs. 22%) and lower extremity amputation (21% vs. 11%) in patients with Rutherford class IV CLI undergoing percutaneous revascu-larization [46]. The duration of DAPT after revasculariza-tion procedures has not been systematically studied in patients with either IC or CLI. A meta-analysis of studies looking at the use of drug-eluting stents for revasculariza-tion of infrapopliteal arteries found that the mean length of DAPT was 1 year [47].

The most effective postoperative antithrombotic regimen is contentious. Platelet inhibition is preferable following PTA when compared to vitamin K antagonists [48]. Currently, long-term low-dose aspirin or clopidogrel is rec-ommended following PTA, as this has been shown to improve

revascularization patency; however, there is no evidence that this regimen improves outcomes in CLI [49]. Higher doses of aspirin failed to significantly improve patency rates and were associated with higher rates of gastrointestinal side effects [50]. Following successful PTA, patients who received 3 months of dalteparin in addition to low-dose aspirin daily exhibited a reduction in restenosis at 1 year compared to those who only received low-dose aspirin (45% vs. 72%; $p=0.01$). However, the addition of dalte-parin only had a beneficial effect when patients had undergone PTA for CLI; in less severe PAD, the addition of dalteparin conferred no benefit [40]. The use of thienopyridines (clopi-dogrel and ticlopidine) as an alternative or in combination with aspirin may be a useful alternative, but data are cur-rently lacking [51]. The optimal antithrombotic medication for surgical bypass patients depends on the type of graft used. Restenosis of venous grafts was best prevented when oral vitamin K antagonists were used (target international normalized ratio, 3.0–4.5), whereas aspirin produced supe-rior results for synthetic grafts [52].

More recently, ticagrelor has been used in patients with CLI who had high on-clopidogrel platelet reactivity (HCPR) undergoing peripheral endovascular interventions. In this small series, it showed to be safe and efficacious [53].

Anticoagulants (Adjuvant)

The evidence for use of adjuvant anticoagulation has been summarized in a recent Cochrane review, which concluded that patients undergoing infrainguinal venous grafts are more likely to benefit from vitamin K antagonists such as warfarin than platelet inhibitors, which did not hold true among patients with prosthetic grafts [54]. However, the evidence was not conclusive, and the authors recommended further RCTs with larger numbers of patients comparing antithrombotic therapies with either placebo or antiplatelet therapies.

Folate and Vitamin B12 (Adjuvant)

In a parallel observational study of 169 patients with CLI undergoing surgical revascularization, 66 had hyperhomo-cysteinemia at baseline. They were treated with vitamin B12 and folate for a mean of 12 days, achieving normalization of their homocysteine levels after 3 weeks. After revasculariza-tion, there was no difference in outcomes between the cohort of patients who had hyperhomocysteinemia at baseline but were treated to normalization of homocysteine levels, com-pared to those who had normal homocysteine levels at base-line. The study also showed, through a multivariate logistic regression analysis, that untreated hyperhomocysteinemia was a strong predictor of graft occlusion and limb loss, sug-gesting that aggressive preoperative treatment of hyperho-mocysteinemia may improve clinical outcomes in patients undergoing surgical revascularization for CLI [55].

Biotherapies

The use of biological therapies to achieve therapeutic neovascularization is an exciting upcoming modality in the treatment of patients with CLI. The term *neovascularization* encompasses *angiogenesis* (sprouting of new capillaries in existing capillary beds), *arteriogenesis* (growth of arterial conduits large enough to be seen on catheter-based angiography), and *vasculogenesis* (formation of blood vessels from vascular or endothelial progenitor cells (EPCs)) [56]. Various types of gene and cell-based therapies that promote neovascularization are being investigated in patients with CLI.

Gene therapy for CLI has primarily focused on genes coding for angiogenic growth factors. In particular, vascular endothelial growth factor (VEGF), fibroblast growth factor (FGF), hepatocyte growth factor (HGF), and hypoxia-inducible factor 1α (HIF-1α) have been studied. Gene transfer to target cells can involve viral and nonviral vectors and intra-arterial, intramuscular, and in vitro routes of delivery. Overall, clinical results have been mixed over a variety of end points including changes in hemodynamics, transcutaneous oxygen tension, pain, ulcer healing, amputation, and survival.

A gelatin hydrogel containing basic FGF was tested in a phase 1 trial and found to be safe [57]. A number of phase 1 clinical trials and long-term follow-up studies have evaluated the safety and potential efficacy of a variety of growth factors including HGF [58–61], VEGF [62], and FGF1 [63] or a combination of growth factors [64]. The majority of these studies have mainly shown safety, and in some, there has been a trend toward potential benefit. A few small RCTs of HGF showed improvements in pain scores and toe–brachial index compared with placebo [65, 66]. However, in a larger RCT ($n=104$), HGF was not associated with significant differences in ankle–brachial or toe–brachial index, pain relief, or wound healing compared with placebo [67]. In an RCT of nonviral 1 (NV1) FGF vs. placebo in patients with CLI, there was no significant difference in the primary end point of ulcer healing, but NV1FGF was associated with a significant reduction in risk of amputation [68]. However, once again, in a larger RCT of the same growth factor, no significant improvement in the time to major amputation was found [69]. Similarly, in a small RCT ($n=54$) of VEGF, no significant difference in amputation rate was demonstrated in patients with CLI and diabetes, although some benefit was seen in a number of secondary outcomes including pressure indices and clinical improvement [70]. Results from several phase 1 and 2 trials were relatively promising; however, evidence of benefit in phase 3 trials is lacking [71]. For example, in the phase 3 trial TAMARIS, there was no difference in the primary outcome of AFS in patients with CLI randomized to treatment with nonviral FGF1 and placebo [72].

More recently, use of bone marrow- or peripheral blood-derived multipotent or pluripotent stem cells as well as endothelial progenitor cells (EPCs) has been employed. Several phase 3 trials have been performed using different bone marrow- and EPC-derived cellular therapies. These therapies are delivered through either direct arterial or intramuscular injection [73]. Earlier this year, autologous cultured adipose-derived stroma/stem cells have been used in a phase 1 study for the treatment of CLI, adding yet another cell line to the armamentarium [74]. Overall, as in the gene therapy studiers, cell therapy appears to have a good safety and tolerability profile. Results have shown variable improvement on ABI measurements, transcutaneous oximetry of the tissues, wound healing, and pain symptoms. In most trials, AFS and overall mortality have not been affected [75–78], although the studies were not powered to show effect on these end points. Several meta-analyses, including a Cochrane review, of phase 1 and 2 trials of cell-based therapies suggest that these treatments are safe and potentially beneficial over a similar spectrum of outcomes as those studied in gene therapy trials for CLI [79, 80]. However, multiple questions remain unanswered regarding the administration of cell-based therapy, including the optimal dosage of cells, the best cell type (CD34+, CD133+, G-CSF mobilized, mesenchymal expanded), the most appropriate cell source (autologous or allogenic, bone marrow derived, or peripheral blood), and the preferred route of administration (intramuscular, intra-arterial, or both) [81]. Several phase 3 randomized trials are underway that will help address these unanswered questions [82].

Hyperbaric Oxygen

There is no proven benefit of hyperbaric oxygen in CLI as primary therapy. A Cochrane review of the effect of hyperbaric oxygen on ulcer healing in patients with diabetes concluded that the therapy increased the rate of ulcer healing at 6 weeks but not at 1 year and there was no significant difference in the risk of major amputation [83]. Studies directed at analyzing the adjuvant role of hyperbaric oxygen combined with wound care and revascularization would likely show faster healing times.

Mechanical Therapies

Spinal cord stimulation (SCS), lumbar sympathectomy, and intermittent pneumatic compression (IPC) have been evaluated as treatment options for CLI patients who are deemed poor candidates for revascularization [84].

Spinal Cord Stimulation (SCS)

SCS improves microcirculatory blood flow, relieves ischemic pain, and reduces amputation rates in patients with CLI. In a retrospective study of 150 patients with CLI who failed conservative and surgical management, SCS increased blood flow and was associated with significant pain relief, improved quality of life, and increase in the transcutaneous pressure of oxygen [85]. A more recent study of 101 consecutive patients with no revascularization options found that a reduced delay between the ulcer onset and implantation of a SCS resulted in improved quality of life and walking distance [86]. In a meta-analysis of six trials comprising 450 patients, those treated with SCS had improved rates of amputation and less pain compared to controls [87]. However, there was no difference in ulcer healing and a relatively high complication rate with SCS, resulting in a number needed to harm of 6.

Intermittent Pneumatic Compression (IPC)

In a small retrospective observational study of 48 patients, improvement in limb salvage and hemodynamics was seen in those treated with IPC compared to unmatched controls [88]. A larger study looked at 189 CLI patients with no revascularization option who underwent treatment with sequential compression biomechanical device and showed this therapy to be a cost- and clinically effective solution in patients with CLI who are not candidates for restoration of flow. This therapy provided adequate limb salvage rates and relief of rest pain without any intervention [89].

Quality of Life

One of the most frequently forgotten aspects of the care of patients with CLI is that these patients are scared and often depressed given their surrounding circumstances. They tend to be facing limb loss and the consequent loss of functionality and independence. They are concerned about becoming a burden to their families and loved ones. Therefore, it is of the essence to keep in mind that our job goes beyond providing the patient with our expertise on whatever our "link" of the chain is. All members of the team should strive to address the psychosocial aspects that are individual to each one of the patients and not assume that another member of the team will do it. Open communication with the patient, the family, and the other members of the team should ensure that if we cannot deal with this aspect of the care, a prompt referral to the adequate member is made. It is clear that the main determinant of their quality of life is related to their ability to maintain their functional and independent status, which is dependent on preservation of the limb. A critical predictor in predicting a patient's mobility post-revascularization is their clinical status at presentation, including their mental function, pre-procedural ambulatory capacity, and independent living status [90, 91]. One year following successful revascularization, 88 % of patients remain ambulatory, 85 % maintain their independence, and 80 % achieve both. At 5 years,

71 % remain ambulatory, and 81 % remain independent [90], illustrating the importance of limb preservation in this patient population.

Surveillance

This is the element that closes "the chain." Post-procedural monitoring focuses on preserving the reestablished and improved arterial flow, along with the consequent improvement or resolution of symptoms: This requires preestablished and scheduled follow-up clinical visits and noninvasive tests to assess the status of the limb and the patency of the vessels. It is important to keep in mind that many of our patients with CLI do not have sensation in their limbs, and symptoms alone may not be an adequate surrogate of the status of the limb. While many would argue that patency is not relevant in CLI, as "you only need 3–6 months for the ulcer to heal," it is clear that these patients have recurrences and that their limbs and lives every day face the fine line that represents the delicate and compromised balance of blood supply and demand. So far our ability to find the right treatment strategy is far from adequate. Numerous studies are enrolling patients and data is being analyzed, looking for therapies that provide better long-term patency in patients with CLI (drug-coated balloons, with and without adjuvant atherectomy). Debates continue to ensue in this regard as clearly seen on the podiums and panels of national and international meetings dedicated to peripheral arterial disease and CLI. The answer is not clear as to which should be the end points to measure outcomes in CLI. Is it limb salvage, amputation-free survival, primary or secondary patency, or "major adverse limb events"? There is no solid scientific data to base decisions on. Only one thing appears clear: We need to educate our patients, families, communities, physicians, and institutions, as we continue to look for more and better answers. The CLI continuum of care should be embraced and instituted. Studies should be designed to assess outcomes obtained with a team approach that includes clinical and noninvasive follow-up and compare it to the current workflow. It appears intuitive that a team approach should be significantly better, but in this era of outcomes research, payers and institutions could argue that there is no data to show that this approach (which sounds expensive) is actually any better than the current one.

Summary

The pathophysiology of CLI is complex and involves both microvascular and macrovascular pathology. Therefore, it is not surprising that therapeutic modalities need be multifold, spanning many health-care specialties and requiring substantial institutional infrastructure to provide optimal patient care. Though challenging, the future of CLI treatment is exciting with increasing focus on optimal wound care and prevention, adherence to proven medical therapies, improving revascularization results with novel endovascular and surgical techniques and devices, and ongoing investigation into promising biotherapies. Of paramount importance is the creation and establishment of the multidisciplinary CLI continuum of care team, with aggressive referral upon identification of skin breakdowns or any other factors that can predispose the patient to a rapid decline and compromised prognosis. Patients with CLI often have chronic wounds, and newer cell-based therapies for chronic wounds show interesting parallels to stem cell therapy for CLI. Several human-derived wound care products and therapies, including human neonatal fibroblast-derived dermis, bilayered bioengineered skin substitute, recombinant human platelet-derived growth factor, and autologous platelet-rich plasma, may provide insight into the mechanisms through which differentiated cells can be used as therapy for chronic wounds and in a similar fashion by which stem cells might have a therapeutic role in the management of patients with CLI. Further studies are needed to assess the cost-efficiency and outcomes of a CLI continuum of care multidisciplinary model and compare it to current standards

References

1. Fernandez N, McEnaney R, Marone LK, et al. Predictors of failure and success of tibial interventions for critical limb ischemia. J Vasc Surg. 2010;52(4):834–42.
2. Karnabatidis D, et al. Incidence, anatomical location, and clinical significance of compressions and fractures in infrapopliteal balloon-expandable metal stents. J Endovasc Ther. 2009;16:15–22.
3. European Working Group on Critical Limb Ischemia. Second European Consensus Document on chronic critical leg ischaemia. Eur J Vasc Surg. 1992;6(Suppl A):1–32.
4. Bosiers M, Scheinert D, Peeters P, et al. Randomized comparison of everolimus-eluting versus bare metal stents in patients with critical limb ischemia and infrapopliteal arterial occlusive disease. The DESTINY study. J Vasc Surg. 2012;55:390–9.
5. Balzer J, Zeller T, Rastan A, et al. Percutaneous interventions below the knee in patients with critical limb ischemia using drug eluting stents. J Cardiovasc Surg. 2010;51:183–91.
6. Siablis D, Karnabatidis D, Katsanos K, et al. Infrapopliteal application of paclitaxel-eluting stents for critical limb ischemia: midterm angiographic and clinical results. J Vasc Interv Radiol. 2007;18:1351–61.
7. Varu V, Hogg M, Kibbe M. Critical limb ischemia. J Vasc Surg. 2010;51:230–41.
8. Norgren L, Hiatt WR, Dormandy JA, Nehler MR, Harris KA, Fowkes FG, On behalf of the TASC II Working Group, et al. Inter-Society Consensus for the management of peripheral arterial disease (TASC II). Eur J Vasc Endovasc Surg. 2007;33 Suppl 1:S1–75.
9. Pipinos I, Judge A, Selsby J, Zhu Z, Swanson S, Nella A, et al. The myopathy of peripheral arterial occlusive disease: part 1. Functional and histomorphological changes and evidence for mitochondrial dysfunction. Vasc Endovascular Surg. 2008;41(6):481–9.
10. Pipinos I, Judge A, Selsby J, Zhu Z, Swanson S, Nella A, et al. The myopathy of peripheral arterial occlusive disease: part 2.Oxidative stress, neuropathy, and shift in muscle fiber type. Vasc Endovascular Surg. 2008;42(2):101–12.
11. Rogers RK, Hiatt WR. Pathophysiology and treatment of critical limb ischemia. 2013. http://www.vascularmed.org/clinical_archive/Pathophysiology-Treatment-of-CLI_11Feb2013.pdf.
12. Becker F, Robert-Ebadi H, Ricco JB, Setacci C, Cao P, de Donato G, et al. Chapter 1: definitions, epidemiology, clinical presentation and prognosis. Eur J Vasc Endovasc Surg. 2011;42(S2):S4–12.
13. Nehler MR, Hiatt WR, Taylor LM. Is revascularization and limb salvage always the best treatment for critical limb ischemia? J Vasc Surg. 2003;37(3):704–8.
14. Valentine RJ, Grayburn PA, Eichhorn EJ, et al. Coronary artery disease is highly prevalent among patients with premature peripheral vascular disease. J Vasc Surg. 1994;19:668–74.
15. Klop RB, Eikelboom BC, Taks AC. Screening of the internal carotid arteries in patients with peripheral vascular disease by colour-flow duplex scanning. Eur J Vasc Surg. 1991;5:41–5.
16. Alexandrova NA, Gibson WC, Norris JW, et al. Carotid artery stenosis in peripheral vascular disease. J Vasc Surg. 1996;23:645–9.
17. Cheng SW, Wu LL, Ting AC, et al. Screening for asymptomatic carotid stenosis in patients with peripheral vascular disease: a prospective study and risk factor analysis. Cardiovasc Surg. 1999;7:303–9.
18. Leng GC, Lee AJ, Fowkes FG, et al. Incidence, natural history and cardiovascular events in symptomatic and asymptomatic peripheral arterial disease in the general population. Int J Epidemiol. 1996;25:1172–81.
19. Kornitzer M, Dramaix M, Sobolski J, Degre S, De Backer G. Ankle/arm pressure index in asymptomatic middle-aged males: an independent predictor of ten-year coronary heart disease mortality. Angiology. 1995;46:211–9.
20. Newman AB, Sutton-Tyrrell K, Vogt MT, Kuller LH. Morbidity and mortality in hypertensive adults with a low ankle/arm blood pressure index. JAMA. 1993;270:487–9.
21. Criqui MH, Langer RD, Fronek A, et al. Mortality over a period of 10 years in patients with peripheral arterial disease. N Engl J Med. 1992;326:381–6.
22. Kaul P, Armstrong PW, Chang WC, Naylor CD, Granger CB, Lee KL, et al. Long-term mortality of patients with acute myocardial infarction in the United States and Canada: comparison of patients enrolled in Global Utilization of Streptokinase and t-PA for Occluded Coronary Arteries (GUSTO)-I. Circulation. 2004;110:1754–60.
23. Diehm N, Baumgartner I, Jaff M, Do DD, Minar E, Schmidli J, et al. A call for uniform reporting standards in studies assessing endovascular treatment for chronic ischaemia of lower limb arteries. Eur Heart J. 2007;28:798–805.
24. Ali FN, Carman TL. Medical management of chronic atherosclerotic peripheral arterial disease. Drugs. 2012;72(16):2073–85.
25. Zhang L, Chen J, Han C. A multicenter clinical trial of recombinant human GM-CSF hydrogel for the treatment of deep second degree burns. Wound Repair Regen. 2009;17:685.
26. Soderstrom M, Aho PS, Lepantalo M, Alback A. The influence of the characteristics of ischemic tissue lesions on ulcer healing time after infrainguinal bypass for critical leg ischemia. J Vasc Surg. 2009;49:932–7.
27. Soderstrom M, Arvela E, Alback A, Aho PS, Lepantalo M. Healing of ischaemic tissue lesions after infrainguinal bypass surgery for critical limb ischaemia. Eur J Vasc Endovasc Surg. 2008;36:90–5.
28. CAPRIE Steering Committee. A randomized, blinded, trial of clopidogrel vs aspirin in patients at risk of ischaemic events (CAPRIE). CAPRIE Steering Committee. Lancet. 1996;348:1329–39.
29. Dean SM, Satiani B. Three cases of digital ischemia successfully treated with cilostazol. Vasc Med. 2001;6(4):245–8.

30. Dean SM, Vaccaro PS. Successful pharmacologic treatment of lower extremity ulcerations in 5 patients with chronic critical limb ischemia. J Am Board Fam Pract. 2002;15(1):55–62.

31. Miyashita Y, Saito S, Miyamoto A, et al. Cilostazol increases skin perfusion pressure in severely ischemic limbs. Angiology. 2011;62(1):15–7.

32. Soga Y, Iida O, Hirano K, et al. Impact of cilostazol after endovascular treatments for infrainguinal disease in patients with critical limb ischemia. J Vasc Surg. 2011;54(6):1659–67.

33. Soga Y, Iida O, Kawasaki D, et al. Impact of cilostazol on angiographic restenosis after balloon angioplasty for infrapopliteal artery disease in patients with critical limb ischemia. Eur J Vasc Endovasc Surg. 2012;44(6):577–81.

34. Norwegian Pentoxifylline Multicenter Trial Group. Efficacy and clinical tolerability of parenteral pentoxifylline in the treatment of critical lower limb ischemia: a placebo controlled multicenter study. Int Angiol. 1996;15(1):75–80.

35. The European Study Group. Intravenous pentoxifylline for the treatment of chronic critical limb ischemia. Eur J Vasc Endovasc Surg. 1995;9(4):426–36.

36. Hirsch AT, Haskal ZJ, Hertzer NR, et al. ACC/AHA 2005 Practice Guidelines for the management of patients with peripheral arterial disease (lower extremity, renal, mesenteric, and abdominal aortic): a collaborative report from the American Association for Vascular Surgery/Society for Vascular Surgery, Society for Cardiovascular Angiography and Interventions, Society for Vascular Medicine and Biology, Society of Interventional Radiology, and the ACC/AHA Task Force on Practice Guidelines (Writing Committee to Develop Guidelines for the Management of Patients With Peripheral Arterial Disease): endorsed by the American Association of Cardiovascular and Pulmonary Rehabilitation; National Heart, Lung, and Blood Institute; Society for Vascular Nursing; TransAtlantic Inter Society Consensus; and Vascular Disease Foundation. Circulation. 2006;113:e463–654.

37. Ruffolo AJ, Romano M, Ciapponi A. Prostanoids for critical limb ischaemia. Cochrane Database Syst Rev. 2010;(1):CD006544.

38. Faglia E, Clerici G, Scatena A, et al. Effectiveness of combined therapy with angiotensin-converting enzyme inhibitors and statins in reducing mortality in diabetic patients with critical limb ischemia: an observational study. Diabetes Res Clin Pract. 2014;103:292–7. doi:10.1016/j.diabres.2013.12.060.

39. Tomoi Y, Soga Y, Iida O, et al. Efficacy of statin treatment after endovascular therapy for isolated below-the-knee disease in patients with critical limb ischemia. Cardiovasc Interv Ther. 2013;28(4):374–82.

40. Koppensteiner R, Spring S, Amann-Vesti BR, et al. Low-molecular-weight heparin for prevention of restenosis after femoropopliteal percutaneous transluminal angioplasty: a randomized controlled trial. J Vasc Surg. 2006;44:1247–53.

41. Tangelder MJ, Lawson JA, Algra A, et al. Systematic review of randomized controlled trials of aspirin and oral anticoagulants in the prevention of graft occlusion and ischemic events after infrainguinal bypass surgery. J Vasc Surg. 1999;30:701–9.

42. Brown J, Lethaby A, Maxwell H, et al. Antiplatelet agents for preventing thrombosis after peripheral arterial bypass surgery. Cochrane Database Syst Rev. 2008;(8):CD000535.

43. Clagett GP, Sobel M, Jackson MR, et al. Antithrombotic therapy in peripheral arterial occlusive disease: the seventh ACCP conference on antithrombotic and thrombolytic therapy. Chest. 2004;126(3 Suppl):609S–26.

44. Belch JJ, Dormandy J, Biasi GM, et al. Results of the randomized, placebo-controlled clopidogrel and acetylsalicylic acid in bypass surgery for peripheral arterial disease (CASPAR) trial. J Vasc Surg 2010;52: 825–33, 833.e1–2.

45. Schanzer A, Hevelone N, Owens CD, Beckman JA, Belkin M, Conte MS. Statins are independently associated with reduced mortality in patients undergoing infrainguinal bypass graft surgery for critical limb ischemia. J Vasc Surg. 2008;47:774–81.

46. Ramo OJ, Juha L, Marti S, Hannu H, Pauliina RM, Risto M. Effects of lovastatin in prevention of restenosis after percutaneous transluminal angioplasty in lower limbs. Int J Angiol. 1995;4:173–6.

47. Fusaro M, Cassese S, Ndrepepa G, et al. Drug-eluting stents for revascularization of infrapopliteal arteries. Updated meta-analysis of randomized trials. J Am Coll Cardiol Intv. 2013;6:1284–93.

48. Arvela E, Dick F. Surveillance after distal revascularization for critical limb ischaemia. Scand J Surg. 2012;101:119–24.

49. Dorffler-Melly J, Koopman MM, Prins MH, Buller HR. Antiplatelet and anticoagulant drugs for prevention of restenosis/reocclusion following peripheral endovascular treatment. Cochrane Database Syst Rev. 2005;1:CD002071.

50. Alonso-Coello P, Bellmunt S, McGorrian C, et al. Antithrombotic therapy in peripheral artery disease: antithrombotic therapy and prevention of thrombosis, 9th ed: American College of Chest Physicians evidence-based clinical practice guidelines. Chest. 2012;141:669–90.

51. Visona A, Tonello D, Zalunardo B, et al. Antithrombotic treatment before and after peripheral artery percutaneous angioplasty. Blood Transfus. 2009;7:18–23.

52. Efficacy of oral anticoagulants compared with aspirin after infrainguinal bypass surgery Aspirin (BOA) Study Group: a randomised trial. Lancet 2000;355:346–51.

53. Spiliopoulos S, Katsanos K, Pastromas G, et al. Initial experience in patients with critical limb ischemia and high on-clopidogrel platelet reactivity undergoing complex peripheral endovascular procedures. Cardiovasc Intervent Radiol. 2014. doi:10.1007/s00270-014-0852-y.

54. Geraghty AJ, Welch K. Antithrombotic agents for preventing thrombosis after infrainguinal arterial bypass surgery. Cochrane Database Syst Rev. 2011;(6):CD000536.

55. Waters PS, Fennessey PJ, Hynes N, et al. The effects of normalizing hyperhomocysteinemia on clinical and operative outcomes in patients with critical limb ischemia. J Endovasc Ther. 2012;19(6):815–25.

56. Attanasio S, Snell J. Therapeutic angiogenesis in the management of critical limb ischemia: current concepts and review. Cardiol Rev. 2009;17(3):115–20.

57. Marui A, Tabata Y, Kojima S, et al. A novel approach to therapeutic angiogenesis for patients with critical limb ischemia by sustained release of basic fibroblast growth factor using biodegradable gelatin hydrogel: an initial report of the phase I–IIa study. Circ J. 2007;71:1181–6.

58. Gu Y, Zhang J, Guo L, et al. A phase I clinical study of naked DNA expressing two isoforms of hepatocyte growth factor to treat patients with critical limb ischemia. J Gene Med. 2011;13:602–10.

59. Henry TD, Hirsch AT, Goldman J, et al. Safety of a non-viral plasmid-encoding dual isoforms of hepatocyte growth factor in critical limb ischemia patients: a phase I study. Gene Ther. 2011;18:788–94.

60. Shigematsu H, Yasuda K, Sasajima T, et al. Transfection of human HGF plasmid DNA improves limb salvage in Buerger's disease patients with critical limb ischemia. Int Angiol. 2011;30:140–9.

61. Morishita R, Makino H, Aoki M, et al. Phase I/IIa clinical trial of therapeutic angiogenesis using hepatocyte growth factor gene transfer to treat critical limb ischemia. Arterioscler Thromb Vasc Biol. 2011;31:713–20.

62. Muona K, Makinen K, Hedman M, Manninen H, Yla-Herttuala S. 10-Year safety follow-up in patients with local VEGF gene transfer to ischemic lower limb. Gene Ther. 2012;19:392–5.

63. Niebuhr A, Henry T, Goldman J, et al. Long-term safety of intramuscular gene transfer of non-viral FGF1 for peripheral artery disease. Gene Ther. 2012;19:264–70.

64. Anghel A, Taranu G, Seclaman E, et al. Safety of vascular endothelial and hepatocyte growth factor gene therapy in patients with critical limb ischemia. Curr Neurovasc Res. 2011;8:183–9.

65. Powell RJ, Goodney P, Mendelsohn FO, Moen EK, Annex BH. Safety and efficacy of patient specific intramuscular injection of HGF plasmid gene therapy on limb perfusion and wound healing in patients with ischemic lower extremity ulceration: results of the HGF-0205 trial. J Vasc Surg. 2010;52:1525–30.

66. Shigematsu H, Yasuda K, Iwai T, et al. Randomized, doubleblind, placebo-controlled clinical trial of hepatocyte growth factor plasmid for critical limb ischemia. Gene Ther. 2010;17:1152–61.

67. Powell RJ, Simons M, Mendelsohn FO, et al. Results of a double-blind, placebo-controlled study to assess the safety of intramuscular injection of hepatocyte growth factor plasmid to improve limb perfusion in patients with critical limb ischemia. Circulation. 2008;118:58–65.

68. Nikol S, Baumgartner I, Van Belle E, et al. Therapeutic angiogenesis with intramuscular NV1FGF improves amputation- free survival in patients with critical limb ischemia. Mol Ther. 2008;16:972–8.

69. Belch J, Hiatt WR, Baumgartner I, et al. Effect of fibroblast growth factor NV1FGF on amputation and death: a randomised placebo-controlled trial of gene therapy in critical limb ischaemia. Lancet. 2011;377:1929–37.

70. Kusumanto YH, van Weel V, Mulder NH, et al. Treatment with intramuscular vascular endothelial growth factor gene compared with placebo for patients with diabetes mellitus and critical limb ischemia: a double-blind randomized trial. Hum Gene Ther. 2006;17:683–91.

71. Tongers J, Roncalli JG, Losordo DW. Therapeutic angiogenesis for critical limb ischemia; microvascular therapies coming of age. Circulation. 2008;118:9–16.

72. Fowkes FG, Price JF. Gene therapy for critical limb ischaemia: the TAMARIS trial. Lancet. 2011;377(9781):1894–6.

73. Lawall H, Bramlage P, Amann B. Treatment of peripheral arterial disease using stem and progenitor cell therapy. J Vasc Surg. 2011;53(2):445–53.

74. Bura A, Planat-Benard V, Bourin P, et al. Phase 1 trial: the use of autologous cultured adipose-derived stroma/stem cells to treat patients with non-revascularizable critical limb ischemia. Cytotherapy. 2014;16(2):245–57.

75. Walter DH, Krankenberg H, Balzer JO, et al. Intraarterial administration of bone marrow mononuclear cells in patients with critical limb ischemia: a randomized-start, placebo controlled pilot trial (PROVASA). Circ Cardiovasc Interv. 2011;4(1):26–37.

76. Lu D, Chen B, Liang Z, et al. Comparison of bone marrow mesenchymal stem cells with bone marrow-derived mononuclear cells for treatment of diabetic critical limb ischemia and foot ulcer: a double-blind, randomized, controlled trial. Diabetes Res Clin Pract. 2011;92(1):26–36.

77. Powell RJ, Comerota AJ, Berceli SA, et al. Interim analysis results from RESTORE-CLI, a randomized, double-blind multicenter phase II trial comparing expanded autologous bone marrow-derived tissue repair cells and placebo in critical limb ischemia. J Vasc Surg. 2011;54(4):1032–41.

78. Perin EC, Silva G, Gahremanpour A, et al. A randomized, controlled study of autologous therapy with bone marrow-derived aldehyde dehydrogenase bright cells in patients with critical limb ischemia. Catheter Cardiovasc Interv. 2011;78(7):1060–7.

79. Fadini GP, Tjwa M. A role for TGF-beta in transforming endothelial progenitor cells into neointimal smooth muscle cells. Atherosclerosis. 2010;211(1):32–5.

80. Moazzami K, Majdzadeh R, Nedjat S. Local intramuscular transplantation of autologous mononuclear cells for critical lower limb ischaemia. Cochrane Database Syst Rev. 2011;(12):CD008347.

81. Sprengers RW, Lips DJ, Moll FL, Verhaar MC. Progenitor cell therapy in patients with critical limb ischemia without surgical options. Ann Surg. 2008;247(3):411–20.

82. Powell RJ. Update on clinical trials evaluating the effect of biologic therapy in patients with critical limb ischemia. J Vasc Surg. 2012;56:264–6.

83. Kranke P, Bennett M, Martyn-St James M, et al. Hyperbaric oxygen therapy for chronic wounds. Cochrane Database Syst Rev. 2012;4:CD004123.

84. Slovut DP, Sullivan TM. Critical limb ischemia: medical and surgical management. Vasc Med. 2008;13(3):281–91.

85. Petrakis IE, Sciacca V. Spinal cord stimulation in critical limb ischemia of the lower extremities: our experience. J Neurosurg Sci. 1999;43(4):285–93.

86. Tshomba Y, Psacharopulo D, Frezza S, et al. Predictors of improved quality of life and claudication in patients undergoing spinal cord stimulation for critical lower limb ischemia. Ann Vasc Surg. 2013. doi:10.1016/j.avsg.2013.06.020.

87. Ubbink DT, Vermeulen H. Spinal cord stimulation for non-reconstructable chronic critical let ischaemia. Cochrane Database Syst Rev. 2003;(3):CD004001.

88. Kovros SJ, Delis KT, Turner NS, et al. Improving limb salvage in critical ischemia with intermittent pneumatic compression: a controlled study with 18-month follow-up. J Vasc Surg. 2008;47:543–9.

89. Tawfick WA, Hamada N, Soylu E, et al. Sequential compression biomechanical device versus primary amputation in patients with critical limb ischemia. Vasc Endovascular Surg. 2013;47(7):532–9.

90. Taylor SM, Kalbaugh CA, Blackhurt DW, Cass AL, Trent EA, Langan 3rd EM, et al. Determinants of functional outcome after revascularization for critical limb ischemia: an analysis of 1000 consecutive vascular interventions. J Vasc Surg. 2006;44:747–55.

91. Goodney PP, Likosky DS, Cronenwett JL. Predicting ambulation status one year after lower extremity bypass. J Vasc Surg. 2009;49(6):1431–9.

Index

A

Abdominal aortic aneurysm, 195
ABI. *See* Ankle brachial index (ABI)
Above-knee amputation (AKA), 612, 614
Accessory saphenous vein, 69
Acute arterial embolus, 34–35
Acute arterial occlusion
    evaluation, 271
    fibrinolytic therapy, 269
    histopathologic assessment, 273
    paradoxic embolism, 273
    thrombophilia, 267
    thrombotic complications, 271
Acute compartment syndrome, 310
Acute critical limb ischemia (aCLI)
    embolism/in situ thrombosis, 37
    lack of collateral blood flow, 37
    measure toe flexor strength, 38
    pain, 37
    paper grip test and intrinsic positive test, 38
    pulses, 38
    symptoms, 37
Acute crush injuries, 484
Acute digital ischemia, 328
Acute embolic occlusion, 162
Acute limb ischemia (ALI), 201
    acute thrombosis, 34
    amputation rate, 1, 4, 5, 443
    angiojet catheter, percutaneous mechanical thrombectomy, 33
    anticoagulation, 5
    arterial embolism (*see* Arterial embolism)
    arterial embolus, right distal common iliac artery, 33
    arterial thrombosis, 29
    atherosclerotic, 442
    cardiac, 442
    categories, 2
    causes, 1
    changing patterns, 3–4
    classification, 2
    CLI, 1
    clinical classification, 31, 164
    clinical evaluation, 162
    clinical findings, 163
    clinical presentation
        embolic ALI, 162
        pain, 163
        pallor, 163
        paralysis, 163
        paresthesia, 163
        poikilothermia, 163
        pulselessness, 163
        thrombotic ALI, 162

comorbidities, 30
conservative management, 5
contralateral, 29
coolness, 30
CTA, 32
data, 3
definition, 1, 159
diabetics, 1
diagnosis (*see* Diagnostic examination)
diagnostic algorithm, 168–169
different stages, severity, 2
differential diagnosis, 3
Doppler effect, 31
double-incision fasciotomy, 36
Duplex ultrasound, 32
echocardiography, 32
embolic, 442
embolism, 1, 160, 161
epidemiological data, 2
etiology, 160
extremity pain, 29
femoral arteries, 446
history, 30, 159
incidence, 1, 2
invasive angiography, 32
loss of sensation, 30
lower extremity (LE), 1, 2, 442
mechanism of, 3
meta-analysis, 443
morbidity and mortality, 5
mortality rates, 1, 4
MRA, 32
muscle necrosis, 160
open surgical thrombectomy, 34–35
physical exam, 29
revascularization, 29
sources, 29
sudden arterial occlusion, 29
surgical, 29
pain, 30
pallor, 30
paradoxical, 442
paralysis, 30
percutaneous *vs.* open surgical revascularization, 35
percutaneous thrombolytic therapy, 32, 34
post-revascularization compartment syndrome, 35
presentation, 2
pulse examination, 31
revascularization, 30
rhabdomyolysis, 35–36
right acute lower extremity ischemia, 31
risk, 5

© Springer International Publishing Switzerland 2017
R.S. Dieter et al. (eds.), *Critical Limb Ischemia*, DOI 10.1007/978-3-319-31991-9

Acute limb ischemia (ALI) (*cont.*)
  rule of Ps, 30
  sensory nerves, 30
  skin and muscle tissue, 30
  smokers, 1
  stroke, 443
  symptoms, 30
  thromboembolectomy, 5, 162
  thrombosis, 442
    atherosclerotic plaque, 161
    healthy artery, 161
    non-atheromatous pathological artery, 161
    trauma, 161, 162
  treatment, 5
    anticoagulation, 32
    catheter and sheath selection, 32
    primary, 32
    revascularization, 32
  upper extremity (UE), 3, 442
  vasoconstriction, 30
Adipose tissue-derived stromal cells (ADSCs), 26
Adjunctive devices
  atherectomy, 403–404
  excisional atherectomy, 404
  orbital atherectomy, 404
Adjunctive management strategies
  amputation, role, 319
  fasciotomy in PCD, 318–319
  periprocedural IVC filters, 318
  venous stents, 318
ADSCs. *See* Adipose tissue-derived stromal cells (ADSCs)
Advanced glycosylation end products (AGEs), 353
Advanced Trauma Life Support (ATLS), 220
AF. *See* Atrial fibrillation (AF)
AKA. *See* Above-knee amputation (AKA)
ALI. *See* Acute limb ischemia (ALI)
American Venous Forum (AVF), 311
Amplatzer PFO/ASD occluder, 116
Amputation, 463
  acute and chronic phase, 252
  cold intolerance, 571
  definitive, 571
  hand salvage, 572
  iatrogenic extremity ischemia (*see* Iatrogenic extremity ischemia)
  MESS, 227
  multiple digit/partial hand, 572–575
  nonurgent, 571
  transhumeral, 581
  transradial, 577, 579
  traumatic, 571
  wrist disarticulation (*see* Wrist disarticulation)
Amputation-free survival (AFS), 375, 631–632
ANCA. *See* Anti-neutrophilic cytoplasmic antibody (ANCA)
Angiogenesis
  neovascularization, 491
  occlusion, artery, 491
  PAD, 492
  process, 491
  therapeutic, 492–493
Angiography, 329
Angiojet percutaneous thrombectomy, 32, 34
AngioJet Rheolytic Thrombectomy System, 315, 316
Angioplasty, 390–391, 429, 455
  balloon, 387
  vs. BMS, 391
  CBA, 398

    excimer laser, 405–406
    PBA, 404
    PELA, 404
    PTA (*see* Percutaneous transluminal angioplasty (PTA))
    SBA, 398
    SIA, 404
    vibrational, 405
AngioSculpt (ASC), 398
Angiosomes, 15, 67, 68, 364, 375
  arteries and foot, 368
  choke vessels, 429
  CLI, 429
  color-coded model, 368
  CRP, 369
  data analysis, 430
  definition, 429
  DR and IR, 369
  infrapopliteal bypass surgery, 430
  meta-analyses, 369
  preoperative angiograms, 368
  revascularization, 367, 429
  tissue loss healing, 429
AngioVac cannula, 312, 313
Ankle-brachial index (ABI), 199, 222, 339, 340, 359, 543, 547, 549, 629, 630
  CLI, 139
  interobserver variability, 139
  limitations, 139, 141
  limited reliability, 140
  medial arterial calcification, 140
  mortality, 139
  occlusive lesion, 139
  PAD, 139
    and claudication, 141
    diagnosis of, 139
  quality, therapeutic intervention, 139
  reduced and noncompressible, 139
  systolic blood pressure, 139
  systolic brachial pressure, 139
Ankle cuff pressure, 200
Anterior humeral circumflex artery, 50
Anterior tibial artery, 64, 65, 67, 68
Anticoagulation
  ACCP anticoagulation guidelines, 319
  lower extremity fasciotomy, 318
  PCDT, 315
  thrombectomy, 312
  venous ischemia, 319
Anti-neutrophilic cytoplasmic antibody (ANCA), 258
Antiphospholipid antibody syndrome
  assay inhibition, 268
  clinical presentation, 268
  diagnosis, 267, 268
  ELISA testing, 268
  laboratory testing, 268
  lupus anticoagulant testing, 268
  management, 269
  pathogenesis, 267–268
Antiphospholipid syndrome (APS), 307
Antithrombotic therapy, 273
Antithrombotic Therapy and Prevention of Thrombosis Guidelines, 311
Aortic abdominal aneurysms (AAA), 74
Aortic/aneurysm surgery, 242
Aortic dissection
  cardiopulmonary bypass, 116
  classification, 116, 117

cocaine, 116
lower limb ischemia, 118
type B dissections, 116, 118
Aortobifemoral bypass, 415
Aortoiliac disease, 246, 375
Arterial access, 359
Arterial circulation, 57–64
Arterial disease management, 341
Arterial dissection. *See* Aortic dissection
Arterial duplex ultrasonography, 147
Arterial duplex ultrasound, 201
accuracy and reliability, 146
anatomic information, 146
B-mode imaging, 146
development, 146
endovascular procedure, 146
lower extremity vasculature, 146
noninvasive and inexpensive imaging, 146
overlying bowel gas, 146
physiologic data, 146
PSV, 146
quality of revascularization, 146
side and degree of calcification, 146
sound waves, 146
stenosis, 146
velocity of blood, 146
Arterial embolism, 3, 29, 114, 261, 273, 285
Arterial insufficiency, 374
Arterial spin labeling (ASL), 191
Arterial thoracic outlet syndrome (aTOS), 79, 81
Arterial thrombosis, 29
Arteriography, 86–87
Arteriotomy, 417
Arteriovenous fistula, 377
Ascending cervical artery, 49
ASD. *See* Atrial septal defect (ASD)
Assay inhibition, 268
Atherectomy
excimer laser, 403–404
excisional and orbital, 404
Atheroembolic episodes
acute limb ischemia, 104
atherosclerotic plaque debris, 104
blue toe syndrome, 104
treatment, 104, 105
Atherosclerosis, 81, 88, 382
Atherosclerotic coronary arteries, 73
Atherosclerotic disease, 641
coronary vessels, 72
diabetics, 72
HF, 71
high blood pressure, 73
IC, 71, 72
long-term survival, 71
SE, 72
stroke, 72, 74
symptoms/carotid bruits, 73
unilateral disease, 72
Atherosclerotic plaque
aortic atherosclerosis, 294
aortic plaques, 295, 297
cholesterol-rich material, 294
conventional arteriography, 297
development, 294
stages, 294

Atrial fibrillation (AF)
acute arterial occlusion, 273, 274
antiplatelet therapy, 274
CHA$_2$DS$_2$-VASc score, 110, 111
echocardiography, 110
non-cerebral embolism, 274
peripheral embolism, 109
stroke and peripheral embolization, 274
valvular atrial fibrillation, 274
warfarin, 110
Atrial septal defect (ASD)
heart failure and symptoms, 115
paradoxical embolization, 115
Autologous cell therapy, 26
Autologous vein grafting, 225
Autonomic dysfunction, 350, 353
Axillary artery, 230
Axillary–bifemoral bypass, 455
Axillo-femoral bypass, 417

B
Balloon angioplasty, 263
BMS, 391, 396
CBA, 398
clinical trials, 392
lower limb ischemia, 390
mechanism, 387
PBA, 404
SBA, 398
Bare-metal stents (BMS) *vs.* angioplasty, 391
Bare-nitinol stent (BNS), 393, 395, 400–402
Basement membrane, 353, 354
BASIL trial, 638
Basilic venous system, 56
BD. *See* Behçet's disease (BD)
Behçet's disease (BD)
aneurysms and thrombus adherent, 287
arterial manifestations, 287
azathioprine, 288
diagnosis, 287
immunosuppressive treatment, 288
micro-and macrovascular system, 26
morphology, 287
mucocutaneous lesions, 287
peripheral arterial lesions, 287
pulmonary arteries, 287
STD, 26
surgical revascularization, 287
vascular complications, 287
Below knee amputation (BKA)
Achilles tendon, 608, 609
anterior skin incision, 605, 607
ERTL technique, 610
osteotomies, 605, 607, 608
posterior flap, 607, 609
tibial osteotomy, 605, 606
Below-the-knee lesions (BTK), 388, 396, 397, 403
Benign endocardial tumor, 325
Benign tumor limb ischemia. *See* Tumor-induced peripheral ischemia
Beta-blockers (BB), 538
Bicipital aponeurosis, 56
BKA. *See* Below knee amputation (BKA)
Blood rheology, 354
Blooming artifact, 177, 179
Blue toe syndrome, 104, 293

Blunt trauma, 217
Botulinum toxin, 262–263
Brachial artery, 50, 52, 56, 231, 233
Brachio-brachial exclusion bypass, 91
Brachiocephalic trunk, 45
Brachiocephalic vein, 56
Brachioradialis muscle, 52
Brown recluse spider bite, 105
Buerger's disease, 79, 81, 84, 90, 249, 251, 253, 471
    CREST syndrome and scleroderma, 102
    diagnosis, 102
    digital ischemia, 102
    TOA, 26
    tobacco usage, 102
    treatment, 102
Bypass grafting (BG), 544, 550–553
Bypass versus angioplasty in severe ischemia of the leg (BASIL), 378,
    379, 382, 391, 424

C
CAD. *See* Coronary artery disease (CAD)
Calcanectomy, 598
Calciphylaxis, 103
Calf vessels, 232
Candidate drugs
    paclitaxel, 394
    rapamycin analogs, 394
    sirolimus (rapamycin), 394
Cannabis-associated arteritis, 250
Carbon dioxide (CO_2) angiography, 153
Carbon dioxide (CO_2)-mediated angiography, 212
Cardiac auscultation, 84
Cardiac tumors, 109, 113, 114, 329, 452
CardioSEAL-STARFlex PFO device, 116
Cardiovascular disease, 641
Cardiovascular magnetic resonance imaging (CMR), 183, 184
Carotid artery stenosis (CAS), 71, 74
CAS. *See* Carotid artery stenosis (CAS)
Catastrophic antiphospholipid antibody syndrome, 268
Catheter-directed thrombolysis (CDT), 92, 313, 314, 441, 442, 448
CDT. *See* Catheter-directed thrombolysis (CDT)
Cell therapy, therapeutic angiogenesis
    advantages, 497
    CLI, 497, 499
    clinical trials, 497
    mobilization of bone marrow stem cells, 497
    mobilization of self stem cells, 497
    modes, 497, 498
    source of stem cells, 497
    treating old diseases, 496
Cephalic system, 56
CES. *See* Cholesterol emboli syndrome (CES)
CHA_2DS_2-VASc score, 110, 111
Charcot foot (CF), 350, 503
Chemotherapeutic agents, 83
Choke vessels', 429
Cholesterol crystals, 293, 294
Cholesterol emboli syndrome (CES)
    atheroma, 293
    atherosclerotic plaque, 294–297
    blue toe syndrome, 293
    diagnosis, 301
    end-organ damage
        central nervous system, 299
        gastrointestinal tract, 300

        kidney, 299–300
        skin, 300–301
    histopathology, 298
    inflammatory response, 298–299
    pathophysiology, 293, 294
    plaque debris, 298
    plaque rupture, 297, 298
    treatment, 301–302
Chronic arterial occlusive disease, 35
Chronic CLI
    amputation, 638
    arterial syndromes, 9
    associated disease, 10
    blood flow, 38
    cannulation, 152
    categories, 10
    claudication, 38, 39
    clinical definition, 10
    continuous Doppler waveforms, 140, 142
    cost, 638
    criteria, 9
    CTA (*see* Computed tomography angiography (CTA))
    definition, 9
    diabetic and nondiabetic patients, 9
    diabetic neuropathy, 12
    diagnosis
        atherosclerotic disease, 137
        complain of rest pain, 137
        etiologies, 137
        etiology, 137
        history examination, 137
        physical examination, 137, 138
        revascularization procedure, 137
        status of tissue loss, 137
        symptoms, 137
        testing, 139
    diagnostic decision, 138
    DSA, 137
    DVT, 39
    epidemiology
        arteriographic progression, 12
        claudication, 12
        heterogeneity, 11
        intermittent claudication, 12
        limitations, 12
        modern risk stratification techniques, 12
        objective parameters, 11
        PAD, 11
        prevalence, 11
        symptomatic disease, 10
        TASC II guidelines, 11, 12
    high risk of limb loss, 137
    intermittent claudication, 38
    invasive imaging
        CO2 angiography, 153
        DSA (*see* Digital subtraction angiography (DSA))
        IVUS, 153
    management, 637
    measurement, 9
    molecular imaging, 154
    MRA, 137, 149–152
    neurospinal compression, 39
    noninvasive anatomic imaging
        arterial Duplex ultrasound, 146, 147
        MRA, 151
    PAD, 9, 13, 137

pain, 38
pedal rubor, 40
peripheral arterial occlusive disease, 12
PET, 153, 154
practice guidelines, 10
prevalence, 9
QISS-MRA, 151
reduction, arterial blood flow, 39
revascularization, 154, 637
risk factors, 12
Rutherford classification system, 9
scope, 13
segmental limb pressures, 140, 143
smokers, 12
socioeconomic impact, 13
symptoms, 10
TASC document, 10
TcPO2, 12, 13
technology, 154
tissue loss, lower extremity, 137
treatment, 637
trials and reporting standards definition, 10
type and severity, 9
ulcer healing, 637
value of ankle pressures, 10
wound care, cost, 638
Chronic kidney disease (CKD)
    contrast-based imaging studies, 566
    drug dose adjustment, 565–566
    pre- and post-kidney transplant care, 566
Chronic limb ischemia (CLI)
    AF, 109–111
    anatomical endpoints
        endovascular and surgical therapy, 629
        graft patency, 630
        symptoms, 629
        target lesion revascularization, 630
        technical success measure, 629–630
    anatomic classifications
        angiosomes, 15, 16
        JENALI, 15
        TASC, 15, 17, 18
    aortic dissection, 116–118
    arterial dissection, 116–118
    cardiac tumors, 113, 114
    endocarditis, 111–112
    functional endpoints
        AFS, 631, 632
        QOL, 633
        quality of life, 631
        return to ambulation, 632–633
        survival and limb salvage, 630
        SVS OPGs, 633
        Wound healing, 631
    iatrogenic, 116
    limb salvage, 629, 634
    LV thrombus, 111
    management, 634
    outcomes, 634
    paradoxical embolism, 114–116
    peripheral arterial atherosclerotic disease, 109
    physiological endpoints
        ABI, 630
        noninvasive testing, 630
        tcPO2 levels, 630
    surgical issues, 629

symptom classifications
    CLI, 16
    Fontaine, 16
    foot infection, 21
    ischemia, 21
    Rutherford, 16
    Wagner ulcer, 21
    WIfI, 16–21
    wound, 21
    wound healing by noninvasive studies, 631
Chronic lymphatic leukemia, 325
Chronic mesenteric ischemia (CMI), 74
Chronic non-healing wounds, 131
Chronic periaortitis (CP)
    diagnosis, 288
    IgG4-related systemic disease, 288
    retroperitoneal fibrosis, 288
    symptoms, 288
Chronic renal insufficiency, 126
Chronic total occlusions (CTOs), 376
    chronic CLI, 404
    crosser CTO recanalization system, 405
    excimer laser angioplasty, 405–406
    Frontrunner CTO catheter, 405
    reentry devices, 406
    SIA, 404
    vibrational angioplasty, 405
Chronic venous ulcers (CVU)
    ESCHAR trial, 627
    negative pressure wound therapy, 627
    prevalence, 627
    risk factors, 627
    surgery, 627
    therapy, 627
    venous ablation, 627
CIN. See Contrast-induced nephropathy (CIN)
Circumflex fibular branch, 66
CKD. See Chronic kidney disease (CKD)
Claw foot, 350
CLI. See Critical limb ischemia (CLI)
CMI. See Chronic mesenteric ischemia (CMI)
Cogan's syndrome (CS), 288
Cold injury, 333
Collagen, wound healing
    bacterial, 133
    deposition
        and formation, extracellular matrix, 132
        and neovascularization, 132
        proliferative phase, 133
    and fibronectin, 133
    growth and deposition, 131
    hemostasis, 131
Collateralization, 177, 179
Color-coded model, 368
Color-coded duplex, 433
Common femoral artery (CFA), 61, 228
Common iliac vessels, 57
Compartment syndrome, 35, 235–237
Complete pedal arch (CPA), 431, 432
Computed tomographic arteriography, 222–223
Computed tomography angiography (CTA), 167, 177, 340, 360, 548
    ALI, 32
    disadvantages, 149
    high accuracy, 147
    ionizing radiation, 149
    left iliac occlusion, 148

Computed tomography angiography (CTA) (*cont.*)
   limitations, 148
   MIP, 148
   modern multi-detector scanners, 147, 148
   and MR angiography, 166
   noninvasive imaging modality, 147
   occlusive arterial disease, 147
   PAD, 148
   primary imaging modality, 148
   primary imaging technique, 147
   quality, 148
   revascularization procedures, 148
   scanning protocols, 171, 172, 174, 175
   sensitivity, 147
Continuous Doppler waveforms, 144
Continuous wave Doppler (CWD), 139
Contralateral dorsalis pedis artery, 376
Contrast-enhanced MRA (CE-MRA)
   advantages, 188
   diagnostic accuracy, 188, 190
   disadvantages, 188, 189
   first pass, 187
   image acquisition, 187
   patient preparation, 185, 186
   peripheral arterial disease, 189
   steady-state, 188
   test bolus method/bolus-tracking method, 187
   time-resolved, 188
Contrast-induced nephropathy (CIN), 212, 360, 566
Contrast venography, 310
Controlled antegrade and retrograde tracking (CART), 377
Coronal gadolinium-enhanced MR angiographic MIP image, 190
Coronary artery disease (CAD), 71
Costocervical trunk, 49
CP. *See* Chronic periaortitis (CP)
C-reactive protein (CRP), 353, 369, 545
Critical colonization, 518
Critical digital ischemia
   and necrosis, 257
   SSc, 260–261
Critical limb ischemia (CLI)
   Ace-I and statins, 644
   aCLI (*see* Acute critical limb ischemia (CLI))
   adequate tissue perfusion, 641
   adjuvant anticoagulation, 539
   AKA, 612–614
   Alprostadil, 491
   amputation, 604
   angiogenesis (*see* Angiogenesis)
   angiography, 211–212
   anticoagulants, 539, 645
   antiplatelet agents, 539
   antiplatelet therapy, 539, 645
   antithrombotic agents, 538–539
   arterial disease, 374–375
   arterial emboli after endovascular procedure, 38
   arteriogenesis, 641, 646
   BKA, 605–611
   Buerger's sign, 40
   cell therapy, 541
   chronic (*see* Chronic limb ischemia (CLI))
   cilostazol, 540, 644
   CKD, 565, 566
   DAASS, 566–568
   diabetes mellitus, 466
   diagnosis, 562–563

   dialysis, 561
   economic cost, 617
   endovascular technologies (*see* Endovascular technologies)
   endovascular treatment, 373
   epidemiology, 543–544
   ERTL technique, 610, 612
   fluorescent angiography, 605
   folate and vitamin B12, 645
   Gaiter area venous ulcer, 41
   gangrene, toe and forefoot, 39
   gastrointestinal side effects, 645
   gene therapy (*see* Gene therapy)
   hyperbaric oxygen, 646
   hyperbaric therapy, 540
   infrapopliteal, 644, 645
   interventional, 643
   intramuscular injection, 646
   IVUS, 214
   kidney disease (*see* Kidney disease)
   lifestyle modification
      evidence-based medicine, 538
      hyperlipidemia, 537
      hypertension, 538
      smoking, 537
   limb loss, 543
   livedo reticularis, 41
   long-term evaluation, 491
   malignancy, 326
   medical history, 37
   mortality rate, 37, 491
   naftidrofuryl, 540
   nonhealing ischemic ulceration, 39
   noninterventional therapies, 643
   OCT, 215
   PAD, 543
   pain relief, 540
   patient evaluation, 37
   pentoxifylline, 539, 644
   pharmacotherapy, 644–645
   physical examination, 40–43
   postoperative care, 614, 615
   Praxilene, 491
   preoperative evaluation, 603
   preoperative medical management, 604
   prevention, 643–644
   prognosis, 555
   prognostic factors, 467
   prostanoids, 539, 644
   pulse examination
      Doppler devices, 42
      Doppler of deep plantar artery, 43
      Doppler of dorsalis pedis artery, 43
      Doppler of posterior tibial artery, 43
      dorsalis pedis, 42
      endovascular interventions, 43
      femoral pulse, 41
      palpation of dorsalis pedis artery, 42
      palpation of popliteal artery, 41
      palpation of posterior tibial artery, 42
      posterior tibial, 42
      upper and lower extremities, 41
   quality of life, 643, 647
   rehabilitation, 615, 617
   revascularization, 641–647
   risk factors, 545–546
   serial debridements, 643

skin barrier, 643
statins, 537
surgical planning, 604
surveillance, 643, 647
symptoms, 647
TASCII guidelines, 561, 562
thienopyridines, 645
through-knee amputation, 610–612, 614, 616
treatment, 467, 491, 642, 648
   amputation, 563
   endovascular revascularization, 563–565
   fluoroscopy, 564, 565
   revascularization, 563
   surgical revascularization, 564–565
   Wagner classification, 563, 564
vasculogenesis, 646
visual inspection, 40–41
wound care, 644
Crosser CTO, 405
CRP. *See* C-reactive protein (CRP)
Cryoglobulinemic vasculitis (CV), 260, 280, 286, 287
Cryoplasty
   femoropopliteal disease, 397
   infrapopliteal disease, 397
   PolarCath system, 397
CS. *See* Cogan's syndrome (CS)
CT evaluation, 180–182
   common artifacts, 177
   CPR, 175, 177
   DSA (*see* Digital subtraction angiography (DSA))
   image acquisition, principle, 173–175
   MIPs, 175
   MPR, 175
   multi-detector CT scanners, 171
   multi-slice CT, 171
   radiation exposure, 175
   vascular stents, 177–180
   volume-rendered images, 175
CTA. *See* Computer tomography angiography (CTA)
Curved multiplanar (CPR) images, 175, 177
Cutting balloon (CB), 397
Cutting balloon angioplasty (CBA), 398
CV. *See* Cryoglobulinemic vasculitis (CV)
Cystic adventitial disease, 99

D

DAASS. *See* Dialysis access-associated steal syndrome (DAASS)
2D angiosome theory, 375
DAPT. *See* Dual antiplatelet therapy (DAPT)
D-Dimer test, 27
Deep brachial artery, 51
Deep cervical arteries, 49
Deep femoral artery, 57, 62
Deep iliac circumflex artery, 59, 62
Deep palmar arch, 52, 55
Deep plantar branch, 67
Deep venous thrombosis (DVT), 305
Descending genicular artery, 64, 69
Diabetes mellitus (DM), 337, 538
   CLI
      clinical presentation, 546–547
      profile, 546
      risk factors, 545–546
   diagnosis
      ABI, 547

      ankle systolic pressures, 547
      color duplex ultrasound, 548
      CTA, 548
      dorsalis pedis and tibialis posterior pulse, 547
      hemodialysis, 548
      hemodynamic tests, 547
      medial arterial calcification, 547
      MRA, 548
      non-invasive and invasive diagnostic, 548
      strain gauge sensor/photoplethysmography, 548
      TBI, 548
      TcPO$_2$, 548
   macrovascular and microvascular disease, 544–545
   PAD, 543
Diabetic foot
   arterial occlusive disease, 349
   catheter-based contrast angiography, 359–360
   classification, 354
   CTA, 360
   diabetes mellitus, 349
   diabetic peripheral neuropathy, 349–351
   individual patient, 360
   infection, 354, 514
   limb salvage team, 365
   medical management, 361–362
   3MRA, 360
   PAD (*see* Peripheral artery disease (PAD))
   pathophysiology, 349–354
   peripheral artery disease, 351–354
   revascularization, 362–364
   screening, 354–359
   surgical bypass options, 364
   surgical management, 362
Diabetic foot ulcers (DFU), 503
Diabetic neuropathy (DN), 349
Diabetic ulcers/neuropathy, 627–628
Diagnostic algorithm, ALI, 168–169
Diagnostic examination
   CTA, 166
   duplex ultrasound, 165
   intraoperative arteriography, 167, 168
   MRA, 166
Dialysis access-associated steal syndrome (DAASS)
   arterial inflow stenosis, 567
   clinical features, 566
   revascularization techniques, 568
   risk factors, 566, 567
Digital-brachial index (DBI), 86
Digital subtraction angiography (DSA), 152, 180–182, 200, 431, 432, 548
Digital sympathectomy, 263
Direct angiosome revascularization (DAR), 436
Distal arm injuries, 232–233
Distal digital ischemia, 87
Distal embolization, 377
Distal radial artery ligation (DRAL), 568
Distal revascularization-interval ligation procedure (DRIL), 567, 568
Distal vein patch (DVP) technique, 364
Distal/ultra-distal bypasses, 433
Doppler indices, 222
Doppler laser image procedures (LDI), 26
Doppler measurements, 329
Doppler spectral analysis, 166
Dorsal carpal network (rete), 54
Dorsal digital veins, 68
Dorsal metacarpal artery, 52

Dorsal metacarpal veins, 68
Dorsal metatarsal arteries, 67
Dorsal scapular artery, 49
Dorsal venous arch, 68
Dorsalis pedis artery, 57, 64, 67
Double-incision (anterolateral and medial) fasciotomy, lower leg, 36
DRAL. *See* Distal radial artery ligation (DRAL)
DRIL. *See* Distal revascularization-interval ligation procedure (DRIL)
Drug-coated balloons, 398
Drug-eluting balloons (DEBs)
    femoropopliteal lesions
        ACC/AHA guidelines, 400
        Bayesian network meta-analysis, 400
        coronary circulation, 399
        DAART, 401, 403
        de novo/restenotic lesions, 399
        DEBATE-SFA, 400
        DEFINITIVE-AR, 401
        FEMPAC study, 399
        IN.PACT Pacific paclitaxel-eluting
            balloon, 399
        IN.PACT SFA trial, 400
        Lutonix Paclitaxel-Coated Balloon, 399
        MAE rate, 399
        PACIFIER, 399
        PCB, 399
        prototype PACCOCATH DEB, 399
        TCT, 399
        THUNDER trial, 399
        TLR rate, 399, 400, 402
        treatment, 399
        UCB, 399
        vascular restenosis, 400, 401
Drug-eluting stents (DES)
    candidate drugs, 393–394
    ideal drug to inhibit restenosis, 393
    infrapopliteal disease, 395–396
DSA. *See* Digital subtraction angiography (DSA)
Dual antiplatelet therapy (DAPT), 645
Dual-source CT (DSCT), 177
Duplex scan, 430
Duplex ultrasonography, 222
Duplex ultrasound (DUS), 165, 166, 208, 310
Dyslipidemia, 125

E
ECCAs. *See* Extracellular contrast agents (ECCAs)
Effort-induced thrombosis, 307
Ehlers-Danlos syndrome, 105, 106
EKOS. *See* EkoSonic Endovascular System (EKOS)
EkoSonic Endovascular System (EKOS), 317
Elbow disarticulation, 579, 580
Embolic and thrombotic disease, 4
Embolic angiosarcoma, 324
Embolic protection devices, 298, 406–407
Embolism, 100, 104
    aCLI, 37
    arterial, 29
    characterization, 160
    healthy artery, 161
    non-cerebral, 274
    paradoxical, 114–116, 273
    pathologic artery, 161
    peripheral, 109
Endarterectomy, 415, 416, 423

Endocarditis
    antimicrobial therapy, 112
    echocardiography, 112
    Staphylococcus/fungal organisms, 111
    surgical intervention, 112
Endothelial dysfunction, 351
Endothelial progenitor cells (EPCs), 646
Endothelial-specific NO synthase (ecNOS), 353
Endovascular technologies
    adjunctive devices, 403–404
    balloon angioplasty, 387
    BMS *vs.* angioplasty, 391
    BTK, 403
    CBA, 398
    cryoplasty, 397
    CTOs (*see* Chronic total occlusions (CTOs))
    DEBs (*see* Drug-eluting balloons (DEBs))
    DES (*see* Drug-eluting stents (DES))
    lower extremity, 388–390
    nitinol self-expanding stents, 391–392
    PTA (*see* Percutaneous transluminal angioplasty (PTA))
    restenosis, 387–388
    SBA, 398
    stent grafts, 392–393
    stenting, 387
    supera peripheral stent system, 392
Endovascular therapy, 225, 369, 370
Endovascular treatment
    abciximab *vs.* control, 383
    access, 376
    aid in healing, 383
    arterial disease, 374–375
    aspirin *vs.* aspirin + dipyridamole, 383
    aspirin + dipyridamole *vs.* vitamin K antagonist, 383
    BASIL trial, 378–379
    cilostazol + aspirin *vs.* ticlopidine + aspirin, 383
    clopidogrel + aspirin *vs.* low molecular weight heparin, 383
    complications of, 377–378
    cost analysis, 382
    Fontaine III, 379
    frequency of, 373–374
    gastrointestinal side effects, 383
    Graziani, 379
    high-dose *vs.* low-dose aspirin, 383
    history of, 373
    lesion crossing, 376–377
    long-term patency, 381
    low molecular weight heparin *vs.* unfractionated
            heparin, 383
    lower extremity interventions, 381–382
    multidisciplinary team, 383
    natural history of, 373
    noninvasive evaluation, 374
    non-revascularized limbs, 379
    OPGs, 379
    patients with renal failure, 379
    plantar arch vessels, 379
    post-intervention surveillance, 382–383
    post-peripheral vascular intervention antiplatelet/anticoagulant
            therapy, 383
    recurrent ulcerations, 380–381
    risk factors, 382
    Rutherford category 4, 379
    technical considerations, 375–376
    upper extremity CLI, 382
    wound healing, 380

Epidemiology, 1–5
  ALI (*see* Acute limb ischemia (ALI))
Ergot derivatives, 106
Escharotomies
  finger, 342
  foot, 344
  forearm, 343
  hand, 342–343
  neck, 343
  thigh, 343
  trunk, 343
  upper arm, 343
EURODIALE Study, 349
Everolimus, 394–396
Excimer laser angioplasty
  CVX-300, 405
  Ocelot, 405–406
  TruePath, 406
  Wildcat and Kittycat, 405
Excimer laser, atherectomy, 403–404
Excisional and orbital atherectomy, 404
Expanded polytetrafluoroethylene (ePTFE), 226, 392
External iliac artery endofibrosis, 99
Extra-anatomic bypass, 415, 423
Extracellular contrast agents (ECCAs), 184
Extracorporeal membrane oxygenation, 116
Extremity ischemia, 323
Extremity trauma, 221

F
Fasciotomy, 306, 457
Femoral aneurysms
  endovascular repairs, 98
  ePTFE, 97
  pseudoaneurysms, 97
Femoral artery, 228
Femoral endarterectomy, 455
Femoral-femoral bypasses, 417
Femoral Paclitaxel (FEMPAC) study, 399
Femoral vein, 69
Femoral vessels, 61–64
Femoropopliteal arteries, 377
Femoropopliteal bypass graft, 194
Femoropopliteal disease, 397
Femoropopliteal occlusive disease, 246
Femoropopliteal lesions, 380
Femoropopliteal segment, 374
FGF gene therapy, 495–496
Fibromuscular dysplasia (FMD), 82
Fibular artery, 57, 64
Flex/carpi radialis tendon, 52
Flow-dependent non-contrast MRA, 191
Flow-spoiled fresh blood imaging (FS-FBI), 190, 191
Fluorescence angiography, 199, 208
FMD. *See* Fibromuscular dysplasia (FMD)
Fontaine classification, 16
Foot and ankle amputations
  anesthetic considerations, 589
  arthroplasty, 589–590
  calcanectomy, 598, 601
  Chopart, 596, 597
  decision making, 588
  factors, 587
  internal, 589–590
  Lisfranc, 594, 596

  long-term care, 598
  mechanical considerations, 589
  nutrition and immunocompetence, 588–589
  physical therapy, 587
  Ray, 591–594
  Syme's, 596, 598, 599
  toe, 590, 591
  transmetatarsal, 594, 595
  vascular perfusion, 588
Foot infection, 21
Foot ulceration, 503, 504 (*see also* Lower extremity ulceration)
Forearm fasciotomy, 237
Frontrunner CTO Catheter, 405
Frostbite
  clinical manifestations, 333
  deeper injury, 335
  history, 333
  intracellular ice crystals, 333
  management, 335
  pathophysiology, 333, 334
  superficial injury, 334

G
Gadolinium-based contrast agents (GBCAs),
    184, 185
Gaiter area venous ulcer, 41
Gangrene
  atherosclerotic, 24, 26
  toe and forefoot, 39
GCA. *See* Giant cell arteritis (GCA)
Gd-BOPTA-enhanced MRA, 433
Gene therapy
  advantages, 493
  CLI
    clinical trials, 499
    development, angiogenesis, 496
    factors with angiogenic potential, 494
    FGF, 495
    growth factors, 494
    HGF, 496
    HIF-1, 496
    methods, 498
    pro-angiogenic growth factors, 494
    therapeutic angiogenesis, 494
    therapeutic transgene of interest, 493
    VEGF, 495
  genetic material, 493
  origin of, 493
  viral and nonviral vectors, 493, 494
General burn approach, 338
Genicular arteries, 64
Giant cell arteritis (GCA), 82
  abundant collateralization, 281, 282
  corticosteroid tapering, 281
  cranial symptoms, 281
  digital subtraction angiography, 282, 283
  external carotid arteries, 281
  ischemic ocular complications, 281
  limb ischemia, 282
  luminal stenosis/occlusion, 281
  peripheral arterial disease, 282
Glomerular filtration rate (eGFR), 212
Gore Helex occluder, 116
Graft failure, 415, 424
Graft patency, 630

H

Hand-held continuous wave Doppler, 419
Hand surgery, 262
HCPR. *See* High on-clopidogrel platelet reactivity
　　(HCPR)
Health-related quality of life (HRQOL), 638
Heparin-induced skin necrosis, 104
Heparin-induced thrombocytopenia (HIT), 307
　　clinical assessment, 270
　　clinical presentation, 269
　　diagnosis, 270
　　isolation, 270
　　management, 271
　　mechanism, 270
　　pathogenesis, 269
　　platelet monitoring, 271
　　pretest probability, 270
　　venous thrombosis, 270
Heparin-induced thrombosis (HIT), 246
Hepatocyte growth factor (HGF),
　　26, 496
Heyde's syndrome, 27
HGF. *See* Hepatocyte growth factor (HGF)
HGF gene therapy, 496
High on-clopidogrel platelet reactivity (HCPR), 645
HIT. *See* Heparin-induced thrombocytopenia (HIT)
　　　(*see* Heparin-induced thrombosis (HIT))
HIV. *See* Human immunodeficiency virus (HIV)
Hollenhorst plaques, 299, 301
HRQOL. *See* Health-related quality of life (HRQOL)
Human immunodeficiency virus (HIV), 289
The Hunting reaction of Lewis, 333
Hybrid approach, 415
Hydrophilic catheter emboli, 242
Hydrophilic polymer emboli
　　angiographic procedure, 244
　　CVA/stroke, 245
　　pulmonary infarct/cavity, 245
　　radiopaque contrast, 244
　　transmetatarsal amputation, 244
Hydrophilic polymer embolus, 245
Hydroxyurea, 272
Hyperbaric oxygen therapy, 253
　　administration, 483
　　cardiac surgery, 483
　　CLI
　　　diabetes mellitus, 486
　　　end-stage nature and complexity, 485
　　　end-stage peripheral arterial disease, 487
　　　guidelines, 485
　　　HBO, 485, 487
　　　limb loss and mortality rates, 485
　　　multilevel arterial occlusive disease, 486
　　　preservation, limbs and functionality, 486
　　　transcutaneous oxygen measurements, 485
　　decompression ill, 483
　　extracorporeal circulation devices, 483
　　physiologic mechanisms, (IR) injury, 483–484
　　wound transcutaneous oxygen algorithm, 486
Hyperbaric oxygen treatment, 362
Hyperglycemia, 354, 504
Hyperhomocysteinemia, 275
Hypothenar hammer syndrome (HHS), 83, 382
Hypothenar/thenar hammer syndrome, 86
Hypothermia, 335

I

Iatrogenic arterial injury, 245
Iatrogenic extremity ischemia
　　amputations, 241
　　aneurysms, 243
　　anticoagulation, 246
　　arterial catheters, 242
　　arterial monitoring line, 243
　　endograft therapy, 245
　　Ethiopia, 242
　　etiology, 241
　　extremity loss, 242
　　graft failure, 242
　　interventional therapy, 241
　　intra-arterial, 242
　　shocklike situation, 242
　　therapeutic procedures, 242
Iatrogenic injury, 83, 116
Iatrogenic limb ischemia, 246
ICG. *See* Indocyanine green angiograms (ICG)
IDSA guidelines. *See* Infectious Disease Society of America (IDSA)
　　　guidelines
Iliac vessels, 57–61, 228
Immediate threatened limb, 2
Incomplete pedal arch (IPA), 431, 432
Indocyanine green angiograms (ICG), 478, 479
Infection
　　CF, 350
　　diabetic foot ulceration, 354
　　diabetic foot ulcers, 362
　　limb-threatening diabetic foot, 361
Infectious Disease Society of America (IDSA) guidelines, 521
Inferior epigastric artery, 59, 62
Inferior gluteal artery, 61, 63
Inferomedial and inferolateral genicular arteries, 64
Inferomedial genicular artery, 64
Inflow operations
　　aortobifemoral bypass, 415
　　arteriotomy, 417
　　definition, 415
　　femoral vessels, 416
　　hybrid approach, 415
　　percutaneous endovascular treatment, 416
　　standard endarterectomy, 416
　　thromboendarterectomy, 417
Infragenicular occlusive disease, 352
Infrainguinal bypass
　　autogenous saphenous vein, 417
　　contralateral saphenous vein, 420
　　cryopreserved cadaveric vein, 421
　　duplex ultrasound, 424
　　non-reversed configuration, 418
　　patency rates, 423
　　popliteal to dorsalis pedis bypass, 420
　　proximal and distal anastomoses, 419
　　PTFE, 421, 423
　　reversed configuration, 418
　　saphenous vein graft, 417
　　short bypass graft, 420
　　vascular disease recognition, 420
Infrainguinal PAD, 378
Infrainguinal vein bypasses, 353
Infrapopliteal angioplasty, 374, 381
Infrapopliteal artery, 375
Infrapopliteal bypass, 429, 430

Infrapopliteal disease
    ACHILLES trial, 396
    coronary stents, 395
    cryoplasty, 397
    DESTINY, 396
    PaRADISE trial, 396
    RCT, 396
    SES, 395
    XIENCE V arm, 396
    YUKON-BTK, 396
Infra-popliteal vasculature, 180
Intermittent claudication (IC), 463, 543
Intermittent pneumatic compression (IPC), 647
Internal and external iliac vessels, 58
Internal iliac artery, 57, 60
Internal pudendal artery, 61
International Working Group of the Diabetic Foot (IWGDF), 521
Interosseous artery, 53, 54
Interosseous branch, 67
Interposition bypass, 455
Intimal ulcer and luminal thrombus, 91
Intra-aortic balloon pumps, 116
Intracellular ice crystals, 333
Intramuscular edema, 160
Intraoperative angiogram, 220
Intravascular ultrasound (IVUS), 153, 212–214
Invasive angiography, 211
Invasive instrumental diagnostics, 167–168
IPC. See Intermittent pneumatic compression (IPC)
Irreversible ischemia, 2
Ischemia-reperfusion (IR) injury
    acute crush Injury, 484–485
    compromised grafts and flaps, 485
    enhanced wound-healing mechanisms, 484
    free radicals, 484
    HBO, 484
    metabolic substrates, 484
    neovascularization, 484
    neutrophils, 484
    nitric oxide (·NO), 484
    tissue, 483
    vasoconstriction, 484
Ischemic limb disease
    aortic arch and brachiocephalic vessels, 23
    arteriosclerotic vascular, 24
    Bechet's disease, 26
    Buerger's disease, 25–26
    coagulation, 27
    D-Dimer test, 27
    gangrene, 26
    Heyde's syndrome, 27
    occlusive arteriosclerotic disease, 23
    Raynaud's disease, 24–25
    vascular dissection, 23
    vascular process, 23, 24
Ischemic paraneoplastic syndrome, 324
Ischemic ulcers, 211
Isolated thrombolysis technique, 316
IWGDF. See International Working Group of the Diabetic Foot (IWGDF)

J
JENALI. See Joint endovascular and noninvasive assessment of limb perfusion (JENALI)
Jetstream systems (Bayer Health System), 404

Joint endovascular and noninvasive assessment of limb perfusion (JENALI), 15
Joint Venous Committee of the Society for Vascular Surgery (SVS), 311

K
Kaplan–Meier analysis, 390
Kaplan–Meier survival curves, 436
KDs. See Knee disarticulations (KDs)
Kidney disease
    epidemiology, 561–562
    limb ischemia, 562
    traditional and novel risk factors, 562
Knee disarticulations (KDs), 610

L
Large vessel vasculitis (LVV)
    diagnosis, 283–284
    epidemiology, 280
    GCA, 281, 282
    limb ischemia, 285
    medical treatment, 284
    pathophysiology, 280
    TA, 282, 283
Larval secretions
    angiogenesis, 532
    antimicrobial peptide, 531
    disrupt bacterial biofilms, 531
    inhibit inflammatory processes, 532
    necrotic tissue, 531
    PI3K/AKT1 protein kinase, 532
    pro-angiogenic effects, 532
    serine protease activity, 532
Lateral anterior malleolar artery, 65
Lateral calcaneal branches, 67
Lateral circumflex artery, 63, 64
Lateral plantar artery, 67
Lateral thoracic artery, 50
LDI. See Doppler laser image procedures (LDI)
LEAD. See Lower extremity arterial disease (LEAD)
Left ventricular (LV) thrombus
    diagnosis, 111
    embolization, 111
    myocardial infarction, 111
Leg ulcers
    causes and treatments, 628
    CLI, 625
        acute/chronic processes, 626
        bypass vs. angioplasty, 626
        comorbidities, 626
        endovascular therapies, 627
        Flush ostial occlusion, 627
        morbidity and mortality, 626
        multidisciplinary approach, 626
        open surgical revascularization, 626
        peripheral arterial occlusive disease, 626
        TASC, 627
    CVU (see Chronic venous ulceration (CVU))
    development, 628
    diabetes mellitus, 627
    endovascular therapies, 626
    etiology, 625
    gene therapy, 628

Limb amputation, 241
Limb ischemia
    antiphospholipid antibody syndrome, 267–269
    atrial fibrillation, 273, 274
    carcinomas, 328
    HIT, 269–271
    hyperhomocysteinemia, 275
    myeloproliferative disorders, 271, 272
    paradoxic embolism, 272–273
    PNH, 275
    symptom, 328
    treatment modalities, 328–329
Limb salvage, 472
    and replantation
        amputated part, 572
        contraindications, 572
        crush and avulsion injuries, 572
        guiding principles, 572
        hand, 572
        indications, 572
        monitoring, 572
        myoglobinuria, 572
        revascularization, 572
        soft tissue coverage, 572
Livedo reticularis, 41
Loop angioplasty, 437
Loop technique recanalization, 370
Lower extremity ALI, 2
Lower extremity amputation prevention (LEAP) project, 361
Lower extremity arterial disease (LEAD), 71
Lower extremity fasciotomy, 236
Lower extremity incidents, 246
Lower extremity ischemia, 2
Lower extremity ischemic venous thrombosis, 309, 310
Lower extremity replantation, 623
Lower extremity ulceration
    Achilles procedure, 512
    ankle mobility, 503
    arthroplasty/amputation, 513
    BATs, 509, 510
    Becaplermin gel, 509
    complications, 514
    compression therapy
        bandages, 507
        devices, 508
        edema and stasis, 507
        four-layer, 508
        limb, 508
        management, 507
        peripheral vascular disease, 508
        predictive factors, 508
        vascular surgery, 507
        vs. standard wound care, 507
        wound closure, 508
        wraps, 508
    debridement, 512, 513
    diabetes, 503
    forefoot ulceration, Achilles, 514
    hyperbaric oxygen therapy, 509
    hypergranular second toe ulcer, 511
    inlay depth shoe with deep toe box, 514
    lateral foot fifth ray amputation site, 511
    long-term care, 514
    NPWT, 509, 510, 512
    off-loading of wounds, 508, 509
    ovine forestomach dressing, 507

University of Texas Diabetic Wound Classification, 504
    vascularity
        and sensation, 503
        and tissue nutrition (see Vascularity and tissue nutrition)
    venous leg ulcer, 510
    Wagner classification, 503
    wound margins/resolution, 503
    wound size and calculation, percent area reduction, 509
Lower limb symptom classification, 10
Lumbar sympathectomy (LS)
    ankle-brachial pressure index, 463
    anterior approach, 460
    anterolateral approach, 460
    arterial occlusive disease, 459
    arterial reconstructive procedures, 459
    arteriovenous anastomoses, 461
    assessment, cutaneous blood flow, 462
    and chemical, 463
    clinical assessment of degree of ischemia, 462
    collateral circulation, 463
    continuous ganglion, 459
    controversial, 462
    failure, 461
    indications, 463
    intermittent claudication, 463
    ischemia and exercise, 461
    lack of objective evidence-based support, 463
    laparoscopic, 461
    lumbar chain, 460
    management, CLI, 462
    muscles splitting, 460
    pain and ischemic ulceration, 462
    peripheral circulation, 463
    peritoneum, 460
    physiological changes, 461
    physiological effect, 463
    posterior approach, 460
    postganglionic fibers, 459
    post-sympathectomy neuralgia, 461
    preganglionic neurons, 459
    refractory ischemic ulceration, 463
    review, 461–462
    sexual dysfunction, 461
    spastic paralysis, 459
    surgical vs. chemical, 461
    symptomatic atherosclerotic occlusive disease, 463
    tactile identification, 460
    transverse incision, 460
    treatment, 459
    vascular and neurological disorders, 459
    vasomotor tone test, 462
LUNA™ parameters, 208
LUNA™ technology, 208
Lung carcinoma, 324
Lupus anticoagulant testing, 268
LVV. See Large vessel vasculitis (LVV)
Lymphomas and leukemias, 328

M
Maggot debridement therapy (MDT)
    angiogenesis, 531
    chronic osteomyelitis, 531
    dipteran flies, 531
    ischemic ulcer, 533
    larval secretions, 531–532

larval therapy, 531
necrotic tissue, 532
necrotic ulcer, 532
non-healing traumatic, 531
peripheral arterial disease, 533
pressure ulcers, 531
treatments, 531
Magnetic resonance angiography (MRA), 200, 223, 360, 548
ALI, 32
CE-MRA, 185
clinical applications, 192–193
Magnetic resonance imaging (MRI), 340
Major amputation rate, 436
Malignancy-associated extremity lymphedema, 329
Malignancy-induced ischemia
case reports
acute left lower extremity ischemia, 324
benign endocardial tumor, 325
chronic lymphatic leukemia, 325
ischemic paraneoplastic syndrome, 324
lung carcinoma, 324
malignancy, 325
primary pulmonary angiosarcoma, 327
squamous cell carcinoma, 325
gangrene, 326
lymphomas and leukemias, 328
Management, diabetic patients
amputation, 553
anti-platelet agents, 551
cardiovascular risk factors, 552
dyslipidemia, 550
glycemic control, 550
hypertension control, 550–551
cilostazol, 551
foot ulceration, 552
graft occlusion, 553
lifestyle modifications, 550
pain control, 552
prostanoids, 551
revascularization procedures, 552–553
therapeutic angiogenesis, 554
therapies, revascularization
lumbar sympathectomy, 553
spinal cord stimulation, 554
Mangled Extremity Severity Score (MESS), 227
Maximal intensity projection (MIP), 175, 177
Maximum intensity projections (MIP), 187
Medial anterior malleolar artery, 65
Medial calcaneal arteries, 66
Medial circumflex artery, 63
Medial epicondyle, 53
Medial plantar artery, 67
Median artery, 54
Mesenteric artery ischemia, 74
Methicillin-resistant *Staphylococcus aureus* (MRSA), 523, 524
Methicillin-susceptible *Staphylococcus aureus* (MSSA),
524, 525
Microvascular, 351, 353
Mid-aortic syndrome, 101
Move during scan (MDS) technique, 188
MRA. *See* Magnetic resonance angiography (MRA)
MRI contrast agents
definition, 184
ECCAs, 184
Gadolinium-based contrast agents, 185
Intravascular/blood pool contrast agents, 184

novel/experimental contrast agents, 184
NSF, 185
MRI safety, 193–195
MRSA. *See* Methicillin-resistant *Staphylococcus aureus*
(MRSA)
MSSA. *See* Methicillin-susceptible *Staphylococcus aureus*
(MSSA)
Multi-detector CT scanners, 171
Multiplanar reformations (MPRs), 175, 177, 187
Multivessel disease, 71
Muscle necrosis, 235
Muscular branches, 61, 63, 64
Musculophrenic arteries, 47
Myeloproliferative disorders
elevated red cell/platelet counts, 271
phenylalanine, 271
polycythemia rubra vera, 272
polycythemia vera, 271
screening, 271
thrombocythemia, 271
vascular surgery, 271
Myoglobinuria, 235

N
National Trauma Data Bank, 218
Natural history
critical limb ischemia without revascularization, 373
non-revascularized limbs, 379
Near-infrared spectroscopy (NIRS), 207
Negative pressure wound therapy, 509
Nephrogenic systemic fibrosis (NSF), 150, 185, 360
Nephrotoxicity, 222
Neurogenic claudication, 106
Neuropathy
diabetic peripheral, 349–351
PAD, 349
Neutrophils, 132
Nitinol self-expanding stents, 391–392
Non-atherosclerotic etiologies
atheroembolic episodes, 104–105
brown recluse spider bite, 105
calciphylaxis, 103
CLI/amputation, 95
cystic adventitial disease, 99
Ehlers-Danlos syndrome, 105–106
ergot derivatives, 106
external iliac artery endofibrosis, 99
femoral aneurysms, 97–98
heparin-induced skin necrosis, 104
lipid hypothesis, 95
macrophages and smooth muscle cells, 95
mid-aortic syndrome, 101
neovascularization, 95
neurogenic claudication, 106
peripheral vascular disease, 96
persistent sciatic artery, 100, 101
popliteal aneurysms, 98–99
popliteal artery entrapment, 100
pseudoxanthoma elasticum, 106
radiation therapy, 105
Raynaud's syndrome, 102–103
TA, 96, 97
thromboangiitis obliterans (*see* Buerger's disease)
vasculitis, 96
warfarin-induced skin necrosis, 103–104

Non-contrast-enhanced MRA (NC-MRA)
    FS-FBI, 190, 191
    phase contrast angiography, 190
    TOF-MRA, 190
Nonhealing ischemic ulceration, 39
Noninvasive imaging
    arterial duplex ultrasonography, 200–206
    laboratory, 199
    plethysmography and segmental Pressures,
            199–200
    SPP, 206
    vascular laboratory, 199
Noninvasive physiologic tests
    ABI (see Ankle-brachial index (ABI))
    CWD, 139
    hyperspectral imaging, 145, 146
    PVR, 141–143
    segmental lime pressure (see Segmental limb pressure)
    skin perfusion pressure, 145
    TcPO2, 144, 145
    tissue perfusion, 143–144
    toe pressure, 143
Non-reversed translocated technique, 417
Nontraumatic lower limb, 349
No pedal arch (NPA), 431, 433
NSF. See Nephrogenic systemic fibrosis (NSF)
Nutrient artery, 61, 66

O
Objective performance goals (OPGs), 379
Obturator artery, 59, 63
Occlusive disease, 79, 81, 90, 92
Off-loading foot wounds, 508, 509
Omental grafting, 329
Omental transplant
    anatomy
        blood supply, 470, 471
        structure, 469–470
    ancient egyptians, 469
    arterialization properties, 469
    biological properties, 470
    gastrointestinal surgery, 480
    inherent properties, 472
    lymphatic drainage, 475
    neovascularization, 470–471
    operative technique, 472–474
    pedicle preparation, 472
    phagocyte cells, 469
    properties, 471–472
    reconstructive surgical procedure, 475–476
    revascularization
        CNS, 480
        ICG, 478, 479
        ischemic conditions, 476–478
        ischemic extremities, 473–475, 477
        myocardium (heart), 479–480
        retina and choroidal capillaries, 478, 479
    spleen trauma, 480
    thoracic surgical procedures, 480
    urogenital surgery, 480
Optical coherence tomography (OCT), 214–215
Osteomyelitis
    clinical and laboratory diagnosis, 526
    culture-guided therapy, 528
    microbiology, 525–526

radiographic diagnosis, 526–527
superficial wound, 525
treatment, 525, 527–528
Osteopontin, 353

P
PACE. See Peripheral arteriopathy and cardiovascular events (PACE)
Paclitaxel, 389, 393–396, 399, 401, 402
PADs. See Peripheral arterial diseases (PADs)
Paget–Schroetter syndrome, 307, 310
Palmar and dorsal carpal network, 54
Palmar sympathectomy, 263
Paradoxical embolism, 161
    arterial embolism, 272, 273
    catheter-based approaches, 115
    cryptogenic stroke, 273
    diagnosis, 115
    ischemic stroke, 272
    mechanism, 272
    medical therapy, 273
    PFO/ASD, 114, 115
    SPARC study, 272
    stroke, 272, 273
    treatment, 115, 116
    variables, 272
    venous thrombosis, 272
Paraneoplastic ischemic manifestations, 328
Paraneoplastic syndrome, 324, 327
Paroxysmal nocturnal thrombophilia (PNH), 275
Patent foramen ovale (PFO)
    CardioSEAL-STARFlex, 116
    cryptogenic strokes/recurrent strokes, 115
    percutaneous devices, 116
    transient ischemic attack/stroke, 115
    warfarin/antiplatelet agents, 115
PAVA. See Proximal arteriovenous anastomoses (PAVA)
Peak ankle velocity (PAV), 339
Peak systolic velocity (PSV), 202
Pedal arch
    anatomy, 427–429
    arcuate artery, 429
    colour-coded duplex, 433–435
    CPA, 431
    DAR, 436
    deep plantar arch, 429
    dorsalis pedis artery, 429
    DSA, 431, 433, 435
    Gd-BOPTA-enhanced MRA, 433
    IPA, 431, 432
    loop angioplasty, 437
    major amputation rate, 436
    non-DAR, 436
    NPA, 431
    pedal bypass patency, 433–436
    pedal bypass tissue loss healing outcome, 436–437
    plantar arch, 428
    venous system, foot, 428
Pedal bypass, 379
Pedal-plantar loop angioplasty, 437
Percutaneous cardiac catheterizations, 116
Percutaneous endovascular treatment, 416
Percutaneous iatrogenic injuries, 245
Percutaneous intentional extraluminal recanalization (PIER), 376
Percutaneous mechanical thrombectomy (PMT), 442
Percutaneous vs. open surgical revascularization, 35

Percutaneous thrombectomy, 312
Percutaneous thrombolytic therapy
    angioplasty, 34
    anticoagulants and antiplatelet medications, 34
    arterial occlusion, 32
    contraindications, 34
    lower extremity angiography, 32
    mechanical thrombectomy, 32
    occlusion, 32
    revascularization, 32
    surgical revascularization, 34
    treating tibial thrombus, 32
Percutaneous transluminal angioplasty (PTA), 544, 552, 553, 555
    adjunctive stenting, 390
    with adjunctive therapies, 390
    ATK, 390
    BTK, 390
    Kaplan–Meier analysis, 390
    success rates, 390
    vs. surgical bypass, 391
Percutaneous vacuum-assisted thrombectomy, 312
Percutaneous vascular interventions, 377
Peripheral academic research consortium (PARC)
    ORC, 21–22
    PAD limb symptoms, 21, 22
Peripheral arterial disease (PAD), 21, 22, 71, 173, 183, 211, 441, 444, 491, 543
    CLI (see Critical limb ischemia (CLI))
    IC, 491, 543
    macrovascular disease, 543
    morbidity and mortality, 543
Peripheral arterial imaging, 201
Peripheral arterial occlusive disease, 30
Peripheral Arteriopathy and Cardiovascular Events (PACE), 72
Peripheral artery disease (PAD), 9, 16, 641
    ABIs, 122
    above-the-knee vessels, 395
    amputations, 122
    chronic renal insufficiency, 126
    claudication symptoms, 122
    CLI, 367
    contrast imaging, 359–360 (see also Critical limb ischemia (CLI))
    CTOs, 406
    data, 122
    description, 367
    diabetes, 352
    development, 126
    dyslipidemia, 125
    effects, 354
    endovascular treatment, 407
    femoropopliteal and aortoiliac disease, 392
    inflammatory markers, 126
    infrapopliteal, 395
    loss of compensatory mechanisms, 121
    macrovascular component, 353
    management of lower extremity, 388
    metabolic supply and demand, lower extremity, 121
    morbidity and mortality, 122
    multifactorial nature, 126
    neuropathy, 349
    noninvasive assessment, 359
    pathophysiology, 121–122
    peripheral neuropathy, 126
    prevalence, 122, 367, 387
    progresses, 123
    progression, 121–123, 126

    with RBC, 395
    revascularization, 370, 399
    risk factor modification and effect
        development, 123
        diagnosis, 124
        DM, 124, 125
        dyslipidemia, 125
        gender differences, 124
        hypertension, 125
        non-modifiable, 123
        racial predispositions, 124
        recommendations, 123
        smoking cessation, 124
        symptom severity, 123
    symptomatic SFA, 392
    symptoms, 122
    thrombosis, 126
    treatment of femoropopliteal, 399, 400
    weight reduction, 125, 126
Peripheral endothelium-dependent vasodilation, 250
Peripheral sympathectomy, 263
Peripheral vascular disease (PVD), 96, 465, 467, 473
Persistent sciatic artery
    atherosclerosis and aneurysm formation, 101
    femoral and popliteal vein, 100
    transgluteal approach, 101
    treatment, 101
PFO. See Patent foramen ovale (PFO)
Pharmacomechanical catheter-directed thrombolysis (PCDT)
    advantage, 316
    AngioJet Rheolytic Thrombectomy system, 316
    ATTRACT trial, 316
    EKOS, 317
    isolated thrombolysis technique, 316
    PCD, 314, 315
    SVS/AVF guidelines, 314
Phase contrast angiography, 190
Phlegmasia alba dolens, 307
Phlegmasia cerulea dolens (PCD)
    ACCP anticoagulation guidelines, 319
    acute compartment syndrome, 310
    adjunctive management strategies (see Adjunctive management strategies)
    anticoagulation, 311
    APS, 307
    canine model, 306
    catheter-directed thrombolysis, 313, 314
    causes, 307
    clinical presentation, 308
    contrast venography, 310
    critical closing pressure, 306
    diagnosis, 310, 311
    duplex ultrasound imaging, 310
    fasciotomy, 306
    fluid sequestration, 308
    grading severity, 308
    hereditary hypercoagulable state, 307
    HIT, 307
    initial management, 311
    PCDT (see Pharmacomechanical catheter-directed thrombolysis (PCDT))
    phlegmasia alba dolens, 308
    PTS, 309
    risk factors, 306, 307
    TF, 307
    thrombectomy, 312, 313

Phlegmasia cerulea dolens (PCD) (*cont.*)
    UEDVT, 307
    venous gangrene, 309
    VTE, 305
Photoplethysmography (PPG), 86
Plain radiographic, 85–86
Plantar arch, 370
Plantar digital branches, 67
Plantar digital veins, 68
Plantar metatarsal arteries, 67
Plantar venous arch, 68, 69
Plaque rupture
    spontaneous atheroembolism, 297
    thrombolytic and anticoagulation
        therapy, 298
    traumatic plaque rupture, 297, 298
Plethysmography, 199, 208
Pneumatic tourniquets, 219
PNH. *See* Paroxysmal nocturnal thrombophilia (PNH)
PolarCath system, 397
Polytetrafluoroethylene (PTFE), 92, 364, 421
Polyvinyl chloride (PVC), 83
Popliteal aneurysms
    endovascular repair, 98
    symptoms, 98
    thrombectomy, 98
    thrombolysis/surgical revascularization, 98
    thrombosis, 98
    vascular ultrasound, 98
Popliteal artery, 57, 61, 64, 69, 228, 230
Popliteal artery entrapment
    arterial occlusion/embolization, 100
    gastrocnemius, 100
    symptoms, 100
Popliteal vein, 69
Posterior humeral circumflex artery, 50
Posterior popliteal approach, 231
Posterior tibial artery, 57, 64–68
Post-thrombotic syndrome (PTS), 309
Pre- and post-revascularization images, 370
Prehospital external hemorrhage control algorithm, 219
Prehospital tourniquet, 218, 220
Preoperative bilateral saphenous vein mapping, 413
Preoperative planning, 413–415
Prevalence, 13
    CLI (*see* Chronic critical limb ischemia (CLI))
PReventing Amputations using Drug eluting StEnts (PaRADISE)
        trial, 396
Primary pulmonary angiosarcoma, 327
Profunda-circumflex trunk, 62
Profunda femoris, 62, 69
Proximal arteriovenous anastomoses (PAVA), 568
Pseudoaneurysm, 224–225, 377
Pseudoxanthoma elasticum, 106
PTFE. *See* Polytetrafluoroethylene (PTFE)
PTS. *See* Post-thrombotic syndrome (PTS)
Pulsatile bleeding, 220
Pulse repetition frequency (PRF), 166
Pulse volume recording (PVR), 141–143, 145, 200,
        359, 374
PVD. *See* Peripheral vascular disease (PVD)

Q
QOL. *See* Quality of life (QOL)
Quality of life (QOL), 465

R
Radial and ulnar exposure, 234
Radial artery, 55
Radiation therapy, 105
Rapamycin analogs, 394
RAS. *See* Renal artery stenosis (RAS)
Raynaud's disease, 24–25
Raynaud's phenomenon (RP), 79, 82, 84
    acute critical ischemia, 261
    analgesia, 259
    anti-phospholipid (Hughes) syndrome, 258
    arterial reconstruction, 264
    balloon angioplasty, 263
    blood investigations, 258
    botulinum toxin injection, 262–263
    cephalic vein, 264
    chronic critical ischemia, 262
    classification, 257
    diagnosis, 257–259
    digital (palmar) sympathectomy, 259
    digital ulceration/critical ischemia, 257, 258
    hand surgery, 262
    nailfold capillaroscopy and thermography, 258, 259
    palmar sympathectomy, 263
    peripheral sympathectomy, 263
    pulmonary hypertension, 261, 262
    SSc (*see* Systemic sclerosis (SSc))
    surgical management, 259, 265
    symptoms, 262
    treatment, 262–263
    venous/arterial grafting, 264
    wound débridement, 262
Raynaud's syndrome, 80, 84
    cold/emotional stimuli, 102
    diagnosis, 103
    digital ulceration and gangrene, 103
    immune disorders, 102
    sympathectomy, 103
REBOA, 225
Receiver operating characteristic (ROC) analysis, 206–207
Reentry devices
    BridgePoint system, 406
    Embolic Protection Devices, 406–407
    Outback, 406
    Pioneer, 406
Refractory ischemic ulceration, 463
Renal artery stenosis (RAS), 71, 72
Repair, wound healing
    factors, 133
    minimal inflammation, 133
    normal, 133
    process, 131
    transforming factor beta, 131
Reperfusion injury, 233–235
Repetitive trauma injury, 83
Restenosis, 380, 387–388
Retinitis pigmentosa, 478
Retroperitoneal iliac vessel, 228
Return to ambulation, 632–633
Revascularization procedures, 362–364, 543, 546, 548, 551–554
    angiosome model, 367
    angiosome-directed interventions, 375
    CLI, 373, 374
    direct and indirect, 375
    endovascular, 374
    non-revascularized limbs, 379

post revascularization limb salvage rate, 377
posterior tibial artery, 375
single tibial artery, 375
surgical *vs.* endovascular, 378
Reverse CART technique, 377
Rhabdomyolysis, 35–36
Risk stratification of CLI, 12, 13
Rutherford classification, 16, 452

S
Safe prehospital tourniquet, 219
Saphenous vein, 69
Saphenous vein bypass, 91
Saphenous vein grafts, 413
Sarcomas, 328
Scapular circumflex artery, 50
Scoring balloon angioplasty (SBA), 398
SCS. *See* Spinal cord stimulation (SCS)
Segmental limb pressure, 141
Segmental pressure, 200
Segmental stenosis, 202
Sexually transmitted disease (STD), 26
Shoulder disarticulation, 581
Sirolimus (Rapamycin), 393–395, 401, 402
Sirolimus for below-the knee (SiroBTK), 395
Sirolimus-eluting stent (SES), 395
Skin and soft-tissue infections
    anatomy, 518, 519
    cellulitis, 518
    diabetic infections, 518
    erysipelas, 518
    impetigo, 518
    surgical site infections, 519
Skin perfusion pressure (SPP), 145, 206–208, 533
Smooth muscle cells, 387, 388
Society for Vascular Surgery's Objective Performance Goals (SVS OPGs), 633
Socioeconomic impact, chronic CLI, 13
Spinal cord stimulation (SCS), 253, 540, 646, 647
    complications, 466
    contraindications, 465
    controversy regarding pain, 467
    electrodes, 466
    implantation, 465
    indications, 465
    limb ischemia, 466
    mechanism, 466
    pain, 465
    pulse generation, 466
    systematic meta-analysis, 467
    transcutaneous oxygen pressure, 467
    treatment, 465
Spiral CT, 171
SPP. *See* skin perfusion pressure (SPP)
Squamous cell carcinoma, 325
SSc. *See* Systemic sclerosis (SSc)
Staphylococcus aureus, wound infections
    MRSA, 523
    MSSA, 524
STD. *See* Sexually transmitted disease (STD)
Stent grafts, 392–393
Stenting
    and balloon angioplasty, 387
    grafts, 392–393

nitinol self-expanding, 391–392
supera peripheral stent system, 392
Sternoclavicular joint, 45
Subclavian aneurysm (UE), 442
Subclavian artery, 45, 224
    axillary artery, 50
    brachial plexus, 47, 49
    brachiocephalic trunk, 45, 47
    carotid sheath, 47
    clavipectoral fascia, 50
    intertubercular groove, 50
    occlusion, 89
    pectoralis minor muscle, 50
    superomedial border, 50
    thyrocervical trunk, 47
    thyroid gland, 48
    upper abdominal wall, 45
Subclavian vein, 56
Subintimal angioplasty (SIA), 374, 376, 404
Supera peripheral stent system, 392
Superficial epigastric artery, 62
Superficial femoral artery (SFA), 228, 391, 446
Superficial palmar arterial arch, 55
Superficial sural artery, 64
Superficial veins, 45, 47, 59, 68–69
Superior gluteal artery, 61, 63
Superomedial and superolateral genicular arteries, 64
Supracondylar humeral fractures, 50
Surgical approach, 369, 370
Surgical revascularization, CLI
    arteriography, 413
    BASIL trial, 425
    diabetic vascular disease, 413
    duplex ultrasound, 413
    foot ulceration, 415
    graft occlusion, 423
    infection, 413, 415
    inflow operations, 415–417
    infrainguinal bypass, 417–421
    lateral and AP arteriogram, 413, 414
    limb salvage, 422
    patency rates, 422
    proximal bypass, 413
    systemic and local complications, 422
    wound infection complications, 422, 424
Surgical treatment, ALI
    angioplasty, 455
    anticoagulation, 456
    aortoiliac occlusion, 451
    axillary–bifemoral bypass, 455
    categorization tool, 452
    classification, 452
    compartment syndrome, 456–457
    criteria, 451
    CTA, 453
    diagnosis, 451
    dissection, 455
    Doppler signals, 454
    duration, location and severity, 451
    electrocardiogram, 453
    embolic and acute thrombotic events, 457
    embolus/thrombosis, 451
    exposure, femoral artery, 454
    fasciotomy, 456, 457
    femoral endarterectomy, 455
    flow-limiting/anastomotic stenosis, 454

Surgical treatment, ALI (*cont.*)
  Fogarty catheter, thromboembolectomy, 454
  four-compartment fasciotomy, 457
  history, 451
  infrainguinal bypass, 454
  interposition bypass, 455
  management, 451
  morbidity and mortality, 457
  MRA, 453
  non-salvageable limb, 456
  nonviable category III limb with tissue loss, 456
  occluded infrainguinal bypass, 453
  percutaneous and open, 455
  physical examination, 451
  reocclusion, 454
  revascularization, 451
  Rutherford classification, 453
  stenosis, 454
  systemic heparinization, 453
  techniques, 453
  thrombectomy, 454
  thromboembolectomy, 453, 454
  thrombosis, 452
  thrombotic events, 452, 453
Sympathectomy, 253, 263
Sympathetic nerve fibers, 47
Symptomatology progression, 323
Systemic lupus erythematosus (SLE), 82
Systemic sclerosis (SSc)
  characterization, 288
  critical digital ischemia, 259–261
  Raynaud's phenomenon, 289
  vascular abnormalities, 259
  vascular hypothesis, 288

T
TA. *See* Takayasu's arteritis (TA)
Takayasu's arteritis (TA), 79, 82
  aortoiliac obstruction, 283, 284
  characterization, 282
  diagnosis, 97
  supraaortic branches, 283
  symptoms, 96
  treatment, 97
Talent® endograft, 195
TAO. *See* Thromboangiitis obliterans (TAO)
Target lesion revascularization (TLR), 392
Targeted muscle reinnervation (TMR)
  amputation, 582
  bilateral shoulder disarticulation injury, 581
  complex and intuitive control of prosthetics, 581
  EMG signals, 581
  median, ulnar and radial nerves, 583
  morbid and debilitating condition, 581
  motor control, 582
  myoelectric designs, 581
  prosthetic function, 583
  sensory, 583
  shoulder disarticulation level, 583
  surgery, 583
  Tinel's sign, 583
  *trans*humeral amputees, 583
TASC. *See* TransAtlantic inter-society consensus (TASC)
TASC II classification, 15
TAVR. *See* Transcatheter aortic valve replacement (TAVR)

TBI. *See* Toe-brachial index (TBI)
Test bolus method/bolus-tracking method, 187
TEVAR. *See* Thoracic endovascular repair (TEVAR)
TF. *See* Tissue factor (TF)
Thermal injury
  ABI, 339
  arterial duplex, 339–340
  associated disease states, 337–338
  burn approach, 338
  case study, 344–346
  classification, 337
  imaging modalities, 340
  pathophysiology, 337
  physical exam, 339
  treatment algorithm, 344, 345
  vascular approach (*see* Vascular approach)
  vascular bed responses, 337
  venous duplex, 340
Thigh compartments, 236
Thoracic endovascular repair (TEVAR), 118
Thoracic outlet syndrome (UE), 88, 442
Thoracoacromial artery, 50, 56
Thoracodorsal artery, 50
Thoracoepigastric vein, 56
Thrombectomy
  open surgical
    acute arterial embolus, 34–35
    chronic arterial occlusive disease, 35
  advantage, 312
  AngioVac cannula, 312
  anticoagulation, 312
Thromboangiitis obliterans (TOA), 81 (*see also* Buerger's disease)
  cannabis and cocaine, 249
  CT angiography, 251, 252
  diagnosis and differential diagnosis, 250, 251
  diagnostic workup, 251–252
  epidemiology, 249
  etiopathogenesis, 249–250
  histology, 250
  intraoperative arteriography, 252, 253
  smoking, 249
  tobacco exposure, 249
  treatment
    acute phase, 252
    amputations, 254
    bosentan, 253
    bypass surgery, 253
    chronic phase, 252
    endovascular therapy, 253
    foot care, 254
    hyperbaric oxygen therapy, 253
    iloprost and aspirin, 252
    inpatient basis, 252
    oral medications, 252–253
    peripheral sympathectomy, 253
    spinal cord stimulation, 253
    thrombolysis, 253
  vasculitis, 249
Thromboembolectomy, 162, 454
Thromboendarterectomy, 417
Thrombophilia, 267
Thrombosis, 1–5, 126
Thrombotic occlusion, 162
Thyrocervical trunk, 47, 48
Tibial artery, 229
Tibial restenosis, 381

Tibial vessels, 375
Time to healing, 380
Tissue factor (TF), 307
TMR, shoulder disarticulation, 584
TOA. *See* Thromboangiitis obliterans (TOA)
Toe amputations
    anatomy, 590
    authors' preferred method, 591, 592
    gangrene, 591
    osteomyelitis, 591
    plantar flaps, 590
Toe-brachial index (TBI), 359, 548
Toe pressure, 143
TransAtlantic Inter-Society Consensus (TASC), 15, 17, 18
TransAtlantic Inter-Society Consensus (TASC) II guidelines, 375,
        561, 562
Transcatheter aortic valve replacement (TAVR), 247
Transcollateral approach, 377
Transcutaneous oximetry, 199, 206
Transcutaneous oxygen pressure (TcPO2), 543, 549
Transcutaneous oxygen tension (TcPO2), 12, 13
Transcutaneous partial pressure of oxygen (TcPO2), 206
    diffuse oxygen, 145
    hyperbaric oxygen therapy, 145
    impact, measurement, 145
    measurements, 144, 145
    normal, 145
    probes, 145
    wound healing, 145
Transhumeral amputations, 581
Transplantation/extremity replantation
    amputated fingertip, distal phalanx/entire digit, 619
    amputated extremity, 620
        condition, injured patient, 620
        factors, survival, 620
        operative management, 620
        postoperative management, 620
        preop management, 620
        salvage, 620
        site of accident, 620
        surgery, 620
    clean-cut injury, 619
    consultation, 620
    crush injury, 619
    crush-amputation injury, 619
    extremity
        cancerous growth, 623
        Canine vascular limb surgery, 623
        challenges, 624
        mid-1960s, 623
        procedures, 623
        programs, 623
        surgery, 623
        tissues, 623
    function and sensation, 619
    larger amputated structures, 619
    patient care
        hospital, 621
        post discharge, 621
        postoperative, 621
        site of injury, 621
        surgical team, 621
    treatment, 619
    upper arm amputation, 620
    wounds, 620
Transradial amputation, 577, 579, 580

Transthoracic echocardiography (TTE), 86
Trauma, 161, 162
Traumatic transhumeral amputation, 582
Traumatic/occupational injuries, 79
Tumor emboli, 246
Tumor-induced extremity ischemia, 328, 329
Tumor-induced peripheral ischemia
    causes, extremity ischemia, 327
    paraneoplastic symptoms, 327
Tumor-induced symptomatology, 327
Tumor-related extremity ischemia, 326

U
UEDVT. *See* Upper extremity deep vein thrombosis (UEDVT)
Ulcer debridement, 512, 513
Ulnar artery, 45, 52, 53, 55, 232, 382
Ulnar collateral artery, 51
Ultrasound technology, 202
Upper extremity, 571
    amputation (*see* Amputation)
    bilateral hand ischemia, diabetic nephropathy and vasculopathy, 577
    bilateral hand loss after farm injury, 579
    chronic progressive disease, 571
    CLI, 571
    digit/partial hand amputation, 572–575
    elbow disarticulation, 579–580
    gunshot wound, 578
    human life, 571
    left thumb amputation, 575
    limb ischemia, 571
    mangling table saw injury, 574
    sarcoma, 576
    severe lawn-mower injury to bilateral hands, 573
    shoulder disarticulation, 581
    TMR, 582, 583
    vascular insufficiency, 571
    wrist disarticulation, 575–577
Upper extremity ALI, 3
Upper extremity arterial disease, 79
Upper extremity deep vein thrombosis (UEDVT), 307
Upper extremity ischemia
    angioplasty, 92
    antiplatelet agents, 90
    aortic arch and cerebral vessels, 81
    arterial embolic, 79
    arterial vasospastic disorders, 80
    atherosclerosis, 79
    axillary artery injury, 82
    cardiac embolism, 79
    chronic injury, 82
    circulation, 243
    connective tissue disorders, 90
    diabetes mellitus, 81
    diagnosis, 80
    diagnostics evaluation, 85–87
    disorders, 79
    ergotamine, 83
    etiologies, 82, 83
    hand/arm ischemia, 243
    iatrogenic injuries, 79
    inflammatory disease, 90
    infrainguinal bypass, 90
    intimal layer injury, 83
    intra-arterial line, 244
    kidney disease, 79

Upper extremity ischemia (*cont.*)
    palpation, 84
    pathophysiology, 80–83
    plain radiograph, 85
    proximal arteries, 79
    pulse deficits, 85
    radial/brachial artery procedure, 243
    reconstruction/bypass, 91
    stenoses/aneurysms, 86
    superficial palmar arch, 85
    surgery, 84
    surgical treatment, 91
    symptoms, 84
    therapeutic procedures, 243
    thrombolysis, 92
    toxins, 83
    trauma, 83, 84
    treatment, 87–93
    vasculitis, 82
    vasospastic disorders, 80, 85
    vasospastic reactions, 85
    venous thrombosis, 309
Upper extremity replantation
    amputation
        children, 622
        crush injuries and prolonged ischemia, 622
        digits, 621
        flexion-contraction, 622
        indications and contraindications, 622
        infections, 622
        joint level, 621
        major extremity, 621
        psychologic, 622
        recovery, 622
        sensation, 622
        survival, 622
        wound and splint care, 622
        wrist, 622
    indications/contraindications, 622

V
Valvular disease/atrioventricular septal defects, 84
Vascular anatomy
    arm, 50, 51
    axillary artery, 45
    cubital fossa, 50
    elbow joint, 51
    forearm and hand, 52–55
    interosseous muscle, 52
    metacarpal bones, 52
    pisiform bone, 53, 54
    radialis indicis, 53
    supracondylar process, 50
    ulnar artery, 51
    ulnar nerve, 51
    veins, 56
Vascular approach
    arterial duplex, 339–340
    arterial insufficiency, 338
    claudication, 338
    diagnostic problem, 339
    disease management
        arterial disease management, 341
        compartment syndrome, 341–342

        escharotomies (*see* Escharotomies)
        venous disease management, 341
    imaging modalities, 340
    physical exam, 339
    predisposing risk factors, 338
    venous disease, 338
    venous duplex, 340
Vascular contusions, 224
Vascular sarcomas, 327
Vascular smooth muscle cells (VSMC), 353
Vascular studies, frequency, 373–374
Vascular trauma
    angiography, 222
    arteriovenous fistulas, 224
    CTA, 222, 223
    distal circulation, 221
    EMS, 218
    endovascular management, 224–225
    ePTFE, 226
    external iliac arteries, 227
    functionality/mortality, 237
    management, 217
    mechanism of Injury, 217
    MESS, 227
    MRA, 223
    nonoperative management, 224
    orthopedic injuries, 226
    prehospital evaluation, 218
    prehospital trauma, 219
    scoring systems, 227
    SFA, 228
    soft tissue injuries, 226
    tissue ischemia, 221
Vasculitis
    cause and pathogenesis, 96
    classification, 279
    CP, 288
    HIV arteriopathy, 289
    immune complex vasculitides, 286–287
    limb ischemia, 289
    LVV (*see* Large vessel vasculitis (LVV))
    necrotizing vasculitides, 285–286
    primary systemic vasculitides, 280
    SSc, 288, 289
    and tissue nutrition
        ankle-brachial index, 504
        BMI, 504
        Doppler pressure, 504
        glycemic control, 504
        hyperglycemia, 504
        nonhealing wounds, 504
        prealbumin levels, 504
        serum albumin, 504
        TLC, 504
        toe brachial index, 504
        transcutaneous partial pressure of oxygen, 504
        wound healing parameters, 504
    treatment, 96
    variable vessel vasculitis
        BD, 287, 288
        CS, 288
VEGF gene therapy, 495
Vein bypass, 418
Vein harvest, 420
Venous disease management, 341

Venous gangrene, 307 (*see also* Phlegmasia cerulea dolens (PCD))
    fasciotomy, 318
    HIT, 307
    limb salvage rates, 306
    PTS, 309
    thrombectomy, 312
Venous injuries, 233
Venous return, 70
Venous system, foot, 428
Venous thromboembolism (VTE), 305
Venous thrombosis, 270
    etiology, 306, 307
    and malignancy, 306
    pathophysiology
        arterial spasm, 305
        canine hind limb model, 305
        gangrene, 305
        venous hydrostatic pressure, 306
    risk factors, 306
Vertebral artery, 47
Viabahn stent graft, 393
Vibrational angioplasty, 405
Video-assisted thoracoscopic (VAT), 324
Volume-rendered images, 175
Volume rendering (VR), 187
VTE. *See* Venous thromboembolism (VTE)

W
Wagner ulcer classification system, 21
Warfarin-induced skin necrosis, 103
Weight reduction, 125, 126
WIfI. *See* Wound, ischemia and foot infection (WIfI)
Wound care
    acute *vs.* chronic ulceration, 504–505
    antimicrobial agents, 505
    antimicrobial topical agents, 505
    autolytic/enzymatic measures, 505
    bactericidal effect, silver, 505
    bioengineered products, 506
    calcium alginates, 506
    debridement, 505
    dressing, 505
    enzymatic agents, 505
    foam dressings, 506
    honey products, 505
    hydrocolloid products, 506
    hydrogels, 506
    Maggot therapy, 505
    newer products, 505
    silver dressing, 505
    specialist, 507
    topical compounding substance, 505
Wound colonization, 518
Wound contamination, 518
Wound healing
    acute, 131
    chronic non-healing wounds, 131
    CLI, 135

    phases
        hemostasis, 131–132
        inflammatory, 132–133
        interaction, 131
        proliferative, 133, 134
        remodeling, 134–135
    repair process, 131
Wound infections
    antibiotic therapy
        conventional teaching, 523
        gram-negative infections, 524, 525
        Staphylococcus aureus, 523–524
    colonization, 518
    contamination and leading, 518
    development, 517
    diabetes, 517
    diagnosis
        clinical signs and symptoms, 521
        culture, 521–522
        IDSA classification system, 521, 522
        IWGDF classification system, 521
        limb ischemia, 521
        moderate infection, 521
        quantitative significance, colonies, 522–523
        types, 522
    diagnostic studies, 523
    microbial contamination/colonization, 517–518
    microbiology
        anaerobes, 520
        comorbidities, 520, 521
        endogenous sources, 519–520
        exogenous sources, 520
        microbial proliferation, 520
        tissue oxygenation and bacterial growth, 520
    microorganisms, 518
    osteomyelitis (*see* Osteomyelitis)
    skin and soft-tissue infections, 518–520
    skin ulcer, 517
    topical antibiotics and antiseptics, 525
Wound-healing mechanisms, 484
Wound, ischemia and foot infection (WIfI), 16–21, 354, 356, 358
Wrist disarticulation
    distal radioulnar joint, 575
    hand prosthetics, 577
    helper hand, 575
    loss of entire hand, 575
    prosthetics, 575
    proximal ligation of radial, median and ulnar nerves, 577
    retention of carpal bones, 577
    salvage procedure, 575
    skin flaps, 577

X
XCELL trial, 380

Z
Zenker's degeneration, 160

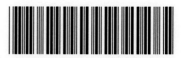